WILEY'S ENGLISH-SPANISH
SPANISH-ENGLISH DICTIONARY OF
PSYCHOLOGY AND PSYCHIATRY

DICCIONARIO DE PSICOLOGÍA Y
PSIQUIATRÍA INGLÉS-ESPAÑOL
ESPAÑOL-INGLÉS WILEY

By the same author

Wiley's English/Spanish and Spanish/English Legal Dictionary

Por el mismo autor

Diccionario jurídico inglés/español y español/inglés Wiley

WILEY'S ENGLISH-SPANISH SPANISH-ENGLISH DICTIONARY OF PSYCHOLOGY AND PSYCHIATRY

DICCIONARIO DE PSICOLOGÍA Y PSIQUIATRÍA INGLÉS-ESPAÑOL ESPAÑOL-INGLÉS WILEY

Steven M. Kaplan
Lexicographer

John Wiley & Sons, Inc.
New York • Chichester • Weinheim • Brisbane • Singapore • Toronto

Library of Congress Cataloging-in-Publication Data:

Kaplan, Steven M.
    Wiley's English-Spanish Spanish-English dictionary of
psychology and psychiatry = Diccionario de psicología y psiquiatría
inglés-español español-inglés Wiley / Steven M. Kaplan.
      p.   cm.
    ISBN 0-471-01460-5 (cloth : alk. paper). — ISBN 0-471-19284-8
(pbk. : alk. paper)
    1. Psychology—Dictionaries—English. 2. Psychiatry—
Dictionaries—English. 3. English language—Dictionaries—Spanish.
4. Psychology—Dictionaries—Spanish. 5. Psychiatry—Dictionaries—
Spanish. 6. Spanish language—Dictionaries—English. I. Title.
II. Title: English-Spanish Spanish-English dictionary of
psychology and psychiatry. III. Title: Diccionario de psicología y
psiquiatría inglés-español español-inglés Wiley.
    BF31.K36 1995
    150-.3—dc20   95–1653

Printed in the United States of America

10 9 8 7 6 5 4 3 2

PREFACE AND NOTES ON THE USE OF THIS DICTIONARY

Throughout the world over 350 million persons speak Spanish, and over 450 million speak English. Most of these are in America, where the ties between Canada, Mexico and the United States have been strengthened by the enactment of the North American Free-Trade Agreement. Most Hispanic nations trade extensively with North America, and in December 1994 the leaders of Western Hemisphere countries agreed in principle to create a free-trade zone encompassing all the Americas. All of which points to the growing need for precise communication between users of the two languages. The realms of psychology and psychiatry are no exception to this trend.

The primary objective of this dictionary is to provide accurate equivalents for the terms found in the disciplines of psychology and psychiatry. There are over 60,000 total entries in the dictionary, more than 30,000 English to Spanish, and over 30,000 more Spanish to English. There are no special rules for the use of this dictionary. The user simply locates the desired entry and reads the equivalent. No entries cross-refer the user to another entry in order to obtain the transliteration.

The entries in the English-to-Spanish section employ spellings which should be consistent with those in the literature. Where alternative English spellings of the same word may be found with some frequency, the variations are provided as separate entries (e.g., *atactic* and *ataxic*). The equivalents offered in Spanish are designed to be understood by the majority of those fluent in the language and specifically in these disciplines. For idiomatic expressions, conceptual equivalents are provided. Equivalents that are used in only a limited geographical region are avoided; inclusion of such regionalisms would add considerable bulk to the dictionary and would not help the majority of users. The same rules apply for entries in the Spanish-to-English section.

Abbreviations and acronyms used in the literature are not included in the dictionary since sequences of letters may have various meanings in different languages, and their equivalents would serve mostly to confuse; the user will find the unabbreviated entry. For example, ICT is not included, but *insulin-coma therapy* is. Trademarked names do not appear, but chemical names of most substances important in these fields do.

Many terms appear in groups of phrasal entries, all of which share the same first word. For such families of phrases, each member is provided as a separate entry, simplifying the search for the desired phrase and its equivalent.

The alphabetization of the entries in the Spanish-to-English portion uses all 29 letters of the Spanish alphabet. Thus, words starting with CH, LL, and Ñ appear, respectively, after words beginning with C, L, and N. Proper names which are not a part of the Spanish lexicon do not follow this rule.

Some words (e.g., *articulate*) have more than one grammatical function. For such terms, in the interest of clarity, each usage is shown as a separate entry, with the part of speech identified by one of the following abbreviations:

(adj) adjective   (n) noun   (v) verb

* * * * * * *

My fullest gratitude goes to John Wiley Senior Editor Herb Reich who, after recognizing the merits of this project, provided guidelines and myriad sources for terms. His constant guidance and understanding, combined with his vast knowledge of the language of these disciplines, greatly benefited my work on this dictionary.

Steven M. Kaplan

PREFACIO Y NOTAS SOBRE EL USO DE ESTE DICCIONARIO

A través del mundo más de 350 millones de personas hablan español, y más de 450 millones hablan inglés. La mayoría de éstas están en América, donde los vínculos entre Canadá, Méjico y los Estados Unidos se han fortalecido por la aprobación del Tratado de Libre Comercio de América del Norte. La mayoría de los países hispanos hacen comercio extenso con América del Norte, y en diciembre de 1994 los líderes de los países del Hemisferio Occidental acordaron en principio para crear una zona de libre comercio abarcando las Américas. Todo lo cual señala hacia la creciente necesidad para comunicación precisa entre los usuarios de las dos lenguas. Los campos de psicología y psiquiatría no son excepciones a esta tendencia.

El objetivo principal de este diccionario es proveer equivalentes precisos para los términos hallados en las disciplinas de psicología y psiquiatría. Hay más de 60,000 voces de entradas en el diccionario, más de 30,000 de inglés a español, y más de 30,000 adicionales de español a inglés. No hay reglas especiales para el uso de este diccionario. El usuario sencillamente localiza la voz de entrada deseada y lee el equivalente. Ninguna voz de entrada refiere a otra para obtener la transliteración.

Las entradas en la sección de inglés a español usan ortografía la cual debe ser consistente con aquella en la literatura. Cuando se encuentran con alguna frecuencia formas diversas de deletrear alguna palabra en inglés, las variaciones se presentan como voces de entrada separadas (p. ej., *atactic* y *ataxic*). Los equivalentes ofrecidos en español están diseñados para ser entendidos por la mayoría de aquellos que dominan el idioma y específicamente estos campos. Para expresiones idiomáticas se proveen equivalentes conceptuales. Se evitan equivalentes que sólo se usan en una zona geográfica limitada; el incluir tales regionalismos añadiría tamaño considerable al diccionario y no ayudaría a la mayoría de los usuarios. Las mismas reglas aplican a las voces de entrada de la sección de español a inglés.

No se incluyen en el diccionario abreviaturas y siglas usadas en la literatura, pues secuencias de letras pueden tener significados diversos en diferentes idiomas, y sus equivalentes servirían mayormente para confundir; el usuario encontrará la voz de entrada sin abreviar. Por ejemplo, ICT no está incluido, pero *insulin-coma therapy* sí lo está. Nombres de marca no aparecen, pero los nombres químicos de la mayoría de las sustancias importantes en estos campos sí aparecen.

Muchas voces de entrada aparecen en grupos de frases, todas las cuales comparten la misma primera palabra. Para dichas familias de frases, cada miembro aparece como una entrada separada, así simplificando la búsqueda de la frase deseada y su equivalente.

La alfabetización de las voces de entrada en la sección de español a inglés usa las 29 letras del abecedario español. Por lo tanto, palabras que empiezan con CH, LL, y Ñ aparecen, respectivamente, tras palabras empezando con C, L, y N. Los nombres propios que no formen parte del lexicón español no siguen esta regla.

Algunas palabras (p. ej., *articulate*) tienen más de una función gramatical. Para dichos términos, con la claridad en mente, cada forma de uso se ofrece como una voz de entrada separada, con la función gramatical identificada por una de las siguientes abreviaturas:

(adj) adjetivo   (n) nombre   (v) verbo

* * * * * * *

Mi más completo agradecimiento va a Herb Reich, editor de John Wiley, quien tras reconocer los méritos de éste proyecto proveyó pautas y variadas fuentes de términos. Su constante asesoría y comprensión, combinadas con su vasto conocimiento del idioma de éstos campos, beneficiaron grandemente mi trabajo en este diccionario.

Steven M. Kaplan

ENGLISH-SPANISH
INGLÉS-ESPAÑOL

A fiber fibra A
a posteriori a posteriori
a posteriori fallacy falacia a posteriori
a posteriori test prueba a posteriori
a priori a priori
a priori test prueba a priori
a priori validity validez a priori
A-type tipo A
A-type personality personalidad tipo A
Abadie's sign signo de Abadie
abaissement depresión
abalienation abalienación
abandonment abandono
abandonment reaction reacción de abandono
abandonment threat amenaza de abandono
abarognosis abarognosis
abasement abatimiento
abasement need necesidad de abatimiento
abasia abasia
abasia-astasia abasia-astasia
abasia atactica abasia atáxica
abasic abásico
abate abatir
abatement abatimiento
abatic abático
abclution abclusión
abdominal abdominal
abdominal bloating hinchazón abdominal
abdominal epilepsy epilepsia abdominal
abdominal melancholia melancolía abdominal
abdominal migraine migraña abdominal
abdominal nephrectomy nefrectomía
    abdominal
abdominal reflex reflejo abdominal
abducens abducente
abducens nerve nervio abducente
abducens nucleus núcleo abducente
abducent abducente
abducent nerve nervio abducente
abduct abducir
abduction abducción
abductor abductor
aberrant aberrante
aberrant energy expression expresión
    aberrante de energía
aberrant ganglion ganglio aberrante
aberrant motivational syndrome síndrome de
    motivación aberrante
aberrant regeneration regeneración aberrante
aberration aberración
abeyance suspensión, espera
abiatrophy abiatrofia
abience abiencia
abient abiente

ability habilidad
ability grouping agrupamiento por habilidades
ability test prueba de habilidad
abiogenetic abiogenético
abionergy abionergia
abiosis abiosis
abiotic abiótico
abiotrophia abiotrofia
abiotrophic atrophic dementia demencia
    atrófica abiotrófica
abiotrophy abiotrofia
abirritant abirritante
abirritative abirritante
ablactation ablactación
ablatio ablación
ablatio penis ablación del pene
ablation ablación
ablepsia ablepsia
ablepsy ablepsia
ablution ablución
ablutomania ablutomanía
abnerval abnerval
abneural abneural
Abney's effect efecto de Abney
Abney's law ley de Abney
abnormal anormal
abnormal behavior conducta anormal
abnormal development desarrollo anormal
abnormal fixation fijación anormal
abnormal impulse to work impulso anormal
    de trabajar
abnormal psychology psicología anormal
abnormality anormalidad
abnormity anormalidad
abomination abominación
aboral aboral
aboriginal therapies terapias aborígenes
abortifacient abortivo
abortion aborto
abortive decision decisión abortiva
abortive neurofibromatosis
    neurofibromatosis abortivo
aboulia abulia
abrasion abrasión
abrasive abrasivo
abreaction abreacción
abrosia abrosia
abscess absceso
abscissa abscisa
absence ausencia
absence seizure acceso de ausencia
absent ausente
absent ejaculation eyaculación ausente
absent state estado ausente
absenteeism ausentismo
absentia ausencia
absentia epileptica ausencia epiléptica
absentmindedness distracción
absinthe absintio
absinthism absintismo
absolute absoluto
absolute accommodation acomodación
    absoluta
absolute agraphia agrafia absoluta
absolute bliss arrobamiento absoluto

absolute error error absoluto
absolute identification identificación absoluta
absolute impression impresión absoluta
absolute inversion inversión absoluta
absolute limen limen absoluto
absolute luminosity luminosidad absoluta
absolute measurement medición absoluta
absolute motion moción absoluta
absolute pitch tono absoluto
absolute rating scale escala de clasificación
    absoluta
absolute refractory period periodo
    refractario absoluto
absolute scale escala absoluta
absolute scotoma escotoma absoluto
absolute sensitivity sensibilidad absoluta
absolute threshold umbral absoluto
absolute value valor absoluto
absolute visual sensitivity sensibilidad visual
    absoluta
absolute zero cero absoluto
absorb absorber
absorbed mania manía absorta
absorption absorción
absorption spectrum espectro de absorción
abstinence abstinencia
abstinence delirium delirio de abstinencia
abstinence rule regla de abstinencia
abstinence symptom síntoma de abstinencia
abstinence syndrome síndrome de abstinencia
abstract abstracto
abstract ability habilidad abstracta
abstract attitude actitud abstracta
abstract attributes atributos abstractos
abstract conceptualization conceptualización
    abstracta
abstract expressionism expresionismo
    abstracto
abstract idea idea abstracta
abstract intelligence inteligencia abstracta
abstract logical thought pensamiento lógico
    abstracto
abstract modeling modelado abstracto
abstract perceptions percepciones abstractas
abstract quality cualidad abstracta
abstract symbolism simbolismo abstracto
abstract thinking pensamiento abstracto
abstracting disabilities discapacidades en
    abstraer
abstraction abstracción
absurdities test prueba de absurdidades
absurdity absurdidad
abterminal abterminal
abulia abulia
abulic abúlico
abulic-akinetic syndrome síndrome
    abúlico-acinético
abulomania abulomanía
abundancy motive motivo de abundancia
abusability abusabilidad
abusable child niño abusable
abuse abuso
abuse liability riesgo de abuso
abused child niño abusado
abusing parent padre abusante, madre

abusante
abusive families familias abusivas
academic académico
academic achievement test prueba de
    aprovechamiento académico
academic abilities grouping agrupamiento
    por habilidades académicas
academic aptitude test prueba de aptitud
    académica
academic functioning funcionamiento
    académico
academic inhibition inhibición académica
academic performance ejecución académica
academic potential potencial académico
academic problem problema académico
academic setting ambiente académico
academic skills disorder trastorno de
    destrezas académicas
academic success éxito académico
academic underachievement subrendimiento
    académico
academic underachievement disorder
    trastorno de subrendimiento académico
acalculia acalculia
acampsia acampsia
acanthamebiasis acantamebiasis
acanthesthesia acantestesia
acarophobia acarofobia
acatalepsia acatalepsia
acatamathesia acatamatesia
acataphasia acatafasia
acathexis acatexia
acathisia acatisia
acathisia paraesthetica acatisia paraestética
acathizia acatisia
accelerated interaction interacción acelerada
acceleration aceleración
accent acento, énfasis
acceptance aceptación
access acceso
access time tiempo de acceso
accessibility accesibilidad
accessibility theory teoría de accesibilidad
accessible accesible
accessory accesorio
accessory catalepsy catalepsia accesoria
accessory cramp calambre accesorio
accessory nerve nervio accesorio
accessory olfactory bulb bulbo olfatorio
    accesorio
accessory symptoms síntomas accesorios
accident accidente
accident behavior conducta que podría
    ocasionar accidentes
accident habit hábito de accidentes
accident neurosis neurosis de accidentes
accident prevention prevención de accidentes
accident-prone propenso a accidentes
accident-prone behavior conducta propensa a
    accidentes
accident-prone personality personalidad
    propensa a accidentes
accident proneness propensión a los
    accidentes
accident reduction reducción de accidentes

accident repeater repetidor de accidentes
accidental accidental
accidental chaining encadenamiento accidental
accidental crisis crisis accidental
accidental error error accidental
accidental homosexuality homosexualidad accidental
accidental hypothermia hipotermia accidental
accidental image imagen accidental
accidental reinforcement refuerzo accidental
accidental stimuli estímulos accidentales
acclimation aclimatación
acclimatization aclimatación
accommodation acomodación
accommodation of nerve acomodación de nervio
accommodation reflex reflejo de acomodación
accommodative acomodativo
accomplishment logro
accomplishment quotient cociente de logro
accoucheur's hand mano de partero
accountability responsabilidad
accreditation acreditación
accretion acrecentamiento
acculturate aculturar
acculturation aculturación
acculturation problem problema de aculturación
accumulation acumulación
accuracy precisión
accuracy compulsion compulsión de precisión
accuracy measures medidas de precisión
accuracy test prueba de precisión
acedia acedia
acenesthesia acenestesia
acerophobia acerofobia
acervuline acervulino
acervulus acérvula
acetaminophen acetaminofeno
acetanilide acetanilida
acetazolamide acetazolamida
acetone acetona
acetophenazine acetofenazina
acetophenetidine acetofenetidina
acetylcholine acetilcolina
acetylcholine receptors receptores de acetilcolina
acetylcholinesterase acetilcolinesterasa
acetylphosphate acetilfosfato
acetylsalicylic acid ácido acetilsalicílico
acetylureas acetilureas
achalasia acalasia
acheiria aqueiria
achieved role papel alcanzado
achievement logro
achievement age edad de logro
achievement battery batería de logro
achievement drive impulso de logro
achievement ethic ética de logro
achievement motivation motivación de logro
achievement motive motivo de logro
achievement need necesidad de logro
achievement quotient cociente de logro

achievement test prueba de aprovechamiento
achievement versus aptitude aprovechamiento contra aptitud
Achilles reflex reflejo de Aquiles
Achilles tendon reflex reflejo del tendón de Aquiles
achiria aquiria
achluophobia acluofobia
achondroplasia acondroplasia
achromat acromático
achromatic acromático
achromatic-chromatic scale escala acromática-cromática
achromatic color color acromático
achromatic color response respuesta a color acromático
achromatic interval intervalo acromático
achromatic response respuesta acromática
achromatism acromatismo
achromatopsia acromatopsia
acid ácido
acid-base disturbance perturbación ácido-base
acidification acidificación
acidification treatment tratamiento de acidificación
acidity acidez
acidophilic adenoma adenoma acidófilo
acidosis acidosis
acme acmé
acmesthesia acmestesia
acne acné
acoasm acusma
acolasia acolasia
aconative aconativo
aconite acónito
aconuresis aconuresis
acoria acoria
Acosta's syndrome síndrome de Acosta
acoumeter acúmetro
acousma acusma
acousmatagnosis acusmatagnosia
acousmatamnesia acusmatamnesia
acoustic acústico
acoustic agraphia agrafia acústica
acoustic aphasia afasia acústica
acoustic confusion confusión acústica
acoustic cue señal acústica
acoustic filter filtro acústico
acoustic generalization generalización acústica
acoustic irritability irritabilidad acústica
acoustic nerve nervio acústico
acoustic neurilemoma neurilemoma acústico
acoustic neurinoma neurinoma acústico
acoustic neuroma neuroma acústico
acoustic papilla papila acústica
acoustic pressure presión acústica
acoustic processing procesamiento acústico
acoustic radiation radiación acústica
acoustic reflex reflejo acústico
acoustic resonance resonancia acústica
acoustic schwannoma schwannoma acústico
acoustic spectrum espectro acústico
acoustic startle reflex reflejo de sobresalto

acústico
acoustic store almacén acústico
acoustic trauma trauma acústico
acoustico-amnestic aphasia afasia
   acusticoamnésica
acousticopalpebral reflex reflejo
   acusticopalpebral
acousticophobia acusticofobia
acoustics acústica
acquaintance rape violación por conocido
acquiescence aquiescencia
acquiescent-response set conjunto de
   respuestas aquiescentes
acquired adquirido
acquired agraphia agrafia adquirida
acquired character carácter adquirido
acquired characteristic característica
   adquirida
acquired discrimination of cues
   discriminación de señales adquirida
acquired drive impulso adquirido
acquired epileptic aphasia afasia epiléptica
   adquirida
acquired equivalence of cues equivalencia de
   señales adquirida
acquired fear temor adquirido
acquired immunodeficiency syndrome
   síndrome de inmunodeficiencia adquirida
acquired motive motivo adquirido
acquired reflex reflejo adquirido
acquired trait rasgo adquirido
acquisition adquisición
acquisition trial ensayo de adquisición
acquisitive spirit espíritu adquisitivo
acquisitiveness adquisitividad
acrai acrai
acrasia acrasia
acrasy acrasia
acroagnosis acroagnosis
acroanesthesia acroanestesia
acroataxia acroataxia
acrobrachycephaly acrobraquicefalia
acrocentric chromosome cromosoma
   acrocéntrico
acrocephalia acrocefalia
acrocephalic acrocefálico
acrocephalous acrocéfalo
acrocephaly acrocefalia
acrocinesia acrocinesia
acrocinesis acrocinesis
acrocyanosis acrocianosis
acrodynia acrodinia
acrodysesthesia acrodisestesia
acroedema acroedema
acroesthesia acroestesia
acrognosis acrognosis
acrohypothermia acrohipotermia
acrohypothermy acrohipotermia
acromegalia acromegalia
acromegaloid acromegaloide
acromegaloid personality personalidad
   acromegaloide
acromegaly acromegalia
acromelalgia acromelalgia
acromial acromial

acromial reflex reflejo acromial
acromicria acromicria
acroneurosis acroneurosis
acronym acrónimo
acroparesthesia acroparestesia
acroparesthesia syndrome síndrome de
   acroparestesia
acrophobia acrofobia
acrosome acrosoma
acrotrophodynia acrotrofodinia
acrotrophoneurosis acrotrofoneurosis
act acto
act ending terminación de acto
act-habit acto-hábito
act psychology psicología de actos
actin actina
acting out descarga involuntaria de impulsos,
   manifestación de emociones previamente
   inhibidas
actinic keratosis queratosis actínica
actinoneuritis actinoneuritis
action acción
action current corriente de acción
action group grupo de acción
action group process proceso de grupo de
   acción
action-instrument acción-instrumento
action interpretation interpretación de acción
action-location acción-ubicación
action potential potencial de acción
action-recipient acción-recipiente
action research investigación de acción
action-specific energy energía de acción
   específica
action stream curso de acción
action system sistema de acción
action tremor temblor de acción
activated epilepsy epilepsia activada
activated sleep sueño activado
activation activación
activation pattern patrón de activación
activation theory of emotion teoría de
   activación de emoción
activator activador
active activo
active analysis análisis activo
active analytic psychotherapy psicoterapia
   analítica activa
active and passive activo y pasivo
active avoidance evitación activa
active castration complex complejo de
   castración activo
active concretization concretización activa
active daydream technique técnica de
   ensueño activo
active euthanasia eutanasia activa
active fantasying fantaseo activo
active immunity inmunidad activa
active introversion introversión activa
active mode of consciousness modo activo de
   conciencia
active negativism negativismo activo
active-passive model modelo activo-pasivo
active processing procesamiento activo
active psychoanalysis psicoanálisis activo

active recreation recreación activa
active short-term memory memoria a corto plazo activo
active sleep sueño activo
active technique técnica activa
active therapist terapeuta activo
active therapy terapia activa
active transport transporte activo
active vocabulary vocabulario activo
actively aggressive reaction type tipo de reacción activamente agresiva
activism activismo
activities of daily living actividades del diario vivir
activity actividad
activity analysis análisis de actividad
activity cage jaula de actividad
activity cycle ciclo de actividad
activity deprivation privación de actividad
activity drive impulso de actividad
activity group psychotherapy psicoterapia de grupo de actividad
activity group therapy terapia de grupo de actividad
activity-interview group psychotherapy psicoterapia de grupo de entrevista de actividad
activity inventory inventario de actividad
activity level nivel de actividad
activity log diario de actividad
activity-play therapy terapia de actividad-juego
activity pleasure placer de actividad
activity quotient cociente de actividad
activity record registro de actividad
activity system sistema de actividad
activity theory of aging teoría de envejecimiento de actividad
activity therapy terapia de actividad
activity wheel rueda de actividad
actograph actógrafo
actomyosin actomiosina
actual actual, real
actual conflict conflicto real
actual neurosis neurosis real
actual self yo real
actualization actualización
actualizing therapy terapia de actualización
actuarial actuarial
acuesthesia acuestesia
acuity agudeza
acuity grating rejilla de agudeza
acuity test prueba de agudeza
aculalia aculalia
acupuncture acupuntura
acute agudo
acute affective reflex reflejo afectivo agudo
acute alcoholic myopathy miopatía alcohólica aguda
acute alcoholism alcoholismo agudo
acute anterior poliomyelitis poliomielitis anterior aguda
acute anxiety ansiedad aguda
acute anxiety attack ataque de ansiedad aguda

acute ascending paralysis parálisis ascendente aguda
acute ataxia ataxia aguda
acute atrophic paralysis parálisis atrófica aguda
acute brachial radiculitis radiculitis braquial aguda
acute brain disorder trastorno cerebral agudo
acute bulbar poliomyelitis poliomielitis bulbar aguda
acute cerebellar ataxia ataxia cerebelosa aguda
acute cerebellar tremor temblor cerebeloso agudo
acute confusional state estado confusional agudo
acute decubitus ulcer úlcera de decúbito aguda
acute delirium delirio agudo
acute delusional psychosis psicosis delusoria aguda
acute depression depresión aguda
acute disseminated encephalomyelitis encefalomielitis diseminada aguda
acute dystonia distonía aguda
acute epidemic leukoencephalitis leucoencefalitis epidémica aguda
acute exercise ejercicio agudo
acute hallucinatory paranoia paranoia alucinatoria aguda
acute hallucinosis alucinosis aguda
acute head trauma trauma de cabeza agudo
acute hemorrhagic encephalitis encefalitis hemorrágica aguda
acute idiopathic polyneuritis polineuritis idiopática aguda
acute illness enfermedad aguda
acute intermittent porphyria porfiria aguda intermitente
acute mania manía aguda
acute myelitis mielitis aguda
acute necrotizing encephalitis encefalitis necrotizante aguda
acute otitis media otitis media aguda
acute pain dolor agudo
acute paranoid disorder trastorno paranoide agudo
acute paranoid reaction reacción paranoide aguda
acute polyneuritis polineuritis aguda
acute porphyria porfiria aguda
acute posttraumatic stress disorder trastorno de estrés postraumático agudo
acute preparation preparación aguda
acute primary hemorrhagic meningoencephalitis meningoencefalitis hemorrágica primaria aguda
acute psychotic break rompimiento psicótico agudo
acute schizophrenia esquizofrenia aguda
acute schizophrenic episode episodio esquizofrénico agudo
acute shock psychosis psicosis de choque agudo
acute situational reaction reacción situacional

aguda
acute stress disorder trastorno de estrés
   agudo
acute stress reaction reacción de estrés aguda
acute stressor estresante agudo
acute tolerance tolerancia aguda
acute transverse myelitis mielitis transversal
   aguda
acute traumatic disorder trastorno traumático
   agudo
acute trypanosomiasis tripanosomiasis aguda
acute undifferentiated schizophrenia
   esquizofrenia indeferenciada aguda
acute viral hepatitis hepatitis viral aguda
ad hoc ad hoc
ad lib ad lib
Adams-Stokes disease enfermedad de
   Adams-Stokes
Adams-Stokes syndrome síndrome de
   Adams-Stokes
adaptability adaptabilidad
adaptation adaptación
adaptation disease enfermedad de adaptación
adaptation level nivel de adaptación
adaptation level theory teoría del nivel de
   adaptación
adaptation mechanisms mecanismos de
   adaptación
adaptation of space perception adaptación de
   percepción de espacio
adaptation period periodo de adaptación
adaptation syndrome síndrome de adaptación
adaptation syndrome of Selye síndrome de
   adaptación de Selye
adaptation time tiempo de adaptación
adaptation to death adaptación a la muerte
adaptational adaptacional
adaptational approach acercamiento
   adaptacional
adaptational dynamics dinámica adaptacional
adapted child niño adaptado
adapted stress theory teoría de estrés
   adaptada
adaptive adaptivo
adaptive act acto adaptivo
adaptive approach acercamiento adaptivo
adaptive behavior conducta adaptiva
adaptive behavior scale escala de conducta
   adaptiva
adaptive control of thought control de
   pensamiento adaptivo
adaptive delinquency delincuencia adaptiva
adaptive function of dreaming función
   adaptiva de soñar
adaptive hypothesis hipótesis adaptiva
adaptive intelligence inteligencia adaptiva
adaptive mechanism mecanismo adaptivo
adaptive processes procesos adaptivos
adaptive skills destrezas adaptivas
adaptive style estilo adaptivo
adaptive technique técnica adaptiva
adaptive test prueba adaptiva
addict adicto
addiction adicción
addiction versus abuse adicción contra abuso

addictive adictivo
addictive alcoholism alcoholismo adictivo
addictive behavior conducta adictiva
addictive personality personalidad adictiva
addictive process proceso adictivo
Addison's disease enfermedad de Addison
additive aditivo
additive burden hypothesis hipótesis de carga
   aditiva
additive color mixture mezcla de colores
   aditiva
additive mixture mezcla aditiva
additive scale escala aditiva
address dirección
adducted aphonia afonía aducida
adduction aducción
adductor aductor
adductor reflex reflejo aductor
ademonia ademonia
ademosyne ademosina
adenine adenina
adenohypophysis adenohipófisis
adenoid type tipo adenoide
adenoma adenoma
adenomatoid adenomatoide
adenoneural adenoneural
adenosine adenosina
adenosine triphosphate trifosfato de
   adenosina
adenyl cyclase adenilciclasa
adenylic acid ácido adenílico
adephagia adefagia
adequate sample muestra adecuada
adequate stimulus estímulo adecuado
adherence adherencia
adherence to medical treatment adherencia a
   tratamiento médico
adhesive arachnoiditis aracnoiditis adhesiva
adhesive otitis media otitis media adhesiva
adiadochocinesia adiadococinesia
adiadochocinesis adiadococinesis
adiadochokinesia adiadococinesia
adiadochokinesis adiadococinesis
adiadokokinesia adiadococinesia
adiadokokinesis adiadococinesis
adiaphoria adiaforia
Adie's pupil pupila de Adie
Adie's syndrome síndrome de Adie
adience adiencia
adient adiente
adipocyte adipocito
adiposalgia adiposalgia
adipose adiposo
adiposis cerebralis adiposis cerebral
adiposogenital adiposogenital
adiposogenital degeneration degeneración
   adiposogenital
adiposogenital dystrophy distrofia
   adiposogenital
adiposogenital syndrome síndrome
   adiposogenital
adipsia adipsia
adjective checklist lista de comprobación de
   adjetivos
adjunctive behavior conducta adjunta

adjunctive skills destrezas adjuntas
adjunctive therapist terapeuta adjunto
adjustment ajuste
adjustment disorder trastorno de ajuste
adjustment disorder with academic inhibition trastorno de ajuste con inhibición académica
adjustment disorder with anxiety trastorno de ajuste con ansiedad
adjustment disorder with anxious mood trastorno de ajuste con humor ansioso
adjustment disorder with atypical features trastorno de ajuste con características atípicas
adjustment disorder with depressed mood trastorno de ajuste con humor deprimido
adjustment disorder with disturbance of conduct trastorno de ajuste con disturbio de conducta
adjustment disorder with mixed emotional features trastorno de ajuste con características emocionales mixtas
adjustment disorder with physical complaints trastorno de ajuste con quejas físicas
adjustment disorder with withdrawal trastorno de ajuste con retirada
adjustment disorder with work inhibition trastorno de ajuste con inhibición de trabajo
adjustment inventory inventario de ajuste
adjustment mechanism mecanismo de ajuste
adjustment method método de ajuste
adjustment of observations ajuste de observaciones
adjustment processes procesos de ajuste
adjustment reaction reacción de ajuste
adjustment reaction of adolescence reacción de ajuste de adolescencia
adjustment reaction of childhood reacción de ajuste de niñez
adjustment reaction of infancy reacción de ajuste de infancia
adjustment reaction of later life reacción de ajuste de la postrimería
adjuvant adyuvante
adjuvant therapy terapia adyuvante
adlerian adleriano
adlerian psychoanalysis psicoanálisis adleriano
adlerian psychology psicología adleriana
administration administración
administrative psychiatry psiquiatría administrativa
admission admisión
admission certification certificación de admisión
admission procedures procedimientos de admisión
adnerval adnerval
adneural adneural
adolescence adolescencia
adolescent adolescente
adolescent affective disorder trastorno afectivo adolescente
adolescent antisocial behavior conducta

antisocial adolescente
adolescent counseling asesoramiento de adolescentes
adolescent crisis crisis adolescente
adolescent development desarrollo adolescente
adolescent father padre adolescente
adolescent homosexuality homosexualidad adolescente
adolescent identity formation formación de identidad adolescente
adolescent mania manía adolescente
adolescent mother madre adolescente
adolescent parent padre adolescente, madre adolescente
adolescent pedophilia pedofilia adolescente
adolescent pregnancy embarazo adolescente
adolescent psychiatry psiquiatría adolescente
adolescent psychotherapy psicoterapia adolescente
adolescent sex changes cambios sexuales de adolescencia
adolescent sex offender ofensor sexual adolescente
adolescent suicide suicidio adolescente
adolescent support group grupo de apoyo adolescente
adolescent turmoil agitación adolescente
adolescent-type behavior conducta tipo adolescente
adopted child niño adoptado
adopted-child studies estudios de niños adoptados
adoption adopción
adoption study estudio de adopción
adoptive adoptivo
adoptive care cuidado adoptivo
adoptive child niño adoptivo
adoptive parent padre adoptivo, madre adoptiva
adrenal adrenal
adrenal cortex corteza adrenal
adrenal gland glándula adrenal
adrenal medulla médula adrenal
adrenalin adrenalina
adrenaline adrenalina
adrenergic adrenérgico
adrenergic blocking agents agentes bloqueadores adrenérgicos
adrenergic circulatory state estado circulatorio adrenérgico
adrenergic drugs drogas adrenérgicas
adrenergic reaction reacción adrenérgica
adrenergic response state estado de respuesta adrenérgica
adrenergic synapse sinapsis adrenérgica
adrenergic system sistema adrenérgico
adrenochrome adrenocromo
adrenocortical insufficiency insuficiencia adrenocortical
adrenocorticotrophic hormone hormona adrenocorticotrópica
adrenogenital syndrome síndrome adrenogenital
adrenoleukodystrophy adrenoleucodistrofia

adrenomyeloneuropathy
   adrenomieloneuropatía
adrenosterone adrenosterona
adromia adromia
adult adulto
adult abuse abuso de adultos
adult antisocial behavior conducta antisocial
   adulta
adult attention-deficit disorder trastorno de
   déficit de atención de adultos
adult children of alcoholics hijos adultos de
   alcohólicos
adult development desarrollo adulto
adult diagnostic and treatment center centro
   de diagnóstico y tratamiento de adultos
adult ego state estado del ego adulto
adult foster home asilo para adultos
adult home hogar de reposo
adult intellectual development desarrollo
   intelectual adulto
adult intelligence inteligencia adulta
adult motivation motivación adulta
**adult pseudohypertrophic muscular
   dystrophy** distrofia muscular
   seudohipertrófica adulta
adult sensorineural lesion lesión
   sensorineural adulta
adult situational reaction reacción situacional
   adulta
adultery adulterio
adulthood adultez
adultomorphism adultomorfismo
advantage by illness ventaja por enfermedad
advantage law ley de ventaja
adventitial cells células adventicias
adventitial neuritis neuritis adventicia
adventitious adventicio
adventitious deafness sordera adventicia
adventitious motor overflow rebosamiento
   motor adventicio
adventitious reinforcement refuerzo
   adventicio
adventurousness audacia
adversary model modelo adverso
adverse adverso
adverse drug reactions reacciones de droga
   adversas
adverse effect efecto adverso
adverse effects of medication efectos
   adversos de medicación
adverse selection selección adversa
advertising publicidad
advertising psychology psicología de anuncios
advertising research investigación de
   anuncios
advice consejo
advocacy apoyo
advocacy research investigación de apoyo
advocate defensor
adynamia adinamia
adynamic adinámico
adynamic ileus íleo adinámico
aelurophobia aelurofobia
aerasthenia aerastenia
aerial perspective perspectiva aérea

aeroacrophobia aeroacrofobia
aeroasthenia aeroastenia
aerobic aeróbico
aerobic capacity capacidad aeróbica
aerobic exercise ejercicio aeróbico
aerobic fitness aptitud aeróbica
aeroneurosis aeroneurosis
aerophagia aerofagia
aerophagy aerofagia
aerophobia aerofobia
aerosialophagy aerosialofagia
affect (n) afecto
affect (v) afectar
affect block bloqueo de afecto
affect displacement desplazamiento de afecto
affect display demostración de afecto
affect energy energía de afecto
affect fantasy fantasía de afecto
affect fixation fijación de afecto
affect hunger hambre de afecto
affect intensity problem problema de
   intensidad de afecto
affect inversion inversión de afecto
affect-laden paranoia paranoia cargada de
   afecto
affect memory memoria afectiva
affect spasm espasmo de afecto
affect within normal range afecto dentro del
   intervalo normal
affectation afectación
affection afección
affectional attachment apego afectivo
affectional bond vínculo afectivo
affectional drive impulso afectivo
affectionate afectuoso
affectionate transference transferencia
   afectuosa
affective afectivo
affective ambivalence ambivalencia afectiva
affective amnesia amnesia afectiva
affective attack ataque afectivo
affective cathexis catexis afectiva
affective-cognitive factors factores
   afectivos-cognitivos
affective decentration descentración afectiva
affective development desarrollo afectivo
affective discharge descarga afectiva
affective disharmony discordia afectiva
affective disorder trastorno afectivo
affective eudemonia eudemonia afectiva
affective experience experiencia afectiva
affective fixation fijación afectiva
affective hallucination alucinación afectiva
affective interaction interacción afectiva
affective monomania monomanía afectiva
affective psychosis psicosis afectiva
affective ratio razón afectiva
affective rigidity rigidez afectiva
affective sensation sensación afectiva
affective separation separación afectiva
affective slumber inercia afectiva
affective state estado afectivo
affective suggestion sugestión afectiva
affective tone tono afectivo
affectivity afectividad

affectomotor afectomotor
affectomotor pattern patrón afectomotor
affectosymbolic afectosimbólico
affectualization afectualización
afference aferencia
afferent aferente
afferent code código aferente
afferent motor aphasia afasia motora aferente
afferent neurons neuronas aferentes
affiliation afiliación
affiliation need necesidad de afiliación
affiliative bonding vinculación afiliativa
affiliative need necesidad afiliativa
affinity afinidad
affinity hypothesis hipótesis de afinidad
affirmation afirmación
affirmative action acción afirmativa
affliction aflicción
affordance funcionalidad
affricate africada
afterbirth secundinas
aftercare asistencia posterior, asistencia postoperatoria
aftercare group grupo de asistencia posterior
aftercontraction poscontracción
aftercurrent poscorriente
afterdischarge descarga persistente
aftereffect efecto posterior
afterexpulsion posexpulsión
afterhearing audición persistente
afterimage imagen persistente
afterimpression sensación persistente
aftermovement movimiento posterior
afterperception percepción persistente
afterpotential pospotencial
aftersensation sensación persistente
aftersound sonido persistente
aftertaste dejo
aftertouch tacto persistente
agamogenesis agamogénesis
agapaxia agapaxia
agapism agapismo
agastroneuria agastroneuria
age edad
age-appropriate maturity madurez apropiada para la edad
age-associated memory decline declinación de memoria asociada con la edad
age critique edad crítica
age de retour edad de retorno
age differences diferencias de edad
age effects efectos de edad
age-equivalent equivalente de edad
age-equivalent scale escala de equivalente de edad
age-grade scaling escalamiento por edad y grado
age norm norma de edad
age ratio razón de edad
age regression regresión de edad
age-related relacionado con la edad
age-related forms of depression formas de depresión relacionadas con la edad
age scale escala de edad

age score puntuación de edad
ageism ageismo
agenesia agenesia
agenesis agenesia
agenetic agenético
agent agente
agent provocateur agente provocador
agerasia agerasia
ageusia ageusia
ageustia ageustia
agglutination aglutinación
aggregation agregación
aggregation problems problemas de agregación
aggression agresión
aggression in attention-deficit disorder agresión en trastorno de déficit de atención
aggression in play agresión en juego
aggression panic pánico de agresión
aggressive agresivo
aggressive behavior conducta agresiva
aggressive behavior during child care conducta agresiva durante cuidado de niños
aggressive conduct conducta agresiva
aggressive conduct disorder trastorno de conducta agresiva
aggressive drive impulso agresivo
aggressive fantasy fantasía agresiva
aggressive instinct instinto agresivo
aggressive-predator type tipo agresivo-predador
aggressive scale escala agresiva
aggressive socialized reaction reacción socializada agresiva
aggressive type tipo agresivo
aggressive undersocialized reaction reacción subsocializada agresiva
aggressiveness agresividad
aggressivity agresividad
aging envejecimiento
aging theory teoría de envejecimiento
agitated agitado
agitated depression depresión agitada
agitation agitación
agitographia agitografía
agitolalia agitolalia
agitophasia agitofasia
aglossia aglosia
agnea agnea
agnosia agnosia
agnosic alexia alexia agnósica
agonist agonista
agonistic behavior conducta agonística
agony agonía
agoraphobia agorafobia
agoraphobia with panic attacks agorafobia con ataques de pánico
agoraphobia without panic attacks agorafobia sin ataques de pánico
agoraphobic agorafóbico
agrammaphasia agramafasia
agrammatica agramatismo
agrammatism agramatismo
agrammatologia agramatología
agranular cortex corteza agranular

agranulocytosis agranulocitosis
agraphia agrafia
agraphic agráfico
agraphognosia agrafognosia
agricultural psychology psicología agrícola
agriothymia agriotimia
agromania agromania
agrypnia agripnia
agrypnocoma agripnocoma
agrypnotic agripnótico
agyiophobia agiofobia
agyria agiria
aha experience experiencia ¡ajá!
ahedonia ahedonia
ahistorical ahistórico
ahylognosia ahilognosia
ahypnia ahipnia
ahypnosia ahipnosia
Aicardi's syndrome síndrome de Aicardi
aichmophobia aicmofobia
aide ayudante
aidoiomania aidoiomanía
AIDS SIDA
AIDS dementia complex complejo de
   demencia de SIDA
ailment dolencia
ailurophobia ailurofobia
aim fin
aim-inhibited inhibido del fin
aim inhibition inhibición del fin
aim transference transferencia del fin
aiming test prueba de puntería
air-bone gap brecha aire-hueso
air conduction conducción de aire
air conduction test prueba de conducción de
   aire
air encephalography encefalografía de aire
air hunger hambre de aire
air phobia fobia de aire
air pollution contaminación del aire
air pollution adaptation adaptación a
   contaminación del aire
air pollution syndrome síndrome de
   contaminación del aire
air pressure effects efectos de presión del
   aire
air swallowing tragado de aire
airsickness mareo aéreo
akatama acatama
akatamathesia acatamatesia
akataphasia acatafasia
akathisia acatisia
akatisia acatisia
Akerfeldt test prueba de Akerfeldt
akinesia acinesia
akinesia algera acinesia álgera
akinesia amnestica acinesia amnésica
akinesis acinesis
akinesthesia acinestesia
akinetic acinético
akinetic-abulic syndrome síndrome
   acinético-abúlico
akinetic apraxia apraxia acinética
akinetic epilepsy epilepsia acinética
akinetic mutism mutismo acinético

akinetic psychosis psicosis acinética
akinetic seizure acceso acinético
akinetic stupor estupor acinético
akoasm acusma
akousticophobia acusticofobia
Akureyri disease enfermedad de Akureyri
Alajouanine's syndrome síndrome de
   Alajouanine
alalia alalia
alalic alálico
alarm alarma
alarm reaction reacción de alarma
alarm reaction stage etapa de reacción de
   alarma
albedo albedo
albedo perception percepción del albedo
albinism albinismo
albino albino
albumin albúmina
albuminocytologic dissociation disociación
   albuminocitológica
alcaptonuria alcaptonuria
alcohol alcohol
alcohol abuse abuso de alcohol
alcohol abuse and dependence abuso de
   alcohol y dependencia
alcohol abuse scale escala de abuso de alcohol
alcohol-addicted adicto al alcohol
alcohol-addicted mother madre adicta al
   alcohol
alcohol amnesic disorder trastorno amnésico
   de alcohol
alcohol amnesic syndrome síndrome
   amnésico de alcohol
alcohol amnestic disorder trastorno amnésico
   de alcohol
alcohol amnestic syndrome síndrome
   amnésico de alcohol
alcohol anxiety disorder trastorno de
   ansiedad de alcohol
alcohol delirium delirio de alcohol
alcohol dementia demencia de alcohol
alcohol dependence dependencia de alcohol
alcohol dependence syndrome síndrome de
   dependencia de alcohol
alcohol derivative derivado del alcohol
alcohol detoxification destoxificación de
   alcohol
alcohol hallucinosis alucinosis de alcohol
alcohol idiosyncratic intoxication
   intoxicación idiosincrásica por alcohol
alcohol-induced mental disorder trastorno
   mental inducido por alcohol
alcohol intoxication intoxicación por alcohol
alcohol-methadone interaction interacción
   alcohol-metadona
alcohol persisting amnestic disorder
   trastorno amnésico persistente de alcohol
alcohol persisting dementia demencia
   persistente de alcohol
alcohol psychosis psicosis de alcohol
alcohol psychotic disorder trastorno psicótico
   de alcohol
alcohol psychotic disorder with delusions
   trastorno psicótico de alcohol con

delusiones

alcohol psychotic disorder with hallucinations trastorno psicótico de alcohol con alucinaciones

alcohol-related relacionado al alcohol

alcohol-related behavior conducta relacionada al alcohol

alcohol sleep disorder trastorno del sueño de alcohol

alcohol tolerance tolerancia de alcohol

alcohol use disorder trastorno de uso de alcohol

alcohol withdrawal retiro de alcohol

alcohol withdrawal delirium delirio del retiro de alcohol

alcohol withdrawal syndrome síndrome del retiro de alcohol

alcoholic alcohólico

alcoholic addiction adicción alcohólica

alcoholic blackout desmayo alcohólico

alcoholic brain syndrome síndrome cerebral alcohólico

alcoholic dementia demencia alcohólica

alcoholic deterioration deterioración alcohólica

alcoholic epilepsy epilepsia alcohólica

alcoholic family familia alcohólica

alcoholic hallucinosis alucinosis alcohólica

alcoholic jealousy celos alcohólicos

alcoholic liver disease enfermedad de hígado alcohólica

alcoholic myopathy miopatía alcohólica

alcoholic neuropathy neuropatía alcohólica

alcoholic organic mental disorders trastornos mentales orgánicos alcohólicos

alcoholic paranoia paranoia alcohólica

alcoholic paranoid state estado paranoide alcohólico

alcoholic parent padre alcohólico, madre alcohólica

alcoholic pseudoparesis seudoparesia alcohólica

alcoholic psychosis psicosis alcohólica

alcoholic twilight state estado crepuscular alcohólico

alcoholism alcoholismo

alcoholism prevention prevención de alcoholismo

alcoholism treatment tratamiento de alcoholismo

alcoholomania alcoholomanía

alcoholophilia alcoholofilia

alcoholophobia alcoholofobia

aldosterone aldosterona

aldosteronism aldosteronismo

alector alector

alert inactivity inactividad alerta

alerting mechanisms mecanismos de alerta

alerting system sistema de alerta

alertness agudeza mental, estado de alerta

alethia aletia

Alexander's disease enfermedad de Alexander

alexia alexia

alexic aléxico

alexithymia alexitimia

algedonic algedónico

algesia algesia

algesic algésico

algesichronometer algesicronómetro

algesimeter algesímetro

algesiogenic algesiogénico

algesiometer algesiómetro

algesthesia algestesia

algesthesis algestesis

algetic algético

algogenesia algogenesia

algogenesis algogénesis

algogenic algogénico

algolagnia algolagnia

algometer algómetro

algometry algometría

algophilia algofilia

algophily algofilia

algophobia algofobia

algopsychalia algopsicalia

algorithm algoritmo

algorithmic-heuristic theory teoría algorítmica-heurística

algospasm algoespasmo

alienation alienación

alienation coefficient coeficiente de alienación

alienist alienista

aliment alimento

alimentary canal canal alimenticio

alimentary orgasm orgasmo alimenticio

alimentary tract tracto alimenticio

aliphatic phenothiazine fenotiazina alifática

alkalinity alcalinidad

alkaloid alcaloide

alkalosis alcalosis

alkaptonuria alcaptonuria

all-or-none todo o nada

all-or-none law ley de todo o nada

all-or-none learning aprendizaje de todo o nada

all-or-none model modelo de todo o nada

all-or-nothing principle principio de todo o nada

all-or-nothing thinking pensamiento de todo o nada

allachesthesia alaquestesia

allele alelo

allelic alélico

allelomorph alelomorfo

allelomorphic alelomórfico

allergen alergeno

allergic alérgico

allergic jaundice ictericia alérgica

allergic potential scale escala de potencial alérgica

allergy alergia

allesthesia alestesia

alliaceous aliáceo

alliance alianza

alliance and splitting alianza y rompimiento

allied aliado

allied health professional profesional aliado a la salud

allied reflex reflejo aliado

alliesthesia aliestesia
alliteration aliteración
allobarbital alobarbital
allocator designante
allocentric alocéntrico
allocheiria aloquiria
allochesthesia aloquestesia
allochiria aloquiria
allocortex alocorteza
allodynia alodinia
alloerotic aloerótico
alloeroticism aloerotismo
alloerotism aloerotismo
alloesthesia aloestesia
allokinesis alocinesia
allolalia alolalia
allomeric function función alomérica
allometry alometría
allomorph alomorfo
allomorphic alomórfico
allonomous alónomo
allopathy alopatía
allophasis alofasis
allophone alófono
alloplasticity aloplasticidad
alloplasty aloplastia
allopsyche alopsiquis
allopsychic alopsíquico
allopsychic delusion delusión alopsíquica
allopsychosis alopsicosis
allotriogeusia alotriogeusia
allotriogeustia alotriogeustia
allotriophagia alotriofagia
allotriophagy alotriofagia
allotriorhexia alotriorhexia
allotriosmia alotriosmia
allotropic alotrópico
allotropic personality personalidad alotrópica
allotropy alotropía
alloxan aloxana
Allport's group relations theory teoría de
   relaciones de grupo de Allport
allusive thinking pensamiento alusivo
Almaric's syndrome síndrome de Almaric
alogia alogia
alopecia alopecia
Alpers' disease enfermedad de Alpers
alpha alfa
alpha adrenergic blocking agent agente de
   bloqueo adrenérgico alfa
alpha adrenergic blocking drug droga de
   bloqueo adrenérgico alfa
alpha adrenergic stimulating drug droga
   estimulante adrenérgico alfa
alpha adrenoceptor adrenoceptor alfa
alpha alcoholism alcoholismo alfa
alpha arc arco alfa
alpha blocking bloqueo alfa
alpha cells células alfa
alpha conditioning condicionamiento alfa
alpha endorphin endorfina alfa
alpha error error alfa
alpha index índice alfa
alpha level nivel alfa
alpha motion moción alfa

alpha movement movimiento alfa
alpha receptor receptor alfa
alpha receptor blocking agent agente de
   bloqueo de receptores alfa
alpha response respuesta alfa
alpha response pathway vía de respuesta alfa
alpha rhythm ritmo alfa
alpha sleep sueño alfa
alpha state estado alfa
alpha wave onda alfa
alpha wave training entrenamiento de ondas
   alfa
alpha hypothesis hipótesis alfa
alphabet alfabeto
alphaprodine alfaprodina
alpinism alpinismo
Alport's syndrome síndrome de Alport
alprazolam alprazolam
Alstrom's syndrome síndrome de Alstrom
Alstrom-Hallgren syndrome síndrome de
   Alstrom-Hallgren
alter alter
alter ego alter ego
altered awareness conciencia alterada
altered awareness during biofeedback
   conciencia alterada durante
   biorretroalimentación
altered state of consciousness estado de
   conciencia alterado
alteregoism alteregoísmo
alternate care cuidado alterno
alternate hemianesthesia hemianestesia
   alternada
alternate forms formas alternas
alternate-response test prueba de respuestas
   alternas
alternate state of consciousness estado de
   conciencia alterno
alternate-uses test prueba de usos alternos
alternating alternante
alternating hemiplegia hemiplejía alternante
alternating mydriasis midriasis alternante
alternating personality personalidad
   alternante
alternating perspective perspectiva alternante
alternating psychosis psicosis alternante
alternating role papel alternante
alternating tremor temblor alternante
alternating vision visión alternante
alternation alternación
alternation method método de alternación
alternation of response theory teoría de
   alternación de respuesta
alternative alternativa
alternative education systems sistemas
   educativos alternativos
alternative group session sesión de grupo
   alternativo
alternative hypothesis hipótesis alternativa
alternative intelligence tests pruebas de
   inteligencia alternativas
alternative psychologies psicologías
   alternativas
alternative psychotherapies psicoterapias
   alternativas

alternative reinforcement refuerzo alternativo
alternative school escuela alternativa
altitude sickness enfermedad de altitud
altricial altricial
altrigenderism atrigenerismo
altruism altruismo
altruistic altruista
altruistic aggression agresión altruista
altruistic behavior conducta altruista
altruistic role papel altruista
altruistic suicide suicidio altruista
alveolar alveolar
alysosis alisosis
Alzheimer's dementia demencia de Alzheimer
Alzheimer's disease enfermedad de Alzheimer
Alzheimer's sclerosis esclerosis de Alzheimer
amacrine cells células amacrinas
amantadine hydrochloride clorhidrato de amantadina
amathophobia amatofobia
amativeness amatividad
amaurosis amaurosis
amaxophobia amaxofobia
ambageusia ambageusia
ambenonium ambenonio
ambidexterity ambidextrismo
ambidextrism ambidextrismo
ambidextrous ambidextro
ambient conditions condiciones ambientales
ambiguity ambigüedad
ambiguity tolerance tolerancia a la ambigüedad
ambiguous ambiguo
ambiguous figure figura ambigua
ambiguous genitalia genitales ambiguos
ambilevous ambilevo
ambisexual ambisexual
ambisexuality ambisexualidad
ambisinister ambisinistro
ambisinistrous ambisinistro
ambitendency ambitendencia
ambition ambición
ambivalence ambivalencia
ambivalence of the intellect ambivalencia del intelecto
ambivalence of the will ambivalencia de la voluntad
ambivalency ambivalencia
ambivalent ambivalente
ambiversion ambiversión
ambivert ambivertido
amblyacousia ambliacusia
amblyaphia ambliafia
amblygeustia ambligeustia
amblyopia ambliopía
amblyoscope amblioscopio
ambrosiac ambrosiaco
ambulation ambulación
ambulatory ambulatorio
ambulatory automatism automatismo ambulatorio
ambulatory care cuidado ambulatorio

ambulatory insulin treatment tratamiento de insulina ambulatoria
ambulatory psychotherapy psicoterapia ambulatoria
ambulatory schizophrenia esquizofrenia ambulatoria
ambulatory services servicios ambulatorios
ambulatory treatment tratamiento ambulatorio
ameboid astrocyte astrocito ameboide
ameboid cell célula ameboide
amelectic ameléctico
ameleia ameleia
ameliorate ameliorar
amenomania amenomanía
amenorrhea amenorrea
amentia amencia
amential amencial
Ames demonstrations demostraciones Ames
Ames room cuarto de Ames
Ames window ventana de Ames
amethopterin ametopterina
amethystic ametístico
ametrophia ametrofia
ametropia ametropía
amiloride hydrochloride clorhidrato de amilorida
amimia amimia
amine amina
amino acid aminoácido
amino acid imbalance desequilibrio aminoácido
amino acid metabolism metabolismo de aminoácidos
aminohydroxybutyric acid ácido aminohidroxibutírico
aminophylline aminofilina
aminopterin aminopterina
aminopyrine aminopirina
amitriptyline amitriptilina
amitriptyline hydrochloride clorhidrato de amitriptilina
ammonium chloride delirium delirio de cloruro de amonio
amnemonic amnemónico
amnemonic agraphia agrafia amnemónica
amnesia amnesia
amnesia after electroconvulsive therapy amnesia tras terapia electroconvulsiva
amnesia after lesions amnesia tras lesiones
amnesia after lobectomies amnesia tras lobectomías
amnesia in Alzheimer's disease amnesia en la enfermedad de Alzheimer
amnesiac amnésico
amnesic amnésico
amnesic aphasia afasia amnésica
amnesic apraxia apraxia amnésica
amnesic confabulation confabulación amnésica
amnesic confabulatory syndrome síndrome confabulatorio amnésico
amnesic disorder trastorno amnnésico
amnesic episode episodio amnésico
amnesic misidentification identificación

errónea amnésica
amnesic psychosis psicosis amnésica
amnesic syndrome síndrome amnésico
amnestic amnésico
amnestic aphasia afasia amnésica
amnestic apraxia apraxia amnésica
amnestic confabulation confabulación
   amnésica
amnestic confabulatory syndrome síndrome
   confabulatorio amnésico
amnestic disorder trastorno amnnésico
amnestic episode episodio amnésico
amnestic misidentification identificación
   errónea amnésica
amnestic psychosis psicosis amnésica
amnestic syndrome síndrome amnésico
amniocentesis amniocentesis
amniography amniografía
amnion amnios
amniotic amniótico
amniotic fluid fluido amniótico
amobarbital amobarbital
amobarbital interview entrevista con
   amobarbital
amok amok
amorous paranoia paranoia amorosa
amorphagnosia amorfagnosia
amorphosynthesis amorfosíntesis
amotivational amotivacional
amotivational syndrome síndrome
   amotivacional
amoxapine amoxapina
amphetamine anfetamina
amphetamine abuse abuso de anfetaminas
amphetamine anxiety disorder trastorno de
   ansiedad anfetamina
amphetamine delirium delirio anfetamina
amphetamine delusional disorder trastorno
   delusorio anfetamina
amphetamine dependence dependencia
   anfetamina
amphetamine disorder trastorno anfetamina
amphetamine effects efectos de anfetaminas
amphetamine-induced mental disorder
   trastorno mental inducido por anfetaminas
amphetamine intoxication intoxicación por
   anfetaminas
amphetamine mood disorder trastorno del
   humor de anfetaminas
amphetamine psychosis psicosis anfetamina
amphetamine psychotic disorder trastorno
   psicótico anfetamina
**amphetamine psychotic disorder with
   delusions** trastorno psicótico anfetamina
   con delusiones
**amphetamine psychotic disorder with
   hallucinations** trastorno psicótico
   anfetamina con alucinaciones
amphetamine sexual dysfunction disfunción
   sexual anfetamina
amphetamine sleep disorder trastorno del
   sueño de anfetaminas
amphetamine tolerance tolerancia de
   anfetaminas
amphetamine use disorder trastorno de uso

de anfetaminas
amphetamine withdrawal retiro de
   anfetaminas
amphicrania anficrania
amphierotism anfierotismo
amphigenesis anfigénesis
amphigenous inversion inversión anfígena
amphimixis anfimixis
amphithymia anfitimia
amphotonia anfotonía
amphotony anfotonía
amplification amplificación
amplification model modelo de amplificación
amplitude amplitud
amplitude distortion distorsión de amplitud
amplitude of response amplitud de respuesta
ampulla ampollita
amputation amputación
amputation doll muñeca de amputación
amputation neuroma neuroma de amputación
amuck amok
amusia amusia
amychophobia amicofobia
amygdala amígdala
amygdaloid amigdaloide
amygdaloid stimulation estimulación
   amigdaloide
amyl nitrite nitrito de amilo
amylase amilasa
amyloid amiloide
amyloidosis amiloidosis
amylophagia amilofagia
amyoesthesia amioestesia
amyoesthesis amioestesia
amyostasia amiostasia
amyosthenia amiostenia
amyotonia amiotonía
amyotonia congenita amiotonía congénita
amyotrophia amiotrofia
amyotrophic lateral sclerosis esclerosis
   lateral amiotrófica
amyotrophy amiotrofia
anabolic anabólico
anabolic phase fase anabólica
anabolic system sistema anabólico
anabolism anabolismo
anacamptometer anacamptómetro
anacatesthesia anacatestesia
anaclisis anaclisis
anaclitic anaclítico
anaclitic choice selección anaclítica
anaclitic depression depresión anaclítica
anaclitic identification identificación
   anaclítica
anaclitic object choice selección de objeto
   anaclítico
anaclitic psychotherapy psicoterapia
   anaclítica
anaclitic therapy terapia anaclítica
anacousia anacusia
anacusia anacusia
anacusis anacusis
anaerobic anaeróbico
anaesthesia anestesia
anaglyph anaglifo

anaglyptoscope anagliptoscopio
anagoge anagogia
anagogic anagógico
anagogic symbolism simbolismo anagógico
anagogic tendency tendencia anagógica
anagogy anagogia
anagram anagrama
anal anal
anal-aggressive character carácter anal-agresivo
anal birth nacimiento anal
anal castration castración anal
anal castration anxiety ansiedad de castración anal
anal character carácter anal
anal-erotic trait rasgo anal-erótico
anal eroticism erotismo anal
anal erotism erotismo anal
anal-expulsive anal-expulsivo
anal-expulsive character carácter anal-expulsivo
anal-expulsive personality personalidad anal-expulsiva
anal-expulsive stage etapa anal-expulsiva
anal fantasies fantasías anales
anal humor humor anal
anal impotence impotencia anal
anal intercourse relación anal
anal masturbation masturbación anal
anal personality personalidad anal
anal phase fase anal
anal rape fantasy fantasía de violación anal
anal reflex reflejo anal
anal retention retención anal
anal-retentive anal-retentivo
anal-retentive character carácter anal-retentivo
anal-retentive personality personalidad anal-retentiva
anal-retentive stage etapa anal-retentiva
anal sadism sadismo anal
anal-sadistic anal-sádico
anal-sadistic stage etapa anal-sádico
anal sphincters esfínteres anales
anal stage etapa anal
anal triad tríada anal
analepsis analepsis
analeptic analéptico
analgesia analgesia
analgesia algera analgesia álgera
analgesia dolorosa analgesia dolorosa
analgesic analgésico
analgesic cuirass coraza analgésica
analgesimeter analgesímetro
analgetic analgético
analgia analgia
anality analidad
analog análogo
analogical reasoning razonamiento analógico
analogies test prueba de analogías
analogous análogo
analogue análogo
analogue experiment experimento análogo
analogue study estudio análogo
analogy analogía

analysand analizando
analysis análisis
analysis by synthesis análisis por síntesis
analysis by synthesis model modelo de análisis por síntesis
analysis in depth análisis a fondo
analysis of covariance análisis de covarianza
analysis of dreams análisis de sueños
analysis of the resistance análisis de la resistencia
analysis of transference análisis de transferencia
analysis of variance análisis de varianza
analysis unit unidad de análisis
analyst analista
analytic analítico
analytic group psychotherapy psicoterapia de grupo analítica
analytic insight penetración analítica
analytic interpretation interpretación analítica
analytic language lenguaje analítico
analytic learning conditions condiciones de aprendizaje analíticas
analytic neurosis neurosis analítica
analytic patient paciente analítico
analytic processing procesamiento analítico
analytic psychiatry psiquiatría analítica
analytic psychology psicología analítica
analytic rules reglas analíticas
analytic stalemate estancamiento analítico
analytic psychotherapy psicoterapia analítica
analytic therapy terapia analítica
analytical analítico
analyzer analizador
anamnesia anamnesia
anamnesis anamnesis
anamnestic anamnésico
anamnestic analysis análisis anamnésico
ananastasia ananastasia
anancasm anancasmo
anancastia anancastia
anancastic anancástico
anancastic personality personalidad anancástica
anandria anandria
anankasm anancasmo
anankastia anancastia
anankastic anancástico
anankastic personality personalidad anancástica
anapeiratic anapeirático
anaphase anafase
anaphia anafia
anaphora anáfora
anaphrodisia anafrodisia
anaphrodisiac anafrodisiaco
anaphylaxis anafilaxis
anaplastic astrocytoma astrocitoma anaplástico
anaptic anáptico
anarchic behavior conducta anárquica
anarithmia anarritmia
anarthria anartria
anastasis anastasis
anastomosis anastomosis

anatomical age edad anatómica
anatomical factors factores anatómicos
anatomy anatomía
anatopism anatopismo
anaudia anaudia
anchor ancla
anchor points puntos de anclaje
anchor test prueba de anclaje
anchorage anclaje
anchoring anclaje
anchoring of ego anclaje del ego
ancillary auxiliar
ancillary care cuidado auxiliar
androgen andrógeno
androgen hormones hormonas andrógenas
androgen hypersecretion hipersecreción
    andrógena
androgen-insensitivity syndrome síndrome
    de insensibilidad a andrógenos
androgen level nivel de andrógeno
androgenic androgénico
androgenization androgenización
androgyneity androginidad
androgynism androginismo
androgynous sex role papel sexual andrógeno
androgyny androginia
androgyny scale escala de androginia
android androide
andromania andromanía
androphile andrófilo
androphilia androfilia
androphobia androfobia
androstenedione androstenediona
androsterone androsterona
anecdotal evidence prueba anecdótica
anecdotal method método anecdótico
anecdotal record registro anecdótico
anechoic anecoico
anechoic chamber cámara anecoica
anejaculatory aneyaculatorio
anejaculatory orgasm orgasmo
    aneyaculatorio
Anel's method método de Anel
anelectronic anelectrónico
anelectrotonus anelectrotono
anemia anemia
anemic anémico
anemic anoxia anoxia anémica
anemophobia anemofobia
anemotropism anemotropismo
anencephalia anencefalia
anencephalic anencefálico
anencephalous anencéfalo
anencephaly anencefalia
anepia anepia
anergasia anergasia
anergastic anergástico
anergia anergia
anergic anérgico
anergic schizophrenia esquizofrenia anérgica
anergic schizophrenic esquizofrénico
    anérgico
anergy anergia
anerotism anerotismo
anesthecinesia anestecinesia

anesthekinesia anestecinesia
anesthesia anestesia
anesthesia dolorosa anestesia dolorosa
anesthesia sexualis anestesia sexual
anesthetic anestésico
anesthetic leprosy lepra anestésica
anethopath anetópata
anethopathy anetopatía
anetopathy anetopatía
aneuploidy aneuploidia
aneurysm aneurisma
aneurysmectomy aneurismectomía
aneuthanasia aneutanasia
Angelucci's syndrome síndrome de Angelucci
anger ira
anger rape violación por ira
angina angina
angina pectoris angina de pecho
anginophobia anginofobia
angioblastoma angioblastoma
angiodysgenetic myelomalacia mielomalacia
    angiodisgenética
angioedema angioedema
angioglioma angioglioma
angiogram angiograma
angiography angiografía
angiolithic sarcoma sarcoma angiolítico
angioma angioma
angiomatosis angiomatosis
angioneurectomy angioneurectomía
angioneuredema angioneuredema
angioneurosis angioneurosis
angioneurotic angioneurótico
angioneurotic edema edema angioneurótico
angioneurotomy angioneurotomía
angioparalytic neurasthenia neurastenia
    angioparalítica
angiopathic angiopático
angiopathic neurasthenia neurastenia
    angiopática
angiopathy angiopatía
angiophacomatosis angiofacomatosis
angiophakomatosis angiofacomatosis
angioscotoma angioscotoma
angiotensin angiotensina
angiotensinogen angiotensinógeno
angor angor
angor animi angor animi
angor pectoris angor pectoris
angry airado
angry aggression agresión airada
angry woman syndrome síndrome de mujer
    airada
angst angustia, ansiedad
angstrom angstrom
angular gyrus circunvolución angular
anhaphia anafia
anhedonia anhedonia
anhidrosis anhidrosis
anhypnia anhipnia
anhypnosis anhipnosis
aniconia aniconia
anilerdine anilerdina
anilinction anilición
anilingus anilingus

anility anilidad
anima anima
animal aggression agresión animal
animal aggressive behavior conducta agresiva
  animal
animal behavior conducta animal
animal cognition cognición animal
animal communication comunicación animal
animal concept learning aprendizaje de
  conceptos animal
animal cruelty crueldad hacia animales
animal hypnosis hipnosis animal
animal intelligence inteligencia animal
animal learning aprendizaje animal
animal magnetism magnetismo animal
animal parental behavior conducta parental
  de animales
animal phobia fobia de animales
animal psychology psicología animal
animal sexual behavior conducta sexual de
  animales
animal sociobiology sociobiología animal
animal studies estudios de animales
animastic animástico
animation animación
animation complex complejo de animación
animatism animatismo
animism animismo
animistic thinking pensamiento animístico
animosity animosidad
animus animus
aniseikonia aniseiconía
anisocoria anisocoria
anisoiconia anisoiconia
anisometropia anisometropía
anisophrenia anisofrenia
anisopia anisopía
anisotropia anisotropía
ankle tobillo
ankle clonus clono del tobillo
ankle jerk sacudida del tobillo
ankle reflex reflejo del tobillo
ankyloglossia anquiloglosia
ankylosing spondylitis espondilitis
  anquilosante
ankylosis anquilosis
ankylostoma ancilostoma
anlage anlaje
annihilation anxiety ansiedad de aniquilación
anniversary excitement excitación de
  aniversario
anniversary hypothesis hipótesis de
  aniversario
anniversary reaction reacción de aniversario
annoyer molestador
annulment anulación
anochlesia anoclesia
anociassociation anociasociación
anodontia anodontia
anodyne anodino
anoesia anoesia
anoesis anoesis
anoetic anoético
anogenital anogenital
anoia anoia

anomalopia anomalopía
anomaloscope anomaloscopio
anomalous anómalo
anomalous contour contorno anómalo
anomalous dichromatism dicromatismo
  anómalo
anomalous sentence oración anómala
anomalous stimulus estímulo anómalo
anomalous trichromatism tricromatismo
  anómalo
anomaly anomalía
anomia anomia
anomic anómico
anomic aphasia afasia anómica
anomic suicide suicidio anómico
anomie anomia
anomie scale escala anomia
anomy anomia
anonymity anonimato
anoopsia anopsia
anophthalmia anoftalmía
anopia anopía
anopsia anopsia
anorectal anorrectal
anorectal spasm espasmo anorrectal
anorectic anorético
anoretic anorético
anorexia anorexia
anorexia nervosa anorexia nerviosa
anorexiant anorexígeno
anorexic anoréxico
anorexigenic anorexígeno
anorgasmia anorgasmia
anorgasmic anorgásmico
anorgasmy anorgasmia
anorthography anortografía
anorthopia anortopía
anorthoscopic anortoscópico
anorthosis anortosis
anosmia anosmia
anosmic anósmico
anosodiaphoria anosodiaforia
anosognosia anosognosia
anosognosic anosognósico
anosognosic epilepsy epilepsia anosognósica
anosognosic seizure acceso anosognósico
anosphresia anosfresia
anovulatory anovulatorio
anovulatory menstrual cycle ciclo menstrual
  anovulatorio
anoxemia anoxemia
anoxia anoxia
antacid antiácido
antagonism antagonismo
antagonism hypothesis hipótesis del
  antagonismo
antagonist antagonista
antagonistic antagónico
antagonistic colors colores antagónicos
antagonistic cooperation cooperación
  antagónica
antagonistic muscles músculos antagónicos
antagonistic reflexes reflejos antagónicos
antaphrodisiac antafrodisiaco
ante partum ante partum

antecedent antecedente
antecedent stimuli estímulos antecedentes
antedating response respuesta adelantada
antephialtic antefiáltico
anterior anterior
anterior cerebral artery arteria cerebral
   anterior
anterior commissure comisura anterior
anterior forceps forceps anterior
anterior horn cuerno anterior
anterior nuclei of thalamus núcleos
   anteriores del tálamo
anterior nucleus núcleo anterior
anterior pituitary pituitaria anterior
anterior pituitary gonadotropin
   gonadotropina pituitaria anterior
anterior-posterior development gradient
   gradiente del desarrollo anterior-posterior
anterior rhizotomy rizotomía anterior
anterior root raíz anterior
anterograde anterógrado
anterograde amnesia amnesia anterógrada
anterograde degeneration degeneración
   anterógrada
anterograde memory memoria anterógrada
anterolateral anterolateral
anterolateral cordotomy cordotomía
   anterolateral
anterolateral system sistema anterolateral
anterolateral tractotomy tractotomía
   anterolateral
anterotic antierótico
anthrax ántrax
anthropocentric antropocéntrico
anthropocentrism antropocentrismo
anthropoid antropoide
anthropology antropología
anthropometry antropometría
anthropomorph antropomorfo
anthropomorphic thinking pensamiento
   antropomórfico
anthropomorphism antropomorfismo
anthroponomy antroponomía
anthropopathy antropopatía
anthropophagy antropofagia
anthropophobia antropofobia
anthroposcopy antroposcopia
anthrotype antrotipo
antiadrenergic antiadrenérgico
antianalytic procedures procedimientos
   antianalíticos
antiandrogen antiandrógeno
antiandrogen therapy terapia antiandrógena
antiandrogenic agent agente antiandrogénico
antianxiety antiansiedad
antianxiety agent agente antiansiedad
antianxiety drug droga antiansiedad
antianxiety medication medicación
   antiansiedad
antibiotic antibiótico
antibody anticuerpo
antibrain antibody anticuerpo anticerebro
anticathexis anticatexis
anticephalagic anticefalágico
anticholinergic anticolinérgico

anticholinergic effect efecto anticolinérgico
anticholinergic syndrome síndrome
   anticolinérgico
anticholinesterase anticolinesterasa
anticipation anticipación
anticipation error error de anticipación
anticipation method método de anticipación
anticipation of role anticipación del papel
anticipatory anticipatorio
anticipatory aggression agresión anticipatoria
anticipatory anxiety ansiedad anticipatoria
anticipatory autocastration autocastración
   anticipatoria
anticipatory error error anticipatorio
anticipatory grief aflicción anticipatoria
anticipatory guidance asesoramiento
   anticipatorio
anticipatory maturation maduración
   anticipatoria
anticipatory-maturation principle principio
   de maduración anticipatoria
anticipatory mourning duelo anticipatorio
anticipatory nausea náusea anticipatoria
anticipatory nausea and vomiting náusea y
   vómitos anticipatorios
anticipatory regret remordimiento
   anticipatorio
anticipatory response respuesta anticipatoria
anticonformity anticonformismo
anticonvulsant anticonvulsivo
anticonvulsive anticonvulsivo
antidepressant antidepresivo
antidepressant drug droga antidepresiva
antidepressive antidepresivo
antidepressive drug droga antidepresiva
antidiuretic antidiurético
antidiuretic hormone hormona antidiurética
antidromic antidrómico
antidromic conduction conducción
   antidrómica
antidromic phenomenon fenómeno
   antidrómico
antiepileptic antiepiléptico
antiepileptic drug droga antiepiléptica
antiestrogenic antiestrogénico
antiexpectation technique técnica
   antiexpectación
antifetishism antifetichismo
antigen antígeno
antigen-antibody reactions reacciones
   antígeno-anticuerpo
antigonadal action acción antigonadal
antihistamine antihistamina
antihypnotic antihipnótico
antiintoxicant antiintoxicante
antiintraception antiintracepción
antilibidinal ego ego antilibidinal
antimania antimanía
antimaniac antimaníaco
antimaniac drug droga antimaníaca
antimaniacal antimaníaco
antimetabolite antimetabolita
antimetropia antimetropía
antimicrobial antimicrobiano
antimotivational syndrome síndrome

antimotivacional
antimyasthenic antimiasténico
antineuralgic antineurálgico
antineuritic antineurítico
antinodal behavior conducta antinodal
antinomy antinomía
antiobsessive antiobsesivo
antiparkinsonian antiparkinsoniano
antiparkinsonian drug droga
   antiparkinsoniana
antiphobic antifóbico
antipraxia antipraxia
antipredator behavior conducta
   antipredadora
antipsychiatry antipsiquiatría
antipsychotic antipsicótico
antipsychotic agent agente antipsicótico
antipsychotic drug droga antipsicótica
antipyretic antipirético
antipyrine antipirina
antireward system sistema antirrecompensa
antirisk factor factor antirriesgo
antiruminant antirrumiante
antisocial antisocial
antisocial activity actividad antisocial
antisocial aggression agresión antisocial
antisocial behavior conducta antisocial
antisocial compulsion compulsión antisocial
antisocial personality personalidad antisocial
antisocial personality disorder trastorno de
   personalidad antisocial
antisocial reaction reacción antisocial
antisocial scale escala antisocial
antisocial spectrum disorder trastorno de
   espectro antisocial
antispasmodic antiespasmódico
antitechnology bias sesgo antitecnología
antitetanic antitetánico
antitonic antitónico
antitrismus antitrismo
antitussive antitusivo
antiviral antiviral
antiviral drug droga antiviral
antivitamin antivitamina
antlophobia antlofobia
Anton's syndrome síndrome de Anton
Antoni type A neurilemoma neurilemoma
   tipo A de Antoni
Antoni type B neurilemoma neurilemoma
   tipo B de Antoni
antonym test prueba de antónimos
antrophose antrofosia
Antyllus' method método de Antyllus
anulospiral ending terminación anuloespiral
anus ano
anvil yunque
anxiety ansiedad
anxiety and sleep problems ansiedad y
   problemas de sueño
anxiety attack ataque de ansiedad
anxiety depersonalization neurosis neurosis
   de despersonalización ansiosa
anxiety depression depresión con ansiedad
anxiety discharge descarga de ansiedad
anxiety disorder trastorno de ansiedad

**anxiety disorder due to general medical
   condition** trastorno de ansiedad debido a
   condición médica general
anxiety disorder of adolescence trastorno de
   ansiedad de adolescencia
anxiety disorder of childhood trastorno de
   ansiedad de niñez
anxiety disturbance disturbio de ansiedad
anxiety dream sueño ansioso
anxiety-elation psychosis psicosis de
   ansiedad-elación
anxiety equivalent equivalente de ansiedad
anxiety fixation fijación de ansiedad
anxiety hierarchy jerarquía de ansiedad
anxiety hysteria histeria ansiosa
anxiety in adolescence ansiedad en
   adolescencia
anxiety management training entrenamiento
   de administración de ansiedad
anxiety neurosis neurosis de ansiedad
anxiety nightmare pesadilla ansiosa
anxiety object objeto de ansiedad
anxiety-prone propenso a ansiedad
anxiety reaction reacción ansiosa
anxiety-relief response respuesta de
   ansiedad-alivio
anxiety resolution resolución de ansiedad
anxiety scale escala de ansiedad
anxiety state estado de ansiedad
anxiety state versus autism estado de
   ansiedad contra autismo
anxiety state versus avoidant disorder estado
   de ansiedad contra trastorno evitante
anxiety state versus schizophrenia estado de
   ansiedad contra esquizofrenia
anxiety syndrome síndrome de ansiedad
anxiety tolerance tolerancia de ansiedad
anxiety typology tipología de ansiedad
anxiety versus fear ansiedad contra temor
anxiolytic ansiolítico
anxiolytic abuse abuso de ansiolítico
anxiolytic anxiety disorder trastorno de
   ansiedad de ansiolítico
anxiolytic delirium delirio de ansiolítico
anxiolytic dependence dependencia de
   ansiolítico
anxiolytic intoxication intoxicación por
   ansiolítico
anxiolytic mood disorder trastorno del humor
   de ansiolítico
anxiolytic persisting amnestic disorder
   trastorno amnésico persistente de ansiolítico
anxiolytic persisting dementia demencia
   persistente de ansiolítico
anxiolytic psychotic disorder trastorno
   psicótico de ansiolítico
anxiolytic psychotic disorder with delusions
   trastorno psicótico de ansiolítico con
   delusiones
**anxiolytic psychotic disorder with
   hallucinations** trastorno psicótico de
   ansiolítico con alucinaciones
anxiolytic sexual dysfunction disfunción
   sexual de ansiolítico
anxiolytic sleep disorder trastorno del sueño

de ansiolítico
anxiolytic use disorder trastorno de uso de
    ansiolítico
anxiolytic withdrawal retiro de ansiolítico
anxious ansioso
anxious-ambivalent child niño
    ansioso-ambivalente
anxious-avoidant child niño ansioso-evitante
anxious delirium delirio ansioso
anxious depression depresión ansiosa
anxious expectation expectación ansiosa
anxious mood humor ansioso
aortic arch syndrome síndrome del cayado
    aórtico
aortic body tumor tumor del cuerpo aórtico
apallesthesia apalestesia
apallic apálico
apallic state estado apálico
apallic syndrome síndrome apálico
apandria apandria
apanthropy apantropía
aparalytic aparalítico
apareunia apareunia
apastia apastia
apathetic apático
apathetic hyperthyroidism hipertiroidismo
    apático
apathetic withdrawal retirada apática
apathism apatismo
apathy apatía
apathy syndrome síndrome de apatía
apeirophobia apeirofobia
aperiodic reinforcement refuerzo aperiódico
aperiodic reinforcement schedule programa
    de refuerzo aperiódico
Apert's syndrome síndrome de Apert
apertural hypothesis hipótesis abertural
aperture abertura
Apgar score puntuación de Apgar
aphagia afagia
aphakia afaquia
aphanisis afanisis
aphasia afasia
aphasiac afásico
aphasic afásico
aphasic disturbance disturbio afásico
aphasiologist afasiólogo
aphasiology afasiología
aphelxia afelxia
aphemesthesia afemestesia
aphemia afemia
aphemic afémico
aphephobia afefobia
aphilopony afiloponia
aphonia afonía
aphonia paralytica afonía paralítica
aphonic afónico
aphonogelia afonogelia
aphonous afónico
aphony afonía
aphoresis aforesis
aphoria aforia
aphrasia afrasia
aphrenia afrenia
aphrodisia afrodisia

aphrodisiac afrodisiaco
aphrodisiomania afrodisiomanía
aphthenxia aftenxia
aphthongia aftongia
apiphobia apifobia
aplasia aplasia
aplastic aplástico
aplestia aplestia
apnea apnea
apneic apneico
apneic pause pausa apneica
apneusis apneusis
apneustic breathing respiración apnéustica
apnoea apnea
apocarteresis apocarteresis
apocleisis apoclesia
apoclesis apoclesia
apodemialgia apodemialgia
apokamnosic apocamnósico
apokamnosis apocamnosis
apolepsis apolepsis
apomorphine apomorfina
aponeurotic reflex reflejo aponeurótico
apopathetic apopatético
apopathetic behavior conducta apopatética
apophysary apofisario
apophysary point punto apofisario
apophysial apofisario
apophysial point punto apofisario
apoplectic apopléctico
apoplectic cyst quiste apopléctico
apoplectic type tipo apopléctico
apoplectiform apoplectiforme
apoplectoid apoplectoide
apoplexy apoplejía
apopnixis apopnixia
aporia aporía
aporioneurosis aporioneurosis
apparatus aparato
apparent aparente
apparent motion moción aparente
apparent movement movimiento aparente
apparent size tamaño aparente
apparition aparición
appeal atractivo
appearance apariencia
appearance-reality discrimination
    discriminación apariencia-realidad
appease apaciguar
appeasement behavior conducta de
    apaciguamiento
apperception apercepción
apperceptive aperceptivo
apperceptive mass masa aperceptiva
appersonation apersonificación
appersonification apersonificación
appestat apestato
appetite apetito
appetite control control de apetito
appetite disorder trastorno de apetito
appetite disturbance disturbio de apetito
appetite suppressant supresor de apetito
appetitive apetitivo
appetitive behavior conducta apetitiva
appetitive conditioning condicionamiento

apetitivo
appetitive learning aprendizaje apetitivo
appetitive phase fase apetitiva
applied anthropology antropología aplicada
applied ethics ética aplicada
applied psychoanalysis psicoanálisis aplicado
applied psychology psicología aplicada
applied research investigación aplicada
apprehension aprehensión
apprehension span lapso de aprehensión
apprehensiveness aprehensión
apprentice complex complejo de aprendiz
apprenticeship noviciado
approach acercamiento
approach-approach conflict conflicto de
    acercamiento-acercamiento
approach-avoidance conflict conflicto de
    acercamiento-evitación
approach gradient gradiente de acercamiento
approach or withdrawal acercamiento o
    retirada
approach response respuesta de acercamiento
appropriate apropiado
appropriate affect afecto apropiado
appropriateness of affect idoneidad de afecto
appropriateness of emotional response
    idoneidad de respuesta emocional
approval aprobación
approval need necesidad de aprobación
approximation aproximación
approximation conditioning
    condicionamiento por aproximación
approximation method método de
    aproximación
appurtenance pertenencia
apractagnosia apractagnosia
apractic apráctico
apragmatism apragmatismo
apraxia apraxia
apraxia algera apraxia álgera
apraxia of gait apraxia de marcha
apraxic apráxico
apraxic dysarthria disartria apráxica
apriorism apriorismo
aprobarbital aprobarbital
aprophoria aproforia
aprosexia aprosexia
aprosodia aprosodia
aprosody aprosodia
apsychia apsiquia
apsychognosia apsicognosia
apsychosis apsicosis
aptitude aptitud
aptitude test prueba de aptitud
apyretic tetanus tétanos apirético
aquaphobia acuafobia
aqueduct of Sylvius acueducto de Silvio
aqueductal intubation intubación acueductal
aqueous humor humor acuoso
arachneophobia aracnofobia
arachnoid aracnoideo
arachnoid cyst quiste aracnoideo
arachnoid granulations granulaciones
    aracnoideas
arachnoid layer capa aracnoidea

arachnoid membrane membrana aracnoidea
arachnoiditis aracnoiditis
arachnophobia aracnofobia
Arago phenomenon fenómeno de Arago
Aran-Duchenne disease enfermedad de
    Aran-Duchenne
araphia arafia
arbitrary arbitrario
arbitrary symbols símbolos arbitrarios
arbitration arbitraje
arbor vitae árbol vital
arborization arborización
arc arco
arc sine transformation transformación arco
    seno
archaic arcaico
archaic brain cerebro arcaico
archaic inheritance herencia arcaica
archaic-paralogical thinking pensamiento
    arcaico-paralógico
archaic residue residuo arcaico
archaic thought pensamiento arcaico
archaism arcaísmo
archetypal form forma arquetípica
archetype arquetipo
archicerebellum arquicerebelo
archicortex arquicorteza
Archimedes spiral espiral de Arquímedes
architectonic arquitectónico
architectural barriers barreras
    arquitectónicas
archival research investigación de archivos
Arctic hysteria histeria ártica
arcuate fasciculus fascículo arqueado
arcuate nucleus núcleo arqueado
arcuate zone of the brain zona arqueada del
    cerebro
ardanesthesia ardanestesia
area área
area diagram diagrama de área
area postrema área postrema
area sampling muestreo por áreas
area striata área estriada
area under the curve área bajo la curva
arecoline arecolina
areflexia arreflexia
areola areola
argentophilic plaques placas argentófilas
argininosuccinic aciduria aciduria
    argininosuccínica
argot argot
argumentativeness argumentatividad
Argyll Robertson pupil pupila de Argyll
    Robertson
argyrophilic plaques placas argirófilas
arhinencephalia arrinencefalia
aristogenics aristogénica
Aristotelian aristotélico
Aristotelian method método aristotélico
Aristotle's illusion ilusión de Aristóteles
arithmetic aritmética
arithmetic disability discapacidad aritmética
arithmetic disorder trastorno aritmético
arithmetic mean media aritmética
arithmetic series serie aritmética

arithmetic word problems problemas de palabras aritméticas
arithmomania aritmomanía
arm extension test prueba de extensión del brazo
arm phenomenon fenómeno del brazo
Arnold-Chiari deformity deformidad de Arnold-Chiari
Arnold-Chiari malformation malformación de Arnold-Chiari
Arnold-Chiari syndrome síndrome de Arnold-Chiari
arousal despertamiento
arousal and emotions despertamiento y emociones
arousal boost aumento de despertamiento
arousal boost mechanism mecanismo de aumento de despertamiento
arousal detection detección de despertamiento
arousal disorder trastorno de despertamiento
arousal function función de despertamiento
arousal reaction reacción de despertamiento
arousal reduction mechanism mecanismo de reducción de despertamiento
arousal state estado de despertamiento
arousal theory teoría de despertamiento
arousal threshold umbral de despertamiento
arranged marriage matrimonio concertado
array ordenación
arrest paro, detención
arrest reaction reacción de detención
arrhigosis arrigosis
arrhinencephalia arrinencefalia
arrhinencephaly arrinencefalia
arrhythmia arritmia
arrhythmokinesis arritmocinesis
arrowhead illusion ilusión de la punta de flecha
arsenic poisoning envenenamiento por arsénico
arsenical tremor temblor arsenical
arsphenamine hemorrhagic encephalitis encefalitis hemorrágica de arsfenamina
art tests pruebas de arte
art therapy terapia artística
arterial circle círculo arterial
arteriogram arteriograma
arteriography arteriografía
arteriole reaction reacción de arteriola
arteriopalmus arteriopalmo
arteriosclerosis arterioesclerosis
arteriosclerotic arterioesclerótico
arteriosclerotic brain disorder trastorno cerebral arterioesclerótico
arteriosclerotic dementia demencia arterioesclerótica
artériosclerotic psychosis psicosis arterioesclerótica
arteritis arteritis
artery arteria
arthresthesia artrestesia
arthritic diathesis diátesis artrítica
arthritic general pseudoparalysis seudoparálisis general artrítica
arthritis artritis

arthritism artritismo
arthrodesis artrodesis
arthrogryposis artrogriposis
arthropathy artropatía
articular articular
articular leprosy lepra articular
articular sensibility sensibilidad articular
articulate (adj) claro
articulate (v) articular
articulate speech habla clara
articulation articulación
articulation disorder trastorno de articulación
articulation error error de articulación
articulation index índice de articulación
articulation speed velocidad de articulación
articulation test prueba de articulación
articulation time tiempo de articulación
articulatory store almacén articulatorio
artifact artefacto
artificial body part parte del cuerpo artificial
artificial disorder trastorno artificial
artificial dream sueño artificial
artificial ear oreja artificial
artificial insemination inseminación artificial
artificial intelligence inteligencia artificial
artificial language lenguaje artificial
artificial neurosis neurosis artificial
artificial penis pene artificial
artificial pupil pupila artificial
artificial selection selección artificial
artificial visual system sistema visual artificial
artificialism artificialismo
artisan's cramp calambre de artesano
arts and crafts artes y oficios
aryepiglottic ariepiglótico
as if como si
as if hypothesis hipótesis como sí
as if performance representación como sí
as if personality personalidad como sí
asapholalia asafolalia
ascendance ascendencia
ascendance-submission ascendencia-sumisión
ascendancy ascendencia
ascending ascendente
ascending degeneration degeneración ascendente
ascending-descending series serie ascendente-descendente
ascending hemiplegia hemiplejía ascendente
ascending myelitis mielitis ascendente
ascending neuritis neuritis ascendente
ascending paralysis parálisis ascendente
ascending reticular system sistema reticular ascendente
asceticism ascetismo
Asch situation situación Asch
ascribed role papel atribuido
asemasia asemasia
asemia asemia
aseptic aséptico
asexual asexual
asitia asitia
asocial asocial
asociality asocialidad

asonia asonia
asoticamania asoticamanía
aspartame aspartama
aspartic acid ácido aspártico
aspartylglycosaminuria
  aspartilglucosaminuria
Asperger's disorder trastorno de Asperger
aspermatism aspermatismo
aspermia aspermia
asphalgesia asfalgesia
asphyxia asfixia
aspiration aspiración
aspiration level nivel de aspiración
aspirational group grupo aspiracional
aspirin effects efectos de la aspirina
aspirin poisoning envenenamiento por
  aspirina
assault asalto
assay ensayo
assertive asertivo
assertive behavior conducta asertiva
assertive behavior facilitation facilitación de
  conducta asertiva
assertive conditioning condicionamiento
  asertivo
assertive training entrenamiento asertivo
assessing children evaluando niños
assessing children for psychotherapy
  evaluando niños para psicoterapia
assessment evaluación
assessment center centro de evaluación
assessment for special education evaluación
  para educación especial
assessment instrument instrumento de
  evaluación
assessment methods métodos de evaluación
assessment of acuity evaluación de agudeza
assessment of anxiety evaluación de ansiedad
assessment of autism evaluación de autismo
assessment of behavior disorders evaluación
  de trastornos de conducta
assessment of communication evaluación de
  comunicación
assessment of competency to stand trial
  evaluación de competencia para someterse
  a juicio
assessment of coordination evaluación de
  coordinación
assessment of criminal responsibility
  evaluación de responsabilidad criminal
assessment of delinquency evaluación de
  delincuencia
assessment of depression evaluación de
  depresión
assessment of eating disorders evaluación de
  trastornos del comer
assessment of emotional dysfunction
  evaluación de disfunción emocional
assessment of language evaluación del
  lenguaje
assessment of learning disabilities evaluación
  de discapacidades de aprendizaje
assessment of social skills evaluación de
  destrezas sociales
assessment team equipo de evaluación

assessment techniques técnicas de evaluación
assets-liabilities technique técnica de
  ventajas-desventajas
assignment asignación
assignment therapy terapia de asignación
assimilable asimilable
assimilate asimilar
assimilation asimilación
assimilation-contrast theory teoría de
  asimilación-contraste
assimilation effect efecto de asimilación
assimilation law ley de asimilación
assimilative illusion ilusión asimilativa
assimilative learning aprendizaje asimilativo
associate asociado
associated movement movimiento asociado
association asociación
association area área de asociación
association by contiguity asociación por
  contigüidad
association coefficient coeficiente de
  asociación
association cortex corteza de asociación
association disturbance disturbio de
  asociación
association experiment experimento de
  asociación
association fibers fibras de asociación
association mechanism mecanismo de
  asociación
association method método de asociación
association neuron neurona de asociación
association neurosis neurosis de asociación
association nuclei núcleos de asociación
association of ideas asociación de ideas
association-reaction time tiempo de
  asociación-reacción
association-sensation ratio razón de
  asociación-sensación
association test prueba de asociación
association theory teoría de asociación
association time tiempo de asociación
associationism asociacionismo
associative asociativo
associative anamnesis anamnesis asociativa
associative aphasia afasia asociativa
associative bond vínculo asociativo
associative-chain theory teoría
  cadena-asociativa
associative conditioning condicionamiento
  asociativo
associative facilitation facilitación asociativa
associative fluency fluidez asociativa
associative illusion ilusión asociativa
associative inhibition inhibición asociativa
associative interference interferencia
  asociativa
associative laws leyes asociativas
associative learning aprendizaje asociativo
associative linkage enlace asociativo
associative memory memoria asociativa
associative networks redes asociativas
associative play juego asociativo
associative shifting cambio asociativo
associative strength fuerza asociativa

associative thinking pensamiento asociativo
assonance asonancia
assortative mating apareamiento selectivo
assortive mating apareamiento selectivo
assumed mean media asumida
assumed similarity parecido asumido
assumption asunción
astasia astasia
astasia-abasia astasia-abasia
astatic astático
astereognosia astereognosia
astereognosis astereognosis
asterixis asterixis
asthenia astenia
asthenic asténico
asthenic feeling sensación asténica
asthenic personality personalidad asténica
asthenic type tipo asténico
asthenology astenología
asthenophobia astenofobia
asthenopia astenopía
asthma asma
astigmatism astigmatismo
astraphobia astrafobia
astrapophobia astrapofobia
astroblastoma astroblastoma
astrocyte astrocito
astrocytoma astrocitoma
astrocytosis astrocitosis
astrocytosis cerebri astrocitosis cerebri
astroependymoma astroependimoma
astroglia astroglia
astrology astrología
asyllabia asilabia
asylum asilo
asymbolia asimbolia
asymmetric asimétrico
asymmetric distribution distribución
    asimétrica
asymmetric motor neuropathy neuropatía
    motora asimétrica
asymmetries in orientation asimetrías en
    orientación
asymmetry asimetría
asymptomatic asintomático
asymptomatic lead-induced neurotoxicity
    neurotoxicidad inducida por el plomo
    asintomática
asymptomatic neurosyphilis neurosífilis
    asintomática
asymptote asíntota
asymptotic asintótico
asynchronous asíncrono
asyndesis asindesis
asyndetic thinking pensamiento asindético
asynergia asinergia
asynergic speech habla asinérgica
asynesia asinesia
asynesis asinesis
asynodia asinodia
at risk a riesgo
atactic atáxico
atactic abasia abasia atáxica
atactic agraphia agrafia atáxica
atactic aphasia afasia atáxica

atactic diplegia diplejía atáxica
atactic dysarthria disartria atáxica
atactic feeling sensación atáxica
atactic gait marcha atáxica
atactic paramyotonia paramiotonía atáxica
atactic paraplegia paraplejía atáxica
atactic speech habla atáxica
atactic writing escritura atáxica
atactilia atactilia
ataractic ataráctico
ataractic drug droga ataráctica
ataraxia ataraxia
ataraxic ataráxico
ataraxy ataraxia
atavism atavismo
ataxia ataxia
ataxia telangiectasia ataxia telangiectasia
ataxiadynamia ataxiadinamia
ataxiagram ataxiagrama
ataxiagraph ataxiágrafo
ataxiameter ataxiámetro
ataxiaphasia ataxiafasia
ataxic atáxico
ataxic abasia abasia atáxica
ataxic agraphia agrafia atáxica
ataxic aphasia afasia atáxica
ataxic diplegia diplejía atáxica
ataxic dysarthria disartria atáxica
ataxic feeling sensación atáxica
ataxic gait marcha atáxica
ataxic paramyotonia paramiotonía atáxica
ataxic paraplegia paraplejía atáxica
ataxic speech habla atáxica
ataxic writing escritura atáxica
ataxiophemia ataxiofemia
ataxiophobia ataxiofobia
ataxophemia ataxofemia
ataxy ataxia
atelesis atelesis
atelia atelia
ateliosis ateliosis
atenolol atenolol
atephobia atefobia
atheromatosis ateromatosis
atherosclerosis ateroesclerosis
athetoid atetoide
athetoid dysarthria disartria atetoide
athetosic atetósico
athetosis atetosis
athetotic atetótico
athetotic dysarthria disartria atetótica
athletic type tipo atlético
athymia atimia
atmosphere atmósfera
atmosphere effect efecto atmosférico
atmospheric conditions condiciones
    atmosféricas
atmospheric perspective perspectiva
    atmosférica
atomism atomismo
atomistic atomístico
atomistic psychology psicología atomística
atonement expiación
atonia atonía
atonic atónico

atonic absence ausencia atónica
atonic bladder vejiga atónica
atonic epilepsy epilepsia atónica
atonic impotence impotencia atónica
atony atonía
atopognosia atopognosia
atopognosis atopognosis
atrabiliary atrabiliario
atresia atresia
atriopeptin atriopeptina
atrophedema atrofedema
atrophic dementia demencia atrófica
atrophoderma atrofoderma
atrophoderma neuriticum atrofoderma
  neurítica
atrophy atrofia
atropine atropina
atropine syndrome síndrome de atropina
attached cranial section sección craneal unida
attached craniotomy craneotomía unida
attachment apego
attachment behavior conducta de apego
attachment behavior in autism conducta de
  apego en autismo
attachment bond vínculo de apego
attachment bond and separation anxiety
  vínculo de apego y ansiedad de separación
attachment disorder trastorno de apego
attachment disorder of infancy trastorno de
  apego de infancia
attachment learning aprendizaje de apego
attachment theory teoría de apego
attack ataque
attack behavior conducta de ataque
attend atender
attendant care cuidado de acompañante
attending behaviors conductas de atención
attensity atensidad
attention atención
attention deficit déficit de atención
attention-deficit disorder trastorno de déficit
  de atención
attention-deficit disorder with hyperactivity
  trastorno de déficit de atención con
  hiperactividad
**attention-deficit disorder without
  hyperactivity** trastorno de déficit de
  atención sin hiperactividad
attention-deficit hyperactivity disorder
  trastorno de déficit de atención hiperactiva
attention disorder trastorno de atención
attention dysfunction disfunción de atención
attention fluctuation fluctuación de atención
attention-focusing procedure procedimiento
  de enfoque de atención
attention-getting atrayente de atención
attention in cognitive functioning atención en
  funcionamiento cognitivo
attention in hypnosis atención en hipnosis
attention level nivel de atención
attention overload sobrecarga de atención
attention reflex reflejo de atención
attention span lapso de atención
attention switching cambio de atención
attention theory teoría de atención

attentive atento
attentiveness atención
attenuation atenuación
attenuator atenuador
attenuator model modelo atenuador
attic child niño de ático
attitude actitud
attitude change cambio de actitudes
attitude cluster grupo de actitudes
attitude measurement medición de actitudes
attitude scale escala de actitudes
attitude survey encuesta de actitudes
attitude theory teoría de actitudes
attitude therapy terapia de actitudes
attitudinal reflex reflejo de actitud
attitudinizine tomar una actitud afectada
attonity atonicidad
attraction atracción
attractiveness atractividad
attributable risk riesgo atribuible
attribute atributo
attribution atribución
attribution error error de atribución
attribution of causality atribución de
  causalidad
attribution of emotion atribución de emoción
attribution of responsibility atribución de
  responsabilidad
attribution theory teoría de atribución
attrition desgaste
atypical atípico
atypical absence ausencia atípica
atypical affective disorder trastorno afectivo
  atípico
atypical antidepressant antidepresivo atípico
atypical anxiety disorder trastorno de
  ansiedad atípico
atypical bipolar disease enfermedad bipolar
  atípica
atypical bipolar disorder trastorno bipolar
  atípico
atypical child niño atípico
atypical childhood psychosis psicosis de
  niñez atípica
atypical conduct disorder trastorno de
  conducta atípica
atypical depression depresión atípica
atypical development desarrollo atípico
atypical disease enfermedad atípica
atypical disorder trastorno atípico
atypical dissociative disorder trastorno
  disociativo atípico
atypical eating disorder trastorno del comer
  atípico
atypical facial neuralgia neuralgia facial
  atípica
atypical factitious disorder trastorno facticio
  atípico
atypical gender identity disorder trastorno
  de identidad de género atípico
atypical impulse control disorder trastorno
  de control de impulsos atípico
atypical mania manía atípica
atypical organic brain syndrome síndrome
  cerebral orgánico atípico

atypical paranoid disorder trastorno
  paranoide atípico
atypical paraphilia parafilia atípica
atypical personality development desarrollo
  de personalidad atípica
atypical personality disorder trastorno de
  personalidad atípica
atypical psychosexual disorder trastorno
  psicosexual atípico
atypical psychosexual dysfunction disfunción
  psicosexual atípica
atypical psychosis psicosis atípica
atypical somatoform disorder trastorno
  somatoforme atípico
atypical stereotyped movement disorder
  trastorno de movimiento estereotipado
  atípico
atypical tic disorder trastorno de tic atípico
atypical trigeminal neuralgia neuralgia
  trigeminal atípica
Aubert-Fleischl paradox paradoja de
  Aubert-Fleischl
Aubert-Forster phenomenon fenómeno de
  Aubert-Forster
Aubert phenomenon fenómeno de Aubert
audibility audibilidad
audibility limit límite de audibilidad
audibility range intervalo de audibilidad
audible audible
audible thought pensamiento audible
audile auditivo
audio brain stimulation estimulación cerebral
  por audio
audioanalgesia audioanalgesia
audiogenic audiogénico
audiogenic epilepsy epilepsia audiogénica
audiogenic seizure acceso audiogénico
audiogram audiograma
audiogyral illusion ilusión audiogiral
audiology audiología
audiometer audiómetro
audiometric zero cero audiométrico
audiometry audiometría
audioverbal amnesia amnesia audioverbal
audiovisual coordination coordinación
  audiovisual
audiovisual training entrenamiento
  audiovisual
audit auditoría
audition audición
auditive auditivo
auditory auditivo
auditory acuity agudeza auditiva
auditory agnosia agnosia auditiva
auditory amnesia amnesia auditiva
auditory aphasia afasia auditiva
auditory arousal threshold umbral de
  despertamiento auditivo
auditory attention atención auditiva
auditory attributes atributos auditivos
auditory behavior conducta auditiva
auditory blending mezcla auditiva
auditory canal canal auditivo
auditory closure cierre auditivo
auditory cortex corteza auditiva

auditory detection detección auditiva
auditory discrimination discriminación
  auditiva
auditory disorder trastorno auditivo
auditory evoked potential potencial evocado
  auditivo
auditory evoked response respuesta evocada
  auditiva
auditory fatigue fatiga auditiva
auditory feedback retroalimentación auditiva
auditory flicker centelleo auditivo
auditory hallucination alucinación auditiva
auditory hyperalgesia hiperalgesia auditiva
auditory hyperesthesia hiperestesia auditiva
auditory image imagen auditiva
auditory localization localización auditiva
auditory masking enmascaramiento auditivo
auditory memory memoria auditiva
auditory memory span lapso de memoria
  auditiva
auditory nerve nervio auditivo
auditory oculogyric reflex reflejo oculógiro
  auditivo
auditory ossicles osículos auditivos
auditory pathology patología auditiva
auditory pathway vía auditiva
auditory perception percepción auditiva
auditory perceptual disorder trastorno
  perceptivo auditivo
auditory preferences preferencias auditivas
auditory processing procesamiento auditivo
auditory projection areas áreas de
  proyección auditiva
auditory reflex reflejo auditivo
auditory sensitivity sensibilidad auditiva
auditory sensory memory memoria sensorial
  auditiva
auditory sequencing encadenamiento auditivo
auditory signals señales auditivas
auditory skills destrezas auditivas
auditory space espacio auditivo
auditory space perception percepción de
  espacio auditivo
auditory span lapso auditivo
auditory spectrum espectro auditivo
auditory stimulation estimulación auditiva
auditory stimulus estímulo auditivo
auditory synesthesia sinestesia auditiva
auditory system sistema auditivo
auditory threshold umbral auditivo
auditory training entrenamiento auditivo
auditory type tipo auditivo
aufgabe predisposición mental
augmentation aumento
aulophobia aulofobia
aura aura
aural aural
aural harmonic armónico aural
auriculopalpebral reflex reflejo
  auriculopalpebral
auriculotemporal nerve syndrome síndrome
  del nervio auriculotemporal
auropalpebral reflex reflejo auropalpebral
auroraphobia aurorafobia
auscultation auscultación

Aussage test prueba de Aussage
Austrian school escuela austríaca
autarchy autarquía
autemesia autemesia
authenticity autenticidad
authoritarian autoritario
authoritarian aggression agresión autoritaria
authoritarian atmosphere atmósfera
  autoritaria
authoritarian character carácter autoritario
authoritarian conscience conciencia
  autoritaria
authoritarian leader líder autoritario
authoritarian parent padre autoritario, madre
  autoritaria
authoritarian personality personalidad
  autoritaria
authoritarian submission sumisión autoritaria
authoritarianism autoritarismo
authority autoridad
authority complex complejo de autoridad
authority confusion confusión de autoridad
authority figure figura de autoridad
authority principle principio de autoridad
autia autía
autism autismo
autism versus attention-deficit disorder
  autismo contra trastorno de déficit de
  atención
autism versus mental retardation autismo
  contra retardo mental
autism versus schizophrenia autismo contra
  esquizofrenia
autistic autista
autistic child niño autista
autistic disorder trastorno autista
autistic fantasy fantasía autista
autistic isolation aislamiento autista
autistic phase fase autista
autistic-presymbiotic adolescent adolescente
  autista-presimbiótico
autistic psychopathy psicopatía autista
autistic psychosis psicosis autista
autistic thinking pensamiento autista
auto shaping condicionamiento por
  aproximación automático
autoaggression autoagresión
autoaggressive activities actividades
  autoagresivas
autoanalysis autoanálisis
autobiographical autobiográfico
autobiographical memory memoria
  autobiográfica
autocastration autocastración
autocatharsis autocatarsis
autocathartic autocatártico
autocentric autocéntrico
autochthonous autóctono
autochthonous activity actividad autóctona
autochthonous delusion delusión autóctona
autochthonous gestalt gestalt autóctono
autochthonous idea idea autóctona
autochthonous variable variable autóctona
autoclitic autoclítico
autocorrelation autocorrelación

autodysosmophobia autodisosmofobia
autoecholalia autoecolalia
autoechopraxia autoecopraxia
autoerotic autoerótico
autoeroticism autoerotismo
autoerotism autoerotismo
autofellatio autofelación
autofetishism autofetichismo
autoflagellation autoflagelación
autogenic autogénico
autogenic reinforcement refuerzo autogénico
autogenic training entrenamiento autogénico
autogenital stimulation estimulación
  autogenital
autogenous autógeno
autognosis autognosis
autographism autografismo
autohypnosis autohipnosis
autohypnotic autohipnótico
autohypnotic amnesia amnesia autohipnótica
autohypnotism autohipnotismo
autoimmune autoinmune
autoimmune disease enfermedad autoinmune
autoimmunity autoinmunidad
autoinstruction autoinstrucción
autoinstructional device aparato
  autoinstructivo
autointoxication autointoxicación
autokinesia autocinesia
autokinesis autocinesis
autokinetic autocinético
autokinetic effect efecto autocinético
autokinetic illusion ilusión autocinética
autokinetic movement movimiento
  autocinético
autolibido autolibido
autology autología
automasochism automasoquismo
automated assessment evaluación
  automatizada
automated clinical records registros clínicos
  automatizados
automated desensitization desensibilización
  automatizada
automatic automático
automatic absence ausencia automática
automatic action acción automática
automatic activation activación automática
automatic anxiety ansiedad automática
automatic chorea corea automática
automatic decision decisión automática
automatic drawing dibujo automático
automatic encoding codificación automática
automatic epilepsy epilepsia automática
automatic judgment juicio automático
automatic memory memoria automática
automatic obedience obediencia automática
automatic perceptual encoding codificación
  perceptiva automática
automatic process proceso automático
automatic processing procesamiento
  automático
automatic seizure acceso automático
automatic speech habla automática
automatic thought pensamiento automático

automatic writing escritura automática
automatism automatismo
automatization automatización
automatization of attention automatización de atención
automatograph automatógrafo
automaton autómata
automaton conformity conformidad de autómata
automnesia automnesia
automorphic automórfico
automorphic perception percepción automórfica
automysophobia automisofobia
autonomasia autonomasia
autonomic autónomo
autonomic-affective law ley autónoma-afectiva
autonomic apparatus aparato autónomo
autonomic arousal despertamiento autónomo
autonomic balance balance autónomo
autonomic conditioning condicionamiento autónomo
autonomic disorder trastorno autónomo
autonomic disorganization desorganización autónoma
autonomic epilepsy epilepsia autónoma
autonomic hyperactivity hiperactividad autónoma
autonomic imbalance desequilibrio autónomo
autonomic-involuntary conditioning condicionamiento autónomo-involuntario
autonomic lability labilidad autónoma
autonomic nerve nervio autónomo
autonomic nervous system sistema nervioso autónomo
autonomic neurogenic bladder vejiga neurogénica autónoma
autonomic reactivity reactividad autónoma
autonomic response respuesta autónoma
autonomic seizure acceso autónomo
autonomic side effect efecto secundario autónomo
autonomotropic autonomotrópico
autonomous autónomo
autonomous activity actividad autónoma
autonomous complex complejo autónomo
autonomous depression depresión autónoma
autonomous ego function función del ego autónomo
autonomous function función autónoma
autonomous morality moralidad autónoma
autonomous psychotherapy psicoterapia autónoma
autonomous stage etapa autónoma
autonomy autonomía
autonomy-heteronomy autonomía-heteronomía
autonomy of motives autonomía de motivos
autonomy versus doubt autonomía contra duda
autonomy versus shame and doubt autonomía contra vergüenza y duda
autopathy autopatía
autophagia autofagia

autophagic autofágico
autophagy autofagia
autophilia autofilia
autophobia autofobia
autophonic response respuesta autofónica
autoplasty autoplastia
autopsy autopsia
autopsy negative death muerte con autopsia negativa
autopsyche autopsiquis
autopsychic autopsíquico
autopsychic delusion delusión autopsíquica
autopsychic orientation orientación autopsíquica
autopsychosis autopsicosis
autoradiography autorradiografía
autosadism autosadismo
autoscopic autoscópico
autoscopic phenomenon fenómeno autoscópico
autoscopic psychosis psicosis autoscópica
autoscopic syndrome síndrome autoscópico
autoscopy autoscopia
autosexualism autosexualismo
autosexuality autosexualidad
autosmia autosmia
autosomal autosómico
autosomal aberrations aberraciones autosómicas
autosomal anomalies anomalías autosómicas
autosomal-dominant autosómico-dominante
autosomal-recessive autosómico-recesivo
autosomatognosis autosomatognosis
autosomatognostic autosomatognóstico
autosome autosoma
autosomnabulism autosonambulismo
autosuggestibility autosugestibilidad
autosuggestion autosugestión
autosymbolism autosimbolismo
autosynnoia autosinoia
autotelic autotélico
autotelik autotélico
autotomia autotomía
autotomy autotomía
autotopagnosia autotopagnosia
auxanology auxanología
auxiliary auxiliar
auxiliary ego ego auxiliar
auxiliary inversion inversión auxiliar
auxiliary solution solución auxiliar
auxiliary therapist terapeuta auxiliar
availability disponibilidad
Avellis' syndrome síndrome de Avellis
average promedio
average deviation desviación promedia
average error error promedio
aversion aversión
aversion conditioning condicionamiento de aversión
aversion learning aprendizaje de aversión
aversion reaction reacción de aversión
aversion response respuesta de aversión
aversion therapy terapia de aversión
aversion therapy and anxiety terapia de aversión y ansiedad

aversion therapy for alcohol abuse terapia de aversión para abuso de alcohol
aversive aversivo
aversive behavior conducta aversiva
aversive conditioning condicionamiento aversivo
aversive control control aversivo
aversive learning aprendizaje aversivo
aversive racism racismo aversivo
aversive stimulus estímulo aversivo
aversive therapy terapia aversiva
aversive training entrenamiento aversivo
aviophobia aviofobia
avoidance evitación
avoidance and escape learning evitación y aprendizaje de escape
avoidance-avoidance conflict conflicto de evitación-evitación
avoidance behavior conducta de evitación
avoidance conditioning condicionamiento de evitación
avoidance gradient gradiente de evitación
avoidance learning aprendizaje de evitación
avoidance response respuesta de evitación
avoidance rituals rituales de evitación
avoidance therapy terapia de evitación
avoidance training entrenamiento de evitación
avoidant evitante
avoidant attachment apego evitante
avoidant disorder trastorno evitante
avoidant disorder of adolescence trastorno evitante de adolescencia
avoidant disorder of childhood trastorno evitante de niñez
avoidant personality personalidad evitante
avoidant personality disorder trastorno de personalidad evitante
avoidant scale escala evitante
avoided relationship relación evitada
avulsion avulsión
awareness conciencia
awareness defect defecto de conciencia
awareness exercise ejercicio de conciencia
awareness training model modelo de entrenamiento de conciencia
axial axial
axial amnesia amnesia axial
axial gradient gradiente axial
axial hyperkinesia hipercinesia axial
axial line línea axial
axial neuritis neuritis axial
axilla axila
axiology axiología
axiom axioma
axis eje
axoaxonic synapse sinapsis axoaxónica
axodendrite axodendrita
axodendritic synapse sinapsis axodendrítica
axolysis axólisis
axon axón
axon hillock montículo axónico
axon reflex reflejo axónico
axon terminal terminal axónico
axonal transport transporte axonal
axone axón

axonopathy axonopatía
axonotmesis axonotmesis
axoplasmic flow flujo axoplásmico
axosomatic synapse sinapsis axosomática
axotomy axotomía
aypnia aipnia
azacyclonol azaciclonol
azaperone azaperona
azathioprine azotioprina
azoospermia azoospermia
azygous ácigos

B

B fiber fibra B
B-type tipo B
B-type personality personalidad tipo B
babble balbuceo
babbling balbuceo
babbling in deaf children balbuceo en niños
  sordos
Babcock sentence oración de Babcock
Babinski's phenomenon fenómeno de
  Babinski
Babinski's sign signo de Babinski
Babinski's syndrome síndrome de Babinski
Babinski-Nageotte syndrome síndrome de
  Babinski-Nageotte
Babinski reflex reflejo de Babinski
Babkin reflex reflejo de Babkin
baby hunger hambre infantil
baby-sitter quien cuida niños
baby talk habla infantil
bacillophobia bacilofobia
back-clipping recorte trasero
back-formation formación hacia atrás
back of foot reflex reflejo del dorso del pie
backache dolor de espalda
backcross retrocruzamiento
backcrossing retrocruzamiento
background fondo, antecedentes
background characteristics características de
  fondo
background intensity intensidad de fondo
background motion moción de fondo
background noise ruido de fondo
backward association asociación hacia atrás
backward chaining encadenamiento hacia
  atrás
backward conditioning condicionamiento
  hacia atrás
backward masking enmascaramiento hacia
  atrás
backward masking technique técnica de
  enmascaramiento hacia atrás
backward reading lectura hacia atrás
backwardness atraso
baclofen baclofeno
bacteremia bacteremia
bacterial bacterial
bacterial cerebral infection infección
  cerebral bacterial
bacterial endocarditis endocarditis bacterial
bacterial infection infección bacterial
bacterial meningitis meningitis bacterial
bad breast pecho malo
bad me yo malo
bad object objeto malo

bad self yo malo
bad trip viaje malo
bahnung bahnung
bait shyness timidez de carnada
balance balance
balance control control de balance
balance theory teoría de balance
balanced bilingual bilingüe balanceado
balanced placebo design diseño de placebo
  balanceado
balanced psychophysical system sistema
  psicofísico balanceado
balanced scale escala balanceada
balbuties balbuceo
Balint's syndrome síndrome de Balint
Ball's operation operación de Ball
ball-and-field test prueba de bola y campo
Ballet's disease enfermedad de Ballet
ballet technique técnica de ballet
ballism balismo
ballismus balismo
ballistic balístico
ballistophobia balistofobia
Balo's disease enfermedad de Balo
Bamatter's syndrome síndrome de Bamatter
Bamberger's disease enfermedad de
  Bamberger
Bamberger's sign signo de Bamberger
band score puntuación de banda
bandage vendaje
bandwagon effect efecto de adhesión
bandwagon technique técnica de adhesión
bandwidth ancho de banda
Bannister's disease enfermedad de Bannister
bar chart gráfic.. de barras
bar diagram diagrama de barras
bar graph gráfica de barras
bar reflex reflejo de palanca
baragnosis baragnosis
Barany's syndrome síndrome de Barany
Barany method método de Barany
Barany test prueba de Barany
barbaralalia barbaralalia
barbital barbital
barbiturate barbiturato
barbiturate abuse abuso de barbituratos
barbiturate addiction adicción de
  barbituratos
barbiturate amnesic disorder trastorno
  amnésico de barbituratos
barbiturate amnestic disorder trastorno
  amnésico de barbituratos
barbiturate intoxication intoxicación por
  barbituratos
barbiturate withdrawal retiro de barbituratos
barbiturate withdrawal delirium delirio del
  retiro de barbituratos
barbituric acid ácido barbitúrico
Bardet-Biedl syndrome síndrome de
  Bardet-Biedl
barefoot doctor doctor descalzo
baresthesia barestesia
baresthesiometer barestesiómetro
baresthesis barestesis
bargaining regateo

bark ladrido
Barkman's reflex reflejo de Barkman
Barnes' dystrophy distrofia de Barnes
Barnum effect efecto de Barnum
barognosis barognosis
barophobia barofobia
baroreceptor barorreceptor
baroreflex barorreflejo
barotaxis barotaxis
barotitis barotitis
Barr body cuerpo de Barr
Barre's sign signo de Barre
Barre-Lieou syndrome síndrome de
   Barre-Lieou
barrier barrera
barrier-free environment ambiente libre de
   barreras
barrier problem problema de barrera
barrier response respuesta de barrera
Bartholin's glands glándulas de Bartholin
bartholinitis bartolinitis
Bartschi-Rochaix's syndrome síndrome de
   Bartschi-Rochaix
baryecoia bariecoia
baryglossia bariglosia
barylalia barilalia
baryphonia barifonía
baryphony barifonía
barythymia baritimia
basal basal
basal age edad basal
basal body temperature temperatura corporal
   basal
basal cell papilloma papiloma de células
   basales
basal ganglia ganglios basales
basal joint reflex reflejo articular basal
basal mental age edad mental basal
basal metabolism metabolismo basal
basal metabolism rate índice de metabolismo
   basal
basal reader approach acercamiento de libros
   de lectura básicos
basal resistance level nivel de resistencia
   basal
basal skull fracture fractura de cráneo basal
base line línea base
base line assessment evaluación de línea base
base rate tasa base
base rate fallacy falacia de tasa base
base rate information información de tasa
   base
Basedow's pseudoparaplegia seudoparaplejía
   de Basedow
Basedowian insanity insania de Basedow
basement effect efecto de sótano
basic básico
basic anxiety ansiedad básica
basic assumptions group grupo de asunciones
   básicas
basic benefit beneficio básico
basic category categoría básica
basic conflict conflicto básico
basic fault falta básica
basic level categorization categorización de

nivel básico
basic level category categoría de nivel básico
basic mistake equivocación básica
basic mistrust desconfianza básica
basic need necesidad básica
basic personality personalidad básica
basic personality type tipo de personalidad
   básica
basic research investigación básica
basic rest-activity cycle ciclo de
   descanso-actividad básico
basic rule regla básica
basic skills destrezas básicas
basic trust confianza básica
basic unit unidad básica
basilar basilar
basilar artery arteria basilar
basilar impression impresión basilar
basilar leptomeningitis leptomeningitis basilar
basilar membrane membrana basilar
basilar meningitis meningitis basilar
basiphobia basifobia
basistasiphobia basistasifobia
basket cell célula en cesta
basket endings terminaciones en cesta
basophil adenoma adenoma basófilo
basophilia basofilia
basophilic adenoma adenoma basófilico
basophilism basofilismo
basophobia basofobia
basostasophobia basostasofobia
Bassen-Kornzweig syndrome síndrome de
   Bassen-Kornzweig
Bastian's law ley de Bastian
bathmotropic batmotrópico
bathophobia batofobia
bathyanesthesia batianestesia
bathyesthesia batiestesia
bathyhyperesthesia batihiperestesia
bathyhypesthia batihipestesia
batophobia batofobia
batrachophobia bratracofobia
battarism batarismo
battarismus batarismo
Batten's disease enfermedad de Batten
Batten-Mayou disease enfermedad de
   Batten-Mayou
Batten-Steinert syndrome síndrome de
   Batten-Steinert
battered golpeado
battered child niño golpeado
battered child syndrome síndrome de niño
   golpeado
battered man hombre golpeado
battered person persona golpeada
battered wife esposa golpeada
battered wife syndrome síndrome de esposa
   golpeada
battered woman mujer golpeada
battering paliza
battery batería
battery of tests batería de pruebas
Battle's sign signo de Battle
battle fatigue fatiga de combate
battle neurosis neurosis de combate

Bayes' theorem teorema de Bayes
Bayesian approach acercamiento de Bayes
Bayle's disease enfermedad de Bayle
Beard's disease enfermedad de Beard
beast fetishism fetichismo bestial
beating azotamiento
beating fantasies fantasias de azotamiento
Bechterew's disease enfermedad de
    Bechterew
Bechterew's sign signo de Bechterew
Bechterew-Mendel reflex reflejo de
    Bechterew-Mendel
Beck's syndrome síndrome de Beck
Becker type tardive muscular dystrophy
    distrofia muscular tardía tipo Becker
Beckwith-Widemann syndrome síndrome de
    Beckwith-Widemann
bedlam manicomio, olla de grillos
bedlamism bedlamismo
bedsore llaga por presión
bedtime rituals rituales a la hora de acostarse
bedwetting enuresis
Beevor's sign signo de Beevor
before-after design diseño antes-después
Begbie's disease enfermedad de Begbie
beginning spurt arranque inicial
behavior conducta
behavior analysis análisis de conducta
behavior assessment evaluación de conducta
behavior chain cadena de conducta
behavior chaining encadenamiento de
    conducta
behavior checklist lista de comprobación de
    conducta
behavior constraint theory teoría de
    constreñimiento de conducta
behavior contract contrato de conducta
behavior control control de conducta
behavior determinant determinante de
    conducta
behavior disorder trastorno de conducta
behavior disorders of childhood trastornos
    de conducta de niñez
behavior episode episodio de conducta
behavior field campo de conducta
behavior genetics genética de conducta
behavior in elevators conducta en ascensores
behavior language lenguaje de conducta
behavior method método de conducta
behavior modeling modelado de conducta
behavior modification modificación de
    conducta
behavior pattern patrón de conducta
behavior problem problema de conducta
behavior problems and child abuse
    problemas de conducta y abuso de niños
behavior rating clasificación de conducta
behavior record registro de conducta
behavior reflex reflejo de conducta
behavior reversal inversión de conducta
behavior sampling muestreo de conducta
behavior setting ambiente de conducta
behavior shaping condicionamiento por
    aproximación
behavior-specimen recording registro de

conducta de espécimen
behavior switching cambio de conducta
behavior system sistema de conducta
behavior theory teoría de conducta
behavior therapy terapia de conducta
behavior therapy for eating problems terapia
    de conducta para problemas del comer
behavior therapy for quitting smoking
    terapia de conducta para dejar de fumar
behavior therapy with type A personalities
    terapia de conducta con personalidades tipo
    A
behavior toxicology toxicología de conducta
behavior type tipo de conducta
behavioral conductual
behavioral approach acercamiento conductual
behavioral approach to abnormal behavior
    acercamiento conductual para conducta
    anormal
behavioral approach to schizophrenia
    acercamiento conductual para esquizofrenia
behavioral assessment evaluación conductual
behavioral assessment procedures
    procedimientos de evaluación conductual
behavioral base line línea base conductual
behavioral clinic clínica conductual
behavioral coding system sistema de
    codificación conductual
behavioral competition theory teoría de
    competencia conductual
behavioral consistency consistencia
    conductual
behavioral contract contrato conductual
behavioral contrast contraste conductual
behavioral control control conductual
behavioral control systems sistemas de
    control conductual
behavioral couples group therapy terapia de
    grupo de parejas conductual
behavioral development desarrollo
    conductual
behavioral diagnosis diagnóstico conductual
behavioral-directive therapy terapia
    conductual-directiva
behavioral disinhibition desinhibición
    conductual
behavioral disorder trastorno conductual
behavioral disposition disposición conductual
behavioral dynamics dinámica conductual
behavioral ecology ecología conductual
behavioral endocrinology endocrinología
    conductual
behavioral-expressive level of emotion nivel
    de emoción conductual-expresiva
behavioral facilitation facilitación conductual
behavioral functionalism funcionalismo
    conductual
behavioral genetics genética conductual
behavioral group therapy terapia de grupo
    conductual
behavioral homology homología conductual
behavioral immunogen inmunógeno
    conductual
behavioral immunology inmunología
    conductual

behavioral inhibition inhibición conductual
behavioral integration integración conductual
behavioral intervention intervención
  conductual
behavioral management administración
  conductual
behavioral management and control
  administración conductual y control
behavioral manifestation manifestación
  conductual
behavioral medicine medicina conductual
behavioral metamorphosis metamorfosis
  conductual
behavioral model modelo conductual
behavioral model of development modelo
  conductual del desarrollo
behavioral modeling modelado conductual
behavioral neurochemistry neuroquímica
  conductual
behavioral neurology neurología conductual
behavioral observation observación
  conductual
behavioral oscillation oscilación conductual
behavioral pathogen patógeno conductual
behavioral pharmacogenetics
  farmacogenética conductual
behavioral plasticity plasticidad conductual
behavioral problem problema conductual
behavioral processes procesos conductuales
behavioral prosthesis prótesis conductual
behavioral psychiatry psiquiatría conductual
behavioral psychology psicología conductual
behavioral psychotherapy psicoterapia
  conductual
behavioral rating scale escala de clasificación
  conductual
behavioral reaction reacción conductual
behavioral rehearsal ensayo conductual
behavioral reorganization reorganización
  conductual
behavioral repertoire repertorio conductual
behavioral research investigación conductual
behavioral response respuesta conductual
behavioral science ciencia conductual
behavioral sink sumidero conductual
behavioral state estado conductual
behavioral system sistema conductual
behavioral technique técnica conductual
behavioral teratogen teratógeno conductual
behavioral teratogenesis teratogénesis
  conductual
behavioral teratogenic susceptibility
  susceptibilidad teratogénica conductual
behavioral theory of depression teoría
  conductual de depresión
behavioral theory of rumination teoría
  conductual de rumiación
behavioral therapy terapia conductual
behavioral therapy for autism terapia
  conductual para autismo
behavioral therapy for mental retardation
  terapia conductual para retardo mental
behavioral toxicity toxicidad conductual
behavioral treatment tratamiento conductual
behavioral variability variabilidad conductual

behaviorism conductismo
behaviorist conductista
behavioristic conductista
Behcet's disease enfermedad de Behcet
Behcet's syndrome síndrome de Behcet
Behr's syndrome síndrome de Behr
being-beyond-the-world
  ser-más-allá-de-la-tierra
being cognition cognición del ser
being-in-the-world ser-en-la-tierra
being love amor del ser
being motivation motivación del ser
being values valores del ser
Bekhterev's nystagmus nistagmo de
  Bekhterev
Bekhterev-Mendel reflex reflejo de
  Bekhterev-Mendel
bel bel
belch eructo
belief creencia
belief systems sistemas de creencias
belief-value matrix matriz de
  creencias-valores
Bell's law ley de Bell
Bell's mania manía de Bell
Bell's palsy parálisis de Bell
Bell's phenomenon fenómeno de Bell
Bell's spasm espasmo de Bell
bell and pad campana y almohadilla
Bell-Magendie law ley de Bell-Magendie
bell-shaped curve curva en forma de campana
belladonna belladona
belladonna delirium delirio de belladona
Bellevue scale escala de Bellevue
belonephobia belonefobia
belonging pertenencia
belongingness pertenencia
bemegride bemegrida
benactyzine benactizina
bends trancazo
beneceptor beneceptor
Benedek's reflex reflejo de Benedek
Benedikt's syndrome síndrome de Benedikt
beneficence beneficiencia
Benham's top trompo de Benham
benign benigno
benign essential tremor temblor esencial
  benigno
benign hereditary tremor temblor hereditario
  benigno
benign myalgic encephalomyelitis
  encefalomielitis miálgica benigna
benign neoplasm neoplasma benigno
benign stupor estupor benigno
benign tetanus tétanos benigno
benperidol benperidol
bentazepam bentazepam
benzaldehyde benzaldehído
benzene benceno
benzoctamine benzoctamina
benzodiazepine benzodiazepina
benzphetamine benzofetamina
benztropine benzotropina
bereavement duelo
bereavement by children duelo por niños

bereavement by infants duelo por infantes
bereavement versus major depression duelo contra depresión mayor
Berger's paresthesia parestesia de Berger
Berger rhythm ritmo de Berger
Berger wave onda de Berger
beriberi beriberi
Bernard's puncture punción de Bernard
Bernard-Horner syndrome síndrome de Bernard-Horner
Bernhardt's disease enfermedad de Bernhardt
Bernhardt-Roth syndrome síndrome de Bernhardt-Roth
Bernoulli distribution distribución de Bernoulli
Bernoulli effect efecto de Bernoulli
berry aneurysm aneurisma en baya
berserk frenético
best answer test prueba de la mejor respuesta
best fit mejor ajuste
best interest doctrine doctrina del mejor interés
best interest of the child doctrine doctrina del mejor interés del niño
best reason test prueba de la mejor razón
bestiality bestialidad
beta beta
beta adrenergic blocker bloqueador adrenérgico beta
beta adrenergic blocking agent agente de bloqueo adrenérgico beta
beta adrenergic blocking drug droga de bloqueo adrenérgico beta
beta alcoholism alcoholismo beta
beta arc arco beta
beta blocker bloqueador beta
beta cells células beta
beta conditioning condicionamiento beta
beta endorphin endorfina beta
beta error error beta
beta hypothesis hipótesis beta
beta level nivel beta
beta motion moción beta
beta movement movimiento beta
beta receptor receptor beta
beta receptor blocking agent agente de bloqueo de receptores beta
beta response respuesta beta
beta rhythm ritmo beta
beta wave onda beta
beta weight peso beta
betahistine betahistina
bethanechol betanecol
between-group variance varianza entre grupos
between-subject variance varianza entre sujetos
Betz cells células de Betz
Beuren syndrome síndrome de Beuren
bewildered perplejo
Bezold-Brucke effect efecto de Bezold-Brucke
Bezold-Jarisch reflex reflejo Bezold-Jarisch
bhang bhang
Bianchi's syndrome síndrome de Bianchi

bias sesgo
biased apperception apercepción sesgada
biased sample muestra sesgada
biased sampling muestreo sesgado
biblioclast biblioclasta
biblioklept biblioclepto
bibliokleptomania bibliocleptomanía
bibliomania bibliomanía
bibliophobia bibliofobia
bibliotherapy biblioterapia
bicarbonate bicarbonato
biceps femoris reflex reflejo de biceps femoral
biceps reflex reflejo del biceps
Bickerstaff's encephalitis encefalitis de Bickerstaff
bicultural bicultural
biculturalism biculturalismo
bidet bidé
bidirectionality of influence bidireccionalidad de influencia
Bidwell's ghost fantasma de Bidwell
Bielschowsky's disease enfermedad de Bielschowsky
Biemond's ataxia ataxia de Biemond
Biemond's syndrome síndrome de Biemond
Biernacki's sign signo de Biernacki
biethnic psychotherapy psicoterapia biétnica
bifactor method método bifactorial
bifactorial theory of conditioning teoría bifactorial de condicionamiento
bifid cranium cráneo bífido
bigamy bigamia
bigeminal pregnancy embarazo bigémino
bilabial bilabial
bilateral bilateral
bilateral hemianopsia hemianopsia bilateral
bilateral lesion lesión bilateral
bilateral speech habla bilateral
bilateral synchrony sincronía bilateral
bilateral transfer transferencia bilateral
bilharziasis bilharziasis
biliary biliar
biliary dyskinesia discinesia biliar
bilingual bilingüe
bilingualism bilingüismo
bilious bilioso
bilious headache dolor de cabeza bilioso
bilirachia bilirraquia
bilirubin bilirrubina
bilirubin encephalopathy encefalopatía por bilirrubina
bill of rights declaración de derechos
bimodal bimodal
bimodal distribution distribución bimodal
bimodality bimodalidad
binary choice selección binaria
binary number system sistema numérico binario
binary relation relación binaria
binasal hemianopsia hemianopsia binasal
binaural binaural
binaural cues señales binaurales
binaural fusion fusión binaural
binaural localization localización binaural

binaural ratio razón binaural
binaural shift cambio binaural
binaural time difference diferencia del
tiempo binaural
Binet age edad Binet
Binet scale escala de Binet
Binet-Simon scale escala de Binet-Simon
Bing's reflex reflejo de Bing
binge hartazgo
binge buying hartazgo del comprar
binge drinking hartazgo del beber
binge eating hartazgo del comer
binge spending hartazgo del gastar
binocular binocular
binocular accommodation acomodación
binocular
binocular cue señal binocular
binocular depth cue señal de profundidad
binocular
binocular disparity disparidad binocular
binocular fixation fijación binocular
binocular fusion fusión binocular
binocular information información binocular
binocular neural field campo neural
binocular
binocular parallax paralaje binocular
binocular perception percepción binocular
binocular rivalry rivalidad binocular
binocular stereoscopic vision visión
estereoscópica binocular
binocular summation sumación binocular
binocular suppression supresión binocular
binocular vision visión binocular
binocularity binocularidad
binomial binomial
binomial distribution distribución binomial
binomial test prueba binomial
Binswanger's dementia demencia de
Binswagner
Binswanger's disease enfermedad de
Binswanger
Binswanger's encephalopathy encefalopatía
de Binswanger
bioacoustics bioacústica
bioanalysis bioanálisis
bioavailability biodisponibilidad
biobehavioral shift cambio bioconductual
biochemical antagonism antagonismo
bioquímico
biochemical approach acercamiento
bioquímico
biochemical defect defecto bioquímico
biochemical pathway vía bioquímica
biochemistry bioquímica
biocybernetics biocibernética
biodynamics biodinámica
bioelectric potential potencial bioeléctrico
bioenergetics bioenergética
bioengineering bioingeniería
bioethics bioética
biofeedback biorretroalimentación
biofeedback for enuresis
biorretroalimentación para enuresis
biofeedback training entrenamiento de
biorretroalimentación

biofeedback treatment of pain tratamiento de
dolor de biorretroalimentación
biofidelity biofidelidad
biofunctional therapy terapia biofuncional
biogenesis biogénesis
biogenetic engineering ingeniería biogenética
biogenetic law ley biogenética
biogenetics biogenética
biogenic biógeno
biogenic amine hypothesis hipótesis de
aminas biógenas
biogenic amines aminas biógenas
biogenic factors factores biógenos
biogenic psychosis psicosis biógena
biogram biograma
biographical data datos biográficos
biographical inventory inventario biográfico
biographical method método biográfico
biography in depth biografía a fondo
biohazard riesgo biológico
biologic biológico
biologic therapy terapia biológica
biologic time tiempo biológico
biological biológico
biological adaptation adaptación biológica
biological aging envejecimiento biológico
biological clock reloj biológico
biological determinism determinismo
biológico
biological drive impulso biológico
biological equilibrium equilibrio biológico
biological factors factores biológicos
biological factors affecting sexuality factores
biológicos que afectan la sexualidad
biological factors in depression factores
biológicos en depresión
biological factors in development factores
biológicos en el desarrollo
biological factors in mood disorders factores
biológicos en trastornos del humor
biological factors in schizophrenia factores
biológicos en esquizofrenia
biological intelligence inteligencia biológica
biological maturity madurez biológica
biological measures medidas biológicas
biological memory memoria biológica
biological model modelo biológico
biological needs necesidades biológicas
biological parent padre biológico, madre
biológica
biological predisposition predisposición
biológica
biological preparedness preparación biológica
biological psychiatry psiquiatría biológica
biological rhythm ritmo biológico
biological sex sexo biológico
biological stress estrés biológico
biological taxonomy taxonomía biológica
biological theory teoría biológica
biological therapy terapia biológica
biological view perspectiva biológica
biological view of delinquency perspectiva
biológica de delincuencia
biological viewpoint punto de vista biológico
biological vulnerability to behavior problems

vulnerabilidad biológica a problemas de
conducta
biologism biologismo
biomechanics biomecánica
biomedical biomédico
biomedical engineering ingeniería biomédica
biomedical ethics ética biomédica
biomedical model modelo biomédico
biomedical therapy terapia biomédica
biomedical treatment tratamiento biomédico
biometrics biometría
biometry biometría
bionegativity bionegatividad
bionic biónico
bionics biónica
bionomics bionómica
biophilia biofilia
biophysical system sistema biofísico
biophysics biofísica
biopsy biopsia
biopsychic biopsíquico
biopsychology biopsicología
biopsychosocial biopsicosocial
biopsychosocial history historial
biopsicosocial
biopsychosocial model modelo biopsicosocial
biopsychosocial response to accidents
respuesta biopsicosocial a los accidentes
biopsychosocial system sistema biopsicosocial
biorhythm biorritmo
biosocial biosocial
biosocial determinism determinismo biosocial
biosocial theory teoría biosocial
biosphere biosfera
biostatistics bioestadística
Biot's breathing respiración de Biot
Biot's respiration respiración de Biot
biotaxis biotaxis
biotechnology biotecnología
biotope biotopo
biotransformation biotransformación
biotransport biotransporte
biotype biotipo
biotypogram biotipograma
biotypology biotipología
biovular twins gemelos biovulares
bipedal locomotion locomoción bipedal
biperiden biperidina
biphasic symptom síntoma bifásico
bipolar bipolar
bipolar affective disorder trastorno afectivo
bipolar
bipolar cell célula bipolar
bipolar disorder trastorno bipolar
bipolar disorder and depression trastorno
bipolar y depresión
bipolar double bind apuro doble bipolar
bipolar I bipolar I
bipolar I disorder trastorno bipolar I
bipolar II bipolar II
bipolar II disorder trastorno bipolar II
bipolar illness enfermedad bipolar
bipolar neuron neurona bipolar
bipolar rating scale escala de clasificación
bipolar

bipolarity bipolaridad
biracial psychotherapy psicoterapia birracial
birth nacimiento
birth adjustment ajuste de nacimiento
birth complications complicaciones de
nacimiento
birth control control de natalidad
birth cry grito de nacimiento
birth defect defecto de nacimiento
birth defects of genitalia defectos de
nacimiento de genitales
birth experience experiencia de nacimiento
birth injury lesión de nacimiento
birth order orden de nacimiento
birth palsy parálisis de nacimiento
birth rate tasa de natalidad
birth trauma trauma de nacimiento
birth weight peso de nacimiento
birthday effect efecto de cumpleaños
birthmark marca de nacimiento
Bischof's myelotomy mielotomía de Bischof
bisensory bisensorial
biserial correlation correlación biserial
bisexual bisexual
bisexual behavior conducta bisexual
bisexual confusion confusión bisexual
bisexual pedophilia pedofilia bisexual
bisexuality bisexualidad
bit bit
bite mordisco
bite bar barra de mordisco
bitemporal hemianopsia hemianopsia
bitemporal
biting attack ataque de morder
biting mania manía de morder
biting stage etapa de morder
bitter amargo
biundulant meningoencephalitis
meningnoencefalitis biondulante
bivalence bivalencia
bivariate bivariado
bizarre estrambótico
bizarre behavior conducta estrambótica
bizarre delusion delusión estrambótica
black box caja negra
black-box approach acercamiento de caja
negra
black-patch syndrome síndrome de placa
negra
blackout desmayo
blackout threshold umbral de desmayo
bladder vejiga
bladder control control de vejiga
bladder reflex reflejo vesical
bladder training entrenamiento de vejiga
blame culpa
blame avoidance evitación de culpa
blame escape escape de culpa
blame need necesidad de culpa
blaming the victim culpando a la víctima
blank experiment experimento en blanco
blank hallucination alucinación en blanco
blank screen pantalla en blanco
blank trial ensayo en blanco
blanket group grupo general

blastomere blastómero
blastophthoria blastoftoria
blastula blástula
blended family familia mezclada
blending mezcla
blepharospasm blefaroespasmo
blepharospasmus blefaroespasmo
blind ciego
blind alley callejón sin salida
blind analysis análisis a ciegas
blind headache dolor de cabeza ciego
blind sight vista ciega
blind spot punto ciego
blind study estudio ciego
blindism manierismo de ciego
blindness ceguera
blink reflex reflejo de parpadeo
blink response respuesta de parpadeo
blinking parpadeo
bliss arrobamiento
bloating abultamiento
block bloque, bloqueo
block-counting test prueba de conteo de bloques
block design diseño en bloque
block-design test prueba de diseños con bloques
block diagram diagrama de bloques
block sampling muestreo en bloques
blockade bloqueo
blocker bloqueador
blocking bloqueo
blocking activity actividad de bloqueo
Blocq's disease enfermedad de Blocq
Blocq's syndrome síndrome de Blocq
blood sangre
blood alcohol concentration concentración de alcohol sanguínea
blood alcohol content contenido de alcohol sanguíneo
blood-brain barrier barrera hematocerebral
blood disorder trastorno sanguíneo
blood level nivel sanguíneo
blood pressure presión sanguínea
blood sugar azúcar sanguínea
blood type tipo sanguíneo
blood urea nitrogen nitrógeno ureico sanguíneo
bloodless decerebration descerebración sin sangre
blue blindness ceguera al azul
blue-collar therapy terapia de trabajador manual
blue edema edema azul
blue-yellow blindness ceguera azul-amarilla
blunted affect afecto rudo
blush ruborizarse
blushing ruborozo
board junta, comida
board and care facility instalación de cuidado y comida
board certified certificado por junta
board certified psychiatrist psiquiatra certificado por junta
boarding home hogar de huéspedes

boarding house casa de huéspedes
bobbing meneo vertical
bodily ego feeling sensación del ego corporal
body cuerpo
body affect afecto corporal
body awareness conciencia del cuerpo
body boundaries límites corporales
body buffer zone zona de amortiguamiento corporal
body build tipo corporal
body-build index índice de tipo corporal
body cathexis catexis corporal
body-centered therapy terapia centrada en el cuerpo
body concept concepto corporal
body conceptualization disturbance disturbio de conceptualización corporal
body contact contacto corporal
body contact and attachment contacto corporal y apego
body dysmorphic disorder trastorno dismórfico corporal
body ego ego corporal
body ego concept concepto del ego corporal
body esteem estima corporal
body ideal ideal corporal
body identity identidad corporal
body image imagen corporal
body image distortion distorsión de imagen corporal
body image disturbance disturbio de imagen corporal
body image hallucinations alucinaciones de imagen corporal
body image therapy terapia de imagen corporal
body language lenguaje corporal
body maintenance mantenimiento corporal
body-mind dichotomy dicotomía cuerpo-mente
body-mind problem problema cuerpo-mente
body monitoring monitorización corporal
body movement movimiento corporal
body narcissism narcisismo corporal
body odor olor corporal
body percept percepto corporal
body protest protesta corporal
body righting reflex reflejo de enderezamiento corporal
body rocking balanceo corporal
body schema esquema corporal
body scheme esquema corporal
body senses sentidos corporales
body temperature temperatura corporal
body therapy terapia corporal
body type tipo corporal
body versus mind cuerpo contra mente
body weight peso corporal
Bogen cage jaula de Bogen
bogeyman cuco
Bogorad's syndrome síndrome de Bogorad
bombesin bombesina
bond vínculo
bondage esclavitud
bondage and discipline esclavitud y disciplina

bonding vinculación
bonding and attachment vinculación y apego
bonding in blended families vinculación en
   familias mezcladas
bonding of parent and child vinculación de
   padre e hijo, vinculación de madre e hijo,
   vinculación de padre e hija, vinculación de
   madre e hija
bonding process proceso de vinculación
bone conduction conducción ósea
bone disease enfermedad ósea
bone flap colgajo óseo
bone marrow médula ósea
bone-pointing apuntamiento de hueso
bone reflex reflejo óseo
bone sensibility sensibilidad ósea
bone wax cera ósea
Bonhoeffer's sign signo de Bonhoeffer
Bonnier's syndrome síndrome de Bonnier
books for the blind libros para los ciegos
Boolean algebra álgebra de Boole
boomerang effect efecto de bumerán
borderline fronterizo
borderline disorder trastorno fronterizo
borderline intellectual functioning
   funcionamiento intelectual fronterizo
borderline intelligence inteligencia fronteriza
borderline mental retardation retardo mental
   fronterizo
borderline personality personalidad
   fronteriza
borderline personality disorder trastorno de
   personalidad fronterizo
borderline personality disorder and schizoid
   personality trastorno de personalidad
   fronterizo y personalidad esquizoide
borderline personality disorder in
   adolescence trastorno de personalidad
   fronterizo en adolescencia
borderline personality disorder in adulthood
   trastorno de personalidad fronterizo en
   adultez
borderline personality disorder in children
   trastorno de personalidad fronterizo en
   niños
borderline personality organization
   organización de personalidad fronteriza
borderline psychosis psicosis fronteriza
borderline scale escala fronteriza
borderline schizophrenia esquizofrenia
   fronteriza
borderline state estado fronterizo
borderline syndrome síndrome fronterizo
boredom aburrimiento
boredom proneness propensión al
   aburrimiento
Borjeson-Forssman-Lehmann syndrome
   síndrome de Borjeson-Forssman-Lehmann
borrowed stress theory teoría del estrés
   prestado
bottle-feeding alimentación por biberón
bottleneck of attention atolladero de atención
bottom-up information información del fondo
   hacia arriba
bottom-up learning aprendizaje del fondo

hacia arriba
bottom-up processing procesamiento del
   fondo hacia arriba
bottom-up solutions soluciones del fondo
   hacia arriba
boulimia bulimia
bound energy energía dirigida
boundary límite
boundary detectors detectores de límites
boundary system sistema de límites
bounded rationality racionalidad limitada
Bourneville's disease enfermedad de
   Bourneville
Bourneville-Pringle disease enfermedad de
   Bourneville-Pringle
bouton botón
bovarism bovarismo
bow motion moción en arco
bow movement movimiento en arco
bow-wow theory teoría de guauguau
bowel control control intestinal
bowel disorder trastorno intestinal
bowel training entrenamiento intestinal
boxer's dementia demencia de boxeador
Boyle's disease enfermedad de Boyle
brace abrazadera
brachial braquial
brachial birth palsy parálisis natal braquial
brachial neuritis neuritis braquial
brachial plexus neuropathy neuropatía del
   plexo braquial
brachial radiculitis radiculitis braquial
brachioradial reflex reflejo braquiorradial
brachybasia braquibasia
brachycephalic braquicefálico
brachycephaly braquicefalia
brachylineal braquilineal
brachymetropia braquimetropía
brachymetropy braquimetropía
brachymorphic braquimórfico
brachyskelic braquisquélico
bradyacusia bradiacusia
bradyarthria bradiartria
bradycardia bradicardia
bradyesthesia bradiestesia
bradyglossia bradiglosia
bradykinesia bradicinesia
bradykinesis bradicinesis
bradykinin bradiquinina
bradylalia bradilalia
bradylexia bradilexia
bradylogia bradilogía
bradyphagia bradifagia
bradyphasia bradifasia
bradyphemia bradifemia
bradyphrasia bradifrasia
bradyphrenia bradifrenia
bradypnea bradipnea
bradypragia bradipragia
bradypsychia bradipsiquia
bradyteleocinesia braditeleocinesia
bradyteleokinesis braditeleocinesis
bradytrophia braditrofia
Braid's strabismus estrabismo de Braid
braid-cutting corte de trenzas

braidsm braidismo
braille braille
brain cerebro
Brain's reflex reflejo de Brain
brain abscess absceso cerebral
brain age quotient cociente de edad cerebral
brain atlas atlas cerebral
brain atrophy atrofia cerebral
brain center centro cerebral
brain cicatrix cicatriz cerebral
brain concussion concusión cerebral
brain congestion congestión cerebral
brain control control cerebral
brain contusion contusión cerebral
brain damage daño cerebral
brain damage and psychiatric disorders daño cerebral y trastornos psiquiátricos
brain-damage behavior syndrome síndrome de conducta por daño cerebral
brain-damage language disorder trastorno del lenguaje por daño cerebral
brain damage prognosis prognosis de daño cerebral
brain damage rehabilitation rehabilitación de daño cerebral
brain death muerte cerebral
brain dimorphism dimorfismo cerebral
brain disease enfermedad cerebral
brain disorder trastorno cerebral
brain dysfunction disfunción cerebral
brain edema edema cerebral
brain electrical activity mapping cartografía de actividad eléctrica cerebral
brain functions funciones cerebrales
brain imaging producción de imagen cerebral
brain-injured child niño lesionado cerebralmente
brain injury lesión cerebral
brain laceration laceración cerebral
brain laterality lateralidad cerebral
brain lateralization lateralización cerebral
brain lesion lesión cerebral
brain metabolism metabolismo cerebral
brain model modelo cerebral
brain murmur murmullo cerebral
brain opioid activity actividad opioide cerebral
brain pathology patología cerebral
brain plasticity plasticidad cerebral
brain potential potencial cerebral
brain research investigación cerebral
brain sand arena cerebral
brain scan exploración cerebral
brain size tamaño cerebral
brain stem tallo cerebral
brain stimulation estimulación cerebral
brain structure estructura cerebral
brain surgery cirugía cerebral
brain swelling tumefacción cerebral
brain syndrome síndrome cerebral
brain transplant transplante cerebral
brain trauma trauma cerebral
brain tumor tumor cerebral
brain wave complex complejo de ondas cerebrales

brain wave cycle ciclo de ondas cerebrales
brain waves ondas cerebrales
brainstem tallo cerebral
brainstem evoked response respuesta evocada del tallo cerebral
brainstem hemorrhage hemorragia del tallo cerebral
brainstorm idea penetrante súbita
brainwashing lavado de cerebro
branching program programa bifurcado
brand loyalty lealtad de marca
brand preference preferencia de marca
Brasdor's method método de Brasdor
Brawner decision decisión de Brawner
break shock choque por interrupción
breakaway phenomenon fenómeno de rompimiento
breakdown colapso
breakoff discontinuación
breakoff phenomenon fenómeno de desprendimiento
breakthrough adelanto
breast pecho
breast complex complejo de pecho
breast envy envidia de pecho
breast-feeding alimentación por pecho
breast-phantom phenomenon fenómeno de pecho fantasma
breath-holding retención de respiración
breathing respiración
breathing-related sleep disorder trastorno del sueño relacionado con la respiración
bredouillement bredouillement
breeder hypothesis hipótesis de criadero
bregma bregma
bregmocardiac reflex reflejo bregmocardíaco
brevilineal brevilineal
bribe soborno
bridge to reality puente hacia la realidad
brief breve
brief dynamic psychotherapy psicoterapia dinámica breve
brief group therapy terapia de grupo breve
brief psychotherapy psicoterapia breve
brief psychotherapy for children psicoterapia breve para niños
brief psychotic disorder trastorno psicótico breve
brief reactive psychosis psicosis reactiva breve
brief separation separación breve
brief-stimuli technique técnica de estímulos breves
brief-stimulus therapy terapia de estímulo breve
Briggs' law ley de Briggs
brightness brillantez
brightness adaptation adaptación a brillantez
brightness constancy constancia de brillantez
brightness contrast contraste de brillantez
brightness discrimination discriminación de brillantez
brightness threshold umbral de brillantez
bril bril
brilliance brillantez

Briquet's ataxia ataxia de Briquet
Briquet's syndrome síndrome de Briquet
Brissaud's disease enfermedad de Brissaud
Brissaud's infantilism infantilismo de
   Brissaud
Brissaud's reflex reflejo de Brissaud
Brissaud-Marie syndrome síndrome de
   Brissaud-Marie
Brissaud-Meige syndrome síndrome de
   Brissaud-Meige
broad affect afecto amplio
Broadbent's apoplexy apoplejía de Broadbent
Broadbent's law ley de Broadbent
Broadbent test prueba de Broadbent
Broca's aphasia afasia de Broca
Broca's area área de Broca
Broca's speech area área del habla de Broca
Brodie's disease enfermedad de Brodie
Brodmann's area área de Brodmann
broken home hogar roto
bromazepam bromazepam
bromhidrosis bromhidrosis
bromide bromuro
bromide hallucinosis alucinosis de bromuro
bromide intoxication intoxicación por
   bromuro
bromidrosiphobia bromidrosifobia
bromidrosis bromidrosis
brominism brominismo
bromisovalum bromisovalum
bromocriptine bromocriptina
bromoglutamate bromoglutamato
bromperidol bromoperidol
bronchial asthma asma bronquial
bronchial spasm espasmo bronquial
bronchodilatation broncodilatación
bronchodilation broncodilación
bronchodilator broncodilatador
bronchodilator medication medicación
   broncodilatador
brontophobia brontofobia
brood meditar ansiosamente
brooding meditación ansiosa
brooding compulsion compulsión de meditar
   ansiosamente
brooding spells rachas de meditación ansiosa
brother complex complejo fraternal
Brown-Sequard's paralysis parálisis de
   Brown-Sequard
Brown-Sequard's syndrome síndrome de
   Brown-Sequard
Brudzinski's sign signo de Brudzinski
Bruns' ataxia ataxia de Bruns
Bruns' sign signo de Bruns
Bruns' syndrome síndrome de Bruns
Brunswik faces caras de Brunswik
Brunswik ratio razón de Brunswik
Brushfield-Wyatt disease enfermedad de
   Brushfield-Wyatt
Brushfield-Wyatt syndrome síndrome de
   Brushfield-Wyatt
brute force fuerza bruta
brute pride orgullo bruto
bruxism bruxismo
bruxomania bruxomanía

bubble concept of personal space concepto
   de burbuja del espacio personal
buccal bucal
buccal intercourse relación bucal
buccal speech habla bucal
buccolingual bucolingual
buccolingual masticatory syndrome
   síndrome masticatorio bucolingual
Buerger's disease enfermedad de Buerger
buffalo neck cuello de búfalo
buffer memoria intermedia, amortiguador
buffer items artículos amortiguadores
buffer memory memoria intermedia
buffering hypothesis hipótesis de
   amortiguamiento
buffoonery psychosis psicosis de bufonería
bufotenin bufotenina
bug error
bulb bulbo
bulbar bulbar
bulbar apoplexy apoplejía bulbar
bulbar myelitis mielitis bulbar
bulbar palsy parálisis bulbar
bulbar paralysis parálisis bulbar
bulbar poliomyelitis poliomielitis bulbar
bulbocapnine bulbocapnina
bulbocavernosus muscle músculo
   bulbocavernoso
bulbocavernosus reflex reflejo
   bulbocavernoso
bulbomimic reflex reflejo bulbomímico
bulbospinal bulboespinal
bulbospinal poliomyelitis poliomielitis
   bulboespinal
bulbospongiosus muscle músculo
   bulboesponjoso
bulbourethral glands glándulas bulbouretrales
bulesis bulesis
bulimia bulimia
bulimia nervosa bulimia nerviosa
bulimic bulímico
bulmorexia bulmorexia
bundle hypothesis hipótesis del montón
Bunsen-Roscoe law ley de Bunsen-Roscoe
Bunyavirus encephalitis encefalitis por
   Bunyavirus
buprenorphine buprenorfina
bupropion bupropiona
bureaucratic leader líder burocrático
Burn and Rand theory teoría de Burn y Rand
burn center centro de quemaduras
burn injuries lesiones de quemaduras
burn unit unidad de quemaduras
burned-out quemado
burned-out schizophrenic esquizofrénico
   quemado
burnout agotamiento
burnout syndrome síndrome de agotamiento
burns quemaduras
burnt quemado
burst estallido
Buschke's disease enfermedad de Buschke
buspirone buspirona
Busse-Buschke disease enfermedad de
   Busse-Buschke

butabarbital butabarbital
butaperazine butaperazina
butethal butetal
butorphanol butorfanol
butriptyline butriptilina
butterfly curve curva en mariposa
butyrophenone butirofenona
Buzzard's maneuver maniobra de Buzzard
by-idea idea secundaria
bypass derivación
bystander effect efecto de circunstantes
bystander involvement envolvimiento de
   circunstantes
byte byte

C

C factor factor C
C fiber fibra C
caapi caapi
cable graft injerto en cable
cable properties propiedades de cables
cacergasia cacergasia
cachectic caquectico
cachexia caquexia
cachexia hypophysiopriva caquexia
   hipofisopriva
cachinnation caquinación
cacodaemonia cacodemonia
cacodemonia cacodemonia
cacodemonomania cacodemonomanía
cacoethes cacoetes
cacogenic cacogénico
cacogeusia cacogeusia
cacolalia cacolalia
cacophoria cacoforia
cacosmia cacosmia
cacosomnia cacosomnia
cacothymia cacotimia
caesarean section sección cesárea
cafard cafard
cafe au lait spot mancha de café con leche
cafeteria feeding alimentación estilo cafetería
caffeine cafeína
caffeine abuse abuso de cafeína
caffeine effects efectos de cafeína
caffeine-induced organic mental disorder
   trastorno mental orgánico inducido por
   cafeína
caffeine intoxication intoxicación por cafeína
caffeine sleep disorder trastorno del sueño de
   cafeína
caffeine use disorder trastorno del uso de
   cafeína
caffeinism cafeinismo
Cain complex complejo de Caín
cainophobia cainofobia
cainotophobia cainotofobia
Cairns' stupor estupor de Cairns
caisson disease enfermedad caison
calamitous relationship relación calamitosa
calcarine area área calcarina
calcarine cortex corteza calcarina
calcarine fissure fisura calcarina
calcitonin calcitonina
calcium bromide bromuro de calcio
calcium deficiency deficiencia de calcio
calcium-deficiency disorders trastornos por
   deficiencia de calcio
calcium regulation regulación de calcio
calculation test prueba de cómputos

calculi calculi
calculus cálculo
calendar age edad calendario
calendar calculation cómputo de calendario
calf love amor juvenil
calibration calibración
call boy chico de cita
call girl chica de cita
callipedia calipedia
callomania calomanía
callosal gyrus circunvolución callosa
callosal sulcus surco calloso
calmative calmante
calomel electrode electrodo de calomel
caloric intake consumo calórico
caloric nystagmus nistagmo calórico
calorie caloría
calvarial hook gancho calvárico
calyx cáliz
camazepam camazepam
camera cámara
camisole camisola
camouflage camuflaje
campimeter campímetro
campimetry campimetría
camptocormia camptocormia
camptospasm camptoespasmo
canal canal
canalization canalización
Canavan's disease enfermedad de Canavan
Canavan's sclerosis esclerosis de Canavan
cancellation cancelación
cancellation discharge descarga de
    cancelación
cancellation mechanism mecanismo de
    cancelación
cancellation test prueba de cancelación
cancellation theory teoría de cancelación
cancer cáncer
cancer pain dolor del cáncer
cancer phobia fobia al cáncer
cancer reactions reacciones al cáncer
cancerophobia cancerofobia
canchasmus cancasmo
candela candela
candidiasis candidiasis
candle candela
cane baston
canine spasm espasmo canino
cannabis cannabis
cannabis abuse abuso de cannabis
cannabis anxiety disorder trastorno de
    ansiedad de cannabis
cannabis delirium delirio de cannabis
cannabis delusional disorder trastorno
    delusorio de cannabis
cannabis dependence dependencia de
    cannabis
cannabis hallucinosis alucinosis de cannabis
cannabis-induced organic mental disorders
    trastornos mentales orgánicos inducidos por
    cannabis
cannabis intoxication intoxicación por
    cannabis
cannabis organic mental disorders trastornos

mentales orgánicos de cannabis
cannabis psychosis psicosis de cannabis
cannabis psychotic disorder trastorno
    psicótico de cannabis
cannabis psychotic disorder with delusions
    trastorno psicótico de cannabis con
    delusiones
**cannabis psychotic disorder with
    hallucinations** trastorno psicótico de
    cannabis con alucinaciones
cannabis use disorder trastorno de uso de
    cannabis
cannabism cannabismo
cannibalism canibalismo
cannibalistic fantasy fantasía canibalística
cannibalistic fixation fijación canibalística
cannibalistic phase fase canibalística
Cannon's theory teoría de Cannon
Cannon-Bard theory teoría de Cannon-Bard
Cannon-Bard theory of emotion teoría de
    emoción de Cannon-Bard
Cannon hypothalamic theory of emotion
    teoría de la emoción hipotalámica de
    Cannon
cannula cánula
Cantelli's sign signo de Cantelli
cantharides cantárida
capacity capacidad
Capgras' phenomenon fenómeno de Capgras
Capgras' syndrome síndrome de Capgras
capillary capilar
capillary fracture fractura capilar
capitium capitium
capping techniques técnicas de
    amortiguamiento
captivation cautivación
captodiam captodiam
captodiamine captodiamina
captopril captopril
caput caput
caput succedaneum caput succedaneum
car controls controles de carro
carbachol carbacol
carbamate carbamato
carbamate psychotherapy psicoterapia con
    carbamatos
carbamazepine carbamazepina
carbidopa carbidopa
carbohydrate metabolism metabolismo de
    carbohidratos
carbon dioxide dióxido de carbono
carbon dioxide inhalation inhalación de
    dióxido de carbono
carbon dioxide inhalation test prueba de
    inhalación de dióxido de carbono
carbon dioxide therapy terapia con dióxido
    de carbono
carbon dioxide withdrawal seizure test
    prueba de acceso por retiro de dióxido de
    carbono
carbon disulfide disulfuro de carbono
carbon disulfide intoxication intoxicación por
    disulfuro de carbono
carbon monoxide monóxido de carbono
carbon monoxide poisoning envenenamiento

por monóxido de carbono
carbon tetrachloride tetracloruro de carbono
carbon tetrachloride poisoning
envenenamiento por tetracloruro de
carbono
carbonic anhydrase anhidrasa carbónica
carbonic anhydrase inhibitors inhibidores de
anhidrasa carbónica
carboxyl group grupo carboxilo
carbromal carbromal
carcinogen carcinógeno
carcinogenic carcinogénico
carcinoma carcinoma
carcinomata carcinomata
carcinomatosis carcinomatosis
carcinomatous carcinomatoso
carcinomatous encephalomyelopathy
encefalomielopatía carcinomatosa
carcinomatous myelopathy mielopatía
carcinomatosa
carcinomatous myopathy miopatía
carcinomatosa
carcinomatous neuromyopathy
neuromiopatía carcinomatosa
carcinophobia carcinofobia
card sorting clasificación de cartas
card-sorting task tarea de clasificar cartas
card-sorting test prueba de clasificar cartas
card-stacking floreo de naipes
cardiac cardíaco
cardiac disorder trastorno cardíaco
cardiac muscle músculo cardíaco
cardiac neurosis neurosis cardíaca
cardiac pacemaker marcapasos cardíaco
cardiac patients pacientes cardíacos
cardiac psychosis psicosis cardíaca
cardiac reactions reacciones cardíacas
cardiac symptoms síntomas cardíacos
cardinal cardenal
cardinal trait rasgo cardenal
cardioexcitatory peptide péptido
cardioexcitatorio
cardiogram cardiograma
cardiomyopathy cardiomiopatía
cardioneural cardioneural
cardioneurosis cardioneurosis
cardiophobia cardiofobia
cardiophrenia cardiofrenia
cardiorespiratory cardiorespiratorio
cardiorespiratory endurance resistencia
cardiorespiratoria
cardiospasm cardioespasmo
cardiotoxic cardiotóxico
cardiovascular cardiovascular
cardiovascular disease enfermedad
cardiovascular
cardiovascular disorder trastorno
cardiovascular
cardiovascular fitness aptitud cardiovascular
cardiovascular function función
cardiovascular
cardiovascular surgery cirugía cardiovascular
cardiovascular system sistema cardiovascular
care cuidado
care and protection cuidado y protección

care and protection proceedings
procedimiento de cuidado y protección
care of elderly cuidado de ancianos
care of young cuidado de la cría
carebaria carebaria
career choice selección de carrera
career conference conferencia de carrera
career counseling asesoramiento de carrera
career decision making toma de decisiones de
carrera
career development desarrollo de carrera
career planning planificación de carrera
career workshop taller de carrera
caregiver cuidante
caregiver in child's social network cuidante
en la red social del niño
caregiver speech habla del cuidante
caretaker custodio
carezza carezza
caricature caricatura
carisoprodol carisoprodol
carnal carnal
carnosine carnosina
carotene caroteno
carotic carótico
carotid carotídeo
carotid body tumor tumor del cuerpo
carotídeo
carotid sinus seno carotídeo
carotid sinus reflex reflejo del seno carotídeo
carotid sinus syncope síncope del seno
carotídeo
carotid sinus syndrome síndrome del seno
carotídeo
carotodynia carotodinia
carpal carpiano
carpal age edad carpiana
carpal tunnel syndrome síndrome del túnel
carpiano
Carpenter's syndrome síndrome de
Carpenter
carphenazine carfenazina
carphologia carfología
carphology carfología
carpopedal carpopedal
carpopedal contraction contracción
carpopedal
carpopedal spasm espasmo carpopedal
carpoptosia carpoptosia
carpoptosis carpoptosis
carrier portador
carrier screening cribado de portadores
Cartesian cartesiano
Cartesian coordinate system sistema de
coordenadas cartesianas
Cartesian coordinates coordenadas
cartesianas
Cartesian dualism dualismo cartesiano
caruncula carúncula
Carus' typology tipología de Carus
case caso
case control study estudio de control de casos
case finding descubrimiento de casos
case history historial de caso
case history study estudio de historiales de

casos
case load carga de casos
case method método de casos
case mix mezcla de casos
case presentation presentación de caso
case register registro de caso
case study estudio de caso
case work trabajo en casos
caseworker trabajador de caso
caste casta
Castellani-Low sign signo de Castellani-Low
castrate castrar
castrating castrante
castrating woman mujer castrante
castration castración
castration anxiety ansiedad de castración
castration complex complejo de castración
castration fear temor de castración
cat's eye syndrome síndrome de ojo de gato
cat-cry syndrome síndrome del maullido de
   gato
cat phobia fobia a los gatos
catabolic catabólico
catabolism catabolismo
cataclonia cataclonia
cataclonus cataclono
catagelophobia catagelofobia
catagenesis catagénesis
catalepsy catalepsia
cataleptic cataléptico
cataleptoid cataleptoide
catalexia catalexia
catalogia catalogía
catalyst catalizador
catalytic agent agente catalítico
catamenia catamenia
catamite catamita
catamnesis catamnesis
cataphasia catafasia
cataphora catáfora
cataphrenia catafrenia
cataplectic catapléctico
cataplectic attack ataque catapléctico
cataplexy cataplejía
cataplexy of awakening cataplejía del
   despertar
cataptosis cataptosis
cataract catarata
catastrophe catástrofe
catastrophe theory teoría de catástrofe
catastrophic catastrófico
catastrophic anxiety ansiedad catastrófica
catastrophic behavior conducta catastrófica
catastrophic expectation expectación
   catastrófica
catastrophic illness enfermedad catastrófica
catastrophic reaction reacción catastrófica
catastrophic schizophrenia esquizofrenia
   catastrófica
catathymia catatimia
catathymic catatímico
catathymic amnesia amnesia catatímica
catathymic crisis crisis catatímica
catathymic violence violencia catatímica
catatonia catatonía

catatoniac catatónico
catatonic catatónico
catatonic cerebral paralysis parálisis cerebral
   catatónica
catatonic dementia demencia catatónica
catatonic excitement excitación catatónica
catatonic negativism negativismo catatónico
catatonic posturing posturación catatónica
catatonic rigidity rigidez catatónica
catatonic schizophrenia esquizofrenia
   catatónica
catatonic state estado catatónico
catatonic stupor estupor catatónico
catatonic type tipo catatónico
catatonic type schizophrenia esquizofrenia
   tipo catatónico
catatonoid catatonoide
catatonoid attitude actitud catatonoide
catatony catatonía
catch trial ensayo de captura
catchment area zona de alcance
catecholamine catecolamina
catecholamine hypothesis hipótesis de las
   catecolaminas
categorical categórico
categorical attitude actitud categórica
categorical concept concepto categórico
categorical imperative imperativo categórico
categorical memory memoria categórica
categorical perception percepción categórica
categorical scale escala categórica
categorical syllogism silogismo categórico
categorical thought pensamiento categórico
categorization categorización
categorization learning aprendizaje de
   categorización
category categoría
category boundaries límites de categorías
category cues señales de categorías
category estimation estimación de categoría
category identification identificación de
   categoría
category mistake equivocación de categoría
category scales escalas de categorías
category test prueba de categorías
catelectrotonus catelectrotono
catharsis catarsis
cathartic catártico
cathectic catéctico
cathectic discharge descarga catéctica
catheter catéter
cathexis catexis
cationic drugs drogas catiónicas
catochus catochus
catotrophobia catotrofobia
Cattell inventories inventarios de Catell
cauda equina cauda equina
cauda equina syndrome síndrome de cauda
   equina
caudal caudal
caudal transtentorial herniation herniación
   transtentorial caudal
caudate nucleus núcleo caudado
caumesthesia caumestesia
causal causal

causal attribution atribución causal
causal connection conexión causal
causal ethological analysis análisis etológico causal
causal inference inferencia causal
causal reasoning razonamiento causal
causal texture textura causal
causalgia causalgia
causality causalidad
causation causalidad
cause-and-effect test prueba de causa y efecto
cause-effect relationship relación causa-efecto
causes of child abuse causas de abuso de niños
caution cautela
cautious shift cambio cauteloso
cavernous-carotid aneurysm aneurisma carotídeo cavernoso
cavernous sinus syndrome síndrome del seno cavernoso
cebocephaly cebocefalia
ceiling tope
ceiling effect efecto de tope
celibacy celibato
cell célula
cell assembly ensamblaje celular
cell body cuerpo celular
cell differentiation diferenciación celular
cell division división celular
cell nucleus núcleo celular
cellular celular
cellular immunity factors factores de inmunidad celular
cellular layers of cortex capas celulares de la corteza
celom celoma
celoma celoma
cenesthesia cenestesia
cenesthesic cenestésico
cenesthesic hallucination alucinación cenestésica
cenesthesis cenestesis
cenesthetic cenestésico
cenesthopathy cenestopatía
cenogamy cenogamia
cenophobia cenofobia
cenotophobia cenotofobia
cenotrope cenotropo
censor censor
censorship censura
census tract tracto del censo
cent centavo
center clipping recorte del centro
centering centraje
centesis centesis
centile centila
centimorgan centimorgan
central central
central anticholinergic syndrome síndrome anticolinérgico central
central aphasia afasia central
central apnea apnea central
central arousal system sistema de despertamiento central

central auditory pathways vías auditivias centrales
central bradycardia bradicardia central
central canal canal central
central chromatolysis cromatólisis central
central conflict conflicto central
central constant constante central
central cord syndrome síndrome del cordón central
central deafness sordera central
central excitatory state estado excitatorio central
central fissure fisura central
central force fuerza central
central ganglioneuroma ganglioneuroma central
central gray gris central
central inhibition inhibición central
central issue cuestión central
central limit theorem teorema del límite central
central nervous system sistema nervioso central
central nervous system depressant depresivo del sistema nervioso central
central nervous system deviation desviación del sistema nervioso central
central nervous system disorder trastorno del sistema nervioso central
central nervous system stimulant estimulante del sistema nervioso central
central neuritis neuritis central
central olfactory pathways vías olfatorias centrales
central pain dolor central
central paralysis parálisis central
central pontine myelinolysis mielinólisis pontina central
central process proceso central
central-processing dysfunction disfunción de procesamiento central
central reflex time tiempo de reflejo central
central sleep apnea apnea del sueño central
central sulcus surco central
central taste pathways vías del gusto centrales
central tegmental nucleus núcleo tegmental central
central tendency tendencia central
central tendency measures medidas de tendencia central
central traits rasgos centrales
central transactional core centro transaccional central
central vision visión central
centralism centralismo
centralist psychology psicología centralista
centration centraje
centrencephalic centrencefálico
centrencephalic epilepsy epilepsia centrencefálica
centrencephalic seizure acceso centrencefálico
centrencephalic system sistema centrencefálico

centrifugal centrífugo
centrifugal nerve nervio centrífugo
centrifugal peripheral pathways vías periféricas centrífugas
centrifugal swing movimiento centrífugo
centripetal centrípeto
centroid centroide
centroid method método centroide
centrokinesia centrocinesia
centrokinetic centrocinético
centromere centrómero
centrophenoxine centrofenoxina
centrosome centrosoma
cephalagia cefalagia
cephalagra cefalagra
cephalalgia cefalalgia
cephalea cefalea
cephalea attonita cefalea atónita
cephaledema cefaledema
cephalemia cefalemia
cephalhematocele cefalhematocele
cephalhematoma cefalhematoma
cephalhydrocele cefalohidrocele
cephalic cefálico
cephalic index índice cefálico
cephalic reflex reflejo cefálico
cephalic tetanus tétanos cefálico
cephalitis cefalitis
cephalocaudal cefalocaudal
cephalocaudal axis eje cefalocaudal
cephalocaudal development desarrollo cefalocaudal
cephalocele cefalocele
cephalocentesis cefalocentesis
cephalodynia cefalodinia
cephalogenesis cefalogénesis
cephalogyric cefalógiro
cephalohematocele cefalohematocele
cephalohematoma cefalohematoma
cephalohemometer cefalohemómetro
cephalomeningitis cefalomeningitis
cephalometry cefalometría
cephalomotor cefalomotor
cephalooculocutaneous telangiectasia telangiectasia cefalooculocutánea
cephalopalpebral reflex reflejo cefalopalpebral
cephalopathy cefalopatía
cephalorrhachidian index índice cefalorraquídeo
cephalotrigeminal angiomatosis angiomatosis cefalotrigeminal
ceptor ceptor
ceramide ceramida
ceraunophobia ceraunofobia
cerea flexibilitas flexibilitas cerea
cerebellar cerebeloso
cerebellar ataxia ataxia cerebelosa
cerebellar atrophy atrofia cerebelosa
cerebellar cortex corteza cerebelosa
cerebellar cyst quiste cerebeloso
cerebellar fit ataque cerebeloso
cerebellar gait marcha cerebelosa
cerebellar rigidity rigidez cerebelosa
cerebellar speech habla cerebelosa

cerebellar syndrome síndrome cerebeloso
cerebellitis cerebelitis
cerebellomedullary malformation syndrome síndrome de malformación cerebelomedular
cerebellopontine cerebelopontino
cerebellopontine angle syndrome síndrome del ángulo cerebelopontino
cerebellopontine angle tumor tumor del ángulo cerebelopontino
cerebellopontine cisternography cisternografía cerebelopontina
cerebellum cerebelo
cerebral cerebral
cerebral abscess absceso cerebral
cerebral agraphia agrafia cerebral
cerebral amyloid angiopathy angiopatía amiloide cerebral
cerebral anemia anemia cerebral
cerebral angiography angiografía cerebral
cerebral angiomatosis angiomatosis cerebral
cerebral anthrax ántrax cerebral
cerebral aqueduct acueducto cerebral
cerebral arteriography arteriografía cerebral
cerebral arteriosclerosis arterioesclerosis cerebral
cerebral blindness ceguera cerebral
cerebral blood flow studies estudios del flujo sanguíneo cerebral
cerebral calculus cálculo cerebral
cerebral cladosporiosis cladosporiosis cerebral
cerebral claudication claudicación cerebral
cerebral commissure comisura cerebral
cerebral compression compresión cerebral
cerebral contusion contusión cerebral
cerebral cortex corteza cerebral
cerebral death muerte cerebral
cerebral decompression descompresión cerebral
cerebral decortication descorticación cerebral
cerebral diataxia diataxia cerebral
cerebral disorganization desorganización cerebral
cerebral dominance dominancia cerebral
cerebral dynamic imaging producción de imagen cerebral dinámica
cerebral dysfunction disfunción cerebral
cerebral dysfunction tests pruebas de disfunción cerebral
cerebral dysplasia displasia cerebral
cerebral dysrhythmia disritmia cerebral
cerebral eclipse eclipse cerebral
cerebral edema edema cerebral
cerebral electrotherapy electroterapia cerebral
cerebral embolism embolismo cerebral
cerebral ganglion ganglio cerebral
cerebral gigantism gigantismo cerebral
cerebral hemisphere hemisferio cerebral
cerebral hemorrhage hemorragia cerebral
cerebral hernia hernia cerebral
cerebral hyperesthesia hiperestesia cerebral
cerebral hyperplasia hiperplasia cerebral
cerebral hypoplasia hipoplasia cerebral
cerebral infarct infarto cerebral

cerebral infection infección cerebral
cerebral injection inyección cerebral
cerebral integration integración cerebral
cerebral intermittent claudication
    claudicación intermitente cerebral
cerebral ischemia isquemia cerebral
cerebral laceration laceración cerebral
cerebral laterality lateralidad cerebral
cerebral lateralization lateralización cerebral
cerebral lipidosis lipidosis cerebral
cerebral localization localización cerebral
cerebral malaria malaria cerebral
cerebral organization organización cerebral
cerebral pacemaker marcapasos cerebral
cerebral palsy parálisis cerebral
cerebral porosis porosis cerebral
cerebral sphingolipidosis esfingolipidosis
    cerebral
cerebral syphilis sífilis cerebral
cerebral tetanus tétanos cerebral
cerebral thrombosis trombosis cerebral
cerebral trauma trauma cerebral
cerebral tuberculosis tuberculosis cerebral
cerebral-vascular accident accidente
    cerebrovascular
cerebral-vascular disease enfermedad
    cerebrovascular
cerebral-vascular insufficiency insuficiencia
    cerebrovascular
cerebralgia cerebralgia
cerebration cerebración
cerebria cerebria
cerebritis cerebritis
cerebroatrophic hyperammonemia
    hiperamonemia cerebroatrófica
cerebrohepatorenal syndrome síndrome
    cerebrohepatorrenal
cerebroma cerebroma
cerebromacular cerebromacular
cerebromacular degeneration degeneración
    cerebromacular
cerebromalacia cerebromalacia
cerebromeningitis cerebromeningitis
cerebropathia cerebropatía
cerebropathy cerebropatía
cerebrosclerosis cerebroesclerosis
cerebroside cerebrósido
cerebroside lipidosis lipidosis cerebrósida
cerebrosidosis cerebrosidosis
cerebrosis cerebrosis
cerebrospinal cerebroespinal
cerebrospinal fever fiebre cerebroespinal
cerebrospinal fluid líquido cerebroespinal
cerebrospinal fluid otorrhea otorrea del
    líquido cerebroespinal
cerebrospinal fluid rhinorrhea rinorrea del
    líquido cerebroespinal
cerebrospinal index índice cerebroespinal
cerebrospinal meningitis meningitis
    cerebroespinal
cerebrospinal pressure presión
    cerebroespinal
cerebrospinal system sistema cerebroespinal
cerebrospinant cerebrospinante
cerebrotendinous cerebrotendinoso

cerebrotendinous cholesterinosis
    colesterinosis cerebrotendinosa
cerebrotendinous xanthomatosis
    xantomatosis cerebrotendinosa
cerebrotomy cerebrotomía
cerebrotonia cerebrotonía
cerebrovascular cerebrovascular
cerebrovascular accident accidente
    cerebrovascular
cerebrovascular disease enfermedad
    cerebrovascular
cerebrovascular insufficiency insuficiencia
    cerebrovascular
cerebrum cerebro
ceremonial ceremonial
ceremony ceremonia
ceroid lipofuscinosis lipofuscinosis ceroide
certainty certidumbre
certainty effect efecto de certidumbre
certainty equivalent equivalente de
    certidumbre
certifiable certificable
certification certificación
certification laws leyes de certificación
certify certificar
ceruloplasmin test prueba ceruloplasmina
cerumen cerumen
ceruminous deafness sordera ceruminosa
cervical cervical
cervical compression syndrome síndrome de
    compresión cervical
cervical disc syndrome síndrome del disco
    cervical
cervical erosion erosión cervical
cervical evaluation evaluación cervical
cervical fibrositis fibrositis cervical
cervical fusion syndrome síndrome de fusión
    cervical
cervical migraine migraña cervical
cervical myositis miositis cervical
cervical myospasm mioespasmo cervical
cervical nerves nervios cervicales
cervical rib syndrome síndrome de costilla
    cervical
cervical spondylosis espondilosis cervical
cervical tension syndrome síndrome de
    tensión cervical
cervicodynia cervicodinia
cervicolumbar phenomenon fenómeno
    cervicolumbar
cervicothoracic cervicotorácico
cervix cérvix
cesarean section sección cesárea
Cestan-Chenais syndrome síndrome de
    Cestan-Chenais
Chaddock reflex reflejo de Chaddock
Chaddock sign signo de Chaddock
chain cadena
chain behavior conducta en cadena
chain reflex reflejo en cadena
chain reproduction reproducción en cadena
chained reinforcement refuerzo encadenado
chained response respuesta encadenada
chained schedule programa encadenado
chaining encadenamiento

chalasis calasis
chalastic fit ataque calástico
challenge strategy estrategia de reto
chance casual
chance action acción casual
chance differences diferencias casuales
chance error error casual
Chance fracture fractura de Chance
chance variation variación casual
chancroid chancroide
change cambio
change agent agente de cambio
change fear temor al cambio
change induction group grupo de inducción
  de cambio
change of behavior cambio de conducta
change of environment cambio de ambiente
change of life cambio de vida
change-over delay demora tras cambio
change point punto de cambio
channel canal
channel capacity capacidad de canal
channels of communication canales de
  comunicación
chaotic caótico
chaotic family familia caótica
character carácter
character analysis análisis de carácter
character armor armadura del carácter
character defense defensa del carácter
character development desarrollo de carácter
character disorder trastorno del carácter
character neurosis neurosis del carácter
character structure estructura del carácter
character trait rasgo del carácter
character type tipo de carácter
characteristic característico
characterization caracterización
characterology caracterología
Charcot's disease enfermedad de Charcot
Charcot's gait marcha de Charcot
Charcot's joint articulación de Charcot
Charcot's syndrome síndrome de Charcot
Charcot's triad triada de Charcot
Charcot's vertigo vértigo de Charcot
Charcot-Bouchard aneurysm aneurisma de
  Charcot-Bouchard
Charcot-Marie-Tooth disease enfermedad de
  Charcot-Marie-Tooth
Charcot-Weiss-Baker syndrome síndrome de
  Charcot-Weiss-Baker
charisma carisma
charismatic carismático
charismatic authority autoridad carismática
charm hechizo
Charpentier's bands bandas de Charpentier
Charpentier's illusion ilusión de Charpentier
Charpentier's law ley de Charpentier
chart esquema
Chaslin's gliosis gliosis de Chaslin
chatterbox effect efecto de papagallo
Chavany-Brunhes syndrome síndrome de
  Chavany-Brunhes
cheating trampa
checking comprobación

checklist lista de comprobación
cheilitis queilitis
cheilophagia queilofagia
cheimaphobia queimafobia
cheirobrachialgia quirobraquialgia
cheirognostic quirognóstico
cheirokinesthesia quirocinestesia
cheirokinesthetic quirocinestésico
cheirospasm quiroespasmo
chelation quelación
chemical químico
chemical abuse abuso de sustancias químicas
chemical antagonism antagonismo químico
chemical aversion therapy terapia de
  aversión química
chemical brain stimulation estimulación
  cerebral química
chemical ceptor ceptor químico
chemical dependence dependencia química
chemical messengers mensajeros químicos
chemical neuroanatomy neuroanatomía
  química
chemical senses sentidos químicos
chemical stimulation estimulación química
chemical sympathectomy simpatectomía
  química
chemical transmission transmisión química
chemical transmitter transmisor químico
chemodectoma quimiodectoma
chemonucleolysis quimionucleólisis
chemopallidectomy quimiopalidectomía
chemopallidothalamectomy
  quimiopalidotalamectomía
chemopallidotomy quimiopalidotomía
chemopsychiatry quimiopsiquiatría
chemoreceptor quimiorreceptor
chemoreceptor trigger zone zona de disparo
  quimiorreceptor
chemoreceptor tumor tumor de
  quimiorreceptor
chemoreflex quimiorreflejo
chemotactic quimiotáctico
chemotaxis quimiotaxis
chemothalamectomy quimiotalamectomía
chemothalamotomy quimiotalamotomía
chemotherapeutic agent agente
  quimioterapéutico
chemotherapy quimioterapia
chemotropism quimiotropismo
cheromania queromanía
cherophobia querofobia
chewing behavior conducta de masticación
chewing method método de masticación
chewing-speech relationship relación
  masticación-habla
Cheyne's disease enfermedad de Cheyne
Cheyne-Stokes breathing respiración de
  Cheyne-Stokes
Cheyne-Stokes psychosis psicosis
  Cheyne-Stokes
Cheyne-Stokes respiration respiración de
  Cheyne-Stokes
chi square ji cuadrada
chi square analysis análisis de ji cuadrada
chi square test prueba de ji cuadrada

Chiari II syndrome síndrome de Chiari II
chiasma quiasma
chiasma syndrome síndrome de quiasma
chicken game juego del gallina
chickenpox varicela
chief complaint queja principal
child niño, hijo, hija
child abuse abuso de niños
child abuse and alcohol use abuso de niños y uso de alcohol
child abuse and suicide abuso de niños y suicidio
child analysis análisis de niños
child assessment evaluación de niños
child beating azotamiento de niño
child-care cuidado de niños
child-care aids ayudas puericulturales
child-care facility instalación para el cuidado de niños
child-care worker trabajador en el cuidado de niños
child-centered centrado en el niño
child-centered family familia centrada en el niño
child development desarrollo de niños
child ego state estado del ego de niño
child guidance asesoramiento de niños
child-guidance clinic clínica de asesoramiento de niños
child-guidance movement movimiento hacia el asesoramiento de niños
child maltreatment maltrato de niños
child molestation abuso sexual de niños
child molesting abuso sexual de niños
child neglect negligencia de niños
child-parent fixation fijación hijo-padre, fijación hijo-madre, fijación hija-padre, fijación hija-madre
child-penis wish deseo hijo-pene
child-placement counseling asesoramiento en la colocación de niños
child pornography pornografía de niños
child prodigy niño prodigio
child prostitution prostitución de niños
child psychiatry psiquiatría de niños
child psychology psicología de niños
child psychotherapy psicoterapia de niños
child-rearing crianza de niños
child-rearing beliefs creencias de la crianza de niños
child-rearing practices prácticas en la crianza de niños
child sexual abuse abuso sexual de niños
childbirth parto
childbirth fear temor al parto
childhood niñez
childhood antisocial behavior conducta antisocial de niñez
childhood anxiety disorder trastorno de ansiedad de niñez
childhood characteristics características de niñez
childhood disintegrative disorder trastorno desintegrante de niñez
childhood fears temores de niñez

childhood gender identity disorder trastorno de identidad de género de niñez
childhood Huntington's chorea corea de Huntington de niñez
childhood land tierra de la niñez
childhood masturbation masturbación de niñez
childhood motivation motivación de niñez
childhood muscular dystrophy distrofia muscular de niñez
childhood neurosis neurosis de niñez
childhood-onset pervasive developmental disorder trastorno penetrante del desarrollo de comienzo en niñez
childhood psychosis psicosis de niñez
childhood schizophrenia esquizofrenia de niñez
childhood sensorineural lesions lesiones sensorineurales de niñez
childhood sleep disorder trastorno del sueño de niñez
childhood trauma trauma de niñez
children's behavioral stages etapas conductuales de niños
children's culture cultura de niños
children's fears temores de niños
children's reaction to amputation reacción de niños a amputación
children's reaction to disasters reacción de niños a desastres
children's reaction to divorce reacción de niños a divorcio
children's reaction to hospitalization reacción de niños a hospitalización
children's reaction to illness reacción de niños a enfermedad
children's rights derechos de niños
children's rights to consent to treatment derechos de niños para consentir a tratamiento
children's rights to refuse treatment derechos de niños para rehusar tratamiento
children as witnesses niños como testigos
children at risk niños a riesgo
children of alcoholics hijos de alcohólicos
chilophagia quilofagia
chimera quimera
chimeric stimulation estimulación quimérica
chin jerk sacudida de la barbilla
chin reflex reflejo de la barbilla
China Syndrome syndrome síndrome del síndrome de la China
chionophobia quionofobia
chirobrachialgia quirobraquialgia
chirocinesthesia quirocinestesia
chirognostic quirognóstico
chirokinesthesia quirocinestesia
chirospasm quiroespasmo
chloral hydrate hidrato de cloral
chloramphenicol cloramfenicol
chlordiazepoxide clordiazepóxido
chloride cloruro
chlorimipramine clorimipramina
chlormezanone clormezanona
chloroquine cloroquina

chlorpromazine clorpromazina
chlorpromazine hydrochloride clorhidrato de clorpromazina
choc choque
Chodzko's reflex reflejo de Chodzko
choice experiment experimento de selección
choice of neurosis selección de neurosis
choice point punto de selección
choice reaction reacción de selección
choice reaction time tiempo de reacción de selección
choice shift cambio de selección
cholecystokinin colecistoquinina
cholecystokinin test prueba de colecistoquinina
cholera cólera
choleric colérico
choleric type tipo colérico
cholesteatoma colesteatoma
cholesterinosis colesterinosis
cholesterol colesterol
choline colina
choline acetylase acetilasa de colina
choline acetyltransferase acetiltransferasa de colina
cholinergic colinérgico
cholinergic drugs drogas colinérgicas
cholinergic neuron neurona colinérgica
cholinergic receptor receptor colinérgico
cholinergic synapse sinapsis colinérgica
cholinergic system sistema colinérgico
cholinergic tract tracto colinérgico
cholinesterase colinesterasa
chorda tympani cuerda del tímpano
chorditis tuberosa corditis tuberosa
chordoma cordoma
chordotomy cordotomía
chorea corea
chorea-acanthocytosis corea-acantocitosis
chorea dimidiata corea dimidiata
chorea festinans corea festinante
chorea gravidarum corea gravídea
chorea major corea mayor
chorea minor corea menor
chorea nutans corea nutans
chorea rotatoria corea rotatoria
chorea saltatoria corea saltatoria
choreal coreal
choreatiform syndrome síndrome coreatiforme
choreic coreico
choreic abasia abasia coreica
choreic movement movimiento coreico
choreiform coreiforme
choreiform movement movimiento coreiforme
choreoathetoid coreoatetoide
choreoathetosis coreoatetosis
choreoid coreoide
choreomania coreomanía
choreophrasia coreofrasia
choriomeningitis coriomeningitis
chorion corion
chorion biopsy biopsia del corion
chorionic villus sampling muestreo de

vellosidades coriónicas
choroid coroides
choroid plexus plexo coroideo
Chotzen's syndrome síndrome de Chotzen
chrematomania crematomanía
chrematophobia crematofobia
chrematorrhea crematorrea
Christensen-Krabbe disease enfermedad de Christensen-Krabbe
chroma croma
chromaffin cromafín
chromaffin tumor tumor cromafín
chromaffinoma cromafinoma
chromaffinopathy cromafinopatía
chromatic cromático
chromatic aberration aberración cromática
chromatic adaptation adaptación cromática
chromatic audition audición cromática
chromatic color color cromático
chromatic contrast contraste cromático
chromatic dimming reducción cromática
chromatic discrimination discriminación cromática
chromatic flicker centelleo cromático
chromatic fusion fusión cromática
chromatic induction inducción cromática
chromatic response respuesta cromática
chromatic scale escala cromática
chromatic valence valencia cromática
chromaticity cromaticidad
chromaticity diagram diagrama de cromaticidad
chromaticness cromaticidad
chromatid cromátide
chromatin cromatina
chromatin-negative cromatina-negativo
chromatin-positive cromatina-positivo
chromatinolysis cromatinólisis
chromatography cromatografía
chromatolysis cromatólisis
chromatolytic cromatolítico
chromatophobia cromatofobia
chromatopsia cromatopsia
chromesthesia cromestesia
chromhidrosis cromhidrosis
chromic myopia miopía crómica
chromidrosis cromidrosis
chromolysis cromólisis
chromomere cromómero
chromophil adenoma adenoma cromófilo
chromophil substance sustancia cromófila
chromophobe adenoma adenoma cromófobo
chromophobia cromofobia
chromopsia cromopsia
chromosomal cromosómico
chromosomal aberration aberración cromosómica
chromosomal abnormality anormalidad cromosómica
chromosomal alteration alteración cromosómica
chromosomal anomaly anomalía cromosómica
chromosome cromosoma
chromosome 13 trisomy trisomia del

cromosoma 13
chromosome 18 trisomy trisomia del
cromosoma 18
chromosome 21 trisomy trisomia del
cromosoma 21
chromosome number número cromosómico
chromosomic cromosómico
chromotherapy cromoterapia
chromotopsia cromotopsia
chronaxia cronaxia
chronaxie cronaxia
chronaxis cronaxis
chronaxy cronaxia
chronic crónico
chronic affective disorder trastorno afectivo
crónico
chronic alcohol abuse abuso de alcohol
crónico
chronic alcoholism alcoholismo crónico
chronic anterior poliomyelitis poliomielitis
anterior crónica
chronic anxiety ansiedad crónica
chronic brain disorder trastorno cerebral
crónico
chronic brain syndrome síndrome cerebral
crónico
chronic bronchitis bronquitis crónica
chronic delusional state of negation estado
de negación delusorio crónico
chronic depression depresión crónica
chronic drug tolerance tolerancia de drogas
crónica
chronic exercise ejercicio crónico
chronic familial polyneuritis polineuritis
familiar crónica
chronic headaches dolores de cabeza crónicos
chronic hyperventilation syndrome síndrome
de hiperventilación crónica
chronic mania manía crónica
chronic mentally ill enfermo mental crónico
chronic mood disorder trastorno del humor
crónico
chronic motor tic disorder trastorno de tic
motor crónico
chronic obstructive pulmonary disease
enfermedad pulmonar obstructiva crónica
chronic pain dolor crónico
chronic preparation preparación crónica
chronic progressive chorea corea progresiva
crónica
chronic schizophrenia esquizofrenia crónica
chronic stress estrés crónico
chronic stressors estresantes crónicos
chronic tolerance tolerancia crónica
chronic traumatic disorder trastorno
traumático crónico
chronic trypanosomiasis tripanosomiasis
crónica
chronic undifferentiated schizophrenia
esquizofrenia indeferenciada crónica
chronic vertigo vértigo crónico
chronic vocal tic disorder trastorno de tic
vocal crónico
chronicity cronicidad
chronobiology cronobiología

chronognosis cronognosis
chronograph cronógrafo
chronologic age edad cronológica
chronological age edad cronológica
chronometric cronométrico
chronometry cronometría
chronophobia cronofobia
chronophysiology cronofisiología
chronoscope cronoscopio
chronotaraxia cronotaraxia
chronotaraxis cronotaraxis
chronotherapy cronoterapia
chthonophagia ctonofagia
chthonophagy ctonofagia
chunk unidad de información
chunking agrupamiento de pensamientos
Chvostek's sign signo de Chvostek
Chvostek's tremor temblor de Chvostek
cibophobia cibofobia
cicatrix cicatriz
cicatrization cicatrización
cigarette-smoke pollution polución del humo
de cigarrillo
cigarette smoking fumar cigarrillos
cilia cilios
ciliary ciliar
ciliary muscle músculo ciliar
ciliospinal reflex reflejo cilioespinal
ciliotomy ciliotomía
cilium cilio
cinaedi cinaedi
cinanesthesia cinanestesia
cinchonism cinconismo
cinclisis cinclisis
cincture sensation sensación de cincho
Cinderella complex complejo de la Cenicienta
cineplasty cineplastia
cineseismography cineseismografía
cingulate cingulado
cingulate cortex corteza cingulada
cingulate gyrus circunvolución cingulada
cingulate herniation herniación cingulada
cingulate sulcus surco cingulado
cingulectomy cingulectomía
cingulotomy cingulotomía
cinnarizine cinarizina
cipher method método de cifra
circadian circadiano
circadian desynchronosis desincronosis
circadiano
circadian realignment realineamiento
circadiano
circadian rhythm ritmo circadiano
circadian rhythm sleep disorder trastorno
del sueño de ritmo circadiano
circannual circanual
circannual rhythm ritmo circanual
circle of Willis círculo de Willis
circuit circuito
circular circular
circular behavior conducta circular
circular illness enfermedad circular
circular insanity insania circular
circular-pattern responses respuestas a
patrones en círculos

circular psychosis psicosis circular
circular reaction reacción circular
circular reasoning razonamiento circular
circulatory circulatorio
circulatory psychosis psicosis circulatoria
circumlocution circunlocución
circumscribed circunscrito
circumscribed amnesia amnesia circunscrita
circumscribed craniomalacia craneomalacia
    circunscrita
circumscribed edema edema circunscrita
circumscribed pyocephalus piocéfalo
    circunscrito
circumscription circunscripción
circumstantial evidence prueba circunstancial
circumstantiality circunstancialidad
circumvallate papilla papila circunvalada
cirrhosis cirrosis
cissa cisa
cisterna cerebellomedullaris cisterna
    cerebellomedularis
cisterna magna cisterna magna
cisternal puncture punción cisternal
cisternography cisternografía
cisvestism cisvestismo
cisvestitism cisvestitismo
Citelli's syndrome síndrome de Citelli
citrate citrato
citta cisa
cittosis citosis
civil commitment confinamiento civil
civil disobedience desobediencia civil
civilian catastrophe reaction reacción de
    catástrofe de civil
civilization civilización
cladosporiosis cladosporiosis
claiming type of depression tipo de depresión
    reclamante
claims review revisión de reclamaciones
clairaudience clariaudición
clairvoyance clarividencia
clan clan
clang association asociación sonora
clarification clarificación
Clarke's column columna de Clarke
clasp-knife navaja
clasp-knife effect efecto de navaja
clasp-knife phenomenon fenómeno de navaja
clasp-knife reflex reflejo de navaja
clasp-knife rigidity rigidez de navaja
clasp-knife spasticity espasticidad de navaja
class clase
class-free test prueba libre de clases
class inclusion inclusión de clase
class interval intervalo de clase
class limits límites de clase
class size tamaño de clase
class structure estructura de clases
classic migraine migraña clásica
classical clásico
classical analysis análisis clásico
classical appetitive conditioning
    condicionamiento apetitivo clásico
classical aversive conditioning
    condicionamiento aversivo clásico

classical conditioning condicionamiento
    clásico
classical depression depresión clásica
classical learning theory teoría del
    aprendizaje clásica
classical paranoia paranoia clásica
classical perception theory teoría de
    percepción clásica
classical psychoanalysis psicoanálisis clásico
classical reflex theory teoría de reflejos
    clásico
classical technique técnica clásica
classical theory teoría clásica
classification clasificación
classification method método de clasificación
classification of abnormal behavior
    clasificación de conducta anormal
classification of anxiety clasificación de
    ansiedad
classification of delinquency clasificación de
    delincuencia
classification test prueba de clasificación
classroom aula
classroom attendance asistencia de aula
classroom discipline disciplina de aula
classroom dynamics dinámica de aula
classroom test prueba de aula
Claude's syndrome síndrome de Claude
claudication claudicación
claustral complex complejo claustral
claustrophilia claustrofilia
claustrophobia claustrofobia
claustrophobic claustrofóbico
claustrum claustro
clava clava
clavus clavo
clawfoot pie en garra
clawhand mano en garra
clawing attack ataque de arañazos
clay-modeling equipment equipo para el
    modelado de arcilla
clay-modeling in hypnosis modelado de
    arcilla en hipnosis
clay-modeling therapy terapia con el
    modelado de arcilla
clear sensorium sensorio claro
clear twilight state estado crepuscular claro
clearness claridad
cleft lip labio hendido
cleft palate paladar hendido
cleft-palate speech habla de paladar hendido
cleft spine espina hendida
Clerambault's syndrome síndrome de
    Clerambault
Clerambault-Kandinski syndrome síndrome
    de Clerambault-Kandinski
clerical-aptitude test prueba de destrezas de
    oficina
cliché cliché
client cliente
client-centered psychotherapy psicoterapia
    centrada en el cliente
client-centered therapy terapia centrada en el
    cliente
climacophobia climacofobia

climacteric climatérico
climacteric melancholia melancolía climatérica
climacteric psychosis psicosis climatérica
climacterium climaterio
climate conformance conformidad del clima
climax clímax
clinging behavior conducta de asirse
clinic clínica
clinical clínico
clinical algorithm algoritmo clínico
clinical application aplicación clínica
clinical assessment evaluación clínica
clinical counseling asesoramiento clínico
clinical diagnosis diagnóstico clínico
clinical group grupo clínico
clinical grouping agrupamiento clínico
clinical hypnotism hipnotismo clínico
clinical judgment juicio clínico
clinical method método clínico
clinical pain dolor clínico
clinical poverty syndrome síndrome de pobreza clínica
clinical prediction predicción clínica
clinical procedure procedimiento clínico
clinical psychiatry psiquiatría clínica
clinical psychologist psicólogo clínico
clinical psychology psicología clínica
clinical psychopharmacology psicofarmacología clínica
clinical sociology sociología clínica
clinical study estudio clínico
clinical teaching enseñanza clínica
clinical trial ensayo clínico
clinical type tipo clínico
clinical versus statistical prediction predicción estadística contra clínica
clinical work trabajo clínico
clinodactyly clinodactilia
clipping recorte
clique peña
clithrophobia clitrofobia
clitoral clitoral
clitoral orgasm orgasmo clitoral
clitoridectomy clitoridectomía
clitoris clítoris
cloaca cloaca
cloaca theory teoría de la cloaca
cloacal theory teoría cloacal
clobazam clobazam
clock reloj
clock-driven behavior conducta accionada por el tiempo
clomipramine clomipramina
clonazepam clonazepam
clone clona
clonic clónico
clonic convulsion convulsión clónica
clonic phase fase clónica
clonic spasm espasmo clónico
clonicity clonicidad
clonicotonic clonicotónico
clonidine clonidina
clonism clonismo
clonospasm clonoespasmo

clonus clono
clorazepic acid ácido clorazépico
closed-ended question pregunta con alternativas fijas
closed figure figura cerrada
closed group grupo cerrado
closed head injury lesión de cabeza cerrada
closed instinct instinto cerrado
closed-loop feedback system sistema de retroalimentación de ciclo cerrado
closed skull fracture fractura de cráneo cerrada
closed system sistema cerrado
closing-in acercamiento
closure cierre
closure principle principio de cierre
clothiapine clotiapina
clotiazepam clotiazepam
clouded enturbado
clouded sensorium sensorio enturbado
clouded state estado enturbado
cloudiness nebulosidad
clouding enturbiamiento
clouding of consciousness enturbiamiento de conciencia
cloverleaf skull cráneo en hoja de trébol
cloverleaf skull syndrome síndrome de cráneo en hoja de trébol
clowning payasadas
clownism clounismo
cloxazolam cloxazolam
clozapine clozapina
clubfoot pie zambo
clue indicio
clumsiness torpeza
clumsy torpe
clumsy-child syndrome síndrome de niño torpe
cluster grupo
cluster analysis análisis de grupos
cluster approach acercamiento de grupos
cluster headaches dolores de cabeza en grupo
cluster marriage matrimonio en grupo
cluster suicides suicidios en grupo
clustering agrupamiento
cluttering agitofasia
Clytemnestra complex complejo de Clytemnestra
co-twin control control de gemelo
coaching entrenamiento
coacting group grupo coactuante
coarctate coartado
coarse tremor temblor grueso
coarticulation coarticulación
Cobb syndrome síndrome de Cobb
coca coca
cocaine cocaína
cocaine abuse abuso de cocaína
cocaine anxiety disorder trastorno de ansiedad de cocaína
cocaine bug hormigueo por cocaína
cocaine delirium delirio de cocaína
cocaine delusional disorder trastorno delusorio de cocaína
cocaine dependence dependencia de cocaína

cocaine habituation habituación de cocaína
cocaine-induced organic mental disorder trastorno mental orgánico inducido por cocaína
cocaine intoxication intoxicación por cocaína
cocaine mood disorder trastorno del humor de cocaína
cocaine psychotic disorder trastorno psicótico de cocaína
cocaine psychotic disorder with delusions trastorno psicótico de cocaína con delusiones
cocaine psychotic disorder with hallucinations trastorno psicótico de cocaína con alucinaciones
cocaine sexual dysfunction disfunción sexual de cocaína
cocaine sleep disorder trastorno del sueño de cocaína
cocaine toxicity toxicidad de cocaína
cocaine use disorder trastorno de uso de cocaína
cocaine withdrawal retiro de cocaína
cocainism cocainismo
cocainomania cocainomanía
cochlea cóclea
cochleagram cocleagrama
cochlear aphasia afasia coclear
cochlear duct conducto coclear
cochlear microphonics microfónicos cocleares
cochlear nerve nervio coclear
cochlear nuclei núcleos cocleares
cochlear recruitment reclutamiento coclear
cochleoorbicular reflex reflejo cocleoorbicular
cochleopalpebral reflex reflejo cocleopalpebral
cochleopalpebral reflex test prueba del reflejo cocleopalpebral
cochleopupillary reflex reflejo cocleopupilar
cochleostapedial reflex reflejo cocleoestapedio
Cockayne's syndrome síndrome de Cockayne
cocktail cóctel
cocktail-party conversationalism conversacionalismo de cóctel
cocktail-party phenomenon fenómeno de cóctel
coconsciousness coconciencia
cocontraction cocontracción
coconut sound sonido de coco
code código
code capacity capacidad de códigos
code of ethics código de ética
code switching cambio de códigos
code test prueba de códigos
codeine codeína
codeine dependence dependencia de codeína
codification codificación
codification of rules stage etapa de codificación de reglas
coding codificación
coding strategies estrategias de codificaciones
coding test prueba de codificaciones

coding theory teoría de codificaciones
codominance codominancia
coefficient coeficiente
coefficient of alienation coeficiente de alienación
coefficient of concordance coeficiente de concordancia
coefficient of correlation coeficiente de correlación
coefficient of determination coeficiente de determinación
coefficient of stability coeficiente de estabilidad
coefficient of variation coeficiente de variación
coelom celoma
coenesthesia coenestesia
coenotrope cenotropo
coercible coercible
coercion coerción
coercive coercitivo
coercive behavior conducta coercitiva
coercive persuasion persuasión coercitiva
coercive philosophy filosofía coercitiva
coercive sex sexo coercitivo
coercive treatment tratamiento coercitivo
coexistence coexistencia
coexistence of neurotransmitters coexistencia de neurotransmisores
coexistent coexistente
coexistent culture cultura coexistente
coexperimenter coexperimentador
coffee consumption consumo de café
cofigurative culture cultura cofigurativa
Cogan's syndrome síndrome de Cogan
cognition cognición
cognition and language cognición y lenguaje
cognition disorder trastorno de cognición
cognitive cognitivo
cognitive abilities habilidades cognitivas
cognitive action acción cognitiva
cognitive anthropology antropología cognitiva
cognitive appraisal evaluación cognitiva
cognitive appraisal theory teoría de evaluación cognitiva
cognitive approach acercamiento cognitivo
cognitive awareness level nivel de conciencia cognitiva
cognitive behavior modification modificación de conducta cognitiva
cognitive behavior therapy terapia de conducta cognitiva
cognitive behavioral psychotherapy psicoterapia conductual cognitiva
cognitive behavioral therapy terapia conductual cognitiva
cognitive behavioral therapy for anxiety terapia conductual cognitiva para ansiedad
cognitive behavioral therapy for child abuse terapia conductual cognitiva para abuso de niños
cognitive behavioral therapy for depression terapia conductual cognitiva para depresión
cognitive behavioral therapy for eating disorders terapia conductual cognitiva

para trastornos del comer
cognitive behavioral therapy for psychosomatic problems terapia conductual cognitiva para problemas psicosomáticos
cognitive capacity capacidad cognitiva
cognitive changes in adulthood cambios cognitivos en adultez
cognitive competence competencia cognitiva
cognitive complexity complejidad cognitiva
cognitive conditioning condicionamiento cognitivo
cognitive contour contorno cognitivo
cognitive control control cognitivo
cognitive decrement decremento cognitivo
cognitive defect defecto cognitivo
cognitive deficit déficit cognitivo
cognitive deficits in abused children déficits cognitivos en niños abusados
cognitive derailment descarrilamiento cognitivo
cognitive determinants of emotion determinantes cognitivos de emoción
cognitive development desarrollo cognitivo
cognitive development and language development desarrollo cognitivo y desarrollo del lenguaje
cognitive development in adults desarrollo cognitivo en adultos
cognitive dissonance disonancia cognitiva
cognitive dissonance theory teoría de la disonancia cognitiva
cognitive economy economía cognitiva
cognitive factor factor cognitivo
cognitive flexibility flexibilidad cognitiva
cognitive function función cognitiva
cognitive function of sleep función cognitiva del sueño
cognitive functioning funcionamiento cognitivo
cognitive growth crecimiento cognitivo
cognitive impairment deterioro cognitivo
cognitive interpretation interpretación cognitiva
cognitive intervention intervención cognitiva
cognitive laterality quotient cociente de lateralidad cognitiva
cognitive learning style estilo de aprendizaje cognitivo
cognitive learning theory teoría del aprendizaje cognitivo
cognitive linguistic treatment tratamiento lingüístico cognitivo
cognitive map mapa cognitivo
cognitive map theory teoría de mapa cognitivo
cognitive marker señal cognitiva
cognitive maturation maduración cognitiva
cognitive mediation mediación cognitiva
cognitive model modelo cognitivo
cognitive need necesidad cognitiva
cognitive operations operaciones cognitivas
cognitive physiological theory teoría fisiológica cognitiva
cognitive procedures procedimientos

cognitivos
cognitive processes procesos cognitivos
cognitive psychology psicología cognitiva
cognitive psychophysiology psicofisiología cognitiva
cognitive rehearsal ensayo cognitivo
cognitive representation representación cognitiva
cognitive restructuring reestructuración cognitiva
cognitive schema esquema cognitivo
cognitive science ciencia cognitiva
cognitive self-reinforcement autorrefuerzo cognitivo
cognitive slippage resbalamiento cognitivo
cognitive stages etapas cognitivas
cognitive state estado cognitivo
cognitive strategy estrategia cognitiva
cognitive structure estructura cognitiva
cognitive style estilo cognitivo
cognitive task tarea cognitiva
cognitive theory teoría cognitiva
cognitive theory of depression teoría de depresión cognitiva
cognitive theory of emotion teoría de emoción cognitiva
cognitive theory of emotional development teoría del desarrollo emocional cognitiva
cognitive theory of learning teoría de aprendizaje cognitiva
cognitive therapy terapia cognitiva
cognitive triad tríada cognitiva
cognitivist cognitivista
cognizance need necesidad de conocimiento
cognization cognización
cognize conocer
cogwheel rueda dentada
cogwheel phenomenon fenómeno de rueda dentada
cogwheel rigidity rigidez en rueda dentada
cohabitation cohabitación
cohesion cohesión
cohesion law ley de cohesión
cohesive self yo cohesivo
cohesiveness cohesividad
cohort cohorte
cohort differences diferencia de cohortes
cohort effect efecto de cohorte
cohort study estudio de cohorte
coin recognition reconocimiento de monedas
coin test prueba de monedas
coital coital
coital headache dolor de cabeza coital
coital position posición coital
coition coito
coitophobia coitofobia
coitus coito
coitus fear temor al coito
coitus interruptus coito interrumpido
coitus representation representación de coito
coitus reservatus coito reservado
colchicine colchicina
cold effects efectos del frío
cold emotion emoción fría
cold pack envoltura fría

cold-pack treatment tratamiento con envolturas frías
cold spot punto frío
coldness frialdad
colic cólico
colitis colitis
collaboration colaboración
collaborative therapy terapia colaboradora
collapse delirium delirio por colapso
collateral colateral
collateral behavior conducta colateral
collateral fiber fibra colateral
colleague-centered consultation consultación centrada en los colegas
collecting coleccionismo
collective colectivo
collective consciousness conciencia colectiva
collective experience experiencia colectiva
collective psychosis psicosis colectiva
collective unconscious inconsciente colectivo
Collet-Sicard syndrome síndrome de Collet-Sicard
colliculus colículo
colligation coligación
collum distortum collum distortum
coloboma coloboma
colony colonia
color adaptation adaptación al color
color agnosia agnosia de color
color antagonism antagonismo de colores
color appearance apariencia de color
color attribute atributo de color
color blindness ceguera al color
color categories categorías de colores
color cells células de color
color circle círculo de color
color cone cono de color
color constancy constancia de color
color contrast contraste de color
color deficiency deficiencia de color
color dreams sueños a colores
color equation ecuación de colores
color fusion fusión de colores
color hearing audición de color
color in dreams colores en sueños
color matching pareo de colores
color mixing mezcla de colores
color mixture mezcla de colores
color perception percepción de color
color preference preferencia de color
color pyramid pirámide de color
color receptors receptores de color
color scale escala de colores
color scotoma escotoma de color
color shades matices de colores
color solid sólido de color
color sorting test prueba de clasificación de colores
color spindle huso de color
color stimuli estímulos de color
color surface superficie de color
color system sistema de colores
color taste gusto de color
color theories teorías de color
color tints tintes de colores

color triangle triángulo de color
color value valor de color
color vision visión de color
color weakness debilidad de color
color wheel rueda de colores
color zones zonas de color
colored audition audición coloreada
colored hearing audición coloreada
colored noise ruido coloreado
colorimeter colorímetro
colorimetry colorimetría
column columna
columnar organization of cortex organización columnar de la corteza
coma coma
coma carcinomatosum coma carcinomatoso
coma scale escala de coma
coma vigil vigilia de coma
comatose comatoso
comatose state estado comatoso
combat fatigue fatiga de combate
combat hysteria histeria de combate
combative combativo
combination combinación
combination law ley de combinación
combination tone tono de combinación
combined sclerosis esclerosis combinada
combined system disease enfermedad de sistemas combinados
combined therapy terapia combinada
combined transcortical aphasia afasia transcortical combinada
combining forms formas de compuestos
comention comención
cometophobia cometofobia
comic cómico
comical cómico
comical nonsense disparates cómicos
coming out declaración
command comando
command automatism automatismo ante mandatos
command negativism negativismo ante mandatos
command style estilo de comando
commensalism comensalismo
comminuted skull fracture fractura de cráneo conminuta
commissural fibers fibras comisurales
commissural myelotomy mielotomía comisural
commissure comisura
commissurotomy comisurotomía
commitment compromiso, confinamiento
commitment laws leyes de confinamiento
common común
common attributes atributos comunes
common chemical sense sentido químico común
common factor factor común
common fate destino común
common-fate law ley del destino común
common migraine migraña común
common phobias fobias comunes
common sense sentido común

common-sense psychiatry psiquiatría de
sentido común
common-sense validity validez de sentido
común
common sensibility sensibilidad común
common trait rasgo común
commotio conmoción
commotio cerebri conmoción cerebral
commotio spinalis conmoción espinal
communal feeling sensación comunal
communal spirit espíritu comunal
commune comuna
communicated psychosis psicosis comunicada
communicating hydrocephalus hidrocefalia
comunicante
communication comunicación
communication channels canales de
comunicación
communication deviance desviación de
comunicación
communication disorder trastorno de
comunicación
communication engineering ingeniería de
comunicación
communication in blind infants
comunicación en infantes ciegos
communication in deaf children
comunicación en niños sordos
communication magic magia de
comunicación
communication network redes de
comunicación
communication pattern patrón de
comunicación
communication processes procesos de
comunicación
communication skills destrezas de
comunicación
communication skills assessment evaluación
de destrezas de comunicación
communication skills training entrenamiento
de destrezas de comunicación
communication styles estilos de comunicación
communication theory teoría de la
comunicación
communication therapy terapia de
comunicación
communication training entrenamiento de
comunicación
communication unit unidad de comunicación
communicative comunicativo
communicative comprehension comprensión
comunicativa
communicative functions funciones
comunicativas
communicology comunicología
communion comunión
communion principle principio de comunión
communiscope comuniscopio
**communities for mentally handicapped
persons** comunidades para personas con
minusvalía mental
community comunidad
community-action group grupo de acción
comunitario

community assessment evaluación
comunitaria
community care cuidado comunitario
community-centered approach acercamiento
centrado en la comunidad
community competence competencia
comunitaria
community divorce divorcio comunitario
community feeling sensación comunitaria
community intervention intervención
comunitaria
community mental health salud mental
comunitaria
community mental health center centro de
salud mental comunitario
community mental health program
programa de salud mental comunitario
community needs necesidades comunitarias
community needs assessment evaluación de
necesidades comunitarias
community organization organización
comunitaria
community program programa comunitario
community psychiatry psiquiatría comunitaria
community psychology psicología
comunitaria
community resources recursos comunitarios
community response to disasters respuesta
de la comunidad a desastres
community role papel comunitario
community services servicios comunitarios
community social worker trabajador social
comunitario
community speech and hearing centers
centros del habla y audición comunitarios
community spirit espíritu comunitario
comorbidity comorbilidad
companion compañero
companion-therapist terapeuta compañero
comparable comparable
comparable forms formas comparables
comparable groups grupos comparables
comparative comparativo
comparative judgment juicio comparativo
comparative psychiatry psiquiatría
comparativa
comparative psychology psicología
comparativa
comparison comparación
comparison level nivel de comparación
comparison procedure procedimiento de
comparación
comparison stimulus estímulo de
comparación
compartmentalization compartimentación
compassion compasión
compatibility compatibilidad
compatible compatible
compeer par
compelled behavior conducta obligada
compensating error error compensatorio
compensation compensación
compensation neurosis neurosis de
compensación
compensatory compensatorio

compensatory education educación compensatoria
compensatory mechanism mecanismo compensatorio
compensatory movement movimiento compensatorio
compensatory nystagmus nistagmo compensatorio
compensatory scoliosis escoliosis compensatoria
compensatory trait rasgo compensatorio
competence competencia
competence knowledge conocimiento de competencia
competence motivation motivación de competencia
competence standards normas de competencia
competency competencia
competency and informed consent competencia y consentimiento informado
competency-based instruction instrucción basada en la competencia
competency in psychology competencia en psicología
competency of child witnesses competencia de niños testigos
competency of minors to consent to treatment competencia de menores para consentir a tratamiento
competency of professionals competencia de profesionales
competency of witness competencia de testigo
competency to make a will competencia para hacer un testamento
competency to stand trial competencia para someterse a juicio
competency to stand trial and insanity competencia para someterse a juicio e insania
competent competente
competition competencia
competition tolerance tolerancia a la competencia
competitive competitivo
competitive anxiety ansiedad competitiva
competitive inhibition inhibición competitiva
competitive motive motivo competitivo
competitive reward structure estructura de recompensa competitiva
complacency complacencia
complaining quejumbroso
complaint queja
complaint habit hábito de quejas
complement complemento
complementarity complementaridad
complementarity of interaction complementaridad de interacción
complementary complementario
complementary color color complementario
complementary instincts instintos complementarios
complementary role papel complementario
complete completo
complete iridoplegia iridoplejía completa

complete-learning method método de aprendizaje completo
complete mother madre completa
complete Oedipus Edipo completo
completely randomized completamente aleatorizado
completion test prueba de terminación
complex complejo
complex absence ausencia compleja
complex indicator indicador de complejos
complex learning aprendizaje complejo
complex learning processes procesos de aprendizaje complejos
complex of ideas complejo de ideas
complex partial seizure acceso parcial complejo
complex person persona compleja
complex precipitated epilepsy epilepsia precipitada compleja
complex reaction reacción compleja
complex reaction time tiempo de reacción compleja
complex tone tono complejo
complex type tipo complejo
complexity factor factor de complejidad
compliance acatamiento, sumisión
compliant character carácter sumiso
complicated fracture fractura complicada
complication complicación
complication experiment experimento de complicación
complications in birth complicaciones en nacimiento
component componente
component instinct instinto componente
componential analysis análisis de componentes
components of emotion componentes de emoción
components of variance model modelo de componentes de varianza
compos mentis compos mentis
composite compuesto
composite figure figura compuesta
composite image imagen compuesta
composite person persona compuesta
composite score puntuación compuesta
composite trait rasgo compuesto
composition of movement composición de movimiento
compound compuesto
compound bilingual bilingüe compuesto
compound conditioning condicionamiento compuesto
compound eye ojo compuesto
compound reaction reacción compuesta
compound reaction time tiempo de reacción compuesta
compound skull fracture fractura de cráneo compuesta
compound stimuli estímulos compuestos
compound task tarea compuesta
compound tone tono compuesto
comprehend comprender
comprehension comprensión

comprehension test prueba de comprensión
comprehensive mental health center centro de salud mental comprensiva
comprehensive solution solución comprensiva
compression compresión
compression anesthesia anestesia por compresión
compression of brain compresión del cerebro
compression paralysis parálisis por compresión
compressive myelopathy mielopatía compresiva
compromise compromiso
compromise activity actividad de compromiso
compromise distortion distorsión de compromiso
compromise formation formación de compromiso
compromiser comprometedor
compulsion compulsión
compulsion neurosis neurosis de compulsión
compulsions versus tics compulsiones contra tics
compulsive compulsivo
compulsive behavior conducta compulsiva
compulsive ceremonial ceremonial compulsivo
compulsive changing cambio compulsivo
compulsive character carácter compulsivo
compulsive coercion coerción compulsiva
compulsive-conduct disorder trastorno de conducta compulsiva
compulsive disorder trastorno compulsivo
compulsive drinker bebedor compulsivo
compulsive eating comer compulsivo
compulsive gambling jugar compulsivo
compulsive idea idea compulsiva
compulsive laughter risa compulsiva
compulsive magic magia compulsiva
compulsive masturbation masturbación compulsiva
compulsive neurosis neurosis compulsiva
compulsive-obsessive psychoneurosis psiconeurosis compulsiva-obsesiva
compulsive orderliness orden compulsivo
compulsive personality personalidad compulsiva
compulsive personality disorder trastorno de personalidad compulsiva
compulsive repetition repetición compulsiva
compulsive restraint control compulsivo
compulsive scale escala compulsiva
compulsive sexual activity actividad sexual compulsiva
compulsive stealing robo compulsivo
compulsiveness carácter compulsivo
computation cómputo
computational metaphor metáfora computacional
compute computar
computed tomography tomografía computerizada
computer computadora
computer-administered test prueba administrada por computadora

computer animation animación de computadora
computer anxiety ansiedad de computadoras
computer-assisted asistido por computadora
computer-assisted assessment evaluación asistida por computadora
computer-assisted instruction instrucción asistida por computadora
computer-generated image imagen generada por computadora
computer graphics gráficos de computadora
computer illiteracy analfabetismo de computadoras
computer-managed instruction instrucción administrada por computadora
computer metaphor metáfora de computadora
computer model modelo de computadora
computer simulation simulación por computadora
computer software programas de computadora
computer thought pensamiento de computadora
computerized computerizado
computerized axial tomography tomografía axial computerizada
computerized diagnosis diagnóstico computerizado
computerized test prueba computerizada
computerized therapy terapia computerizada
computerized tomography tomografía computerizada
conarium conario
conation conación
conative conativo
conatus conato
concatenation concatenación
concealed antisocial activity actividad antisocial oculta
conceive concebir
conceived values valores concebidos
concentration concentración
concentration difficulty dificultad de concentración
concentration span lapso de concentración
concentration test prueba de concentración
concept concepto
concept acquisition adquisición de concepto
concept-attainment model modelo del logro de conceptos
concept categorization categorización de concepto
concept discovery descubrimiento de concepto
concept formation formación de concepto
concept-formation test prueba de formación de conceptos
concept identification identificación de concepto
concept induction inducción de concepto
concept learning aprendizaje de conceptos
concept representation representación de concepto
concept use uso de concepto

conception concepción
conception age edad de concepción
conceptual conceptual
conceptual development desarrollo
  conceptual
conceptual disorder trastorno conceptual
conceptual disorganization desorganización
  conceptual
conceptual disturbance disturbio conceptual
conceptual field campo conceptual
conceptual learning aprendizaje conceptual
conceptual model modelo conceptual
conceptual nervous system sistema nervioso
  conceptual
conceptual replication replicación conceptual
conceptual systems sistemas conceptuales
conceptual tempo tempo conceptual
conceptualization conceptualización
conceptually guided control control guiado
  conceptualmente
concomitant concomitante
concomitant variation variación concomitante
concordance concordancia
concordance coefficient coeficiente de
  concordancia
concordance rate tasa de concordancia
concrete concreto
concrete attitude actitud concreta
concrete image imagen concreta
concrete intelligence inteligencia concreta
concrete operations operaciones concretas
concrete operations level nivel de
  operaciones concretas
concrete operations period periodo de
  operaciones concretas
concrete operations stage etapa de
  operaciones concretas
concrete operatory thought pensamiento
  operatorio concreto
concrete picture imagen concreta
concrete thinking pensamiento concreto
concreteness concreticidad
concretism concretismo
concretistic thinking pensamiento concreto
concretization concretización
concretize concretar
concretizing attitude actitud concretante
concurrent concurrente
concurrent medical audit auditoría médica
  concurrente
concurrent reaction time tiempo de reacción
  concurrente
concurrent reinforcement refuerzo
  concurrente
concurrent review revisión concurrente
concurrent schedules programas concurrentes
concurrent tasks tareas concurrentes
concurrent therapy terapia concurrente
concurrent validity validez concurrente
concussion concusión
concussion myelitis mielitis por concusión
condemnation condenación
condensation condensación
condition condición
condition not attributable to a mental

disorder condición no atribuible a un
  trastorno mental
conditionability condicionabilidad
conditional assignment asignación
  condicional
conditional discrimination discriminación
  condicional
conditional love amor condicional
conditional positive regard estimación
  positiva condicional
conditional probability probabilidad
  condicional
conditional reflex reflejo condicional
conditional release libertad condicional
conditional response respuesta condicional
conditional statement declaración condicional
conditionalism condicionalismo
conditioned condicionado
conditioned anxiety ansiedad condicionada
conditioned appetitive response respuesta
  apetitiva condicionada
conditioned aversion aversión condicionada
conditioned avoidance evitación condicionada
conditioned avoidance response respuesta de
  evitación condicionada
conditioned cues señales condicionadas
conditioned drug tolerance tolerancia de
  drogas condicionada
conditioned emotional response respuesta
  emocional condicionada
conditioned emotions emociones
  condicionadas
conditioned escape escape condicionado
conditioned escape response respuesta de
  escape condicionado
conditioned fear temor condicionado
conditioned inhibition inhibición
  condicionada
conditioned reflex reflejo condicionado
conditioned-reflex therapy terapia de reflejos
  condicionados
conditioned reinforcer reforzador
  condicionado
conditioned response respuesta condicionada
conditioned response learning aprendizaje de
  respuesta condicionada
conditioned stimulus estímulo condicionado
conditioned suppression supresión
  condicionada
conditioned taste aversion aversión de gusto
  condicionada
conditioned toxicosis toxicosis condicionada
conditioning condicionamiento
conditioning by successive approximations
  condicionamiento por aproximaciones
  sucesivas
conditioning during sleep condicionamiento
  durante el sueño
conditioning of compensatory reactions
  condicionamiento de reacciones
  compensatorias
conditioning therapy terapia de
  condicionamiento
conditions of worth condiciones de mérito
condom condón

conduct conducta
conduct disorder trastorno de conducta
conduct disorder versus affective disorder
   trastorno de conducta contra trastorno
   afectivo
conduct disturbance disturbio de conducta
conduction conducción
conduction aphasia afasia de conducción
conduction deafness sordera de conducción
conductivity conductividad
cones conos
confabulation confabulación
confabulosis confabulosis
confederate confederado
conference conferencia
conference method método de conferencias
confession confesión
confidence confianza
confidence interval intervalo de confianza
confidence limits límites de confianza
confidentiality confidencialidad
confidentiality and consent to treatment
   confidencialidad y consentimiento a
   tratamiento
confidentiality and informed consent
   confidencialidad y consentimiento
   informado
configuration configuración
configurational configuracional
configurational effects efectos
   configuracionales
configurational tendency tendencia
   configuracional
confinement confinamiento
confinement effects efectos de confinamiento
confinement fear temor al confinamiento
confirmation confirmación
confirmation bias sesgo de confirmación
confirming reaction reacción confirmante
conflict conflicto
conflict avoidance evitación de conflicto
conflict behavior conducta de conflicto
conflict detouring desviación de conflicto
conflict displacement desplazamiento de
   conflicto
conflict-free area área libre de conflictos
conflict-free function función libre de
   conflictos
conflict-free sphere esfera libre de conflictos
conflict mediation mediación de conflicto
conflict of interest conflicto de intereses
conflict resolution resolución de conflicto
conflict resolution therapy terapia de
   resolución de conflicto
confluence confluencia
confluence model modelo de confluencia
conformance conformidad
conformity conformidad
conformity in cults conformidad en cultos
confound confundir
confrontation confrontación
confrontational confrontante
confrontational methods métodos
   confrontantes
confusion confusión

confusion errors errores de confusión
confusion lines líneas de confusión
confusion of values confusión de valores
confusion psychosis psicosis de confusión
confusional confusional
confusional automatism automatismo
   confusional
confusional state estado confusional
confusionism confusionismo
congenital congénito
congenital acromicria acromicria congénita
congenital adrenal hyperplasia hiperplasia
   adrenal congénita
congenital alexia alexia congénita
congenital anomaly anomalía congénita
congenital aphasia afasia congénita
congenital atonic pseudoparalysis
   seudoparálisis atónica congénita
congenital cerebral aneurysm aneurisma
   cerebral congénito
congenital cytomegalovirus infection
   infección con citomegalovirus congénita
congenital deafness sordera congénita
congenital defect defecto congénito
congenital deformity deformidad congénita
congenital dysplastic angiomatosis
   angiomatosis displástica congénita
congenital dysplastic angiopathy angiopatía
   displástica congénita
congenital facial diplegia diplejía facial
   congénita
congenital hip subluxation subluxación de
   cadera congénita
congenital hydrocephalus hidrocefalia
   congénita
congenital hypothyroidism hipotiroidismo
   congénito
congenital infection infección congénita
congenital malformation malformación
   congénita
congenital nystagmus nistagmo congénito
congenital orthopedic condition condición
   ortopédica congénita
congenital paramyotonia paramiotonía
   congénita
congenital rubella syndrome síndrome de
   rubéola congénita
congenital sensory neuropathy with
   anhidrosis neuropatía sensorial congénita
   con anhidrosis
congenital spastic paraplegia paraplejía
   espástica congénita
congenital syphilis sífilis congénita
congenital toxoplasmosis toxoplasmosis
   congénita
congenital word blindness ceguera de
   palabras congénita
congestion congestión
congophilic congófilo
congruence congruencia
congruence principle principio de
   congruencia
congruent congruente
congruent attitude change cambio de actitud
   congruente

congruent points puntos congruentes
congruent retinal points puntos retinales
  congruentes
congruity theory teoría de congruencia
conjoint conjunto
conjoint counseling asesoramiento conjunto
conjoint interview entrevista conjunta
conjoint marital therapy terapia marital
  conjunta
conjoint measurement medición conjunta
conjoint therapy terapia conjunta
conjugal conyugal
conjugal paranoia paranoia conyugal
conjugal psychosis psicosis conyugal
conjugal unit unidad conyugal
conjugate movement movimiento conjugado
conjugate paralysis parálisis conjugada
conjugate reinforcement refuerzo conjugado
conjugation conjugación
conjunctiva conjuntiva
conjunctival reflex reflejo conjuntival
conjunctive conjuntivo
conjunctive concept concepto conjuntivo
conjunctive motivation motivación conjuntiva
conjunctive reinforcement refuerzo
  conjuntivo
conjunctive schedule programa conjuntivo
conjunctivity conjuntividad
Conn's syndrome síndrome de Conn
connate connato
connection conexión
connectionism conexionismo
connector conector
connotation connotación
connotative meaning significado connotativo
conquering-hero daydream ensueño de héroe
  triunfador
Conradi's disease enfermedad de Conradi
consanguine consanguíneo
consanguineous matings apareamientos
  consanguíneos
consanguinity consanguinidad
conscience conciencia
conscious consciente
conscious perception percepción consciente
conscious processes procesos conscientes
conscious resistance resistencia consciente
conscious state estado consciente
consciousness conocimiento, conciencia
consciousness disturbances disturbios de
  conciencia
consciousness expansion expansión de
  conciencia
consciousness raising levantamiento de
  conciencia
consensual consensual
consensual eye reflex reflejo de ojos
  consensual
consensual light reflex reflejo de luz
  consensual
consensual reflex reflejo consensual
consensual validation validación consensual
consensual validity validez consensual
consensus consenso
consent consentimiento

consequences consecuencias
consequent consecuente
conservation conservación
conservation-withdrawal
  conservación-retirada
conservatism conservatismo
conservative conservativo
conservator conservador
consideration consideración
consistency consistencia
consistency principle principio de la
  consistencia
consistency theory teoría de la consistencia
consolation consolación
consolation dream sueño de consolación
consolidation consolidación
consolidation gradient gradiente de
  consolidación
consolidation hypothesis hipótesis de
  consolidación
consolidation time tiempo de consolidación
consonance consonancia
consonant consonante
consonant trigram trigrama consonante
conspecific de la misma especie
constancy constancia
constancy hypothesis hipótesis de constancia
constancy of conditions constancia de
  condiciones
constancy of internal environment
  constancia del ambiente interno
constancy of the intelligence quotient
  constancia del cociente de inteligencia
constancy of the organism constancia del
  organismo
constancy phenomenon fenómeno de
  constancia
constant constante
constant error error constante
constant stimuli estímulos constantes
constant-stimuli method método de estímulos
  constantes
constellation constelación
constellatory construct constructo
  constelatorio
constipation constipación
constituent constitutivo
constitution constitución
constitutional constitucional
constitutional depressive disposition
  disposición depresiva constitucional
constitutional factors factores
  constitucionales
constitutional insanity insania constitucional
constitutional mania manía constitucional
constitutional manic disposition disposición
  maníaca constitucional
constitutional medicine medicina
  constitucional
constitutional psychology psicología
  constitucional
constitutional psychopath psicópata
  constitucional
constitutional psychosis psicosis
  constitucional

constitutional theory teoría constitucional
constitutional type tipo constitucional
constrained association asociación constreñida
constraint constreñimiento
constraint of movement constreñimiento de movimiento
constraint of thought constreñimiento de pensamientos
constricted restringido
constricted affect afecto restringido
constriction constricción
constrictor vaginae constrictor de la vagina
construct constructo
construct validity validez del constructo
construction need necesidad de construcción
constructional apraxia apraxia de construcción
constructionism construccionismo
constructive constructivo
constructive approach acercamiento constructivo
constructive apraxia apraxia constructiva
constructive memory memoria constructiva
constructivism constructivismo
consultant consultor
consultation consultación
consultation-liaison psychiatry psiquiatría de consultación-coordinación
consulting consultor
consulting psychologist psicólogo consultor
consulting psychology psicología consultora
consumer consumidor
consumer behavior conducta del consumidor
consumer characteristics características del consumidor
consumer education educación del consumidor
consumer-jury technique técnica del jurado de consumidores
consumer psychology psicología del consumidor
consumer research investigación del consumidor
consumer survey encuesta de consumidores
consumerism consumerismo
consummatory consumatorio
consummatory act acto consumatorio
consummatory communication comunicación consumatoria
consummatory response respuesta consumatoria
consummatory stimulus estímulo consumatorio
contact contacto
contact behavior conducta de contacto
contact ceptor ceptor de contacto
contact comfort comodidad de contacto
contact dermatitis dermatitis por contacto
contact desensitization desensibilización de contacto
contact hypothesis hipótesis de contacto
contact lenses lentes de contacto
contact with reality contacto con la realidad
contagion contagio

contamination contaminación
contamination obsession obsesión de contaminación
contemplation contemplación
contemporaneity contemporaneidad
contemporaneous contemporáneo
contemporaneous explanation principle principio de la explicación contemporánea
contempt desprecio
contemptuous despreciativo
content contenido
content-addressable store almacén de contenido direccionable
content analysis análisis de contenido
content psychology psicología de contenido
content-thought disorder trastorno del contenido de pensamientos
content validity validez de contenido
content word palabra de contenido
contentious contencioso
contentiousness carácter contencioso
contentive contentivo
context contexto
context bias sesgo del contexto
context clues indicios del contexto
context effects efectos del contexto
context flexibility flexibilidad del contexto
context-independent independiente del contexto
context shifting cambio del contexto
context theory teoría del contexto
context theory of meaning teoría del contexto del significado
contextual contextual
contextual association asociación contextual
contextual cue señal contextual
contextual discrimination discriminación contextual
contextual fluctuation fluctuación contextual
contextual information información contextual
contextualism contextualismo
contiguity contigüidad
contiguity of associations contigüidad de las asociaciones
contiguity principle principio de la contigüidad
contiguity theory teoría de la contigüidad
continence continencia
continent continente
contingency contingencia
contingency analysis análisis de contingencias
contingency awareness conciencia de contingencias
contingency coefficient coeficiente de contingencia
contingency contract contrato con contingencias
contingency contracting contratación con contingencias
contingency management administración de contingencias
contingency model modelo de contingencia
contingency reinforcement refuerzo de contingencia

contingency table tabla de contingencias
contingency theory teoría de contingencias
contingency theory of leadership teoría de
   liderazgo de contingencias
contingent contingente
contingent negative variation variación
   negativa contingente
contingent punishment castigo contingente
contingent relationship relación contingente
contingent suggestion sugestión contingente
continuant continuante
continuation continuación
continuation maintenance therapy terapia de
   mantenimiento de continuación
continued learning aprendizaje continuado
continued reinforcement refuerzo continuado
continued stay review revisión de estadía
   continuada
continuing-care unit unidad de cuidado
   continuado
continuing education educación continuada
continuing medical education educación
   médica continuada
continuity continuidad
continuity hypothesis hipótesis de continuidad
continuity hypothesis of dreams hipótesis de
   continuidad de sueños
continuity of care continuidad del cuidado
continuity theory teoría de continuidad
continuity theory of aging teoría de
   continuidad del envejecimiento
continuity theory of learning teoría de
   continuidad del aprendizaje
continuous continuo
continuous amnesia amnesia continua
continuous-bath treatment tratamiento de
   baño continuo
continuous group grupo continuo
continuous growth crecimiento continuo
continuous model modelo continuo
continuous narcosis narcosis continua
continuous panel panel continuo
continuous positive airway pressure presión
   en las vías aéreas positiva continua
continuous random variable variable
   aleatoria continua
continuous reinforcement refuerzo continuo
continuous reinforcement schedule programa
   de refuerzo continuo
continuous scale escala continua
continuous sleep therapy terapia de sueño
   continuo
continuous tasks tareas continuas
continuous tremor temblor continuo
continuous variable variable continua
continuum continuo
contour contorno
contraception contracepción
contraceptive contraceptivo
contraceptive pill píldora contraceptiva
contract contrato
contractibility contractibilidad
contractility contractilidad
contraction contracción
contractual contractual

contractual psychiatry psiquiatría contractual
contractual psychology psicología contractual
contractual psychotherapy psicoterapia
   contractual
contractural contractural
contractural diathesis diátesis contractural
contracture contractura
contradictory contradictorio
contrafissura contrafisura
contraindication contraindicación
contralateral contralateral
contralateral hearing aid audífono
   contralateral
contralateral hemiplegia hemiplejía
   contralateral
contralateral reflex reflejo contralateral
contralateral sign signo contralateral
contrasexual contrasexual
contrast contraste
contrast effect efecto de contraste
contrast effects in interviewing efectos de
   contraste al entrevistar
contrast sensitivity sensibilidad de contraste
contrast sensitivity function función de
   sensibilidad de contraste
contrast threshold umbral de contraste
contrasuggestibility contrasugestibilidad
contrecoup contragolpe
contrecoup injury of brain lesión cerebral
   por contragolpe
contrectation contrectación
control control
control adoptees adoptados control
control analysis análisis control
control condition condición control
control-devices research investigación de
   aparatos de control
control experiment experimento control
control group grupo control
control of obesity control de obesidad
control of variables control de variables
control system sistema de control
control theory teoría control
control training entrenamiento de control
control variable variable control
controlled controlado
controlled analysis análisis controlado
controlled association asociación controlada
controlled attention atención controlada
controlled breathing respiración controlada
controlled clinical trial ensayo clínico
   controlado
controlled drinking beber controlado
controlled-drinking therapy terapia de beber
   controlado
controlled-exposure technique técnica de
   exposición controlada
controlled processing procesamiento
   controlado
controlled sampling muestreo controlado
controlled substance sustancia controlada
controlled variable variable controlada
controlling controlador
contusion contusión
convalescent convaleciente

convalescent center centro de convalecientes
convenience dreams sueños de conveniencia
convention convención
conventional convencional
conventional level nivel convencional
conventional level of moral development
    nivel convencional del desarrollo moral
conventional need necesidad convencional
conventional role conformity conformidad
    con papel convencional
conventional signs signos convencionales
conventional virus virus convencional
conventionalism convencionalismo
conventionality convencionalismo
convergence convergencia
convergence angle ángulo de convergencia
convergence parallax paralaje de
    convergencia
convergent convergente
convergent evolution evolución convergente
convergent strabismus estrabismo
    convergente
convergent thinking pensamiento convergente
convergent validity validez convergente
conversational conversacional
conversational catharsis catarsis
    conversacional
conversational maxims máximas
    conversacionales
conversational postulates postulados
    conversacionales
converse converso
conversion conversión
conversion disorder trastorno de conversión
conversion hysteria histeria de conversión
conversion hysteria neurosis neurosis de
    histeria de conversión
conversion of emotion conversión de emoción
conversion paralysis parálisis de conversión
conversion reaction reacción de conversión
conversion seizure acceso de conversión
conversion symptom síntoma de conversión
convexity convexidad
convexity syndrome síndrome de convexidad
convexobasia convexobasia
convolution convolución
convulsant convulsivante
convulsant threshold umbral de convulsivante
convulsion convulsión
convulsive convulsivo
convulsive disorder trastorno convulsivo
convulsive reflex reflejo convulsivo
convulsive shock therapy terapia de choques
    convulsivos
convulsive state estado convulsivo
convulsive therapy terapia convulsiva
convulsive tic tic convulsivo
Cooley's anemia anemia de Cooley
Coolidge effect efecto de Coolidge
cooling of affect enfriamiento de afecto
Coombs' test prueba de Coombs
cooperation cooperación
cooperative cooperativo
cooperative education educación cooperativa
cooperative motive motivo cooperativo

cooperative play juego cooperativo
cooperative reward structure estructura de
    recompensa cooperativa
cooperative therapy terapia cooperativa
cooperative training entrenamiento
    cooperativo
cooperative urban house casa urbana
    cooperativa
cooperators cooperadores
coordinate (adj) coordinado
coordinate (n) coordenada
coordinate (v) coordinar
coordinate bilingual bilingüe coordinado
coordinate convulsion convulsión coordinada
coordinate morality moralidad coordinada
coordinated coordinado
coordinated reflex reflejo coordinado
coordination coordinación
coordination disorder trastorno de
    coordinación
coordination of secondary schemes
    coordinación de proyectos secundarios
coparental divorce divorcio coparental
cope bregar
coping ability habilidad para bregar
coping behavior conducta para bregar
coping mechanism mecanismo para bregar
coping mechanisms in borderline personality
    disorder mecanismos para bregar en
    trastorno de personalidad fronterizo
coping skills destrezas para bregar
coping strategy estrategia para bregar
coping style estilo para bregar
coping styles of children estilos para bregar
    de niños
coprolagnia coprolagnia
coprolalia coprolalia
coprology coprología
coprophagia coprofagia
coprophagy coprofagia
coprophemia coprofemia
coprophil coprófilo
coprophilia coprofilia
coprophilic coprofílico
coprophobia coprofobia
coprophrasia coprofrasia
copropraxia copropraxia
copulation copulación
copulatory behavior conducta copulatoria
copycat copión
copycat suicide suicidio copión
copying behavior conducta de copiarse
copying mania manía de copiarse
cord bladder vejiga en cuerda
cordectomy cordectomía
cordopexy cordopexia
cordotomy cordotomía
core gender identity identidad de género
    núcleo
core sex identity identidad de sexo núcleo
corium corium
cornea córnea
corneal reflection technique técnica de
    reflexión corneal
corneal transplant transplante corneal

Cornelia de Lange syndrome síndrome de Cornelia de Lange
Cornell technique técnica de Cornell
corollary corolario
coronal coronal
coronal section sección coronal
coronary coronario
coronary artery disease enfermedad arterial coronaria
coronary-prone propenso a coronaria
coronary risk riesgo coronario
corpora arenacea cuerpos arenáceos
corpora cavernosa cuerpo cavernoso
corpora quadrigemina cuerpos cuadrigéminos
corporal corporal
corporate class clase corporativa
corpus cuerpo
corpus callosum cuerpo calloso
corpus callosum syndrome síndrome del cuerpo calloso
corpus luteum cuerpo lúteo
corpus spongiosum cuerpo esponjoso
corpus striatum cuerpo estriado
corpuscle corpúsculo
correction corrección
correction for chance corrección para casualidad
correction for continuity corrección para continuidad
correction for guessing corrección para barruntamiento
correctional community psychology psicología comunitaria correccional
correctional institution institución correccional
correctional mental health services servicios de salud mental correccionales
correctional psychiatrist psiquiatra correccional
correctional psychiatry psiquiatría correccional
correctional psychologist psicólogo correccional
correctional psychologists as consultants psicólogos correccionales como consultores
correctional psychology psicología correccional
corrective correctivo
corrective emotional experience experiencia emocional correctiva
corrective therapist terapeuta correctivo
correlate correlacionar
correlated correlacionado
correlated axes ejes correlacionados
correlation correlación
correlation and regression correlación y regresión
correlation cluster grupo de correlaciones
correlation coefficient coeficiente de correlación
correlation matrix matriz de correlación
correlation method método de correlación
correlation model modelo de correlación
correlation ratio razón de correlación

correlation table tabla de correlación
correlational correlacional
correlational method método correlacional
correlational redundancy redundancia correlacional
correlational statistics estadística correlacional
correlational studies estudios correlacionales
correlative correlativo
correspondence correspondencia
corresponding retinal points puntos retinales correspondientes
cortex corteza
Corti's membrane membrana de Corti
cortical cortical
cortical amnesia amnesia cortical
cortical apraxia apraxia cortical
cortical arousal factor factor de despertamiento cortical
cortical blindness ceguera cortical
cortical center centro cortical
cortical control control cortical
cortical deafness sordera cortical
cortical dominance dominancia cortical
cortical epilepsy epilepsia cortical
cortical-evoked response respuesta evocada cortical
cortical induction inducción cortical
cortical inhibition inhibición cortical
cortical lesion lesión cortical
cortical localization of function localización de función cortical
cortical motor aphasia afasia motora cortical
cortical potentials potenciales corticales
cortical processes procesos corticales
cortical sensibility sensibilidad cortical
cortical sensory aphasia afasia sensorial cortical
cortical zones zonas corticales
corticalization corticalización
corticectomy corticectomía
corticobulbar corticobulbar
corticobulbar fibers fibras corticobulbares
corticobulbar nucleus núcleo corticobulbar
corticofugal corticófugo
corticofugal nerve fibers fibras nerviosas corticófugas
corticoid corticoide
corticoid therapy terapia de corticoides
corticonuclear corticonuclear
corticonuclear fibers fibras corticonucleares
corticopontine corticopontino
corticopontine nucleus núcleo corticopontino
corticospinal corticoespinal
corticospinal tract tracto corticoespinal
corticosteroid corticosteroide
corticosteroid therapy terapia corticosteroide
corticosterone corticosterona
corticotrophic hormone hormona corticotrópica
corticotropine corticotropina
corticotropine-releasing factor factor liberador de corticotropina
corticotropine-releasing hormone hormona liberadora de corticotropina

cortin cortina
cortisol cortisol
cortisone cortisona
coruscation coruscación
corybantic rites ritos coribantes
cosmic consciousness conciencia cósmica
cosmic identification identificación cósmica
cosmic sensitivity sensibilidad cósmica
cosmology cosmología
cost-benefit analysis análisis de
    costo-beneficio
cost containment contención de costos
cost-effectiveness analysis análisis de
    costo-efectividad
cost-reward analysis análisis de
    costo-recompensa
cost-reward model modelo de
    costo-recompensa
cost shifting desplazamiento de costos
costal arch reflex reflejo del arco costal
costoclavicular syndrome síndrome
    costoclavicular
costopectoral reflex reflejo costopectoral
Cotard's syndrome síndrome de Cotard
cotherapy coterapia
cottage plan sistema de casitas de campo
Cotte's operation operación de Cotte
Cottunius disease enfermedad de Cottunius
coumarin cumarina
counseling asesoramiento
counseling interview entrevista de
    asesoramiento
counseling ladder escalera de asesoramiento
counseling of survivors asesoramiento de
    sobrevivientes
counseling of victims asesoramiento de
    víctimas
counseling process proceso de asesoramiento
counseling psychologist psicólogo de
    asesoramiento
counseling psychology psicología de
    asesoramiento
counseling relationship relación de
    asesoramiento
counseling services servicios de
    asesoramiento
counselor asesor
counselor-centered therapy terapia centrada
    en el asesor
counselor education educación de asesor
counter (adj) contrario
counter (n) contador
counter (v) contrarrestar
counter ego contraego
counter-wish dream sueño contra deseo
counteraction need necesidad de contrarrestar
counteraffect contraafecto
counterbalancing contrabalanceo
countercathexis contracatexis
countercompulsion contracompulsión
counterconditioning contracondicionamiento
counterconditioning with hypnotism
    contracondicionamiento con hipnotismo
counterconformity contraconformidad
counterculture contracultura

counterfactual contrahechos
counterfeit role papel falso
counterformula contrafórmula
counteridentification contraidentificación
counterinvestment contrainversión
counterirritant contrairritante
counterphobia contrafobia
counterphobic contrafóbico
counterphobic character carácter
    contrafóbico
countershock contrachoque
countershock phase fase contrachoque
countersuggestion contrasugestión
countertransference contratransferencia
countertransference neurosis neurosis de
    contratransferencia
countervolition contravolición
counterwill contravoluntad
counting obsession obsesión de contar
coup injury of brain lesión de golpe del
    cerebro
couple pareja
couples group therapy terapia de grupo de
    parejas
couples sex therapy terapia sexual de parejas
couples therapy terapia de parejas
coupling acoplamiento
court-ordered treatment tratamiento
    ordenado por tribunal
courtesan fantasy fantasía de cortesana
courtroom psychology psicología de la sala
    del tribunal
courtship cortejo
courtship behavior conducta de cortejo
courtship display exhibición de cortejo
cousin marriage matrimonio de primos
couvade covada
couvade syndrome síndrome de covada
covariance covarianza
cover memory memoria cubriente
covert encubierto
covert behavior conducta encubierta
covert conditioning condicionamiento
    encubierto
covert extinction extinción encubierta
covert modeling modelado encubierto
covert reinforcement refuerzo encubierto
covert response respuesta encubierta
covert sensitization sensibilización encubierta
covert speech habla encubierta
Coxsackie encephalitis encefalitis por
    Coxsackie
crack crack
craft palsy parálisis ocupacional
cramp calambre
cramp neurosis neurosis de calambre
cranial craneal
cranial anomaly anomalía craneal
cranial arteritis arteritis craneal
cranial capacity capacidad craneal
cranial division división craneal
cranial index índice craneal
cranial nerves nervios craneales
cranial pia mater piamadre craneal
cranial reflex reflejo craneal

craniamphitomy craneoanfitomía
craniectomy craniectomía
craniocardiac reflex reflejo craneocardíaco
craniocele craneocele
craniofacial craneofacial
craniofacial anomalies anomalías craneofaciales
craniofacial dysostosis disostosis craneofacial
craniofacial surgery cirugía craneofacial
craniognomy craneognomia
craniograph craneógrafo
craniology craneología
craniomalacia craneomalacia
craniomeningocele craneomeningocele
craniometry craneometría
craniopathy craneopatía
craniopharyngioma craneofaringioma
cranioplasty craneoplastia
craniopuncture craneopunción
craniorrhachischisis craneorraquisquisis
craniosacral craneosacra
craniosacral division división craneosacra
craniosacral system sistema craneosacro
cranioschisis craneosquisis
craniosclerosis craneoesclerosis
cranioscopy craneoscopia
craniosinus fistula fístula craneosinusal
craniostenosis craneoestenosis
craniosynostosis craneosinostosis
craniosynostosis syndrome síndrome de craneosinostosis
craniotabes craneotabes
craniotomy craneotomía
craniotonoscopy craneotonoscopia
craniotrypesis craneotripesis
cranium cráneo
cranium bifidum cráneo bífido
craving antojo
crawling gateamiento
craze manía
creatine phosphokinase fosfocinasa de creatina
creatinine creatinina
creative creativo
creative imagination imaginación creativa
creative resultants resultantes creativos
creative self yo creativo
creative synthesis síntesis creativa
creative thinking pensamiento creativo
creativity creatividad
creativity measures medidas de creatividad
creativity test prueba de creatividad
credibility credibilidad
credulity credulidad
creeping and crawling aids ayudas para gatear
creeping palsy parálisis progresiva
cremasteric reflex reflejo cremastérico
cremnophobia cremnofobia
crepuscular crepuscular
crescendo sleep sueño en crescendo
Crespi effect efecto de Crespi
cretinism cretinismo
Creutzfeldt-Jakob disease enfermedad de Creutzfeldt-Jakob

cri-du-chat syndrome síndrome del maullido de gato
crib death muerte en cuna
cribiform plate placa cribiforme
Crichton-Browne's sign signo de Crichton-Browne
Crigler-Najjar disease enfermedad de Crigler-Najjar
Crigler-Najjar syndrome síndrome de Crigler-Najjar
crime from sense of guilt crimen por sentimiento de culpabilidad
crime prevention prevención de crímenes
crime prevention by counseling prevención de crímenes mediante asesoramiento
crime prevention by punishing prevención de crímenes mediante castigo
criminal criminal
criminal anthropology antropología criminal
criminal commitment confinamiento criminal
criminal hygiene higiene criminal
criminal insanity insania criminal
criminal intent intención criminal
criminal irresponsibility irresponsabilidad criminal
criminal justice justicia criminal
criminal psychiatry psiquiatría criminal
criminal psychology psicología criminal
criminal psychopath psicópata criminal
criminal responsibility responsabilidad criminal
criminal responsibility and insanity defense responsabilidad criminal y defensa de insania
criminal type tipo criminal
criminalism criminalismo
criminality criminalidad
criminally insane insano criminalmente
criminology criminología
criminosis criminosis
crisis crisis
crisis center centro de crisis
crisis effect efecto de crisis
crisis group grupo de crisis
crisis intervention intervención de crisis
crisis intervention group grupo de intervención de crisis
crisis-intervention group psychotherapy psicoterapia de grupo de intervención de crisis
crisis management administración de crisis
crisis management of self-destructive behavior administración de crisis de conducta autodestructiva
crisis management of violent behavior administración de crisis de conducta violenta
crisis resolution resolución de crisis
crisis rites ritos de crisis
crisis team equipo de crisis
crisis theory teoría de crisis
crisis therapy terapia de crisis
crispation crispación
criteria criterios
criterion criterio

criterion behavior conducta de criterio
criterion dimensions dimensiones de criterio
criterion group grupo de criterio
criterion measures medidas de criterio
criterion score puntuación de criterio
criterion validity validez de criterio
criterion variable variable de criterio
critical crítico
critical area área crítica
critical bandwidth ancho de banda crítico
critical common-sense approach
  acercamiento de sentido común crítico
critical duration duración crítica
critical flicker frequency frecuencia de
  centelleo crítica
critical fusion frequency frecuencia de fusión
  crítica
critical incident technique técnica de
  incidentes críticos
critical interval intervalo crítico
critical judgment juicio crítico
critical period periodo crítico
critical point punto crítico
critical ratio razón crítica
critical region región crítica
critical score puntuación crítica
critical thinking pensamiento crítico
critical value valor crítico
criticizing faculty facultad de criticar
crocidismus crocidismo
Crocker-Henderson system sistema de
  Crocker-Henderson
crocodile tears lágrimas de cocodrilo
crocodile tears syndrome síndrome de
  lágrimas de cocodrilo
Crooke's granules gránulos de Crooke
cross-adaptation adaptación cruzada
cross-addiction adicción cruzada
cross-association asociación cruzada
cross-conditioning condicionamiento cruzado
cross-correlation correlación cruzada
cross-correlation mechanism mecanismo de
  correlación cruzada
cross-correspondence correspondencia
  cruzada
cross-cultural transcultural
cross-cultural approach acercamiento
  transcultural
cross-cultural assessment evaluación
  transcultural
cross-cultural comparison comparación
  transcultural
cross-cultural counseling asesoramiento
  transcultural
cross-cultural method método transcultural
cross-cultural psychiatry psiquiatría
  transcultural
cross-cultural psychological assessment
  evaluación psicológica transcultural
cross-cultural psychology psicología
  transcultural
cross-cultural psychotherapy psicoterapia
  transcultural
cross-cultural test prueba transcultural
cross-cultural training program programa de

  entrenamiento transcultural
cross-dependence dependencia cruzada
cross-dependence of hallucinogens
  dependencia cruzada de alucinógenos
cross-dressing transvestismo
cross-fostering crianza cruzada
cross-gender behavior conducta de género
  cruzado
cross-gender disorder trastorno de género
  cruzado
cross-gender identification identificación de
  género cruzado
cross-linkage theory teoría de enlaces
  cruzados
cross-modal transmodal
cross-modal abilities habilidades transmodales
cross-modal transfer transferencia transmodal
cross-modality matching pareo de
  modalidades cruzadas
cross-parental identification identificación
  parental cruzada
cross-section sección transversal
cross-sectional method método transversal
cross-sectional prevalence prevalencia
  transversal
cross-sectional research investigación
  transversal
cross-sectional study estudio transversal
cross-tabulations tabulaciones cruzadas
cross-tolerance tolerancia cruzada
cross-tolerance of drugs tolerancia cruzada
  de drogas
cross-validation validación cruzada
crossed cruzado
crossed adductor jerk sacudida del aductor
  cruzada
crossed adductor reflex reflejo del aductor
  cruzado
crossed anesthesia anestesia cruzada
crossed dominance dominancia cruzada
crossed extension reflex reflejo de extensión
  cruzada
crossed hemianesthesia hemianestesia
  cruzada
crossed jerk sacudida cruzada
crossed knee jerk sacudida de rodilla cruzada
crossed knee reflex reflejo de rodilla cruzado
crossed laterality lateralidad cruzada
crossed-nerve experiments experimentos de
  nervios cruzados
crossed paralysis parálisis cruzada
crossed perception percepción cruzada
crossed phrenic phenomenon fenómeno
  frénico cruzado
crossed reflex reflejo cruzado
crossed reflex of pelvis reflejo cruzado del
  pelvis
crossed spino-adductor reflex reflejo
  espinoaductor cruzado
crossing-over entrecruzamiento
crossover entrecruzamiento
Crouzon's disease enfermedad de Crouzon
Crow type I schizophrenia esquizofrenia tipo
  I de Crow
Crow type II schizophrenia esquizofrenia

tipo II de Crow
crowd multitud
crowd behavior conducta de multitud
crowd consciousness conciencia de multitud
crowding apiñamiento
crucial crucial
crucial experiment experimento crucial
crude score puntuación en bruto
crus penis raíz del pene
crush syndrome síndrome de aplastamiento
crusotomy crusotomía
crutch muleta
crutch palsy parálisis por muletas
crutch paralysis parálisis por muletas
Cruveilhier's disease enfermedad de
   Cruveilhier
cry grito, llanto
cry for help grito para socorro
cry reflex reflejo de llanto
cryalgesia crialgesia
cryanesthesia crianestesia
cryesthesia criestesia
crying llanto
crymodynia crimodinia
cryogenic criogénico
cryogenic methods métodos criogénicos
cryogenic surgery cirugía criogénica
cryohypophysectomy criohipofisectomía
cryopallidectomy criopalidectomía
cryophobia criofobia
cryoprobe criosonda
cryopulvinectomy criopulvinectomía
cryospasm crioespasmo
cryosurgery criocirugía
cryothalamectomy criotalamectomía
cryptesthesia criptestesia
cryptococcoma criptococoma
cryptococcosis criptococosis
Cryptococcus Cryptococcus
cryptogenic symbolism simbolismo
   criptogénico
cryptography criptografía
cryptomnesia criptomnesia
cryptophasia criptofasia
cryptophoric symbolism simbolismo
   criptofórico
cryptophthalmos syndrome síndrome
   criptoftálmico
cryptorchid criptórquido
cryptorchidism criptorquidismo
cryptorchism criptorquismo
cryptotia criptotia
crystal gazing contemplación de cristal
crystallization cristalización
crystallized abilities habilidades cristalizadas
crystallized intelligence inteligencia
   cristalizada
crystallophobia cristalofobia
cuboidodigital reflex reflejo cuboidodigital
cuddling arrimo
cuddling behavior conducta de arrimo
cue señal
cue ambiguity ambigüedad de señal
cue function función de señal
cue reduction reducción de señal

cue reversal inversión de señal
cued memory memoria señalada
cues to localization señales de localización
cuirass coraza
culmen culmen
cult culto
cult of personality culto de personalidad
cultural cultural
cultural absolute absoluto cultural
cultural absolutism absolutismo cultural
cultural adaptability adaptabilidad cultural
cultural adaptation adaptación cultural
cultural anthropology antropología cultural
cultural area área cultural
cultural artifact artefacto cultural
cultural assimilation asimilación cultural
cultural bias sesgo cultural
cultural bias in tests sesgo cultural en
   pruebas
cultural blindness ceguera cultural
cultural conserve conserva cultural
cultural considerations in assessment
   consideraciones culturales en evaluación
cultural deprivation privación cultural
cultural determinism determinismo cultural
cultural differences diferencias culturales
cultural diversity diversidad cultural
cultural drift rumbo cultural
cultural factors factores culturales
cultural factors in behavior factores
   culturales en conducta
cultural factors in depression factores
   culturales en depresión
cultural factors in emotion factores culturales
   en emoción
cultural-familial mental retardation retardo
   mental cultural-familiar
cultural identity identidad cultural
cultural integration integración cultural
cultural items artículos culturales
cultural lag atraso cultural
cultural monism monismo cultural
cultural norms normas culturales
cultural parallelism paralelismo cultural
cultural pluralism pluralismo cultural
cultural process proceso cultural
cultural psychiatry psiquiatría cultural
cultural relativism relativismo cultural
cultural residue residuo cultural
cultural shock choque cultural
cultural transmission transmisión cultural
cultural values valores culturales
culturalists culturalistas
culturally deprived desaventajado
   culturalmente
culturally different diferente culturalmente
culturally disadvantaged desaventajado
   culturalmente
culture cultura
culture area área cultural
culture-bound limitado a una cultura
culture-bound disorder trastorno limitado a
   una cultura
culture-bound syndrome síndrome limitado a
   una cultura

culture-bound variable variable limitada a una cultura
culture clash choque cultural
culture complex complejo cultural
culture conflict conflicto cultural
culture contact contacto cultural
culture-epoch theory teoría de épocas culturales
culture-fair test prueba sin sesgo cultural
culture-free test prueba sin sesgo cultural
culture island isla cultural
culture lag atraso cultural
culture lead adelanto cultural
culture pattern patrón cultural
culture shock choque cultural
culture-specific específico de cultura
culture-specific psychological motive motivo psicológico específico de cultura
culture-specific syndrome síndrome específico de cultura
culture trait rasgo cultural
culturgen unidad cultural
cumulative cumulativo
cumulative frequency curve curva de frecuencias cumulativas
cumulative frequency distribution distribución de frecuencias cumulativas
cumulative record registro cumulativo
cumulative recorder registrador cumulativo
cumulative response curve curva de respuestas cumulativas
cumulative score puntuación cumulativa
cumulative tests pruebas cumulativas
cuneate cuneiforme
cuneate nucleus núcleo cuneiforme
cunnilinctio cunilición
cunnilinction cunilición
cunnilinctus cunilición
cunnilinguist cunilingüista
cunnilingus cunilingus
cunnus vulva
curare curare
curbing of aggression contención de agresión
curiosity curiosidad
curiosity drive impulso de curiosidad
curiosity instinct instinto de curiosidad
current corriente
current material material corriente
current of injury corriente de lesión
curriculum currículo
curriculum development desarrollo de currículo
Curschmann-Batten-Steinert syndrome síndrome de Curschmann-Batten-Steinert
curse maldición
cursing imprecación
cursing magic magia de imprecación
curve curva
curve fitting ajuste de curvas
curvilinear curvilíneo
curvilinear correlation correlación curvilínea
curvilinear regression regresión curvilínea
curvilinear relationship relación curvilínea
Cushing's basophilism basofilismo de Cushing

Cushing's disease enfermedad de Cushing
Cushing's syndrome síndrome de Cushing
Cushing effect efecto de Cushing
Cushing phenomenon fenómeno de Cushing
Cushing response respuesta de Cushing
cushingoid cushingoide
custodial care cuidado custodial
custodial parent padre custodial, madre custodial
custody custodia
custody dispute disputa de custodia
custody quotient cociente de custodia
cutaneomeningospinal angiomatosis angiomatosis cutaneomeningoespinal
cutaneous cutáneo
cutaneous albinism albinismo cutáneo
cutaneous anesthesia anestesia cutánea
cutaneous experience experiencia cutánea
cutaneous meningioma meningioma cutáneo
cutaneous pain dolor cutáneo
cutaneous perception percepción cutánea
cutaneous pupil reflex reflejo de pupila cutáneo
cutaneous pupillary reflex reflejo pupilar cutáneo
cutaneous receptors receptores cutáneos
cutaneous reflex reflejo cutáneo
cutaneous sense sentido cutáneo
cutaneous sensitivity sensibilidad cutánea
cutting corte
cutting score puntuación cortante
cyamemazine ciamemazina
cyanosis cianosis
cyanotic syndrome of Scheid síndrome cianótico de Scheid
cybernetic theory of aging teoría cibernética del envejecimiento
cybernetics cibernética
cyberphobia ciberfobia
cyclandelate ciclandelato
cyclazocine ciclazocina
cycle ciclo
cycle length duración de ciclo
cycle per second ciclo por segundo
cycle test prueba cíclica
cyclencephaly ciclencefalia
cyclic cíclico
cyclic disorder trastorno cíclico
cyclic illness enfermedad cíclica
cyclic insanity insania cíclica
cyclobarbital ciclobarbital
cycloid cicloide
cycloid psychosis psicosis cicloide
cyclopean eye ojo de cíclope
cyclopentolate ciclopentolato
cyclophoria cicloforia
cyclophosphamide ciclofosfamida
cyclophrenia ciclofrenia
cycloplegia cicloplejía
cycloplegic ciclopléjico
cyclopropane ciclopropano
cycloserine cicloserina
cyclothymia ciclotimia
cyclothymiac ciclotímico
cyclothymic ciclotímico

cyclothymic-depressive behavior conducta
   depresiva ciclotímica
cyclothymic disorder trastorno ciclotímico
cyclothymic personality personalidad
   ciclotímica
cyclothymic personality disorder trastorno de
   personalidad ciclotímica
cyclothymosis ciclotimosis
cycrimine hydrochloride clorhidrato de
   cicrimina
cyesis ciesis
cynanthropy cinantropía
cynic cínico
cynic spasm espasmo cínico
cynicism cinismo
cynophobia cinofobia
cynorexia cinorexia
cypridophobia cipridofobia
cypriphobia ciprifobia
cyproheptadine ciproheptadina
cyproterone acetate acetato de ciproterona
cyst quiste
cystathioninuria cistationinuria
cysteine cisteína
cystic fibrosis fibrosis quística
cystic papillomatous craniopharyngioma
   craneofaringioma papilomatoso quístico
cytheromania citeromanía
cytoarchitecture citoarquitectura
cytogenetics citogenética
cytogenic citogénico
cytoid bodies cuerpos citoides
cytology citología
cytomegalic disease enfermedad citomegálica
cytomegalovirus citomegalovirus
cytoplasm citoplasma
cytosine citosina
cytotoxic citotóxico

D

D'Acosta's syndrome síndrome de D'Acosta
d'Ocagne nomogram nomograma de
   d'Ocagne
D sleep sueño D
D value valor D
Da Costa's syndrome síndrome de Da Costa
dactylology dactilología
dactylospasm dactiloespasmo
daemonophobia demonofobia
daily living diario vivir
daily living aids ayudas para el diario vivir
daily living skills destrezas del diario vivir
Dale's law ley de Dale
daltonism daltonismo
damming-up represamiento
damned-up represado
damned-up libido libido represado
damping amortiguamiento
damping effect efecto de amortiguamiento
Dana's operation operación de Dana
Dana's syndrome síndrome de Dana
dance education educación de danza
dance epidemic epidemia de danza
dance therapy terapia de danza
dancing chorea corea danzante
dancing disease enfermedad danzante
dancing eyes ojos danzantes
dancing madness locura de danza
dancing mania manía de danza
dancing spasm espasmo danzante
Dandy operation operación de Dandy
Dandy-Walker syndrome síndrome de
   Dandy-Walker
danger peligro
danger situation situación de peligro
dangerousness peligrosidad
dangers of hypnotism peligros de hipnotismo
Danielssen's disease enfermedad de
   Danielssen
Danielssen-Boeck disease enfermedad de
   Danielssen-Boeck
dantrolene dantroleno
dapsone dapsona
dark adaptation adaptación a la obscuridad
dark light luz obscura
darkness fear temor a la obscuridad
darkness studies estudios en la obscuridad
dart and dome dardo y cúpula
darwinian fitness aptitud darwiniana
darwinian reflex reflejo darwiniano
darwinism darwinismo
Dasein Dasein
data datos
data base base de datos

data-based basado en datos
data collection recolección de datos
data limitation limitación de datos
data snooping husmeo de datos
data structure estructura de datos
date rape violación por acompañante
datum dato
Dauerschlaf Dauerschlaf
Dawson's encephalitis encefalitis de Dawson
day blindness ceguera duirna
day camp campamento diurno
day care cuidado diurno
day care in the child's home cuidado diurno en el hogar del niño
day care personnel personal de cuidado diurno
day care program programa de cuidado diurno
day care residential treatment tratamiento residencial de cuidado diurno
day center centro diurno
day hospital hospital diurno
day residue residuos del día
day treatment tratamiento diurno
daydream ensueño
daylight vision visión de luz del día
daymare pesadilla despierta
de Clerambault's syndrome síndrome de de Clerambault
de Lange syndrome síndrome de de Lange
de Morsier's syndrome síndrome de de Morsier
de Sanctis-Cacchione syndrome síndrome de de Sanctis-Cacchione
deadly mortal
deadly catatonia catatonía mortal
deaf sordo
deaf-blind sordo-ciego
deaf-mute sordo-mudo
deafferentation desaferentación
deafness sordera
deaggressivization desagresivización
deanalize desanalizar
death muerte
death anxiety ansiedad de muerte
death criteria criterios de muerte
death expectation expectación de muerte
death feigning fingimiento de muerte
death instinct instinto de muerte
death neurosis neurosis de muerte
death of loved one muerte de ser querido
death of spouse muerte de cónyuge
death rate tasa de mortalidad
death resulting from child abuse muerte resultante de abuso de niños
death resulting from child neglect muerte resultante de negligencia de niños
death trance trance de muerte
death wish deseo de muerte
debility debilidad
Debre-Semelaigne syndrome síndrome de Debre-Semelaigne
debriefing informe posterior al sujeto
debrisoquin debrisoquina
debug depurar

decadence decadencia
decalage decalaje
decanoate decanoato
decathexis descatexis
decay deterioro
decay theory teoría del deterioro
decay theory of forgetting teoría del deterioro de olvidar
deceleration deceleración
deceleration techniques técnicas de deceleración
decenter descentrar
decentering descentramiento
decentralization descentralización
decentration descentración
deception decepción
decerebrate descerebrardo
decerebrate plasticity plasticidad de descerebración
decerebrate rigidity rigidez de descerebración
decerebration descerebración
decerebrize descerebrizar
decibel decibel
decibel scale escala de decibelios
decile decil
decision decisión
decision analysis análisis de decisiones
decision balance sheet hoja de balance de decisiones
decision effects efectos de decisiones
decision environment ambiente de decisiones
decision factors factores de decisiones
decision making toma de decisiones
decision making by groups toma de decisiones por grupos
decision making under stress toma de decisiones bajo estrés
decision matrix matriz de decisiones
decision rules reglas de decisiones
decision strategies estrategias de decisiones
decision support system sistema de apoyo de decisiones
decision theory teoría de decisiones
decision tree árbol de decisiones
decision uncertainty incertidumbre de decisiones
declarative declarativo
declarative knowledge conocimiento declarativo
decode descodificar
decoding descodificación
decompensation descompensación
decompensative neurosis neurosis descompensativa
decompose descomponer
decomposition descomposición
decomposition of ego descomposición del ego
decomposition of movement descomposición de movimiento
decompression descompresión
decompression operation operación de descompresión
decompression sickness enfermedad de descompresión

deconditioning descondicionamiento
decontextualization descontextualización
decorticate descorticar
decortication descorticación
decortization descortización
decrement decremento
decrypt descriptar
decubitus decúbito
decubitus paralysis parálisis por decúbito
decussation decusación
dedifferentiation desdiferenciación
deduction deducción
deductive deductivo
deductive logic lógica deductiva
deductive reasoning razonamiento deductivo
deductive thinking pensamiento deductivo
deep profundo
deep abdominal reflex reflejo abdominal
  profundo
deep depression depresión profunda
deep interpretation interpretación profunda
deep-pressure sensitivity sensibilidad de
  presión profunda
deep reflex reflejo profundo
deep sensibility sensibilidad profunda
deep sensitivity sensibilidad profunda
deep sleep sueño profundo
deep-sleep state estado de sueño profundo
deep structure estructura profunda
deep trance trance profundo
deerotize deserotizar
defaulter faltante
defecation reflex reflejo de defecación
defect defecto
defective defectivo
defemination desfeminación
defendance defendencia
defense defensa
defense hysteria histeria de defensa
defense interpretation interpretación de
  defensa
defense mechanism mecanismo de defensa
defense neuropsychosis neuropsicosis de
  defensa
defense psychoneurosis psiconeurosis de
  defensa
defense reaction reacción de defensa
defense reflex reflejo de defensa
defense strategies estrategias de defensa
defensible defendible
defensive defensivo
defensive avoidance reaction reacción de
  evitación defensiva
defensive behavior conducta defensiva
defensive emotion emoción defensiva
defensive exclusion exclusión defensiva
defensive identification identificación
  defensiva
defensive reaction reacción defensiva
defensive strategy estrategia defensiva
defensiveness estado defensivo
deference deferencia
deference behavior conducta de deferencia
deference need necesidad de deferencia
deferred diferido

deferred diagnosis diagnóstico diferido
deferred obedience obediencia diferida
deferred reaction reacción diferida
deferred shock choque diferido
defiance desafío
deficiency deficiencia
deficiency love amor por deficiencia
deficiency motivation motivación por
  deficiencia
deficiency motive motivo por deficiencia
deficiency needs necesidades por deficiencia
deficit déficit
deficit model modelo de déficit
deficit symptoms síntomas de déficit
definition definición
definitive definitivo
deflection deflexión
deformation deformación
deformation of the self deformación del yo
deformity deformidad
defusion desfusión
deganglionate desganglionar
degeneracy degeneración
degeneracy theory teoría de la degeneración
degenerate degenerado
degenerated degenerado
degeneratio degeneración
degeneration degeneración
degeneration psychosis psicosis de
  degeneración
degenerative degenerativo
degenerative chorea corea degenerativa
degenerative dementia demencia
  degenerativa
degenerative psychosis psicosis degenerativa
degenerative status estado degenerativo
degenitalization desgenitalización
deglutition reflex reflejo de deglución
degradation degradación
degraded degradado
degraded stimulus estímulo degradado
degree grado
degree of freedom grado de libertad
degustation degustación
dehoaxing informe posterior al sujeto
dehumanization deshumanización
dehydration deshidratación
dehydration reactions reacciones de
  deshidratación
dehydroisoandrosterone
  dehidroisoandrosterona
dehypnotize deshipnotizar
deindividuation desindividuación
deindividuation in groups desindividuación
  en grupos
deinstinctualization desinstintualización
deinstitutionalization desinstitucionalización
Deiters' cells células de Deiters
deixis deixis
déjà entendu déjà entendu
déjà eprouvé déjà eprouvé
déjà fait déjà fait
déjà pensé déjà pensé
déjà raconté déjà raconté
déjà vécu déjà vécu

déjà voulu déjà voulu
déjà vu déjà vu
déjà vu phenomenon fenómeno de déjà vu
dejection desaliento
Dejerine's disease enfermedad de Dejerine
Dejerine's hand phenomenon fenómeno de la
mano de Dejerine
Dejerine's peripheral neurotabes neurotabes
periférico de Dejerine
Dejerine's reflex reflejo de Dejerine
Dejerine's sign signo de Dejerine
Dejerine-Klumpke syndrome síndrome de
Dejerine-Klumpke
Dejerine-Lichtheim phenomenon fenómeno
de Dejerine-Lichtheim
Dejerine-Roussy syndrome síndrome de
Dejerine-Roussy
Dejerine-Sottas disease enfermedad de
Dejerine-Sottas
Dejerine-Thomas syndrome síndrome de
Dejerine-Thomas
delay conditioning condicionamiento de
demora
delay interval intervalo de demora
delay of gratification demora de gratificación
delay of reinforcement demora de refuerzo
delay of reward demora de recompensa
delay of reward gradient gradiente de
demora de recompensa
delay therapy terapia de demora
delayed demorado
delayed alternation alternación demorada
delayed-alternation test prueba de alternación
demorada
delayed auditory feedback retroalimentación
auditiva demorada
delayed conditioned response respuesta
condicionada demorada
delayed conditioning condicionamiento
demorado
delayed discharge descarga demorada
delayed ejaculation eyaculación demorada
delayed grief aflicción demorada
delayed instinct instinto demorado
delayed-matching test prueba de pareo
demorado
delayed procedure procedimiento demorado
delayed reaction reacción demorada
delayed reaction experiment experimento de
reacción demorada
delayed recall recordación demorada
delayed reflex reflejo demorado
delayed reinforcement refuerzo demorado
delayed response respuesta demorada
delayed reward recompensa demorada
delayed sensation sensación demorada
delayed shock choque demorado
delayed sleep-onset insomnia insomnio de
comienzo de sueño demorado
delayed sleep phase syndrome síndrome de
fase del sueño demorado
delayed speech habla demorada
delayed stress syndrome síndrome de estrés
demorado
delayed walking andar demorado

deletion deleción
deliberate deliberado
deliberate self-harm daño propio deliberado
delibidinization deslibidinización
Delilah syndrome síndrome de Dalila
delinquency delincuencia
delinquency prevention prevención de
delincuencia
delinquent delincuente
delinquent behavior conducta delincuente
deliriant delirante
deliriant confusion confusión delirante
delirious delirante
delirious mania manía delirante
delirious reaction reacción delirante
delirious shock choque delirante
delirious state estado delirante
delirium delirio
delirium due to general medical condition
delirio debido a condición médica general
delirium grave delirio grave
delirium in acute illness delirio en
enfermedad aguda
delirium mussitans delirio musitante
delirium of metamorphosis delirio de
metamorfosis
delirium of persecution delirio de
persecución
delirium tremens delirium tremens
delirium verborum delirium verborum
delivery parto
delorazepam delorazepam
Delphi method método de Delfos
Delphi technique técnica de Delfos
delta delta
delta alcoholism alcoholismo delta
delta motion moción delta
delta movement movimiento delta
delta rhythm ritmo delta
delta sleep sueño delta
delta wave onda delta
delta-wave sleep sueño de ondas delta
delusion delusión
delusion of being controlled delusión de estar
controlado
delusion of control delusión de control
delusion of grandeur delusión de grandeza
delusion of impoverishment delusión de
empobrecimiento
delusion of infidelity delusión de infidelidad
delusion of influence delusión de influencia
delusion of jealousy delusión de celos
delusion of negation delusión de negación
delusion of observation delusión de
observación
delusion of passivity delusión de pasividad
delusion of persecution delusión de
persecución
delusion of poverty delusión de pobreza
delusion of reference delusión de referencia
delusion of self-accusation delusión de
autoacusación
delusion of sin and guilt delusión de pecado y
culpabilidad
delusion system sistema de delusiones

delusional delusorio
delusional depression depresión delusoria
delusional disorder trastorno delusorio
delusional jealousy celos delusorios
delusional loving amor delusorio
delusional mania manía delusoria
delusional misidentification identificación errónea delusoria
delusional mood humor delusorio
delusional paranoid disorder trastorno paranoide delusorio
delusional speech habla delusoria
delusional syndrome síndrome delusorio
delusional system sistema delusorio
demand character carácter de exigencia
demand characteristics características de exigencia
demand feeding alimentación a petición
demarcation demarcación
demarcation current corriente de demarcación
demarcation potential potencial de demarcación
demented demente
dementia demencia
dementia apoplectica demencia apopléctica
dementia associated with alcoholism demencia asociada con alcoholismo
dementia dialytica demencia dialítica
dementia of Alzheimer type demencia de tipo Alzheimer
dementia paralytica demencia paralítica
dementia paranoides demencia paranoide
dementia praecox demencia precoz
dementia praesenilis demencia presenil
dementia precox demencia precoz
dementia presenilis demencia presenil
dementia pugilistica demencia pugilística
democratic atmosphere atmósfera democrática
demographic demográfico
demographic analysis análisis demográfico
demographic pattern patrón demográfico
demography demografía
demoniac demoníaco
demonic demoníaco
demonic character carácter demoníaco
demonic possession posesión demoníaca
demonologic demonológico
demonologic concept of illness concepto demonológico de enfermedad
demonology demonología
demonomania demonomanía
demonophobia demonofobia
demonstration demostración
demophobia demofobia
demoralization desmoralización
demoralized desmoralizado
demorphinization desmorfinización
Demosthenes complex complejo de Demóstenes
demyelinating desmielinizante
demyelinating disease enfermedad desmielinizante
demyelinating encephalopathy encefalopatía

desmielinizante
demyelination desmielinación
demyelinization desmielinización
denarcissism desnarcisismo
dendrite dendrita
dendritic spine espina dendrítica
dendritic zone zona dendrítica
dendrophilia dendrofilia
dendrophily dendrofilia
denervate desnervar
denervation desnervación
denervation hypersensitivity hipersensibilidad de desnervación
deneutralization desneutralización
denial negación
denial of facts negación de hechos
denial of implications negación de implicaciones
denial of reality negación de la realidad
denial visual hallucination syndrome síndrome de alucinación visual de negación
denied grief aflicción negada
denotation denotación
denotative denotativo
denotative meaning significado denotativo
density densidad
density function función de densidad
dental dental
dental age edad dental
dental care cuidado dental
dental patient reactions reacciones de pacientes dentales
dental work with hypnotism trabajo dental con hipnotismo
dentate gyrus circunvolución dentada
dentate nucleus núcleo dentado
dentatectomy dentatectomía
deontology deontología
deorality desoralidad
deoxyribonucleic acid ácido desoxirribonucleico
dependence dependencia
dependence disorder trastorno de dependencia
dependence on therapy dependencia de terapia
dependency dependencia
dependency needs necesidades de dependencia
dependency syndrome síndrome de dependencia
dependent dependiente
dependent model modelo dependiente
dependent personality personalidad dependiente
dependent personality disorder trastorno de personalidad dependiente
dependent scale escala dependiente
dependent variable variable dependiente
depersonalization despersonalización
depersonalization disorder trastorno de despersonalización
depersonalization neurosis neurosis de despersonalización
depersonalization syndrome síndrome de

despersonalización
depersonification despersonificación
depletive depletivo
depletive treatment tratamiento depletivo
depolarization despolarización
depopulation despoblación
depravation depravación
depraved depravado
depravity depravación
depressant depresivo
depressant drug droga depresiva
depressed deprimido
depressed bipolar disorder trastorno bipolar
 deprimido
depressed fracture fractura deprimida
**depressed mother and infant's affective
 development** madre deprimida y el
 desarrollo afectivo de infante
depressed skull fracture fractura de cráneo
 deprimida
depression depresión
depression and anxiety depresión y ansiedad
depression and anxiety disorders depresión y
 trastornos de ansiedad
depression and learned helplessness
 depresión e impotencia aprendida
depression and suicidal behavior depresión y
 conducta suicida
depression and suicide depresión y suicidio
depression caused by separation depresión
 causada por separación
depression following parental death
 depresión tras muerte parental
depression in abused children depresión en
 niños abusados
depression in adolescents depresión en
 adolescentes
depression in adulthood depresión en adultez
depression in preadolescents depresión en
 preadolescentes
depression prevalence prevalencia de
 depresión
depression scale escala de depresión
depression versus anxiety disorder depresión
 contra trastorno de ansiedad
depression versus organic mental syndrome
 depresión contra síndrome mental orgánico
depression versus schizophrenia depresión
 contra esquizofrenia
depressive depresivo
depressive adjustment disorder trastorno de
 ajuste depresivo
depressive anxiety ansiedad depresiva
depressive character carácter depresivo
depressive crash choque depresivo
depressive disorder trastorno depresivo
depressive episode episodio depresivo
depressive hebephrenia hebefrenia depresiva
depressive mania manía depresiva
depressive neurosis neurosis depresiva
depressive personality personalidad depresiva
depressive position posición depresiva
depressive psychosis psicosis depresiva
depressive reaction reacción depresiva
depressive spectrum espectro depresivo

depressive spectrum disorder trastorno de
 espectro depresivo
depressive stupor estupor depresivo
depressomotor depresomotor
depressor depresor
depressor nerve nervio depresor
deprivation privación
deprivation dwarfism enanismo por privación
deprivation effects efectos de privación
deprivation experiment experimento de
 privación
deprivation index índice de privación
deprivation of privileges privación de
 privilegios
deprivation of sleep privación de sueño
deprogramming desprogramación
depth profundidad
depth analysis análisis profundo
depth interview entrevista profunda
depth of mood profundidad del humor
depth of processing profundidad de
 procesamiento
depth perception percepción de profundidad
depth psychology psicología profunda
depth recording registro en profundidad
depth therapy terapia profunda
derailment descarrilamiento
derailment of volition descarrilamiento de
 volición
derangement trastorno mental
Dercum's syndrome síndrome de Dercum
derealization desrealización
dereism dereísmo
dereistic dereístico
dereistic thinking pensamiento dereístico
derivation derivación
derivative derivado
derivative insight penetración derivada
derived derivado
derived need necesidad derivada
derived property propiedad derivada
derived scale escala derivada
derived score puntuación derivada
dermal sense sentido dermal
dermal sensitivity sensibilidad dermal
dermatitis dermatitis
dermatogenic torticollis tortícolis
 dermatógeno
dermatoglyphics dermatoglifo
dermatome dermatoma
dermatoneurosis dermatoneurosis
dermatophobia dermatofobia
dermatosiophobia dermatosiofobia
dermatothlasia dermatotlasia
dermatozoic dermatozoico
dermographia dermografía
dermoneurosis dermoneurosis
dermooptical perception percepción
 dermoóptica
descending descendiente
descending degeneration degeneración
 descendiente
descending neuritis neuritis descendiente
descending pathways vías descendientes
descending reticular system sistema reticular

descendiente
description descripción
description of behavior descripción de conducta
descriptive descriptivo
descriptive approach acercamiento descriptivo
descriptive average promedio descriptivo
descriptive behaviorism conductismo descriptivo
descriptive era era descriptiva
descriptive ethics ética descriptiva
descriptive principle principio descriptivo
descriptive psychiatry psiquiatría descriptiva
descriptive psychology psicología descriptiva
descriptive responsibility responsabilidad descriptiva
descriptive statistics estadística descriptiva
descriptive unconscious inconsciente descriptivo
desensitization desensibilización
desensitization procedure procedimiento de desensibilización
desensitization therapy terapia de desensibilización
deserpidine deserpidina
desexualization desexualización
design diseño
design cycle ciclo de diseños
design of experimental methods diseño de métodos experimentales
designer drugs drogas modificadas
desipramine desipramina
desire deseo
desmethyldiazepam desmetildiazepam
desmethylimipramine desmetilimipramina
desmodynia desmodinia
desmopressin desmopresina
desocialization desocialización
despair desesperación
despairing desesperado
despeciation despeciación
desperation desesperación
destination destino
destiny neurosis neurosis de destino
destruction method método de destrucción
destructive destructivo
destructive behavior conducta destructiva
destructive drive impulso destructivo
destructive instinct instinto destructivo
destructive obedience obediencia destructiva
destructiveness destructividad
destructiveness in play behavior destructividad en conducta de juego
destrudo destrudo
desymbolization desimbolización
desynchronization desincronización
desynchronized desincronizado
desynchronized sleep sueño desincronizado
desynchronosis desincronosis
desynchronous desincrónico
detached desprendido
detached affect afecto desprendido
detached cranial section sección craneal desprendida

detached craniotomy craneotomía desprendida
detached retina retina desprendida
detachment desprendimiento
detection detección
detection and recognition detección y reconocimiento
detection experiment experimento de detección
detection task tarea de detección
detection theory teoría de detección
detection threshold umbral de detección
detention detención
deterioration deterioración
deterioration effect efecto de deterioración
deterioration index índice de deterioración
deterioration of attention deterioración de atención
deterioration quotient cociente de deterioración
deterioration scale escala de deterioración
deteriorative deteriorativo
deteriorative psychosis psicosis deteriorativa
determinant determinante
determinant need necesidad de determinante
determination determinación
determination coefficient coeficiente de determinación
determinative determinativo
determinative idea idea determinativa
determiner determinador
determining determinante
determining quality cualidad determinante
determining set predisposición determinante
determining tendency tendencia determinante
determinism determinismo
deterrent disuasivo
deterrent therapy terapia disuasiva
dethroning destronamiento
detour problem problema de desvíos
detoxication destoxicación
detoxification destoxificación
detoxification center centro de destoxificación
detumescence detumescencia
deuteranomaly deuteranomalía
deuteranopia deuteranopía
deuteropathy deuteropatía
deuterophallic stage etapa deuterofálica
devaluation devaluación
development desarrollo
development and environment desarrollo y ambiente
development of attention desarrollo de atención
development of cognition desarrollo de cognición
development of ego support desarrollo de apoyo del ego
development of emotions desarrollo de emociones
development of fear desarrollo de temor
development of human behavior desarrollo de la conducta humana
development of language desarrollo del

lenguaje

development of perception desarrollo de percepción

developmental acceleration aceleración del desarrollo

developmental age edad del desarrollo

developmental amentia amencia del desarrollo

developmental aphasia afasia del desarrollo

developmental arithmetic disorder trastorno aritmético del desarrollo

developmental articulation disorder trastorno de articulación del desarrollo

developmental aspects of anxiety aspectos del desarrollo de ansiedad

developmental assessment evaluación del desarrollo

developmental borderline personality disorder trastorno de personalidad fronterizo del desarrollo

developmental coordination disorder trastorno de coordinación del desarrollo

developmental counseling asesoramiento del desarrollo

developmental crisis crisis del desarrollo

developmental deficit déficit del desarrollo

developmental deficits in borderline personality disorder déficits del desarrollo en trastorno de personalidad fronteriza

developmental delay demora del desarrollo

developmental disability discapacidad del desarrollo

developmental disorder trastorno del desarrollo

developmental disorders and child abuse trastornos del desarrollo y abuso de niños

developmental disorders of the brain injured trastornos del desarrollo de aquellos con lesiones cerebrales

developmental dyslexia dislexia del desarrollo

developmental dysphasia disfasia del desarrollo

developmental expressive language disorder trastorno del lenguaje expresivo del desarrollo

developmental expressive writing disorder trastorno del escribir expresivo del desarrollo

developmental factors factores del desarrollo

developmental follow-up seguimiento del desarrollo

developmental homeostasis homeostasis del desarrollo

developmental hyperactivity hiperactividad del desarrollo

developmental imbalance desequilibrio del desarrollo

developmental immaturity inmadurez del desarrollo

developmental injury lesión del desarrollo

developmental lag atraso del desarrollo

developmental landmark hito del desarrollo

developmental language and speech disorder trastorno del lenguaje y habla del

desarrollo

developmental language disorder trastorno del lenguaje del desarrollo

developmental levels niveles del desarrollo

developmental milestone hito del desarrollo

developmental norm norma del desarrollo

developmental pattern patrón del desarrollo

developmental period periodo del desarrollo

developmental phase fase del desarrollo

developmental phonologic disorder trastorno fonológico del desarrollo

developmental psychobiology psicobiología del desarrollo

developmental psycholinguistics psicolingüística del desarrollo

developmental psychologist psicólogo del desarrollo

developmental psychology psicología del desarrollo

developmental psychopathology psicopatología del desarrollo

developmental quotient cociente del desarrollo

developmental readiness disposición del desarrollo

developmental reading lectura del desarrollo

developmental reading disorder trastorno de lectura del desarrollo

developmental receptive language disorder trastorno del lenguaje receptivo del desarrollo

developmental retardation retardo del desarrollo

developmental scales escalas del desarrollo

developmental school escuela del desarrollo

developmental sequence secuencia del desarrollo

developmental stage etapa del desarrollo

developmental stressor estresante del desarrollo

developmental stressors in adolescence estresantes del desarrollo en adolescencia

developmental stressors in preschool children estresantes del desarrollo en niños preescolares

developmental task tarea del desarrollo

developmental teaching model modelo de enseñanza del desarrollo

developmental theories teorías del desarrollo

developmental theorist teorizante del desarrollo

developmental variance varianza del desarrollo

developmental word blindness ceguera de palabras del desarrollo

developmental zero cero del desarrollo

deviance desviación

deviancy desviación

deviant desviado

deviant behavior conducta desviada

deviant maturation maduración desviada

deviant sexual behavior conducta sexual desviada

deviant thinking pattern in delinquency patrón de pensamiento desviado en

delincuencia
deviate desviado
deviation desviación
deviation-amplification feedback
retroalimentación de ampliación de
desviación
deviation intelligence quotient cociente de
inteligencia de desviación
deviation score puntuación de desviación
Devic's disease enfermedad de Devic
device aparato
device for automatic desensitization aparato
para desensibilización automática
devolution devolución
dexamethasone dexametasona
dexamethasone suppression test prueba de
supresión de dexametasona
**dexamethasone suppression test and
depression diagnosis** prueba de supresión
de dexametasona y diagnóstico de
depresión
dexamethasone suppression test and suicide
prueba de supresión de dexametasona y
suicidio
dexamphetamine dexanfetamina
dexter diestro
dexterity destreza
dexterity test prueba de destreza
dextrad dextrado
dextral diestro
dextrality dextralidad
dextrality-sinistrality dextralidad-sinistralidad
dextran dextran
dextroamphetamine dextroanfetamina
dextrocerebral dextrocerebral
dextromanual dextromanual
dextropedal dextropedal
dextrophobia dextrofobia
dextrosinistral dextrosinistral
diabetes diabetes
diabetes insipidus diabetes insípida
diabetes mellitus diabetes mellitus
diabetic diabético
diabetic acidosis acidosis diabética
diabetic arthropathy artropatía diabética
diabetic coma coma diabético
diabetic mother madre diabética
diabetic myelopathy mielopatía diabética
diabetic neuropathy neuropatía diabética
diabetic puncture punción diabética
diabetic reaction reacción diabética
diabetic retinopathy retinopatía diabética
diacetylmorphine diacetilmorfina
diachronic diacrónico
diachronic study estudio diacrónico
diachronic versus synchronic models
modelos diacrónicos contra sincrónicos
diacritical marking system sistema de signos
diacríticos
diad díada
diadic diádico
diadochokinesis diadococinesis
diagnosis diagnóstico
diagnosis of anxiety diagnóstico de ansiedad
diagnosis of borderline personality disorder

diagnóstico de trastorno de personalidad
fronteriza
diagnosis of elimination disorders
diagnóstico de trastornos de eliminación
diagnostic diagnóstico
diagnostic anesthesia anestesia diagnóstica
diagnostic audiometry audiometría
diagnóstica
diagnostic axes ejes diagnósticos
diagnostic center centro diagnóstico
diagnostic confidence confianza diagnóstica
diagnostic educational test prueba educativa
diagnóstica
diagnostic formulation formulación
diagnóstica
diagnostic interview entrevista diagnóstica
diagnostic label etiqueta diagnóstica
diagnostic-prescriptive educational approach
acercamiento educativo
diagnóstico-prescriptivo
diagnostic procedure procedimiento
diagnóstico
diagnostic test prueba diagnóstica
diagnostic value valor diagnóstico
diagnostician diagnosticador
diagram diagrama
dialect dialecto
dialectic dialéctico
dialectical dialéctico
dialectical behavior therapy terapia de
conducta dialéctica
dialectical method método dialéctico
dialectical psychology psicología dialéctica
dialectical reasoning razonamiento dialéctico
dialectical teaching enseñanza dialéctica
dialogue diálogo
dialysis diálisis
dialysis dementia demencia por diálisis
dialysis encephalopathy syndrome síndrome
de encefalopatía por diálisis
diamine diamina
Diana complex complejo de Diana
dianoetic dianoético
diaphemetric diafemétrico
diaphoresis diaforesis
diarrhea diarrea
diary method método de diario
diaschisis diasquisis
diastatic skull fracture fractura de cráneo
diastática
diastematocrania diastematocrania
diastematomyelia diastematomielia
diastole diástole
diastolic blood pressure presión sanguínea
diastólica
diastrophic dwarfism enanismo diastrófico
diataxia diataxia
diathermy diatermia
diathesis diátesis
diathesis-stress hypothesis hipótesis
diátesis-estrés
diathesis-stress paradigm paradigma
diátesis-estrés
diathesis-stress theory of schizophrenia
teoría diátesis-estrés de la esquizofrenia

diazepam diazepam
diazoxide diazóxido
dibenzepin dibenzepina
dichloralphenazone dicloralfenazona
dichotic dicótico
dichotic listening audición dicótica
dichotic listening studies estudios de audición dicótica
dichotomous tactile test prueba táctil dicotómica
dichotomous thinking pensamiento dicotómico
dichotomy dicotomía
dichromacy dicromacia
dichromasy dicromacia
dichromat dicrómata
dichromatism dicromatismo
dichromatopsia dicromatopsia
dichromia dicromia
dichromic dicrómico
dichromopsia dicromopsia
dictator dictador
didactic didáctico
didactic analysis análisis didáctico
didactic group therapy terapia de grupo didáctica
didactic interaction interacción didáctica
didactic therapy terapia didáctica
diencephalic diencefálico
diencephalic epilepsy epilepsia diencefálica
diencephalic stupor estupor diencefálico
diencephalic syndrome of infancy síndrome diencefálico de infancia
diencephalon diencéfalo
diencephalosis diencefalosis
diet dieta
dietary dietético
dietary chaos syndrome síndrome de caos dietético
dietary deficiency deficiencia dietética
dietary neophobia neofobia dietética
diethylpropion dietilpropion
diethylstilbestrol dietilestilbestrol
diethyltryptamine dietiltriptamina
difference diferencia
difference limen limen de diferencia
difference threshold umbral de diferencia
difference tone tono de diferencia
differential diferencial
differential accuracy precisión diferencial
differential amplifier amplificador diferencial
differential conditioning condicionamiento diferencial
differential diagnosis diagnóstico diferencial
differential diagnosis of depression diagnóstico diferencial de depresión
differential diagnosis of eating disorders diagnóstico diferencial de trastornos del comer
differential emotions theory teoría de emociones diferencial
differential extinction extinción diferencial
differential fertility fertilidad diferencial
differential growth crecimiento diferencial
differential inhibition inhibición diferencial

differential limen limen diferencial
differential psychology psicología diferencial
differential rate reinforcement refuerzo de ritmo diferencial
differential reinforcement refuerzo diferencial
differential reinforcement of high rate refuerzo diferencial de ritmo alto
differential reinforcement of low rate refuerzo diferencial de ritmo bajo
differential reinforcement of other behavior refuerzo diferencial de otras conductas
differential reinforcement of paced responses refuerzo diferencial de respuestas en ritmo
differential reinforcement techniques técnicas de refuerzo diferencial
differential relaxation relajación diferencial
differential response respuesta diferencial
differential scoring tanteo diferencial
differential sensitivity sensibilidad diferencial
differential stimulus estímulo diferencial
differential threshold umbral diferencial
differential validity validez diferencial
differentiation diferenciación
differentiation of cells diferenciación de células
differentiation theory teoría de diferenciación
difficult child niño difícil
difficulty dificultad
difficulty scale escala de dificultad
difficulty value valor de dificultad
diffraction difracción
diffuse difuso
diffuse infantile familial sclerosis esclerosis familiar infantil difusa
diffuse reflection reflexión difusa
diffuse sclerosis esclerosis difusa
diffuse thalamic projection system sistema de proyección talámica difusa
diffused reflex reflejo difuso
diffusion difusión
diffusion of responsibility difusión de responsabilidad
diffusion process proceso de difusión
diffusion respiration respiración por difusión
digestive system sistema digestivo
digestive type tipo digestivo
digit-span test prueba de lapso de dígitos
digital digital
digital angiography angiografía digital
digital reflex reflejo digital
digitalgia paresthetica digitalgia parestésica
digraph dígrafo
dihydrocodeine dihidrocodeína
dihydroergotoxine dihidroergotoxina
dihydromorphine dihidromorfina
dihydroxyphenylalanine dihidroxifenilalanina
dikephobia diquefobia
dilapidation dilapidación
dilatation dilatación
dilation dilatación
dildo dildo
dilemma dilema
diltiazem diltiazem
dilution effect efecto de dilución

dimenhydrinate dimenhidrinato
dimension dimensión
dimercaprol dimercaprol
dimethoxyamphetamine dimetoxianfetamina
dimethylamphetamine dimetilanfetamina
dimethyltryptamine dimetiltriptamina
diminished capacity capacidad disminuida
diminished libido libido disminuido
diminishing returns utilidad decreciente
diminishing returns law ley de utilidad
  decreciente
diminutive visual hallucination alucinación
  visual diminutiva
dimming atenuación
dimorphism dimorfismo
dinomania dinomanía
Diogenes syndrome síndrome de Diógenes
dionism dionismo
Dionysian attitude actitud dionisiaca
diopter dioptría
dioptric aberration aberración dióptrica
diotic diótico
diphasic milk fever fiebre de leche difásica
diphenhydramine difenhidramina
diphenoxylate difenoxilato
diphenylhydantoin difenilhidantoína
diphtheria difteria
diphtheritic diftérico
diphtheritic neuropathy neuropatía diftérica
diphtheritic paralysis parálisis diftérica
diphthong diptongo
dipipanone dipipanona
diplacusis diplacusia
diplegia diplejía
diploid diploide
diploid number número diploide
diploidy diploidia
diplomyelia diplomielia
diplopia diplopía
dippoldism dippoldismo
dipsesis dipsesis
dipsomania dipsomanía
dipsosis dipsosis
dipyridamole dipiridamol
direct directo
direct aggression agresión directa
direct analysis análisis directo
direct apprehension aprehensión directa
direct association asociación directa
direct-contact group grupo de contacto
  directo
direct correlation correlación directa
direct decision therapy terapia de decisiones
  directas
direct effect efecto directo
direct fracture fractura directa
direct instruction instrucción directa
direct interview entrevista directa
direct measurement medición directa
direct method método directo
direct observation observación directa
direct perception percepción directa
direct psychoanalysis psicoanálisis directo
direct realism realismo directo
direct reflex reflejo directo

direct suggestion sugestión directa
directed dirigido
directed analysis análisis dirigido
directed attention atención dirigida
directed thinking pensamiento dirigido
direction prognosis prognosis de dirección
directional direccional
directional confusion confusión direccional
directional sensitivity sensibilidad direccional
directional test of hypothesis prueba
  direccional de hipótesis
directionality direccionalidad
directionality problem problema de
  direccionalidad
directions test prueba de direcciones
directive directivo
directive counseling asesoramiento directivo
directive fiction ficción directiva
directive group psychotherapy psicoterapia
  de grupo directiva
directive-play therapy terapia de juego
  directivo
directive psychotherapy psicoterapia
  directiva
directive therapy terapia directiva
dirhinic dirrínico
dirigation dirigación
dirigomotor dirogomotor
dirt eating comer tierra
dirty urine orina sucia
disability discapacidad
disability syndrome síndrome de discapacidad
disabled incapacitado
disadvantaged desaventajado
disaggregation desagregación
disambiguation desambiguación
disarranged sentence test prueba de oración
  desarreglada
disassociation disasociación
disaster desastre
disaster adaptation adaptación de desastre
disaster analysis análisis de desastre
disaster syndrome síndrome de desastre
disavowal repudiación
discectomy discectomía
discharge descarga, dada de alta
discharge of affect descarga de afecto
discharge procedure procedimiento de dar de
  alta
discharge rate proporción de dadas de alta
dischronation discronación
discipline disciplina
disclosure divulgación
disclosure of deceptions divulgación de
  decepciones
discogenic discogénico
discogram discograma
discography discografía
discomfort incomodidad
discomfort-relief quotient cociente de
  incomodidad-alivio
disconnection desconexión
disconnection syndrome síndrome de
  desconexión
discontinuity discontinuidad

discontinuity hypothesis hipótesis de la discontinuidad
discontinuity theory teoría de la discontinuidad
discontinuity theory of learning teoría de la discontinuidad de aprendizaje
discontinuous discontinuo
discopathy discopatía
discord discordia
discordance discordancia
discotomy discotomía
discourse discurso
discourse analysis análisis de discurso
discovery descubrimiento
discovery learning aprendizaje de descubrimiento
discovery method método de descubrimiento
discovery risk riesgo de descubrimiento
discrepancy discrepancia
discrepancy evaluation evaluación de discrepancias
discrepant discrepante
discrepant stimulus estímulo discrepante
discrete discreto
discrete emotions emociones discretas
discrete measure medida discreta
discrete variable variable discreta
discriminability discriminabilidad
discriminal dispersion dispersión discriminal
discriminant discriminante
discriminant analysis análisis discriminante
discriminant function función discriminante
discriminant stimulus estímulo discriminante
discriminant validation validación discriminante
discriminant validity validez de discriminante
discriminated discriminado
discriminated operant operante discriminado
discriminating discriminante
discriminating power poder discriminante
discriminating range intervalo discriminante
discrimination discriminación
discrimination in classical conditioning discriminación en condicionamiento clásico
discrimination in psychiatric services discriminación en servicios psiquiátricos
discrimination index índice de discriminación
discrimination learning aprendizaje de discriminación
discrimination model modelo de discriminación
discrimination range intervalo de discriminación
discrimination-reaction time tiempo de discriminación-reacción
discrimination task tarea de discriminación
discrimination value valor de discriminación
discriminative discriminativo
discriminative control control discriminativo
discriminative learning aprendizaje discriminativo
discriminative stimulus estímulo discriminativo
discussion discusión
discussion group grupo de discusión

discussion leader líder de discusión
discussion method método de discusión
disease enfermedad
disease and life changes enfermedades y cambios de vida
disease and stress enfermedad y estrés
disease fear temor a enfermedades
disease model modelo de enfermedad
disease narcissism narcisismo por enfermedad
disease phobia fobia a enfermedades
diseases of adaptation enfermedades de adaptación
disengagement rompimiento
disengagement theory teoría del rompimiento
disengagement theory of aging teoría del rompimiento de envejecimiento
disequilibrium desequilibrio
disfigurement desfiguración
disgust repugnancia
dishabituation deshabituación
disillusionment desilusión
disincentive desincentivo
disinhibition desinhibición
disinhibition syndrome síndrome de desinhibición
disintegration desintegración
disintegration of personality desintegración de personalidad
disintegrative desintegrante
disintegrative disorder trastorno desintegrante
disintegrative psychosis psicosis desintegrante
disjoint inconexo
disjoint sets conjuntos inconexos
disjunction disyunción
disjunctive disyuntivo
disjunctive concept concepto disyuntivo
disjunctive motivation motivación disyuntiva
disjunctive reaction reacción disyuntiva
disjunctive rule regla disyuntiva
disjunctive syllogism silogismo disyuntivo
disjunctive therapy terapia disyuntiva
disk disco
disk syndrome síndrome del disco
dismemberment desmembración
dismemberment complex complejo de desmembración
disobedience desobediencia
disobedient desobediente
disorder trastorno
disorder of affect trastorno de afecto
disorder of communication trastorno de comunicación
disorder of excessive somnolence trastorno de somnolencia excesiva
disorder of impulse control trastorno de control de impulsos
disorder of impulse control not elsewhere classified trastorno de control de impulsos no clasificado en otra parte
disorder of initiating and maintaining sleep trastorno de iniciar y mantener el sueño
disorder of written expression trastorno de expresión escrita
disordered trastornado

disordered behavior conducta trastornada
disorders of the self trastornos del yo
disorganization desorganización
disorganized desorganizado
disorganized behavior conducta desorganizada
disorganized schizophrenia esquizofrenia desorganizada
disorganized type schizophrenia esquizofrenia de tipo desorganizada
disorientation desorientación
disparagement menoscabo
disparate retinal points puntos retinales dispares
disparity disparidad
dispersion dispersión
dispersion circle círculo de dispersión
displaced desplazado
displaced aggression agresión desplazada
displaced child syndrome síndrome de niño desplazado
displaced vision visión desplazada
displacement desplazamiento
displacement activity actividad de desplazamiento
displacement behavior conducta de desplazamiento
displacement in language desplazamiento en el lenguaje
displacement of affect desplazamiento del afecto
display despliegue
display behavior conducta de despliegue
display design diseño de despliegue
display rules reglas de despliegue
disposition disposición
dispositional disposicional
dispositional attribution atribución disposicional
disruption disrupción
disruptive disruptivo
disruptive behavior conducta disruptiva
disruptive behavior disorder trastorno de conducta disruptiva
disseminated diseminado
disseminated sclerosis esclerosis diseminada
dissimilation disimilación
dissimulation disimulación
dissimulator disimulador
dissociate disociar
dissociated disociado
dissociated anesthesia anestesia disociada
dissociated learning aprendizaje disociado
dissociation disociación
dissociation sensibility sensibilidad de disociación
dissociation syndrome síndrome de disociación
dissociative disociativo
dissociative amnesia amnesia disociativa
dissociative anesthesia anestesia disociativa
dissociative disorder trastorno disociativo
dissociative disorders and conversion reaction trastornos disociativos y reacción de conversión

dissociative fugue fuga disociativa
dissociative group grupo disociativo
dissociative hysteria histeria disociativa
dissociative identity identidad disociativa
dissociative identity disorder trastorno de identidad disociativa
dissociative reaction reacción disociativa
dissociative syndrome síndrome disociativo
dissonance disonancia
distal distal
distal dystrophy distrofia distal
distal effect efecto distal
distal response respuesta distal
distal stimulus estímulo distal
distal variable variable distal
distance distancia
distance ceptor ceptor a distancia
distance cues señales de distancia
distance hypnotherapy hipnoterapia de distancia
distance perception percepción de distancia
distance receptor receptor a distancia
distance vision visión de distancia
distance zones zonas de distancia
distinctive distintivo
distinctive feature característica distintiva
distorted distorsionado
distorted room cuarto distorsionado
distortion distorsión
distortion by transference distorsión por transferencia
distractibility distractibilidad
distractible distraíble
distractible speech habla distraíble
distraction distracción
distraction hypothesis hipótesis de distracción
distractor distractor
distractor technique técnica de distractor
distress angustia
distress-relief quotient cociente de angustia-alivio
distributed effort esfuerzo distribuido
distributed practice práctica distribuida
distributed processing procesamiento distribuido
distribution distribución
distribution curve curva de distribución
distribution-free libre de distribuciones
distribution-free statistics estadística libre de distribuciones
distribution of practice distribución de práctica
distributional redundancy redundancia distribucional
distributive distributivo
distributive analysis análisis distributivo
distributive analysis and synthesis análisis distributivo y síntesis
distributive justice justicia distributiva
disturbance disturbio
disturbance associated with conversion phenomena disturbio asociado con fenómenos de conversión
disturbance associated with organic mental disease disturbio asociado con enfermedad

mental orgánica
disturbance in content of thought disturbio en contenido de pensamientos
disturbance in form of thinking disturbio en la forma de pensar
disturbance in speech disturbio en el habla
disturbance in suggestibility disturbio en sugestibilidad
disturbance of associations disturbio de asociaciones
disturbance of attention disturbio de atención
disturbance of consciousness disturbio de conciencia
disturbance of memory disturbio de memoria
disturbing perturbador
disturbing event evento perturbador
disturbing memory memoria perturbadora
disulfiram disulfiram
disuse desuso
disuse hypothesis of forgetting hipótesis del desuso de olvidar
disuse principle principio del desuso
disutility desutilidad
diuresis diuresis
diuretic diurético
diurnal diurno
diurnal cycle ciclo diurno
diurnal rhythm ritmo diurno
diurnal variation variación diurna
divagation divagación
divergence divergencia
divergent divergente
divergent strabismus estrabismo divergente
divergent thinking pensamiento divergente
diversive diversivo
diversive exploration exploración diversiva
divided dividido
divided brain cerebro dividido
divided consciousness conciencia dividida
divination adivinación
diving reflex reflejo de zambullida
divorce divorcio
divorce adjustment ajuste de divorcio
divorce counseling asesoramiento de divorcio
dixyrazine dixirazina
dizygotic dizigótico
dizygotic twins gemelos dicigóticos
dizziness mareamiento
docile dócil
docility docilidad
doctor game juego del doctor
doctor-patient relationship relación doctor-paciente
doctrine doctrina
documentation documentación
documentation of child abuse documentación de abuso de niños
Dogiel's corpuscle corpúsculo de Dogiel
dogma dogma
dol dol
dolichocephalic dolicocefálico
dolichocephaly dolicocefalia
dolichoectatic artery arteria dolicoectática
dolichomorphic dolicomórfico
doll's eye sign signo de ojos de muñeca

doll play juego con muñecas
Dollinger-Bielschowsky syndrome síndrome de Dollinger-Bielschowsky
dolorific dolorífico
dolorimetry dolorimetría
dolorogenic zone zona dolorogénica
dolorology dolorología
domal sampling muestreo doméstico
domatophobia domatofobia
domestic doméstico
domestic violence violencia doméstica
domestic violence and child abuse violencia doméstica y abuso de niños
domestic violence and incest violencia doméstica e incesto
domestic violence and sexual abuse violencia doméstica y abuso sexual
domestic violence and spouse abuse violencia doméstica y abuso del cónyuge
domesticated domesticado
domesticated pride orgullo domesticado
domicile domicilio
domiciliary domiciliario
domiciliary care cuidado domiciliario
domiciliary care home hogar de cuidado domiciliario
dominance dominancia
dominance aggression agresión de dominancia
dominance hierarchy jerarquía de dominancia
dominance need necesidad de dominancia
dominance-submission dominancia-sumisión
dominance-subordination relationships relaciones de dominancia-subordinación
dominance test prueba de dominancia
dominant dominante
dominant determinant determinante dominante
dominant frequency frecuencia dominante
dominant gene gen dominante
dominant genotype genotipo dominante
dominant hemisphere hemisferio dominante
dominant idea idea dominante
dominant inheritance herencia dominante
dominant mentality mentalidad dominante
dominant trait rasgo dominante
dominant wavelength longitud de onda dominante
dominator dominador
domperidone domperidona
donatism donatismo
Donders' law ley de Donders
Donders' method método de Donders
door-in-the-face effect efecto de la puerta en la cara
door-in-the-face technique técnica de la puerta en la cara
Doose syndrome síndrome de Doose
dopa dopa
dopamine dopamina
dopamine and affective state dopamina y estado afectivo
dopamine and depression dopamina y depresión

dopamine hypothesis hipótesis de dopamina
dopamine hypothesis of schizophrenia
   hipótesis de dopamina de esquizofrenia
dopamine receptor receptor de dopamina
dopamine receptor sensitivity sensibilidad de
   receptor de dopamina
dopaminergic dopaminérgico
dopaminergic activity actividad
   dopaminérgica
dopaminergic drug droga dopaminérgica
dopaminergic neuron neurona dopaminérgica
dopaminergic pathway vía dopaminérgica
dopaminergic synapse sinapsis dopaminérgica
dopaminergic tract tracto dopaminérgico
Doppelganger phenomenon fenómeno de
   Doppelganger
Doppler effect efecto de Doppler
Doppler shift desplazamiento de Doppler
doraphobia dorafobia
Dorian love amor dorio
doromania doromanía
dorsal dorsal
dorsal column columna dorsal
dorsal column stimulation estimulación de
   columna dorsal
dorsal reflex reflejo dorsal
dorsal root raíz dorsal
dorsal tegmental bundle fascículo tegmental
   dorsal
dorsolateral dorsolateral
dorsolateral convexity syndrome síndrome
   de convexidad dorsolateral
dorsolateral nucleus núcleo dorsolateral
dorsomedial dorsomedial
dorsomedial nucleus núcleo dorsomedial
dorsum of foot reflex reflejo del dorso del pie
dorsum pedis reflex reflejo del dorso del pie
dosage dosis
dose dosis
dose-response relationship relación de
   dosis-respuesta
dotting test prueba de punteo
double doble
double-alternation learning aprendizaje de
   alternación doble
double-alternation problem problema de
   alternación doble
double approach-avoidance conflict conflicto
   de acercamiento-evitación doble
double approach conflict conflicto de
   acercamiento doble
double aspect theory teoría de doble aspecto
double athetosis atetosis doble
double avoidance conflict conflicto de
   evitación doble
double bind apuro doble
double bind theory of schizophrenia teoría
   de apuro doble de esquizofrenia
double-blind doble ciego
double-blind crossover entrecruzamiento
   doble ciego
double-blind research investigación doble
   ciego
double-blind study estudio doble ciego
double cancellation cancelación doble

double compartment hydrocephalus
   hidrocefalia de compartimiento doble
double congenital athetosis atetosis congénita
   doble
double consciousness conciencia doble
double depression depresión doble
double dissociation disociación doble
double entendre equívoco
double-entry table tabla de doble entrada
double hemiplegia hemiplejía doble
double images imágenes dobles
double insanity insania doble
double meaning doble sentido
double orientation orientación doble
double personality personalidad doble
double-point threshold umbral de punto doble
double representation representación doble
double sampling muestreo doble
double simultaneous stimulation estimulación
   simultánea doble
double simultaneous tactile sensation
   sensación táctil simultánea doble
double standard rasero doble
double superego superego doble
double variation variación doble
double vision visión doble
double-Y condition condición de Y doble
doubt duda
doubting incrédulo
doubting mania manía incrédula
doubting spell racha incrédula
Down's disease enfermedad de Down
Down's syndrome síndrome de Down
down-beat nystagmus nistagmo hacia abajo
downward mobility movilidad hacia abajo
dowsing rabdomancia
doxapram doxapram
doxepin hydrochloride clorhidrato de
   doxepina
doxogenic doxogénico
doxylamine doxilamina
drama therapy terapia de drama
dramatic dramático
dramatic personality personalidad dramática
dramatic play juego dramático
dramatic speech habla dramática
dramatism dramatismo
dramatization dramatización
dramatogenic dramatogénico
drapetomania drapetomanía
drawing dibujo
drawing disability discapacidad de dibujo
drawing in hypnosis dibujo en hipnosis
drawing test prueba de dibujo
dread terror
dream sueño
dream analysis análisis de sueños
dream anxiety attack ataque de ansiedad de
   sueños
dream anxiety disorder trastorno de ansiedad
   de sueños
dream association asociación de sueños
dream censorship censura de sueños
dream content contenido de sueños
dream determinant determinante de sueño

dream ego ego de sueños
dream enhancement realzado de sueños
dream formation formación de sueños
dream function función de sueños
dream illusion ilusión de sueño
dream induction inducción de sueño
dream instigator instigador de sueño
dream interpretation interpretación de sueños
dream pain dolor en sueños
dream recall recordación de sueños
dream recall and anxiety recordación de
    sueños y ansiedad
dream reporting reportaje de sueños
dream screen pantalla de sueños
dream-series method método de serie de
    sueños
dream state estado de sueño
dream stimulus estímulo de sueño
dream suggestion sugestión de sueño
dream symbolism simbolismo de sueños
dream within a dream sueño dentro de un
    sueño
dream-work trabajo del sueño
dreamlike state estado como de sueño
dreams and time of night sueños y hora de la
    noche
dreams compared to fairy tales sueños
    comparados con cuentos de hadas
dreams of children sueños de niños
dreams of death sueños de muerte
dreams of homosexuality sueños de
    homosexualidad
dreams of the blind sueños de los ciegos
dreams of the deaf sueños de los sordos
dreams of the physically disabled sueños de
    los incapacitados físicamente
dreamy state estado soñador
dress vestimenta
dressing vestir
dressing apraxia apraxia del vestir
dressing behavior conducta del vestir
drill practicar repetidamente
drinking beber
drinking aids ayudas para beber
drinking behavior conducta del beber
drinking bout juerga de borrachera
drive impulso
drive arousal despertamiento de impulso
drive-arousal stimulus estímulo de
    despertamiento de impulso
drive-discharge hypothesis hipótesis de
    descarga de impulso
drive displacement desplazamiento de
    impulso
drive reduction reducción de impulso
drive-reduction hypothesis hipótesis de
    reducción de impulso
drive-reduction theory teoría de reducción de
    impulso
drive regulation regulación de impulso
drive specificity especificidad de impulso
drive state estado de impulso
drive stimuli estímulos de impulso
drive theory teoría de impulsos
driver's thigh muslo de conductor

driver education educación de conductor
driving conducción
dromic drómico
dromolepsy dromolepsia
dromomania dromomanía
dromophobia dromofobia
drop caída
drop attack ataque de caída
droperidol droperidol
drowsiness modorra
drowsiness in infancy modorra en infancia
drug droga
drug abuse abuso de drogas
drug abuse in adolescence abuso de drogas
    en adolescencia
drug abuse scale escala de abuso de drogas
drug addiction drogadicción
drug antagonism antagonismo de drogas
drug counselor asesor de drogas
drug culture cultura de drogas
drug defaulter faltante de drogas
drug dementia demencia por drogas
drug dependence dependencia de drogas
drug education educación de drogas
drug effects efectos de drogas
drug effects in lie detection efectos de drogas
    en detección de mentiras
drug holiday día libre de droga
drug-induced inducido por drogas
drug-induced parkinsonism parkinsonismo
    inducido por drogas
drug-induced psychosis psicosis inducida por
    drogas
drug interaction interacción de drogas
drug level nivel de droga
drug of choice droga de predilección
drug psychosis psicosis por drogas
drug tetanus tétanos por drogas
drug therapy terapia de drogas
drug tolerance tolerancia de drogas
drug use uso de drogas
drugs for pain drogas para el dolor
drugs for treating mental illness drogas para
    tratar enfermedad mental
drugs for treating pain drogas para tratar el
    dolor
drunkenness embriaguez
dry beriberi beriberi seco
dry leprosy lepra seca
dry mouth boca seca
dry orgasm orgasmo seco
dual doble
dual ambivalence ambivalencia doble
dual-arousal theory teoría de despertamiento
    doble
dual-code hypothesis hipótesis de código
    doble
dual encoding codificación doble
dual-instinct theory teoría de instinto doble
dual leadership liderazgo doble
dual-leadership therapy terapia de liderazgo
    doble
dual masturbation masturbación doble
dual-memory theory teoría de memoria doble
dual personality personalidad doble

dual-process theory teoría de proceso doble
dual-sex therapy terapia de sexo doble
dual therapy terapia doble
dual threshold umbral doble
dual transference transferencia doble
dual-transference therapy terapia de
    transferencia doble
dualism dualismo
Dubini's disease enfermedad de Dubini
Duchenne's disease enfermedad de Duchenne
Duchenne's dystrophy distrofia de Duchenne
Duchenne's paralysis parálisis de Duchenne
Duchenne's sign signo de Duchenne
Duchenne's syndrome síndrome de Duchenne
Duchenne-Aran disease enfermedad de
    Duchenne-Aran
Duchenne-Erb paralysis parálisis de
    Duchenne-Erb
Duckworth's phenomenon fenómeno de
    Duckworth
ductus deferens ductus deferens
dull normal lerdo normal
dumb mudo
dummy muñeco, placebo
Duncan test prueba de Duncan
duplex transmission transmisión doble
duplicative duplicativo
duplicative reaction reacción duplicativa
duplicity duplicidad
duplicity theory teoría de la duplicidad
dura mater duramadre
Durante's disease enfermedad de Durante
duraplasty duraplastia
duration duración
duration of breast-feeding duración de
    alimentación por pecho
duration of coma duración de coma
duration tetany tetania duradera
Durck's nodes nódulos de Durck
Duret's lesion lesión de Duret
Durham rule regla de Durham
Durham test prueba de Durham
duty deber
duty to warn deber de advertir
dwarfism enanismo
dyad díada
dyadic diádico
dyadic psychotherapy psicoterapia diádica
dyadic relationship relación diádica
dyadic session sesión diádica
dyadic symbiosis simbiosis diádica
dyadic therapy terapia diádica
dying phobia fobia de morir
dynamic dinámico
dynamic approach acercamiento dinámico
dynamic apraxia apraxia dinámica
dynamic disease enfermedad dinámica
dynamic equilibrium equilibrio dinámico
dynamic formulation formulación dinámica
dynamic psychiatry psiquiatría dinámica
dynamic psychology psicología dinámica
dynamic psychotherapy psicoterapia
    dinámica
dynamic reasoning razonamiento dinámico
dynamic-situations principle principio de

situaciones dinámicas
dynamic system sistema dinámico
dynamic theory teoría dinámica
dynamic unconscious inconsciente dinámico
dynamical system theory teoría de sistema
    dinámico
dynamics dinámica
dynamism dinamismo
dynamogenesis dinamogénesis
dynamometer dinamómetro
dyne dina
dysacousia disacusia
dysacusia disacusia
dysacusis disacusis
dysantigraphia disantigrafia
dysaphia disafia
dysaphic disáfico
dysarthria disartria
dysarthria literalis disartria literal
dysarthria syllabaris spasmodica disartria
    silábica espasmódica
dysarthric disártrico
dysarthrosis disartrosis
dysautonomia disautonomía
dysbasia disbasia
dysbasia lordotica progressiva disbasia
    lordótica progresiva
dysboulia disbulia
dysbulia disbulia
dysbulic disbúlico
dyscalculia discalculia
dyscheiral disquirial
dyscheiria disquiria
dyschezia disquecia
dyschiral disquiral
dyschiria disquiria
dyschromatopsia discromatopsia
dyschronism discronismo
dyscinesia discinesia
dyscoimesis discoimesis
dyscontrol descontrol
dyscontrol syndrome síndrome de descontrol
dyscrasia discrasia
dysdiadochocinesia disdiadococinesia
dysdiadochokinesia disdiadococinesia
dysdiadochokinesis disdiadococinesis
dyseneia diseneia
dyserethism diseretismo
dysergasia disergasia
dysergia disergia
dysesthesia disestesia
dysfluency disfluidez
dysfunction disfunción
dysfunctional disfuncional
dysfunctional family familia disfuncional
dysgenesia disgenesia
dysgenesis disgenesia
dysgenic disgénico
dysgeusia disgeusia
dysglucosis disglucosis
dysgnosia disgnosia
dysgrammatism disgramatismo
dysgraphia disgrafia
dyshomophilia dishomofilia
dysidentity disidentidad

dyskinesia discinesia
dyskinesia algera discinesia álgera
dyskinesis discinesis
dyskinetic discinético
dyslalia dislalia
dyslexia dislexia
dyslexic disléxico
dyslogia dislogia
dysmegalopsia dismegalopsia
dysmenorrhea dismenorrea
dysmentia dismencia
dysmetria dismetría
dysmetropsia dismetropsia
dysmimia dismimia
dysmnesia dismnesia
dysmnesic dismnésico
dysmnesic psychosis psicosis dismnésica
dysmnesic syndrome síndrome dismnésico
dysmorphic dismórfico
dysmorphic delusion delusión dismórfica
dysmorphic somatoform disorder trastorno
    somatoforme dismórfico
dysmorphobia dismorfobia
dysmorphomania dismorfomanía
dysmorphophobia dismorfofobia
dysmyelination dismielinación
dysmyotonia dismiotonía
dysnystaxis disnistaxis
dysorexia disorexia
dysosmia disosmia
dysostosis disostosis
dyspallia dispalia
dyspareunia dispareunia
dysperception dispercepción
dysphagia disfagia
dysphagia spastica disfagia espástica
dysphagy disfagia
dysphasia disfasia
dysphemia disfemia
dysphonia disfonía
dysphonia spastica disfonía espástica
dysphonic disfónico
dysphoria disforia
dysphoria nervosa disforia nerviosa
dysphoric disfórico
dysphoric mood humor disfórico
dysphrasia disfrasia
dysphrenia disfrenia
dysphylaxia disfilaxia
dysplasia displasia
dysplastic displástico
dysplastic type tipo displástico
dyspnea disnea
dysponesis disponesis
dyspraxia dispraxia
dysprosody disprosodia
dysrhythmia disritmia
dyssocial disocial
dyssocial behavior conducta disocial
dyssocial drinking beber disocial
dyssocial personality personalidad disocial
dyssocial reaction reacción disocial
dyssomnia disomnia
dyssomnia in childhood disomnia en niñez
dysspermia dispermia

dysstasia distasia
dyssymbiosis disimbiosis
dyssynergia disinergia
dyssynergia cerebellaris disinergia cerebelosa
dyssynergia cerebellaris myoclonica
    disinergia cerebelosa mioclónica
dyssynergia cerebellaris progressiva
    disinergia cerebelosa progresiva
dystaxia distaxia
dysthymia distimia
dysthymia scale escala de distimia
dysthymic distímico
dysthymic disorder trastorno distímico
dystocia distocia
dystonia distonía
dystonia lenticularis distonía lenticular
dystonia musculorum deformans distonía
    muscular deformante
dystonic distónico
dystonic movement movimiento distónico
dystonic reaction reacción distónica
dystonic torticollis tortícolis distónico
dystrophia distrofia
dystrophia adiposogenitalis distrofia
    adiposogenital
dystrophia myotonica distrofia miotónica
dystrophoneurosis distrofoneurosis
dystrophy distrofia
dystropy distropía
dystychia distiquia
dysuria disuria

E

e scale escala e
E trisomy trisomia E
Eagle syndrome síndrome de Eagle
ear drum tambor del oído
ear pulling tironeo de oreja
early temprano
early adolescence adolescencia temprana
early adulthood adultez temprana
early childhood niñez temprana
early childhood development desarrollo de
    niñez temprana
early childhood education educación de niñez
    temprana
early experiences experiencias tempranas
early infantile autism autismo infantil
    temprano
early intervention intervención temprana
early learning aprendizaje temprano
early life experiences experiencias de vida
    temprana
early posttraumatic epilepsy epilepsia
    postraumática temprana
early recollection memoria temprana
early trauma hypothesis of autistic disorder
    hipótesis de trauma temprano de trastorno
    autista
early versus late maturation maduración
    temprana contra tarde
earphone audífono
earth-eating comer tierra
eastern equine encephalomyelitis
    encefalomielitis equina del este
easy child niño fácil
eating aids ayudas del comer
eating and hunger comer y hambre
eating behavior conducta del comer
eating compulsion compulsión del comer
eating disorder trastorno del comer
eating disorder in adolescence trastorno del
    comer en adolescencia
eating disorder in infancy trastorno del
    comer en infancia
eating disturbance disturbio del comer
eating epilepsy epilepsia del comer
eating habits hábitos del comer
eating without saturation comer sin
    saturación
Eaton-Lambert syndrome síndrome de
    Eaton-Lambert
Ebbinghaus curve curva de Ebbinghaus
Ebbinghaus curve of retention curva de
    retención de Ebbinghaus
Ebbinghaus test prueba de Ebbinghaus
ebriecation ebriecación

eccentric excéntrico
eccentric projection proyección excéntrica
ecchondrosis econdrosis
ecchondrosis physaliformis econdrosis
    fisaliforme
ecchondrosis physaliphora econdrosis
    fisalífora
eccyesis ecciesis
ecdemomania ecdemomanía
ecdemonomania ecdemonomanía
ecdysiasm ecdisiasmo
echeosis equeosis
echo eco
echo phenomenon fenómeno de eco
echo principle principio de eco
echo reaction reacción de eco
echo sign signo de eco
echo speech habla de eco
echoacousia ecoacusia
echocardiogram ecocardiograma
echocardiography ecocardiografía
echoencephalograph ecoencefalógrafo
echoencephalography ecoencefalografía
echographia ecografía
echoic ecoico
echoic behavior conducta ecoica
echoic memory memoria ecoica
echokinesia ecocinesia
echokinesis ecocinesis
echolalia ecolalia
echolalia and language ecolalia y lenguaje
echolalia and language acquisition ecolalia y
    adquisición del lenguaje
echolalia and language disorders ecolalia y
    trastornos del lenguaje
echolalia in autism ecolalia en autismo
echolocation ecoubicación
echomatism ecomatismo
echomimia ecomimia
echomotism ecomotismo
echopalilalia ecopalilalia
echopathy ecopatía
echophotony ecofotonía
echophrasia ecofrasia
echopraxia ecopraxia
eclactisma eclactisma
eclampsia eclampsia
eclampsia nutans eclampsia nutans
eclamptic eclámptico
eclamptic symptoms síntomas eclámpticos
eclamptogenic eclamptogénico
eclamptogenous eclamptógeno
eclectic ecléctico
eclectic approach acercamiento ecléctico
eclectic behaviorism conductismo ecléctico
eclectic counseling asesoramiento ecléctico
eclectic hypnotherapy hipnoterapia ecléctica
eclectic psychotherapy psicoterapia ecléctica
eclecticism eclecticismo
eclimia eclimia
ecmnesia ecmnesia
ecnoia ecnoia
ecological ecológico
ecological approach acercamiento ecológico
ecological inventory inventario ecológico

ecological model modelo ecológico
ecological niche nicho ecológico
ecological optics ópitca ecológica
ecological perception percepción ecológica
ecological perspective perspectiva ecológica
ecological perspective of development
    perspectiva ecológica del desarrollo
ecological psychiatry psiquiatría ecológica
ecological psychology psicología ecológica
ecological realism realismo ecológico
ecological study estudio ecológico
ecological systems model modelo de sistemas
    ecológicos
ecological theory teoría ecológica
ecological theory of perception teoría
    ecológica de percepción
ecological validity validez ecológica
ecology ecología
ecomania ecomanía
economic económico
economic approach acercamiento económico
economic divorce divorcio económico
economic hardship penuria económica
economic issues of divorce cuestiones
    económicas del divorcio
economic stress estrés económico
Economo's disease enfermedad de Economo
economy principle principio de la economía
ecopharmacology ecofarmacología
ecophobia ecofobia
ecopsychiatry ecopsiquiatría
ecopsychology ecopsicología
ecosphere ecosfera
ecosystem ecosistema
ecouteur ecouteur
ecouteurism ecouteurismo
ecphoria ecforia
ecphorize ecforizar
ecstasy éxtasis
ecstatic extático
ecstatic state estado extático
ectoderm ectodermo
ectogenous ectógeno
ectomorph ectomorfo
ectomorphic ectomórfico
ectomorphy ectomorfia
ectopia pupillae ectopia pupilar
ectopic ectópico
ectopic pinealoma pinealoma ectópico
ectopic pregnancy embarazo ectópico
ectopic testis testículo ectópico
ectoplasm ectoplasma
ectype ectipo
eczema eccema
edema edema
edge effect efecto de borde
edge perception percepción de borde
Edinger-Westphal nucleus núcleo de
    Edinger-Westphal
edipism edipismo
Edipus complex complejo de Edipo
educability educabilidad
educable educable
educable mentally retarded retardado mental
    educable

education educación
education-socialization model modelo de
    educación-socialización
education stage etapa de educación
educational educacional
educational acceleration aceleración
    educacional
educational achievement aprovechamiento
    educacional
educational age edad educacional
educational approach acercamiento
    educacional
educational assessment evaluación
    educacional
educational counseling asesoramiento
    educacional
educational guidance asesoramiento
    educacional
educational history historial educacional
educational intervention intervención
    educacional
educational mainstreaming traslación a la
    corriente principal educacional
educational measurement medición
    educacional
educational opportunities oportunidades
    educacionales
educational placement colocación
    educacional
educational program programa educacional
educational psychologist psicólogo
    educacional
educational psychology psicología
    educacional
educational quotient cociente educacional
educational services servicios educacionales
educational test prueba educacional
educational therapist terapeuta educacional
educationally subnormal subnormal
    educativamente
educative educativo
educative intervention intervención educativa
Edward's syndrome síndrome de Edward
effect efecto
effect gradient gradiente de efecto
effect law ley de efecto
effect spread extensión de efecto
effectance efectancia
effectance motive motivo de efectancia
effective efectivo
effective habit strength fuerza del hábito
    efectiva
effective reaction potential potencial de
    reacción efectivo
effective stimulus estímulo efectivo
effective temperature temperatura efectiva
effective weight peso efectivo
effectiveness efectividad
effector efector
effects of caffeine efectos de cafeína
effects of child abuse efectos de abuso de
    niños
effects of child sexual abuse efectos de abuso
    sexual de niños
effects of hospitalization efectos de

hospitalización
effects of stress efectos de estrés
effeminate afeminado
effeminate homosexuality homosexualidad
  afeminada
effeminated man hombre afeminado
efferent eferente
efferent motor aphasia afasia motora eferente
efficacy eficacia
efficient eficiente
efficient cause causa eficiente
effort esfuerzo
effort-shape technique técnica
  esfuerzo-forma
effort syndrome síndrome de esfuerzo
egersis egersis
ego ego
ego-alien ajeno al ego
ego-alter theory teoría del álter ego
ego alteration alteración del ego
ego analysis análisis del ego
ego anxiety ansiedad del ego
ego block bloqueador del ego
ego boundary límite del ego
ego-boundary loss pérdida del límite del ego
ego cathexis catexis del ego
ego center centro del ego
ego complex complejo del ego
ego control control del ego
ego-coping skill destreza para bregar del ego
ego defense defensa del ego
ego defense mechanism mecanismo de
  defensa del ego
ego defenses and violent behavior defensas
  del ego y conducta violenta
ego development desarrollo del ego
ego deviation desviación del ego
ego distortion distorsión del ego
ego drive impulso del ego
ego duplication duplicación del ego
ego-dystonic egodistónico
ego-dystonic behavior conducta egodistónica
ego-dystonic homosexuality homosexualidad
  egodistónica
ego erotism erotismo del ego
ego failure fracaso del ego
ego formation formación del ego
ego function función del ego
ego functioning in preschoolers
  funcionamiento del ego en preescolares
ego ideal ego ideal
ego identity identidad del ego
ego instinct instinto del ego
ego integration integración del ego
ego-integrative egointegrativo
ego integrity integridad del ego
ego integrity versus despair integridad del
  ego contra desesperación
ego involvement envolvimiento del ego
ego libido libido del ego
ego maximization maximización del ego
ego mechanism mecanismo del ego
ego model modelo del ego
ego narcissism narcisismo del ego
ego needs necesidades del ego

ego neurosis neurosis del ego
ego nuclei núcleos del ego
ego-object polarity polaridad ego-objeto
ego psychology psicología del ego
ego psychotherapy psicoterapia del ego
ego resistance resistencia del ego
ego retrenchment reducción del ego
ego splitting rompimiento del ego
ego stability estabilidad del ego
ego state estado del ego
ego strength fuerza del ego
ego strength scale escala de fuerza del ego
ego strengthening techniques técnicas para
  fortalecimiento del ego
ego stress estrés del ego
ego structure estructura del ego
ego subject sujeto del ego
ego suffering sufrimiento del ego
ego support apoyo del ego
ego support from family apoyo del ego de
  familia
ego support from friends apoyo del ego de
  amigos
ego support from groups apoyo del ego de
  grupos
ego-syntonic egosintónico
ego-syntonic homosexuality homosexualidad
  egosintónica
ego threat amenaza al ego
ego transcendence trascendencia del ego
ego weakness debilidad del ego
egocentric egocéntrico
egocentric judgment juicio egocéntrico
egocentric localization ubicación egocéntrica
egocentric speech habla egocéntrica
egocentric thinking pensamiento egocéntrico
egocentricity egocentrismo
egocentrism egocentrismo
egocentrism during adolescence
  egocentrismo durante adolescencia
egoism egoísmo
egoistic egoísta
egoistic model of altruism modelo egoísta de
  altruísmo
egoistic suicide suicidio egoísta
egomania egomanía
egomorphism egomorfismo
egopathy egopatía
egotheism egoteísmo
egotic egótico
egotism egotismo
egotistic egotista
egotistic suicide suicidio egotista
egotistical egotista
egotization egotización
egotropic egotrópico
egotropy egotropía
egregorsis egregorsis
Ehret's syndrome síndrome de Ehret
Eichhorst's neuritis neuritis de Eichhorst
eidetic eidético
eidetic image imagen eidética
eidetic imagery imaginería eidética
eidetic personification personificación
  eidética

eidetic psychotherapy psicoterapia eidética
eidetic type tipo eidético
eidoptometry eidoptometría
Eigenwelt Eigenwelt
eighth nerve tumor tumor del octavo nervio
Einstellung Einstellung
Eisenlohr's syndrome síndrome de Eisenlohr
eisoptrophobia eisoptrofobia
ejaculatio eyaculación
ejaculatio praecox eyaculación precoz
ejaculatio retardata eyaculación retardada
ejaculation eyaculación
ejaculation disorder trastorno de eyaculación
ejaculation physiology fisiología de
    eyaculación
ejaculatory eyaculatorio
ejaculatory duct conducto eyaculatorio
ejaculatory incompetence incompetencia
    eyaculatoria
ejaculatory pain dolor eyaculatorio
Ekbom syndrome síndrome de Ekbom
ekphorize ecforizar
elaborated code código complicado
elaboration elaboración
elaborative rehearsal ensayo complicado
elation elación
elbow jerk sacudida del codo
elbow reflex reflejo del codo
elder mayor
elder abuse abuso de mayores
elderly anciano
elderly abuse abuso de ancianos
elderly antidepressants antidepresivos de
    ancianos
elderly anxiety ansiedad de ancianos
elderly dementia demencia de ancianos
elderly depression depresión de ancianos
elderly insomnia insomnio de ancianos
elderly psychosis psicosis de ancianos
elective electivo
elective anorexia anorexia electiva
elective mutism mutismo electivo
Electra complex complejo de Electra
electric aversion therapy terapia de aversión
    eléctrica
electric chorea corea eléctrica
electric convulsion therapy terapia de
    convulsión eléctrica
electric ophthalmia oftalmía eléctrica
electric senses sentidos eléctricos
electric shock choque eléctrico
electric shock therapy terapia de choques
    eléctricos
electric skin shock choque de piel eléctrico
electric sleep sueño eléctrico
electrical activity of the brain actividad
    eléctrica del cerebro
electrical brain stimulation estimulación
    cerebral eléctrica
electrical habituation habituación eléctrica
electrical intracranial stimulation
    estimulación intracraneal eléctrica
electrical nervous system stimulation
    estimulación del sistema nervioso eléctrico
electrical sleep sueño eléctrico

electrical stimulation estimulación eléctrica
electrical stimulation of cortex estimulación
    eléctrica de la corteza
electrical transcranial stimulation
    estimulación transcraneal eléctrica
electroanalgesia electroanalgesia
electrocardiogram electrocardiograma
electrocardiograph electrocardiógrafo
electrocardiographic effect efecto
    electrocardiográfico
electrocerebral electrocerebral
electrocerebral silence silencio
    electrocerebral
electrocontractility electrocontractilidad
electroconvulsive electroconvulsivo
electroconvulsive shock choque
    electroconvulsivo
electroconvulsive therapy terapia
    electroconvulsiva
electroconvulsive treatment tratamiento
    electroconvulsivo
electrocorticogram electrocorticograma
electrocorticography electrocorticografía
electrocutaneous electrocutáneo
electrocutaneous stimulation estimulación
    electrocutánea
electrode electrodo
electrode placement colocación de electrodo
electrodermal electrodérmico
electrodermal activity actividad
    electrodérmica
electrodermal activity in sleep actividad
    electrodérmica durante el sueño
electrodermal response respuesta
    electrodérmica
electrodiagnosis electrodiagnóstico
electroencephalic audiometry audiometría
    electroencefálica
electroencephalogram electroencefalograma
electroencephalograph electroencefalógrafo
electroencephalographic
    electroencefalográfico
electroencephalographic dysrhythmia
    disritmia electroencefalográfica
electroencephalography electroencefalografía
electrographic electrográfico
electrographic features of the sleep cycle
    características electrográficas del ciclo de
    sueño
electrolepsy electrolepsia
electrolyte electrólito
electrolyte balance balance de electrólito
electrolyte imbalance desequilibrio de
    electrólito
electromagnetic electromagnético
electromagnetic radiation radiación
    electromagnética
electromagnetic spectrum espectro
    electromagnético
electromicturition electromicturición
electromuscular electromuscular
electromuscular sensibility sensibilidad
    electromuscular
electromyogram electromiograma
electromyograph electromiógrafo

electronarcosis electronarcosis
electroneurography electroneurografía
electroneurolysis electroneurólisis
electroneuromyography
    electroneuromiografía
electronic electrónico
electronic aids ayudas electrónicas
electronic monitoring monitorización
    electrónica
electronystagmography electronistagmografía
electrooculogram electrooculograma
electroolfactogram electroolfatograma
electropathology electropatología
electrophobia electrofobia
electrophoresis electroforesis
electrophrenic electrofrénico
electrophrenic respiration respiración
    electrofrénica
electrophysiology electrofisiología
electroplexy electroplejía
electroretinogram electrorretinograma
electroshock electrochoque
electroshock therapy terapia de
    electrochoques
electrosleep electrosueño
electrosleep therapy terapia de electrosueño
electrospectrography electroespectrografía
electrospinogram electroespinograma
electrospinography electroespinografía
electrostimulation electroestimulación
electrotherapeutic electroterapéutico
electrotherapeutic sleep sueño
    electroterapéutico
electrotherapeutic sleep therapy terapia de
    sueño electroterapéutico
electrotherapy electroterapia
electrotonic electrotónico
electrotonic conduction conducción
    electrotónica
electrotonus electrotono
element elemento
elemental elemental
elemental anxiety ansiedad elemental
elementarism elementarismo
elementary elemental
elementary anxiety ansiedad elemental
elementary hallucination alucinación
    elemental
elementary partial seizure acceso parcial
    elemental
elementary process proceso elemental
elements of language elementos del lenguaje
elements of thought elementos de
    pensamiento
elephantiasis elefantiasis
elephantiasis neuromatosa elefantiasis
    neuromatosa
eleutheromania eleuteromanía
elevated mood humor elevado
elevation elevación
elfin facies facies de duende
elicit evocar
elicited evocado
elicited behavior conducta evocada
elimination eliminación

elimination disorder trastorno de eliminación
elimination drive impulso de eliminación
Elithorn maze laberinto de Elithorn
ellipsis elipsis
Ellis-van Creveld syndrome síndrome de
    Ellis-van Creveld
elopement fuga
elucidation elucidación
emancipated emancipado
emancipated minor menor emancipado
emancipation emancipación
emancipation disorder trastorno de
    emancipación
emasculation emasculación
embarrassment vergüenza
embarrassment dream sueño de vergüenza
embarrassment psychosis psicosis de
    vergüenza
embedded figure figura encerrada
embedded-figures test prueba de figuras
    encerradas
emblem emblema
embolalia embolalia
embolic apoplexy apoplejía embólica
embolism embolismo
embolization embolización
embololalia embololalia
embolophasia embolofasia
embolophrasia embolofrasia
embrace abrazo
embrace reflex reflejo de abrazo
embracing abrazante
embracing behavior conducta abrazante
embryo embrión
embryology embriología
embryonic embriónico
embryonic period periodo embriónico
emergence emergencia
emergence of empathy emergencia de
    empatía
emergency emergencia
emergency contagion contagio de emergencia
emergency dyscontrol descontrol de
    emergencia
emergency intervention intervención de
    emergencia
emergency psychotherapy psicoterapia de
    emergencia
emergency room sala de emergencia
emergency services servicios de emergencia
emergency theory teoría de emergencia
emergency theory of emotions teoría de
    emergencia de emociones
emergent emergente
emergent evolution evolución emergente
emergentism emergentismo
emesis emesis
emetomania emetomanía
emetophobia emetofobia
emic émico
emission emisión
emit emitir
emitted behavior conducta emitida
emmenia emenia
emmeniopathy emeniopatía

Emmert's law ley de Emmert
emmetropia emetropía
emotion emoción
emotional emocional
emotional abuse abuso emocional
emotional adjustment ajuste emocional
emotional age edad emocional
emotional amenorrhea amenorrea emocional
emotional anesthesia anestesia emocional
emotional appeal apelación emocional
emotional appeals in advertising apelaciones
  emocionales en anuncios
emotional arousal despertamiento emocional
emotional attitude actitud emocional
emotional beggar mendigo emocional
emotional behavior conducta emocional
emotional bias sesgo emocional
emotional blocking bloqueo emocional
emotional conflict conflicto emocional
emotional contagion contagio emocional
emotional dependence dependencia
  emocional
emotional deprivation privación emocional
emotional deterioration deterioración
  emocional
emotional development desarrollo emocional
emotional disease enfermedad emocional
emotional disorder trastorno emocional
emotional disturbance disturbio emocional
emotional divorce divorcio emocional
emotional dysfunction disfunción emocional
emotional dysfunction in adolescence
  disfunción emocional en adolescencia
emotional expression expresión emocional
emotional expression in blind infants
  expresión emocional en infantes ciegos
emotional expression in preschoolers
  expresión emocional en preescolares
emotional flooding inundación emocional
emotional functioning funcionamiento
  emocional
emotional handicap minusvalía emocional
emotional illness enfermedad emocional
emotional immaturity inmadurez emocional
emotional indicator indicador emocional
emotional inoculation inoculación emocional
emotional insight penetración emocional
emotional instability inestabilidad emocional
emotional insulation aislamiento emocional
emotional lability labilidad emocional
emotional leukocytosis leucocitosis emocional
emotional maturity madurez emocional
emotional nutriment nutrimento emocional
emotional overlay sobreposición emocional
emotional reaction reacción emocional
emotional reaction of children to divorce
  reacción emocional de niños al divorcio
emotional reeducation reeducación emocional
emotional release descarga emocional
emotional response respuesta emocional
emotional security seguridad emocional
emotional speech habla emocional
emotional stability estabilidad emocional
emotional storm tormenta emocional
emotional stress estrés emocional

emotional stupor estupor emocional
emotional supplies suministros emocionales
emotional support apoyo emocional
emotional tension tensión emocional
emotional threshold umbral emocional
emotional tone tono emocional
emotionality emocionalidad
emotionally emocionalmente
emotionally handicapped minusválido
  emocionalmente
emotionally unstable inestable
  emocionalmente
emotionally unstable personality
  personalidad inestable emocionalmente
emotiovascular emotiovascular
emotive emotivo
emotive imagery imaginería emotiva
emotive processes procesos emotivos
emotive therapy terapia emotiva
empathetic empático
empathic empático
empathic index índice empático
empathic understanding entendimiento
  empático
empathize empatizar
empathy empatía
empathy-altruism hypothesis hipótesis de
  empatía-altruismo
empathy training entrenamiento de empatía
emphatic enfático
emphysema enfisema
empiric empírico
empiric-risk figure cifra de riesgo empírico
empirical empírico
empirical construct constructo empírico
empirical equation ecuación empírica
empirical law ley empírica
empirical law of effect ley de efecto empírica
empirical-rational strategy estrategia
  empírica-racional
empirical research investigación empírica
empirical research methods métodos de
  investigación empírica
empirical risk riesgo empírico
empirical self yo empírico
empirical test prueba empírica
empirical validity validez empírica
empiricism empirismo
employee empleado
employee attitude survey encuesta de
  actitudes de empleados
employee evaluation evaluación de empleado
employee productivity productividad de
  empleado
employment empleo
employment interview entrevista de empleo
employment patterns patrones de empleo
employment practices prácticas de empleo
employment test prueba de empleo
employment workshop taller de empleo
emprosthotonos emprostótonos
empty-chair technique técnica de silla vacía
empty nest nido vacío
empty-nest syndrome síndrome de nido vacío
empty organism organismo vacío

empty set conjunto vacío
empty word palabra vacía
emulation emulación
emylcamate emilcamato
enabler habilitador
enactive representation representación
  representativa
enanthate enantato
enantiobiosis enantiobiosis
enantiodromia enantiodromia
enantiopathic enantiopático
encapsulated encapsulado
encapsulated delusion delusión encapsulada
encapsulated end organ órgano terminal
  encapsulado
encapsulated nerve endings terminaciones
  nerviosas encapsuladas
encapsulation encapsulación
encatalepsis encatalepsia
encephalalgia encefalalgia
encephalasthenia encefalastenia
encephalatrophic encefalatrófico
encephalatrophy encefalatrofía
encephalauxe encefalauxa
encephalemia encefalemia
encephalic encefálico
encephalic angioma angioma encefálico
encephalitic encefalítico
encephalitis encefalitis
encephalitis hemorrhagica encefalitis
  hemorrágica
encephalitis lethargica encefalitis letárgica
encephalitis neonatorum encefalitis neonatal
encephalitis periaxialis concentrica
  encefalitis periaxial concéntrica
encephalitis periaxialis diffusa encefalitis
  periaxial difusa
encephalitis pyogenica encefalitis piogénica
encephalitis subcorticalis chronica encefalitis
  subcortical crónica
encephalitogen encefalitógeno
encephalitogenic encefalitogénico
encephalization encefalización
encephalocele encefalocele
encephaloclastic microcephaly microcefalia
  encefaloclástica
encephalodynia encefalodinia
encephalodysplasia encefalodisplasia
encephalofacial angiomatosis angiomatosis
  encefalofacial
encephalogram encefalograma
encephalography encefalografía
encephaloid encefaloide
encephalolith encefalolito
encephalology encefalología
encephaloma encefaloma
encephalomalacia encefalomalacia
encephalomeningitis encefalomeningitis
encephalomeningocele encefalomeningocele
encephalomeningopathy
  encefalomeningopatía
encephalometer encefalómetro
encephalomyelitis encefalomielitis
encephalomyelocele encefalomielocele
encephalomyeloneuropathy

encefalomieloneuropatía
encephalomyelopathy encefalomielopatía
encephalomyeloradiculitis
  encefalomielorradiculitis
encephalomyeloradiculopathy
  encefalomielorradiculopatía
encephalomyocarditis encefalomiocarditis
encephalon encéfalo
encephalonarcosis encefalonarcosis
encephalopathia encefalopatía
encephalopathy encefalopatía
encephalopsy encefalopsia
encephalopsychosis encefalopsicosis
encephalopyosis encefalopiosis
encephalorrhagia encefalorragia
encephaloschisis encefalosquisis
encephalosclerosis encefaloesclerosis
encephaloscope encefaloscopio
encephaloscopy encefaloscopia
encephalosis encefalosis
encephalothlipsis encefalotlipsis
encephalotome encefalótomo
encephalotomy encefalotomía
encephalotrigeminal encefalotrigeminal
encephalotrigeminal angiomatosis
  angiomatosis encefalotrigeminal
encephalotrigeminal vascular syndrome
  síndrome vascular encefalotrigeminal
encode codificar
encoding codificación
encopresis encopresis
encounter encuentro
encounter group grupo de encuentro
encounter movement movimiento de
  encuentro
encouragement aliento
encryption encripción
enculturation enculturación
end brush cepillo terminal
end button botón terminal
end foot pie terminal
end organ órgano terminal
end plate placa terminal
end-plate potential potencial de placa
  terminal
end pleasure placer final
end spurt arranque final
end state estado final
end test prueba final
endarterectomy endarterectomía
endemic endémico
endemic neuritis neuritis endémica
endemic paralytic vertigo vértigo paralítico
  endémico
endoaneurysmoplasty endoaneurismoplastía
endoaneurysmorrhaphy endoaneurismorrafia
endocarditis endocarditis
endocathection endocatección
endocept endocepto
endocrine endocrino
endocrine disorder trastorno endocrino
endocrine gland glándula endocrina
endocrinism endocrinismo
endocrinological endocrinológico
endocrinological disorder trastorno

endocrinológico
endocrinology endocrinología
endocrinopathy endocrinopatía
endoderm endodermo
endogamy endogamia
endogenesis endogénesis
endogenetic endogenético
endogenetic factors factores endogenéticos
endogenic endogénico
endogenic factors factores endogénicos
endogenomorphic endogenomórfico
endogenomorphic depression depresión
  endogenomórfica
endogenomorphic syndrome síndrome
  endogenomórfico
endogenous endógeno
endogenous clock reloj endógeno
endogenous depression depresión endógena
endogenous factors factores endógenos
endogenous opioid opioide endógeno
endogenous rhythm ritmo endógeno
endogenous smile sonrisa endógena
endogenous stimulation estimulación
  endógena
endogenous thyrotoxicosis tirotoxicosis
  endógena
endogeny endogenia
endolymph endolinfa
endolymphatic potential potencial
  endolinfático
endometrial cycle ciclo endometrial
endometritis endometritis
endometrium endometrio
endomorph endomorfo
endomorphic endomórfico
endomorphy endomorfia
endomusia endomusia
endoneuritis endoneuritis
endonuclease endonucleasa
endoperineuritis endoperineuritis
endophasia endofasia
endoplasmic reticulum retículo endoplásmico
endopsychic endopsíquico
endopsychic censor censor endopsíquico
endopsychic perception percepción
  endopsíquica
endopsychic structure estructura
  endopsíquica
endoreactive endoreactivo
endorphin endorfina
endorphin hypothesis hipótesis de endorfinas
enduring perdurable
enelicomorphism enelicomorfismo
enema enema
enema addiction adicción a enemas
enema drug administration administración de
  drogas por enema
energizer energizador
energy energía
energy lack falta de energía
enervation enervación
enforced treatment tratamiento forzado
Engelmann's disease enfermedad de
  Engelmann
engineering model modelo de ingeniería

engineering psychologist psicólogo de
  ingeniería
engineering psychology psicología de
  ingeniería
engram engrama
engraphia engrafia
engross absorber
engrossment absorción
enissophobia enisofobia
enjoyment disfrute
enkephalin encefalina
enmeshment enredamiento
enomania enomanía
enosimania enosimanía
enosiophobia enosiofobia
enriched enriquecido
enriched environment ambiente enriquecido
enrichment enriquecimiento
enrichment program programa de
  enriquecimiento
entasia entasia
entasis entasis
entatic entático
entelechy entelequia
enteric virus virus entérico
enteric virus infection infección por virus
  entérico
enteroceptor enteroceptor
enterogastric reflex reflejo enterogástrico
enthlasis entlasis
entitlement derecho
entity entidad
entoderm entodermo
entomophobia entomofobia
entoptic entóptico
entrapment entrampamiento
entrapment neuropathy neuropatía de
  entrampamiento
entropy entropía
entry behavior conducta de entrada
enuresis enuresis
enuretic enurético
enuretic absence ausencia enurética
environment ambiente
environment-centered services servicios
  centrados en el ambiente
environment modification modificación de
  ambiente
environmental ambiental
environmental approach acercamiento
  ambiental
environmental assessment evaluación
  ambiental
environmental attribution atribución
  ambiental
environmental change cambio ambiental
environmental demand exigencia ambiental
environmental deprivation privación
  ambiental
environmental design diseño ambiental
environmental determinant determinante
  ambiental
environmental determination determinación
  ambiental
environmental disadvantage desventaja

ambiental
environmental education educación ambiental
environmental effects efectos ambientales
environmental effects on cognitive development efectos ambientales en el desarrollo cognitivo
environmental enhancement realzado ambiental
environmental enrichment enriquecimiento ambiental
environmental enrichment model modelo de enriquecimiento ambiental
environmental esthetics estética ambiental
environmental experimentation experimentación ambiental
environmental hazards riesgos ambientales
environmental instability inestabilidad ambiental
environmental-learning theory teoría de aprendizaje ambiental
environmental-load theory teoría de carga ambiental
environmental manipulation manipulación ambiental
environmental measures medidas ambientales
environmental modification modificación ambiental
environmental-mold trait rasgo de molde ambiental
environmental noise ruido ambiental
environmental privation privación ambiental
environmental psychology psicología ambiental
environmental stimulation estimulación ambiental
environmental stress estrés ambiental
environmental-stress theory teoría de estrés ambiental
environmental therapy terapia ambiental
environmental toxins toxinas ambientales
environmentalism ambientalismo
environmentalist ambientalista
envy envidia
enzygotic encigótico
enzygotic twins gemelos encigóticos
enzyme enzima
enzyme genes genes de enzimas
enzyme induction inducción de enzimas
eonism eonismo
eosinophil adenoma adenoma eosinófilo
eosinophilic meningoencephalitis meningoencefalitis eosinófila
eosophobia eosofobia
ependyma epéndimo
ependymal cyst quiste ependimario
ependymitis ependimitis
ependymoblastoma ependimoblastoma
ependymoma ependimoma
ephebiatrics efebiatría
ephedrine efedrina
ephemeral efímero
ephemeral mania manía efímera
epicritic epicrítico
epicritic sensation sensación epicrítica
epicritic sensibility sensibilidad epicrítica

epicritic system sistema epicrítico
epidemic epidemia
epidemic catalepsy catalepsia epidémica
epidemic cerebrospinal meningitis meningitis cerebroespinal epidémica
epidemic encephalitis encefalitis epidémica
epidemic hysteria histeria epidémica
epidemic myalgic encephalomyelitis encefalomielitis miálgica epidémica
epidemic myalgic encephalomyelopathy encefalomielopatía miálgica epidémica
epidemic neuromyasthenia neuromiastenia epidémica
epidemic tetany tetania epidémica
epidemic vertigo vértigo epidémico
epidemiology epidemiología
epidemiology of mental disorders epidemiología de trastornos mentales
epidermis epidermis
epididymis epidídimo
epididymitis epididimitis
epidural epidural
epidural block bloqueo epidural
epidural hematoma hematoma epidural
epidural meningitis meningitis epidural
epidurography epidurografía
epigastric epigástrico
epigastric reflex reflejo epigástrico
epigenesis epigénesis
epigenetic epigenético
epigenetic principle principio epigenético
epigenetic theory teoría epigenética
epiglottis epiglotis
epilempsis epilempsia
epilepsia nutans epilepsia nutatoria
epilepsia partialis continua epilepsia parcial continua
epilepsy epilepsia
epileptic epiléptico
epileptic absence ausencia epiléptica
epileptic aura aura epiléptica
epileptic cephalea cefalea epiléptica
epileptic character carácter epiléptico
epileptic clouded state estado enturbado epiléptico
epileptic cry grito epiléptico
epileptic dementia demencia epiléptica
epileptic deterioration deterioración epiléptica
epileptic disorder trastorno epiléptico
epileptic equivalent equivalente epiléptico
epileptic furor furor epiléptico
epileptic personality personalidad epiléptica
epileptic psychopathic constitution constitución psicopática epiléptica
epileptic psychosis psicosis epiléptica
epileptiform epileptiforme
epileptiform neuralgia neuralgia epileptiforme
epileptiform seizure acceso epileptiforme
epileptogenic epileptogénico
epileptogenic encephalopathy encefalopatía epileptogénica
epileptogenic foci focos epileptogénicos
epileptogenic lesion lesión epileptogénica

epileptogenic zone zona epileptogénica
epileptogenous epileptógeno
epileptoid epileptoide
epiloia epiloia
epimenorrhagia epimenorragia
epinephrine epinefrina
epinosic epinósico
epinosic gain ganancia epinósica
epinosis epinosis
epiphenomenalism epifenomenalismo
epiphenomenon epifenómeno
epiphysiopathy epifisiopatía
epiphysis epífisis
episode episodio
episodic episódico
episodic amnesia amnesia episódica
episodic-behavior disorder trastorno de conducta episódica
episodic disorder trastorno episódico
episodic dyscontrol descontrol episódico
episodic dyscontrol syndrome síndrome de descontrol episódico
episodic memory memoria episódica
episodic memory and Alzheimer's disease memoria episódica y enfermedad de Alzheimer
episodic processes procesos episódicos
epispadias epispadias
epistasis epistasis
epistemic epistémico
epistemology epistemología
epistemophilia epistemofilia
epithalamus epitálamo
epithelioma epitelioma
epithelium epitelio
epoch época
epochal amnesia amnesia de época
eponym epónimo
epsilon épsilon
epsilon alcoholism alcoholismo épsilon
epsilon motion moción épsilon
epsilon movement movimiento épsilon
Epstein's symptom síntoma de Epstein
Epstein-Barr virus virus de Epstein-Barr
equal and unequal cases method método de casos iguales y desiguales
equal-appearing-intervals method método de intervalos aparentemente iguales
equal-interval scale escala de intervalos iguales
equality igualdad
equality law ley de igualdad
equality stage etapa de igualdad
equalization igualación
equalization of excitation igualación de excitación
equated scores puntuaciones igualadas
equation ecuación
equatorial plane plano ecuatorial
equilibration equilibración
equilibrium equilibrio
equine encephalitis encefalitis equina
equine gait marcha equina
equinophobia equinofobia
equipment equipo

equipment design diseño de equipo
equipotentiality equipotencialidad
equipotentiality law ley de equipotencialidad
equipotentiality of cues equipotencialidad de señales
equity equidad
equity stage etapa de equidad
equity theory teoría de equidad
equity theory of attraction teoría de equidad de atracción
equivalence equivalencia
equivalence belief creencia de equivalencia
equivalence coefficient coeficiente de equivalencia
equivalence of cues equivalencia de señales
equivalent equivalente
equivalent form forma equivalente
equivalent form reliability confiabilidad de forma equivalente
equivalent groups grupos equivalentes
equivalent groups procedure procedimiento de grupos equivalentes
equivalents method método de equivalentes
Erb's atrophy atrofia de Erb
Erb's disease enfermedad de Erb
Erb's palsy parálisis de Erb
Erb's paralysis parálisis de Erb
Erb's sign signo de Erb
Erb's spinal paralysis parálisis espinal de Erb
Erb-Charcot disease enfermedad de Erb-Charcot
Erb-Goldflam syndrome síndrome de Erb-Goldflam
Erb-Westphal sign signo de Erb-Westphal
Erdheim tumor tumor de Erdheim
erect erecto
erectile eréctil
erectile dysfunction disfunción eréctil
erection erección
erector-spinal reflex reflejo erector-espinal
eremiophobia eremiofobia
eremophilia eremofilia
eremophobia eremofobia
erethism eretismo
erethismic eretísmico
erethistic eretístico
erethistic shock choque eretístico
erethitic eretítico
erethizophrenia eretizofrenia
erethizophrenic eretizofrénico
ereuthophobia ereutofobia
erg ergio
ergasia ergasia
ergasiomania ergasiomanía
ergasiophobia ergasiofobia
ergastic ergástico
ergastoplasm ergastoplasma
ergic érgico
ergic trait rasgo érgico
ergodialepsis ergodialepsia
ergograph ergógrafo
ergomania ergomanía
ergonomics ergonomía
ergophobia ergofobia
ergopsychometry ergopsicometría

ergot cornezuelo de centeno
ergotamine ergotamina
ergotherapy ergoterapia
ergotism ergotismo
ergotropic ergotrópico
ergotropic process proceso ergotrópico
ergotropic system sistema ergotrópico
Erichsen's disease enfermedad de Erichsen
erogeneity erogeneidad
erogenous erógeno
erogenous zone zona erógena
Eros Eros
erosion erosión
erotic erótico
erotic apathy apatía erótica
erotic-arousal pattern patrón de despertamiento erótico
erotic character carácter erótico
erotic delusion delusión erótica
erotic instinct instinto erótico
erotic paranoia paranoia erótica
erotic pyromania piromanía erótica
erotic seizure acceso erótico
erotic transference transferencia erótica
erotic type tipo erótico
erotic zoophilism zoofilismo erótico
eroticism erotismo
eroticize erotizar
eroticized erotizado
eroticized fantasy fantasía erotizada
erotism erotismo
erotization erotización
erotized erotizado
erotized anxiety ansiedad erotizada
erotized hanging ahorcadura erotizada
erotocrat erotócrata
erotogenesis erotogénesis
erotogenetic erotogenético
erotogenic erotogénico
erotogenic masochism masoquismo erotogénico
erotogenic zone zona erotogénica
erotographomania erotografomanía
erotolalia erotolalia
erotomania erotomanía
erotomanic erotomaníaco
erotomanic delusional state estado delusorio erotomaníaca
erotomanic type tipo erotomaníaco
erotopathic erotopático
erotopathy erotopatía
erotophobia erotofobia
erratic errático
error error
error analysis análisis de errores
error attribution atribución de error
error of estimate error de estimado
error of measurement error de medición
error of variance error de varianza
eructation eructación
erythermalgia eritermalgia
erythralgia eritralgia
erythredema eritredema
erythredema polyneuritis polineuritis eritredema

erythrism eritrismo
erythrocyte sedimentation rate tasa de sedimentación de eritrocitos
erythroleukoblastosis eritroleucoblastosis
erythromelalgia eritromelalgia
erythrophobia eritrofobia
erythroprosopalgia eritroprosopalgia
erythropsia eritropsia
escape escape
escape-avoidance learning aprendizaje de escape-evitación
escape behavior conducta de escape
escape conditioning condicionamiento de escape
escape drinking beber de escape
escape from freedom escape de libertad
escape from reality escape de la realidad
escape into illness escape a enfermedad
escape learning aprendizaje de escape
escape mechanism mecanismo de escape
escape phenomenon fenómeno de escape
escape training entrenamiento de escape
escapism escapismo
Escherich's sign signo de Escherich
eserine eserina
esoethmoiditis esoetmoiditis
esophageal achalasia acalasia esofagal
esophageal neurosis neurosis esofagal
esophageal voice voz esofagal
esophagosalivary reflex reflejo esofagosalival
esophoria esoforia
esotropia esotropía
essay test prueba de ensayo
essence esencia
essential esencial
essential alcoholism alcoholismo esencial
essential anosmia anosmia esencial
essential dysmenorrhea dismenorrea esencial
essential hypertension hipertensión esencial
essential tremor temblor esencial
establishment establecimiento
esteem estima
esteem need necesidad de estima
esthematology estematología
esthesia estesia
esthesiodic estesiódico
esthesiodic system sistema estesiódico
esthesiogenesis estesiogénesis
esthesiogenic estesiogénico
esthesiography estesiografía
esthesiology estesiología
esthesiometer estesiómetro
esthesiometry estesiometría
esthesioneuroblastoma estesioneuroblastoma
esthesioneurocytoma estesioneurocitoma
esthesioneurosis estesioneurosis
esthesionosus estesionosis
esthesiophysiology estesiofisiología
esthesioscopy estesioscopia
esthesodic estesódico
esthetic estético
esthetic pleasure placer estético
esthetic value valor estético
esthetics estética
estimate estimado

estimation estimación
estradiol estradiol
estrangement alienación
estriol estriol
estrogen estrógeno
estromania estromanía
estrone estrona
estrous behavior conducta estrual
estrus estro
estrus cycle ciclo estrual
état état
état crible état crible
eternal suckling amamantamiento eterno
ethambutol etambutol
ethanol etanol
ethanol intoxication intoxicación por etanol
ethanolism etanolismo
ethchlorvynol etclorvinol
ether éter
ether convulsion convulsión por éter
ether effects efectos del éter
etheromania eteromanía
ethical ético
ethical approach acercamiento ético
ethical conflict conflicto ético
ethical imperative imperativo ético
ethical issues cuestiones éticas
ethical issues and informed consent
cuestiones éticas y consentimiento
informado
ethical issues in classification cuestiones
éticas en la clasificación
ethical issues in correctional psychology
cuestiones éticas en la psicología
correccional
ethical issues in education cuestiones éticas
en la educación
ethical issues in malpractice cuestiones éticas
en la negligencia profesional
ethical issues in psychiatry cuestiones éticas
en la psiquiatría
ethical issues in psychology cuestiones éticas
en la psicología
ethical issues in right to treatment cuestiones
éticas en el derecho a tratamiento
ethical principles principios éticos
ethical problems problemas éticos
ethical risk hypothesis hipótesis de riesgo
ético
ethical theories teorías éticas
ethical treatment tratamiento ético
ethical treatment of animals tratamiento ético
de animales
ethics ética
ethinamate etinamato
ethmocephaly etmocefalia
ethnic étnico
ethnic factors factores étnicos
ethnic group grupo étnico
ethnic psychosis psicosis étnica
ethnocentrism etnocentrismo
ethnocentrism scale escala de etnocentrismo
ethnographic etnográfico
ethnographic approach acercamiento
etnográfico

ethnography etnografía
ethnological etnológico
ethnological study estudio etnológico
ethnology etnología
ethnomethodology etnometodología
ethnopsychiatry etnopsiquiatría
ethnopsychology etnopsicología
ethnopsychopharmacology
etnopsicofarmacología
ethnoscience etnociencia
ethnosemantics etnosemántica
ethogram etograma
ethological etológico
ethological model of personal space modelo
etológico del espacio personal
ethologist etólogo
ethology etología
ethopharmacology etofarmacología
ethopropazine etopropazina
ethosuximide etosuximida
ethyl alcohol alcohol etílico
ethylamine etilamina
ethylphenacemide etilfenacemida
etic ético
etiologic etiológico
etiologic factors factores etiológicos
etiologic factors in accidents factores
etiológicos en accidentes
etiological etiológico
etiological validity validez etiológica
etiology etiología
etiology of depression etiología de depresión
etiology of eating disorders etiología de
trastornos del comer
etryptamine etriptamina
eudemonia eudemonia
euergasia euergasia
eufunction eufunción
eugenic eugénico
eugenics eugenesia
eugenism eugenismo
eugnosia eugnosia
Eulenburg's disease enfermedad de
Eulenburg
eumetria eumetría
eumorphic eumórfico
eunoia eunoia
eunuch eunuco
eunuchoid eunucoide
eunuchoidism eunucoidismo
euosmia euosmia
euphoretic euforético
euphoria euforia
euphoriant euforígeno
euphoric eufórico
euphoric apathy apatía eufórica
euphoric mood humor eufórico
euphorohallucinogen euforoalucinógeno
eupraxia eupraxia
eurhythmia euritmia
eurotophobia eurotofobia
eurymorph eurimorfo
euryplastic euriplástico
eusthenic eusténico
eustress euestrés

eutelegenesis eutelegenesia
euthanasia eutanasia
euthenics euténica
euthymia eutimia
euthymic eutímico
euthymic mood humor eutímico
eutonic eutónico
eutychia eutiquia
evaluated evaluado
evaluated time tiempo evaluado
evaluation evaluación
evaluation apprehension aprehensión de
 evaluación
evaluation contract contrato de evaluación
evaluation dissemination diseminación de
 evaluación
evaluation interview entrevista de evaluación
evaluation of research evaluación de
 investigación
evaluation of training evaluación de
 entrenamiento
evaluation research investigación de
 evaluación
evaluation utilization utilización de
 evaluación
evaluative evaluativo
evaluative ratings clasificaciones evaluativas
evaluative reasoning razonamiento evaluativo
evaluator evaluador
evasion evasión
evasive evasivo
event evento
event-related brain potential potencial
 cerebral relacionado a evento
event-related euphoria euforia relacionada a
 evento
event-related potential potencial relacionado
 a evento
event sequence secuencia de eventos
event uncertainty incertidumbre de eventos
eversion eversión
eversion theory teoría de eversión
eversion theory of aging teoría de eversión de
 envejecimiento
evil eye mal de ojo
eviration eviración
evisceroneurotomy evisceroneurotomía
evocative evocador
evocative memory memoria evocadora
evocative therapy terapia evocadora
evoke evocar
evoked evocado
evoked potential potencial evocado
evoked response respuesta evocada
evolutility evolutilidad
evolution evolución
evolution of brain evolución del cerebro
evolution theory teoría de evolución
evolutionary theory teoría evolutiva
ex-patient ex paciente
ex-patient club club de ex pacientes
ex post facto ex post facto
ex post facto research investigación ex post
 facto
exacerbate exacerbar

exact replication replicación exacta
exafference exaferencia
exaggeration exageración
exaggeration in wit exageración en gracia
exaltation exaltación
exalted exaltado
exalted paranoia paranoia exaltada
examination examinación
examination anxiety ansiedad de examinación
examination dream sueño de examinación
exception excepción
exceptional excepcional
exceptional child niño excepcional
exceptional memory memoria excepcional
excessive excesivo
excessive daytime sleepiness somnolencia
 diurna excesiva
excessive somnolence somnolencia excesiva
excessively excesivamente
excessively loud speech habla excesivamente
 alta
excessively soft speech habla excesivamente
 suave
exchange theory teoría de intercambio
excitability excitabilidad
excitability of neuron excitabilidad de
 neurona
excitable excitable
excitant excitante
excitation excitación
excitation and conduction excitación y
 conducción
excitation gradient gradiente de excitación
excitatory excitatorio
excitatory agent agente excitatorio
excitatory conditioning condicionamiento
 excitatorio
excitatory field campo excitatorio
excitatory-inhibitory processes procesos
 excitatorios-inhibitorios
excitatory irradiation irradiación excitatoria
excitatory-postsynaptic potential potencial
 postsináptico excitatorio
excitatory potential potencial excitatorio
excitatory state estado excitatorio
excitatory synapse sinapsis excitatoria
excitatory threshold umbral excitatorio
excited excitado
excited catatonia catatonía excitada
excitement excitación
excitement-calm excitación-calma
excitement phase fase de excitación
excitement phase of sexual response fase de
 excitación de respuesta sexual
excitomotor excitomotor
exclamation exclamación
exclamation theory teoría de exclamación
exclusion exclusión
exclusion criteria criterios de exclusión
excoriation excoriación
excrement excremento
executive ejecutivo
executive area área ejecutiva
executive ego function función del ego
 ejecutivo

executive information system sistema de información ejecutiva
executive organ órgano ejecutivo
executive selection selección ejecutiva
executive stress estrés ejecutivo
exencephalia exencefalia
exencephalic exencefálico
exencephalocele exencefalocele
exencephalous exencéfalo
exencephaly exencefalia
exercise ejercicio
exercise activity actividad de ejercicio
exercise as coping behavior ejercicio como conducta para bregar
exercise as distraction ejercicio como distracción
exercise cycle ciclo de ejercicio
exercise frequency frecuencia de ejercicio
exercise intensity intensidad de ejercicio
exercise law ley de ejercicio
exercise psychology psicología de ejercicio
exhaustion agotamiento
exhaustion death muerte por agotamiento
exhaustion delirium delirio de agotamiento
exhaustion phase fase de agotamiento
exhaustion psychosis psicosis de agotamiento
exhaustion stage etapa de agotamiento
exhaustion state estado de agotamiento
exhaustive exhaustivo
exhaustive search búsqueda exhaustiva
exhaustive stupor estupor exhaustivo
exhibitionism exhibicionismo
exhibitionist exhibicionista
exhibitionistic exhibicionista
exhibitionistic need necesidad exhibicionista
exhilarant exhilarante
existence existencia
existence need necesidad de existencia
existential existencial
existential analysis análisis existencial
existential anxiety ansiedad existencial
existential crisis crisis existencial
existential ego function función del ego existencial
existential-humanistic therapy terapia existencial-humanística
existential living vivir existencial
existential neurosis neurosis existencial
existential phenomenology fenomenología existencial
existential psychiatry psiquiatría existencial
existential psychoanalysis psicoanálisis existencial
existential psychology psicología existencial
existential psychotherapy psicoterapia existencial
existential school escuela existencial
existential therapy terapia existencial
existential vacuum vacío existencial
existentialism existencialismo
exit event evento de salida
exit interview entrevista de salida
exocathection exocatección
exocrine exocrino
exocrine gland glándula exocrina

exocytosis exocitosis
exogamy exogamia
exogenesis exogénesis
exogenetic exogenético
exogenic exogénico
exogenous exógeno
exogenous depression depresión exógena
exogenous factors factores exógenos
exogenous smile sonrisa exógena
exogenous stimulation estimulación exógena
exogenous stress estrés exógeno
exon exón
exonerative exonerativo
exonerative moral reasoning razonamiento moral exonerativo
exophoria exoforia
exophthalmia exoftalmía
exophthalmos exoftalmos
exophthalmus exoftalmos
exopsychic exopsíquico
exorcism exorcismo
exosomatic exosomático
exosomatic method método exosomático
exosomatic technique técnica exosomática
exotic exótico
exotic bias sesgo exótico
exotic psychosis psicosis exótica
exotropia exotropía
expanded consciousness conciencia expandida
expansion expansión
expansive expansivo
expansive delusion delusión expansiva
expansive ideas ideas expansivas
expansive mood humor expansivo
expansiveness expansividad
expectancy expectación
expectancy chart gráfica de expectación
expectancy theory teoría de expectación
expectancy-value theory teoría de expectaciones-valores
expectation expectación
expectation neurosis neurosis de expectación
expected frequency frecuencia esperada
expected value valor esperado
expediter coordinador
experience experiencia
experiential experiencial
experiential group grupo experiencial
experiential psychotherapy psicoterapia experiencial
experiment experimento
experimental experimental
experimental aesthetics estética experimental
experimental allergic encephalitis encefalitis alérgica experimental
experimental allergic encephalomyelitis encefalomielitis alérgica experimental
experimental analysis análisis experimental
experimental analysis of behavior análisis de conducta experimental
experimental bias sesgo experimental
experimental condition condición experimental
experimental control control experimental
experimental design diseño experimental

experimental disorder trastorno experimental
experimental error error experimental
experimental esthetics estética experimental
experimental extinction extinción experimental
experimental factor factor experimental
experimental group grupo experimental
experimental hypothesis hipótesis experimental
experimental marriage matrimonio experimental
experimental method método experimental
experimental neurasthenia neurastenia experimental
experimental neurosis neurosis experimental
experimental pain dolor experimental
experimental psychology psicología experimental
experimental psychotherapy psicoterapia experimental
experimental realism realismo experimental
experimental series serie experimental
experimental variable variable experimental
experimental variables in sleep studies variables experimentales en estudios de sueño
experimentally induced conflicts conflictos inducidos experimentalmente
experimenter experimentador
experimenter bias sesgo del experimentador
experimenter effects efectos del experimentador
experimenter-expectancy effect efecto de las expectaciones del experimentador
expert witness testigo perito
expiation expiación
expiatory expiatorio
expiatory punishment castigo expiatorio
explanation explicación
explanation of behavior explicación de conducta
explicit explícito
explicit behavior conducta explícita
explicit role papel explícito
exploitation explotación
exploitation of children explotación de niños
exploitative explotador
exploitative character carácter explotador
exploitative-manipulative behavior conducta explotadora-manipulativa
exploitative orientation orientación explotadora
exploitative personality personalidad explotadora
exploiting explotador
exploiting type tipo explotador
exploration exploración
exploration drive impulso de exploración
exploratory exploratorio
exploratory behavior conducta exploratoria
exploratory drive impulso exploratorio
exploratory insight-oriented psychotherapy psicoterapia orientada a la penetración exploratoria
exploratory study estudio exploratorio

explosion readiness disposición de explosión
explosive explosivo
explosive aggressive behavior conducta agresiva explosiva
explosive disorder trastorno explosivo
explosive personality personalidad explosiva
explosive personality disorder trastorno de personalidad explosiva
explosive speech habla explosiva
exposition exposición
exposition attitude actitud de exposición
exposition need necesidad de exposición
exposure exposición
exposure deafness sordera por exposición
exposure learning aprendizaje por exposición
exposure to aggression and imitation exposición a agresión e imitación
expressed emotion emoción expresada
expressed emotionality emocionalidad expresada
expression expresión
expression method método de expresión
expression of affect expresión de afecto
expression of anger expresión de ira
expression of disgust expresión de repugnancia
expression of enjoyment expresión de disfrute
expression of fear expresión de temor
expressive expresivo
expressive amimia amimia expresiva
expressive amusia amusia expresiva
expressive aphasia afasia expresiva
expressive arts artes expresivas
expressive behavior conducta expresiva
expressive dysphasia disfasia expresiva
expressive language disorder trastorno del lenguaje expresivo
expressive language skills destrezas del lenguaje expresivas
expressive methods métodos expresivos
expressive movements movimientos expresivos
expressive pattern patrón expresivo
expressive therapy terapia expresiva
expressivity expresividad
extended care cuidado extendido
extended family familia extendida
extended-family therapy terapia de familia extendida
extended stay estadía extendida
extended-stay review revisión de estadía extendida
extension extensión
extension reflex reflejo de extensión
extensor extensor
extensor tetanus tétanos extensor
exteriorization exteriorización
exteriorize exteriorizar
external externo
external aim fin externo
external auditory meatus meato auditivo externo
external boundary límite externo
external capsule cápsula externa

external chemical messenger mensajero
  químico externo
external ear oído externo
external factors factores externos
external factors in aggression factores
  externos en agresión
external genitalia genitales externos
external granular layer capa granular externa
external hair cells of ear células pilosas
  externas del oído
external hydrocephalus hidrocefalia externa
external inhibition inhibición externa
external malleolar sign signo maleolar
  externo
external meningitis meningitis externa
external oblique reflex reflejo oblicuo
  externo
external pyocephalus piocefalia externa
external sense sentido externo
external stimuli estímulos externos
external stimuli during sleep estímulos
  externos durante el sueño
external stimuli prior to sleep estímulos
  externos antes del sueño
external trauma trauma externo
external validity validez externa
externalization externalización
externalization of problems externalización
  de problemas
externalizing externalizante
externalizing behavior conducta
  externalizante
externalizing-internalizing
  externalizante-internalizante
exteroceptive exteroceptivo
exteroceptive conditioning condicionamiento
  exteroceptivo
exteroceptor exteroceptor
exterofective exterofectivo
exteropsychic exteropsíquico
extinction extinción
extinction in learning extinción en
  aprendizaje
extinction inhibition inhibición de extinción
extinction of behavior extinción de conducta
extinction of behavior with hypnotism
  extinción de conducta con hipnotismo
extinction of ego extinción del ego
extinction phenomena fenómenos de
  extinción
extinction ratio razón de extinción
extinction techniques técnicas de extinción
extinction trial ensayo de extinción
extinguish extinguir
extinguished extinguido
extirpation extirpación
extracellular thirst sed extracelular
extraception extracepción
extracranial extracraneal
extracranial pneumatocele neumatocele
  extracraneal
extracranial pneumocele neumocele
  extracraneal
extractive extractivo
extractive disorder trastorno extractivo

extradimensional extradimensional
extradimensional shift cambio
  extradimensional
extradural extradural
extradural hematorrhachis hematorraquis
  extradural
extradural hemorrhage hemorragia
  extradural
extraindividual extraindividual
extraindividual behavior conducta
  extraindividual
extraintracranial bypass derivación
  extraintracraneal
extrajection extrayección
extramarital extramarital
extramarital intercourse relación
  extramarital
extramarital sex sexo extramarital
extrapineal pinealoma pinealoma extrapineal
extrapolate extrapolar
extrapsychic extrapsíquico
extrapsychic conflict conflicto extrapsíquico
extrapunitive extrapunitivo
extrapyramidal extrapiramidal
extrapyramidal disease enfermedad
  extrapiramidal
extrapyramidal dyskinesia discinesia
  extrapiramidal
extrapyramidal effect efecto extrapiramidal
extrapyramidal involvement envolvimiento
  extrapiramidal
extrapyramidal motor system sistema motor
  extrapiramidal
extrapyramidal syndrome síndrome
  extrapiramidal
extrapyramidal system sistema
  extrapiramidal
extrapyramidal tract tracto extrapiramidal
extrasensory extrasensorial
extrasensory perception percepción
  extrasensorial
extrasensory thought transference
  transferencia de pensamientos
  extrasensorial
extraspective extraspectivo
extraspective perspective perspectiva
  extraspectiva
extraspectral extraespectral
extraspectral hue matiz extraespectral
extrauterine pregnancy embarazo
  extrauterino
extraversion extraversión
extraversion-introversion
  extraversión-introversión
extravert extravertido
extraverted extravertido
extraverted type tipo extravertido
extreme extremo
extreme somatosensory evoked potential
  potencial evocado somatosensorial extremo
extremity extremidad
extrinsic extrínseco
extrinsic asthma asma extrínseca
extrinsic cortex corteza extrínseca
extrinsic eye muscles músculos de ojo

extrínsecos
extrinsic interest interés extrínseco
extrinsic motivation motivación extrínseca
extrinsic reward recompensa extrínseca
extrinsic thalamus tálamo extrínseco
extropunitive extropunitivo
extrospection extrospección
extroversion extroversión
extrovert extrovertido
eye bank banco de ojos
eye-closure reflex reflejo del cierre de ojo
eye contact contacto ocular
eye dominance dominancia de ojo
eye field campo de ojo
eye-hand coordination coordinación
  ojo-mano
eye-hand preference preferencia ojo-mano
eye movements movimientos de ojo
eye muscles músculos de ojo
eye position posición de ojo
eye preference preferencia de ojo
eye-roll sign signo del rodado de ojo
eye span lapso de ojo
eye structure estructura del ojo
eye-voice span lapso ojo-voz
eyeglasses espejuelos
eyelash sign signo de pestañas
eyelid conditioning condicionamiento de
  párpado
eyes versus cameras ojos contra cámaras
eyewitness testigo ocular
eyewitness testimony testimonio de testigo
  ocular

F

F body cuerpo F
F distribution distribución F
F ratio razón F
F scale escala F
F test prueba F
fable fábula
fables test prueba de fábulas
fabrication invención
Fabry's disease enfermedad de Fabry
fabulation fabulación
face-hand test prueba cara-mano
face recognition reconocimiento de caras
face saving salvamento de apariencias
face-saving behavior conducta de salvamento
  de apariencias
face-to-face cara a cara
face-to-face group grupo de cara a cara
face validity validez aparente
facial diplegia diplejía facial
facial disfigurement desfiguración facial
facial display demostración facial
facial expression expresión facial
facial hemiatrophy hemiatrofia facial
facial hemiplegia hemiplejía facial
facial nerve nervio facial
facial neuralgia neuralgia facial
facial palsy parálisis facial
facial paralysis parálisis facial
facial perception percepción facial
facial reflex reflejo facial
facial spasm espasmo facial
facial talk habla facial
facial tic tic facial
facial trophoneurosis trofoneurosis facial
facial vision visión facial
facialis phenomenon fenómeno facial
facies facies
facies dolorosa facies dolorosa
facilitation facilitación
facilitator facilitador
faciocephalalgia faciocefalalgia
faciolingual faciolingual
facioplegia facioplejía
facioscapulohumeral facioescapulohumeral
facioscapulohumeral atrophy atrofia
  facioescapulohumeral
facioscapulohumeral muscular dystrophy
  distrofia muscular facioescapulohumeral
fact-giver dador de datos
fact-seeker buscador de datos
factitial facticio
factitious facticio
factitious disorder trastorno facticio
factitious disorder with physical symptoms

trastorno facticio con síntomas físicos
factitious disorder with psychological symptoms trastorno facticio con síntomas psicológicos
factor factor
factor analysis análisis factorial
factor axes ejes factoriales
factor coefficient coeficiente factorial
factor-comparison method método de comparación factorial
factor configuration configuración factorial
factor loading carga factorial
factor matrix matriz factorial
factor of uniform density factor de densidad uniforme
factor reflection reflexión factorial
factor resolution resolución factorial
factor rotation rotación factorial
factor space espacio factorial
factor structure estructura factorial
factor theory teoría factorial
factor theory of learning teoría factorial de aprendizaje
factor theory of personality teoría factorial de personalidad
factor weight peso factorial
factorial design diseño factorial
factorial experiment experimento factorial
factorial invariance invarianza factorial
factoring factorización
factors influencing attachment factores que influencian el apego
factors influencing development factores que influencian el desarrollo
facts of life hechos de la vida
factual verídico
factual knowledge conocimiento verídico
facultative facultativo
faculty facultad
faculty psychology psicología de facultades
fad novedad
fading desvanecimiento
Fahr's disease enfermedad de Fahr
Fahr's syndrome síndrome de Fahr
failure fracaso
failure through success fracaso a través del éxito
failure to grow syndrome síndrome de fracaso en crecer
failure to mourn fracaso en enlutar
failure to thrive fracaso en medrar
failure to thrive syndrome síndrome de fracaso en medrar
failure to warn fracaso en avisar
faint (n) desmayo
faint (v) desmayarse
fainting desmayo
fairy tale cuento de hadas
faith cure cura por fe
faith healing curación por fe
fake fingir
faking fingimiento
fall chronometer cronómetro de caída
fallacy falacia
fallectomy falectomía

falling sickness enfermedad de caerse
Fallopian neuritis neuritis de Falopio
Fallopian-tube pregnancy embarazo de trompa de Falopio
Fallopian tubes trompas de Falopio
Falret's disease enfermedad de Falret
false falso
false alarm falsa alarma
false association asociación falsa
false conditioning condicionamiento falso
false confession confesión falsa
false-consensus bias sesgo de consenso falso
false euphoria euforia falsa
false masturbation masturbación falsa
false negative falsonegativo
false neuroma neuroma falso
false positive falsopositivo
false pregnancy embarazo falso
false recognition reconocimiento falso
false self yo falso
false transmitter transmisor falso
falsehood falsedad
falsetto falsete
falsifiable falsificable
falsifiable hypothesis hipótesis falsificable
falsification falsificación
falx cerebelli falx cerebelli
falx cerebri falx cerebri
familial familiar
familial amyloid neuropathy neuropatía amiloide familiar
familial amyloidosis amiloidosis familiar
familial bipolar disorder trastorno bipolar familiar
familial dysautonomia disautonomía familiar
familial encephalopathy encefalopatía familiar
familial factor factor familiar
familial hormonal disorder trastorno hormonal familiar
familial mental retardation retardo mental familiar
familial microcephaly microcefalia familiar
familial periodic paralysis parálisis periódica familiar
familial psychosis psicosis familiar
familial retardation retardo familiar
familial spinal muscular atrophy atrofia muscular espinal familiar
familial splenic anemia anemia esplénica familiar
familial unconscious inconsciente familiar
familianism familianismo
familiar familiar
familiar color color familiar
family familia
family and substance abuse familia y abuso de sustancias
family assessment evaluación familiar
family autonomy autonomía familiar
family care cuidado familiar
family circumstances circunstancias familiares
family conflict conflicto familiar
family constellation constelación familiar

family counseling asesoramiento familiar
family court corte familiar
family crisis crisis familiar
family culture cultura familiar
family discord discordia familiar
family education educación familiar
family environment ambiente familiar
family evaluation evaluación familiar
family friends amistades familiares
family functioning funcionamiento familiar
family group grupo familiar
family group intake entrevista inicial de grupo familiar
family group therapy terapia de grupo familiar
family history historial familiar
family history and psychosis historial familiar y psicosis
family identity identidad familiar
family incubus íncubo familiar
family instability inestabilidad familiar
family instability and suicidal behavior inestabilidad familiar y conducta suicida
family interaction method método de interacción familiar
family intervention intervención familiar
family law derecho familiar
family method método familiar
family neurosis neurosis familiar
family pattern patrón familiar
family planning planificación familiar
family resemblance semejanza familiar
family risk study estudio de riesgo familiar
family romance romance familiar
family social work trabajo social familiar
family structure estructura familiar
family studies estudios de familias
family support group grupo de apoyo familiar
family systems interview entrevista de sistemas de familia
family systems theory teoría de sistemas de familia
family therapy terapia familiar
family therapy for child abuse terapia familiar para abuso de hijos
family therapy for delinquency terapia familiar para delincuencia
family therapy for eating disorders terapia familiar para trastornos del comer
family therapy for psychosomatic problems terapia familiar para problemas psicosomáticos
family therapy for sexual problems terapia familiar para problemas sexuales
family type tipo familiar
family violence violencia familiar
fan sign signo de abanico
fanaticism fanatismo
Fanconi's anemia anemia de Fanconi
fantasm fantasma
fantasmic thinking pensamiento fantásmico
fantasy fantasía
fantasy absence ausencia de fantasía
fantasy cathexis catexis de fantasía

fantasy life vida de fantasía
fantasy period periodo de fantasía
far-field evoked potential potencial evocado de campo lejano
far point punto lejano
Farber's lipogranulomatosis lipogranulomatosis de Farber
farsightedness vista lejana
fascicular fascicular
fascicular degeneration degeneración fascicular
fascicular graft injerto fascicular
fascicular ophthalmoplegia oftalmoplejía fascicular
fasciculation fasciculación
fasciculi fascículos
fasciculi proprii fascículos propios
fasciculus fascículo
fasciculus cuneatus fascículo cuneiforme
fasciculus gracilis fascículo gracilis
fascinating fascinante
fascinating gaze mirada fija fascinante
fascination fascinación
fascinum mal de ojo
fasciolar gyrus circunvolución fasciolar
fashion moda
fashioning effect efecto formativo
fast rhythm ritmo rápido
fastidium cibi fastidium cibi
fastidium potus fastidium potus
fasting phase fase de ayuno
fatal fatal
fatal accident accidente fatal
fatal illness enfermedad fatal
fatalism fatalismo
fate destino
fate analysis análisis de destino
fate neurosis neurosis de destino
father's involvement with breast-feeding envolvimiento del padre con alimentación por pecho
father absence ausencia del padre
father blues depresión del padre
father-child relationship relación padre-hijo, relación padre-hija
father complex complejo paterno
father-daughter incest incesto padre-hija
father figure figura paterna
father fixation fijación en el padre
father hypnosis hipnosis paterna
father ideal ideal paterna
father imago imago paterno
father-infant interaction interacción de padre-infante
father substitute sustituto del padre
father surrogate sustituto del padre
fatigue fatiga
fatigue state estado de fatiga
fatigue studies estudios de fatiga
fatiguing vigil vigilia fatigante
fatuity fatuidad
faucial faucial
faucial paralysis parálisis faucial
faucial reflex reflejo faucial
fault falta

fausse reconnaissance fausse reconnaissance
faux de mieux faux de mieux
favoritism favoritismo
fear temor
fear appeal atracción por temor
fear conditioning condicionamiento de temor
fear drive impulso de temor
fear hypnosis hipnosis por temor
fear-induced inducido por temor
fear-induced aggression agresión inducida
  por temor
fear induction inducción de temor
fear of animals temor a animales
fear of being alone temor a estar solo
fear of being buried alive temor a ser
  enterrado vivo
fear of being enclosed temor a ser encerrado
fear of being touched temor a ser tocado
fear of blood temor a la sangre
fear of brain disease temor a enfermedad
  mental
fear of burglars temor a ladrones
fear of cats temor a gatos
fear of change temor al cambio
fear of childbirth temor al parto
fear of confinement temor a confinamiento
fear of contamination temor a contaminación
fear of corpses temor a cadáveres
fear of crowds temor a multitudes
fear of darkness temor a la obscuridad
fear of death temor a la muerte
fear of deformity temor a deformidad
fear of demons temor a demonios
fear of disease temor a enfermedad
fear of dismemberment temor de
  desmembración
fear of dogs temor a perros
fear of eating temor a comer
fear of eternity temor a la eternidad
fear of everything temor a todo
fear of failure temor al fracaso
fear of female genitals temor a genitales
  femeninos
fear of fire temor al fuego
fear of flying temor a volar
fear of food temor a comida
fear of ghosts temor a fantasmas
fear of heights temor a alturas
fear of injury temor a lesión
fear of innovation temor a innovación
fear of insanity temor a insania
fear of insects temor a insectos
fear of justice temor a justicia
fear of lightning temor a relámpagos
fear of loneliness temor a la soledad
fear of male genitals temor a genitales
  masculinos
fear of marriage temor al matrimonio
fear of medicine temor a la medicina
fear of men temor a hombres
fear of mice temor a ratones
fear of naked bodies temor a cuerpos
  desnudos
fear of night temor a la noche
fear of odors temor a olores

fear of pain temor al dolor
fear of people temor a gente
fear of pleasure temor al placer
fear of poison temor al veneno
fear of punishment temor al castigo
fear of rejection temor al rechazo
fear of sex temor al sexo
fear of sleep temor al sueño
fear of strangers temor a extraños
fear of success temor al éxito
fear of venereal disease temor a enfermedad
  venérea
fear of women temor a mujeres
fear response respuesta de temor
fear versus anxiety temor contra ansiedad
feasibility factibilidad
feasibility test prueba de factibilidad
feature característica
feature analysis análisis de características
feature comparison comparación de
  características
feature detector detector de características
feature indicator indicador de características
feature integration integración de
  características
feature model modelo de características
feature-profile test prueba de
  características-perfil
febrile febril
febrile convulsion convulsión febril
febrile psychosis psicosis febril
febriphobia febrifobia
feces heces
feces-child-penis concept concepto de
  heces-niño-pene
Fechner's approach acercamiento de Fechner
Fechner's colors colores de Fechner
Fechner's law ley de Fechner
Fechner's paradox paradoja de Fechner
fecundate fecundar
fecundation fecundación
fecundity fecundidad
fee-for-service plan plan de precio por
  servicio
feeble-mindedness debilidad mental
feedback retroalimentación
feedback control control de retroalimentación
feedback evaluation evaluación de
  retroalimentación
feedback loop ciclo de retroalimentación
feedback mechanism mecanismo de
  retroalimentación
feedback system sistema de retroalimentación
feeding alimentación
feeding behavior conducta de alimentación
feeding center centro de alimentación
feeding difficulty dificultad de alimentación
feeding disorder trastorno de alimentación
feeding habits hábitos de alimentación
feeding pattern patrón de alimentación
feeding problem problema de alimentación
feeding system sistema de alimentación
feeding technique técnica de alimentación
feeling sentimiento
feeling apperception apercepción de

sentimiento
feeling-talk habla de sentimientos
feeling theory of three dimensions teoría de sentimientos de tres dimensiones
feeling tone tono de sentimientos
feelings analysis análisis de sentimientos
feelings of unreality sentimientos de irrealidad
Feer's disease enfermedad de Feer
feign fingir
feigned fingido
feigned bereavement duelo fingido
Feingold hypothesis hipótesis de Feingold
fellatio felación
fellatio fantasy fantasía de felatorismo
fellation felación
fellator felator
fellatorism felatorismo
fellatrice felatriz
fellatrix felatriz
female femenino
female circumcision circuncisión femenina
female climacterium climaterio femenino
female dyspareunia dispareunia femenina
female dyspareunia due to general medical condition dispareunia femenina debido a condición médica general
female ejaculation eyaculación femenina
female genitalia genitales femeninos
female-genitals fear temor a los genitales femeninos
female hypoactive sexual desire disorder trastorno de deseo sexual hipoactivo femenino
female hypoactive sexual desire disorder due to general medical condition trastorno de deseo sexual hipoactivo femenino debido a condición médica general
female impersonator imitador de mujeres
female orgasmic disorder trastorno orgásmico femenino
female sexual arousal disorder trastorno de despertamiento sexual femenino
female sexual dysfunction disfunción sexual femenina
femaleness feminidad
feminine femenino
feminine identification identificación femenina
feminine identity identidad femenina
feminine masochism masoquismo femenino
femininity feminidad
femininity complex complejo de feminidad
feminism feminismo
feminist feminista
feminist psychotherapy psicoterapia feminista
feminist therapy terapia feminista
feminization feminización
femoral reflex reflejo femoral
femoroabdominal reflex reflejo femoroabdominal
fenestra ovalis fenestra ovalis
fenestra rotunda fenestra rotunda
fenestration fenestración
fenethylline fenetilina

fenfluramine fenfluramina
fenfluramine in autism fenfluramina en autismo
feral feral
feral child niño feral
Fere method método de Fere
Fere phenomenon fenómeno de Fere
Fereol-Graux palsy parálisis de Fereol-Graux
Fernald method método de Fernald
ferning cristalización en helecho
ferric chloride test prueba de cloruro férrico
ferrugination ferruginación
Ferry-Porter law ley de Ferry-Porter
fertility fertilidad
fertility rate tasa de fertilidad
fertilization fertilización
festinant festinante
festinant gait marcha festinante
festination festinación
fetal fetal
fetal activity actividad fetal
fetal adenoma adenoma fetal
fetal alcohol effect efecto del alcohol fetal
fetal alcohol syndrome síndrome del alcohol fetal
fetal attachment apego fetal
fetal barbital syndrome síndrome barbital fetal
fetal cephalometry cefalometría fetal
fetal death muerte fetal
fetal development desarrollo fetal
fetal distress angustia fetal
fetal infection infección fetal
fetal learning aprendizaje fetal
fetal malnutrition desnutrición fetal
fetal-maternal exchange intercambio fetal-maternal
fetal period periodo fetal
fetal response respuesta fetal
fetal screening cribado fetal
fetal stage etapa fetal
fetalism fetalismo
fetation fetación
fetish fetiche
fetishism fetichismo
fetishistic fetichístico
fetishistic cross-dressing transvestismo fetichístico
fetology fetología
fetus feto
fetus at risk feto a riesgo
fever fiebre
Fiamberti hypothesis hipótesis de Fiamberti
fiber fibra
fibril fibrilla
fibrillary fibrilar
fibrillary astrocyte astrocito fibrilar
fibrillary chorea corea fibrilar
fibrillary myoclonia mioclonía fibrilar
fibrillary neuroma neuroma fibrilar
fibrillary tremor temblor fibrilar
fibrillation fibrilación
fibriophobia fibriofobia
fibrogliosis fibrogliosis
fibroma fibroma

fibroneuroma fibroneuroma
fibropsammoma fibropsamoma
fibrosis fibrosis
fibrositic fibrosítico
fibrositic headache dolor de cabeza fibrosítico
fibrositis fibrositis
fibrous fibroso
fibrous astrocyte astrocito fibroso
fiction ficción
fictional ficticio
fictional finalism finalismo ficticio
fictitious ficticio
fictitious feeding alimentación ficticia
fidget inquietarse
fidgetiness inquietud
fidgety inquieto
fiducial fiduciario
fiducial limits límites fiduciarios
fiduciary fiduciario
fiduciary relation relación fiduciaria
field campo
field-cognition mode modo de cognición de campo
field defect defecto de campo
field dependence dependencia de campo
field experiment experimento de campo
field experimentation experimentación de campo
field force fuerza de campo
field independence independencia de campo
field independence-dependence independencia-dependencia de campo
field investigation investigación de campo
field of consciousness campo de conciencia
field of regard campo de mirada
field properties propiedades de campo
field research investigación de campo
field space espacio de campo
field structure estructura de campo
field teacher maestro de campo
field theory teoría de campo
field work trabajo de campo
fields of Forel campos de Forel
fight-flight assumption asunción de pelea-fuga
fight-flight reaction reacción de pelea-fuga
Figueira's syndrome síndrome de Figueira
figural figural
figural aftereffects efectos posteriores figurales
figural cohesion cohesión figural
figural synthesis síntesis figural
figurative figurativo
figurative knowledge conocimiento figurativo
figurative language lenguaje figurativo
figure figura
figure and ground figura y fondo
figure-drawing test prueba de dibujo de figuras
figure-ground figura-fondo
figure-ground distortion distorsión de figura-fondo
figure-ground perception percepción de figura-fondo

filial filial
filial generation generación filial
filial regression regresión filial
filial regression law ley de regresión filial
filicide filicidio
filiform papilla papila filiforme
filioparental filioparental
filled pause pausa rellenada
filler relleno
filler material material de relleno
film película
film color color de película
filter filtro
filter theory teoría de filtro
fimbria fimbria
final common path vía común final
final tendency tendencia final
finalism finalismo
Finckh test prueba de Finckh
fine motor motor fino
fine motor activity actividad de motor fino
fine motor coordination coordinación de motor fino
fine motor movement movimiento de motor fino
fine motor skills destrezas de motor fino
fine tremor temblor fino
finger agnosia agnosia digital
finger-biting morder de dedos
finger-biting behavior conducta del morder de dedos
finger-nose test prueba de dedo-nariz
finger painting pintura con dedos
finger phenomenon fenómeno del dedo
finger spelling deletreo con dedos
finger-thumb reflex reflejo dedo-pulgar
fire-setting behavior conducta del prender fuegos
first admission primera admisión
first aid primeros auxilios
first attack primer ataque
first cause primera causa
first-degree burn quemadura de primer grado
first impression primera impresión
first moment primer momento
first negative phase primera fase negativa
first-order correlation correlación de primera orden
first-order factor factor de primer orden
first phase of repression primera fase de represión
first-rank symptoms síntomas de primer rango
first-signal system sistema de primera señal
first signaling system primer sistema de señalamiento
first words primeras palabras
Fisch-Renwick syndrome síndrome de Fisch-Renwick
Fisher's syndrome síndrome de Fisher
Fisher's test prueba de Fisher
Fisher's Z-transformation transformación Z de Fisher
Fisher exact test prueba exacta de Fisher
fission fisión

fissure fisura
fissure of Rolando fisura de Rolando
fissure of Sylvius fisura de Silvio
fistula fístula
fit ajuste, ataque
fitness aptitud
fitness for trial aptitud para juicio
fitness level nivel de aptitud
fits of horrendous temptation ataques de
   tentación horrenda
Fitt's law ley de Fitt
five-day hospital hospital de cinco días
five-to-seven shift cambio de cinco a siete
fixate fijar
fixated fijo
fixated response respuesta fija
fixation fijación
fixation hysteria histeria de fijación
fixation line línea de fijación
fixation of affect fijación de afecto
fixation of attention fijación de atención
fixation pause pausa de fijación
fixation point punto de fijación
fixed fijo
fixed-action pattern patrón de acción fija
fixed alternative alternativa fija
fixed-effects fallacy falacia de efectos fijos
fixed factor factor fijo
fixed idea idea fija
fixed image imagen fija
fixed interval intervalo fijo
fixed-interval reinforcement schedule
   programa de refuerzo de intervalo fijo
fixed-interval schedule programa de intervalo
   fijo
fixed model modelo fijo
fixed pupil pupila fija
fixed ratio razón fija
fixed-ratio reinforcement schedule programa
   de refuerzo de razón fija
fixed-ratio schedule programa de razón fija
fixed reinforcement refuerzo fijo
fixed role papel fijo
fixed-role therapy terapia de papel fijo
fixed torticollis tortícolis fijo
fixedly fijamente
fixedness fijeza
fixity fijeza
flaccid fláccido
flaccid paralysis parálisis fláccida
flagellantism flagelantismo
flagellation flagelación
flagellomania flagelomanía
flap colgajo
flapping tremor temblor de aleteo
flashback escena retrospectiva
flashback hallucinosis alucinosis de escena
   retrospectiva
flashbulb memory memoria de lámpara de
   destello
flasher exhibicionista
flashing pain dolor relampagueante
flashing pain syndrome síndrome de dolor
   relampagueante
flat affect afecto insulso

flat electroencephalogram
   electroencefalograma plano
flat foot pie plano
flat top waves ondas de tope plano
Flatau's law ley de Flatau
Flatau-Schilder disease enfermedad de
   Flatau-Schilder
flattened affect afecto aplanado
flattening aplanamiento
flattening of affect aplanamiento de afecto
flavism flavismo
flavor sabor
Flesch formula fórmula de Flesch
Flesch index índice de Flesch
flexibilitas cerea flexibilitas cerea
flexible flexible
flexible work hours horas de trabajo flexibles
flexion flexión
flexion reflex reflejo de flexión
flexitime horario flexible
flexor flexor
flexor muscle músculo flexor
flexor reflex reflejo flexor
flexor tetanus tétanos flexor
flicker centelleo
flicker discrimination discriminación de
   centelleo
flicker frequency frecuencia de centelleo
flicker fusion point punto de fusión de
   centelleo
flicker sensitivity sensibilidad de centelleo
flicker stimulus estímulo de centelleo
flight fuga
flight from reality fuga de la realidad
flight into disease fuga a enfermedad
flight into fantasy fuga a fantasía
flight into health fuga a salud
flight into illness fuga a enfermedad
flight into reality fuga a realidad
flight of colors fuga de colores
flight of ideas fuga de ideas
flight or fight fuga o pelea
flight or fight response respuesta de fuga o
   pelea
flippancy ligereza
flippant ligero
floating flotante
floating affect afecto flotante
floating transference transferencia flotante
floccillation flocilación
flogger azotador
flogging the dead horse technique técnica de
   azotar al caballo muerto
flooding inundación
floor effect efecto de suelo
Flourens' theory teoría de Flourens
flow chart organigrama
flowery florido
fluanisone fluanisona
fluctuating ego states estados del ego
   fluctuantes
fluctuation fluctuación
fluctuation of attention fluctuación de
   atención
fluctuations of mood fluctuaciones del humor

fluency fluidez
fluency disorder trastorno de fluidez
fluent fluente
fluent aphasia afasia fluente
fluid fluido
fluid abilities habilidades fluidas
fluid intelligence inteligencia fluida
fluidazepam fluidazepam
fluidity fluidez
flunitrazepam flunitrazepam
fluoxetine fluoxetina
flupentixol flupentixol
fluphenazine flufenacina
flurazepam flurazepam
fluspirilene fluspirileno
flutazolam flutazolam
flutter aleteo
flying saucer platillo volador
Flynn-Aird syndrome síndrome de
    Flynn-Aird
focal focal
focal attention atención focal
focal-conflict theory teoría de conflictos
    focales
focal degeneration degeneración focal
focal dermal hypoplasia hipoplasia dermal
    focal
focal epilepsy epilepsia focal
focal length longitud focal
focal pathology patología focal
focal psychotherapy psicoterapia focal
focal sclerosis esclerosis focal
focal stress estrés focal
focal suicide suicidio focal
focal therapy terapia focal
focus foco
focus of attention foco de atención
focused enfocado
focused analysis análisis enfocado
focused delirium delirio enfocado
focusing enfoque
focusing disturbance disturbio de enfoque
focusing mechanism mecanismo de enfoque
Foix-Alajouanine myelitis mielitis de
    Foix-Alajouanine
folate folato
folic acid ácido fólico
folie folie
folie à cinq folie à cinq
folie à deux folie à deux
folie à double forme folie à double forme
folie à famille folie à famille
folie à pleusirs folie à pleusirs
folie à quatre folie à quatre
folie à trois folie à trois
folie circulaire folie circulaire
folie collective folie collective
folie communiquée folie communiquée
folie d'action folie d'action
folie démonomaniaque folie démonomaniaque
folie des grandeurs folie des grandeurs
folie des persécutions folie des persécutions
folie du doute folie du doute
folie du pourquoi folie du pourquoi
folie gémellaire folie gémellaire

folie hypocondriaque folie hypocondriaque
folie imitative folie imitative
folie imposée folie imposée
folie instantanée folie instantanée
folie morale folie morale
folie paralytique folie paralytique
folie pénitentiare folie pénitentiare
folie raisonnante folie raisonnante
folie simulée folie simulée
folie simultanè folie simultanè
folie systématisée folie systématisée
folie utérine folie utérine
folie vaniteuse folie vaniteuse
folium folium
folk healer curandero popular
folk healing curación popular
folk mind mente popular
folk psychiatry psiquiatría popular
folk psychology psicología popular
folk soul alma popular
folklore folclor
folkways cultura popular
follicle folículo
follicle-stimulating hormone hormona
    estimulante de folículos
Folling's disease enfermedad de Folling
Folling's test prueba de Folling
follow-through continuación
follow-up seguimiento
follow-up counseling asesoramiento de
    seguimiento
follow-up examination examinación de
    seguimiento
follow-up history historial de seguimiento
follow-up study estudio de seguimiento
following behavior conducta de seguir
following reaction reacción de seguir
fontanel fontanela
fontanelle fontanela
food additives aditivos de comida
food allergy alergia de comida
food aversion aversión de comida
food craving antojo de comidas
food deprivation privación de comidas
food faddism manía de comidas
food-intake regulation regulación de consumo
    de comida
food intolerance intolerancia de comida
food preferences preferencias de comida
food-satiation theory teoría de saciedad de
    comida
food self-selection autoselección de comida
food therapy terapia de comida
foot anesthesia anestesia de pie
foot-candle bujía-pie
foot-dragging arrastramiento de pie
foot drop caída de pie
foot fetishism fetichismo de pies
foot-in-the-door effect efecto del pie en la
    puerta
foot-in-the-door technique técnica del pie en
    la puerta
foot-lambert lambert-pie
for-profit hospital hospital con fines de lucro
foramen foramen

foramen magnum foramen magno
foraminal herniation herniación foraminal
foraminotomy foraminotomía
force fuerza
force field campo de fuerza
forced forzado
forced choice selección forzada
forced-choice technique técnica de
    selecciones forzadas
forced-choice test prueba de selecciones
    forzadas
forced displacement desplazamiento forzado
forced fantasy fantasía forzada
forced feeding alimentación forzada
forced grasping reflex reflejo de agarre
    forzado
forced impulses impulsos forzados
forced-response test prueba de respuestas
    forzadas
forced sex sexo forzado
forced treatment tratamiento forzado
forceps injury lesión por fórceps
forceps major fórceps mayor
forceps minor fórceps menor
forebrain cerebro anterior
forecasting pronosticación
forecasting efficiency eficiencia de
    pronosticación
foreconscious preconsciente
foredispleasure desplacer previo
foreground primer plano
foregrounding poner en primer plano
foreign accent acento extranjero
foreign language lenguaje extranjero
forensic forense
forensic assessment evaluación forense
forensic evaluation evaluación forense
forensic medicine medicina forense
forensic psychiatry psiquiatría forense
forensic psychology psicología forense
forensic uses of hypnotism usos forenses del
    hipnotismo
foreperiod preperiodo
foreplay excitación sexual previa
forepleasure placer previo
foreshortening escorzo
forget olvidar
forgetfulness olvido
forgetting olvidar
forgetting curve curva de olvido
form constancy constancia de forma
form discrimination discriminación de formas
form-function distinction distinción de
    forma-función
form-function relation relación de
    forma-función
form perception percepción de formas
form word palabra de forma
formal discipline disciplina formal
formal operations operaciones formales
formal operations stage etapa de operaciones
    formales
formal operatory level nivel operatorio
    formal
formal operatory period periodo operatorio

formal
formal operatory stage etapa operatoria
    formal
formal operatory thought pensamiento
    operatorio formal
formal organization organización formal
formal parallelism paralelismo formal
formal thought pensamiento formal
formal thought disorder trastorno de
    pensamiento formal
formalism formalismo
formant formante
format formato
format of treatment formato de tratamiento
formation formación
formation of attitudes formación de actitudes
formative formativo
formative evaluation evaluación formativa
formative theory teoría formativa
formative theory of personality teoría
    formativa de personalidad
formboard tabla de formas
formboard test prueba de tabla de formas
formed visual hallucination alucinación
    visual formada
formication formicación
formula fórmula
fornicate fornicar
fornication fornicación
fornix fórnix
fortification fortificación
fortification figure figura de fortificación
fortification spectrum espectro de
    fortificación
forward association asociación hacia adelante
fossa fosa
fossula fossula
foster care cuidado adoptivo
foster child hijo adoptivo, hija adoptiva
foster-child fantasy fantasía de hijo adoptivo,
    fantasía de hija adoptiva
foster family familia adoptiva
foster-family care cuidado de familia adoptiva
foster home hogar adoptivo
Foster Kennedy's syndrome síndrome de
    Foster Kennedy
foster placement colocación adoptiva
Fothergill's disease enfermedad de Fothergill
Fothergill's neuralgia neuralgia de Fothergill
four-day workweek semana de trabajo de
    cuatro días
four phases of medical practice cuatro fases
    de la práctica médica
Fourier's law ley de Fourier
Fourier analysis análisis de Fourier
Fournier tests pruebas de Fournier
fourth moment cuarto momento
fovea fovea
fovea centralis fovea centralis
foveal foveal
foveal vision visión foveal
Foville's syndrome síndrome de Foville
fractional fraccional
fractional analysis análisis fraccional
fractional antedating goal response respuesta

de fin adelantado fraccional
fractionation fraccionamiento
fracture fractura
fracture by contrecoup fractura por contragolpe
fragile frágil
fragile X chromosome cromosoma X frágil
fragile X syndrome síndrome de X frágil
fragmentary fragmentado
fragmentary delusion delusión fragmentado
fragmentary seizures accesos fragmentados
fragmentation fragmentación
fragmentation of thinking fragmentación de pensamiento
frame marco
frame analysis análisis de marco
frame of orientation marco de orientación
frame of orientation need necesidad de marco de orientación
frame of reference marco de referencia
Frankenstein factor factor de Frankenstein
fraternal twins gemelos fraternos
Frazier's needle aguja de Frazier
Frazier-Spiller operation operación de Frazier-Spiller
free-access environment ambiente de libre acceso
free association asociación libre
free-association in hypnosis asociación libre en hipnosis
free bone flap colgajo óseo libre
free-floating anxiety ansiedad flotante
free-floating attention atención flotante
free-floating fear temor flotante
free nerve endings terminaciones nerviosas libres
free operant operante libre
free-operant avoidance evitación de operante libre
free play juego libre
free recall recordación libre
free-recall task tarea de recordación libre
free response respuesta libre
free-response test prueba de respuestas libres
free will libre albedrío
freedom libertad
freedom of will libertad de voluntad
freedom to choose libertad de seleccionar
freezing congelación
freezing behavior conducta de congelación
Fregoli's phenomenon fenómeno de Fregoli
frenetic frenético
Frenkel's symptom síntoma de Frenkel
frenulum frenillo
frenzy frenesí
frequency frecuencia
frequency curve curva de frecuencias
frequency discrimination discriminación de frecuencias
frequency distribution distribución de frecuencias
frequency judgment juicio de frecuencias
frequency law ley de frecuencias
frequency method método de frecuencias
frequency polygon polígono de frecuencias

frequency theory teoría de frecuencias
frequency theory of hearing teoría de frecuencias de audición
Freud's theory teoría de Freud
freudian freudiano
freudian approach acercamiento freudiano
freudian fixation fijación freudiana
freudian psychoanalysis psicoanálisis freudiano
freudian slip desliz freudiano
freudian theory teoría freudiana
freudian theory of personality teoría freudiana de personalidad
Frey's irritation hairs pelos de irritación de Frey
Frey's syndrome síndrome de Frey
fricative fricativo
friction-conformity model modelo de conformidad a fricción
Friedmann's complex complejo de Friedmann
Friedmann's disease enfermedad de Friedmann
Friedreich's ataxia ataxia de Friedreich
Friedreich's disease enfermedad de Friedreich
friendly amistoso
friendship amistad
friendship model modelo de amistad
friendship relationships relaciones de amistad
fright espanto
frightened espantado
frightened to death espantado a muerte
frightening espantoso
frightening experience experiencia espantosa
frightful espantoso
frigid frígido
frigidity frigidez
fringe margen
fringe of consciousness margen de conciencia
Frohlich's syndrome síndrome de Frohlich
Froin's syndrome síndrome de Froin
Froment's sign signo de Froment
Fromm's theory teoría de Fromm
front-clipping recorte delantero
front-tap reflex reflejo de golpecito frontal
frontal frontal
frontal cortex corteza frontal
frontal eye-field lesion lesión de campo de ojo frontal
frontal gyrectomy girectomía frontal
frontal lobe lóbulo frontal
frontal lobe dysfunction disfunción de lóbulo frontal
frontal lobe injury lesión de lóbulo frontal
frontal lobe syndrome síndrome de lóbulo frontal
frontal lobotomy lobotomía frontal
frontal perceptual disorder trastorno perceptivo frontal
frontalis muscle músculo frontal
frottage frotación
frotteur frotador
frotteurism frotación
frozen noise ruido congelado

frozen watchfulness vigilancia congelada
fructosuria fructosuria
fruity frutal
frustration frustración
frustration-aggression hypothesis hipótesis de frustración-agresión
frustration and aggression frustración y agresión
frustration from punishment frustración de castigo
frustration-regression hypothesis hipótesis de frustración-regresión
frustration response respuesta de frustración
frustration tolerance tolerancia de frustración
frustrative frustratorio
fucosidosis fucosidosis
Fuerstner's disease enfermedad de Fuerstner
fugue fuga
fugue state estado de fuga
fulfillment realización
fulgurant fulgurante
fulgurating fulgurante
fulgurating migraine migraña fulgurante
full remission remisión completa
full word palabra completa
Fullerton-Cattell law ley de Fullerton-Cattell
fully functioning person persona completamente en funcionamiento
fulminant fulminante
function función
function complex complejo de funciones
function engram engrama de funciones
function of dreams función de sueños
function pleasure placer de función
function types tipos de funciones
function word palabra de función
functional funcional
functional activities actividades funcionales
functional aids ayudas funcionales
functional ailment dolencia funcional
functional analysis análisis funcional
functional analysis of environments análisis funcional de ambientes
functional anosmia anosmia funcional
functional antagonism antagonismo funcional
functional aphasia afasia funcional
functional aphonia afonía funcional
functional apoplexy apoplejía funcional
functional assessment evaluación funcional
functional asymmetry asimetría funcional
functional autonomy autonomía funcional
functional blindness ceguera funcional
functional bradykinesia bradicinesia funcional
functional budgeting presupuestación funcional
functional conformance conformidad funcional
functional contracture contractura funcional
functional deafness sordera funcional
functional disease enfermedad funcional
functional disorder trastorno funcional
functional distance distancia funcional
functional dysmenorrhea dismenorrea funcional

functional dyspareunia dispareunia funcional
functional dysphonia disfonía funcional
functional encopresis encopresis funcional
functional enuresis enuresis funcional
functional fixedness firmeza funcional
functional fixity fijeza funcional
functional hyperinsulinism hiperinsulinismo funcional
functional illness enfermedad funcional
functional inferiority inferioridad funcional
functional integration integración funcional
functional invariant invariante funcional
functional knowledge conocimiento funcional
functional leadership liderazgo funcional
functional moneme monema funcional
functional neurosurgery neurocirugía funcional
functional pain dolor funcional
functional plasticity plasticidad funcional
functional psychology psicología funcional
functional psychosis psicosis funcional
functional reasoning razonamiento funcional
functional relation relación funcional
functional skills destrezas funcionales
functional spasm espasmo funcional
functional speech disorder trastorno del habla funcional
functional stimulus estímulo funcional
functional task tarea funcional
functional type tipo funcional
functional unity unidad funcional
functional vaginismus vaginismo funcional
functional voice disorder trastorno de voz funcional
functionalism funcionalismo
functions of family funciones de familia
fund of information fondo de información
fund of intelligence fondo de inteligencia
fundamental fundamental
fundamental attribution error error de atribución fundamental
fundamental color color fundamental
fundamental emotion emoción fundamental
fundamental needs necesidades fundamentales
fundamental response processes procesos de respuesta fundamentales
fundamental rule regla fundamental
fundamental skill destreza fundamental
fundamental symptom síntoma fundamental
fundamental tone tono fundamental
fungiform papillae papilas fungiformes
fungus hongo
fungus cerebri hongo cerebral
funicular funicular
funicular graft injerto funicular
funicular myelitis mielitis funicular
funicular myelosis mielosis funicular
funiculitis funiculitis
Funkenstein test prueba de Funkenstein
funnel sequence secuencia de embudo
funnel technique técnica de embudo
furor furor
furor epilepticus furor epilepticus
furthest neighbor analysis análisis de vecino

    más lejano
fusiform gyrus circunvolución fusiforme
fusion fusión
fusion frequency frecuencia de fusión
fusion state estado de fusión
futile fútil
future shock choque del futuro
futuristics futurística
fuzzy logic lógica indistinta
fuzzy set conjunto indistinto

G

G factor factor G
gag reflex reflejo de ahogamiento
gain ganancia
gain by illness ganancia por enfermedad
gain-loss theory of attraction teoría de
    atracción de ganancia-pérdida
Gairdner's disease enfermedad de Gairdner
gait marcha
gait disorder trastorno de marcha
galactorrhea galactorrea
galactosemia galactosemia
Galant's reflex reflejo de Galant
Galassi's pupillary phenomenon fenómeno
    pupilar de Galassi
galea galea
galeanthropy galeantropía
galeatomy galeatomía
galeophobia galeofobia
Gall's craniology craneología de Gall
gallows humor humor de patíbulo
Galton bar barra de Galton
Galton whistle pito de Galton
galvanic galvánico
galvanic skin reaction reacción de piel
    galvánica
galvanic skin reflex reflejo de piel galvánico
galvanic skin response respuesta de piel
    galvánica
galvanic vertigo vértigo galvánico
galvanometer galvanómetro
galvanotropism galvanotropismo
gambler jugador
gambler's fallacy falacia del jugador
gambling jugar
gambling behavior conducta de jugar
game juego
game theory teoría del juego
games people play juegos que juega la gente
gamete gameto
gamma gama
gamma alcoholism alcoholismo gama
gamma-aminobutyric acid ácido
    gama-aminobutírico
gamma hypothesis hipótesis gama
gamma motion moción gama
gamma motor neuron neurona motora gama
gamma movement movimiento gama
gamma waves ondas gama
gammacism gamacismo
gamonomania gamonomanía
gamophobia gamofobia
gang pandilla
gang behavior conducta de pandilla
ganglia ganglios

gangliectomy gangliectomía
gangliitis ganglitis
gangliocytoma gangliocitoma
ganglioglioma ganglioglioma
gangliolysis gangliólisis
ganglioma ganglioma
ganglion ganglio
ganglion cell célula ganglionar
ganglion trigeminale ganglio trigeminal
ganglionectomy ganglionectomía
ganglioneuroma ganglioneuroma
ganglioneuromatosis ganglioneuromatosis
ganglionic ganglionar
ganglionic blocking agents agentes
  bloqueadores ganglionares
ganglionic layer capa ganglionar
ganglionitis ganglionitis
ganglionostomy ganglionostomía
ganglioplegic gangliopléjico
ganglioside lipidosis lipidosis gangliósida
gangliosidosis gangliosidosis
gangrene gangrena
Ganser's syndrome síndrome de Ganser
Ganzfeld Ganzfeld
gap junction unión de brecha
García effect efecto de García
Gardner-Diamond syndrome síndrome de
  Gardner-Diamond
gargalanesthesia gargalanestesia
gargalesthesia gargalestesia
gargoylism gargolismo
gas poisoning envenenamiento por gas
gasoline intoxication intoxicación por gasolina
Gasserian ganglion ganglio de Gasser
gastric gástrico
gastric crisis crisis gástrica
gastric motility movilidad gástrica
gastric neurasthenia neurastenia gástrica
gastric neuropathy neuropatía gástrica
gastric tetany tetania gástrica
gastric vertigo vértigo gástrico
gastrin gastrina
gastrocolic reflex reflejo gastrocólico
gastroduodenal ulceration ulceración
  gastroduodenal
gastroenteritis gastroenteritis
gastroesophageal reflux reflujo
  gastroesofágico
gastroileal reflex reflejo gastroileal
gastrointestinal gastrointestinal
gastrointestinal disorder trastorno
  gastrointestinal
gastrointestinal motility movilidad
  gastrointestinal
gastrointestinal problem problema
  gastrointestinal
gastroparalysis gastroparálisis
gastroparesis gastroparesia
gastrulation gastrulación
gate-control hypothesis hipótesis de control
  de puerta
gate-control theory teoría de control de
  puerta
gate-control theory of pain teoría de control
  de puerta del dolor

gatekeeper portero
gateway drugs drogas de entrada
gating desconexión periódica
gating mechanism mecanismo de desconexión
  periódica
gating model modelo de desconexión
  periódica
gatophobia gatofobia
Gaucher's disease enfermedad de Gaucher
Gault decision decisión de Gault
gaussian gauseano
gaussian curve curva gauseana
gaussian distribution distribución gauseana
gay gay
Gayet-Wernicke's encephalopathy
  encefalopatía de Gayet-Wernicke
gaze mirada fija
Gedanken experiment experimento Gedanken
Gegenhalten Gegenhalten
Geigel's reflex reflejo de Geigel
gelasmus gelasmo
gelastic epilepsy epilepsia gelástica
Gelineau's syndrome síndrome de Gelineau
gelotripsy gelotripsia
gemastete cell célula gemastete
gemellology gemelología
gemistocyte gemistocito
gemistocytic gemistocítico
gemistocytic astrocyte astrocito gemistocítico
gemistocytic astrocytoma astrocitoma
  gemistocítico
gemistocytic cell célula gemistocítica
gemistocytic reaction reacción gemistocítica
gemistocytoma gemistocitoma
gender género
gender ambiguity psychosis psicosis de
  ambigüedad de género
gender constancy constancia de género
gender development desarrollo de género
gender differences diferencias de género
gender dysphoria disforia de género
gender identity identidad de género
gender-identity disorder trastorno de
  identidad de género
gender-identity disorder of adolescence
  trastorno de identidad de género de
  adolescencia
gender-identity disorder of adulthood
  trastorno de identidad de género de adultez
gender-identity disorder of childhood
  trastorno de identidad de género de niñez
gender-identity formation formación de
  identidad de género
gender nonconformity inconformismo de
  género
gender orientation orientación de género
gender preference preferencia de género
gender reassignment reasignación de género
gender role papel de género
gender-role development desarrollo de papel
  de género
gender-role disorder trastorno de papel de
  género
gender-role disorder of childhood trastorno
  de papel de género de niñez

gender-role stress estrés de papel de género
gender theory teoría de género
gene gen
gene expression expresión de genes
gene frequency frecuencia de genes
gene marker marcador de genes
gene mutation mutación de gen
gene pair par de genes
gene-splicing empalme de genes
genealogy genealogía
general ability habilidad general
general adaptation reaction reacción de
adaptación general
general adaptational syndrome síndrome
adaptacional general
general anesthetic anestésico general
general aptitude aptitud general
general aptitude test prueba de aptitud
general
general arousal despertamiento general
general factor factor general
general image imagen general
general language disability discapacidad del
lenguaje general
general medical condition condición médica
general
general memory capacity capacidad de
memoria general
general paralysis parálisis general
general paresis paresia general
general principles transfer transferencia de
principios generales
general psychology psicología general
general reasoning razonamiento general
general semantics semántica general
general sensation sensación general
general systems theory teoría de sistemas
generales
general transfer transferencia general
generality generalidad
generalization generalización
generalization gradient gradiente de
generalización
generalization in learning generalización en
aprendizaje
generalized generalizado
generalized amnesia amnesia generalizada
generalized anxiety ansiedad generalizada
generalized anxiety disorder trastorno de
ansiedad generalizada
generalized gangliosidosis gangliosidosis
generalizada
generalized inhibitory potential potencial
inhibitorio generalizado
generalized other otro generalizado
generalized reinforcer reforzador
generalizado
generalized seizure acceso generalizado
generalized tetanus tétanos generalizado
generalized tonic-clonic epilepsy epilepsia
tónica-clónica generalizada
generalized tonic-clonic seizure acceso
tónico-clónico generalizado
generalizing assimilation asimilación
generalizante

generation generación
generation gap brecha generacional
generative generativo
generative empathy empatía generativa
generative grammar gramática generativa
generative semantics semántica generativa
generativity generatividad
generativity versus self-absorption
generatividad contra absorción propia
generativity versus stagnation generatividad
contra estancación
generator potential potencial de generador
generic genérico
generic name nombre genérico
generic skills destrezas genéricas
genetic genético
genetic block bloqueo genético
genetic code código genético
genetic counseling asesoramiento genético
genetic counselor asesor genético
genetic defect defecto genético
genetic determination determinación genética
genetic directive directivo genético
genetic disorder trastorno genético
genetic dominance dominancia genética
genetic drift rumbo genético
genetic endowment dotación genética
genetic engineering ingeniería genética
genetic epistemology epistemología genética
genetic error error genético
genetic factors factores genéticos
genetic factors in affective disorders factores
genéticos en trastornos afectivos
genetic factors in aggression factores
genéticos en agresión
genetic factors in altruism factores genéticos
en altruismo
genetic factors in Alzheimer's disease
factores genéticos en la enfermedad de
Alzheimer
genetic factors in autism factores genéticos
en autismo
genetic factors in eating disorders factores
genéticos en trastornos del comer
genetic factors in emotions factores genéticos
en emociones
genetic factors in epilepsy factores genéticos
en epilepsia
genetic factors in hypertension factores
genéticos en hipertensión
genetic factors in intelligence factores
genéticos en inteligencia
genetic factors in memory factores genéticos
en memoria
genetic factors in mental disorders factores
genéticos en trastornos mentales
genetic factors in personality factores
genéticos en personalidad
genetic factors in schizophrenia factores
genéticos en esquizofrenia
genetic fitness aptitud genética
genetic guidance asesoramiento genético
genetic influence influencia genética
genetic influence in autism influencia
genética en autismo

genetic influence in behavior influencia
  genética en conducta
genetic influence in depression influencia
  genética en depresión
genetic influence in development influencia
  genética en el desarrollo
genetic influence in mental disorders
  influencia genética en trastornos mentales
genetic linkage enlace genético
genetic map mapa genético
genetic marker marcador genético
genetic material material genético
genetic mediation mediación genética
genetic memory memoria genética
genetic method método genético
genetic predisposition predisposición genética
genetic programming programación genética
genetic psychology psicología genética
genetic recessiveness recesividad genética
genetic redundancy redundancia genética
genetic screening cribado genético
genetic sequence secuencia genética
genetic storage almacenamiento genético
genetic structure estructura genética
genetic technology tecnología genética
genetic theory teoría genética
genetic transmission transmisión genética
genetic transmission of depression
  transmisión genética de depresión
genetic vulnerability vulnerabilidad genética
geneticism geneticismo
geneticist genetista
genetics genética
genetophobia genetofobia
genetotrophic genetotrófico
genetotrophic disease enfermedad
  genetotrófica
Genevan school escuela ginebrina
genial genial
genic génico
geniculate geniculado
geniculate bodies cuerpos geniculados
geniculate neuralgia neuralgia geniculada
geniculate otalgia otalgia geniculada
genidentic genidéntico
genital genital
genital character carácter genital
genital development desarrollo genital
genital eroticism erotismo genital
genital-femoral nerve nervio genital-femoral
genital herpes herpes genital
genital intercourse relación genital
genital level nivel genital
genital love amor genital
genital maturity madurez genital
genital mutilation mutilación genital
genital phase fase genital
genital play juego genital
genital primacy primacía genital
genital sex sexo genital
genital stage etapa genital
genital stimulation estimulación genital
genital structure estructura genital
genital zone zona genital
genitalia genitales

genitality genitalidad
genitalize genitalizar
genitourinary genitourinario
genius genio
genocopy genocopia
genogram genograma
genome genoma
genophobia genofobia
genotype genotipo
genotypic genotípico
genotypic programming programación
  genotípica
genotypical genotípico
gens gens
genu genu
genus género
geographical change cambio geográfico
geometric illusion ilusión geométrica
geometric mean media geométrica
geometric series serie geométrica
geophagia geofagia
geophagism geofagismo
geophagy geofagia
geotaxis geotaxis
geotropism geotropismo
gephyrophobia gefirofobia
Gerhardt's disease enfermedad de Gerhardt
Gerhardt-Semon law ley de Gerhardt-Semon
geriatric geriátrico
geriatric delinquency delincuencia geriátrica
geriatric disorder trastorno geriátrico
geriatric psychiatry psiquiatría geriátrica
geriatric psychology psicología geriátrica
geriatric psychopharmacology
  psicofarmacología geriátrica
geriatric rehabilitation rehabilitación
  geriátrica
geriatric screening and evaluation center
  centro de evaluación y cribado geriátrico
geriatrics geriatría
geriopsychosis geriopsicosis
Gerlier's disease enfermedad de Gerlier
germ cell célula germinativa
germ plasm plasma germinativo
germ theory teoría germinativa
German measles sarampión alemán
germinal germinativo
germinal period periodo germinativo
germinal stage etapa germinativa
germinally affected afectado germinalmente
germinoma germinoma
gerocomy gerocomía
geromorphism geromorfismo
gerontological gerontológico
gerontological psychiatry psiquiatría
  gerontológica
gerontological psychology psicología
  gerontológica
gerontology gerontología
gerontophilia gerontofilia
gerontophobia gerontofobia
gerophilia gerofilia
gerophobia gerofobia
geropsychiatry geropsiquiatría
geropsychology geropsicología

Gerstmann's syndrome síndrome de Gerstmann
Gerstmann-Straussler syndrome síndrome de Gerstmann-Straussler
gestagen gestágeno
gestalt gestalt
gestalt factor factor gestalt
gestalt laws of organization leyes de organización gestalt
gestalt phenomenon fenómeno gestalt
gestalt psychology psicología gestalt
gestalt theory teoría gestalt
gestalt therapy terapia gestalt
gestaltism gestaltismo
gestation gestación
gestation period periodo de gestación
gestational age edad gestacional
gestational psychosis psicosis gestacional
gesticulation gesticulación
gestural gestual
gestural automatism automatismo gestual
gestural communication comunicación gestual
gestural language lenguaje gestual
gestural-postural language lenguaje gestual-postural
gesture gesto
geumaphobia geumafobia
geusis geusia
Gheel colony colonia de Gheel
ghost image imagen de fantasma
giant axonal neuropathy neuropatía axonal gigante
giant cell arteritis arteritis de células gigantes
giant follicular lymphadenopathy linfadenopatía folicular gigante
giant hives urticaria gigante
giant urticaria urticaria gigante
gibberish galimatías
Gifford's reflex reflejo de Gifford
gifted dotado
gifted child niño dotado
gigantism gigantismo
gigantocellular glioma glioma gigantocelular
gigantocellular tegmental field campo tegmental gigantocelular
Gigli's saw sierra de Gigli
Gilles de la Tourette's disease enfermedad de Gilles de la Tourette
Gilles de la Tourette's syndrome síndrome de Gilles de la Tourette
ginger paralysis parálisis de jengibre
girdle anesthesia anestesia en cinturón
girdle pain dolor en cinturón
girdle sensation sensación en cinturón
githagism gitagismo
give-and-take dar y tomar
give-and-take process proceso de dar y tomar
given-new distinction distinción dado-nuevo
Gjessing's syndrome síndrome de Gjessing
glabrous glabro
gland glándula
glans glande
glans clitoris glande del clítoris
glans penis glande del pene

glaucoma glaucoma
glia glia
glial cell célula glial
glial insufficiency insuficiencia glial
Glick effect efecto de Glick
glioblastoma glioblastoma
glioblastosis cerebri glioblastosis cerebral
glioma glioma
glioma of optic chiasm glioma de quiasma óptico
glioma of the spinal cord glioma de la médula espinal
glioma telangiectodes glioma telangiectodes
gliomatosis gliomatosis
gliomatous gliomatoso
gliomyxoma gliomixoma
glioneuroma glioneuroma
gliosarcoma gliosarcoma
gliosis gliosis
glissando glisando
global global
global amnesia amnesia global
global aphasia afasia global
global crisis crisis global
global dreaming soñar global
global experiment experimento global
global paralysis parálisis global
global preference preferencia global
global processing procesamiento global
global rating clasificación global
globoid cell célula globoide
globoid cell leukodystrophy leucodistrofia de célula globiode
globus globo
globus hystericus globo histérico
globus pallidus globo pálido
glomectomy glomectomía
glorified self yo glorificado
glossal glosal
glossocinesthetic glosocinestésico
glossodontotropism glosodontotropismo
glossodynia glosodinia
glossodyniotropism glosodiniotropismo
glossokinesthetic glosocinestésico
glossolabiolaryngeal glosolabiolaríngeo
glossolabiolaryngeal paralysis parálisis glosolabiolaríngeo
glossolabiopharyngeal glosolabiofaríngeo
glossolabiopharyngeal paralysis parálisis glosolabiofaríngea
glossolalia glosolalia
glossolysis glosólisis
glossopharyngeal glosofaríngeo
glossopharyngeal nerve nervio glosofaríngeo
glossopharyngeal neuralgia neuralgia glosofaríngea
glossopharyngeal tic tic glosofaríngeo
glossophobia glosofobia
glossoplegia glosoplejía
glossospasm glosoespasmo
glossosynthesis glososíntesis
glossy skin piel brillante
glottal glotal
glottal stop oclusión glotal
glottidospasm glotidoespasmo

glottis glotis
glove anesthesia anestesia en guante
glucagon glucagón
glucocorticoid glucocorticoide
glucogenosis glucogenosis
glucose glucosa
glucose-tolerance test prueba de tolerancia de glucosa
glucostatic theory teoría glucoestática
glue-sniffing inhalación de pega
glutamate glutamato
glutamic acid ácido glutámico
glutamyl glutamilo
gluteal reflex reflejo glúteo
glutethimide glutetimida
glycinate glicinato
glycine glicina
glycogen glucógeno
glycogenolysis glucogenólisis
glycogenosis glucogenosis
glycogeusia glucogeusia
glycorrhachia glucorraquia
GM1 gangliosidosis gangliosidosis GM1
GM2 gangliosidosis gangliosidosis GM2
GM3 gangliosidosis gangliosidosis GM3
gnashing rechinamiento
gnosia gnosia
gnostic gnóstico
gnostic function función gnóstica
go-around circular
goal fin
goal-attainment model modelo de logro de fin
goal-directed behavior conducta dirigida a un fin
goal gradient gradiente de fin
goal-limited adjustment therapy terapia de ajuste limitado a fin
goal-limited therapy terapia limitada a fin
goal model of evaluation modelo de fin de evaluación
goal object objeto fin
goal orientation orientación de fin
goal response respuesta de fin
goal setting establecimiento de fin
goal stimulus estímulo de fin
golden mean media dorada
golden section sección dorada
Goldenhar's syndrome síndrome de Goldenhar
Goldflam disease enfermedad de Goldflam
Goldscheider's disease enfermedad de Goldscheider
Goldscheider's test prueba de Goldscheider
Goldstein's toe sign signo de los dedos del pie de Goldstein
Golgi apparatus aparato de Golgi
Golgi corpuscles corpúsculos de Golgi
Golgi-Mazzoni corpuscles corpúsculos de Golgi-Mazzoni
Golgi neuron neurona de Golgi
Golgi stain colorante de Golgi
Golgi tendon organ órgano tendinoso de Golgi
Golgi type I neuron neurona tipo I de Golgi
Golgi type II neuron neurona tipo II de Golgi

Goltz syndrome síndrome de Goltz
Gompertz curve curva de Gompertz
gonad gónada
gonadal gonadal
gonadal cycle ciclo gonadal
gonadal dysgenesis disgenesia gonadal
gonadal hormone hormona gonadal
gonadocentric gonadocéntrico
gonadotrophic gonadotrófico
gonadotrophic hormone hormona gonadotrófica
gonadotropin gonadotropina
gonadotropin-producing adenoma adenoma productor de gonadotropinas
gonadotropin-releasing hormone hormona liberadora de gonadotropinas
gonococcus gonococo
gonorrhea gonorrea
good-and-evil test prueba de bien y mal
good breast pecho bueno
good continuation continuación buena
good-enough mothering cuidados maternales suficientemente buenos
good gestalt gestalt bueno
good-me yo bueno
good object objeto bueno
good shape forma buena
goodness of fit precisión del ajuste
Gordon's sign signo de Gordon
Gordon's symptom síntoma de Gordon
Gordon reflex reflejo de Gordon
gorge engullir
gorger engullidor
gorger-vomiter engullidor-vomitador
Gorlin's sign signo de Gorlin
Gottschaldt figures figuras de Gottschaldt
Gowers disease enfermedad de Gowers
Gowers syndrome síndrome de Gowers
Graafian follicle folículo de de Graaf
gracile tubercule tubérculo grácil
gracilis nucleus núcleo grácil
gradation method método de graduación
grade equivalent equivalente de grado
grade I astrocytoma astrocitoma grado I
grade II astrocytoma astrocitoma grado II
grade III astrocytoma astrocitoma grado III
grade IV astrocytoma astrocitoma grado IV
grade norm norma de grado
grade scale escala de grado
graded activity actividad graduada
graded potential potencial graduado
Gradenigo's syndrome síndrome de Gradenigo
gradient gradiente
gradient of effect gradiente de efecto
gradient of generalization gradiente de generalización
gradient of reinforcement gradiente de refuerzo
gradient of response generalization gradiente de generalización de respuestas
gradient of stimulus generalization gradiente de generalización de estímulo
gradient of texture gradiente de textura
grading calificación

grading in education calificación en educación
graduate education educación graduada
Graefe's disease enfermedad de Graefe
Graefe's sign signo de Graefe
Graefe's spot mancha de Graefe
graft injerto
graft rejection rechazo de injerto
grammar gramática
grammar development stage etapa del desarrollo de gramática
grammar formation stage etapa de formación de gramática
grammatical word palabra gramatical
grand crisis gran crisis
grand mal gran mal
grand mal epilepsy epilepsia de gran mal
grandfather complex complejo de abuelo
grandiose grandioso
grandiose delusion delusión de grandeza
grandiosity grandiosidad
grandmother complex complejo de abuela
Granit theory of color vision teoría de visión de color de Granit
granular cell célula granular
granular cell myoblastoma mioblastoma de células granulares
granular cell tumor tumor de células granulares
granular cortex corteza granular
granular layer capa granular
granule gránulo
granuloma granuloma
granuloma inguinale granuloma inguinal
granulomatous granulomatoso
granulomatous arteritis arteritis granulomatoso
granulomatous encephalomyelitis encefalomielitis granulomatosa
granulovacuolar degeneration degeneración granulovacuolar
graph gráfica
graphanesthesia grafanestesia
grapheme grafema
graphesthesia grafestesia
graphic gráfico
graphic analysis análisis gráfico
graphic aphasia afasia gráfica
graphic-arts therapy terapia de artes gráficas
graphic individuality individualidad gráfica
graphic language lenguaje gráfico
graphic rating scale escala de clasificación gráfica
graphodyne grafodina
graphology grafología
graphomania grafomanía
graphometry grafometría
graphomotor grafomotor
graphomotor aphasia afasia grafomotora
graphomotor technique técnica grafomotora
graphopathology grafopatología
graphophobia grafofobia
graphorrhea graforrea
graphospasm grafoespasmo
grasp agarre

grasp reflex reflejo de agarre
grasping reflex reflejo de agarre
Grasset's law ley de Grasset
Grasset's phenomenon fenómeno de Grasset
Grasset's sign signo de Grasset
Grasset-Gaussel phenomenon fenómeno de Grasset-Gaussel
Grassmann's laws leyes de Grassmann
gratification gratificación
gratification of instincts gratificación de instintos
Graves' disease enfermedad de Graves
gravidity gravidez
gray commissure comisura gris
gray degeneration degeneración gris
gray market mercado gris
gray matter sustancia gris
gray-out desmayo parcial
gray-out syndrome síndrome de desmayo parcial
great toe reflex reflejo del dedo gordo del pie
Greek love amor griego
Greenfield's disease enfermedad de Greenfield
Greenspoon effect efecto de Greenspoon
greeting behavior conducta de saludo
gregarious gregario
gregariousness gregarismo
grief aflicción
grief management administración de aflicción
grief reaction reacción de aflicción
grief therapy terapia de aflicción
grief work trabajo de aflicción
Grieg's disease enfermedad de Grieg
grievance queja
grimace mueca
Griselda complex complejo de Griselda
grooming acicaladura
grooming behavior conducta de acicaladura
groove surco
gross motor activity actividad de motor grueso
gross motor movement movimiento de motor grueso
gross motor skills destrezas de motor grueso
gross motor skills learning aprendizaje de destrezas de motor grueso
gross score puntuación bruta
gross stress reaction reacción de estrés enorme
ground fondo, base
group grupo
group acceptance aceptación de grupo
group analysis análisis de grupo
group analytic psychotherapy psicoterapia analítica de grupo
group atmosphere atmósfera de grupo
group behavior conducta de grupo
group boundary límite de grupo
group career counseling asesoramiento de carrera de grupo
group-centered leader líder centrado en el grupo
group climate clima de grupo
group cohesion cohesión de grupo

group consciousness conciencia de grupo
group contagion contagio de grupo
group control control de grupo
group counseling asesoramiento de grupo
group decision decisión de grupo
group differences diferencias de grupos
group dimension dimensión de grupo
group dynamics dinámica de grupo
group experience experiencia de grupo
group experiment experimento de grupo
group factor factor de grupo
group feeling sentimiento de grupo
group G monosomy monosomía de grupo G
group harmony harmonía de grupo
group home hogar de grupo
group hypnotherapy hipnoterapia de grupo
group hysteria histeria de grupo
group identification identificación de grupo
group influence influencia de grupo
group influence on aggression influencia de
    grupo en agresión
group influence on aggressive behavior
    influencia de grupo en conducta agresiva
group integration integración de grupo
group intelligence test prueba de inteligencia
    de grupo
group interview entrevista de grupo
group locomotion locomoción de grupo
group marriage matrimonio de grupo
group mind mente de grupo
group morale moral de grupo
group norm norma de grupo
group practice práctica de grupo
group pressure presión de grupo
group problem-solving resolución de
    problemas de grupo
group process proceso de grupo
group psychosis psicosis de grupo
group psychotherapy psicoterapia de grupo
group relations relaciones de grupo
group-relations theory teoría de relaciones de
    grupo
group residence residencia de grupo
group rigidity rigidez de grupo
group risk-taking toma de riesgos de grupo
group role papel de grupo
group sex sexo de grupo
group solidarity solidaridad de grupo
group space espacio de grupo
group structure estructura de grupo
group superego superego de grupo
group tension tensión de grupo
group territorial behavior conducta
    territorial de grupo
group test prueba de grupo
group therapy terapia de grupo
group therapy for autism terapia de grupo
    para autismo
group therapy for children terapia de grupo
    para niños
group therapy for children of divorced
    parents terapia de grupo para niños de
    padres divorciados
group therapy for learning disorders terapia
    de grupo para trastornos de aprendizaje

group therapy for parents terapia de grupo
    para padres
group type tipo de grupo
group type conduct disorder trastorno de
    conducta de tipo de grupo
group work trabajo de grupo
grouped frequency distribution distribución
    de frecuencias agrupadas
grouping agrupamiento
grouping error error de agrupamiento
growing fracture fractura de crecimiento
growing pains dolores del crecimiento
growth crecimiento
growth center centro de crecimiento
growth curve curva de crecimiento
growth hormone hormona del crecimiento
growth hormone producing adenoma
    adenoma productor de hormona del
    crecimiento
growth hormone releasing factor factor
    liberador de hormona del crecimiento
growth motivation motivación de crecimiento
growth needs necesidades del crecimiento
growth principle principio del crecimiento
growth spurt arranque de crecimiento
grumble refunfuñar
grumbling refunfuñon
grumbling mania manía de refunfuñar
guanine guanina
guarded cauteloso
guardianship tutela
Gubler's hemiplegia hemiplejía de Gubler
Gubler's line línea de Gubler
Gubler's paralysis parálisis de Gubler
Gubler's syndrome síndrome de Gubler
guess barrunto
guess-who technique técnica de adivina quien
guessing barruntamiento
guessing bias sesgo por barruntamiento
guidance asesoramiento
guidance-cooperation model modelo de
    asesoramiento-cooperación
guidance program programa de
    asesoramiento
guidance specialist especialista en
    asesoramiento
guide dog perro guía
guideline pauta
guidelines for use of hypnosis pautas para el
    uso de hipnosis
Guillain-Barre reflex reflejo de
    Guillain-Barre
Guillain-Barre syndrome síndrome de
    Guillain-Barre
guilt culpabilidad
guilt feelings sentimientos de culpabilidad
guilty culpable
Guinon's disease enfermedad de Guinon
Gunn's syndrome síndrome de Gunn
Gunn's synkinetic syndrome síndrome
    sincinético de Gunn
Gunn phenomenon fenómeno de Gunn
Gunther's disease enfermedad de Gunther
Gunther-Waldenstrom syndrome síndrome
    de Gunther-Waldenstrom

gust gusto
gustation gustación
gustatism gustatismo
gustatory gustatorio
gustatory anesthesia anestesia gustatoria
gustatory audition audición gustatoria
gustatory hallucination alucinación gustatoria
gustatory hyperesthesia hiperestesia
    gustatoria
gustatory nerve nervio gustatorio
gustatory seizure acceso gustatorio
gustatory-sudorific reflex reflejo
    gustatorio-sudorífico
gustatory sweating syndrome síndrome de
    sudación gustatoria
Guthrie's contiguous conditioning
    condicionamiento contiguo de Guthrie
Guthrie test prueba de Guthrie
gutter fracture fractura en canaleta
Guttman scaling escalamiento de Guttman
guttural gutural
gutturotetany guturotetania
gymnophobia gimnofobia
gynander ginandro
gynandromorph ginandromorfo
gynandry ginandria
gynecology ginecología
gynecomania ginecomanía
gynecomastia ginecomastia
gynephobia ginefobia
gynomonoecism ginomonoecismo
gynophobia ginofobia
gyrectomy girectomía
gyrospasm giroespasmo
gyrus circunvolución

H cells células H
H reflex reflejo H
Haab's pupillary reflex reflejo pupilar de
    Haab
habeas corpus hábeas corpus
habenular ganglion ganglión habenular
habilitation habilitación
habit hábito
habit chorea corea habitual
habit complaint queja de hábito
habit deterioration deterioración de hábito
habit disorder trastorno de hábito
habit disturbance disturbio de hábito
habit family hierarchy jerarquía de familia de
    hábitos
habit formation formación de hábitos
habit-forming que forma hábito
habit hierarchy jerarquía de hábitos
habit interference interferencia de hábito
habit memory memoria de hábitos
habit reversal inversión de hábito
habit spasm espasmo habitual
habit strength fuerza de hábito
habit tic tic habitual
habit training entrenamiento de hábito
habitat hábitat
habituated habituado
habituated response respuesta habituada
habituation habituación
habituation in animal learning habituación
    en aprendizaje animal
habituation in learning habituación en
    aprendizaje
habitus hábito
habitus apoplecticus hábito apopléctico
habitus phthisicus hábito tísico
habromania habromanía
hadephobia hadefobia
Haeckel's biogenetic law ley biogenética de
    Haeckel
Haenel's symptom síntoma de Haenel
hagiotherapy hagioterapia
hair cell célula pilosa
hair follicle folículo piloso
hair pulling tironeo de pelo
hairline fracture fractura capilar
Hakim's disease enfermedad de Hakim
halazepam halazepam
half-life media vida
half-show medio espectáculo
halfway children niños intermedios
halfway house casa de transición
Hallermann-Streiff syndrome síndrome de
    Hallermann-Streiff

Hallervorden-Spatz disease enfermedad de
    Hallervorden-Spatz
Hallervorden-Spatz syndrome síndrome de
    Hallervorden-Spatz
Hallervorden syndrome síndrome de
    Hallervorden
hallucinate alucinar
hallucination alucinación
hallucination of conception alucinación de
    concepción
hallucination of perception alucinación de
    percepción
hallucinatory alucinatorio
hallucinatory epilepsy epilepsia alucinatoria
hallucinatory game juego alucinatorio
hallucinatory image imagen alucinatoria
hallucinatory neuralgia neuralgia alucinatoria
hallucinatory verbigeration verbigeración
    alucinatoria
hallucinogen alucinógeno
hallucinogen abuse abuso de alucinógenos
hallucinogen-affective disorder trastorno
    alucinógeno-afectivo
hallucinogen anxiety disorder trastorno de
    ansiedad de alucinógeno
hallucinogen cross dependence dependencia
    cruzada de alucinógenos
hallucinogen delirium delirio de alucinógeno
hallucinogen delusional disorder trastorno
    delusorio de alucinógeno
hallucinogen dependence dependencia de
    alucinógeno
hallucinogen hallucinosis alucinosis de
    alucinógeno
hallucinogen-induced organic mental
    disorder trastorno mental orgánico
    inducido por alucinógenos
hallucinogen intoxication intoxicación por
    alucinógeno
hallucinogen mood disorder trastorno del
    humor de alucinógeno
hallucinogen persisting perception disorder
    trastorno de percepción persistente de
    alucinógeno
hallucinogen psychotic disorder trastorno
    psicótico de alucinógeno
hallucinogen psychotic disorder with
    delusions trastorno psicótico de
    alucinógeno con delusiones
hallucinogen psychotic disorder with
    hallucinations trastorno psicótico de
    alucinógeno con alucinaciones
hallucinogen use disorder trastorno del uso
    de alucinógenos
hallucinogenic alucinogénico
hallucinogenic drug droga alucinogénica
hallucinosis alucinosis
halo effect efecto de halo
haloperidol haloperidol
haloperidol in autism haloperidol en autismo
haloperidol in Tourette's syndrome
    haloperidol en síndrome de Tourette
haloxazolam haloxazolam
halving method método de bisección
hamartophobia hamartofobia

hamaxophobia hamaxofobia
hammock bandage vendaje en hamaca
Hammond's disease enfermedad de
    Hammond
Hand-Christian-Schuller syndrome síndrome
    de Hand-Christian-Schuller
hand controls controles de mano
hand-to-mouth reaction reacción de mano a
    boca
hand-to-mouth reflex reflejo de mano a boca
hand-washing obsession obsesión de lavarse
    las manos
handedness utilización preferencial de mano
handicap minusvalía
handwriting escritura
handwriting analysis análisis de escritura
handwriting problems problemas de escritura
hangman's fracture fractura de verdugo
hangover resaca
Hansen's disease enfermedad de Hansen
haphalgesia hafalgesia
haphazard fortuito
haphazard sampling muestreo fortuito
haphephobia hafefobia
haploid haploide
haploid cell célula haploide
haploid number número haploide
haploidy haploidia
haplology haplología
happiness felicidad
happy puppet syndrome síndrome de muñeco
    feliz
haptephobia haptefobia
haptic háptico
haptic hallucination alucinación háptica
haptic perception percepción háptica
haptics háptica
haptodysphoria haptodisforia
haptometer haptómetro
haptophonia haptofonía
hard palate paladar duro
hardiness resistencia
hardness dureza
hardness of hearing dureza de audición
hardware equipo
Hardy-Weinberg law ley de Hardy-Weinberg
harelip labio leporino
harm-avoidance need necesidad de evitación
    de daño
harmine harmina
harmonic armónico
harmonic analysis análisis armónico
harmonic mean media armónica
harmonizer armonista
harmony armonía
harp theory teoría de arpa
harpaxophobia harpaxofobia
harria harria
Harris' formula fórmula de Harris
Harris' migraine migraña de Harris
Harris' syndrome síndrome de Harris
Hartel technique técnica de Hartel
Hartnup disease enfermedad de Hartnup
hashish hachís
hassle jaleo

hatred odio
Hawthorne effect efecto de Hawthorne
hazard riesgo
hazardous arriesgado
hazardous treatment tratamiento arriesgado
Head's lines líneas de Head
Head's zones zonas de Head
head-banging golpeamiento de cabeza
head-bobbing doll syndrome síndrome de
  muñeca con meneo vertical de cabeza
head consciousness conciencia de cabeza
head-dropping test prueba de caída de cabeza
head injury lesión de cabeza
head-knocking golpeteo de cabeza
head movements movimientos de cabeza
head-rolling rodado de cabeza
head rotation rotación de cabeza
head-shrinking encogimiento de cabezas
head start ventaja inicial
head tetanus tétanos de cabeza
head-tilt inclinación de cabeza
head trauma trauma de cabeza
headache dolor de cabeza
heal curar
healer curador
healing curación
health salud
health care cuidado de salud
health care provider proveedor de cuidado de
  salud
health care system sistema de cuidado de
  salud
health insurance seguro de salud
health law derecho de salud
health maintenance mantenimiento de salud
health maintenance organization
  organización de mantenimiento de salud
health policy política de salud
health professional profesional de salud
health psychologist psicólogo de salud
health psychology psicología de salud
health visitor visitante de salud
healthy saludable
healthy identification identificación saludable
healthy personality personalidad saludable
hearing audición
hearing acuity agudeza de audición
hearing aid audífono
hearing changes cambios de audición
hearing changes in adulthood cambios de
  audición en adultez
hearing disorder trastorno de audición
hearing impaired de audición deteriorada
hearing impairment deterioro de audición
hearing in infants audición en infantes
hearing loss pérdida de audición
hearing problems problemas de audición
hearing test prueba de audición
hearing theories teorías de audición
hearsay prueba por referencia
heart attack ataque cardíaco
heart block bloqueo cardíaco
heart disease enfermedad cardíaca
heart disorder trastorno cardíaco
heart rate ritmo cardíaco

heart rate in infants sleep ritmo cardíaco en
  el sueño de infantes
heart reflex reflejo del corazón
heat effects efectos del calor
heat exhaustion agotamiento por calor
heat hyperpyrexia hiperpirexia por calor
heat-induced asthenia astenia inducida por
  calor
heat stress estrés por calor
heat stroke golpe de calor
heavy metal intoxication intoxicación por
  metal pesado
Hebb's theory teoría de Hebb
Hebb's theory of perceptual learning teoría
  de Hebb de aprendizaje perceptivo
hebephilia hebefilia
hebephrenia hebefrenia
hebephrenic hebefrénico
hebephrenic dementia demencia hebefrénica
hebephrenic schizophrenia esquizofrenia
  hebefrénica
hebetic hebético
hebetude hebetud
hedge rodeo
hedonic hedónico
hedonic diet dieta hedónica
hedonic level nivel hedónico
hedonic rating clasificación hedónica
hedonic tone tono hedónico
hedonic-tone factor factor de tono hedónico
hedonism hedonismo
hedonistic hedonístico
hedonistic orientation orientación hedonística
hedonistic utilitarianism utilitarismo
  hedonístico
hedonophobia hedonofobia
heel talón
heel jar sacudida del talón
heel tap golpecito de talón
heel-tap reaction reacción de golpecito de
  talón
heel-tap test prueba de golpecito de talón
heel-to-knee test prueba de talón a rodilla
Heidenheim's disease enfermedad de
  Heidenheim
height vertigo vértigo de alturas
Heilbronner's thigh muslo de Heilbronner
Heine-Medin disease enfermedad de
  Heine-Medin
Heinis constant constante de Heinis
Hejna test prueba de Hejna
helicine artery arteria helicina
helicopod gait marcha helicópoda
helicopodia helicopodia
helicotrema helicotrema
heliencephalitis heliencefalitis
heliophobia heliofobia
heliotropism heliotropismo
Hellenic love amor helénico
hellenologomania helenologomanía
hellenologophobia helenologofobia
hellenomania helenomanía
Heller's disease enfermedad de Heller
Heller's syndrome síndrome de Heller
helminthophobia helmintofobia

helper therapy terapia de ayudante
helpful figure figura socorrante
helping behavior conducta de ayuda
helping model modelo de ayuda
helping profession profesión de ayuda
helping relationship relación de ayuda
helplessness impotencia
hemangioblastoma hemangioblastoma
hematencephalon hematencéfalo
hematidrosis hematidrosis
hematocephaly hematocefalia
hematocrit hematócrito
hematocyte hematocito
hematoencephalic hematoencefálico
hematoencephalic barrier barrera
    hematoencefálica
hematoma hematoma
hematophobia hematofobia
hematuria hematuria
hemeralopia hemeralopía
hemeraphonia hemerafonía
hemiacrosomia hemiacrosomía
hemiakinesia hemiacinesia
hemialgia hemialgia
hemiamyosthenia hemiamiostenia
hemianalgesia hemianalgesia
hemianesthesia hemianestesia
hemianopia hemianopía
hemianopic hemianópico
hemianopsia hemianopsia
hemiapraxia hemiapraxia
hemiasomatagnosia hemiasomatagnosia
hemiasomatognosia hemiasomatognosia
hemiasynergia hemiasinergia
hemiataxia hemiataxia
hemiathetosis hemiatetosis
hemiatrophy hemiatrofia
hemiballism hemibalismo
hemiballismus hemibalismo
hemibulbar syndrome síndrome hemibulbar
hemicephalalgia hemicefalalgia
hemichorea hemicorea
hemicrania hemicrania
hemicraniectomy hemicraniectomía
hemicraniosis hemicraniosis
hemicraniotomy hemicraniotomía
hemidecortication hemidescorticación
hemidepersonalization
    hemidespersonalización
hemidysesthesia hemidisestesia
hemiepilepsy hemiepilepsia
hemifacial hemifacial
hemifacial spasm espasmo hemifacial
hemihydranencephaly hemihidranencefalia
hemihypalgesia hemihipalgesia
hemihyperesthesia hemihiperestesia
hemihypertonia hemihipertonía
hemihypertrophy hemihipertrofia
hemihypesthesia hemihipestesia
hemihypoesthesia hemihipoestesia
hemihypotonia hemihipotonía
hemilaminectomy hemilaminectomía
hemilateral hemilateral
hemilateral chorea corea hemilateral
hemiopalgia hemiopalgia

hemiopia hemiopía
hemiparanesthesia hemiparanestesia
hemiparaplegia hemiparaplejía
hemiparesis hemiparesia
hemiplegia hemiplejía
hemiplegia alternans hemiplejía alternante
hemiplegia cruciata hemiplejía cruzada
hemiplegic hemipléjico
hemiplegic amyotrophy amiotrofia
    hemipléjica
hemiplegic gait marcha hemipléjica
hemiplegic migraine migraña hemipléjica
hemisensory hemisensorial
hemisensory loss pérdida hemisensorial
hemisomatognosis hemisomatognosis
hemispasm hemiespasmo
hemispatial hemiespacial
hemispatial neglect desatención hemiespacial
hemisphere hemisferio
hemisphere deficiency deficiencia de
    hemisferio
hemisphere specialization especialización de
    hemisferio
hemispherectomy hemisferectomía
hemispheric hemisférico
hemispheric asymmetries asimetrías
    hemisféricas
hemispheric dominance dominancia
    hemisférica
hemispheric response respuesta hemisférica
hemispheric specialization especialización
    hemisférica
hemithermoanesthesia hemitermoanestesia
hemitonia hemitonía
hemitremor hemitemblor
hemizygote hemicigoto
hemizygous hemicigótico
hemlock cicuta
hemocyte hemocito
hemoglobin hemoglobina
hemophilia hemofilia
hemophobia hemofobia
hemorrhachis hemorraquis
hemorrhage hemorragia
hemorrhagic hemorrágico
hemorrhagic pachymeningitis
    paquimeningitis hemorrágica
hemosiderosis hemosiderosis
hemothymia hemotimia
Henning's prism prisma de Henning
Henning's tetrahedron tetraedro de Henning
Henoch's chorea corea de Henoch
heparitinuria heparitinuria
hepatic hepático
hepatic coma coma hepático
hepatic encephalopathy encefalopatía
    hepática
hepatic porphyria porfiria hepática
hepatitis hepatitis
hepatolenticular hepatolenticular
hepatolenticular degeneration degeneración
    hepatolenticular
hepatolenticular disease enfermedad
    hepatolenticular
herbalist herbolario

Herbartian psychology psicología herbartiana
Herbartianism herbartianismo
herbivorous herbívoro
herd instinct instinto de manada
herding gregarismo
here-and-now approach acercamiento de aquí
   y ahora
hereditarial hereditario
hereditarianism hereditarismo
hereditary hereditario
hereditary angioneurotic edema edema
   angioneurótico hereditario
hereditary ataxia ataxia hereditaria
hereditary cerebellar ataxia ataxia cerebelosa
   hereditaria
hereditary cerebellar ataxia of Marie ataxia
   cerebelosa hereditaria de Marie
hereditary chorea corea hereditaria
hereditary choreoathetosis coreoatetosis
   hereditaria
hereditary disorder trastorno hereditario
hereditary factor factor hereditario
hereditary hypertrophic neuropathy
   neuropatía hipertrófica hereditaria
hereditary myokymia mioquimia hereditaria
hereditary myopathy miopatía hereditaria
hereditary photomyoclonus fotomioclono
   hereditario
hereditary predisposition predisposición
   hereditaria
hereditary sensory radicular neuropathy
   neuropatía radicular sensorial hereditaria
hereditary spastic paraplegia paraplejía
   espástica hereditaria
hereditary spinal ataxia ataxia espinal
   hereditaria
heredity herencia
heredity-environment controversy
   controversia herencia-ambiente
heredoataxia heredoataxia
heredofamilial heredofamiliar
heredofamilial psychosis psicosis
   heredofamiliar
heredofamilial tremor temblor heredofamiliar
heredopathia heredopatía
heredopathia atactica polyneuritiformis
   heredopatía atáxica polineuritiforme
Hering afterimage imagen persistente de
   Hering
Hering-Breuer reflex reflejo de
   Hering-Breuer
Hering grays grises de Hering
Hering illusion ilusión de Hering
Hering theory teoría de Hering
Hering theory of color vision teoría de
   Hering de visión de colores
heritability heredabilidad
heritability of personality heredabilidad de
   personalidad
heritability ratio razón de heredabilidad
heritable heredable
heritage herencia
hermaphrodism hermafrodismo
hermaphrodite hermafrodita
hermaphroditism hermafroditismo

hermeneutics hermenéutica
hermetic hermético
hernia hernia
herniated disk disco herniado
herniation herniación
hero daydream ensueño de héroe
hero worship culto de héroes
heroin heroína
heroin-addicted mother madre adicta a la
   heroína
heroin addiction adicción de heroína
heroin overdose sobredosis de heroína
heroinomania heroinomanía
herpes herpes
herpes encephalitis encefalitis por herpes
herpes infection infección por herpes
herpes simplex encephalitis encefalitis por
   herpes simple
herpes simplex type 1 herpes simple tipo 1
herpes simplex type 2 herpes simple tipo 2
herpes simplex virus virus del herpes simple
herpetic herpético
herpetic meningoencephalitis
   meningoencefalitis herpética
Herrmann's disease enfermedad de
   Herrmann
Herrmann's syndrome síndrome de
   Herrmann
hersage hersaje
Hertwig-Magendie phenomenon fenómeno
   de Hertwig-Magendie
hertz hertz
Herxheimer reaction reacción de Herxheimer
Heschl gyrus circunvolución de Heschl
hesitant speech habla hesitante
hesitation pause pausa de hesitación
Hess image imagen de Hess
hetaeral fantasy fantasía heteral
heterarchy heterarquía
heteresthesia heterestesia
heterocentric heterocéntrico
heterochrony heterocronía
heteroclite heteroclito
heterocyclic antidepressant drug droga
   antidepresiva heterocíclica
heteroerotic heteroerótico
heteroeroticism heteroerotismo
heteroerotism heteroerotismo
heterogamous heterógamo
heterogeneity heterogeneidad
heterogeneous heterogéneo
heterogeneous grouping agrupamiento
   heterogéneo
heterogeny heterogeneidad
heterohypnosis heterohipnosis
heterokinesia heterocinesia
heterokinesis heterocinesis
heterolalia heterolalia
heteroliteral heteroliteral
heterologous heterólogo
heterologous artificial insemination
   inseminación artificial heteróloga
heterologous stimulus estímulo heterólogo
heteromorphous heteromorfo
heteronomous heterónomo

heteronomous psychotherapy psicoterapia
   heterónoma
heteronomous stage etapa heterónoma
heteronomous superego superego heterónomo
heteronomy heteronomía
heteronymous heterónimo
heteronymous hemianopia hemianopía
   heterónima
heteronymous reflex reflejo heterónimo
heteropathy heteropatía
heterophasia heterofasia
heterophemia heterofemia
heterophemy heterofemia
heterophonia heterofonía
heterophoria heteroforia
heteropsychologic heteropsicológico
heterorexia heterorexia
heteroscedasticity heterosedasticidad
heterosexual heterosexual
heterosexual anxiety ansiedad heterosexual
heterosexual pedophilia pedofilia
   heterosexual
heterosexuality heterosexualidad
heterosis heterosis
heterosociality heterosociabilidad
heterosome heterosoma
heterosuggestibility heterosugestibilidad
heterosuggestion heterosugestión
heterosynaptic facilitation facilitación
   heterosináptica
heterotopia heterotopia
heterotopic heterotópico
heterotopic pain dolor heterotópico
heterotropia heterotropía
heterozygosis heterocigosis
heterozygosity heterocigosidad
heterozygote heterocigoto
heterozygous heterocigótico
heterozygousness heterocigosidad
heuristic heurística
hexamethonium hexametonio
hexobarbital hexobarbital
hexosaminidase A hexosaminidasa A
Heyer-Pudenz valve válvula de Heyer-Pudenz
Heymans' law ley de Heymans
hibernation hibernación
Hick's law ley de Hick
Hick-Hyman law ley de Hick-Hyman
hidden camera cámara escondida
hidden-clue test prueba de indicios
   escondidos
hidden figure figura escondida
hidden-figure test prueba de figuras
   escondidas
hidden learning aprendizaje escondido
hidden observer observador escondido
hidden self yo escondido
hidden surface superficie escondida
hidrosis hidrosis
hierarchical jerárquico
hierarchical analysis análisis jerárquico
hierarchical arrangement arreglo jerárquico
hierarchical classification clasificación
   jerárquica
hierarchical organization organización
   jerárquica
hierarchical theory teoría jerárquica
hierarchical theory of instinct teoría
   jerárquica del instinto
hierarchy jerarquía
hierarchy of motives jerarquía de motivos
hierarchy of needs jerarquía de necesidades
hieromania hieromanía
hierophobia hierofobia
hierotherapy hieroterapia
high blood pressure presión sanguínea alta
high-frequency deafness sordera de
   frecuencias altas
high-intensity transition transición de
   intensidad alta
high-risk de riesgo alto
high-risk approach acercamiento de alto
   riesgo
high-risk infant infante de alto riesgo
high-steppage gait marcha de estepaje alto
high-volume hospital hospital de alto volumen
higher brain centers centros cerebrales
   superiores
higher-level skills destrezas de nivel superior
higher mental processes procesos mentales
   superiores
higher-order conditioning condicionamiento
   de orden superior
higher-order constructs constructos de orden
   superior
higher-order interaction interacción de orden
   superior
higher response unit unidad de respuesta
   superior
higher states of consciousness estados
   superiores de conciencia
highway hypnosis hipnosis de carretera
hillock montículo
Hilton's law ley de Hilton
Hilton's method método de Hilton
hindbrain cerebro posterior
Hinman syndrome síndrome de Hinman
hip dislocation dislocación de cadera
hip dysplasia displasia de cadera
hip-flexion phenomenon fenómeno de flexión
   de cadera
hip phenomenon fenómeno de cadera
hip replacement reemplazo de cadera
hippanthropy hipantropía
Hippel's disease enfermedad de Hippel
Hippel-Landau disease enfermedad de
   Hippel-Landau
hippocampal commissure comisura del
   hipocampo
hippocampal sclerosis esclerosis hipocámpica
hippocampus hipocampo
hippophobia hipofobia
hippus hippus
Hirshsprung's disease enfermedad de
   Hirshsprung
histamine histamina
histamine headache dolor de cabeza
   histamínico
histaminic histamínico
histaminic cephalagia cefalagia histamínica

histaminic headache dolor de cabeza histamínico
histiocytosis histiocitosis
histogram histograma
histologic histológico
histologic technician técnico histológico
histology histología
histonectomy histonectomía
historical method método histórico
historical psychoanalysis psicoanálisis histórico
history historial
history of present illness historial de la enfermedad presente
history taking toma de historial
histrionic histriónico
histrionic personality personalidad histriónica
histrionic personality disorder trastorno de personalidad histriónica
histrionic personality traits rasgos de personalidad histriónica
histrionic scale escala histriónica
histrionic spasm espasmo histriónico
Hitzig's girdle cinturón de Hitzig
hives urticaria
hoarding acaparamiento
hoarding character carácter acaparador
hoarding personality personalidad acaparadora
hoarding type tipo acaparador
Hobson's choice selección forzada
hodological space espacio hodológico
hodophobia hodofobia
Hoffding step paso de Hoffding
Hoffmann's muscular atrophy atrofia muscular de Hoffmann
Hoffmann's phenomenon fenómeno de Hoffmann
Hoffmann's reflex reflejo de Hoffmann
Hoffmann's sign signo de Hoffmann
holergasia holergasia
holiday syndrome síndrome de feriado
holism holismo
holistic holísitco
holistic healing curación holísitica
holistic medicine medicina holísitica
holistic psychology psicología holísitca
holistic treatment tratamiento holísitco
Hollander test prueba de Hollander
Holmes-Adie pupil pupila de Holmes-Adie
Holmes-Adie syndrome síndrome de Holmes-Adie
Holmes-Rahe questionnaire cuestionario de Holmes-Rahe
Holmgren test prueba de Holmgren
holocord holocordón
holographic holográfico
holographic memory memoria holográfica
holography holografía
holophrase holofrase
holophrastic holofrástico
holophrastic stage etapa holofrástica
holoprosencephaly holoprosencefalia
holorachischisis holorraquisquisis
holotelencephaly holotelencefalia

Holt system sistema de Holt
Holter monitor test prueba de monitor de Holter
home care cuidado en el hogar
home environment ambiente del hogar
home health aide ayudante de salud en el hogar
home instruction instrucción en el hogar
home-service agency agencia de servicios en el hogar
home visit visita al hogar
homebound limitado al hogar
homeless sin hogar
homeopathic homeopático
homeopathic principle principio homeopático
homeopathy homeopatía
homeostasis homeostasis
homeostatic homeostático
homeostatic equilibrium equilibrio homeostático
homeostatic model modelo homeostático
homeostatic principle principio homeostático
homeostenosis homeostenosis
homesickness añoranza
homework tareas
homichlophobia homiclofobia
homicidal homicida
homicidal behavior conducta homicida
homicidal monomania monomanía homicida
homicide homicidio
homicidomania homicidiomanía
homilopathy homilopatía
homilophobia homilofobia
homing habilidad de retornar al hogar
homoclite homoclito
homocystinuria homocistinuria
homoerotic homoerótico
homoeroticism homoerotismo
homoerotism homoerotismo
homogamy homogamia
homogeneity homogeneidad
homogeneity of variance homogeneidad de varianza
homogeneous homogéneo
homogeneous grouping agrupamiento homogéneo
homogeneous reinforcement refuerzo homogéneo
homogenic homogénico
homogenic love amor homogénico
homogenitality homogenitalidad
homogeny homogeneidad
homograph homógrafo
homolateral homolateral
homologous homólogo
homologous artificial insemination inseminación artificial homóloga
homologous stimulus estímulo homólogo
homologue homólogo
homology homología
homonomy drive impulso de homonomía
homonym homónimo
homonym symptom síntoma de homónimo
homonymous homónimo
homonymous hemianopia hemianopia

homónima
homonymous quadrantic field defect defecto
de campo cuadrántico homónimo
homonymous reflex reflejo homónimo
homophile homófilo
homophobia homofobia
homophone homófono
homoscedasticity homosedasticidad
homosexual homosexual
homosexual behavior conducta homosexual
homosexual community comunidad
homosexual
homosexual marriage matrimonio
homosexual
homosexual panic pánico homosexual
homosexual pedophilia pedofilia homosexual
homosexual rape violación homosexual
homosexuality homosexualidad
homosocial homosocial
homosocial peer group grupo paritario
homosocial
homosociality homosocialidad
homotopic homotópico
homotopic pain dolor homotópico
homovanillic acid ácido homovanílico
homozygocity homocigosidad
homozygosis homocigosis
homozygote homocigoto
homozygous homocigoto
homozygousness homocigosidad
homunculus homúnculo
honesty honradez
honesty test prueba de honradez
honeymoon luna de miel
Honi phenomenon fenómeno de Honi
Hooke's law ley de Hooke
Hoover's signs signos de Hoover
hopelessness desesperación
Hoppe-Goldflam disease enfermedad de
Hoppe-Goldflam
horizon horizonte
horizontal horizontal
horizontal cells células horizontales
horizontal decalage decalaje horizontal
horizontal group grupo horizontal
horizontal growth crecimiento horizontal
horizontal mobility movilidad horizontal
horizontal plane plano horizontal
horizontal sampling muestreo horizontal
horizontal section sección horizontal
horizontal transmission transmisión
horizontal
horizontal-vertical illusion ilusión
horizontal-vertical
horizontal vertigo vértigo horizontal
hormephobia hormefobia
hormic psychology psicología hórmica
hormism hormismo
hormonal hormonal
hormonal gender género hormonal
hormone hormona
Horner's law ley de Horner
Horner's syndrome síndrome de Horner
horopter horóptero
horrific temptations tentaciones horrendas

Horton's arteritis arteritis de Horton
Horton's cephalagia cefalagia de Horton
Horton's headache dolor de cabeza de
Horton
hospice hospicio
hospice movement movimiento de hospicios
hospital hospital
hospital design diseño de hospital
hospital-induced insomnia insomnio inducido
por hospital
hospitalism hospitalismo
hospitalitis hospitalitis
hospitalization hospitalización
hospitalization for psychosis hospitalización
para psicosis
host mother madre hospedante
hostile hostil
hostile aggression agresión hostil
hostile-aggressive response to stress
respuesta hostil-agresiva al estrés
hostile-aggressive responses in children
respuestas hostiles-agresivas en niños
hostile transference transferencia hostil
hostility hostilidad
hostility in play hostilidad en juego
hot flash rubor caliente
hot-line línea de emergencia
hot-line service servicio de línea de
emergencia
hot pack envoltura caliente
hot-pack treatment tratamiento con
envolturas calientes
hottentotism hotentotismo
housebound limitado a la casa
household familia
household move mudanza de familia
housewife's neurosis neurosis de ama de casa
housewife's syndrome síndrome de ama de
casa
hue matiz
hue discrimination discriminación de matices
huffing resollar
Hughlings Jackson's syndrome síndrome de
Hughlings Jackson
human behavior conducta humana
human behavioral rhythms ritmos
conductuales humanos
human chorionic gonadotropin
gonadotropina coriónica humana
human companionship compañía humana
human courtship patterns patrones de
cortejo humanos
human development desarrollo humano
human ecology ecología humana
human engineering ingeniería humana
human factors factores humanos
human-factors psychology psicología de
factores humanos
human-growth movement movimiento de
crecimiento humano
human immunodeficiency virus virus de
inmunodeficiencia humana
human information processing
procesamiento de información humano
human intelligence inteligencia humana

human menopausal gonadotropin
gonadotropina menopáusica humana
human-motivation theory teoría de
motivación humana
human movement movimiento humano
human nature naturaleza humana
human potential potencial humano
human-potential growth center centro de
crecimiento de potencial humano
human-potential model modelo de potencial
humano
human-potential movement movimiento de
potencial humano
human relations relaciones humanas
human-relations group grupo de relaciones
humanas
human-relations training entrenamiento en
relaciones humanas
human services servicios humanos
human sexuality sexualidad humana
human surrogate sustituto de humano
human therapeutic experience experiencia
terapéutica humana
humanism humanismo
humanistic humanístico
humanistic conscience conciencia humanística
humanistic-existential therapy terapia
humanística-existencial
humanistic perspective perspectiva
humanística
humanistic psychology psicología humanística
humanistic school escuela humanística
humanistic theory teoría humanística
humanistic therapy terapia humanística
humidity effects efectos de la humedad
humiliation humillación
humor humor
humoral humoral
humoral immunity factors factores de
inmunidad humoral
humoral theory teoría humoral
hunger hambre
hunger and anorexia nervosa hambre y
anorexia nerviosa
hunger awareness conciencia de hambre
hunger drive impulso de hambre
hunger strike huelga de hambre
Hunt's atrophy atrofia de Hunt
Hunt's neuralgia neuralgia de Hunt
Hunt's paradoxical phenomenon fenómeno
paradójico de Hunt
Hunt's syndrome síndrome de Hunt
Hunt's tremor temblor de Hunt
Hunter's operation operación de Hunter
Hunter's syndrome síndrome de Hunter
Huntington's chorea corea de Huntington
Huntington's disease enfermedad de
Huntington
Hurler's syndrome síndrome de Hurler
hurry sickness enfermedad de prisa
Hutchinson's facies facies de Hutchinson
Hutchinson's mask máscara de Hutchinson
Hutchinson's pupil pupila de Hutchinson
hyaline membrane membrana hialina
hyaline-membrane disease enfermedad de

membrana hialina
hyalophagia hialofagia
hyalophagy hialofagia
hyalophobia hialofobia
hybrid híbrido
hybrid vigor vigor de híbridos
hybridization hibridación
hydantoin hidantoína
hydralazine hidralazina
hydranencephaly hidranencefalia
hydration hidración
hydraulic model modelo hidraulico
hydraulic theory teoría hidraulica
hydraulic theory of hearing teoría hidraulica
de audición
hydrencephalocele hidrencefalocele
hydrencephalomeningocele
hidrencefalomeningocele
hydrencephalus hidrencéfalo
hydrocele hidrocele
hydrocele spinalis hidrocele espinal
hydrocephalic hidrocefálico
hydrocephalocele hidrocefalocele
hydrocephaloid hidrocefaloide
hydrocephalus hidrocefalia
hydrocephalus ex vacuo hidrocefalia ex
vacuo
hydrocephaly hidrocefalia
hydrochloride clorhidrato
hydrocodone hidrocodona
hydrocortisone hidrocortisona
hydrodipsomania hidrodipsomanía
hydroencephalocele hidroencefalocele
hydromeningocele hidromeningocele
hydromicrocephaly hidromicrocefalia
hydromyelia hidromielia
hydromyelocele hidromielocele
hydrophobia hidrofobia
hydrophobic hidrofóbico
hydrophobic tetanus tétanos hidrofóbico
hydrophobophobia hidrofobofobia
hydrophorograph hidroforógrafo
hydrosyringomyelia hidrosiringomielia
hydrotherapy hidroterapia
hydroxide hidróxido
hydroxytryptamine hidroxitriptamina
hydroxytryptophan hidroxitriptófano
hydroxyzine hidroxicina
hyelophobia hielofobia
hygieiolatry higieiolatría
hygiene higiene
hygroma higroma
hygrophobia higrofobia
hylephobia hilefobia
hylophobia hilofobia
hymen himen
hyoscine hioscina
hyoscyamine hiosciamina
hypacusia hipacusia
hypalgesia hipalgesia
hypalgesic hipalgésico
hypalgetic hipalgésico
hypalgia hipalgia
hypengyophobia hipengiofobia
hyperabduction syndrome síndrome de

hiperabducción
hyperactive hiperactivo
hyperactive child syndrome síndrome de niño hiperactivo
hyperactive sexual arousal despertamiento sexual hiperactivo
hyperactive sexual desire deseo sexual hiperactivo
hyperactivity hiperactividad
hyperacusia hiperacusia
hyperacusis hiperacusia
hyperadrenal constitution constitución hiperadrenal
hyperadrenocorticism hiperadrenocorticismo
hyperaesthetic personality personalidad hiperestética
hyperageusia hiperageusia
hyperaggressivity hiperagresividad
hyperaldosternism hiperaldosternismo
hyperalert hiperalerto
hyperalgesia hiperalgesia
hyperalgesic hiperalgésico
hyperalgetic hiperalgésico
hyperalgia hiperalgia
hyperammonemia hiperamonemia
hyperammoniemia hiperamoniemia
hyperaphia hiperafia
hyperaphic hiperáfico
hyperbolic hiperbólico
hyperbolic misidentification identificación errónea hiperbólica
hyperbulimia hiperbulimia
hypercalcemia hipercalcemia
hypercalcemia syndrome síndrome de hipercalcemia
hypercapnia hipercapnia
hypercarbia hipercarbia
hypercathexis hipercatexis
hypercenesthesia hipercenestesia
hypercinesia hipercinesia
hypercinesis hipercinesis
hypercoenesthesia hipercenestesia
hypercognization hipercognización
hypercompensatory hipercompensatorio
hypercompensatory type tipo hipercompensatorio
hypercryalgesia hipercrialgesia
hypercryesthesia hipercriestesia
hyperdynamia hiperdinamia
hyperdynamic hiperdinámico
hyperechema hiperequema
hyperemia hiperemia
hyperephidrosis hiperefidrosis
hyperepithymia hiperepitimia
hyperergasia hiperergasia
hyperergic encephalitis encefalitis hiperérgica
hypereridic hipererídico
hypereridic state estado hipererídico
hyperesthesia hiperestesia
hyperesthesia olfactoria hiperestesia olfatoria
hyperesthesia optica hiperestesia óptica
hyperesthetic hiperestético
hyperesthetic memory memoria hiperestética
hyperexcitability hiperexcitabilidad
hyperextension-hyperflexion injury lesión de

hiperextensión-hiperflexión
hyperfemininity hiperfeminidad
hyperfunction hiperfunción
hypergargalesthesia hipergargalestesia
hypergasia hipergasia
hypergenital hipergenital
hypergenital type tipo hipergenital
hypergenitalism hipergenitalismo
hypergeometric distribution distribución hipergeométrica
hypergeusia hipergeusia
hyperglycemia hiperglucemia
hyperglycemic hiperglucémico
hyperglycemic index índice hiperglucémico
hyperglycorrhachia hiperglucorraquia
hypergnosis hipergnosis
hyperhedonia hiperhedonia
hyperhedonism hiperhedonismo
hyperhidrosis hiperhidrosis
hyperindependence hiperindependencia
hyperingestion hiperingestión
hyperinsulinism hiperinsulinismo
hyperkalemia hipericalemia
hyperkalemic periodic paralysis parálisis periódica hiperpotasémica
hyperkinesia hipercinesia
hyperkinesis hipercinesis
hyperkinesis with developmental delay hipercinesis con demora del desarrollo
hyperkinesthesia hipercinestesia
hyperkinetic hipercinético
hyperkinetic encephalopathy encefalopatía hipercinética
hyperkinetic impulse disorder trastorno de impulsos hipercinéticos
hyperkinetic reaction of childhood reacción hipercinética de niñez
hyperkinetic syndrome síndrome hipercinético
hyperlexia hiperlexia
hyperlipidemia hiperlipidemia
hyperlipoproteinemia hiperlipoproteinemia
hyperlogia hiperlogia
hyperlordosis hiperlordosis
hyperlysinemia hiperlisinemia
hypermania hipermanía
hypermanic hipermaníaco
hypermasculinity hipermasculinidad
hypermenorrhea hipermenorrea
hypermetamorphosis hipermetamorfosis
hypermetria hipermetría
hypermetropia hipermetropía
hypermimia hipermimia
hypermnesia hipermnesia
hypermotility hipermovilidad
hypermyesthesia hipermiestesia
hypermyotonia hipermiotonía
hypernatremic encephalopathy encefalopatía hipernatrémica
hypernoia hipernoia
hypernomic hipernómico
hyperobesity hiperobesidad
hyperontomorph hiperontomorfo
hyperopia hiperopía
hyperopic vision visión hiperópica

hyperorality hiperoralidad
hyperorexia hiperorexia
hyperosmia hiperosmia
hyperosmolar hyperglycemic nonketonic
    coma coma no cetónico hiperglucémico
    hiperosmolar
hyperosphresia hiperosfresia
hyperostotic spondylosis espondilosis
    hiperostótica
hyperparathyroidism hiperparatiroidismo
hyperparesthesia hiperparestesia
hyperpathia hiperpatía
hyperphagia hiperfagia
hyperphasia hiperfasia
hyperphoria hiperforia
hyperphrasia hiperfrasia
hyperphrenia hiperfrenia
hyperpipecolatemia hiperpipecolatemia
hyperpituitary hiperpituitario
hyperpituitary constitution constitución
    hiperpituitaria
hyperplasia hiperplasia
hyperpnea hiperpnea
hyperpnoea hiperpnea
hyperpolarization hiperpolarización
hyperponesis hiperponesis
hyperpragia hiperpragia
hyperpragic hiperprágico
hyperpraxia hiperpraxia
hyperprosessis hiperprosesis
hyperprosexia hiperprosexia
hyperpsychosis hiperpsicosis
hyperquantivalent idea idea
    hipercuantivalente
hyperreflexia hiperreflexia
hypersensitivity hipersensibilidad
hypersensitivity reaction reacción de
    hipersensibilidad
hypersensitivity theory teoría de
    hipersensibilidad
hypersexuality hipersexualidad
hypersomnia hipersomnia
hypersomnia disorder trastorno de
    hipersomnia
hypersomnic encephalitis encefalitis
    hipersómnica
hypersomnolence hipersomnolencia
hypersomnolence disorder trastorno de
    hipersomnolencia
hypersthenic hipersténico
hypertarachia hipertaraquia
hypertelorism hipertelorismo
hypertension hipertensión
hypertension and stress hipertensión y estrés
hypertensive hipertensivo
hypertensive crisis crisis hipertensiva
hypertensive encephalopathy encefalopatía
    hipertensiva
hyperthermalgesia hipertermalgesia
hyperthermia hipertermia
hyperthermoesthesia hipertermoestesia
hyperthymia hipertimia
hyperthymic hipertímico
hyperthyroid hipertiroide
hyperthyroid constitution constitución

    hipertiroide
hyperthyroidism hipertiroidismo
hypertonia hipertonía
hypertonic hipertónico
hypertonic absence ausencia hipertónica
hypertonic-dyskinetic syndrome síndrome
    hipertónico-discinético
hypertonic type tipo hipertónico
hypertonicity hipertonicidad
hypertransfusion treatment tratamiento de
    hipertransfusión
hypertrichophobia hipertricofobia
hypertrophic hipertrófico
hypertrophic cervical pachymeningitis
    paquimeningitis cervical hipertrófica
hypertrophic interstitial neuropathy
    neuropatía intersticial hipertrófica
hypertrophic obesity obesidad hipertrófica
hypertrophy hipertrofia
hypertropia hipertropía
hypertychia hipertiquia
hyperuricemia hiperuricemia
hyperuricosuria hiperuricosuria
hypervegetative type tipo hipervegetativo
hyperventilation hiperventilación
hyperventilation syndrome síndrome de
    hiperventilación
hyperventilation test prueba de
    hiperventilación
hyperventilation tetany tetania por
    hiperventilación
hypervigilance hipervigilancia
hypervigilant hipervigilante
hypervitaminosis hipervitaminosis
hypervolemia hipervolemia
hypesthesia hipestesia
hyphedonia hifedonia
hypnagogic hipnagógico
hypnagogic hallucination alucinación
    hipnagógica
hypnagogic image imagen hipnagógica
hypnagogic intoxication intoxicación
    hipnagógica
hypnagogic reverie ensueño hipnagógico
hypnagogic state estado hipnagógico
hypnagogue hipnagogo
hypnalgia hipnalgia
hypnapagogic hipnapagógico
hypnesthesia hipnestesia
hypnic hípnico
hypnoanalysis hipnoanálisis
hypnobat hipnóbata
hypnocatharsis hipnocatarsis
hypnocinematograph hipnocinematógrafo
hypnodelic therapy terapia hipnodélica
hypnodontics hipnodóntica
hypnodrama hipnodrama
hypnogenesis hipnogénesis
hypnogenic hipnogénico
hypnogenic spot mancha hipnogénica
hypnogenous hipnogénico
hypnogogic hipnogógico
hypnogogic image imagen hipnogógica
hypnogogic state estado hipnogógico
hypnograph hipnógrafo

hypnoid hipnoideo
hypnoid state estado hipnoideo
hypnoidal hipnoideo
hypnoidization hipnoidización
hypnolepsy hipnolepsia
hypnologist hipnólogo
hypnology hipnología
hypnonarcosis hipnonarcosis
hypnopaedia hipnopedia
hypnopathy hipnopatía
hypnophobia hipnofobia
hypnophrenosis hipnofrenosis
hypnoplasty hipnoplastia
hypnopompic hipnopómpico
hypnopompic hallucination alucinación
    hipnopómpica
hypnopompic image imagen hipnopómpica
hypnosedative hipnosedante
hypnosigenesis hipnosigénesis
hypnosis hipnosis
hypnosis as treatment for chronic pain
    hipnosis como tratamiento para dolor
    crónico
hypnosis in memory enhancement hipnosis
    en realzado de memoria
hypnosis in research hipnosis en
    investigación
hypnosuggestion hipnosugestión
hypnotherapy hipnoterapia
hypnotic hipnótico
hypnotic abuse abuso de hipnótico
hypnotic analgesia analgesia hipnótica
hypnotic anxiety disorder trastorno de
    ansiedad de hipnótico
hypnotic delirium delirio de hipnótico
hypnotic dependence dependencia de
    hipnótico
hypnotic drug droga hipnótica
hypnotic induction inducción hipnótica
hypnotic intoxication intoxicación por
    hipnótico
hypnotic mood disorder trastorno del humor
    de hipnótico
hypnotic persisting amnestic disorder
    trastorno amnésico persistente de hipnótico
hypnotic persisting dementia demencia
    persistente de hipnótico
hypnotic psychotherapy psicoterapia
    hipnótica
hypnotic psychotic disorder trastorno
    psicótico de hipnótico
hypnotic psychotic disorder with delusions
    trastorno psicótico de hipnótico con
    delusiones
**hypnotic psychotic disorder with
    hallucinations** trastorno psicótico de
    hipnótico con alucinaciones
hypnotic reeducation reeducación hipnótica
hypnotic regression regresión hipnótica
hypnotic relationship relación hipnótica
hypnotic rigidity rigidez hipnótica
hypnotic-sedative drug droga
    hipnótica-sedante
hypnotic sexual dysfunction disfunción
    sexual de hipnótico

hypnotic sleep sueño hipnótico
hypnotic sleep disorder trastorno del sueño
    de hipnótico
hypnotic state estado hipnótico
hypnotic susceptibility susceptibilidad
    hipnótica
hypnotic susceptibility scale escala de
    susceptibilidad hipnótica
hypnotic trance trance hipnótico
hypnotic use disorder trastorno de uso de
    hipnótico
hypnotic withdrawal retiro de hipnótico
hypnotism hipnotismo
hypnotism in education hipnotismo en
    educación
hypnotism in therapy hipnotismo en terapia
hypnotist hipnotista
hypnotizability hipnotizabilidad
hypnotization hipnotización
hypnotize hipnotizar
hypnotized witness testigo hipnotizado
hypnotoid hipnotoide
hypoactive hipoactivo
hypoactive sexual arousal despertamiento
    sexual hipoactivo
hypoactive sexual desire deseo sexual
    hipoactivo
hypoactive sexual desire disorder trastorno
    de deseo sexual hipoactivo
hypoactivity hipoactividad
hypoacusia hipoacusia
hypoadrenal constitution constitución
    hipoadrenal
hypoaffective hipoafectivo
hypoaffective type tipo hipoafectivo
hypoageusia hipoageusia
hypoalgesia hipoalgesia
hypobaropathy hipobaropatía
hypoboulia hipobulia
hypobulia hipobulia
hypocalcemia hipocalcemia
hypocathexis hipocatexis
hypochondria hipocondria
hypochondriac hipocondríaco
hypochondriac language lenguaje
    hipocondríaco
hypochondriacal hipocondríaco
hypochondriacal delusion delusión
    hipocondríaca
hypochondriacal melancholia melancolía
    hipocondríaca
hypochondriacal neurosis neurosis
    hipocondríaca
hypochondriacal psychosis psicosis
    hipocondríaca
hypochondrial hipocondrial
hypochondrial reflex reflejo hipocondrial
hypochondriasis hipocondriasis
hypochondriasis scale escala de
    hipocondriasis
hypochoresis hipocoresis
hypocognization hipocognización
hypocrisy hipocresía
hypodepression hipodepresión
hypodermic hipodérmico

hypodermic injection inyección hipodérmica
hypodontia hipodoncia
hypoemotionality hipoemocionalidad
hypoendocrinism hipoendocrinismo
hypoergasia hipoergasia
hypoergastia hipoergastia
hypoergia hipoergia
hypoergy hipoergia
hypoesthesia hipoestesia
hypoevolutism hipoevolutismo
hypofrontality hypothesis hipótesis de hipofrontalidad
hypofunction hipofunción
hypoganglionosis hipoganglionosis
hypogastric hipogástrico
hypogastric nerve nervio hipogástrico
hypogastric reflex reflejo hipogástrico
hypogenital hipogenital
hypogenital temperament temperamento hipogenital
hypogenital type tipo hipogenital
hypogenitalism hipogenitalismo
hypogeusia hipogeusia
hypoglossal nerve nervio hipogloso
hypoglycemia hipoglucemia
hypoglycemic hipoglucémico
hypoglycemic coma coma hipoglucémico
hypoglycorrhachia hipoglucorraquia
hypogonadism hipogonadismo
hypogonadism with anosmia hipogonadismo con anosmia
hypohypnotic hipohipnótico
hypokalemic periodic paralysis parálisis periódica hipopotasémica
hypokinesia hipocinesia
hypokinesis hipocinesis
hypokinesthesia hipocinestesia
hypokinetic hipocinético
hypokinetic syndrome síndrome hipocinético
hypolepsiomania hipolepsiomanía
hypolexia hipolexia
hypolipemia hipolipemia
hypologia hipologia
hypomania hipomanía
hypomania scale escala de hipomanía
hypomanic hipomaníaco
hypomanic disorder trastorno hipomaníaco
hypomanic episode episodio hipomaníaco
hypomanic personality personalidad hipomaníaca
hypomanic scale escala hipomaníaca
hypomanic state estado hipomaníaco
hypomelancholia hipomelancolía
hypomenorrhea hipomenorrea
hypometamorphosis hipometamorfosis
hypometria hipometría
hypometropia hipometropía
hypomnesia hipomnesia
hypomotility hipomovilidad
hypomyelination hipomielinación
hypomyelinogenesis hipomielinogénesis
hyponoia hiponoia
hyponoic hiponoico
hypoparathyroid constitution constitución hipoparatiroidea

hypoparathyroid tetany tetania hipoparatiroidea
hypoparathyroidism hipoparatiroidismo
hypophagia hipofagia
hypophoria hipoforia
hypophosphatasia hipofosfatasia
hypophrasia hipofrasia
hypophrenia hipofrenia
hypophrenosis hipofrenosis
hypophysectomize hipofisectomizar
hypophysectomy hipofisectomía
hypophysial hipofisario
hypophysial cachexia caquexia hipofisaria
hypophysial fossa fosa hipofisaria
hypophysial syndrome síndrome hipofisario
hypophysio-sphenoidal syndrome síndrome hipofisioesfenoidal
hypophysis hipófisis
hypopituitarism hipopituitarismo
hypopituitary hipopituitario
hypopituitary constitution constitución hipopituitaria
hypoplasia hipoplasia
hypoplastic hipoplástico
hypopraxia hipopraxia
hypoprosessis hipoprosesis
hypoprosexia hipoprosexia
hypopsychosis hipopsicosis
hyporeflexia hiporreflexia
hyposensitivity hiposensibilidad
hyposexuality hiposexualidad
hyposmia hiposmia
hyposomnia hiposomnia
hyposomniac hiposomníaco
hyposophobia hiposofobia
hypospadias hipospadias
hyposphresia hiposfresia
hypostasis hipostasis
hyposthenia hipostenia
hypostheniant hiposteniante
hyposthenic hiposténico
hypotaxia hipotaxia
hypotaxis hipotaxis
hypotension hipotensión
hypotensive hipotensivo
hypothalamic hipotalámico
hypothalamic hormone hormona hipotalámica
hypothalamic-hypophysial portal system sistema portal hipotalámico-hipofisario
hypothalamic obesity obesidad hipotalámica
hypothalamic-pituitary axis eje hipotalámico-pituitario
hypothalamic-pituitary axis dysfunction disfunción de eje hipotalámico-pituitario
hypothalamic sulcus surco hipotalámico
hypothalamic syndrome síndrome hipotalámico
hypothalamic theory of Cannon teoría hipotalámica de Cannon
hypothalamotomy hipotalamotomía
hypothalamus hipotálamo
hypothemic hipotémico
hypothemic disorder trastorno hipotémico
hypothermesthesia hipotermestesia

hypothermia hipotermia
hypothesis hipótesis
hypothesis behavior conducta de hipótesis
hypothesis generation generación de hipótesis
hypothesis testing comprobación de hipótesis
hypothetical hipotético
hypothetical construct constructo hipotético
hypothetical-deductive method método
    hipotético-deductivo
hypothetical-deductive reasoning
    razonamiento hipotético-deductivo
hypothetical imperative imperativo hipotético
hypothetical syllogism silogismo hipotético
hypothetico-deductive reasoning
    razonamiento hipotético-deductivo
hypothymia hipotimia
hypothymic hipotímico
hypothyroid hipotiroideo
hypothyroidism hipotiroidismo
hypotonia hipotonía
hypotonic hipotónico
hypotonicity hipotonicidad
hypotonous hipotono
hypotony hipotonía
hypotrophy hipotrofia
hypotropia hipotropía
hypovegetative hipovegetativo
hypovigility hipovigilancia
hypovolemia hipovolemia
hypoxemia hipoxemia
hypoxia hipoxia
hypoxic hipóxico
hypoxic drive impulso hipóxico
hypoxyphilia hipoxifilia
hypsarrhythmia hipsarritmia
hypsicephalic hipsicefálico
hypsicephaly hipsicefalia
hypsocephaly hipsocefalia
hypsophobia hipsofobia
hysterectomy histerectomía
hysteresis histéresis
hysteria histeria
hysteria scale escala de histeria
hysteric histérico
hysterical histérico
hysterical amaurosis amaurosis histérica
hysterical amnesia amnesia histérica
hysterical anesthesia anestesia histérica
hysterical aphonia afonía histérica
hysterical ataxia ataxia histérica
hysterical blindness ceguera histérica
hysterical character carácter histérico
hysterical chorea corea histérica
hysterical convulsion convulsión histérica
hysterical deafness sordera histérica
hysterical disorder trastorno histérico
hysterical hiccough hipo histérico
hysterical hypalgia hipalgia histérica
hysterical imitation imitación histérica
hysterical joint articulación histérica
hysterical materialization materialización
    histérica
hysterical neurosis neurosis histérica
hysterical paralysis parálisis histérica
hysterical paresis paresia histérica

hysterical personality personalidad histérica
hysterical personality disorder trastorno de
    personalidad histérica
hysterical polydipsia polidipsia histérica
hysterical pregnancy embarazo histérico
hysterical pseudodementia seudodemencia
    histérica
hysterical psychosis psicosis histérica
hysterical reaction reacción histérica
hysterical seizure acceso histérico
hysterical state estado histérico
hysterical stupor estupor histérico
hysterical syncope síncope histérico
hysterical vomiting vómitos histéricos
hystericoneuralgic histericoneurálgico
hysterics histerismo
hysteriform histeriforme
hysteriosis histeriosis
hysterocatalepsy histerocatalepsia
hysteroepilepsy histeroepilepsia
hysterofrenic histerofrénico
hysterogenic histerogénico
hysterogenic spot punto histerogénico
hysterogenic zones zonas histerogénicas
hysterogenous histerógeno
hysteroid histeroide
hysteroid convulsion convulsión histeroide
hysteroid dysphoria disforia histeroide
hysteronarcolepsy histeronarcolepsia
hysterophilia histerofilia
hysteropia histeropía
hysterosalpingography histerosalpingografía
hysteroscopy histeroscopia
hysterosyntonic histerosintónico
hysterotrismus histerotrismo

I

I-cell disease enfermedad de células I
iatric iátrico
iatrogenesis iatrogénesis
iatrogenic iatrogénico
iatrogenic disorder trastorno iatrogénico
iatrogenic homosexuality homosexualidad
    iatrogénica
iatrogenic illness enfermedad iatrogénica
iatrogenic psychosis psicosis iatrogénica
iatrogeny iatrogenia
iatrotropic stimulus estímulo iatrotrópico
Icarus complex complejo de Icaro
iceblock theory teoría de bloque de hielo
ichthyophobia ictiofobia
ichthyosis-hypogonadism syndrome
    síndrome de ictiosis-hipogonadismo
icon icono
iconic icónico
iconic content contenido icónico
iconic memory memoria icónica
iconic mode modo icónico
iconic representation representación icónica
iconic sign signo icónico
iconic stage etapa icónica
iconic storage almacenamiento icónico
iconicity iconicidad
iconomania iconomanía
iconophobia iconofobia
ictal ictal
ictal emotions emociones ictales
icterus icterus
icterus gravis neonatorum icterus grave
    neonatal
ictus ictus
ictus epilepticus ictus epilepticus
ictus paralyticus ictus paralyticus
id id
id anxiety ansiedad del id
id-ego id-ego
id interpretation interpretación del id
id omnipotence omnipotencia del id
id psychology psicología del id
id resistance resistencia del id
id sadism sadismo del id
id wish deseo del id
idea chase persecución de ideas
idea of influence idea de influencia
idea of reference idea de referencia
idea of unreality idea de irrealidad
ideal ideal
ideal detector detector ideal
ideal ego ego ideal
ideal masochism masoquismo ideal
ideal observer observador ideal

ideal parent padre ideal, madre ideal
idealism idealismo
idealization idealización
idealization and disillusionment idealización
    y desilusión
idealize idealizar
idealized idealizado
idealized image imagen idealizada
idealized self yo idealizado
ideation ideación
ideational ideacional
ideational agnosia agnosia ideacional
ideational apraxia apraxia ideacional
ideational fluency fluidez ideacional
ideational learning aprendizaje ideacional
ideational shield escudo ideacional
ideatory ideatorio
ideatory apraxia apraxia ideatoria
idee fixe idea fija
identical idéntico
identical-direction law ley de dirección
    idéntica
identical elements theory teoría de elementos
    idénticos
identical points puntos idénticos
identical retinal points puntos retinales
    idénticos
identical twins gemelos idénticos
identification identificación
identification figure figura de identificación
identification of spatial patterns
    identificación de patrones espaciales
identification phenomenon fenómeno de
    identificación
identification test prueba de identificación
identification transference transferencia de
    identificación
identification with the aggressor
    identificación con el agresor
identify identificar
identifying data datos de identificación
identity identidad
identity confusion confusión de identidad
identity crisis crisis de identidad
identity development desarrollo de identidad
identity diffusion difusión de identidad
identity disorder trastorno de identidad
identity disorder of childhood trastorno de
    identidad de niñez
identity disturbance disturbio de identidad
identity formation formación de identidad
identity formation in adolescence formación
    de identidad en adolescencia
identity integration integración de identidad
identity need necesidad de identidad
identity problem problema de identidad
identity theory teoría de identidad
identity versus role confusion identidad
    contra confusión de papel
ideodynamics ideodinámica
ideogenetic ideogenético
ideoglandular ideoglandular
ideogram ideograma
ideographic ideográfico
ideographic psychology psicología

ideográfica
ideokinetic ideocinético
ideokinetic apraxia apraxia ideocinética
ideokinetic praxis praxis ideocinética
ideological ideológico
ideological commitment compromiso
   ideológico
ideology ideología
ideomotion ideomoción
ideomotor ideomotor
ideomotor act acto ideomotor
ideomotor apraxia apraxia ideomotora
ideomotor signaling señalamiento ideomotor
ideophobia ideofobia
ideophrenia ideofrenia
ideoplastia ideoplastia
ideoplastic ideoplástico
ideoplasty ideoplastia
ideosensory ideosensorial
ideosensory signaling señalamiento
   ideosensorial
idiodynamic idiodinámico
idiodynamic control control idiodinámico
idiodynamics idiodinámica
idiogamist idiogamista
idioglossia idioglosia
idiogram idiograma
idiographic idiográfico
idiographic approach acercamiento
   idiográfico
idiohypnotism idiohipnotismo
idiolalia idiolalia
idiom modismo
idiomuscular idiomuscular
idioneurosis idioneurosis
idiopathic idiopático
idiopathic autoscopy autoscopia idiopática
idiopathic epilepsy epilepsia idiopática
idiopathic muscular atrophy atrofia muscular
   idiopática
idiopathic neuralgia neuralgia idiopática
idiophrenia idiofrenia
idiophrenic idiofrénico
idioplasm idioplasma
idioplasma idioplasma
idiopsychologic idiopsicológico
idioreflex idiorreflejo
idioretinal idiorretinal
idioretinal light luz idiorretinal
idiosome idiosoma
idiospasm idioespasmo
idiosyncrasia olfactoria idiosincrasia olfatoria
idiosyncrasy idiosincrasia
idiosyncrasy-credit model modelo de
   idiosincrasia-crédito
idiosyncratic idiosincrásico
idiosyncratic intoxication intoxicación
   idiosincrásica
idiosyncratic reaction reacción idiosincrásica
idiotropic idiotrópico
idiovariation idiovariación
ignipedites ignipedites
ignore ignorar
ikonic icónico
ikonic representation representación icónica

ikota ikota
ileostomy ileostomía
Ilheus encephalitis encefalitis por Iheus
iliohypogastric nerve nervio iliohipogástrico
ilioinguinal nerve nervio ilioinguinal
illegal source fuente ilegal
illicit ilícito
illiteracy analfabetismo
illness enfermedad
illness as self-punishment enfermedad como
   autocastigo
illness behavior conducta de enfermedad
illogical ilógico
illogicality falta de lógica
illuminance iluminancia
illumination iluminación
illumination conditions condiciones de
   iluminación
illumination standards normas de
   iluminación
illumination unit unidad de iluminación
illuminism iluminismo
illusion ilusión
illusion of doubles ilusión de dobles
illusion of motion ilusión de moción
illusion of negative doubles ilusión de dobles
   negativos
illusion of orientation ilusión de orientación
illusion of positive doubles ilusión de dobles
   positivos
illusion of size ilusión de tamaño
illusional ilusional
illusory ilusorio
illusory contour contorno ilusorio
illusory correlation correlación ilusoria
illusory motion moción ilusoria
illusory movement movimiento ilusorio
illustrator ilustrador
image imagen
image agglutinations aglutinaciones de
   imágenes
imageless sin imagen
imageless thought pensamiento sin imagen
imagery imaginería
imagery and emotions imaginería y
   emociones
imagery code código de imaginería
imagery therapy terapia de imaginería
imaginal imaginal
imaginal desensitization desensibilización
   imaginal
imaginal exposure exposición imaginal
imaginal flooding inundación imaginal
imaginary imaginario
imaginary companion compañero imaginario
imagination imaginación
imaginative play juego imaginativo
imagine imaginar
imaging producción de imagen
imago imago
imbalance desequilibrio
imidazole imidazol
imidazole syndrome síndrome de imidazol
imipramine imipramina
imitation imitación

imitation and learning imitación y
aprendizaje
imitation and social development imitación y
desarrollo social
imitation in infants imitación en infantes
imitative imitativo
imitative learning aprendizaje imitativo
imitative processes procesos imitativos
imitative speech habla imitativa
imitative tetanus tétanos imitativo
immanent inmanente
immanent justice justicia inmanente
immature inmaduro
immature personality personalidad inmadura
immature personality disorder trastorno de
personalidad inmadura
immediacy inmediación
immediacy behavior conducta de proximidad
immediate inmediato
immediate association asociación inmediata
immediate constituent constitutivo inmediato
immediate experience experiencia inmediata
immediate memory memoria inmediata
immediate posttraumatic automatism
automatismo postraumático inmediato
immediate posttraumatic convulsion
convulsión postraumática inmediata
immobility inmovilidad
immobilization inmovilización
immobilization paralysis parálisis de
inmovilización
immobilizing inmovilizante
immobilizing activity actividad inmovilizante
immoral inmoral
immoral imperative imperativo inmoral
immorality inmoralidad
immune deficiency syndrome síndrome de
deficiencia inmune
immune system sistema inmune
immune system and stress sistema inmune y
estrés
immune system regulation regulación del
sistema inmune
immunity inmunidad
immunity factors factores de inmunidad
immunization inmunización
immunogen inmunógeno
immunoglobulin inmunoglobulina
immunological inmunológico
immunological functioning funcionamiento
inmunológico
immunological paralysis parálisis
inmunológica
immunology inmunología
immunosuppresive inmunosupresivo
immunosuppresive drug droga
inmunosupresiva
immunosuppression inmunosupresión
impact impacto
impact analysis análisis de impacto
impaired deteriorado
impaired insight penetración deteriorada
impaired judgment juicio deteriorado
impaired sexual desire deseo sexual
deteriorado

impairment deterioro
impairment index índice de deterioro
impairment of academic functioning
deterioro de funcionamiento académico
impasse atolladero
impatience impaciencia
impedance impedancia
impedance method método de impedancia
impediment impedimento
imperative imperativo
imperative attitude actitud imperativa
imperative conception concepción imperativa
imperceptible imperceptible
imperception impercepción
impersonal impersonal
impersonal projection proyección impersonal
impersonal relationship relación impersonal
impersonation imitación
impetus ímpetu
implant implante
implantation implantación
implication implicación
implicit implícito
implicit behavior conducta implícita
implicit learning aprendizaje implícito
implicit memory memoria implícita
implicit personality theory teoría de
personalidad implícita
implicit response respuesta implícita
implicit role papel implícito
implicit speech habla implícita
implied implícito
implied directive directivo implícito
implosion implosión
implosion therapy terapia de implosión
implosive implosivo
implosive therapy terapia implosiva
impossible figure figura imposible
impostor impostor
impostor syndrome síndrome de impostor
impotence impotencia
impotency impotencia
impregnation impregnación
impression impresión
impression formation formación de impresión
impression management administración de
impresiones
impression method método de impresión
impression of universality impresión de
universalidad
impressive aphasia afasia impresiva
imprinting impronta
improvement mejora
improvement rate tasa de mejora
improvisation improvisación
impuberism impuberismo
impuberty impubertad
impulse impulso
impulse control control de impulsos
impulse control disorder trastorno de control
de impulsos
impulse disorder trastorno de impulsos
impulse interpretation interpretación de
impulsos
impulse neurosis neurosis de impulsos

impulsion impulsión
impulsive impulsivo
impulsive behavior conducta impulsiva
impulsive character carácter impulsivo
impulsive obsession obsesión impulsiva
impulsive personality personalidad impulsiva
impulsive tempo tempo impulsivo
impulsiveness impulsividad
impulsivity impulsividad
impulsivity and eating disorders
    impulsividad y trastornos del comer
impulsivity and language disorders
    impulsividad y trastornos del lenguaje
impulsivity and suicidal behavior
    impulsividad y conducta suicida
impunitive impunitivo
impunitive response respuesta impunitiva
in-between intermedio
in-group grupo exclusivo
in-group favoritism favoritismo en grupo
    exclusivo
in-house interno
in-house evaluation evaluación interna
in loco parentis in loco parentis
in utero in utero
in vitro in vitro
in vivo in vivo
inability inhabilidad
inaccessibility inaccesibilidad
inaccessible inaccesible
inaccessible memory memoria inaccesible
inadequacy insuficiencia
inadequate inadecuado
inadequate personality personalidad
    inadecuada
inadequate stimulus estímulo inadecuado
inanimate inanimado
inanition inanición
inappetence inapetencia
inappropriate inapropiado
inappropriate affect afecto inapropiado
inappropriate behavior conducta inapropiada
inappropriateness impropiedad
inappropriateness of affect impropiedad de
    afecto
inarticulate inarticulado
inassimilable inasimilable
inattention inatención
inborn ingénito
inborn error of metabolism error de
    metabolismo ingénito
inbred engendrado por reproducción
    consanguínea, ingénito
inbreeding reproducción consanguínea
incendiarism incendiarismo
incentive incentivo
incentive system sistema de incentivos
incentive theory teoría de incentivos
incest incesto
incest barrier barrera al incesto
incest fantasy fantasía de incesto
incest taboo tabú de incesto
incest wish deseo de incesto
incestuous incestuoso
incestuous desire deseo incestuoso

incestuous ties vínculos incestuosos
incidence incidencia
incidence of child abuse incidencia de abuso
    de niños
incidence rate tasa de incidencia
incident incidente
incident region región incidente
incidental incidental
incidental image imagen incidental
incidental learning aprendizaje incidental
incidental memory memoria incidental
incidental stimulus estímulo incidental
incipient incipiente
incipient psychosis psicosis incipiente
inclusion inclusión
inclusion-body encephalitis encefalitis de
    cuerpos de inclusión
inclusion-cell disease enfermedad de células
    de inclusión
inclusion criteria criterios de inclusión
inclusive inclusivo
inclusive fitness aptitud inclusiva
incoercible incoercible
incoherence incoherencia
incoherent incoherente
incommensurable inconmensurable
incompatibility incompatibilidad
incompatible incompatible
incompatible response respuesta incompatible
incompetence incompetencia
incompetence plea alegación de
    incompetencia
incompetency incompetencia
incompetent incompetente
incomplete incompleto
incomplete alexia alexia incompleta
incomplete neurofibromatosis
    neurofibromatosis incompleta
incomplete pictures test prueba de pinturas
    incompletas
incomplete sentences oraciones incompletas
incomplete sentences test prueba de
    oraciones incompletas
incongruity incongruencia
inconstancy inconstancia
incontinence incontinencia
incontinent incontinente
incontinentia incontinencia
incoordination incoordinación
incorporation incorporación
increment incremento
increment threshold umbral de incremento
incremental incremental
incremental validity validez incremental
incubation incubación
incubation of avoidance incubación de
    evitación
incubus íncubo
incus incus
indecency indecencia
indeloxazine indeloxazina
indemnity neurosis neurosis de indemnidad
independence independencia
independent independiente
independent events eventos independientes

independent living vivir independiente
independent-living aids ayudas para vivir independiente
independent personality personalidad independiente
independent play juego independiente
independent practice práctica independiente
independent variable variable independiente
indeterminate indeterminado
indeterminism indeterminismo
index índice
index adoptees adoptados índice
index case caso índice
index number número índice
index of body build índice de tipo corporal
index of difficulty índice de dificultad
index of discrimination índice de discriminación
index of forecasting efficiency índice de eficiencia de pronóstico
index of refraction índice de refracción
index of reliability índice de confiabilidad
index of sexuality índice de sexualidad
index of variability índice de variabilidad
index variable variable índice
indexical communication comunicación indicativa
indexical sign signo indicativo
indicant indicante
indicator indicador
indifference indiferencia
indifference point punto de indiferencia
indifference to pain syndrome síndrome de indiferencia al dolor
indifferent indiferente
indifferent stimulus estímulo indiferente
indigenous indígena
indigenous family culture cultura familiar indígena
indigenous worker trabajador indígeno
indigestion indigestión
indirect indirecto
indirect association asociación indirecta
indirect correlation correlación indirecta
indirect directive directivo indirecto
indirect effects efectos indirectos
indirect fracture fractura indirecta
indirect measurement medición indirecta
indirect method of therapy método indirecto de terapia
indirect scaling escalamiento indirecto
indirect speech habla indirecta
indirect speech act acto del habla indirecta
indirect survey encuesta indirecta
indirect theory of perception teoría de percepción indirecta
indirect vision visión indirecta
indissociation indisociación
individual individual
individual differences diferencias individuales
individual differences in language development diferencias individuales en el desarrollo del lenguaje
individual differences in perception diferencias individuales en percepción

individual differences in personality diferencias individuales en personalidad
individual education educación individual
individual program programa individual
individual psychological motives motivos psicológicos individuales
individual psychology psicología individual
individual psychotherapy psicoterapia individual
individual reactions to disasters reacciones individuales a desastres
individual response respuesta individual
individual-response specificity especificidad de respuesta individual
individual symbol símbolo individual
individual test prueba individual
individual therapy terapia individual
individualism individualismo
individuality individualidad
individuality theory teoría de individualidad
individualized individualizado
individualized assessment evaluación individualizada
individualized education plan plan de educación individualizada
individualized education plans and mainstreaming planes de educación individualizada y traslación a la corriente principal
individualized education program programa de educación individualizada
individualized education programs and mainstreaming programas de educación individualizada y traslación a la corriente principal
individualized instruction instrucción individualizada
individualized reading lectura individualizada
individuation individuación
individuation stage etapa de individuación
individuation techniques técnicas de individuación
indoctrination adoctrinamiento
indolamine indolamina
indole indol
indole derivative derivado del indol
induced inducido
induced abortion aborto inducido
induced aggression agresión inducida
induced color color inducido
induced compliance acatamiento inducido
induced hallucination alucinación inducida
induced hypothermia hipotermia inducida
induced motion moción inducida
induced movement movimiento inducido
induced psychosis psicosis inducida
induced psychotic disorder trastorno psicótico inducido
induced tonus tono inducido
induced trance trance inducido
induction inducción
induction test prueba de inducción
inductive inductivo
inductive problem solving resolución de problemas inductiva

inductive reasoning razonamiento inductivo
inductive teaching method método de
    enseñanza inductivo
indulgence indulgencia
indusium griseum indusium griseum
industrial industrial
industrial consultant consultor industrial
industrial-organizational psychology
    psicología industrial-organizacional
industrial psychiatry psiquiatría industrial
industrial psychology psicología industrial
industrial rehabilitation counselor asesor de
    rehabilitación industrial
industrial therapy terapia industrial
industry industria
industry versus inferiority industria contra
    inferioridad
inebriation inebriación
inebriety inebriedad
ineffability inefabilidad
ineffable inefable
ineffective ineficaz
ineffective stimulus estímulo ineficaz
inertia inercia
inertia principle principio de inercia
inertia time tiempo de inercia
infancy infancia
infancy research investigación de infancia
infant infante
infant and preschool tests pruebas de infantes
    y preescolares
infant at risk infante a riesgo
infant behavior conducta de infantes
infant behavior and breast-feeding conducta
    de infantes y alimentación por pecho
infant development desarrollo de infantes
infant learning aprendizaje de infantes
infant mental health salud mental de infantes
infant mortality mortalidad de infantes
infant narcotic withdrawal retiro narcótico
    de infante
infant perception percepción de infantes
infant perception of color percepción de
    color de infantes
infant perceptual ability habilidad perceptiva
    de infantes
infant play juego de infantes
infant play behavior conducta de juego de
    infantes
infant psychiatry psiquiatría de infantes
infant reactions to hospitalization reacciones
    de infantes a hospitalización
infant reactions to illness reacciones de
    infantes a enfermedad
infant reactions to parental divorce
    reacciones de infantes a divorcio parental
infant scale escala de infante
infant socialization socialización de infantes
infant-stimulation program programa de
    estimulación de infantes
infant studies estudios de infantes
infant test prueba de infante
infanticide infanticidio
infantile infantil
infantile amnesia amnesia infantil

infantile articulation articulación infantil
infantile atrophy atrofia infantil
infantile autism autismo infantil
infantile autism and childhood schizophrenia
    autismo infantil y esquizofrenia de niñez
infantile-birth theories teorías infantiles de
    nacimiento
infantile convulsion convulsión infantil
infantile diplegia diplejía infantil
infantile dynamics dinámica infantil
infantile hemiplegia hemiplejía infantil
infantile hyperkinetic syndrome síndrome
    hipercinético infantil
infantile masturbation masturbación infantil
infantile muscular atrophy atrofia muscular
    infantil
infantile myxedema mixedema infantil
infantile neuroaxonal dystrophy distrofia
    neuroaxonal infantil
infantile neuronal degeneration degeneración
    neuronal infantil
infantile osteopetrosis osteopetrosis infantil
infantile paralysis parálisis infantil
infantile paresis paresia infantil
infantile perseveration perseveración infantil
infantile personality personalidad infantil
infantile polycystic disease enfermedad
    poliquística infantil
infantile progressive spinal muscular atrophy
    atrofia muscular espinal progresiva infantil
infantile sadism sadismo infantil
infantile seduction seducción infantil
infantile sexuality sexualidad infantil
infantile spasm espasmo infantil
infantile spastic paraplegia paraplejía
    espástica infantil
infantile speech habla infantil
infantile tetany tetania infantil
infantilism infantilismo
infantilistic infantilístico
infantilization infantilización
infarct infarto
infarction infarto
infatuation amartelamiento
infection infección
infection-exhaustion psychosis psicosis de
    infección-agotamiento
infection theory teoría de infección
infectious infeccioso
infectious disease enfermedad infecciosa
infectious-exhaustive syndrome síndrome
    infeccioso-exhaustivo
infectious hepatitis hepatitis infecciosa
infectious mononucleosis mononucleosis
    infecciosa
infectious ophthalmoplegia oftalmoplejía
    infecciosa
infectious polyneuritis polineuritis infecciosa
infecundity infecundidad
inference inferencia
inferential inferencial
inferential bias in memory sesgo inferencial
    en memoria
inferential statistics estadística inferencial
inferential strategies estrategias inferenciales

inferior inferior
inferior colliculus colículo inferior
inferior function función inferior
inferior longitudinal fasciculus fascículo longitudinal inferior
inferior oblique oblicuo inferior
inferior polioencephalitis polioencefalitis inferior
inferior rectus recto inferior
inferiority inferioridad
inferiority complex complejo de inferioridad
inferiority feelings sentimientos de inferioridad
inferotemporal inferotemporal
inferotemporal cortex corteza inferotemporal
infertility infertilidad
infestation infestación
infestation delusion delusión de infestación
infibulation infibulación
infidelity infidelidad
infidelity delusion delusión de infidelidad
infiltration infiltración
infinity neurosis neurosis de lo infinito
infirmity achaque
inflammation inflamación
inflammatory inflamatorio
inflammatory dysmenorrhea dismenorrea inflamatoria
inflection inflexión
inflection point punto de inflexión
influence influencia
influencing influyente
influencing machine máquina influyente
influenza influenza
informal informal
informal admission admisión informal
informal organization organización informal
informal source fuente informal
informal support system sistema de apoyo informal
informal test prueba informal
information información
information acquisition adquisición de información
information feedback retroalimentación de información
information gathering recolección de información
information-input process proceso de entrada de información
information-optimization position posición de optimización de información
information overload sobrecarga de información
information processing procesamiento de información
information-processing ability habilidad de procesamiento de información
information processing and cognition procesamiento de información y cognición
information processing and perception procesamiento de información y percepción
information-processing theory teoría de procesamiento de información
information science ciencia de la información

information system sistema de información
information theory teoría de información
information transfer transferencia de información
information transmission transmisión de información
informed informado
informed consent consentimiento informado
informed consent and child abuse consentimiento informado y abuso de niños
informed consent and competency consentimiento informado y competencia
informed consent and comprehension of information consentimiento informado y comprensión de información
informed consent and confidentiality consentimiento informado y confidencialidad
informed consent and patient decision making consentimiento informado y toma de decisiones de pacientes
informed consent and treatment consentimiento informado y tratamiento
informed consent in research consentimiento informado en investigación
infraclinoid aneurysm aneurisma infraclinoideo
infradian infradiano
infradian rhythm ritmo infradiano
infrahuman infrahumano
infrapsychic infrapsíquico
infrared infrarrojo
infrared spectrophotometer espectrofotómetro infrarrojo
infrared theory of smell teoría infrarroja del olfato
infrequency infrecuencia
infrequency scale escala de infrecuencia
infundibuloma infundibuloma
infundibulum infundibulum
infusion infusión
ingestive ingestivo
ingestive behavior conducta ingestiva
ingratiating congraciador
ingratiation congraciamiento
ingravescent ingravescente
ingravescent apoplexy apoplejía ingravescente
inguinal inguinal
inguinal adenopathy adenopatía inguinal
inhalant inhalante
inhalant abuse abuso de inhalante
inhalant anxiety disorder trastorno de ansiedad de inhalante
inhalant delirium delirio de inhalante
inhalant dependence dependencia de inhalante
inhalant-induced organic mental disorder trastorno mental orgánico inducido por inhalante
inhalant intoxication intoxicación por inhalante
inhalant mood disorder trastorno del humor de inhalante
inhalant persistent dementia demencia

persistente de inhalante
inhalant psychotic disorder trastorno
  psicótico de inhalante
inhalant psychotic disorder with delusions
  trastorno psicótico de inhalante con
  delusiones
inhalant psychotic disorder with
  hallucinations trastorno psicótico de
  inhalante con alucinaciones
inhalant use disorder trastorno de uso de
  inhalante
inhalation inhalación
inhalation convulsive treatment tratamiento
  convulsivo de inhalación
inhalation of drugs inhalación de drogas
inhalation therapy terapia de inhalación
inherent inherente
inherit heredar
inheritable heredable
inheritance herencia
inheritance of acquired characteristics
  legado de características adquiridas
inherited heredado
inherited disorder trastorno heredado
inherited releasing mechanism mecanismo
  liberador heredado
inherited trait rasgo heredado
inhibit inhibir
inhibited inhibido
inhibited female orgasm orgasmo femenino
  inhibido
inhibited grief aflicción inhibida
inhibited male orgasm orgasmo masculino
  inhibido
inhibited mania manía inhibida
inhibited sexual arousal despertamiento
  sexual inhibido
inhibited sexual desire deseo sexual inhibido
inhibited sexual excitement excitación sexual
  inhibida
inhibition inhibición
inhibition mechanism mecanismo de
  inhibición
inhibition of delay inhibición de demora
inhibition of inhibition inhibición de
  inhibición
inhibition of reinforcement inhibición de
  refuerzo
inhibition with reinforcement inhibición con
  refuerzo
inhibitor inhibidor
inhibitory inhibitorio
inhibitory conditioning condicionamiento
  inhibitorio
inhibitory maturation maduración inhibitoria
inhibitory obsession obsesión inhibitoria
inhibitory postsynaptic potential potencial
  postsináptico inhibitorio
inhibitory potential potencial inhibitorio
inhibitory process proceso inhibitorio
inhibitory reflex reflejo inhibitorio
inhibitory synapse sinapsis inhibitoria
iniencephaly iniencefalia
initial inicial
initial cry llanto inicial

initial insomnia insomnio inicial
initial interview entrevista inicial
initial spurt arranque inicial
initiating iniciador
initiating structure estructura iniciadora
initiation iniciación
initiative iniciativa
initiative versus guilt iniciativa contra
  culpabilidad
initiator iniciador
injection inyección
injection administration administración de
  inyección
injury lesión
injury of intervertebral disk lesión de disco
  intervertebral
injury potential potencial de lesión
inkblot test prueba de manchas de tinta
innate innato
innate behavior conducta innata
innate ideas ideas innatas
innate reflex reflejo innato
innate releasing mechanism mecanismo
  liberador innato
innate response system sistema de respuesta
  innata
innate versus learned innato contra aprendido
innate versus learned behavior conducta
  innata contra aprendida
inner interno
inner boundary límite interno
inner conflict conflicto interno
inner controls controles internos
inner-directed dirigido hacia lo interno
inner-directed behavior conducta dirigida
  hacia lo interno
inner ear oído interno
inner estrangement alienación interna
inner language lenguaje interno
inner-personal region región personal interna
inner speech habla interna
innervation inervación
innervation apraxia apraxia de inervación
innocent inocente
innovation innovación
innovation processes procesos de innovación
innovative innovador
innovative psychotherapies psicoterapias
  innovadoras
innovative therapies terapias innovadoras
inoculate inocular
inoculation inoculación
inoculation hypothesis hipótesis de
  inoculación
inpatient paciente internado
inpatient services servicios de pacientes
  internados
inpatient treatment tratamiento de pacientes
  internados
input entrada
input disorder trastorno de entrada
input-output entrada-salida
input-output mechanism mecanismo de
  entrada-salida
inquiry indagación, pregunta

inquiry training model modelo de
entrenamiento de indagación
insane insano
insane asylum asilo de insanos
insanity insania
insanity defense defensa de insania
insanity of negation insania de negación
insanity panic pánico de insania
insect society sociedad de insectos
insecticides as behavioral teratogens
insecticidas como teratógenos conductuales
insecure inseguro
insecure attachment apego inseguro
insecurity inseguridad
insemination inseminación
insensible insensible
insensitivity insensibilidad
insertion inserción
inside density densidad interna
insight penetración
insight-oriented psychotherapy psicoterapia
orientada a la penetración
insight therapy terapia de penetración
insolation insolación
insomnia insomnio
insomnia and anxiety insomnio y ansiedad
insomnia disorder trastorno de insomnio
insomniac insomne
inspection inspección
inspectionalism inspeccionalismo
inspectionism inspeccionismo
inspiration inspiración
inspiration-expiration inspiración-expiración
inspiration-expiration ratio razón de
inspiración-expiración
inspiration group therapy terapia de grupo
de inspiración
instability inestabilidad
instant instante
instigation instigación
instigation therapy terapia de instigación
instigator instigador
instinct instinto
instinct eruption erupción de instinto
instinct need necesidad de instinto
instinct presentation presentación de instinto
instinct-ridden acosado por instintos
instinctive instintivo
instinctive behavior conducta instintiva
instinctive monomania monomanía instintiva
instinctoid needs necesidades instintoides
instinctual instintivo
instinctual aggression agresión instintiva
instinctual aim fin instintivo
instinctual anxiety ansiedad instintiva
instinctual drive impulso instintivo
instinctual dyscontrol descontrol instintivo
instinctual fusion fusión instintiva
instinctual impulse impulso instintivo
instinctual renunciation renunciación
instintiva
instinctualization instintualización
instinctualization of smell instintualización
del olfato
institution institución

institutional institucional
institutional care cuidado institucional
institutional neurosis neurosis institucional
institutional peonage peonaje institucional
institutional relocation reubicación
institucional
institutional review board junta de revisión
institucional
institutional transference transferencia
institucional
institutional treatment tratamiento
institucional
institutionalism institucionalismo
institutionalization institucionalización
institutionalization and legal rights
institucionalización y derechos legales
institutionalize institucionalizar
instruction instrucción
instructional instruccional
instructional plan plan instruccional
instructional theory teoría instruccional
instrument instrumento
instrument design diseño de instrumento
instrumental instrumental
instrumental act acto instrumental
instrumental aggression agresión
instrumental
instrumental behavior conducta instrumental
instrumental conditioning condicionamiento
instrumental
instrumental dependence dependencia
instrumental
instrumental-relativist orientation
orientación instrumental-relativista
instrumental response respuesta instrumental
instrumentalism instrumentalismo
instrumentality medio
instrumentality theory teoría del medio
insufficiency insuficiencia
insufficiency of eyelids insuficiencia de
párpados
insula ínsula
insular insular
insular sclerosis esclerosis insular
insularity insularidad
insulin insulina
insulin abnormality anormalidad insulínica
insulin coma coma insulínico
insulin-coma therapy terapia de coma
insulínico
insulin-coma treatment tratamiento de coma
insulínico
insulin-dependent diabetes diabetes
dependiente de insulina
insulin hypoglycemia test prueba de
hipoglucemia insulínica
insulin lipodystrophy lipodistrofia insulínica
insulin shock choque insulínico
insulin-shock therapy terapia de choque
insulínico
insulin treatment tratamiento de insulina
insult insulto
intake admisión
intake-orientation group grupo de
orientación de admisión

integrate integrar
integrated integrado
integrated model modelo integrado
integration integración
integrative integrante
integrative capacities capacidades integrantes
integrative learning aprendizaje integrante
integrative properties propiedades integrantes
integrity integridad
integrity group grupo de integridad
integrity versus despair integridad contra
　　desesperación
intellect intelecto
intellectual intelectual
intellectual assessment evaluación intelectual
**intellectual assessment of developmental
　　disorders** evaluación intelectual de
　　trastornos del desarrollo
intellectual aura aura intelectual
intellectual detachment desprendimiento
　　intelectual
intellectual deterioration deterioración
　　intelectual
intellectual development desarrollo intelectual
intellectual functioning funcionamiento
　　intelectual
intellectual functions funciones intelectuales
intellectual impoverishment empobrecimiento
　　intelectual
intellectual inadequacy insuficiencia
　　intelectual
intellectual insight penetración intelectual
intellectual maturity madurez intelectual
intellectual monomania monomanía
　　intelectual
intellectual operations operaciones
　　intelectuales
intellectual rigidity rigidez intelectual
intellectual subaverage functioning
　　funcinonamiento bajo promedio intelectual
intellectualism intelectualismo
intellectualization intelectualización
intelligence inteligencia
intelligence and environment inteligencia y
　　ambiente
intelligence and heredity inteligencia y
　　herencia
intelligence assessment evaluación de
　　inteligencia
intelligence measures medidas de inteligencia
intelligence quotient cociente de inteligencia
intelligence quotient test prueba de cociente
　　de inteligencia
intelligence scale escala de inteligencia
intelligence test prueba de inteligencia
intemperance intemperancia
intensity intensidad
intensity discrimination discriminación de
　　intensidad
intensity of affect intensidad de afecto
intensity of mood intensidad del humor
intensity of reaction intensidad de reacción
intensive intensivo
intensive care cuidado intensivo
intensive-care syndrome síndrome de cuidado

intensivo
intensive-care unit unidad de cuidado
　　intensivo
intensive psychotherapy psicoterapia
　　intensiva
intent intención
intention intención
intention spasm espasmo de intención
intention tremor temblor de intención
intentional intencional
intentional accident accidente intencional
intentional behavior conducta intencional
intentional death muerte intencional
intentional forgetting olvidar intencional
intentional learning aprendizaje intencional
intentional state estado intencional
intentional unvoluntary behavior conducta
　　involuntaria intencional
intentionality intencionalidad
interaction interacción
interaction effect efecto de interacción
interaction process analysis análisis del
　　proceso de interacción
interaction territory territorio de interacción
interaction theory of personality teoría de
　　personalidad de interacción
interaction variance varianza de interacción
interactional interactivo
interactional contract contrato interactivo
interactional psychotherapy psicoterapia
　　interactiva
interactional synchrony sincronía interactiva
interactionism interaccionismo
interactions and habits interacciones y
　　hábitos
interactive interactivo
interactive disturbance disturbio interactivo
interactive dualism dualismo interactivo
interactive measurement medición interactiva
interaural interaural
interaural differences diferencias interaurales
interaural rivalry rivalidad interaural
interbehavioral interconductual
interbehavioral psychology psicología
　　interconductual
interbody intercuerpo
interbrain cerebro intermedio
intercalated intercalado
intercalation intercalación
intercerebral intercerebral
intercerebral fibers fibras intercerebrales
intercorrelation intercorrelación
intercortical intercortical
intercostal neuralgia neuralgia intercostal
intercourse relación
interdental sigmatism sigmatismo interdental
interdisciplinary interdisciplinario
interdisciplinary approach acercamiento
　　interdisciplinario
interdisciplinary environmental design
　　diseño ambiental interdisciplinario
interdisciplinary treatment tratamiento
　　interdisciplinario
interego interego
interest interés

interest factors factores de interés
interest inventory inventario de intereses
interest test prueba de intereses
interested interesado
interface interfase
interface accentuation acentuación de '
　interfase
interference interferencia
interference effects efectos de interferencia
interference theory teoría de interferencia
interference theory of forgetting teoría de
　interferencia de olvidar
intergenerational intergeneracional
intergenerational mobility movilidad
　intergeneracional
intergroup intergrupo
intergroup conflict conflicto intergrupo
intergroup-contact hypothesis hipótesis de
　contacto de intergrupo
intergroup exercises ejercicios intergrupales
interhemispheric interhemisférico
interhemispheric transfer transferencia
　interhemisférica
interictal interictal
interindividual interindividual
interindividual differences diferencias
　interindividuales
interiorized imitation imitación interiorizada
interjection theory teoría de interjección
interjectional theory teoría interjeccional
interjudge reliability confiabilidad interjueces
interlocking entrelazado
interlocking reinforcement refuerzo
　entrelazado
interlocking schedule programa entrelazado
intermarriage matrimonio mixto, matrimonio
　entre parientes
intermediate intermedio
intermediate-acting barbiturates barbituratos
　de acción intermedia
intermediate brain syndrome due to alcohol
　síndrome cerebral intermedio debido al
　alcohol
intermediate-care facility instalación de
　cuidado intermedio
intermediate gene gen intermedio
intermediate needs necesidades intermedias
intermediate precentral area área precentral
　intermedia
intermediate sex sexo intermedio
intermetamorphosis intermetamorfosis
intermission intermisión
intermittence intermitencia
intermittence tone tono de intermitencia
intermittent intermitente
intermittent acute porphyria porfiria aguda
　intermitente
intermittent cramp calambre intermitente
intermittent explosive disorder trastorno
　explosivo intermitente
intermittent insomnia insomnio intermitente
intermittent processing procesamiento
　intermitente
intermittent psychosis psicosis intermitente
intermittent reinforcement refuerzo

intermitente
intermittent schedule programa intermitente
intermittent tetanus tétanos intermitente
intermittent torticollis tortícolis intermitente
intermodal intermodal
intermodal fluency fluidez intermodal
intermodal integration integración intermodal
intermodal perception percepción intermodal
internal interno
internal aim fin interno
internal boundary límite interno
internal capsule cápsula interna
internal capsule syndrome síndrome de
　cápsula interna
internal carotid artery arteria carótida
　interna
internal conflict conflicto interno
internal consistency consistencia interna
internal decompression descompresión
　interna
internal ear oído interno
internal environment ambiente interno
internal-external scale escala interna-externa
internal factors factores internos
internal factors in aggression factores
　internos en agresión
internal feedback retroalimentación interna
internal granular layer capa granular interna
internal hair cells células pilosas internas
internal hydrocephalus hidrocefalia interna
internal inhibition inhibición interna
internal locus of control locus de control
　interno
internal meningitis meningitis interna
internal pyocephalus piocefalia interna
internal rectus recto interno
internal representation representación interna
internal respiration respiración interna
internal rhythm ritmo interno
internal secretion gland glándula de
　secreción interna
internal senses sentidos internos
internal state estado interno
internal validity validez interna
internalization internalización
internalized internalizado
internalized sentences oraciones
　internalizadas
internalized speech habla internalizada
internalizing internalizante
internalizing behavior conducta internalizante
international candle bujía internacional
interneuron interneurona
interneurosensory interneurosensorial
interneurosensory learning aprendizaje
　interneurosensorial
internship internado
internuncial internuncial
internuncial neuron neurona internuncial
interobserver interobservador
interobserver reliability confiabilidad de
　interobservador
interoception interocepción
interoceptive interoceptivo
interoceptive conditioning condicionamiento

interoceptivo
interoceptive sense sentido interoceptivo
interoceptor interoceptor
interocular interocular
interocular distance distancia interocular
interosystem interosistema
interpenetration interpenetración
interpersonal interpersonal
interpersonal accommodation acomodación
   interpersonal
interpersonal attraction atracción
   interpersonal
interpersonal boundary regulation
   regulación de límites interpersonales
interpersonal communication comunicación
   interpersonal
interpersonal concordance concordancia
   interpersonal
interpersonal conflict conflicto interpersonal
interpersonal control control interpersonal
interpersonal distance distancia interpersonal
interpersonal morality moralidad
   interpersonal
interpersonal perception percepción
   interpersonal
interpersonal problem problema
   interpersonal
interpersonal process proceso interpersonal
interpersonal psychiatry psiquiatría
   interpersonal
interpersonal psychotherapy psicoterapia
   interpersonal
interpersonal relations relaciones
   interpersonales
interpersonal relationship relación
   interpersonal
interpersonal relationship deficit déficit de
   relaciones interpersonales
interpersonal role conflict conflicto de papel
   interpersonal
interpersonal skills destrezas interpersonales
interpersonal skills development desarrollo
   de destrezas interpersonales
interpersonal theory teoría interpersonal
interpersonal therapy terapia interpersonal
interpersonal trust confianza interpersonal
interpersonal trust scale escala de confianza
   interpersonal
interpolate interpolar
interpolated interpolado
interpolated reinforcement refuerzo
   interpolado
interposition interposición
interpretation interpretación
interpretation delusion delusión de
   interpretación
interpretation of dreams interpretación de
   sueños
interpretative interpretativo
interpretative therapy terapia interpretativa
interpsychology interpsicología
interquartile range intervalo intercuartil
interresponse time tiempo entre respuestas
interrogative interrogativo
interrupted interrumpido

interrupted dream sueño interrumpido
interruption interrupción
interruption tone tono de interrupción
interscapular reflex reflejo interescapular
intersegmental intersegmentario
intersegmental tract tracto intersegmentario
intersensory intersensorial
intersensory bias sesgo intersensorial
intersensory disorder trastorno intersensorial
intersensory integration integración
   intersensorial
intersensory interactions interacciones
   intersensoriales
intersensory perception percepción
   intersensorial
intersex intersexo
intersexuality intersexualidad
interstice intersticio
interstimulation interestimulación
interstimulus interestímulo
interstimulus interval intervalo de
   interestímulo
interstitial intersticial
interstitial cell stimulating hormone
   hormona estimulante de células
   intersticiales
interstitial cells células intersticiales
interstitial nephritis nefritis intersticial
interstitial neuritis neuritis intersticial
interstitial neurosyphilis neurosífilis
   intersticial
intersubjective intersubjetivo
interthalamic intertalámico
interthalamic adhesions adhesiones
   intertalámicas
intertrial interval intervalo entre ensayos
interval intervalo
interval estimate estimado de intervalo
interval of uncertainty intervalo de
   incertidumbre
interval psychosis psicosis de intervalo
interval reinforcement refuerzo de intervalo
interval scale escala de intervalos
interval schedule programa de intervalos
intervening interviniente
intervening act acto interviniente
intervening variable variable interviniente
intervention intervención
intervention for delinquency intervención
   para delincuencia
intervention research investigación de
   intervención
intervention technique técnica de
   intervención
interventricular foramen of Monro foramen
   interventricular de Monro
intervertebral foramen foramen
   intervertebral
interview entrevista
interview content contenido de entrevista
interview contrast effect efecto de contraste
   de entrevistas
interview group psychotherapy psicoterapia
   de grupo de entrevista
interview process proceso de entrevista

interview therapy terapia de entrevista
interviewer entrevistador
interviewer bias sesgo del entrevistador
interviewer effects efectos del entrevistador
interviewer stereotype estereotipo del entrevistador
interviewer training entrenamiento del entrevistador
intestinal intestinal
intestinal lipodystrophy lipodistrofia intestinal
intestinal sepsis sepsis intestinal
intimacy intimidad
intimacy disorder trastorno de intimidad
intimacy principle principio de intimidad
intimacy versus isolation intimidad contra aislamiento
intimacy versus self-absorption intimidad contra absorción propia
intimate íntimo
intimate relationship relación íntima
intimate zone zona íntima
intimidate intimidar
intimidation intimidación
intolerance intolerancia
intolerance of ambiguity intolerancia de ambigüedad
intonation entonación
intonation contour contorno de entonación
intoxication intoxicación
intraception intracepción
intraceptive intraceptivo
intraceptive signaling señalamiento intraceptivo
intracerebral intracerebral
intracerebral hemorrhage hemorragia intracerebral
intracisternal intracisternal
intraconscious intraconsciente
intraconscious personality personalidad intraconsciente
intracranial intracraneal
intracranial aneurysm aneurisma intracraneal
intracranial gumma goma intracraneal
intracranial hematoma hematoma intracraneal
intracranial hemorrhage hemorragia intracraneal
intracranial hypotension hipotensión intracraneal
intracranial pneumatocele neumatocele intracraneal
intracranial pneumocele neumocele intracraneal
intracranial pressure presión intracraneal
intracranial stimulation estimulación intracraneal
intracranial tumor tumor intracraneal
intractable intratable
intractable pain dolor intratable
intrafusal intrafusal
intrafusal fibers fibras intrafusales
intrafusal motoneurons motoneuronas intrafusales
intragroup intragrupo
intragroup territorial behavior conducta

territorial intragrupal
intraindividual intraindividual
intraindividual differences diferencias intraindividuales
intralaminar system sistema intralaminar
intramedullary tractotomy tractotomía intramedular
intramodal intramodal
intramodal abilities habilidades intramodales
intramural intramural
intramuscular intramuscular
intramuscular injection inyección intramuscular
intraneurosensory intraneurosensorial
intraneurosensory learning aprendizaje intraneurosensorial
intransitivity intransitividad
intraocular intraocular
intraocular modification modificación intraocular
intraocular neuritis neuritis intraocular
intraocular pressure presión intraocular
intrapersonal intrapersonal
intrapersonal conflict conflicto intrapersonal
intrapsychic intrapsíquico
intrapsychic ataxia ataxia intrapsíquica
intrapsychic censorship censura intrapsíquica
intrapsychic conflict conflicto intrapsíquico
intrapsychic society sociedad intrapsíquica
intraserial intraserial
intraserial learning aprendizaje intraserial
intrasubject intrasujeto
intrauterine intrauterino
intrauterine device dispositivo intrauterino
intravascular intravascular
intravascular ligature ligadura intravascular
intravenous intravenoso
intravenous injection inyección intravenosa
intraventricular intraventricular
intraventricular hemorrhage hemorragia intraventricular
intraventricular injection inyección intraventricular
intraverbal intraverbal
intrinsic intrínseco
intrinsic behavior conducta intrínseca
intrinsic cortex corteza intrínseca
intrinsic eye muscles músculos oculares intrínsecos
intrinsic factor factor intrínseco
intrinsic interest interés intrínseco
intrinsic motivation motivación intrínseca
intrinsic reflex reflejo intrínseco
intrinsic reward recompensa intrínseca
intrinsic validity validez intrínseca
introitus introito
introjection introyección
intromission intromisión
intron intrón
intropunitive intropunitivo
intropunitive response respuesta intropunitiva
introspection introspección
introspectionism introspeccionismo
introspective introspectivo
introspective method método introspectivo

introversion introversión
introversion-extraversion
  introversión-extraversión
introversion-extraversion continuum
  continuo introversión-extraversión
introversion-extroversion
  introversión-extroversión
introversion-extroversion continuum
  continuo introversión-extroversión
introvert introvertido
introverted introvertido
introverted personality personalidad
  introvertida
introverted personality disorder trastorno de
  personalidad introvertida
introverted type tipo introvertido
intrusion intrusión
intrusion error error de intrusión
intrusion response respuesta de intrusión
intrusive intrusivo
intrusive treatment tratamiento intrusivo
intubation intubación
intuition intuición
intuitive intuitivo
intuitive behavior conducta intuitiva
intuitive sociogram sociograma intuitivo
intuitive stage etapa intuitiva
intuitive type tipo intuitivo
invalid inválido
invalidate invalidar
invalidism invalidismo
invariable invariable
invariable hues matices invariables
invariance invarianza
invasion of privacy invasión de privacidad
invasive invasor
invasive treatment tratamiento invasor
inventory inventario
inventory test prueba de inventario
inverse inverso
inverse agonist agonista inverso
inverse correlation correlación inversa
inverse derivation derivación inversa
inverse factor analysis análisis factorial
  inverso
inverse hypothesis hipótesis inversa
inverse nystagmus nistagmo inverso
inverse relationship relación inversa
inverse-square law ley inversa de cuadrados
inversion inversión
inversion of affect inversión de afecto
inversion relationship relación de inversión
invert invertido
inverted invertido
inverted factor analysis análisis factorial
  invertido
inverted Oedipus complex complejo de Edipo
  invertido
inverted radial reflex reflejo radial invertido
inverted reflex reflejo invertido
inverted sadism sadismo invertido
inverted-U curve curva en U invertida
inverted-U distribution distribución en U
  invertida
inverted-U function función en U invertida

investigation investigación
investigation of child abuse investigación de
  abuso de niños
investigatory investigador
investigatory reflex reflejo investigador
investment inversión
inveterate inveterado
inveterate drinking beber inveterado
invisible college colegio invisible
invisible playmate compañero de juego
  invisible
involuntary involuntario
involuntary admission admisión involuntaria
involuntary discharge dada de alta
  involuntaria
involuntary eye movements movimientos de
  ojo involuntarios
involuntary hospitalization hospitalización
  involuntaria
involuntary movement movimiento
  involuntario
involuntary muscles músculos involuntarios
involuntary response respuesta involuntaria
involuntary treatment tratamiento
  involuntario
involution involución
involutional involutivo
involutional depression depresión involutiva
involutional melancholia melancolía
  involutiva
involutional paranoid state estado paranoide
  involutivo
involutional paraphrenia parafrenia
  involutiva
involutional period periodo involutivo
involutional psychosis psicosis involutiva
involutional psychotic reaction reacción
  psicótica involutiva
involvement envolvimiento
inward interno
inward picture imagen interna
ion pump bomba de iones
ionizing radiation radiación ionizante
iontophoresis iontoforesis
iophobia iofobia
iota iota
iproniazid iproniazida
ipsation ipsación
ipsative ipsativo
ipsative scale escala ipsativa
ipsative scaling escalamiento ipsativo
ipsative score puntuación ipsativa
ipsilateral ipsilateral
ipsilateral deficit déficit ipsilateral
ipsilateral reflex reflejo ipsilateral
ipsolateral ipsolateral
iridocyclitis iridociclitis
iridoparalysis iridoparálisis
iridoplegia iridoplejía
iris iris
iris reflex reflejo del iris
iritic irítico
iritic reflex reflejo irítico
iron lung pulmón de hierro
iron overloading sobrecarga de hierro

irradiation irradiación
irradiation effects efectos de irradiación
irradiation theory teoría de irradiación
irradiation theory of learning teoría de
   aprendizaje de irradiación
irrational irracional
irrational action acción irracional
irrational belief creencia irracional
irrational desire deseo irracional
irrational type tipo irracional
irrationality irracionalidad
irreality irrealidad
irreality level nivel de irrealidad
irrelevant irrelevante
irrelevant answer respuesta irrelevante
irrelevant attributes atributos irrelevantes
irrelevant language lenguaje irrelevante
irresistible irresistible
irresistible apprehension aprehensión
   irresistible
irresistible impulse impulso irresistible
irresistible impulse test prueba de impulsos
   irresistibles
irresponsibility irresponsabilidad
irreversible irreversible
irreversible shock choque irreversible
irritability irritabilidad
irritability of cell irritabilidad de célula
irritable irritable
irritable bladder vejiga irritable
irritable bowel syndrome síndrome de
   intestino irritable
irritable heart corazón irritable
irritable mood humor irritable
irritable testis testículo irritable
irritation irritación
irrumation irrumación
Isakower phenomenon fenómeno de
   Isakower
ischemia isquemia
ischemic isquémico
ischemic lumbago lumbago isquémico
ischemic muscular atrophy atrofia muscular
   isquémica
ischemic optic neuropathy neuropatía óptica
   isquémica
ischialgia isquialgia
ischiodynia isquiodinia
ischioneuralgia isquioneuralgia
ischnophonia iscnofonía
ischophonia iscofonía
Ishihara test prueba de Ishihara
island of Reil isla de Reil
islands of Langerhans islas de Langerhans
isocarboxazid isocarboxazida
isochromosome isocromosoma
isochronal isocronal
isocoria isocoria
isocortex isocorteza
isoelectric isoeléctrico
isoelectric electroencephalogram
   electroencefalograma isoeléctrico
isoelectric encephalogram encefalograma
   isoeléctrico
isogamous isógamo

isolate aislar
isolated aislado
isolated brain cerebro aislado
isolated delusion delusión aislada
isolated environment ambiente aislado
isolated explosive disorder trastorno
   explosivo aislado
isolation aislamiento
isolation amentia amencia por aislamiento
isolation effect efecto de aislamiento
isolation experiment experimento de
   aislamiento
isolation of affect aislamiento de afecto
isomeric function función isomérica
isometric contraction contracción isométrica
isomorphism isomorfismo
isomorphous isomorfo
isomorphous gliosis gliosis isomorfa
isoniazid isoniazida
isoniazid neuropathy neuropatía por
   isoniazida
isopathic principle principio isopático
isophilia isofilia
isophilic isofílico
isophonic isofónico
isophonic contour contorno isofónico
isopropanol isopropanol
isoproterenol isoproterenol
isosexual isosexual
isotonic isotónico
isotonic contraction contracción isotónica
isozyme isozima
issue cuestión
isthmoparalysis istmoparálisis
isthmoplegia istmoplejía
itch comezón
itching comezón
item artículo
item analysis análisis de artículos
item difficulty dificultad de artículo
item response respuesta de artículo
item scaling escalamiento de artículo
item selection selección de artículo
item validity validez de artículo
item weighting ponderación de artículo
itemized rating scale escala de clasificación
   detallada
ithycyphosis iticifosis
ithykyphosis iticifosis
ithylordosis itilordosis
itinerant itinerante
itinerant teacher maestro itinerante
ixomielitis ixomielitis

J

J coefficient coeficiente J
J curve curva en J
J-sella deformity deformidad selar en J
Jackson's law ley de Jackson
Jackson's principle principio de Jackson
Jackson's rule regla de Jackson
Jackson's sign signo de Jackson
Jackson's syndrome síndrome de Jackson
jacksonian epilepsy epilepsia jacksoniana
jacksonian march marcha jacksoniana
Jacobson's organ órgano de Jacobson
Jacobson's reflex reflejo de Jacobson
jactatio capitis nocturna jactación de cabeza
    nocturna
jactation jactación
jactitation jactitación
Jahnke's syndrome síndrome de Jahnke
Jakob-Creutzfeldt disease enfermedad de
    Jakob-Creutzfeldt
jamais phenomenon fenómeno de jamais
jamais vu jamais vu
James-Lange theory teoría de James-Lange
James-Lange theory of emotion teoría de
    emoción de James-Lange
Janet's disease enfermedad de Janet
Janet's psychology psicología de Janet
Janet's test prueba de Janet
Jansky-Bielschowsky disease enfermedad de
    Jansky-Bielschowsky
Janusian thinking pensamiento janoniano
jar sacudida
jargon jerga
jargon aphasia afasia de jerga
Jarisch-Herxheimer reaction reacción de
    Jarisch-Herxheimer
jaundice ictericia
jaw mandíbula
jaw-grinding rechinamiento
jaw jerk sacudida mandibular
jaw reflex reflejo mandibular
jaw-winking phenomenon fenómeno de guiño
    mandibular
jaw-winking sign signo de guiño mandibular
jaw-winking syndrome síndrome de guiño
    mandibular
jealous celoso
jealous spouse cónyuge celoso
jealous type tipo celoso
jealousy celos
Jellinek's formula fórmula de Jellinek
Jendrassik's maneuver maniobra de
    Jendrassik
Jendrassik reinforcement refuerzo de
    Jendrassik

jerk sacudida
jerk finger dedo en gatillo
jet-lag desincronosis circadiano
jet-lag phenomenon fenómeno de
    desincronosis circadiano
jitter fluctuación
job analysis análisis de trabajo
job-characteristics model modelo de
    características de trabajo
job-component method método de
    componentes de trabajo
job design diseño de trabajo
job dimensions dimensiones de trabajo
job enrichment enriquecimiento de trabajo
job evaluation evaluación de trabajo
job information información de trabajo
job interview entrevista de trabajo
job performance ejecución de trabajo
job placement colocación de trabajo
job-related displacement desplazamiento
    relacionado al trabajo
job requirements requisitos de trabajo
job satisfaction satisfacción de trabajo
job security seguridad de trabajo
job stress estrés de trabajo
Jocasta complex complejo de Yocasta
Joffroy's reflex reflejo de Joffroy
Joffroy's sign signo de Joffroy
joint custody custodia conjunta
joint event evento conjunto
joint play juego conjunto
joint probability probabilidad conjunta
joint sense sentido articular
joking relationship relación de relajar
Jolly's reaction reacción de Jolly
Jost's law ley de Jost
Joubert's syndrome síndrome de Joubert
joy felicidad
judgment juicio
Julesz's stereogram estereograma de Julesz
jumper saltador
jumper disease enfermedad de saltador
juncture coyuntura
jungian jungiano
jungian psychoanalysis psicoanálisis jungiano
jungian psychology psicología jungiana
juror bias sesgo de jurado
juror competence competencia de jurado
jury psychology psicología de jurado
jury selection selección de jurado
just noticeable difference diferencia
    escasamente notable
just noticeable differences method método
    de diferencias escasamente notables
justice justicia
justification justificación
juvenescence juventud
juvenile juvenil
juvenile chorea corea juvenil
juvenile delinquency delincuencia juvenil
juvenile era era juvenil
juvenile general paralysis parálisis general
    juvenil
juvenile impostor impostor juvenil
juvenile muscular atrophy atrofia muscular

juvenil
juvenile myoclonic epilepsy epilepsia
   mioclónica juvenil
juvenile paresis paresia juvenil
juvenile period periodo juvenil
juvenile tabes tabes juvenil
juvenilism juvenilismo
juxtaposition yuxtaposición

K

K complex complejo K
K scale escala K
K strategy estrategia K
Kahlbaum-Wernicke syndrome síndrome de
   Kahlbaum-Wernicke
Kahn test prueba de Kahn
kainophobia cainofobia
kainotophobia cainotofobia
kakorrhaphiophobia cacorrafiofobia
kakosmia cacosmia
Kallmann's syndrome síndrome de Kallmann
Kandinsky-Clerambault complex complejo
   de Kandinsky-Clerambault
Kanner's syndrome síndrome de Kanner
kappa kappa
kappa waves ondas kappa
karezza carezza
karyotype cariotipo
katasexual catasexual
katasexuality catasexualidad
katatonia catatonía
kathisophobia catisofobia
Kayser-Fleischer ring anillo de
   Kayser-Fleischer
Kearns-Sayre syndrome síndrome de
   Kearns-Sayre
Keeler polygraph polígrafo de Keeler
Keen's operation operación de Keen
Kegel exercises ejercicios de Kegel
keirospasm queiroespasmo
Keller plan plan de Keller
Kempf's disease enfermedad de Kempf
Kendall tests pruebas de Kendall
Kennedy's syndrome síndrome de Kennedy
kenophobia quenofobia
Kerandel's symptom síntoma de Kerandel
kerasin histiocytosis histiocitosis de querasina
keratitis queratitis
keratosis queratosis
keraunoneurosis queraunoneurosis
keraunophobia queraunofobia
kernicterus kernicterus
Kernig's sign signo de Kernig
kernikterus kernicterus
Kernohan's notch escotadura de Kernohan
ketosteroid cetoesteriode
key concept concepto clave
key question pregunta clave
key-word method método de palabra clave
kid's culture cultura de niños
kidnapping secuestro
kidnapping by parent secuestro por padre,
   secuestro por madre
kilobytophobia kilobitofobia

kin parentela
kinanesthesia cinanestesia
kindling kindling
kinematics cinemática
kinemorph cinemorfo
kinephantom cinefantasma
kinesalgia cinesalgia
kinesia cinesia
kinesics cinésica
kinesiology cinesiología
kinesioneurosis cinesioneurosis
kinesipathy cinesipatía
kinesitherapy cinesiterapia
kinesophobia cinesofobia
kinesthesia cinestesia
kinesthesiometer cinestesiómetro
kinesthetic cinestésico
kinesthetic apraxia apraxia cinestésica
kinesthetic aura aura cinestésica
kinesthetic hallucination alucinación
    cinestésica
kinesthetic method método cinestésico
kinesthetic sense sentido cinestésico
kinetic cinético
kinetic ataxia ataxia cinética
kinetic depth effect efecto de profundidad
    cinético
kinetic drive impulso cinético
kinetic information información cinética
kinetic tremor temblor cinético
kinky-hair disease enfermedad de cabello
    ensortijado
kinky-hair syndrome síndrome de cabello
    ensortijado
kinohapt cinohapto
kinship parentesco
Kisch's reflex reflejo de Kisch
kissing behavior conducta de besar
Kjersted-Robinson law ley de
    Kjersted-Robinson
klazomania clazomanía
Klebedenken Klebedenken
Klebenbleiben Klebenbleiben
Kleine-Levin syndrome síndrome de
    Kleine-Levin
kleptolagnia cleptolagnia
kleptomania cleptomanía
kleptomaniac cleptomaníaco
kleptophobia cleptofobia
Klinefelter's syndrome síndrome de
    Klinefelter
klinotaxis clinotaxis
Klippel's disease enfermedad de Klippel
Klippel-Feil syndrome síndrome de
    Klippel-Feil
klismaphilia clismafilia
Klumpke's paralysis parálisis de Klumpke
Klumpke-Dejerine syndrome síndrome de
    Klumpke-Dejerine
Kluver-Bucy syndrome síndrome de
    Kluver-Bucy
knee-jerk sacudida de rodilla
knee-jerk reflex reflejo de sacudida de rodilla
knee phenomenon fenómeno de rodilla
knee reflex reflejo de rodilla

knowledge conocimiento
knowledge by acquaintance conocimiento por
    familiaridad
knowledge of results conocimiento de
    resultados
knowledge test prueba de conocimientos
Kocher-Debre-Semelaigne syndrome
    síndrome de Kocher-Debre-Semelaigne
Koenig cylinders cilindros de Koenig
Koerber-Salus-Elschnig syndrome síndrome
    de Koerber-Salus-Elschnig
Koerte-Ballance operation operación de
    Koerte-Ballance
Kohler-Restorff phenomenon fenómeno de
    Kohler-Restorff
Kohnstamm's phenomenon fenómeno de
    Kohnstamm
Kohnstamm maneuver maniobra de
    Kohnstamm
Kohnstamm test prueba de Kohnstamm
koinotropy coinotropia
Kojewnikoff's epilepsy epilepsia de
    Kojewnikoff
Kolomogorov-Smirnov test prueba de
    Kolomogorov-Smirnov
kolyphrenia colifrenia
kolytic colítico
Konig bars barras de Konig
kopophobia copofobia
koprolagnia coprolagnia
koprolalia coprolalia
koprophagia coprofagia
koprophemia coprofemia
koprophilia coprofilia
koprophobia coprofobia
koro koro
Korsakoff's psychosis psicosis de Korsakoff
Korsakoff's syndrome síndrome de
    Korsakoff
Korte's laws leyes de Korte
Krabbe's disease enfermedad de Krabbe
Krabbe's syndrome síndrome de Krabbe
Kraepelin's disease enfermedad de Kraepelin
Krause end bulb bulbo terminal de Krause
Kretschmer types tipos de Kretschmer
Kretschmer typology tipología de Kretschmer
Kruskal-Shepard scaling escalamiento de
    Kruskal-Shepard
Kruskal-Wallis test prueba de Kruskal-Wallis
kubisagari kubisagari
kubisagaru kubisagaru
Kuder-Richardson formulas fórmulas de
    Kuder-Richardson
Kufs disease enfermedad de Kufs
Kugelberg-Welander disease enfermedad de
    Kugelberg-Welander
Kuhne's phenomenon fenómeno de Kuhne
Kummell's spondylitis espondilitis de
    Kummell
Kundt's rules reglas de Kundt
kurtosis curtosis
Kussmaul's aphasia afasia de Kussmaul
Kussmaul's coma coma de Kussmaul
Kussmaul-Landry paralysis parálisis de
    Kussmaul-Landry

kwashiorkor kwashiorkor
kymatism cimatismo
kymograph cimógrafo
kyphoscoliosis cifoescoliosis
kyphosis cifosis

L

la belle indifference la belle indifference
Labbe's neurocirculatory syndrome
    síndrome neurocirculatorio de Labbe
labeling etiquetaje
labeling theory teoría de etiquetaje
labia labios
labia majora labios mayores
labia minora labios menores
labial labial
labial paralysis parálisis labial
labile lábil
labile affect afecto lábil
labile mood humor lábil
labile personality disorder trastorno de
    personalidad lábil
lability labilidad
lability-stability labilidad-estabilidad
labiochorea labiocorea
labiodental labiodental
labioglossolaryngeal labioglosolaríngeo
labioglossopharyngeal labioglosofaríngeo
labiolabial labiolabial
labium labio
labium majus labio mayor
labium minus labio menor
laboratory laboratorio
laboratory investigation investigación de
    laboratorio
laboratory method model modelo de método
    de laboratorio
laboratory test prueba de laboratorio
laboratory training entrenamiento de
    laboratorio
labyrinth laberinto
labyrinthine laberíntico
labyrinthine reflex reflejo laberíntico
labyrinthine righting reflex reflejo de
    enderezamiento laberíntico
labyrinthine sense sentido laberíntico
labyrinthine torticollis tortícolis laberíntico
laceration laceración
lachrymal lagrimal
lack of empathy falta de empatía
lack of involvement falta de envolvimiento
lack of motivation falta de motivación
lack of penetrance falta de penetrancia
laconic lacónico
laconic speech habla lacónica
lacrimal lagrimal
lacrimal gland glándula lagrimal
lacrimal reflex reflejo lagrimal
lacrimation lacrimación
lacrimo-gustatory reflex reflejo
    lagrimo-gustatorio

lactate (n) lactato
lactate (v) lactar
lactate challenge reto de lactato
lactate threshold umbral de lactato
lactation lactación
lactogenic hormone hormona lactogénica
lacuna laguna
lacuna cerebri laguna cerebral
lacunar lagunar
lacunar amnesia amnesia lagunar
Ladd-Franklin theory teoría de
  Ladd-Franklin
Lafora's disease enfermedad de Lafora
Lafora body cuerpo de Lafora
Lafora body disease enfermedad de cuerpos
  de Lafora
lag atraso
lagophthalmos lagoftalmos
lagophthalmus lagoftalmos
Laingian view perspectiva de Laingian
laissez-faire laissez-faire
laissez-faire atmosphere atmósfera
  laissez-faire
laissez-faire group grupo laissez-faire
laissez-faire leader líder laissez-faire
laliophobia laliofobia
lallation lalación
lalling laleo
lalochezia laloquezia
lalognosis lalognosis
laloneurosis laloneurosis
lalopathy lalopatía
lalophobia lalofobia
laloplegia laloplejía
lalorrhea lalorrea
lamarckian theory teoría lamarckiana
Lamaze method método de Lamaze
lambda lambda
lambert lambert
Lambert's law ley de Lambert
Lambert cosine law ley de cosenos de
  Lambert
Lambert-Eaton syndrome síndrome de
  Lambert-Eaton
lambitus lambitus
lamina lámina
laminar laminar
laminar cortical necrosis necrosis cortical
  laminar
laminar cortical sclerosis esclerosis cortical
  laminar
laminectomy laminectomía
laminotomy laminotomía
lancinating lancinante
Land effect efecto de Land
land of childhood tierra de niñez
Land theory of color vision teoría de Land de
  visión de color
Landau-Kleffner syndrome síndrome de
  Landau-Kleffner
Landau reflex reflejo de Landau
landmark hito
Landolt circle círculo de Landolt
Landolt ring anillo de Landolt
Landouzy-Dejerine dystrophy distrofia de

Landouzy-Dejerine
Landouzy-Grasset law ley de
  Landouzy-Grasset
Landry's paralysis parálisis de Landry
Landry's syndrome síndrome de Landry
Landry-Guillain-Barre syndrome síndrome
  de Landry-Guillain-Barre
Langdon Down's disease enfermedad de
  Langdon Down
Lange's test prueba de Lange
language lenguaje
language acquisition adquisición del lenguaje
language acquisition device aparato de
  adquisición del lenguaje
language acquisition system sistema de
  adquisición del lenguaje
language and perception lenguaje y
  percepción
language and speech disorder trastorno del
  lenguaje y habla
language arts artes del lenguaje
language centers centros del lenguaje
language comprehension comprensión del
  lenguaje
language deficit déficit del lenguaje
language deficit and brain damage déficit
  del lenguaje y daño cerebral
language deficit and child abuse déficit del
  lenguaje y abuso de niños
language deficit and intelligence tests déficit
  del lenguaje y pruebas de inteligencia
language development desarrollo del lenguaje
language development in babbling desarrollo
  del lenguaje en balbuceo
language disability discapacidad del lenguaje
language disorder trastorno del lenguaje
language-experience approach to reading
  acercamiento a la lectura de experiencias
  del lenguaje
language game juego lingüístico
language in animals lenguaje en animales
language in autism lenguaje en autismo
language in play lenguaje en juego
language localization ubicación del lenguaje
language origin origen del lenguaje
language pathology patología del lenguaje
language problem problema del lenguaje
language retardation retardo del lenguaje
language score puntuación del lenguaje
language skills destrezas del lenguaje
language test prueba del lenguaje
language theories teorías del lenguaje
language therapy terapia del lenguaje
language zone zona del lenguaje
lanugo lanugo
laparoscopy laparoscopia
lapse lapso
lapsus lapsus
lapsus calami lapsus calami
lapsus linguae lapsus linguae
lapsus memoriae lapsus memoriae
larval sadism sadismo larval
larval schizophrenia esquizofrenia larval
laryngeal cancer cáncer laríngeo
laryngeal chorea corea laríngea

laryngeal crisis crisis laríngea
laryngeal epilepsy epilepsia laríngea
laryngeal reflex reflejo laríngeo
laryngeal syncope síncope laríngeo
laryngeal vertigo vértigo laríngeo
laryngectomy laringectomía
laryngoparalysis laringoparálisis
laryngopharynx laringofaringe
laryngoplegia laringoplejía
laryngospasm laringoespasmo
laryngospastic laringoespástico
laryngospastic reflex reflejo laringoespástico
larynx laringe
lascivia lascivia
lasciviency lascivia
lascivus lascivo
Lasegue's disease enfermedad de Lasegue
Lasegue's sign signo de Lasegue
Lasegue's syndrome síndrome de Lasegue
laser light luz lasérica
Lashley jumping stand plataforma de saltos
    de Lashley
lassitude lasitud
latah lata
late adolescence adolescencia tardía
late adulthood adultez tardía
late epilepsy epilepsia tardía
late infantile systemic lipidosis lipidosis
    sistémica infantil tardía
late life forgetting olvidar en la vida tardía
late luteal phase dysphoric disorder
    trastorno disfórico de fase lútea tardía
late-onset schizophrenia esquizofrenia de
    comienzo tardío
late paraphrenia parafrenia tardía
latency latencia
latency of reply latencia de respuesta
latency of response latencia de respuesta
latency period periodo de latencia
latency phase fase de latencia
latency stage etapa de latencia
latency stage of psychosexual development
    etapa de latencia del desarrollo psicosexual
latent latente
latent additional period periodo adicional
    latente
latent content contenido latente
latent dream content contenido de sueños
    latente
latent extinction extinción latente
latent goal fin latente
latent homosexual homosexual latente
latent homosexuality homosexualidad latente
latent inhibition inhibición latente
latent learning aprendizaje latente
latent period periodo latente
latent process proceso latente
latent psychosis psicosis latente
latent reflex reflejo latente
latent schizophrenia esquizofrenia latente
latent social identity identidad social latente
latent tetany tetania latente
latent trait rasgo latente
latent trait theory teoría de rasgo latente
latent zone zona latente

lateral lateral
lateral bundle fascículo lateral
lateral cervical nucleus núcleo cervical lateral
lateral confusion confusión lateral
lateral corticospinal tract tracto
    corticoespinal lateral
lateral differences diferencias laterales
lateral dominance dominancia lateral
lateral dorsal nucleus núcleo dorsal lateral
lateral fissure fisura lateral
lateral geniculate body cuerpo geniculado
    lateral
lateral geniculate nucleus núcleo geniculado
    lateral
lateral gyrus circunvolución lateral
lateral horn cuerno lateral
lateral hypothalamic syndrome síndrome
    hipotalámico lateral
lateral hypothalamus hipotálamo lateral
lateral inhibition inhibición lateral
lateral lemniscus lemnisco lateral
lateral masking enmascaramiento lateral
lateral medullary syndrome síndrome
    medular lateral
lateral olfactory tract tracto olfatorio lateral
lateral orbital gyrus circunvolución orbital
    lateral
lateral posterior nucleus núcleo posterior
    lateral
lateral preoptic area área preóptica lateral
lateral rectus recto lateral
lateral section sección lateral
lateral specialization especialización lateral
lateral spinal sclerosis esclerosis espinal
    lateral
lateral spinothalamic tract tracto
    espinotalámico lateral
lateral sulcus surco lateral
lateral thalamic nucleus núcleo talámico
    lateral
lateral thinking pensamiento lateral
lateral ventricle ventrículo lateral
lateral vertigo vértigo lateral
laterality lateralidad
lateralization lateralización
lateropulsion lateropulsión
lathyrism latirismo
Latin square cuadrado latino
latitude latitud
lattah lata
laudanum laúdano
laughing disease enfermedad de la risa
laughing sickness enfermedad de la risa
laughter risa
laughter reflex reflejo de la risa
Laurence-Biedl syndrome síndrome de
    Laurence-Biedl
Laurence-Moon-Bardet-Biedl syndrome
    síndrome de Laurence-Moon-Bardet-Biedl
Laurence-Moon-Biedl syndrome síndrome de
    Laurence-Moon-Biedl
Laurence-Moon syndrome síndrome de
    Laurence-Moon
law ley
law-and-order orientation orientación de ley

y orden
law of advantage ley de ventaja
law of assimilation ley de asimilación
law of association ley de asociación
law of avalanche ley de avalancha
law of average localization ley de
  localización promedia
law of Bichat ley de Bichat
law of cohesion ley de cohesión
law of combination ley de combinación
law of common fate ley de destino común
law of constancy ley de constancia
law of contiguity ley de contigüidad
law of contrast ley de contraste
law of denervation ley de desnervación
law of diminishing returns ley de utilidad
  decreciente
law of effect ley de efecto
law of equality ley de igualdad
law of equipotentiality ley de
  equipotencialidad
law of exercise ley de ejercicio
law of filial regression ley de regresión filial
law of forward conduction ley de conducción
  hacia adelante
law of frequency ley de frecuencia
law of identical direction ley de dirección
  idéntica
law of initial value ley de valor inicial
law of isochronism ley de isocronismo
law of large numbers ley de números grandes
law of least action ley de acción mínima
law of mass action ley de acción en masa
law of parsimony ley de parsimonia
law of Pragnanz ley de Pragnanz
law of precision ley de precisión
law of primacy ley de primacía
law of prior entry ley de entrada previa
law of progression ley de progresión
law of proximity ley de proximidad
law of readiness ley de disposición
law of recency ley de lo más reciente
law of referred pain ley de dolor referido
law of repetition ley de repetición
law of retrogenesis ley de retrogénesis
Lawford's syndrome síndrome de Lawford
laws of color preference leyes de
  preferencias de colores
laws of learning leyes del aprendizaje
laws of organization leyes de organización
lax laxo
laxative laxante
laxative abuse abuso de laxantes
laxative addiction adicción a laxantes
lay no profesional
layer capa
lead plomo
lead-cap headache dolor de cabeza de capa
  de plomo
lead encephalitis encefalitis por plomo
lead encephalopathy encefalopatía por plomo
lead exposure and cognitive development
  exposición a plomo y desarrollo cognitivo
lead neuropathy neuropatía por plomo
lead palsy parálisis por plomo

lead paralysis parálisis por plomo
lead-pipe rigidity rigidez de tubo de plomo
lead poisoning envenenamiento por plomo
leader líder
leaderless sin líder
leaderless group grupo sin líder
leaderless-group therapy terapia de grupo sin
  líder
leadership liderazgo
leadership effectiveness efectividad de
  liderazgo
leadership role papel de liderazgo
leadership style estilo de liderazgo
leadership theory teoría de liderazgo
leadership training entrenamiento de
  liderazgo
leading dominante
leading eye ojo dominante
leading hemisphere hemisferio dominante
Lear complex complejo de Lear
learn aprender
learn-to-learn concept concepto de aprender
  a aprender
learned aprendido
learned autonomic control control
  autonómico aprendido
learned behavior conducta aprendida
learned discrimination discriminación
  aprendida
learned drive impulso aprendido
learned helplessness impotencia aprendida
learned helplessness and apathy impotencia
  aprendida y apatía
learned helplessness theory of depression
  teoría de depresión de impotencia
  aprendida
learned motivation motivación aprendida
learned response respuesta aprendida
learned tolerance tolerancia aprendida
learning aprendizaje
learning ability habilidad de aprendizaje
learning and cognitive development
  aprendizaje y desarrollo cognitivo
learning and cues aprendizaje y señales
learning and memory aprendizaje y memoria
learning and retention aprendizaje y
  retención
learning and rewards aprendizaje y
  recompensas
learning anxiety ansiedad de aprendizaje
learning aversion aversión de aprendizaje
learning curve curva de aprendizaje
learning disabilities in child abuse victims
  discapacidades de aprendizaje en víctimas
  de abuso de niños
learning disability discapacidad de
  aprendizaje
learning disability specialist especialista de
  discapacidades de aprendizaje
learning during sleep aprendizaje durante
  sueño
learning from experience aprendizaje de
  experiencias
learning model modelo de aprendizaje
learning of language aprendizaje del lenguaje

learning paradigm paradigma de aprendizaje
learning potential potencial de aprendizaje
learning problem problema de aprendizaje
learning session sesión de aprendizaje
learning set predisposición para aprendizaje
learning strategy estrategia de aprendizaje
learning style estilo de aprendizaje
learning theory teoría de aprendizaje
learning to learn aprendiendo a aprender
learning trial ensayo de aprendizaje
learning without awareness aprendizaje sin
  conciencia
least-effort principle principio del esfuerzo
  mínimo
least resistance resistencia mínima
least-resistance site sitio de resistencia
  mínima
least restrictive alternative alternativa menos
  restrictiva
least restrictive environment ambiente menos
  restrictivo
least-squares cuadrados mínimos
least-squares criterion criterio de cuadrados
  mínimos
least-squares principle principio de cuadrados
  mínimos
leaving the field abandonando el campo
Leber's disease enfermedad de Leber
Leboyer method método de Leboyer
Leboyer technique técnica de Leboyer
lecanomancy lecanomancia
lecheur lecheur
lecture method método de conferencia
left-footed sinistropedal
left-handed zurdo
left hemisphere hemisferio izquierdo
leg phenomenon fenómeno de pierna
legal legal
legal authority autoridad legal
legal capacity capacidad legal
legal custody custodia legal
legal divorce divorcio legal
legal medicine medicina legal
legal psychiatry psiquiatría legal
legal psychology psicología legal
legal rights derechos legales
legalistic orientation orientación legalista
legasthenia legastenia
Legendre's sign signo de Legendre
Leichtenstern's phenomenon fenómeno de
  Leichtenstern
Leichtenstern's sign signo de Leichtenstern
Leigh's disease enfermedad de Leigh
leipolalia leipolalia
leisure ocio
lemma lema
lemniscal lemniscal
lemniscal system sistema lemniscal
lemniscus lemnisco
length duración
length of dreams duración de sueños
length of stay duración de estadía
lengthening reaction reacción de
  alargamiento
Lenhossek's processes procesos de Lenhossek

Lennox-Gastaut syndrome síndrome de
  Lennox-Gastaut
Lennox syndrome síndrome de Lennox
lens lente
lens of eye lente del ojo
lenticular lenticular
lenticular-fasciculus stimulation estimulación
  lenticular-fascículo
lenticular nucleus núcleo lenticular
lenticular progressive degeneration
  degeneración progresiva lenticular
leprechaunism leprecaunismo
leprosy lepra
leprous leproso
leprous neuropathy neuropatía leprosa
leptokurtic leptocúrtico
leptokurtosis leptocurtosis
leptomeningeal leptomeníngeo
leptomeningeal carcinoma carcinoma
  leptomeníngeo
leptomeningeal carcinomatosis
  carcinomatosis leptomeníngea
leptomeningeal fibrosis fibrosis
  leptomeníngea
leptomeninges leptomeninges
leptomeningitis leptomeningitis
leptomorph leptomorfo
leptoprosophia leptoprosofia
leptosomal leptosomal
leptosome leptosoma
leptosomic leptosómico
Leri's sign signo de Leri
Leriche's operation operación de Leriche
Leroy's disease enfermedad de Leroy
lesbian lesbiana
lesbianism lesbianismo
Lesch-Nyhan syndrome síndrome de
  Lesch-Nyhan
lesion lesión
lethal letal
lethal catatonia catatonía letal
lethality letalidad
lethality scale escala de letalidad
lethargic letárgico
lethargic hypnosis hipnosis letárgica
lethargy letargia
letheomania leteomanía
lethologica letológica
letter blindness ceguera literal
letter reversal inversión de letras
leucocyte leucocito
leucoencephalitis leucoencefalitis
leucotomy leucotomía
leuenkephalin leuencefalina
leukemia leucemia
leukocyte leucocito
leukocytic leucocítico
leukocytic sarcoma sarcoma leucocítico
leukocytosis leucocitosis
leukodystrophia leucodistrofia
leukodystrophia cerebri progressiva
  leucodistrofia cerebral progresiva
leukodystrophy leucodistrofia
leukoencephalitis leucoencefalitis
leukoencephalopathy leucoencefalopatía

leukomyelopathy leucomielopatía
leukotome leucotomo
leukotomy leucotomía
levator elevador
levee effect efecto de dique
level nivel
level of achievement nivel de logro
level of aspiration nivel de aspiración
level of attachment nivel de apego
level of care nivel de cuidado
level of confidence nivel de confianza
level of consciousness nivel de conciencia
level of decentration nivel de descentración
level of development nivel del desarrollo
level of risk nivel de riesgo
level of significance nivel de significación
leveling nivelación
leveling effect efecto de nivelación
leveling-sharpening nivelación-agudización
levels of processing niveles de procesamiento
leverage apalancamiento
levirate levirato
levitation levitación
levoamphetamine levoanfetamina
levodopa levodopa
levomepromazine levomepromazina
levophobia levofobia
levopromazine levopromazina
levorphanol levorfanol
Lewy body cuerpo de Lewy
lex talionis ley del talión
lexical léxico
lexical comprehension comprensión léxica
lexical-decision task tarea de decisión léxica
lexical memory memoria léxica
lexicology lexicología
lexicon lexicón
lexicostatistics lexicoestadística
Leyden's ataxia ataxia de Leyden
Leyden's neuritis neuritis de Leyden
Leyden-Mobius muscular dystrophy
    distrofia muscular de Leyden-Mobius
Lhermitte's sign signo de Lhermitte
Lhermitte-Duclos disease enfermedad de
    Lhermitte-Duclos
liability responsabilidad
liability insurance seguro de responsabilidad
    civil
liaison coordinación
liaison nursing enfermería de coordinación
liaison psychiatry psiquiatría de coordinación
liar mentiroso
libidinal libidinal
libidinal cathexis catexis libidinal
libidinal object constancy constancia de
    objeto libidinal
libidinal phase fase libidinal
libidinal transference transferencia libidinal
libidinal type tipo libidinal
libidinization libidinización
libidinize libidinizar
libidinous libidinoso
libido libido
libido analog análogo de libido
libido-binding activity actividad de ligadura

de libido
libido fixation fijación de libido
libido organization organización de libido
libido theory teoría de libido
libido wish deseo de libido
lice piojos
Lichtheim's sign signo de Lichtheim
Lichtheim's test prueba de Lichtheim
licking behavior conducta de lamedura
Liddell-Sherrington reflex reflejo de
    Liddell-Sherrington
lidocaine lidocaína
lie mentira
lie detection detección de mentiras
lie detector detector de mentiras
lie scale escala de mentiras
life chance oportunidad de vida
life change cambio de vida
life-change rating scale escala de
    clasificación de cambios de vida
life-change units unidades de cambio de vida
life circumstance problem problema de
    circunstancia de vida
life course curso de vida
life crisis crisis de vida
life crisis and health crisis de vida y salud
life-crisis unit unidad de crisis de vida
life cycle ciclo de vida
life cycle theory teoría de ciclos de vida
life energy energía de vida
life-event stress estrés de eventos de la vida
life-event stress theory teoría de estrés de
    eventos de la vida
life events eventos de la vida
life expectancy expectativa de vida
life fear temor de vida
life goal fin de la vida
life history historial de vida
life history model modelo de historial de vida
life instinct instinto de vida
life lie mentira de vida
life plan plan de vida
life rhythm ritmo de vida
life script libreto de vida
life space espacio de vida
life span lapso de vida
life-span development desarrollo de lapso de
    vida
life stage etapa de vida
life stress estrés de vida
life table tabla de vida
lifestyle estilo de vida
lifestyle assessment evaluación de estilo de
    vida
lifetime vida
lifetime personality personalidad de vida
lifetime prevalence prevalencia de vida
ligand ligando
ligature ligadura
light adaptation adaptación a luz
light induction inducción de luz
light reflex reflejo de luz
light sensitivity sensibilidad de luz
light sleep sueño liviano
light sleeper durmiente liviano

light sleeper versus deep sleeper durmiente
liviano contra durmiente profundo
light trance trance liviano
lightness claridad
lightning calculator calculador relámpago
likelihood probabilidad
likelihood ratio razón de probabilidad
Likert scale escala de Likert
liking scale escala de preferencia
Lilliputian hallucination alucinación
liliputiense
limb miembro
limb-girdle muscular dystrophy distrofia
muscular de cinturones de miembros
limb-kinetic apraxia apraxia limbocinética
limbic límbico
limbic cortex corteza límbica
limbic lobe lóbulo límbico
limbic system sistema límbico
limen limen
liminal liminal
liminal stimulus estímulo liminal
liminometer liminómetro
limit límite
limit setting establecimiento de límites
limitation limitación
limitations of intelligence tests limitaciones
de pruebas de inteligencia
limited limitado
limited-capacity retrieval recuperación de
capacidad limitada
limited responsibility responsabilidad limitada
limited-symptom attack ataque de síntomas
limitados
limophoitas limofoitas
limophthisis limotisis
limosis limosis
limulus límulo
Lindau's disease enfermedad de Lindau
Lindau's tumor tumor de Lindau
line línea
line of fixation línea de fijación
linear lineal
linear correlation correlación lineal
linear craniectomy craniectomía lineal
linear-operator model modelo de operador
lineal
linear perspective perspectiva lineal
linear program programa lineal
linear regression regresión lineal
linear skull fracture fractura de cráneo lineal
linear system sistema lineal
linear type tipo lineal
lingam lingam
linguadental linguadental
lingual lingual
lingual gyrus circunvolución lingual
lingual nerve nervio lingual
lingual papilla papila lingual
lingual trophoneurosis trofoneurosis lingual
linguistic lingüístico
linguistic approach acercamiento lingüístico
linguistic-kinesic approach acercamiento
lingüístico-cinésico
linguistic relativity relatividad lingüística

linguistic stage etapa lingüística
linguistic universals universales lingüísticos
linguistics lingüística
lingula lingula
link enlace
linkage enlace
linonophobia linonofobia
lip-biting morder de labios
lip eroticism erotismo labial
lip-reading lectura labial
lip reflex reflejo labial
lipidosis lipidosis
lipochondrodystrophia lipocondrodistrofia
lipochondystrophia lipocondistrofia
lipochondystrophy lipocondistrofia
lipofuscin lipofuscina
lipofuscinosis lipofuscinosis
lipoid lipoide
lipomeningocele lipomeningocele
liquidation of attachment liquidación de
apego
lisp (n) ceceo
lisp (v) cecear
lisping ceceo
Lissajou's figures figuras de Lissajou
Lissauer's dementia paralytica demencia
paralítica de Lissauer
Lissauer's tract tracto de Lissauer
Lissauer type paresis paresia tipo Lissauer
lissencephalia lisencefalia
lissencephalic lisencefálico
lissencephaly lisencefalia
lissencephaly syndrome síndrome de
lisencefalia
lissophobia lisofobia
listening attitude actitud de escuchar
listening with the third ear escuchar con el
tercer oído
literacy alfabetismo
literacy test prueba de alfabetismo
literal literal
literal agraphia agrafia literal
literal alexia alexia literal
literal paraphasia parafasia literal
literalism literalismo
lithiasis litiasis
lithic lítico
lithic diathesis diátesis lítica
lithium litio
lithium carbonate carbonato de litio
lithium therapy terapia de litio
litigious litigioso
litigious delusional state estado delusorio
litigioso
litigious paranoia paranoia litigiosa
Litten's sign signo de Litten
Little's disease enfermedad de Little
Littre's glands glándulas de Littre
Lloyd Morgan's canon canon de Lloyd
Morgan
loading carga
lobar lobar
lobar sclerosis esclerosis lobar
lobe lóbulo
lobectomy lobectomía

lobotomy lobotomía
local epilepsy epilepsia local
local excitatory state estado excitatorio local
local potential potencial local
local sign signo local
local syncope síncope local
local tetanus tétanos local
local theory of thirst teoría local de sed
local tic tic local
localization localización
localization agnosia agnosia de localización
localization of function localización de
   función
localization of symptoms localización de
   síntomas
localized localizado
localized amnesia amnesia localizada
localized function función localizada
location ubicación
location bias sesgo de ubicación
location constancy constancia de ubicación
location error error de ubicación
locked ward pabellón cerrado con llave
lockjaw mandíbula trabada
locomotion locomoción
locomotor locomotor
locomotor activity actividad locomotora
locomotor arrest paro locomotor
locomotor ataxia ataxia locomotora
locomotor-genital stage etapa locomotora
   genital
locomotor maze laberinto locomotor
loculation loculación
loculation syndrome síndrome de loculación
locus locus
locus coeruleus locus coeruleus
locus minoris resistentiae locus minoris
   resistentiae
locus of control locus de control
Loeffler's syndrome síndrome de Loeffler
log diario, logaritmo
log law ley de logaritmo
logagnosia logagnosia
logagraphia logagrafia
logamnesia logamnesia
logaphasia logafasia
logarithm logaritmo
logarithmic logarítmico
logarithmic curve curva logarítmica
logarithmic mean media logarítmica
logarithmic relationship relación logarítmica
logasthenia logastenia
logic lógica
logical lógico
logical inference inferencia lógica
logical positivism positivismo lógico
logical reasoning razonamiento lógico
logicogrammatical logicogramatical
logicogrammatical disorder trastorno
   logicogramatical
logistic logístico
logistic curve curva logística
logistics logística
logoclonia logoclonia
logodiarrhea logodiarrea

logography logografía
logomania logomanía
logomonomania logomonomanía
logoneurosis logoneurosis
logopathy logopatía
logopedics logopedia
logophasia logofasia
logoplegia logoplejía
logorrhea logorrea
logospasm logoespasmo
logotherapy logoterapia
loneliness soledad
long-term a largo plazo
long-term care cuidado a largo plazo
long-term memory memoria a largo plazo
long-term potentiation potenciación a largo
   plazo
long-term psychotherapy psicoterapia a largo
   plazo
longevity longevidad
longilineal longilineal
longitudinal longitudinal
longitudinal fissure fisura longitudinal
longitudinal method método longitudinal
longitudinal study estudio longitudinal
longitudinal sulcus surco longitudinal
longitypical longitípico
looking-glass self yo de espejo
looming inminente
loosening aflojamiento
loosening of association aflojamiento de
   asociación
loprazolam loprazolam
lorazepam lorazepam
lordosis lordosis
loss pérdida
loss and grief pérdida y aflicción
loss and suicidal behavior pérdida y conducta
   suicida
loss of affect pérdida de afecto
loss of control pérdida de control
loss of personal identity pérdida de identidad
   personal
lost-letter technique técnica de cartas
   perdidas
Lou Gehrig's disease enfermedad de Lou
   Gehrig
loud speech habla alta
loudness sonoridad
loudness adaptation adaptación a sonoridad
Louis-Bar syndrome síndrome de Louis-Bar
louse piojo
love need necesidad de amor
love object objeto de amor
love scale escala de amor
Loven reflex reflejo de Loven
low delirium delirio bajo
low fever fiebre baja
low-pressure hydrocephalus hidrocefalia de
   presión baja
low tension glaucoma glaucoma de baja
   tensión
low-volume hospital hospital de bajo volumen
lower inferior
lower abdominal periosteal reflex reflejo

perióstico abdominal inferior
lower motor neuron neurona motora inferior
loxapine loxapina
loxia loxia
lucid lúcido
lucid dream sueño lúcido
lucid interval intervalo lúcido
lucid sleep sueño lúcido
lucidification lucidificación
lucidity lucidez
ludic lúdico
ludic activity actividad lúdica
ludotherapy ludoterapia
lues lúes
Luft's disease enfermedad de Luft
lumbago lumbago
lumbar lumbar
lumbar nerve nervio lumbar
lumbar puncture punción lumbar
lumbar puncture needle aguja de punción
    lumbar
lumbar rheumatism reumatismo lumbar
lumbarization lumbarización
lumen lumen
luminance luminancia
luminosity luminosidad
luminosity coefficient coeficiente de
    luminosidad
luminosity curve curva de luminosidad
luminous luminoso
luminous flux flujo luminoso
luminous intensity intensidad luminosa
lump in the throat nudo en la garganta
lumpectomy lumpectomía
lunacy locura
lunatic lunático
lung pulmón
lupinosis lupinosis
lupus lupus
lupus erythematosus lupus eritematoso
Luria technique técnica de Luria
lust lujuria
lust dynamism dinamismo de lujuria
luteal lúteo
luteal phase fase lútea
luteinizing hormone hormona luteinizante
lux lux
lycanthropy licantropía
lycomania licomanía
lycorexia licorexia
lygophilia ligofilia
lying mentir
lymph linfa
lymphocyte linfocito
lymphocytic linfocítico
lymphocytic adenohypophysitis
    adenohipofisitis linfocítica
lymphocytic choriomeningitis coriomeningitis
    linfocítica
lymphoid linfoide
lymphoid hypophysitis hipofisitis linfoide
lysatotherapy lisatoterapia
lysergic acid ácido lisérgico
lysergic acid amide amida de ácido lisérgico
lysergic acid diethylamide dietilamida de

ácido lisérgico
lysergic acid diethylamide psychotherapy
    psicoterapia de dietilamida de ácido
    lisérgico
lysergic acid monoethylamide monoetilamida
    de ácido lisérgico
lysinuria lisinuria
lyssa lisa
lyssophobia lisofobia
lytic cocktail cóctel lítico

M'Naghten rule regla de M'Naghten
MacBeth illuminometer iluminómtero de
    MacBeth
Macewen's sign signo de Macewen
Macewen's symptom síntoma de Macewen
Mach bands bandas de Mach
Mach scale escala de Mach
Machado-Joseph disease enfermedad de
    Machado-Joseph
Machiavellism maquiavelismo
machine fever fiebre de máquina
machine intelligence inteligencia de máquina
machine translation traducción por máquina
MacLean's theory of emotion teoría de
    emoción de MacLean
macrencephalia macrencefalia
macrencephaly macrencefalia
macroadenoma macroadenoma
macrobiotic macrobiótico
macrobiotic diet dieta macrobiótica
macrocephalia macrocefalia
macrocephalic macrocefálico
macrocephalous macrocéfalo
macrocephaly macrocefalia
macrocosm macrocosmo
macrocranium macrocráneo
macroelectrode macroelectrodo
macroencephalon macroencéfalo
macroesthesia macroestesia
macrogenitosomia macrogenitosomía
macroglobulinemia macroglobulinemia
macroglossia macroglosia
macrography macrografía
macrogyria macrogiria
macrology macrología
macromania macromanía
macromastia macromastia
macrophage macrófago
macropsia macropsia
macroskelic macrosquélico
macrosomatognosia macrosomatognosia
macrosplanchnic build tipo macroesplácnico
macrostereognosis macroestereognosis
macula acusticae mácula acústica
macula lutea mácula lútea
maculocerebral maculocerebral
Mad Hatter syndrome síndrome de
    sombrero loco
Maddox rod test prueba de varillas de
    Maddox
madness locura
Madonna complex complejo de Madona
Madonna-prostitute complex complejo de
    Madona-prostituta

Maerz and Paul color dictionary diccionario
    de colores de Maerz y Paul
magazine cargador
magazine training entrenamiento de cargador
Magendie's law ley de Magendie
Magendie-Hertwig sign signo de
    Magendie-Hertwig
Magendie-Hertwig syndrome síndrome de
    Magendie-Hertwig
magic magia
magic bone hueso mágico
magic helper ayudante mágico
magic omnipotence omnipotencia mágica
magic phase fase mágica
magical mágico
magical thinking pensamiento mágico
Magna Mater Magna Mater
magnacide magnacidio
Magnan's sign signo de Magnan
Magnan's trombone movement movimiento
    de trombón de Magnan
magnesium magnesio
magnet reaction reacción de imán
magnet reflex reflejo de imán
magnetic apraxia apraxia magnética
magnetic resonance imaging producción de
    imagen por resonancia magnética
magnetic sense sentido magnético
magnetism magnetismo
magnetoencephalogram
    magnetoencefalograma
magnetoencephalography
    magnetoencefalografía
magnetometer magnetómetro
magnetotropism magnetotropismo
magnitude estimation estimación de magnitud
magnitude of response magnitud de respuesta
magnitude production producción de
    magnitud
Magnus de Kleyn postural reflexes reflejos
    posturales de Magnus de Kleyn
Maier's law ley de Maier
maieusiophobia mayeusiofobia
main principal
Main's syndrome síndrome de Main
main d'accoucheur main d'accoucheur
main effect efecto principal
main en crochet main en crochet
main en griffe main en griffe
mainstreaming traslación a la corriente
    principal
mainstreaming and curriculum traslación a
    la corriente principal y currículo
mainstreaming and individualized education
    traslación a la corriente principal y
    educación individualizada
mainstreaming and social skills traslación a
    la corriente principal y destrezas sociales
maintaining cause causa mantenedora
maintaining stimulus estímulo mantenedor
maintenance mantenimiento
maintenance drug droga de mantenimiento
maintenance drug therapy terapia de droga
    de mantenimiento
maintenance functions funciones de

mantenimiento
maintenance level nivel de mantenimiento
maintenance minimum mínimo de
mantenimiento
maintenance schedule programa de
mantenimiento
maintenance therapy terapia de
mantenimiento
major mayor
major affective disorder trastorno afectivo
mayor
major asynergia of Babinski asinergia mayor
de Babinski
major depression depresión mayor
major depression episode episodio de
depresión mayor
major depressive disorder trastorno
depresivo mayor
major depressive episode episodio depresivo
mayor
major dysrhythmia disritmia mayor
major epilepsy epilepsia mayor
major hypnosis hipnosis mayor
major hysteria histeria mayor
major motor seizure acceso motor mayor
major role therapy terapia de papel mayor
major solution solución mayor
major tranquilizer tranquilizante mayor
maladaptation inadaptación
maladaptive inadaptivo
maladaptive behavior conducta inadaptiva
maladaptive mechanism mecanismo
inadaptivo
maladaptive response respuesta inadaptiva
maladjusted inadaptado
maladjusted child niño inadaptado
maladjustment inadaptación
malaise malestar
malapropism malapropismo
malaria malaria
male alcoholism subtype subtipo de
alcoholismo masculino
male climacterium climaterio masculino
male continence continencia masculina
**male dyspareunia due to general medical
condition** dispareunia masculina debido a
condición médica general
male ejaculation eyaculación masculina
male erectile disorder trastorno eréctil
masculino
**male erectile disorder due to general medical
condition** trastorno eréctil masculino
debido a condición médica general
male genitalia genitales masculinos
male homosexual prostitution prostitución de
homosexuales masculinos
male hypoactive sexual desire disorder
trastorno de deseo sexual hipoactivo
masculino
male member miembro masculino
male menopause menopausia masculina
male orgasmic disorder trastorno orgásmico
masculino
male sexual dysfunction disfunción sexual
masculina

maleate maleato
maleness masculinidad
malevolent malévolo
malevolent transformation transformación
malévola
malformation malformación
malfunction disfunción
malign (adj) maligno
malign (v) difamar
malignancy malignidad
malignant maligno
malignant alcoholism alcoholismo maligno
malignant identity diffusion difusión de
identidad maligna
malignant neoplasm neoplasma maligno
malignant neuroleptic syndrome síndrome
neuroléptico maligno
malignant neurosis neurosis maligna
malignant psychosis psicosis maligna
malignant stupor estupor maligno
malignant syndrome síndrome maligno
Malin syndrome síndrome de Malin
malinger simularse enfermo
malingerer enfermo simulado
malingering simulación de enfermo
malleation maleación
malleus martillo
malnutrition desnutrición
malonic acid ácido malónico
malpractice negligencia profesional
Malthusian theory teoría de Malthus
malum malum
malum minus malum minus
malum vertebrale suboccipitale malum
vertebrale suboccipitale
mammalingus mamalingus
mammary mamaria
mammary glands glándulas mamarias
mammary neuralgia neuralgia mamaria
mammillary body cuerpo mamilar
mammotropic hormone hormona
mamotrópica
managed care cuidado administrado
managed mental health care cuidado de
salud mental administrado
management administración
management by objectives administración
por objetivos
management decision making toma de
decisiones de administración
management risk riesgo de administración
manager disease enfermedad de
administrador
managerial administrativo
managerial psychology psicología
administrativa
managerial role papel administrativo
managing emotions administrando emociones
managing stress administrando estrés
mand interpelación
mandibular mandibular
mandibular reflex reflejo mandibular
maneuver maniobra
mania manía
mania of recommencement manía de

recomenzar
mania phantastica infantilis manía fantástica
   infantil
mania transitoria manía transitoria
maniac maníaco
maniacal maníaco
maniacal exaltation exaltación maníaca
maniacal grief reaction reacción de aflicción
   maníaca
maniaphobia maniafobia
manic maníaco
manic bipolar disorder trastorno bipolar
   maníaco
manic-depressive maniacodepresivo
manic-depressive disorder trastorno
   maniacodepresivo
manic-depressive illness enfermedad
   maniacodepresivo
manic-depressive personality personalidad
   maniacodepresiva
manic-depressive psychosis psicosis
   maniacodepresiva
manic-depressive reaction reacción
   maniacodepresiva
manic disorder trastorno maníaco
manic episode episodio maníaco
manic excitement excitación maníaca
manic hebephrenia hebefrenia maníaca
manic mood humor maníaco
manic state estado maníaco
manic stupor estupor maníaco
manic syndrome síndrome maníaco
manicy manicia
manifest manifiesto
manifest anxiety ansiedad manifiesta
manifest content contenido manifiesto
manifest goal fin manifiesto
manifest tetany tetania manifiesta
manifestation manifestación
manipulation manipulación
manipulative manipulativo
manipulative behavior conducta manipulativa
manipulative drive impulso manipulativo
manipulative techniques técnicas
   manipulativas
manipulatory drive impulso manipulativo
mannerism manierismo
mannitol manitol
Mannkopf's sign signo de Mannkopf
mannosidosis manosidosis
manoptoscope manoptoscopio
mantle layer capa del manto
mantle sclerosis esclerosis del manto
mantra mantra
manual manual
manual alphabet alfabeto manual
manual arts therapist terapeuta de artes
   manuales
manual babbling in deaf children balbuceo
   manual en niños sordos
manual dexterity destreza manual
manual dominance dominancia manual
manual language lenguaje manual
manual method método manual
manualism manualismo

map-reading test prueba de lectura de mapa
maple syrup urine disease enfermedad de
   orina de jarabe de arce
maplike skull cráneo en mapa
maprotiline maprotilina
marasmic marásmico
marasmic state estado marásmico
marasmus marasmo
marathon maratón
marathon group grupo de maratón
marathon group psychotherapy psicoterapia
   de grupo de maratón
marathon session sesión de maratón
Marbe's law ley de Marbe
Marchant's zone zona de Marchant
Marchi stain colorante de Marchi
Marchiafava-Bignami disease enfermedad de
   Marchiafava-Bignami
Marcus Gunn phenomenon fenómeno de
   Marcus Gunn
Marcus Gunn sign signo de Marcus Gunn
Marcus Gunn syndrome síndrome de Marcus
   Gunn
Marfan's syndrome síndrome de Marfan
margin margen
margin of attention margen de atención
margin of consciousness margen de
   conciencia
marginal marginal
marginal consciousness conciencia marginal
marginal frequency frecuencia marginal
marginal group grupo marginal
marginal individual individuo marginal
marginal intelligence inteligencia marginal
marginal psychosis psicosis marginal
marginal sulcus surco marginal
marginal total total marginal
marginal transvestite transvestista marginal
Marie's ataxia ataxia de Marie
Marie-Robinson syndrome síndrome de
   Marie-Robinson
Marie-Strumpell disease enfermedad de
   Marie-Strumpell
marihuana marihuana
marijuana marijuana
Marin Amat's syndrome síndrome de Marin
   Amat
Marinesco's succulent hand mano suculenta
   de Marinesco
Marinesco-Garland syndrome síndrome de
   Marinesco-Garland
Marinesco-Sjogren syndrome síndrome de
   Marinesco-Sjogren
mariposia mariposia
marital marital
marital adjustment ajuste marital
marital conflict conflicto marital
marital counseling asesoramiento marital
marital couples group therapy terapia de
   grupo de parejas maritales
marital discord discordia marital
marital history historial marital
marital infidelity infidelidad marital
marital interaction interacción marital
marital problems problemas maritales

marital relationship relación marital
marital schism cisma marital
marital status estado marital
marital therapy terapia marital
marker marcador
market basket cesta de compras
market research investigación de mercado
marketing mercadeo
marketing orientation orientación de mercadeo
marketing personality personalidad de mercadeo
marketing type tipo de mercadeo
Markoff chain cadena de Markoff
Markoff chaining encadenamiento de Markoff
Markov chain cadena de Markov
Markov chaining encadenamiento de Markov
Markov process proceso de Markov
Maroteaux-Lamy syndrome síndrome de Maroteaux-Lamy
marriage matrimonio
marriage contract contrato matrimonial
marriage counseling asesoramiento matrimonial
marriage counseling in groups asesoramiento matrimonial en grupos
marriage therapy terapia matrimonial
Martinotti cells células de Martinotti
masculine masculino
masculine identity identidad masculina
masculine protest protesta masculina
masculinity masculinidad
masculinity-femininity scale escala de masculinidad-feminidad
masculinity-femininity tests pruebas de masculinidad-feminidad
masculinize masculinizar
Masini's sign signo de Masini
mask máscara
masked affection afección enmascarada
masked depression depresión enmascarada
masked disorder trastorno enmascarado
masked epilepsy epilepsia enmascarada
masked homosexuality homosexualidad enmascarada
masked obsession obsesión enmascarada
masking enmascaramiento
Maslow's hierarchy jerarquía de Maslow
Maslow's motivational hierarchy jerarquía motivacional de Maslow
Maslow's theory of human motivation teoría de Maslow de motivación humana
masochism masoquismo
masochist masoquista
masochistic masoquista
masochistic character carácter masoquista
masochistic fantasy fantasía masoquista
masochistic personality personalidad masoquista
masochistic personality disorder trastorno de personalidad masoquista
masochistic sabotage sabotaje masoquista
masochistic wish-dream deseo-sueño masoquista

mass masa
mass action acción en masa
mass action theory teoría de acción en masa
mass behavior conducta en masa
mass contagion contagio en masa
mass hysteria histeria en masa
mass masochism masoquismo en masa
mass media medios de comunicación
mass method método en masa
mass movement movimiento en masa
mass observation observación en masa
mass polarization polarización en masa
mass psychology psicología en masa
mass reflex reflejo en masa
massa intermedia masa intermedia
massage masaje
masseter reflex reflejo masetérico
massive masivo
massive seizure acceso masivo
Masson disk disco de Masson
massotherapy masoterapia
Mast syndrome síndrome de Mast
mastectomy mastectomía
mastery dominio
mastery instinct instinto de dominio
mastery motive motivo de dominio
mastery test prueba de dominio
mastery training entrenamiento de dominio
masticatory masticatorio
masticatory diplegia diplejía masticatoria
masticatory spasm espasmo masticatorio
mastigophobia mastigofobia
mastodynia mastodinia
masturbate masturbar
masturbation masturbación
masturbation and guilt masturbación y culpabilidad
masturbation equivalent equivalente de masturbación
Matas' operation operación de Matas
matched group grupo apareado
matched-group design diseño de grupo apareado
matched-group procedure procedimiento de grupo apareado
matched pair par apareado
matched sample muestra apareada
matching pareo
matching hypothesis hipótesis de pareo
matching law ley de pareo
matching test prueba de pareo
matching to sample pareo a muestra
materialism materialismo
maternal maternal
maternal age edad maternal
maternal aggression agresión maternal
maternal attachment apego maternal
maternal attitudes actitudes maternales
maternal behavior conducta maternal
maternal depression depresión maternal
maternal deprivation privación maternal
maternal deprivation syndrome síndrome de privación maternal
maternal diabetes diabetes maternal
maternal drive impulso maternal

maternal impression impresión maternal
maternal neglect negligencia maternal
maternal rejection rechazo maternal
maternal role papel maternal
maternal stress estrés maternal
maternal substance abuse abuso de
  sustancias maternal
maternity maternidad
maternity blues depresión de maternidad
mathemagenic matemagénico
mathematical matemático
mathematical anxiety ansiedad matemática
mathematical biology biología matemática
mathematical learning theory teoría de
  aprendizaje matemática
mathematical model modelo matemático
mathematical psychology psicología
  matemática
mathematico-deductive method método
  deductivo matemático
mathematics disorder trastorno matemático
mating apareamiento
mating behavior conducta de apareamiento
matriarchal matriarcal
matriarchal family familia matriarcal
matriarchy matriarcado
matricide matricidio
matrilineal matrilineal
matrilineal descent descendencia matrilineal
matrilocal matrilocal
matrix matriz
mattoid matoide
maturation maduración
maturation-degeneration hypothesis
  hipótesis de maduración-degeneración
maturation hypothesis hipótesis de
  maduración
maturational maduracional
maturational crisis crisis maduracional
maturational lag atraso maduracional
mature maduro
mature defense defensa madura
maturity madurez
maturity-onset diabetes diabetes de comienzo
  en madurez
maturity rating clasificación de madurez
matutinal epilepsy epilepsia matutina
maudlin drunkenness embriaguez sensiblera
maximal máximo
maximal age edad máxima
maximal stimulus estímulo máximo
maximum máximo
maximum allowable cost costo máximo
  permisible
maximum likelihood probabilidad máxima
maximum-likelihood estimator estimador de
  probabilidad máxima
maximum-security unit unidad de seguridad
  máxima
Maxwell disks discos de Maxwell
May-White syndrome síndrome de
  May-White
Mayer's reflex reflejo de Mayer
maze laberinto
maze behavior conducta de laberinto

maze learning aprendizaje de laberinto
McCarthy's reflex reflejo de McCarthy
McCollough afterimage imagen persistente
  de McCollough
McCollough effect efecto de McCollough
McNemar test prueba de McNemar
mean media
mean deviation desviación media
mean length of utterance longitud media de
  expresión
mean square media cuadrática
meaning significado
meaning in language significado en el
  lenguaje
meaning of dreams significado de sueños
meaning of words significado de palabras
meaningful significativo
meaningful learning aprendizaje significativo
meaningful memory memoria significativa
means medios
means-end capacity capacidad medios-fin
means-end relations relaciones medios-fin
means-ends expectation expectación
  medios-fines
means-ends readiness disposición
  medios-fines
means object objeto de medios
means situation situación de medios
measure medida
measure of central tendency medida de
  tendencia central
measure of dispersion medida de dispersión
measure of variation medida de variación
measured intelligence inteligencia medida
measurement medición
measurement of affective disorders medición
  de trastornos afectivos
measurement scale escala de medición
measurement techniques técnicas de
  medición
meatus meato
mechanical mecánico
mechanical ability habilidad mecánica
mechanical anosmia anosmia mecánica
mechanical aptitude aptitud mecánica
mechanical-aptitude test prueba de aptitud
  mecánica
mechanical causality causalidad mecánica
mechanical intelligence inteligencia mecánica
mechanical vertigo vértigo mecánico
mechanism mecanismo
mechanisms of group psychotherapy
  mecanismos de psicoterapia en grupo
mechanistic mecanístico
mechanistic approach acercamiento
  mecanístico
mechanistic theory teoría mecanística
mechanophobia mecanofobia
mechanoreceptor mecanorreceptor
mechanoreflex mecanorreflejo
Meckel's syndrome síndrome de Meckel
meclofenoxate meclofenoxato
meclozine meclozina
meconism meconismo
medazepam medazepam

Medea complex complejo de Medea
medial medial
medial bundle fascículo medial
medial dorsal nucleus núcleo dorsal medial
medial forebrain bundle fascículo del
   cerebro anterior medial
medial geniculate body cuerpo geniculado
   medial
medial geniculate nucleus núcleo geniculado
   medial
medial lemniscus lemnisco medial
medial olfactory stria estrías olfatorias
   mediales
medial orbital gyrus circunvolución orbital
   medial
medial phoneme fonema medial
medial plane plano medial
medial rectus recto medial
medial syllable sílaba medial
median mediana
median group grupo medio
median interval intervalo medio
median plane plano medio
mediate (adj) mediato
mediate (v) mediar
mediate association asociación mediata
mediation mediación
mediation mechanisms mecanismos de
   mediación
mediation processes procesos de mediación
mediation theory teoría de mediación
mediator mediador
medical médico
medical anthropology antropología médica
medical assessment evaluación médica
medical audit auditoría médica
medical care cuidado médico
medical care evaluation evaluación de
   cuidado médico
medical diagnosis diagnóstico médico
medical ethics ética médica
medical history historial médico
medical jurisprudence jurisprudencia médica
medical laboratory technician técnico de
   laboratorio médico
medical model modelo médico
medical model of disease modelo médico de
   enfermedad
medical model of psychotherapy modelo
   médico de psicoterapia
medical psychology psicología médica
medical psychotherapy psicoterapia médica
medical record registro médico
medical review revisión médica
medical social worker trabajador social
   médico
medical syndrome síndrome médico
medication medicación
medication for chronic pain medicación para
   dolor crónico
medication-induced movement disorder
   trastorno de movimientos inducido por
   medicación
medication-induced postural tremor temblor
   postural inducido por medicación

medicine medicina
medicolegal medicolegal
medicopsychology medicopsicología
medieval thinking pensamiento medieval
mediopubic reflex reflejo mediopúbico
meditation meditación
medium medio
medium trance trance mediano
mediumistic hypothesis hipótesis
   mediumística
medulla médula
medulla oblongata médula oblonga
medullary medular
medullary cystic disease enfermedad quística
   medular
medullary pyramidotomy piramidotomía
   medular
medullary tegmental paralysis parálisis
   tegmental medular
medullectomy medulectomía
medulloblastoma meduloblastoma
medulloepithelioma meduloepitelioma
medullomyoblastoma medulomioblastoma
mefexamide mefexamida
megacephalia megacefalia
megacephalic megacefálico
megacephalous megacéfalo
megacephaly megacefalia
megadose megadosis
megadose pharmacotherapy farmacoterapia
   de megadosis
megalgia megalgia
megalocephalia megalocefalia
megalocephaly megalocefalia
megaloencephalic megaloencefálico
megaloencephalon megaloencéfalo
megaloencephaly megaloencefalia
megalographia megalografía
megalomania megalomanía
megalomaniac megalomaníaco
megalophobia megalofobia
megalopia megalopia
megalopia hysterica megalopia histérica
megalopsia megalopsia
megalosplanchnic megaloesplácnico
megavitamin megavitamina
megavitamin therapy terapia de
   megavitamina
Meige syndrome síndrome de Meige
meiosis meiosis
meiotic meiótico
Meissner's corpuscles corpúsculos de
   Meissner
mel mel
melancholia melancolía
melancholia agitata melancolía agitada
melancholic melancólico
melancholic mood humor melancólico
melancholic personality personalidad
   melancólica
melancholic type tipo melancólico
melancholy melancolía
melanocyte melanocito
melanocyte-stimulating hormone hormona
   melanocitoestimulante

melanoma melanoma
melanosis melanosis
melatonin melatonina
melatonin test prueba de melatonina
melioristic meliorístico
melissophobia melisofobia
melitracen melitracen
Melkersson-Rosenthal syndrome síndrome
    de Melkersson-Rosenthal
melody perception percepción de melodía
melomania melomanía
member miembro
membership group grupo de miembros
membrane membrana
membrane growth crecimiento de membrana
membranectomy membranectomía
membranous dysmenorrhea dismenorrea
    membranosa
membrum virile miembro viril
memorize memorizar
memory memoria
memory afterimage imagen persistente de
    memoria
memory aids ayudas de memoria
memory and Alzheimer's disease memoria y
    enfermedad de Alzheimer
memory and amnesia memoria y amnesia
memory and attention memoria y atención
memory and brain damage memoria y daño
    cerebral
memory capacity capacidad de memoria
memory color color de memoria
memory consolidation consolidación de
    memoria
memory cramp calambre de memoria
memory curve curva de memoria
memory defect defecto de memoria
memory disorder trastorno de memoria
memory distortion distorsión de memoria
memory drum cilindro de memoria
memory during sleep memoria durante sueño
memory experiment experimento de memoria
memory falsification falsificación de memoria
memory illusion ilusión de memoria
memory image imagen de memoria
memory impairment deterioro de memoria
memory reference referencia de memoria
memory retention retención de memoria
memory romance romance de memoria
memory span lapso de memoria
memory storage almacenamiento de memoria
memory system sistema de memoria
memory trace rastro de memoria
memory training entrenamiento de memoria
memory transfer transferencia de memoria
ménage à trois ménage à trois
menarche menarca
mendacity mendacidad
Mendel's instep reflex reflejo del empeine de
    Mendel
Mendel's reflex reflejo de Mendel
Mendel-Bechterew reflex reflejo de
    Mendel-Bechterew
mendelian mendeliano
mendelian laws leyes mendelianas

mendelian modes of inheritance modos de
    herencia mendelianos
mendelian ratio razón mendeliana
mendelian rules of inheritance reglas de
    herencia mendelianas
mendelism mendelismo
Mengo encephalitis encefalitis por Mengo
meningeal meníngeo
meningeal carcinoma carcinoma meníngeo
meningeal carcinomatosis carcinomatosis
    meníngea
meningeal hernia hernia meníngea
meningeal syphilis sífilis meníngea
meningeorrhaphy meningeorrafia
meninges meninges
meningioma meningioma
meningiomatosis meningiomatosis
meningism meningismo
meningismus meningismo
meningitic meningítico
meningitic curve curva meningítica
meningitic streak estría meningítica
meningitis meningitis
meningitophobia meningitofobia
meningocele meningocele
meningocerebral cicatrix cicatriz
    meningocerebral
meningococcal meningitis meningitis
    meningocócica
meningoencephalitis meningoencefalitis
meningoencephalocele meningoencefalocele
meningoencephalomyelitis
    meningoencefalomielitis
meningoencephalopathy
    meningoencefalopatía
meningomyelitis meningomielitis
meningomyelocele meningomielocele
meningoradiculitis meningorradiculitis
meningorrhagia meningorragia
meningotyphoid fever fiebre meningotifoidea
meningovascular syphilis sífilis
    meningovascular
Menkes' syndrome síndrome de Menkes
menopausal menopáusico
menopausal depression depresión
    menopáusica
menopausal myopathy miopatía menopáusica
menopause menopausia
menorrhagia menorragia
mens rea mens rea
menses menstruo
menstrual menstrual
menstrual age edad menstrual
menstrual cycle ciclo menstrual
menstrual disorder trastorno menstrual
menstrual molimen molimen menstrual
menstruation menstruación
mensuration mensuración
mental mental
mental aberration aberración mental
mental ability habilidad mental
mental abuse abuso mental
mental age edad mental
mental agraphia agrafia mental
mental apparatus aparato mental

mental arithmetic aritmética mental
mental asthenia astenia mental
mental asymmetry asimetría mental
mental ataxia ataxia mental
mental blind spot punto ciego mental
mental chemistry química mental
mental chronometrics cronométrica mental
mental chronometry cronometría mental
mental claudication claudicación mental
mental confusion confusión mental
mental content contenido mental
mental deficiency deficiencia mental
mental deterioration deterioración mental
mental development desarrollo mental
mental discipline disciplina mental
mental disease enfermedad mental
mental disorder trastorno mental
mental disorder due to general medical condition trastorno mental debido a condición médica general
mental disturbance disturbio mental
mental dynamism dinamismo mental
mental eclipse eclipse mental
mental element elemento mental
mental evolution evolución mental
mental examination examinación mental
mental experiment experimento mental
mental faculty facultad mental
mental fog niebla mental
mental function función mental
mental growth crecimiento mental
mental handicap minusvalía mental
mental healing curación mental
mental health salud mental
mental-health clinic clínica de salud mental
mental-health counselor asesor de salud mental
mental-health program programa de salud mental
mental-health worker trabajador de salud mental
mental hospital hospital mental
mental hygiene higiene mental
mental illness enfermedad mental
mental image imagen mental
mental imagery imaginería mental
mental impairment deterioro mental
mental impression impresión mental
mental institution institución mental
mental level nivel mental
mental masochism masoquismo mental
mental maturity madurez mental
mental measurement medición mental
mental mechanism mecanismo mental
mental metabolism metabolismo mental
mental paper-folding test prueba de doblar papel mental
mental patient paciente mental
mental patient organization organización de pacientes mentales
mental process proceso mental
mental representation representación mental
mental resource recurso mental
mental retardation retardo mental
mental retardation and brain dysfunction

retardo mental y disfunción cerebral
mental retardation and cognitive function retardo mental y función cognitiva
mental retardation and language retardo mental y lenguaje
mental retardation and learning retardo mental y aprendizaje
mental retardation and legal rights retardo mental y derechos legales
mental retardation versus autism retardo mental contra autismo
mental rotation rotación mental
mental scale escala mental
mental scotoma escotoma mental
mental set predisposición mental
mental status estado mental
mental-status examination examinación del estado mental
mental structure estructura mental
mental synthesis síntesis mental
mental telepathy telepatía mental
mental tension tensión mental
mental test prueba mental
mental topography topografía mental
mentalism mentalismo
mentality mentalidad
mentally mentalmente
mentally handicapped minusválido mentalmente
mentally retarded retardado mentalmente
mentally retarded persons' rights derechos de personas retardadas mentalmente
mentation mentación
mentation scale escala de mentación
menticide menticidio
mentism mentismo
meperidine meperidina
meperidine hydrochloride clorhidrato de meperidina
mephenesin mefenesina
mephenoxalone mefenoxalona
mephenytoin mefenitoína
mephobarbital mefobarbital
meprobamate meprobamato
meralgia meralgia
meralgia paraesthetica meralgia paraestésica
mercurial tremor temblor mercurial
mercury encephalopathy encefalopatía por mercurio
mercy killing eutanasia
merergasia merergasia
merger state estado de fusión
merit rating clasificación por mérito
Merkel's corpuscles corpúsculos de Merkel
Merkel's law ley de Merkel
Merkel's tactile disk disco táctil de Merkel
merogony merogonia
merorachischisis merorraquisquisis
merorrhachischisis merorraquisquisis
merosmia merosmia
merycism mericismo
Merzbacher-Pelizaeus disease enfermedad de Merzbacher-Pelizaeus
mescaline mescalina
mesencephalic mesencefálico

mesencephalic nucleus núcleo mesencefálico
mesencephalic tegmentum tegmento
  mesencefálico
mesencephalitis mesencefalitis
mesencephalon mesencéfalo
mesencephalotomy mesencefalotomía
mesial mesial
mesmerism mesmerismo
mesmerize mesmerizar
mesoblastic sensibility sensibilidad
  mesoblástica
mesocephalic mesocefálico
mesocephaly mesocefalia
mesoderm mesodermo
mesokurtic mesocúrtico
mesokurtosis mesocurtosis
mesolimbic-mesocortical tract tracto
  mesolímbico mesocortical
mesomorph mesomorfo
mesomorphic mesomórfico
mesomorphic body type tipo corporal
  mesomórfico
mesomorphy mesomorfia
mesoneuritis mesoneuritis
mesopic mesópico
mesopic luminosity luminosidad mesópica
mesopic vision visión mesópica
mesoridazine mesoridazina
mesoridazine besylate besilato de
  mesoridazina
mesorrhachischisis mesorraquisquisis
mesoskelic mesoesquélico
mesosomatic mesosomático
message mensaje
messenger mensajero
messenger ribonucleic acid ácido
  ribonucleico mensajero
mesylate mesilato
meta-analysis metaanálisis
metabolic metabólico
metabolic anomaly anomalía metabólica
metabolic anoxia anoxia metabólica
metabolic coma coma metabólico
metabolic defect defecto metabólico
metabolic dysperception dispercepción
  metabólica
metabolic encephalitis encefalitis metabólica
metabolic encephalopathy encefalopatía
  metabólica
metabolic-nutritional model modelo
  metabólico-nutricional
metabolic screening cribado metabólico
metabolism metabolismo
metacarpohypothenar reflex reflejo
  metacarpohipotenar
metacarpothenar reflex reflejo
  metacarpotenar
metachromatic leukodystrophy leucodistrofia
  metacromática
metacommunication metacomunicación
metacontrast metacontraste
metaerotism metaerotismo
metaesthetic metaestético
metaesthetic range intervalo metaestético
metaevaluation metaevaluación

metagnosis metagnosis
metal intoxication intoxicación por metal
metalanguage metalenguaje
metalinguistics metalingüística
metallic metálico
metallic tremor temblor metálico
metallophobia metalofobia
metalloscopy metaloscopia
metameric metamérico
metameric match apareamiento metamérico
metamers metámeros
metamorphopsia metamorfopsia
metamorphosis metamorfosis
metamorphosis sexualis paranoica
  metamorfosis sexual paranoide
metamotivation metamotivación
metaneeds metanecesidades
metapathology metapatología
metaphase metafase
metaphor metáfora
metaphoric metafórico
metaphoric language lenguaje metafórico
metaphoric matching pareo metafórico
metaphoric paralogia paralogía metafórica
metaphoric symbolism simbolismo
  metafórico
metaphrenia metafrenia
metaphysical metafísico
metaphysics metafísica
metapramine metapramina
metapsychiatry metapsiquiatría
metapsychoanalysis metapsicoanálisis
metapsychological metapsicológico
metapsychological profile perfil
  metapsicológico
metapsychology metapsicología
metastasis metástasis
metatarsal reflex reflejo metatarsiano
metatarsalgia metatarsalgia
metathalamus metatálamo
metatheory metateoría
metathetic metatético
metatropism metatropismo
metempirical metempírico
metempsychosis metempsicosis
metencephalon metencéfalo
metenkephalin metencefalina
meteorophobia meteorofobia
methacholine infusion test prueba de infusión
  de metacolina
methadone metadona
methadone center centro de metadona
methadone hydrochloride clorhidrato de
  metadona
methadone maintenance mantenimiento de
  metadona
methadone maintenance treatment
  tratamiento de mantenimiento de metadona
methamphetamine mentanfetamina
methamphetamine abuse abuso de
  mentanfetaminas
methamphetamine hydrochloride clorhidrato
  de mentanfetamina
methapyrilene metapirileno
methaqualone metacualona

methilepsia metilepsia
methocarbamol metocarbamol
method método
method of approximations método de
    aproximaciones
method of constant stimuli método de
    estímulos constantes
method of limits método de límites
method of successive approximations método
    de aproximaciones sucesivas
methodical chorea corea metódica
methodology metodología
methods analysis análisis de métodos
methotrimeprazine metotrimeprazina
methoxamine metoxamina
methsuximide metsuximida
methyldopa metildopa
methylphenidate metilfenidato
methylphenobarbital metilfenobarbital
methyprylon metiprilona
methysergide metisergida
metoclopramide metoclopramida
metonymic distortion distorsión metonímica
metonymy metonimia
metopon metopón
metopoplasty metopoplastia
metoprolol metoprolol
metric métrico
metric methods métodos métricos
metric ophthalmoscopy oftalmoscopia
    métrica
metric system sistema métrico
metromania metromanía
metronoscope metronoscopio
Meyer-Archambault loop asa de
    Meyer-Archambault
mianserin mianserina
micosis micosis
micrencephalia micrencefalia
micrencephalous micrencéfalo
micrencephaly micrencefalia
microadenoma microadenoma
microangiopathy microangiopatía
microbiophobia microbiofobia
microcephalia microcefalia
microcephalic microcefálico
microcephaly microcefalia
microcosm microcosmo
microdysgenesia microdisgenesia
microelectrode microelectrodo
microelectrode technique técnica de
    microelectrodo
microencephaly microencefalia
microgeny microgenia
microglia microglia
microglioma microglioma
microgliomatosis microgliomatosis
microgliosis microgliosis
microglossia microglosia
micrognathia micrognatia
micrography micrografía
microgyria microgiria
micromania micromanía
micromastia micromastia
micromelia micromelia

micromillimeter micromilímetro
micron micrón
microneurovascular anastomosis anastomosis
    microneurovascular
microorchidism microorquidismo
microorganism microorganismo
microphobia microfobia
microphonia microfonía
microphonic microfónico
micropsia micropsia
micropsychophysiology micropsicofisiología
micropsychosis micropsicosis
microptic hallucination alucinación
    micróptica
microscope microscopio
microscopic microscópico
microscopic level nivel microscópico
microseme microsemo
microsleep microsueño
microsocial microsocial
microsocial engineering ingeniería
    microsocial
microsomatic microsomático
microsomatognosia microsomatognosia
microsome microsoma
microsomia microsomía
microsplanchnic microesplácnico
microsplanchnic type tipo microesplácnico
microsurgery microcirugía
microsuture microsutura
microtome micrótomo
microtraining microentrenamiento
microvascular microvascular
microvascular anastomosis anastomosis
    microvascular
micrurgical micrúrgico
micturition micturición
micturition reflex reflejo de micturición
micturition syncope síncope de micturición
Midas punishment castigo de Midas
Midas syndrome síndrome de Midas
midazolam midazolam
midbrain mesencéfalo
midbrain deafness sordera mesencefálica
middle adolescence adolescencia mediana
middle adulthood adultez mediana
middle age edad madura
middle age pedophilia pedofilia en edad
    madura
middle cerebral artery arteria cerebral media
middle class clase media
middle commissure comisura media
middle ear oído medio
middle fossa fosa media
middle insomnia insomnio mediano
midlife edad mediana
midlife crisis crisis de edad mediana
midparent media parental
midpoint punto medio
midscore puntuación media
Mignon delusion delusión de Mignon
migraine migraña
migraine headache dolor de cabeza de
    migraña
migraine personality personalidad de migraña

migration migración
migration adaptation adaptación de migración
migration behavior conducta de migración
migration psychosis psicosis de migración
Mikulicz operation operación de Mikulicz
mild depression depresión leve
mild mental retardation retardo mental leve
miliary aneurysm aneurisma miliar
milieu ambiente
milieu therapy terapia ambiental
milk-ejection reflex reflejo de eyección de leche
Millard-Gubler syndrome síndrome de Millard-Gubler
Milles' syndrome síndrome de Milles
millilambert mililambert
millimicron milimicrón
Milton's disease enfermedad de Milton
mimesis mimesis
mimetic mimético
mimetic chorea corea mimética
mimetic paralysis parálisis mimética
mimic mímico
mimic convulsion convulsión mímica
mimic spasm espasmo mímico
mimic tic tic mímico
mimicry mímica
Minamata disease enfermedad de Minamata
mind mente
mind-altering drugs drogas alterantes de mente
mind blindness ceguera mental
mind-body perception percepción mente-cuerpo
mind-body problem problema mente-cuerpo
mind control control de mente
mind pain dolor de mente
mind-reading lectura de pensamientos
miner's cramp calambre de minero
mineralocorticoid mineralocorticoide
miniature miniatura
miniature end-plate potential potencial de placa terminal miniatura
miniature experiment experimento miniatura
miniature mind mente miniatura
miniature system sistema miniatura
minimal mínimo
minimal audible field campo audible mínimo
minimal audible pressure presión audible mínima
minimal brain damage daño cerebral mínimo
minimal brain dysfunction disfunción cerebral mínima
minimal cerebral dysfunction disfunción cerebral mínima
minimal-change method método de cambio mínimo
minimal cue señal mínima
minimal pair par mínimo
minimal risk riesgo mínimo
minimization minimización
minimum mínimo
minimum absolute threshold umbral absoluto mínimo

minimum audible field campo audible mínimo
minimum audible pressure presión audible mínima
minimum-change therapy terapia de cambio mínimo
minimum distance principle principio de distancia mínima
minor menor
minor analysis análisis menor
minor epilepsy epilepsia menor
minor hemisphere hemisferio menor
minor hypnosis hipnosis menor
minor hysteria histeria menor
minor tranquilizer tranquilizante menor
minority group grupo minoritario
minority-group psychiatry psiquiatría de grupo minoritario
miopragia miopragia
miosis miosis
mirror-drawing dibujo con espejo
mirror-drawing test prueba de dibujo con espejo
mirror-reading lectura en espejo
mirror sign signo de espejo
mirror technique técnica de espejo
mirror transference transferencia de espejo
mirror-writing escritura en espejo
misandry misandria
misanthropy misantropía
miscarriage aborto espontaneo
misdirection phenomenon fenómeno de dirección errada
miserliness tacañería
miserotia miserotia
misidentification identificación errónea
misocainia misocainia
misogamy misogamia
misogyny misoginia
misologia misología
misology misología
misoneism misoneísmo
misopedia misopedia
misopedy misopedia
missing-parts test prueba de partes faltantes
mistake equivocación
mistrust desconfianza
mistrust versus trust desconfianza contra confianza
misuse of intelligence quotient scores mal uso de puntuaciones de cociente de inteligencia
Mitchell's disease enfermedad de Mitchell
Mitchell's treatment tratamiento de Mitchell
mitochondria mitocondria
mitosis mitosis
mitral mitral
mitral cell célula mitral
mitral stenosis estenosis mitral
mixed mixto
mixed aphasia afasia mixta
mixed bipolar disorder trastorno bipolar mixto
mixed cerebral dominance dominancia cerebral mixta

mixed deafness sordera mixta
mixed design diseño mixto
mixed disturbance disturbio mixto
mixed dominance dominancia mixta
mixed emotional features características
    emocionales mixtas
mixed glioma glioma mixto
mixed laterality lateralidad mixta
mixed model modelo mixto
mixed-motive game juego de motivos mixtos
mixed-motive task tarea de motivos mixtos
mixed neurosis neurosis mixta
mixed paralysis parálisis mixta
mixed phobic fóbico mixto
mixed receptive-expressive language
    disorder trastorno del lenguaje
    receptivo-expresivo mixto
mixed reinforcement refuerzo mixto
mixed sampling muestreo mixto
mixed schedule programa mixto
mixed schizophrenia esquizofrenia mixta
mixed specific developmental disorder
    trastorno del desarrollo específico mixto
mixed transcortical aphasia afasia
    transcortical mixta
mixoscopia mixoscopia
mixoscopia bestialis mixoscopia bestial
mixovariation mixovariación
mneme mnema
mnemenic mneménico
mnemic mnémico
mnemic hypothesis hipótesis mnémica
mnemic theory teoría mnémica
mnemism mnemismo
mnemonic mnemónico
mnemonic device aparato mnemónico
mnemonic meaning of dreams significado
    mnemónico de sueños
mnemonic strategy estrategia mnemónica
mnemonic trace rastro mnemónico
mnemonics mnemónica
mnemonist mnemonista
mob muchedumbre
mob behavior conducta de muchedumbre
mob psychology psicología de muchedumbre
mobile móvil
mobile clinic clínica móvil
mobile spasm espasmo móvil
mobility movilidad
mobility of libido movilidad de libido
mobilization movilización
mobilization reaction reacción de
    movilización
Mobius' syndrome síndrome de Mobius
Mobius disease enfermedad de Mobius
modal modal
modal adaptive task tarea adaptiva modal
modality modalidad
modality profile perfil de modalidad
mode modo
mode of inheritance modo de herencia
model modelo
model game juego modelo
model of development modelo del desarrollo
model of illness modelo de enfermedad

model psychosis psicosis modelo
modeling modelado
moderate moderado
moderate depression depresión moderada
moderate mental retardation retardo mental
    moderado
moderate retardation retardo moderado
moderator moderador
moderator variable variable moderadora
modification modificación
modification of aggression modificación de
    agresión
modified modificado
modified replication replicación modificada
modified simple mastectomy mastectomía
    simple modificada
modifier modificador
modulation transfer function función de
    transferencia de modulación
modulator modulador
modulator curve curva de moduladores
module módulo
modulus módulo
modus operandi modus operandi
mogiarthria mogiartría
mogigraphia mogigrafía
mogilalia mogilalia
mogiphonia mogifonía
molar molar
molar approach acercamiento molar
molar behavior conducta molar
molar rating scale escala de clasificación
    molar
molecular molecular
molecular approach acercamiento molecular
molecular behavior conducta molecular
molecular psychiatry psiquiatría molecular
molecularism molecularismo
molestation vejación
molilalia molilalia
molimen molimen
molindone molindona
molluscum molusco
molluscum fibrosum molusco fibroso
Molyneux's question pregunta de Molyneux
molysmophobia molismofobia
molysophobia molisofobia
moment momento
monad mónada
Monakow's syndrome síndrome de Monakow
monathetosis monatetosis
monaural monaural
Mondonesi's reflex reflejo de Mondonesi
monesthetic monoestético
moniliasis moniliasis
monism monismo
monistic monístico
monitor (n) monitor
monitor (v) monitorizar
monitoring monitorización
monkey love amor de mono
monkey-paw pata de mono
monkey psychiatrist psiquiatra mono
monkey therapist terapueta mono
monoamine monoamina

monoamine hypothesis hipótesis monoamina
monoamine oxidase monoamina oxidasa
monoamine oxidase inhibitor inhibidor de monoamina oxidasa
monoblepsia monoblepsia
monochorea monocorea
monochorionic twins gemelos monocoriónicos
monochromacy monocromacia
monochromasy monocromacia
monochromat monocromato
monochromatism monocromatismo
monochromia monocromia
monocular monocular
monocular cue señal monocular
monocular depth cue señal de profundidad monocular
monocular suppression supresión monocular
monocular vision visión monocular
monogamy monogamia
monogony monogonia
monohybrid monohíbrido
monoideism monoideísmo
monomania monomanía
monomaniac monomaníaco
monomatric monomátrico
monomyoplegia monomioplejía
mononeuralgia mononeuralgia
mononeuritis mononeuritis
mononeuritis multiplex mononeuritis múltiple
mononeuropathy mononeuropatía
mononeuropathy multiplex mononeuropatía múltiple
mononoea mononoea
monopagia monopagia
monoparesis monoparesia
monoparesthesia monoparestesia
monopathophobia monopatofobia
monophagism monofagismo
monophasia monofasia
monophasic monofásico
monophasic sleep rhythm ritmo de sueño monofásico
monophobia monofobia
monoplegia monoplejía
monoplegia masticatoria monoplejía masticatoria
monopolar depression depresión monopolar
monoptic monóptico
monorchid monórquido
monorhinic monorrínico
monosodium glutamate glutamato monosódico
monosomy monosomía
monospasm monoespasmo
monosymptomatic monosintomático
monosymptomatic circumscription circunscripción monosintomática
monosymptomatic hypochondriacal psychosis psicosis hipocondríaca monosintomática
monosymptomatic hypochondriasis hipocondriasis monosintomática
monosymptomatic neurosis neurosis monosintomática

monosymptomatic psychosis psicosis monosintomática
monosynaptic monosináptico
monosynaptic arc arco monosináptico
monosynaptic reflex arc arco reflejo monosináptico
monotic monótico
monotonic monotónico
monotonous monótono
monotonous speech habla monótona
monotropic monotrópico
monovular twins gemelos monoovulares
monozygocity monocigosidad
monozygosity monocigosidad
monozygote monocigoto
monozygotic monocigótico
monozygotic twins gemelos monocigóticos
Monte Carlo method método de Monte Carlo
Monte Carlo procedure procedimiento de Monte Carlo
Montessori method método de Montessori
mood humor
mood-altering drugs drogas alterantes del humor
mood-congruent delusion delusión del humor congruente
mood-congruent hallucination alucinación del humor congruente
mood-congruent psychotic feature característica psicótica del humor congruente
mood disorder trastorno del humor
mood disorder due to general medical condition trastorno del humor debido a condición médica general
mood-incongruent delusion delusión del humor incongruente
mood-incongruent hallucination alucinación del humor incongruente
mood-incongruent psychotic feature característica psicótica del humor incongruente
mood induction inducción del humor
mood stabilizer estabilizador del humor
mood-stabilizing drug droga estabilizante del humor
mood swing viraje del humor
moodiness humor caprichoso
moon illusion ilusión de la luna
Moore's method método de Moore
moral moral
moral anxiety ansiedad moral
moral ataxia ataxia moral
moral behavior conducta moral
moral behavior in children conducta moral en niños
moral code código moral
moral conduct conducta moral
moral consistency consistencia moral
moral development desarrollo moral
moral dilemma dilema moral
moral education educación moral
moral hazard riesgo moral
moral independence independencia moral
moral independence stage etapa de

independencia moral
moral judgment juicio moral
moral masochism masoquismo moral
moral obligation obligación moral
moral philosophy filosofía moral
moral pride orgullo moral
moral principle principio moral
moral realism realismo moral
moral realism stage etapa de realismo moral
moral reasoning razonamiento moral
moral reasoning during adolescence
　razonamiento moral durante adolescencia
moral relativism relativismo moral
moral right derecho moral
moral treatment tratamiento moral
moral turpitude vileza moral
morale moral
morality moralidad
morality of constraint moralidad de
　constreñimiento
morality of cooperation moralidad de
　cooperación
moratorium moratoria
morbid mórbido
morbid dependency dependencia mórbida
morbid impulse impulso mórbido
morbid jealousy celos mórbidos
morbid perplexity perplejidad mórbida
morbid thirst sed mórbida
morbidity morbilidad
morbidity rate tasa de morbilidad
Morel's syndrome síndrome de Morel
mores costumbres
Morgagni's disease enfermedad de Morgagni
Morgagni's syndrome síndrome de Morgagni
Morgagni-Adams-Stokes syndrome síndrome
　de Morgagni-Adams-Stokes
Morgan's canon canon de Morgan
Morgan's principle principio de Morgan
moria moria
Morita therapy terapia de Morita
morning sickness enfermedad matutina
Moro reflex reflejo de Moro
Moro response respuesta de Moro
morpheme morfema
morphine morfina
morphine dependence dependencia de
　morfina
morphine withdrawal retiro de morfina
morphinism morfinismo
morphinomania morfinomanía
morphogenesis morfogénesis
morphological morfológico
morphological index índice morfológico
morphology morfología
morphophonemics morfofonémica
morphosynthesis morfosíntesis
morsicatio buccarum morsicatio buccarum
morsicatio labiorum morsicatio labiorum
mortality mortalidad
mortality rate tasa de mortalidad
mortido mortido
Morton's neuralgia neuralgia de Morton
morula mórula
Morvan's chorea corea de Morvan

Morvan's disease enfermedad de Morvan
mosaic mosaico
mosaic test prueba de mosaico
mosaic theory of perception teoría de
　mosaico de percepción
mosaicism mosaiquismo
Moschowitz's disease enfermedad de
　Moschowitz
most comfortable loudness sonoridad más
　cómoda
mother's response to crying respuesta de la
　madre al llanto
mother archetype arquetipo materno
mother-child relationship relación
　madre-hijo, relación madre-hija
mother complex complejo materno
mother figure figura materna
mother fixation fijación en la madre
mother hypnosis hipnosis materna
mother image imagen materna
mother-infant interactions interacciones
　madre-infante
mother-infant proximity proximidad
　madre-infante
mother-son incest incesto madre-hijo
mother substitute sustituta de madre
mother superior complex complejo de madre
　superiora
mother surrogate sustituta de madre
mothering cuidados maternales
motile móvil
motilin motilina
motility movilidad
motility disorder trastorno de movilidad
motility psychosis psicosis de movilidad
motion moción
motion aftereffects efectos posteriores de
　moción
motion detection detección de moción
motion economy economía de moción
motion parallax paralaje de moción
motion perception percepción de moción
motion perspective perspectiva de moción
motion sickness enfermedad de moción
motion study estudio de moción
motivate motivar
motivated motivado
motivated error error motivado
motivated forgetting olvidar motivado
motivation motivación
motivation research investigación de
　motivación
motivational motivacional
motivational factor factor motivacional
motivational hierarchy jerarquía motivacional
motivational selectivity selectividad
　motivacional
motive motivo
motive hierarchy jerarquía de motivos
motokinesthetic motocinestésico
motokinesthetic method método
　motocinestésico
motoneuron motoneurona
motor motor
motor abreaction abreacción motora

motor agraphia agrafia motora
motor alexia alexia motora
motor amimia amimia motora
motor amusia amusia motora
motor aphasia afasia motora
motor apraxia apraxia motora
motor area área motora
motor ataxia ataxia motora
motor behavior conducta motora
motor compliance acatamiento motor
motor conversion symptom síntoma de conversión motor
motor coordination coordinación motora
motor cortex corteza motora
motor dapsone neuropathy neuropatía motora por dapsona
motor development desarrollo motor
motor disability discapacidad motora
motor disorder trastorno motor
motor disturbance disturbio motor
motor end plate placa terminal motora
motor equivalence equivalencia motora
motor function función motora
motor habit hábito motor
motor homunculus homúnculo motor
motor image imagen motora
motor imitation imitación motora
motor impersistence impersistencia motora
motor inhibition inhibición motora
motor-kinesthetic method método motocinestésico
motor learning aprendizaje motor
motor memory memoria motora
motor milestone hito motor
motor nerve nervio motor
motor neuron neurona motora
motor neuron disease enfermedad de neuronas motoras
motor neuron lesion lesión de neuronas motoras
motor neurosis neurosis motora
motor paralysis parálisis motora
motor perseveration perseveración motora
motor persistence persistencia motora
motor point punto motor
motor projection area área de proyección motora
motor reaction type tipo de reacción motora
motor response respuesta motora
motor sense sentido motor
motor set predisposición motora
motor skills destrezas motoras
motor skills disorder trastorno de destrezas motoras
motor system sistema motor
motor tension tensión motora
motor test prueba motora
motor theory teoría motora
motor theory of consciousness teoría motora de conciencia
motor theory of speech perception teoría motora de percepción del habla
motor theory of thought teoría motora del pensamiento
motor unit unidad motora

motor zone zona motora
mourn enlutar
mourning luto
mourning by children luto por niños
movement movimiento
movement afterimage imagen persistente de movimiento
movement control control de movimiento
movement disorder trastorno de movimiento
movement disturbance disturbio de movimiento
movement education educación de movimiento
movement illusion ilusión de movimiento
movement in sleep movimiento en sueño
movement learning aprendizaje de movimiento
movement perspective perspectiva de movimiento
movement sense sentido de movimiento
movement-sensitive retinal cells células retinales sentitivas al movimiento
movement therapy terapia de movimiento
moving of household mudanza de familia
mucopolysaccharide mucopolisacárido
mucopolysaccharidosis mucopolisacaridosis
mucous mucoso
mucous membrane membrana mucosa
mucoviscidosis mucoviscidosis
mucus moco
Muller's fibers fibras de Muller
Muller's law ley de Muller
Muller-Lyer illusion ilusión de Muller-Lyer
Muller-Schumann law ley de Muller-Schumann
Muller-Urban method método de Muller-Urban
Mullerian ducts conductos de Muller
Mullerian system sistema de Muller
multiaxial multiaxial
multiaxial assessment evaluación multiaxial
multiaxial classification clasificación multiaxial
multicultural multicultural
multicultural counseling asesoramiento multicultural
multidetermination multideterminación
multidetermined multideterminado
multidetermined behavior conducta multideterminada
multidimensional multidimensional
multidimensional analysis análisis multidimensional
multidimensional pain management administración de dolor multidimensional
multidimensional scaling escalamiento multidimensional
multidimensional variable variable multidimensional
multidisciplinary multidisciplinario
multidisciplinary approach acercamiento multidisciplinario
multifactorial multifactorial
multifactorial inheritance herencia multifactorial

multifactorial model modelo multifactorial
multihandicapped multiminusválido
multiinfarct dementia demencia multiinfarto
multimodal multimodal
multimodal assessment evaluación multimodal
multimodal behavior therapy terapia de conducta multimodal
multimodal distribution distribución multimodal
multimodal perception percepción multimodal
multimodal theory of intelligence teoría multimodal de inteligencia
multimodal therapy terapia multimodal
multinomial distribution distribución multinomial
multiparous multípara
multiphasic multifásico
multiple múltiple
multiple-aptitude test prueba de aptitudes múltiples
multiple causation causalidad múltiple
multiple-choice experiment experimento de selección múltiple
multiple correlation correlación múltiple
multiple delusions delusiones múltiples
multiple ego states estados del ego múltiples
multiple-factor inheritance herencia de factores múltiples
multiple family therapy terapia de familia múltiple
multiple identification identificación múltiple
multiple loss pérdida múltiple
multiple mothering cuidados maternos múltiples
multiple mucosal neuroma syndrome síndrome de neuroma mucoso múltiple
multiple myeloma mieloma múltiple
multiple myositis miositis múltiple
multiple neuritis neuritis múltiple
multiple personality personalidad múltiple
multiple personality disorder trastorno de personalidad múltiple
multiple regression regresión múltiple
multiple reinforcement refuerzo múltiple
multiple-reinforcement schedule programa de refuerzo múltiple
multiple-role playing desempeño de papeles múltiples
multiple sclerosis esclerosis múltiple
multiple-spike recording registro de puntas múltiples
multiple therapy terapia múltiple
multiple tics with coprolalia tics múltiples con coprolalia
multiplication of personality multiplicación de personalidad
multiplication table test prueba de tabla de multiplicación
multiplicity multiplicidad
multipolar cell célula multipolar
multipolar neuron neurona multipolar
multipolarity multipolaridad
multisensory multisensorial

multisensory method método multisensorial
multistage theory teoría de etapas múltiples
multisynaptic arc arco multisináptico
multisynaptic reflex arc arco de reflejo multisináptico
multivariate multivariado
multivariate analysis análisis multivariado
multivariate analysis of variance análisis multivariado de variancia
multivariate study estudio multivariado
mumbling musitación
mummy attitude actitud de momia
mumps meningoencephalitis meningoencefalitis de paperas
Munchausen syndrome síndrome de Munchausen
mundane realism realismo mundano
Munsell color system sistema de colores de Munsell
murder asesinato
murmur murmullo
muscarine muscarina
muscle músculo
muscle-action potential potencial de acción muscular
muscle contraction contracción muscular
muscle fiber fibra muscular
muscle-reading lectura muscular
muscle relaxant relajante muscular
muscle relaxation relajamiento muscular
muscle sensation sensación muscular
muscle spasm espasmo muscular
muscle spindle huso muscular
muscle tone tono muscular
muscular muscular
muscular-anal stage etapa muscular-anal
muscular anesthesia anestesia muscular
muscular atrophy atrofia muscular
muscular dystrophy distrofia muscular
muscular hyperesthesia hiperestesia muscular
muscular insufficiency insuficiencia muscular
muscular reflex reflejo muscular
muscular sense sentido muscular
muscular trophoneurosis trofoneurosis muscular
muscular type tipo muscular
musculoskeletal musculoesquelético
musculoskeletal pain dolor musculoesquelético
musculoskeletal system sistema musculoesquelético
musculospiral musculoespiral
musculospiral paralysis parálisis musculoespiral
music blindness ceguera de música
music therapy terapia de música
musical agraphia agrafia musical
musical alexia alexia musical
musical therapy terapia musical
musician's cramp calambre de músico
musicogenic epilepsy epilepsia musicogénica
musicotherapy musicoterapia
musophobia musofobia
mussitation musitación
mutagen mutágeno

mutagenic mutagénico
mutant mutante
mutation mutación
mutation rate tasa de mutación
mute mudo
mutilating leprosy lepra mutilante
mutilation mutilación
mutism mutismo
muttering delirium delirio murmurante
mutual mutuo
mutual aid group grupo de ayuda mutua
mutual-help services servicios de ayuda
   múltiple
mutual lateral masking enmascaramiento
   lateral mutuo
mutual masturbation masturbación mutua
mutual participation model modelo de
   participación mutua
mutualism mutualismo
mutuality mutualidad
mutually mutuamente
mutually exclusive mutuamente exclusivo
mutually exclusive events eventos
   mutuamente exclusivos
myalgia mialgia
myasthenia miastenia
myasthenia gravis miastenia grave
myasthenic miasténico
myasthenic facies facies miasténica
myasthenic reaction reacción miasténica
myatonia miatonía
myatonia congenita miatonía congénita
myatony miatonía
mycetism micetismo
mycetismus micetismo
mycetismus cerebralis micetismo cerebral
Mycobacterium leprae Mycobacterium leprae
mycoplasma micoplasma
mydriasis midriasis
mydriatic midriático
mydriatic rigidity rigidez midriática
myelapoplexy mielapoplejía
myelatelia mielatelia
myelauxe mielauxia
myelencephalon mielencéfalo
myelin mielina
myelin sheath vaina de mielina
myelinated axon axón mielinizado
myelination mielinación
myelinization mielinización
myelinoclasis mielinoclasis
myelinolysis mielinólisis
myelitic mielítico
myelitis mielitis
myeloarchitecture mieloarquitectura
myelocele mielocele
myelocyst mieloquiste
myelocystic mieloquístico
myelocystocele mielocistocele
myelocystomeningocele
   mielocistomeningocele
myelodiastasis mielodiastasia
myelodysplasia mielodisplasia
myelogram mielograma
myelography mielografía

myeloid mieloide
myelolysis mielólisis
myelomalacia mielomalacia
myelomeningocele mielomeningocele
myelon mielón
myeloneuritis mieloneuritis
myeloparalysis mieloparálisis
myelopathic mielopático
myelopathy mielopatía
myelopetal mielópeto
myelophthisic mielotísico
myelophthisis mielotisis
myeloplegia mieloplejía
myeloradiculitis mielorradiculitis
myeloradiculodysplasia
   mielorradiculodisplasia
myeloradiculopathy mielorradiculopatía
myeloradiculopolyneuronitis
   mielorradiculopolineuronitis
myelorrhagia mielorragia
myelorrhaphy mielorrafia
myeloschisis mielosquisis
myelosis mielosis
myelosyphilis mielosífilis
myelosyringosis mielosiringosis
myelotome mielótomo
myelotomography mielotomografía
myelotomy mielotomía
myesthesia miestesia
myoblastoma mioblastoma
myobradia miobradia
myocelialgia miocelialgia
myoclonia mioclonía
myoclonic mioclónico
myoclonic absence ausencia mioclónica
myoclonic astatic epilepsy epilepsia astática
   mioclónica
myoclonic dementia demencia mioclónica
myoclonic encephalitis encefalitis mioclónica
myoclonic epilepsy epilepsia mioclónica
myoclonic movement movimiento mioclónico
myoclonic seizure acceso mioclónico
myoclonic sleep disorder trastorno del sueño
   mioclónico
myoclonus mioclono
myoclonus epilepsy epilepsia mioclónica
myoclonus multiplex mioclono múltiple
myodynia miodinia
myodystony miodistonía
myodystrophia miodistrofia
myodystrophy miodistrofia
myoedema mioedema
myoelectric arm brazo mioeléctrico
myoesthesia mioestesia
myoesthesis mioestesis
myofascia miofascia
myogenic miogénico
myogenic paralysis parálisis miogénica
myoglobin mioglobina
myoglobinuria mioglobinuria
myogram miograma
myograph miógrafo
myography miografía
myokymia mioquimia
myoneural junction unión mioneural

myoneuralgia mioneuralgia
myoneurasthenia mioneurastenia
myoneuroma mioneuroma
myopalmus miopalmo
myoparalysis mioparálisis
myoparesis mioparesia
myopathic miopático
myopathic atrophy atrofia miopática
myopathic facies facies miopática
myopathy miopatía
myopia miopía
myorhythmia miorritmia
myosalgia miosalgia
myoseism mioseísmo
myosin miosina
myosis miosis
myositis miositis
myospasm mioespasmo
myospasmus mioespasmo
myotactic miotáctico
myotatic reflex reflejo miotático
myotenotomy miotenotomía
myotonia miotonía
myotonia acquisita miotonía adquirida
myotonia atrophica miotonía atrófica
myotonia congenita miotonía congénita
myotonia dystrophica miotonía distrófica
myotonia neonatorum miotonía neonatal
myotonic miotónico
myotonic disorder trastorno miotónico
myotonic dystrophy distrofia miotónica
myotonic pupillary reaction reacción pupilar
    miotónica
myotonoid miotonoide
myotonus miotono
myotony miotonía
myotypical response respuesta miotípica
myriachit miriaquita
myringotomy miringotomía
mysophilia misofilia
mysophobia misofobia
mysticism misticismo
myth mito
mythomania mitomanía
mythophobia mitofobia
myths about hypnotism mitos sobre
    hipnotismo
myxedema mixedema
myxoneuroma mixoneuroma
myxoneurosis mixoneurosis
myxopapillary ependymoma ependimoma
    mixopapilar

N

nadolol nadolol
naevus nevo
Naffziger syndrome síndrome de Naffziger
nail-biting comer de uñas
naive ingenuo
naive observer observador ingenuo
naive realism realismo ingenuo
naive subjects sujetos ingenuos
nalbuphine nalbufina
Nalline test prueba de Nalline
nalorphine nalorfina
naloxone naloxona
naltrexone naltrexona
naming nombramiento
Nancy school escuela de Nancy
nanism nanismo
nanny niñera
nanocephalic dwarfism enanismo
    nanocefálico
nanometer nanómetro
Napalkov phenomenon fenómeno de
    Napalkov
naphtha nafta
naproxen naproxeno
napsylate napsilato
narcism narcisismo
narcissism narcisismo
narcissistic narcisista
narcissistic character carácter narcisista
narcissistic equilibrium equilibrio narcisista
narcissistic gain ganancia narcisista
narcissistic libido libido narcisista
narcissistic neurosis neurosis narcisista
narcissistic object-choice objeto de selección
    narcisista
narcissistic oral fixation fijación oral
    narcisista
narcissistic personality personalidad
    narcisista
narcissistic personality disorder trastorno de
    personalidad narcisista
narcissistic scale escala narcisista
narcissistic scar cicatriz narcisista
narcissistic type tipo narcisista
narcissistic wound herida narcisista
narcoanalysis narcoanálisis
narcocatharsis narcocatarsis
narcohypnia narcohipnia
narcohypnosis narcohipnosis
narcolepsy narcolepsia
narcolepsy-catalepsy syndrome síndrome de
    narcolepsia-catalepsia
narcoleptic narcoléptico
narcoleptic tetrad tétrada narcoléptica

narcomania narcomanía
narcosis narcosis
narcosuggestion narcosugestión
narcosynthesis narcosíntesis
narcotherapy narcoterapia
narcotic narcótico
narcotic addiction adicción narcótica
narcotic analgesic analgésico narcótico
narcotic analgesic addiction adicción de
    analgésico narcótico
narcotic antagonist antagonista narcótico
narcotic blockade bloqueo narcótico
narcotic blocking agent agente bloqueador
    narcótico
narcotic dependence dependencia narcótica
narcotic drug droga narcótica
narcotic hunger hambre narcótica
narcotic stupor estupor narcótico
narcotism narcotismo
narcotization narcotización
nares nares
narratophilia narratofilia
nasal nasal
nasal glioma glioma nasal
nascent naciente
nasomental nasomental
nasomental reflex reflejo nasomental
nasopharynx nasofaringe
native nativo
nativism nativismo
nativistic theory teoría nativista
natural natural
natural aptitude aptitud natural
natural category categoría natural
natural childbirth parto natural
natural cues señales naturales
natural disaster desastre natural
natural group grupo natural
natural homosexual period periodo
    homosexual natural
natural language lenguaje natural
natural monism monismo natural
natural selection selección natural
natural study estudio natural
naturalistic naturalista
naturalistic approach acercamiento
    naturalista
naturalistic assessment evaluación naturalista
naturalistic observation observación
    naturalista
nature naturaleza
nature-nurture controversy controversia
    naturaleza-crianza
nature-nurture issue cuestión
    naturaleza-crianza
nature of relationships naturaleza de
    relaciones
nature versus nurture naturaleza contra
    crianza
nausea náusea
nautilus eye ojo de nautilo
nautomania nautomanía
near point punto cercano
near-point of convergence punto cercano de
    convergencia

near vision visión cercana
nearsightedness vista cercana
neck cuello
neck reflex reflejo de cuello
neck sign signo de cuello
Necker cube cubo de Necker
necromania necromanía
necromimesis necromimesis
necrophilia necrofilia
necrophilic necrofílico
necrophilic fantasy fantasía necrofílica
necrophilism necrofilismo
necrophobia necrofobia
necropsy necropsia
necrosadism necrosadismo
necrosis necrosis
necrotizing necrotizante
necrotizing encephalitis encefalitis
    necrotizante
necrotizing encephalomyelopathy
    encefalomielopatía necrotizante
need necesidad
need arousal despertamiento de necesidades
need cathexis catexis de necesidad
need-drive-incentive model modelo de
    necesidad-impulso-incentivo
need-fear dilemma dilema necesidad-temor
need for achievement necesidad de logro
need for affiliation necesidad de afiliación
need for approval necesidad de aprobación
need for dreams necesidad de sueños
need for non-rapid eye movement sleep
    necesidad de sueño de movimientos
    oculares no rápidos
need for punishment necesidad de castigo
need for sleep necesidad de sueño
need gratification gratificación de
    necesidades
need hierarchy jerarquía de necesidades
need-hierarchy theory teoría de jerarquía de
    necesidades
need-press method método de necesidades y
    factores ambientales apremiantes
need-press theory teoría de necesidades y
    factores ambientales apremiantes
need reduction reducción de necesidad
need state estado de necesidad
need tension tensión de necesidad
needle aguja
needs assessment evaluación de necesidades
needs-assessment survey encuesta de
    evaluación de necesidades
neencephalon neoencéfalo
Neftel's disease enfermedad de Neftel
negation negación
negation insanity insania de negación
negative negativo
negative acceleration aceleración negativa
negative adaptation adaptación negativa
negative afterimage imagen persistente
    negativa
negative ambition ambición negativa
negative attitude actitud negativa
negative attitude change cambio de actitud
    negativo

negative cathexis   catexis negativa
negative contrast   contraste negativo
negative correlation   correlación negativa
negative diagnosis   diagnóstico negativo
negative discriminative stimulus   estímulo discriminativo negativo
negative eugenics   eugenesia negativa
negative example   ejemplo negativo
negative feedback   retroalimentación negativa
negative hallucination   alucinación negativa
negative identity   identidad negativa
negative incentive   incentivo negativo
negative induction   inducción negativa
negative law of effect   ley de efecto negativo
negative Oedipus complex   complejo de Edipo negativo
negative period   periodo negativo
negative practice   práctica negativa
negative punishment   castigo negativo
negative reaction   reacción negativa
negative reinforcement   refuerzo negativo
negative reinforcer   reforzador negativo
negative response   respuesta negativa
negative reward   recompensa negativa
negative sensation   sensación negativa
negative suggestion   sugestión negativa
negative symptom   síntoma negativo
negative-symptom schizophrenia   esquizofrenia de síntomas negativos
negative therapeutic reaction   reacción terapéutica negativa
negative transfer   transferencia negativa
negative transference   transferencia negativa
negative tropism   tropismo negativo
negative utilitarianism   utilitarismo negativo
negative valence   valencia negativa
negatively   negativamente
negatively bathmotropic   negativamente batmotrópico
negativism   negativismo
neglect   negligencia
neglect of child   negligencia de niño
neglect of duty   negligencia del deber
negotiation   negociación
Negro's phenomenon   fenómeno de Negro
neighboring region   región vecina
Nelson syndrome   síndrome de Nelson
Nelson tumor   tumor de Nelson
nemaline myopathy   miopatía nemalínica
neo-freudian   neo-freudiano
neoanalyst   neoanalista
neoassociationism   neoasociacionismo
neoatavism   neoatavismo
neobehavioral   neoconductual
neobehavioral viewpoint   punto de vista neoconductual
neobehaviorism   neoconductismo
neocerebellum   neocerebelo
neoconnectionism   neoconexionismo
neocortex   neocorteza
neographism   neografismo
neography   neografía
neolalia   neolalia
neolallism   neolalismo
neolocal   neolocal

neologism   neologismo
neologistic jargon   jerga neologística
neology   neología
neomimism   neomimismo
neomnesis   neomnesis
neonatal   neonatal
neonatal abstinence syndrome   síndrome de abstinencia neonatal
neonatal apoplexy   apoplejía neonatal
neonatal asphyxia   asfixia neonatal
neonatal death   muerte neonatal
neonatal development   desarrollo neonatal
neonatal intensive care unit   unidad de cuidado intensivo neonatal
neonatal period   periodo neonatal
neonatal separation   separación neonatal
neonatal tetany   tetania neonatal
neonate   neonato
neonate differences   diferencias entre neonatos
neopallium   neopalio
neophasia   neofasia
neophilia   neofilia
neophobia   neofobia
neophrenia   neofrenia
neoplasm   neoplasma
neoplastic   neoplásico
neoplastic arachnoiditis   aracnoiditis neoplásica
neoplastic disease   enfermedad neoplásica
neoplastic meningitis   meningitis neoplásica
neopsychic   neopsíquico
neopsychoanalysis   neopsicoanálisis
neopsychoanalytical   neopsicoanalítico
neosleep   neosueño
neostriatum   neoestriado
neoteny   neotenia
nephrogenic diabetes insipidus   diabetes insípida nefrógena
nephron   nefrona
Neri's sign   signo de Neri
nerve   nervio
nerve avulsion   avulsión nerviosa
nerve block   bloqueo nervioso
nerve cell   célula nerviosa
nerve center   centro nervioso
nerve conduction   conducción de nervio
nerve conduction velocity   velocidad de conducción de nervio
nerve current   corriente nerviosa
nerve deafness   sordera nerviosa
nerve decompression   descompresión nerviosa
nerve ending   terminación nerviosa
nerve fiber   fibra nerviosa
nerve graft   injerto nervioso
nerve implantation   implantación de nervio
nerve impulse   impulso nervioso
nerve-muscle preparation   preparación nervio-músculo
nerve pain   dolor nervioso
nerve pathway   vía nerviosa
nerve-point massage   masaje de puntas de nervios
nerve process   proceso nervioso
nerve root   raíz nerviosa

nerve suture sutura de nervio
nerve tissue tejido nervioso
nerve trunk tronco nervioso
nervimotility nervimovilidad
nervimotion nervimoción
nervimotor nervimotor
nervine nervina
nervous nervioso
nervous asthma asma nerviosa
nervous bladder vejiga nerviosa
nervous breakdown colapso nervioso
nervous current corriente nerviosa
nervous disease enfermedad nerviosa
nervous energy energía nerviosa
nervous exhaustion agotamiento nervioso
nervous habit hábito nervioso
nervous hunger hambre nerviosa
nervous impulse impulso nervioso
nervous indigestion indigestión nerviosa
nervous system sistema nervioso
nervous tissue tejido nervioso
nervous vomiting vómitos nerviosos
nervousness nerviosidad
nest-building construcción de nido
net fertility fertilidad neta
network red
network-analysis evaluation evaluación de
    análisis de red
network biotaxis biotaxis de red
network model modelo de red
network therapy terapia de red
neuradynamia neuradinamia
neuragmia neuragmia
neural neural
neural arc arco neural
neural circuitry circuitos neurales
neural conduction conducción neural
neural crest cresta neural
neural crest syndrome síndrome de cresta
    neural
neural current corriente neural
neural cyst quiste neural
neural deafness sordera neural
neural discharge descarga neural
neural excitation excitación neural
neural facilitation facilitación neural
neural fibril fibrilla neural
neural fold pliege neural
neural groove surco neural
neural growth factor factor de crecimiento
    neural
neural impulse impulso neural
neural induction inducción neural
neural irritability irritabilidad neural
neural mechanism mecanismo neural
neural mechanisms of learning mecanismos
    neurales de aprendizaje
neural network red neural
neural parenchyma parénquima neural
neural pathway vía neural
neural plate placa neural
neural process proceso neural
neural reinforcement refuerzo neural
neural reorganization reorganización neural
neural retina retina neural

neural reverberation reverberación neural
neural system sistema neural
neural transmission transmisión neural
neural trauma trauma neural
neural tube tubo neural
neural-tube defect defecto de tubo neural
neuralgia neuralgia
neuralgic neurálgico
neuralgic amyotrophy amiotrofia neurálgica
neuralgiform neuralgiforme
neuranagenesis neuranagénesis
neurapraxia neurapraxia
neurasthenia neurastenia
neurasthenia gravis neurastenia grave
neurasthenia precox neurastenia precoz
neurasthenic neurasténico
neurasthenic helmet casco neurasténico
neurasthenic neurosis neurosis neurasténica
neurasthenoid neurastenoide
neuraxis neuraxis
neuraxon neuraxón
neurectasia neurectasia
neurectasis neurectasis
neurectasy neurectasia
neurectomy neurecotmía
neurectopia neurectopia
neurectopy neurectopia
neuremia neuremia
neurergic neurérgico
neurexeresis neurexéresis
neuriatria neuriatría
neuriatry neuriatría
neurilemma neurilema
neurilemoma neurilemoma
neurility neurilidad
neurimotility neurimovilidad
neurimotor neurimotor
neurin neurina
neurinoma neurinoma
neurinomatosis neurinomatosis
neuritic neurítico
neuritic atrophy atrofia neurítica
neuritic plaque placa neurítica
neuritis neuritis
neuroadaptation neuroadaptación
neuroallergy neuroalergia
neuroanalysis neuroanálisis
neuroanastomosis neuroanastomosis
neuroanatomy neuroanatomía
neuroarthritism neuroartritismo
neuroarthropathy neuroartropatía
neuroaugmentation neuroaumento
neuroaxonal neuroaxonal
neuroaxonal degeneration degeneración
    neuroaxonal
neurobehavioral neuroconductual
neurobehavioral syndrome síndrome
    neuroconductual
neurobiotactic neurobiotáctico
neurobiotactic movement movimiento
    neurobiotáctico
neurobiotaxis neurobiotaxis
neuroblast neuroblasto
neuroblastoma neuroblastoma
neurocardiac neurocardíaco

neurocentral neurocentral
neurochemical neuroquímico
neurochemistry neuroquímica
neurochemistry of sleep neuroquímica del sueño
neurochorioretinitis neurocoriorretinitis
neurochoroiditis neurocoroiditis
neurocirculatory neurocirculatorio
neurocirculatory asthenia astenia neurocirculatoria
neurocladism neurocladismo
neurocristopathy neurocristopatía
neurocutaneous neurocutáneo
neurocutaneous melanosis melanosis neurocutánea
neurocutaneous syndrome síndrome neurocutáneo
neurocyte neurocito
neurocytolysis neurocitólisis
neurocytoma neurocitoma
neurodermatitis neurodermatitis
neurodynia neurodinia
neuroectomy neuroectomía
neuroeffector neuroefector
neuroeffector junction unión de neuroefector
neuroeffector transmission transmisión neuroefectora
neuroencephalomyelopathy neuroencefalomielopatía
neuroendocrine neuroendocrino
neuroendocrine dysfunction disfunción neuroendocrina
neuroendocrinology neuroendocrinología
neuroethology neuroetología
neurofibril neurofibrilla
neurofibrillary neurofibrilar
neurofibrillary degeneration degeneración neurofibrilar
neurofibroma neurofibroma
neurofibromatosis neurofibromatosis
neurogenesis neurogénesis
neurogenetic neurogenético
neurogenic neurogénico
neurogenic atrophy atrofia neurogénica
neurogenic bladder vejiga neurogénica
neurogenic drive impulso neurogénico
neurogenic fracture fractura neurogénica
neurogenous neurógeno
neuroglia neuroglia
neuroglial neuroglial
neuroglial sclerosis esclerosis neuroglial
neurogliomatosis neurogliomatosis
neurogram neurograma
neurography neurografía
neurohormone neurohormona
neurohumor neurohumor
neurohumoral neurohumoral
neurohumoral transmission transmisión neurohumoral
neurohypnosis neurohipnosis
neurohypophysis neurohipófisis
neuroinduction neuroinducción
neurolemma neurolema
neuroleptic neuroléptico
neuroleptic drug droga neuroléptica

neuroleptic-induced acute akathisia acatisia aguda inducida por neuroléptico
neuroleptic-induced acute dystonia distonía aguda inducida por neuroléptico
neuroleptic-induced parkinsonism parkinsonismo inducido por neuroléptico
neuroleptic-induced tardive dyskinesia discinesia tardía inducida por neuroléptico
neuroleptic malignant syndrome síndrome maligno neuroléptico
neuroleptic syndrome síndrome neuroléptico
neurolinguistic neurolingüítico
neurolinguistics neurolingüística
neurologic neurológico
neurologic disorder trastorno neurológico
neurological neurológico
neurological amnesia amnesia neurológica
neurological correlation correlación neurológica
neurological defect defecto neurológico
neurological deterioration deterioración neurológica
neurological development desarrollo neurológico
neurological disorder trastorno neurológico
neurological evaluation evaluación neurológica
neurological examination examinación neurológica
neurological impairment deterioro neurológico
neurological impairment and child abuse deterioro neurológico y abuso de niños
neurological maturation maduración neurológica
neurologist neurólogo
neurology neurología
neurolymphomatosis neurolinfomatosis
neurolysis neurólisis
neurolytic neurolítico
neuroma neuroma
neuroma cutis neuroma cutáneo
neuroma telangiectodes neuroma telangiectásico
neuromalacia neuromalacia
neuromatosis neuromatosis
neuromelanin neuromelanina
neuromessenger neuromensajero
neurometrics neurométrica
neuromimesis neuromimesis
neuromodulator neuromodulador
neuromuscular neuromuscular
neuromuscular disease enfermedad neuromuscular
neuromuscular disorder trastorno neuromuscular
neuromuscular junction unión neuromuscular
neuromuscular system sistema neuromuscular
neuromyasthenia neuromiastenia
neuromyelitis neuromielitis
neuromyelitis optica neuromielitis óptica
neuromyopathy neuromiopatía
neuromyositis neuromiositis
neuron neurona

neuronal neuronal
neuronal degeneration degeneración neuronal
neuronal lipidosis lipidosis neuronal
neuronal membrane membrana neuronal
neuronal plasticity plasticidad neuronal
neuronal polypeptide polipéptido neuronal
neurone neurona
neuronitis neuronitis
neuronopathy neuronopatía
neuronophage neuronófago
neuronophagia neuronofagia
neuronophagy neuronofagia
neuronyxis neuronixis
neurooncology neurooncología
neuroopthalmalogy neurooftalmología
neurootology neurootología
neuropapillitis neuropapilitis
neuroparalysis neuroparálisis
neuroparalytic neuroparalítico
neuroparalytic keratitis queratitis
    neuroparalítica
neuroparalytic ophthalmia oftalmía
    neuroparalítica
neuropath neurópata
neuropathic neuropático
neuropathic arthritis artritis neuropática
neuropathic arthropathy artropatía
    neuropática
neuropathic joint articulación neuropática
neuropathic traits rasgos neuropáticos
neuropathogenesis neuropatogénesis
neuropathological neuropatológico
neuropathology neuropatología
neuropathy neuropatía
neuropeptide neuropéptido
neuropharmacology neurofarmacología
neurophillic neurofílico
neurophrenia neurofrenia
neurophthalmology neuroftalmología
neurophysins neurofisinas
neurophysiological neurofisiológico
neurophysiological effects of exercise efectos
    neurofisiológicos del ejercicio
neurophysiology neurofisiología
neuropil neurópilo
neuroplasm neuroplasma
neuroplasty neuroplastia
neuroplegic neuroplégico
neuroplexus neuroplexo
neuropsychiatry neuropsiquiatría
neuropsychodiagnosis neuropsicodiagnóstico
neuropsychologic neuropsicológico
neuropsychologic disorder trastorno
    neuropsicológico
neuropsychological neuropsicológico
neuropsychological assessment evaluación
    neuropsicológica
neuropsychological development desarrollo
    neuropsicológico
neuropsychological dysfunction disfunción
    neuropsicológica
neuropsychology neuropsicología
neuropsychopathic neuropsicopático
neuropsychopathy neuropsicopatía
neuropsychopharmacology

neuropsicofarmacología
neuropsychosis neuropsicosis
neuropsychotropic neuropsicotrópico
neuropsychotropic agent agente
    neuropsicotrópico
neuroreceptor neurorreceptor
neurorecidive neurorrecidiva
neurorecurrence neurorrecurrencia
neurorelapse neurorrelapso
neuroretinitis neurorretinitis
neurorrhaphy neurorrafia
neurosarcocleisis neurosarcocleisis
neurosarcoidosis neurosarcoidosis
neuroschwannoma neuroschwannoma
neuroscience neurociencia
neurosecretory neurosecretorio
neurosecretory cell célula neurosecretoria
neurosis neurosis
neurosis tarda neurosis tardía
neurospasm neuroespasmo
neurosthenia neurostenia
neurostimulator neuroestimulador
neurosurgeon neurocirujano
neurosurgery neurocirugía
neurosuture neurosutura
neurosyphilis neurosífilis
neurotabes neurotabes
neurotendinal spindle huso neurotendinal
neurotensin neurotensina
neurotension neurotensión
neurothekeoma neurotequeoma
neurotherapeutics neuroterapéutica
neurotherapy neuroterapia
neurothlipsia neurotlipsia
neurothlipsis neurotlipsis
neurotic neurótico
neurotic anxiety ansiedad neurótica
neurotic arrangement arreglo neurótico
neurotic breakthrough adelanto neurótico
neurotic character carácter neurótico
neurotic claim reclamación neurótica
neurotic compliance acatamiento neurótico
neurotic conflict conflicto neurótico
neurotic defense defensa neurótica
neurotic defense system sistema de defensas
    neurótico
neurotic depression depresión neurótica
neurotic-depressive reaction reacción
    neurótica-depresiva
neurotic disorder trastorno neurótico
neurotic excoriation excoriación neurótica
neurotic fiction ficción neurótica
neurotic guilt culpabilidad neurótica
neurotic hunger strike huelga de hambre
    neurótica
neurotic insanity panic pánico de insania
    neurótica
neurotic inventory inventario neurótico
neurotic manifestation manifestación
    neurótica
neurotic needs necesidades neuróticas
neurotic nucleus núcleo neurótico
neurotic paradox paradoja neurótica
neurotic personality personalidad neurótica
neurotic pride orgullo neurótico

neurotic process proceso neurótico
neurotic rebelliousness rebeldía neurótica
neurotic resignation resignación neurótica
neurotic-sleep attack ataque de sueño
   neurótico
neurotic sociopath sociópata neurótico
neurotic solution solución neurótica
neurotic syndrome síndrome neurótico
neurotic trait rasgo neurótico
neurotic trend tendencia neurótica
neuroticism neuroticismo
neurotigenesis neurotigénesis
neurotigenic neurotigénico
neurotization neurotización
neurotize neurotizar
neurotmesis neurotmesis
neurotology neurotología
neurotome neurótomo
neurotomy neurotomía
neurotonic neurotónico
neurotony neurotonía
neurotoxic neurotóxico
neurotoxic substance sustancia neurotóxica
neurotoxin neurotoxina
neurotransmission neurotransmisión
neurotransmitter neurotransmisor
neurotransmitter metabolite metabolito
   neurotransmisor
neurotransmitter receptor receptor
   neurotransmisor
neurotrauma neurotrauma
neurotripsy neurotripsia
neurotrophic neurotrófico
neurotrophic atrophy atrofia neurotrófica
neurotrophic factor factor neurotrófico
neurotrophy neurotrofia
neurotropic neurotrópico
neurotropism neurotropismo
neurotropy neurotropía
neurotrosis neurotrosis
neurovaricosis neurovaricosis
neurovaricosity neurovaricosidad
neurovascular neurovascular
neurovascular flap colgajo neurovascular
neurovegetative system sistema
   neurovegetativo
neurulation neurulación
neutral neutral
neutral color color neutral
neutral environment ambiente neutral
neutral gray gris neutral
neutral stimulus estímulo neutral
neutrality neutralidad
neutralization neutralización
neutralizer neutralizador
nevoid nevoide
nevoid amentia amencia nevoide
nevus nevo
newborn recién nacido
newborn screening cribado de recién nacidos
nexus nexo
niacin niacina
nialamide nialamida
nicotine nicotina
nicotine dependence dependencia de nicotina

nicotine-induced organic mental disorder
   trastorno mental orgánico inducido por
   nicotina
nicotine test prueba de nicotina
nicotine use disorder trastorno de uso de
   nicotina
nicotine withdrawal retiro de nicotina
nicotinic nicotínico
nicotinic acid ácido nicotínico
nicotinic acid deficiency deficiencia de ácido
   nicotínico
nictation nictación
nictitating nictitante
nictitating spasm espasmo nictitante
nictitation nictitación
Nielsen's disease enfermedad de Nielsen
Niemann-Pick disease enfermedad de
   Niemann-Pick
night blindness ceguera nocturna
night-care program programa de cuidado
   nocturno
night-eating comer nocturno
night-eating syndrome síndrome de comer
   nocturno
night fantasy fantasía nocturna
night hospital hospital nocturno
night pain dolor nocturno
night palsy parálisis nocturna
night residue residuo nocturno
night terror pavor nocturno
night vision visión nocturna
nightmare pesadilla
nightmare disorder trastorno de pesadillas
nightshade poisoning envenenamiento por
   solano
nigrostriatal nigroestriado
nihilism nihilismo
nihilistic nihilístico
nihilistic delusion delusión nihilística
nimetazepam nimetazepam
ninth cranial nerve noveno nervio craneal
nirvana nirvana
nirvana principle principio de nirvana
Nissl bodies cuerpos de Nissl
Nissl method método de Nissl
Nissl stain colorante de Nissl
nit nit
nitrazepam nitrazepam
nitrogen narcosis narcosis por nitrógeno
nitrogen poisoning envenenamiento por
   nitrógeno
nitrous oxide óxido nitroso
no reflow phenomenon fenómeno de no
   reflujo
nociceptive nociceptivo
nociceptive reflex reflejo nociceptivo
nociceptor nociceptor
nocifensor nocifensor
nocifensor reflex reflejo nocifensor
nociinfluence nociinfluencia
nociperception nocipercepción
noctambulation noctambulación
noctiphobia noctifobia
nocturia nocturia
nocturnal nocturno

nocturnal diarrhea diarrea nocturna
nocturnal emission emisión nocturna
nocturnal enuresis enuresis nocturna
nocturnal epilepsy epilepsia nocturna
nocturnal hemiplegia hemiplejía nocturna
nocturnal myoclonus mioclono nocturno
nocturnal paralysis parálisis nocturna
nocturnal penile tumescence tumescencia
 peniana nocturna
nocturnal penile tumescence test prueba de
 tumescencia peniana nocturna
nocturnal rhythms ritmos nocturnos
nocturnal vertigo vértigo nocturno
nodal nodal
nodal behavior conducta nodal
nodal point punto nodal
nodding cabeceo
nodding spasm espasmo de cabeceo
node nódulo
nodes of Ranvier nódulos de Ranvier
nodular nodular
nodular headache dolor de cabeza nodular
nodular mesoneuritis mesoneuritis nodular
nodular panencephalitis panencefalitis
 nodular
nodule nódulo
noematic noemático
noesis noesis
noetic noético
noetic anxiety ansiedad noética
noise ruido
noise conditions condiciones de ruido
noise effects efectos de ruido
noise pollution contaminación de ruido
nomadism nomadismo
nomatophobia nomatofobia
nomenclature nomenclatura
nomifensine nomifensina
nominal nominal
nominal aphasia afasia nominal
nominal definition definición nominal
nominal realism realismo nominal
nominal scale escala nominal
nominal weight peso nominal
nominalism nominalismo
nominating technique técnica de nominación
nomogram nomograma
nomograph nomógrafo
nomological nomológico
nomothetic nomotético
nomothetic approach acercamiento
 nomotético
non compos mentis non compos mentis
non-existence inexistencia
non-rapid eye movement movimientos
 oculares no rápidos
non-rapid eye movement sleep sueño de
 movimientos oculares no rápidos
non sequitur non sequitur
nonadditive no aditivo
nonaffective no afectivo
nonaffective hallucination alucinación no
 afectiva
nonaggressive no agresivo
nonaggressive socialized reaction reacción

socializada no agresiva
nonaggressive society sociedad no agresiva
nonaggressive undersocialized reaction
 reacción subsocializada no agresiva
nonalcoholic Korsakoff psychosis psicosis de
 Korsakoff no alcohólica
nonaversive no aversivo
nonaversive behavior modification
 modificación de conducta no aversiva
nonbarbiturate sedative sedante no
 barbiturato
nonchromaffin paraganglioma
 paraganglioma no cromafínico
noncommunicating no comunicante
noncommunicating hydrocephalus
 hidrocefalia incomunicante
noncomplementary no complementario
noncomplementary role papel no
 complementario
noncompliance incumplimiento
noncompliance with medical treatment
 incumplimiento con tratamiento médico
noncompliance with treatment
 incumplimiento con tratamiento
**noncompliance with treatment for mental
 disorder** incumplimiento con tratamiento
 para trastorno mental
nonconformity inconformismo
nonconscious inconsciente
nonconscious process proceso inconsciente
noncontingent no contingente
noncontingent reinforcement refuerzo no
 contingente
nondestructive aggression agresión no
 destructiva
nondirectional test of hypothesis prueba de
 hipótesis no direccional
nondirective no directivo
nondirective approach acercamiento no
 directivo
nondirective interview entrevista no directiva
nondirective play therapy terapia de juego no
 directivo
nondirective psychoanalysis psicoanálisis no
 directivo
nondirective psychotherapy psicoterapia no
 directiva
nondirective teaching model modelo de
 enseñanza no directivo
nondirective therapy terapia no directiva
nondisjunction no disyunción
nondominant no dominante
nonexperimental no experimental
nonexperimental method método no
 experimental
nonfluent no fluente
nonfluent aphasia afasia no fluente
nonintermittent no intermitente
nonintermittent reinforcement schedule
 programa de refuerzo no intermitente
noninvasive no invasor
nonketonic no cetónico
nonketonic hyperglycemia hiperglucemia no
 cetónica
nonlegitimate authority autoridad ilegítima

nonlinear no lineal
nonlinear correlation correlación no lineal
nonlinear relationship relación no lineal
nonmetric no métrico
nonmetric scaling escalamiento no métrico
nonnutritive sucking procedures
  procedimientos de mamar no nutritivos
nonorganic failure to thrive fracaso en
  medrar no orgánico
nonorganic failure to thrive and child abuse
  fracaso en medrar no orgánico y abuso de
  niños
nonorganic hearing loss pérdida de audición
  no organica
nonorganic speech impairment deterioro del
  habla no organico
nonparametric no paramétrico
nonparametric statistics estadística no
  paramétrica
nonparticipant no participante
nonparticipant observer observador no
  participante
nonpathological no patológico
nonpathological lying mentir no patológico
nonphobic no fóbico
nonphobic anxiety behavior therapy terapia
  de conducta de ansiedad no fóbica
nonpreferred no preferido
nonpsychotic no psicótico
nonpsychotic mental disorder trastorno
  mental no psicótico
nonpsychotropic no psicotrópico
nonpsychotropic drug droga no psicotrópica
nonrational no racional
nonreactive no reactivo
nonreactive depression depresión no reactiva
nonrecognition no reconocimiento
nonrecombinant no recombinante
nonregressive schizophrenia esquizofrenia no
  regresiva
nonreproductive no reproductivo
nonsense disparate
nonsense figure figura disparatada
nonsense syllable sílaba disparatada
nonsense syndrome síndrome de disparates
nonsocial no social
nonspecific no específico
nonspecific effect efecto no específico
nonspecific encephalomyeloneuropathy
  encefalomieloneuropatía inespecífica
nonspecific research investigación no
  específica
nonspecific system sistema no específico
nonspecific urethritis uretritis no específica
nonstriate visual cortex corteza visual no
  estriada
nonsystematic no sistemático
nonsystematic schizophrenia esquizofrenia
  no sistemática
nontraditional no tradicional
nontraditional hypnotism hipnotismo no
  tradicional
nontranssexual cross-gender disorder
  trastorno de género cruzado no transexual
nonverbal no verbal

nonverbal behavior conducta no verbal
nonverbal communication comunicación no
  verbal
nonverbal communication in infants
  comunicación no verbal en infantes
nonverbal intelligence inteligencia no verbal
nonverbal language lenguaje no verbal
nonverbal test prueba no verbal
nonverbal therapy terapia no verbal
nonvoluntary involuntario
noogenic noogénico
noogenic neurosis neurosis noogénica
noology noología
Noonan's syndrome síndrome de Noonan
nootropic nootrópico
nootropic drug dementia of Alzheimer type
  demencia de droga nootrópica de tipo de
  Alzheimer
noradrenaline noradrenalina
noradrenaline dementia of Alzheimer type
  demencia de noradrenalina de tipo de
  Alzheimer
noradrenergic noradrenérgico
noradrenergic neuron neurona
  noradrenérgica
noradrenergic synapse sinapsis
  noradrenérgica
nordazepam nordazepam
norepinephrine norepinefrina
norepinephrine receptor receptor de
  norepinefrina
norm norma
norm group grupo de norma
normal adolescence adolescencia normal
normal autism autismo normal
normal curve curva normal
normal delivery parto normal
normal development desarrollo normal
normal distribution distribución normal
normal fears of infants temores normales de
  infantes
normal pregnancy embarazo normal
normal pressure hydrocephalus hidrocefalia
  de presión normal
normal probability curve curva de
  probabilidades normal
normality normalidad
normalization normalización
normalize normalizar
normative normativo
normative compliance acatamiento normativo
normative crisis crisis normativa
normative ethics ética normativa
normative-reeducative strategy estrategia
  normativa-reeducativa
normative research methods métodos de
  investigación normativos
normative science ciencia normativa
normative score puntuación normativa
normative survey encuesta normativa
normokalemic periodic paralysis parálisis
  periódica normopotasémica
normosplanchnic type tipo normoesplácnico
normotensive normotenso
normotensive individual individuo

normotenso
normothymotic normotimótico
normotonic normotónico
normotype normotipo
normotypical normotípico
Norrie's disease enfermedad de Norrie
nortriptyline nortriptilina
nortriptyline hydrochloride clorhidrato de
  nortriptilina
nose-bridge-lid reflex reflejo de
  nariz-puente-párpado
nose distance distancia entre narices
nose-eye reflex reflejo de nariz-ojo
nosocomial nosocomial
nosocomiom nosocomio
nosocomium nosocomio
nosogenesis nosogénesis
nosogeny nosogenia
nosography nosografía
nosological nosológico
nosological approach acercamiento
  nosológico
nosology nosología
nosomania nosomanía
nosophilia nosofilia
nosophobia nosofobia
nostalgia nostalgia
nostomania nostomanía
nostophobia nostofobia
not elsewhere classified no clasificado en otra
  parte
not-for-profit hospital hospital sin fines de
  lucro
not me no yo
not otherwise specified no especificado de
  otra manera
notanencephalia notanencefalia
notch escotadura
note blindness ceguera para las notas
Nothnagel's syndrome síndrome de
  Nothnagel
notochord notocordio
notogenesis notogénesis
noumenal noumenal
nous nous
novelty novedad
noxa noxa
noxious nocivo
nuclear nuclear
nuclear complex complejo nuclear
nuclear conflict conflicto nuclear
nuclear family familia nuclear
nuclear imaging producción de imágenes
  nuclear
nuclear jaundice ictericia nuclear
nuclear magnetic resonance resonancia
  magnética nuclear
nuclear-medical technologist tecnólogo
  nuclear-médico
nuclear neurosis neurosis nuclear
nuclear ophthalmoplegia oftalmoplejía
  nuclear
nuclear problem problema nuclear
nuclear schizophrenia esquizofrenia nuclear
nuclear transsexual transexual nuclear

nuclear transvestite transvestista nuclear
nucleic acid ácido nucleico
nucleofugal nucleófugo
nucleolus nucléolo
nucleopetal nucleópeto
nucleotide nucleótido
nucleus núcleo
nucleus globosus núcleo globoso
nucleus of the raphe núcleo del rafe
nucleus pulposus núcleo pulposo
nucleus ruber núcleo rojo
nucleus thoracicus núcleo torácico
nudism nudismo
null nulo
null-cell adenoma ademoma de células nulas
null hypothesis hipótesis nula
null result resultado nulo
null set conjunto nulo
nulliparous nulípara
number completion test prueba de
  terminación de números
number factor factor numérico
numbness entumecimiento
numerical numérico
numerical ability habilidad numérica
numerical value valor numérico
nursing behavior conducta de lactancia
nursing home hogar de cuidados médicos
nurturance crianza
nurturance need necesidad de crianza
nurture crianza
nutation nutación
nutrition nutrición
nutritional nutricional
nutritional assessment evaluación nutricional
nutritional deficiency deficiencia nutricional
nutritional disorder trastorno nutricional
nutritional factor factor nutricional
nutritional polyneuropathy polineuropatía
  nutricional
nutritional therapy terapia nutricional
nutritional type cerebellar atrophy atrofia
  cerebelosa tipo nutricional
nyctalgia nictalgia
nyctalopia nictalopía
nyctophilia nictofilia
nyctophobia nictofobia
nyctophonia nictofonía
nympholepsy ninfolepsia
nymphomania ninfomanía
nymphomaniac ninfomaníaca
nymphomaniacal ninfomaníaco
nystagmus nistagmo

O element elemento O
O technique técnica O
obdormition obdormición
obedience obediencia
obedience to authority obediencia a la
  autoridad
obesity obesidad
obesity treatment tratamiento de obesidad
obfuscation ofuscación
object objeto
object addiction adicción a objetos
object-assembly test prueba de ensamblaje de
  objetos
object assimilation asimilación de objeto
object attitude actitud de objeto
object blindness ceguera de objetos
object cathexis catexis de objeto
object choice selección de objeto
object color color de objeto
object concept concepto de objeto
object constancy constancia de objeto
object discrimination discriminación de
  objetos
object exploration exploración de objetos
object identification identificación de objeto
object libido libido de objetos
object loss pérdida de objeto
object love amor de objeto
object of instinct objeto de instinto
object permanence permanencia de objeto
object relations relaciones de objetos
object relations theory teoría de relaciones de
  objetos
object relationship relación de objeto
object representation representación de
  objeto
object reversal test prueba de inversión de
  objetos
object size tamaño de objeto
object sorting test prueba de clasificación de
  objetos
object test prueba de objetos
objectivation objetivación
objective objetivo
objective anxiety ansiedad objetiva
objective assessment evaluación objetiva
objective examination examinación objetiva
objective orientation orientación objetiva
objective psychology psicología objetiva
objective psychotherapy psicoterapia objetiva
objective reality realidad objetiva
objective scoring tanteo objetivo
objective self-awareness conciencia propia
  objetiva

objective sensation sensación objetiva
objective set predisposición objetiva
objective sociogram sociograma objetivo
objective test prueba objetiva
objective type tipo objetivo
objective vertigo vértigo objetivo
objectivism objetivismo
objectivity objetividad
oblativity oblatividad
obligatory obligatorio
obligatory perception percepción obligatoria
oblique oblicuo
oblique decalage decalaje oblicuo
oblique rotation rotación oblicua
oblique solution solución oblicua
obliterative arachnoiditis aracnoiditis
  obliterativa
oblongata oblongo
obnubilation obnubilación
obscenity obscenidad
obscenity-purity complex complejo de
  obscenidad-pureza
obscurantism obscurantismo
observation observación
observation commitment confinamiento para
  observación
observation delusion delusión de observación
observation technique técnica de observación
observation trial ensayo de observación
observational observacional
observational learning aprendizaje
  observacional
observational learning and aggression
  aprendizaje observacional y agresión
observational learning in children
  aprendizaje observacional en niños
observational learning theory teoría de
  aprendizaje observacional
observational method método observacional
observed behavior conducta observada
observer observador
observer drift tendencia de observadores
observer reliability confiabilidad de
  observador
observer sociogram sociograma de
  observador
obsession obsesión
obsessional brooding meditación ansiosa
  obsesiva
obsessional character carácter obsesivo
obsessional disorder trastorno obsesivo
obsessional neurosis neurosis obsesiva
obsessional personality personalidad obsesiva
obsessional thoughts pensamientos obsesivos
obsessional type tipo obsesivo
obsessions and compulsions obsesiones y
  compulsiones
obsessive obsesivo
obsessive attack ataque obsesivo
obsessive behavior conducta obsesiva
obsessive-compulsive obsesivo-compulsivo
obsessive-compulsive disorder trastorno
  obsesivo-compulsivo
obsessive-compulsive disorder versus
  schizophrenia trastorno

obsesivo-compulsivo contra esquizofrenia
obsessive-compulsive neurosis neurosis obsesiva-compulsiva
obsessive-compulsive personality personalidad obsesiva-compulsiva
obsessive-compulsive personality disorder trastorno de personalidad obsesivo-compulsivo
obsessive-compulsive psychoneurosis psiconeurosis obsesiva-compulsiva
obsessive doubt duda obsesiva
obsessive fantasy fantasía obsesiva
obsessive fear temor obsesivo
obsessive impulse impulso obsesivo
obsessive personality personalidad obsesiva
obstacle sense sentido de obstáculos
obstetrical obstétrico
obstetrical hand mano obstétrica
obstetrical optimality score puntuación de optimidad obstétrica
obstetrical optimality score and cognitive development puntuación de optimidad obstétrica y desarrollo cognitivo
obstetrical paralysis parálisis obstétrica
obstetrical scale escala obstétrica
obstinate obstinado
obstinate progression progresión obstinada
obstinately obstinadamente
obstipation obstipación
obstruction obstrucción
obstruction box caja de obstrucción
obstruction method método de obstrucción
obstructive obstructivo
obstructive apnea apnea obstructiva
obstructive disease enfermedad obstructiva
obstructive dysmenorrhea dismenorrea obstructiva
obstructive hydrocephalus hidrocefalia obstructiva
obstructive sleep apnea apnea del sueño obstructiva
obtained obtenido
obtained frequency frecuencia obtenida
obtained mean media obtenida
obtained score puntuación obtenida
obtrusive intruso
obtrusive idea idea intrusa
obturation obturación
obturator obturador
obtuse obtuso
obtusion obtusión
Occam's razor navaja de Occam
occasional ocasional
occasional inversion inversión ocasional
occipital occipital
occipital lobe lóbulo occipital
occipital neuralgia neuralgia occipital
occipital neuritis neuritis occipital
occlusal neurosis neurosis oclusal
occlusion oclusión
occlusive oclusivo
occlusive meningitis meningitis oclusiva
occult oculto
occult hydrocephalus hidrocefalia oculta
occult myelodysplasia mielodisplasia oculta

occultism ocultismo
occupation ocupación
occupational ocupacional
occupational ability habilidad ocupacional
occupational adjustment ajuste ocupacional
occupational analysis análisis ocupacional
occupational choice selección ocupacional
occupational clinical psychology psicología clínica ocupacional
occupational counseling asesoramiento ocupacional
occupational cramp calambre ocupacional
occupational delirium delirio ocupacional
occupational drinking beber ocupacional
occupational family familia ocupacional
occupational group grupo ocupacional
occupational hierarchy jerarquía ocupacional
occupational history historial ocupacional
occupational inhibition inhibición ocupacional
occupational interest inventory inventario de intereses ocupacionales
occupational interests intereses ocupacionales
occupational level nivel ocupacional
occupational neurosis neurosis ocupacional
occupational norm norma ocupacional
occupational problem problema ocupacional
occupational psychiatry psiquiatría ocupacional
occupational rehabilitation rehabilitación ocupacional
occupational spasm espasmo ocupacional
occupational stability estabilidad ocupacional
occupational stress estrés ocupacional
occupational test prueba ocupacional
occupational therapist terapeuta ocupacional
occupational therapy terapia ocupacional
oceanic feeling sensación oceánica
ochlophobia oclofobia
octave octava
ocular ocular
ocular albinism albinismo ocular
ocular bobbing meneo vertical ocular
ocular dominance dominancia ocular
ocular flutter aleteo ocular
ocular hypertelorism hipertelorismo ocular
ocular motor apraxia apraxia motora ocular
ocular myopathy miopatía ocular
ocular paralysis parálisis ocular
ocular pursuit rastreo ocular
ocular torsional movement movimiento torsional ocular
ocular torticollis tortícolis ocular
oculist oculista
oculocardiac reflex reflejo oculocardíaco
oculocephalic oculocefálico
oculocephalic reflex reflejo oculocefálico
oculocephalogyric oculocefalógiro
oculocephalogyric reflex reflejo oculocefalógiro
oculocerebral oculocerebral
oculocerebral-hypopigmentation syndrome síndrome de hipopigmentación oculocerebral
oculocerebrorenal oculocerebrorrenal

oculocerebrorenal syndrome síndrome oculocerebrorrenal
oculoencephalic oculoencefálico
oculoencephalic angiomatosis angiomatosis oculoencefálica
oculogyral oculógiro
oculogyral crisis crisis oculógira
oculogyral illusion ilusión oculógira
oculogyric oculógiro
oculogyric crisis crisis oculógira
oculogyric spasm espasmo oculógiro
oculomotor oculomotor
oculomotor apraxia apraxia oculomotora
oculomotor nerve nervio oculomotor
oculomotor nucleus núcleo oculomotor
oculomotor response respuesta oculomotora
odaxesmus odaxesmo
odaxetic odaxético
odd-even reliability confiabilidad de pares-nones
odd-even technique técnica de pares-nones
oddities of behavior rarezas de conducta
oddity rareza
oddity problem problema de rareza
odogenesis odogénesis
odonterism odonterismo
odontoneuralgia odontoneuralgia
odontophobia odontofobia
odor olor
odor identification identificación de olores
odor prism prisma de olores
odoriferous odorífero
odorimetry odorimetría
odynometer odinómetro
odynophobia odinofobia
oedipal edípico
oedipal complex complejo edípico
oedipal conflict conflicto edípico
oedipal neurosis neurosis edípica
oedipal period periodo edípico
oedipal phase fase edípica
oedipal situation situación edípica
oedipal stage etapa edípica
oedipism edipismo
Oedipus complex complejo de Edipo
oestrus estro
ogive ojiva
Ogura operation operación de Ogura
Ohm's law ley de Ohm
oikiophobia oiquiofobia
oikofugic oicofugaz
oikomania oicomanía
oikophobia oicofobia
oikotropic oicotrópico
oinomania oinomanía
old age vejez
olecranon reflex reflejo del olécranon
olfaction olfacción
olfactometer olfatómetro
olfactometry olfatometría
olfactophobia olfatofobia
olfactory olfatorio
olfactory anesthesia anestesia olfatoria
olfactory areas áreas olfatorias
olfactory brain cerebro olfatorio

olfactory bulbs bulbos olfatorios
olfactory epithelium epitelio olfatorio
olfactory eroticism erotismo olfartorio
olfactory esthesioneuroblastoma estesioneuroblastoma olfatorio
olfactory hallucination alucinación olfatoria
olfactory hyperesthesia hiperestesia olfatoria
olfactory hypesthesia hipestesia olfatoria
olfactory nerve nervio olfatorio
olfactory neuroblastoma neuroblastoma olfatorio
olfactory reference syndrome síndrome de referencia olfatoria
olfactory sensitivity sensibilidad olfatoria
olfactory stimulation estimulación olfatoria
olfactory sulcus surco olfatorio
olfactory system sistema olfatorio
olfactory tract tracto olfatorio
oligodactyly oligodactilia
oligodendroblastoma oligodendroblastoma
oligodendrocyte oligodendrocito
oligodendroglia oligodendroglia
oligodendroglioma oligodendroglioma
oligoencephaly oligoencefalia
oligohydramnios oligohidramnios
oligologia oligologia
oligomenorrhea oligomenorrea
oligophrenia oligofrenia
oligoria oligoria
oligospermia oligospermia
oligothymia oligotimia
olivary olivar
olivary body cuerpo olivar
olivary nucleus núcleo olivar
olivocochlear bundle fascículo olivococlear
olivopontocerebellar olivopontocerebeloso
olivopontocerebellar atrophy atrofia olivopontocerebelosa
olivopontocerebellar degeneration degeneración olivopontocerebelosa
olophonia olofonía
ombrophobia ombrofobia
ombudsman ombudsman
omega omega
omicron ómicron
omission omisión
omission of duty omisión del deber
ommatidium omatidio
ommatophobia omatofobia
Ommaya reservoir reservorio de Ommaya
omnibus test prueba colectiva
omnipotence omnipotencia
omnipotence of thought omnipotencia de pensamiento
omophagia omofagia
on-the-job training entrenamiento en el trabajo
onanism onanismo
oncocytoma oncocitoma
oncogene oncogen
oncology oncología
Ondine's curse maldición de Ondine
one-tailed probability probabilidad de una cola
one-tailed test prueba de una cola

one trial learning aprendizaje de un ensayo
one-way mirror espejo unidireccional
Oneida community comunidad de Oneida
oneiric onírico
oneirism onirismo
oneirocritical onirocrítico
oneirodelirium onirodelirio
oneirodynia onirodinia
oneirodynia activa onirodinia activa
oneirodynia gravis onirodinia grave
oneirogmus onirogma
oneirogonorrhea onirogonorrea
oneirology onirología
oneiromancy oniromancia
oneironosus onironoso
oneirophrenia onirofrenia
oneiroscopy oniroscopia
oniomania oniomanía
onion bulb neuropathy neuropatía en bulbo
    de cebolla
onlooker play juego de espectador
only child hijo único, hija única
onology onología
onomatomania onomatomanía
onomatophobia onomatofobia
onomatopoeia onomatopeya
onomatopoesis onomatopoyesis
onomatopoiesis onomatopoyesis
onset comienzo
ontoanalysis ontoanálisis
ontoanalytic ontoanalítico
ontoanalytic model modelo ontoanalítico
ontogenesis ontogénesis
ontogenetic ontogenético
ontogeny ontogenia
ontology ontología
onychophagia onicofagia
onychophagy onicofagia
oocyte oocito
oogenesis oogénesis
oogonuim oogonio
oophorectomy ooforectomía
opacity opacidad
Opalski cell célula de Opalski
opaque opaco
open classroom aula abierta
open-classroom design diseño de aula abierta
open cordotomy cordotomía abierta
open-cue situation situación de señales
    abiertas
open-door hospital hospital de puertas
    abiertas
open-door policy política de puertas abiertas
open education educación abierta
open-ended question pregunta sin alternativas
    fijas
open fracture fractura abierta
open group grupo abierto
open head injury lesión de cabeza abierta
open hospital hospital abierto
open instinct instinto abierto
open marriage matrimonio abierto
open skull fracture fractura de cráneo abierta
open study estudio abierto
open system sistema abierto

open trial ensayo abierto
open ward pabellón abierto
open words palabras abiertas
operant operante
operant aggression agresión operante
operant behavior conducta operante
operant behaviorism conductismo operante
operant conditioning condicionamiento
    operante
operant learning aprendizaje operante
operant level nivel operante
operant reserve reserva operante
operant response respuesta operante
operating microscope microscopio operatorio
operation operación
operational operacional
operational definition definición operacional
operational evaluation evaluación operacional
operational planning planificación
    operacional
operational research investigación
    operacional
operational thought pensamiento operacional
operationalism operacionalismo
operationism operacionismo
operations research investigación de
    operaciones
operative operativo
operative behavior conducta operativa
operative knowledge conocimiento operativo
operator operador
operatory operatorio
operatory stage etapa operatoria
operatory thought pensamiento operatorio
ophidiophilia ofidiofilia
ophidiophobia ofidiofobia
ophryosis ofriosis
ophthalmia oftalmía
ophthalmia neonatorum oftalmía neonatal
ophthalmic oftálmico
ophthalmic artery arteria oftálmica
ophthalmic migraine migraña oftálmica
ophthalmology oftalmología
ophthalmometer oftalmómetro
ophthalmoplegia oftalmoplejía
ophthalmoplegia externa oftalmoplejía
    externa
ophthalmoplegia interna oftalmoplejía interna
ophthalmoplegia internuclearis oftalmoplejía
    internuclear
ophthalmoplegia orbital oftalmoplejía
    orbitaria
ophthalmoplegia partialis oftalmoplejía
    parcial
ophthalmoplegia progressiva oftalmoplejía
    progresiva
ophthalmoplegia totalis oftalmoplejía total
ophthalmoplegic oftalmopléjico
ophthalmoplegic dystrophy distrofia
    oftalmopléjica
ophthalmoplegic migraine migraña
    oftalmopléjica
ophthalmoscope oftalmoscopio
ophthalmoscopy oftalmoscopia
opiate opiáceo

opiate addiction adicción a opiáceos
opiate antagonist antagonista opiáceo
opiate receptor receptor de opiáceos
opinion opinión
opinion poll encuesta de opiniones
opinionaire cuestionario de opiniones
opioid opioide
opioid abuse abuso de opioide
opioid delirium delirio de opioide
opioid dependence dependencia de opioide
opioid-induced organic mental disorder
   trastorno mental orgánico inducido por
   opioide
opioid intoxication intoxicación por opioide
opioid mood disorder trastorno del humor de
   opioide
opioid psychotic disorder trastorno psicótico
   de opioide
opioid psychotic disorder with delusions
   trastorno psicótico de opioide con
   delusiones
opioid psychotic disorder with hallucinations
   trastorno psicótico de opioide con
   alucinaciones
opioid receptor receptor de opioide
opioid sexual dysfunction disfunción sexual
   de opioide
opioid sleep disorder trastorno del sueño de
   opioide
opioid use disorder trastorno de uso de
   opioide
opioid withdrawal retiro de opioide
opiomania opiomanía
opipramol opipramol
opisthoporeia opistoporeia
opisthotonic opistotónico
opisthotonoid opistotonoide
opisthotonos opistótonos
opisthotonus opistótonos
opium opio
opium addiction adicción a opio
opium alkaloid alcaloide de opio
opium dependence dependencia de opio
opotherapy opoterapia
Oppenheim's disease enfermedad de
   Oppenheim
Oppenheim's reflex reflejo de Oppenheim
Oppenheim's syndrome síndrome de
   Oppenheim
Oppenheimer treatment tratamiento de
   Oppenheimer
opponent process procesos de oponentes
**opponent-process theory of acquired
   motivation** teoría de procesos de
   oponentes de motivación adquirida
opponent-process theory of color vision
   teoría de procesos de oponentes de visión
   de color
opponent-process theory of motivation teoría
   de procesos de oponentes de motivación
opposites test prueba de opuestos
oppositional oposicional
oppositional defiant disorder trastorno
   desafiante oposicional
oppositional disorder trastorno oposicional

oppositional personality disorder trastorno
   de personalidad oposicional
oppositional thinking pensamiento
   oposicional
opsin opsina
opsoclonus opsoclono
opsomania opsomanía
optic óptico
optic agnosia agnosia óptica
optic atrophy atrofia óptica
optic atrophy-ataxia syndrome síndrome de
   atrofia-ataxia óptico
optic chiasm quiasma óptico
optic disk disco óptico
optic fiber regeneration regeneración de
   fibras ópticas
optic nerve nervio óptico
optic neuritis neuritis óptica
optic papilla papila óptica
optic radiation radiación óptica
optic tract tracto óptico
optical óptico
optical alexia alexia óptica
optical axis eje óptico
optical defect defecto óptico
optical illusion ilusión óptica
optical image imagen óptica
optical imaging producción de imagen óptica
optical projection proyección óptica
optical righting reflex reflejo de
   enderezamiento óptico
optician óptico
opticofacial opticofacial
opticofacial reflex reflejo opticofacial
optics óptica
optimal óptimo
optimal functioning funcionamiento óptimo
optimal group size tamaño de grupo óptimo
optimal interpersonal distance distancia
   interpersonal óptima
optimal-stimulation principle principio de
   estimulación óptima
optimism optimismo
optimum óptimo
optional stopping terminación opcional
optional-stopping fallacy falacia de
   terminación opcional
optogram optograma
optokinetic optocinético
optokinetic nystagmus nistagmo optocinético
optometrist optometrista
optometry optometría
oral administration administración oral
oral-aggressive oral-agresivo
oral-aggressive character carácter
   oral-agresivo
oral anxiety ansiedad oral
oral behavior conducta oral
oral-biting period periodo de morder oral
oral cavity cavidad oral
oral character carácter oral
oral coitus coito oral
oral contraceptive pill píldora contraceptiva
   oral
oral dependence dependencia oral

oral dependency dependencia oral
oral drive impulso oral
oral dynamism dinamismo oral
oral dyskinesia discinesia oral
oral eroticism erotismo oral
oral-eroticism stage etapa de erotismo oral
oral-facial-digital syndrome síndrome
   oral-facial-digital
oral fixation fijación oral
oral-genital contact contacto oral-genital
oral gratification gratificación oral
oral impregnation impregnación oral
oral-incorporative oral-incorporativo
oral-incorporative phase fase incorporativa
   oral
oral method método oral
oral neurosis neurosis oral
oral orientation orientación oral
oral-passive oral-pasivo
oral-passive type tipo oral-pasivo
oral personality personalidad oral
oral pessimism pesimismo oral
oral phase fase oral
oral primacy primacía oral
oral reading lectura oral
oral-receptive oral-receptivo
oral-receptive character carácter
   oral-receptivo
oral regression regresión oral
oral sadism sadismo oral
oral-sadistic stage etapa oral-sádica
oral-sensory stage etapa oral-sensorial
oral stage etapa oral
oral stereotypy estereotipia oral
oral sucking period periodo de mamar oral
oral test prueba oral
oral triad tríada oral
oralism oralismo
orality oralidad
Orbeli effect efecto de Orbeli
orbicularis orbicular
orbicularis oculi reflex reflejo orbicular de
   los ojos
orbicularis pupillary reflex reflejo pupilar
   orbicular
Orbison figure figura de Orbison
orbital orbital
orbital decompression descompresión orbital
orbitomedial orbitomedial
orbitomedial syndrome síndrome
   orbitomedial
orchiectomy orquiectomía
order orden
order effect efecto del orden
order of magnitude orden de magnitud
order of merit orden de mérito
ordinal ordinal
ordinal position posición ordinal
ordinal scale escala ordinal
ordinate ordenada
orectic oréctico
Orestes complex complejo de Orestes
orexia orexia
orexis orexis
organ órgano

organ eroticism erotismo orgánico
organ inferiority inferioridad orgánica
organ language lenguaje orgánico
organ libido libido orgánico
organ neurosis neurosis orgánica
organ of Corti órgano de Corti
organ pleasure placer orgánico
organ speech habla orgánica
organ transplant trasplante de órgano
organelle organelo
organic orgánico
organic affective syndrome síndrome afectivo
   orgánico
organic aggressive syndrome síndrome
   agresivo orgánico
organic amnesia amnesia orgánica
organic amnestic disorder trastorno amnésico
   orgánico
organic anxiety ansiedad orgánica
organic anxiety disorder trastorno de
   ansiedad orgánica
organic anxiety syndrome síndrome de
   ansiedad orgánica
organic approach acercamiento orgánico
organic brain syndrome síndrome cerebral
   orgánico
organic contracture contractura orgánica
organic defect defecto orgánico
organic defect of the central nervous system
   defecto orgánico del sistema nervioso
   central
organic delirium delirio orgánico
organic delusional disorder trastorno
   delusorio orgánico
organic delusional syndrome síndrome
   delusorio orgánico
organic dementia demencia orgánica
organic depressive syndrome síndrome
   depresivo orgánico
organic disorder trastorno orgánico
organic hallucination alucinación orgánica
organic hallucinosis alucinosis orgánica
organic headache dolor de cabeza orgánico
organic integrity test prueba de integridad
   orgánica
organic manic syndrome síndrome maníaco
   orgánico
organic mental disorder trastorno mental
   orgánico
organic mental syndrome síndrome mental
   orgánico
organic mood disorder trastorno del humor
   orgánico
organic mood syndrome síndrome del humor
   orgánico
organic pain dolor orgánico
organic paralysis parálisis orgánica
organic personality disorder trastorno de
   personalidad orgánico
organic personality syndrome síndrome de
   personalidad orgánico
organic psychosis psicosis orgánica
organic reaction reacción orgánica
organic repression represión orgánica
organic retardation retardo orgánico

organic sensation sensación orgánica
organic speech impairment deterioro del
 habla orgánico
organic syndrome síndrome orgánico
organic therapy terapia orgánica
organic variable variable orgánica
organic vertigo vértigo orgánico
organic viewpoint punto de vista orgánico
organicism organicismo
organicist organicista
organicity organicidad
organicity assessment evaluación de
 organicidad
organicity test prueba de organicidad
organism organismo
organismic organísmico
organismic determinant determinante
 organísmico
organismic psychology psicología
 organísmica
organismic variable variable organísmica
organization organización
organizational organizativo
organizational climate clima organizativo
organizational diagnosis diagnóstico
 organizativo
organizational dynamics dinámica
 organizativa
organizational psychology psicología
 organizativa
organized play juego organizado
organogenesis organogénesis
organogenetic organogenético
organogenic organogénico
organoleptic organoléptico
organotherapy organoterapia
orgasm orgasmo
orgasm disorder trastorno de orgasmo
orgasmic orgásmico
orgasmic cephalgia cefalgia orgásmica
orgasmic dysfunction disfunción orgásmica
orgasmic impotence impotencia orgásmica
orgasmic phase fase orgásmica
orgasmic platform plataforma orgásmica
orgasmic reconditioning recondicionamiento
 orgásmico
orgastic orgástico
orgastic impotence impotencia orgástica
orgastic potency potencia orgástica
orgiastic orgiástico
orgone orgón
orgone accumulator acumulador de orgón
orgone box caja de orgón
orgone therapy terapia de orgón
orgonomy orgonomía
orgy orgía
orientation orientación
orientation disorder trastorno de orientación
orientation illusion ilusión de orientación
orienting reflex reflejo de orientación
orienting response respuesta de orientación
origin-of-language theory teoría de origen del
 lenguaje
original original
original response respuesta original

original score puntuación original
originality originalidad
ornithinemia ornitinemia
ornithophobia ornitofobia
orofacial orofacial
orofacial dyskinesia discinesia orofacial
orogenital orogenital
orogenital activity actividad orogenital
oropharynx orofaringe
orphan huérfano
orphan drug droga huérfana
orphan virus virus huérfano
orthergasia ortergasia
orthobiosis ortobiosis
orthochorea ortocorea
orthodox psychoanalysis psicoanálisis
 ortodoxo
orthodox sleep sueño ortodoxo
orthogenesis ortogénesis
orthogenics ortogénica
orthogenital ortogenital
orthognathia ortognatia
orthogonal ortogonal
orthogonal rotation rotación ortogonal
orthogonal solution solución ortogonal
orthogonal trait rasgo ortogonal
orthograde ortógrado
orthograde degeneration degeneración
 ortógrada
orthography ortografía
orthomolecular ortomolecular
orthomolecular psychiatry psiquiatría
 ortomolecular
orthomolecular therapy terapia
 ortomolecular
orthomolecular treatment tratamiento
 ortomolecular
orthonasia ortonasia
orthopedic ortopédico
orthopedic disorder trastorno ortopédico
orthophrenia ortofrenia
orthopnea ortopnea
orthopsychiatry ortopsiquiatría
orthoptics ortóptica
orthostatic ortostático
orthostatic hypertension hipertensión
 ortostática
orthostatic hypotension hipotensión
 ortostática
orthosympathetic ortosimpático
orthotics-prosthetics ortótica-prostética
orthotonos ortótonos
orthotonus ortótonos
oscillation oscilación
oscillograph oscilógrafo
oscillometer oscilómetro
oscilloscope osciloscopio
osmoceptor osmoceptor
osmodysphoria osmodisforia
osmophobia osmofobia
osmoreceptor osmorreceptor
osmotherapy osmoterapia
osphresia osfresia
osphresiolagnia osfresiolagnia
osphresiophilia osfresiofilia

osphresiophobia osfresiofobia
osphresis osfresis
ossicle osículo
ossify osificar
osteitis osteítis
osteitis deformans osteítis deformante
osteitis fibrosa cystica osteítis fibrosa quística
ostensive ostensivo
osteoarthritis osteoartritis
osteodiastasis osteodiastasis
osteogenesis osteogénesis
osteogenesis imperfecta osteogénesis
 imperfecta
osteoma osteoma
osteomalacia osteomalacia
osteomyelitis osteomielitis
osteopathic osteopático
osteopathic scoliosis escoliosis osteopática
osteopetrosis osteopetrosis
osteoplastic osteoplástico
osteoplastic craniotomy craneotomía
 osteoplástica
osteoporosis osteoporosis
osteoporosis circumscripta cranii
 osteoporosis craneal circunscripta
osteosarcoma osteosarcoma
osteotomy osteotomía
ostomy ostomía
Ostwald color system sistema de colores de
 Ostwald
Ostwald scale escala de Ostwald
otalgia otalgia
Othello syndrome síndrome de Otelo
other behavior otra conducta
other-directed dirigido hacia otros
other-directed person persona dirigida hacia
 otros
other disorder otro trastorno
other female sexual dysfunction otra
 disfunción sexual femenina
other interpersonal problems otros
 problemas interpersonales
other male sexual dysfunction otra
 disfunción sexual masculina
other psychosexual disorder otro trastorno
 psicosexual
other sexual disorder otro trastorno sexual
other specified affective disorder otro
 trastorno afectivo especificado
other specified family circumstance otra
 circunstancia familiar especificada
other specified substance dependence otra
 dependencia de sustancia especificada
other substance abuse abuso de otra sustancia
other substance anxiety disorder trastorno de
 ansiedad de otra sustancia
other substance delirium delirio de otra
 sustancia
other substance dependence dependencia de
 otra sustancia
other substance intoxication intoxicación por
 otra sustancia
other substance mood disorder trastorno del
 humor de otra sustancia
other substance persisting amnestic disorder

trastorno amnésico persistente de otra
 sustancia
other substance persisting dementia
 demencia persistente de otra sustancia
other substance psychotic disorder trastorno
 psicótico de otra sustancia
other substance psychotic disorder with
 delusions trastorno psicótico de otra
 sustancia con delusiones
other substance psychotic disorder with
 hallucinations trastorno psicótico de otra
 sustancia con alucinaciones
other substance sexual dysfunction
 disfunción sexual de otra sustancia
other substance sleep disorder trastorno del
 sueño de otra sustancia
other substance use disorder trastorno de uso
 de otra sustancia
other substance withdrawal retiro de otra
 sustancia
otic ótico
otic abscess absceso ótico
otitic otítico
otitic hydrocephalus hidrocefalia otítica
otitic meningitis meningitis otítica
otitis otitis
otitis externa otitis externa
otitis interna otitis interna
otitis media otitis media
otocerebritis otocerebritis
otoencephalitis otoencefalitis
otogenic otogénico
otogenic tone tono otogénico
otohemineurasthenia otohemineurastenia
otolaryngology otolaringología
otolith otolito
otology otología
otoneuralgia otoneuralgia
otopalatodigital otopalatodigital
otopalatodigital syndrome síndrome
 otopalatodigital
otorrhea otorrea
otosclerosis otoesclerosis
out-group grupo excluído
out-of-body experience experiencia fuera del
 cuerpo
outbreeding reproducción no consanguínea
outcome resultado
outcome evaluation evaluación de resultados
outcome research investigación de resultados
outcome variable variable de resultados
outer boundary límite exterior
outer-directed dirigido hacia el exterior
outer-directed person persona dirigida hacia
 el exterior
outer hair cells células pilosas externas
outlet salida
outpatient paciente externo
outpatient clinic clínica de pacientes externos
outpatient services servicios de pacientes
 externos
outpatient treatment tratamiento de pacientes
 externos
output salida
outreach services servicios de extensión

outside density densidad externa
oval window ventana oval
ovarian ovárico
ovarian cycle ciclo ovárico
ovarian dysgenesis disgenesia ovárica
ovarian follicle folículo ovárico
ovariectomy ovariectomía
ovariotomy ovariotomía
ovary ovario
over-the-counter drugs drogas de mostrador
overachievement sobrerrendimiento
overactivity sobreactividad
overanxious sobreansioso
overanxious disorder trastorno sobreansioso
overanxious disorder of childhood trastorno
    sobreansioso de niñez
overbreathing sobreventilación
overcome superar
overcoming superación
overcoming of fear superación del temor
overcompensation sobrecompensación
overcontrolled sobrecontrolado
overcorrection sobrecorrección
overcrowding sobreapiñamiento
overdependent sobredependiente
overdependent behavior conducta
    sobredependiente
overdetermination sobredeterminación
overdose sobredosis
overexclusion sobreexclusión
overextension sobreextensión
overflow rebosamiento
overflow activity actividad de rebosamiento
overflow incontinence incontinencia por
    rebosamiento
overgeneralization sobregeneralización
overheating sobrecalentamiento
overinclusion sobreinclusión
overlapping factor factor solapante
overlapping groups grupos solapantes
overlay sobreposición
overlearning sobreaprendizaje
overload sobrecarga
overload model of stress modelo de
    sobrecarga de estrés
overload theory teoría de sobrecarga
overmobilization sobremovilización
overpopulation superpoblación
overproduction sobreproducción
overprotection sobreprotección
overreaction sobrerreacción
overresponse sobrerrespuesta
overstimulation sobreestimulación
overt manifiesto
overt homosexuality homosexualidad
    manifiesta
overt response respuesta manifiesta
overt sensitization sensibilización manifiesta
overtone armónico
overvalued idea idea sobrevalorada
overweight sobrepeso
ovulation ovulación
ovum óvulo
oxazepam oxazepam
oxazolam oxazolam

oxyacoia oxiacoia
oxyakoia oxiacoia
oxyaphia oxiafia
oxycephalia oxicefalia
oxycephalic oxicefálico
oxycephalous oxicéfalo
oxycephaly oxicefalia
oxycodone oxicodona
oxyesthesia oxiestesia
oxygen debt deuda de oxígeno
oxygen regulation regulación de oxígeno
oxygeusia oxigeusia
oxyosmia oxiosmia
oxyosphresia oxiosfresia
oxypertine oxipertina
oxytocic oxitócico
oxytocin oxitocina

P

P technique técnica P
pacemaker marcapasos
Pachon's test prueba de Pachon
pachygyria paquigiria
pachyleptomeningitis paquileptomeningitis
pachymeningitis paquimeningitis
pachymeningitis externa paquimeningitis
   externa
pachymeningitis interna paquimeningitis
   interna
pachymeningopathy paquimeningopatía
pachymeninx paquimeninge
pacification pacificación
pacifier chupete
pacinian corpuscle corpúsculo de Pacini
pack envoltura
padded cell celda acolchada
Paget's disease enfermedad de Paget
pagophagia pagofagia
paidology paidología
pain dolor
pain agnosia agnosia de dolor
pain behavior conducta de dolor
pain clinic clínica de dolor
pain conduction conducción de dolor
pain disorder trastorno de dolor
pain disorder associated with psychological
   factors trastorno de dolor asociado con
   factores psicológicos
pain endurance resistencia de dolor
pain in dreams dolor en sueños
pain management administración de dolor
pain mechanism mecanismo de dolor
pain pathways vías de dolor
pain phobia fobia al dolor
pain-pleasure principle principio de
   dolor-placer
pain principle principio de dolor
pain-prone disorder trastorno propenso al
   dolor
pain reaction reacción de dolor
pain receptor receptor de dolor
pain sense sentido de dolor
pain spot punto de dolor
pain syndrome síndrome de dolor
pain threshold umbral de dolor
pain tolerance tolerancia de dolor
painful doloroso
painful anesthesia anestesia dolorosa
painful intercourse relación dolorosa
painful paraplegia paraplejía dolorosa
painful point punto doloroso
paired associates pares asociados
paired-associates learning aprendizaje de

pares asociados
paired-associates method método de pares
   asociados
paired comparison comparación emparejada
paired-comparisons method método de
   comparaciones emparejadas
palatal palatal
palatal myoclonus mioclono palatal
palatal nystagmus nistagmo palatal
palatal reflex reflejo palatal
palate paladar
palatine palatino
palatine reflex reflejo palatino
palatoplegia palatoplejía
paleencephalon paleoencéfalo
paleocerebellum paleocerebelo
paleocortex paleocorteza
paleologic paleológico
paleologic thinking pensamiento paleológico
paleomnesis paleomnesis
paleophrenia paleofrenia
paleopsychic paleopsíquico
paleopsychology paleopsicología
paleosensation paleosensación
paleospinothalamic paleoespinotalámico
paleospinothalamic tract tracto
   paleoespinotalámico
paleostriatal paleoestriatal
paleostriatal syndrome síndrome
   paleoestriatal
paleostriatum paleoestriado
paleosymbol paleosímbolo
palicinesia palicinesia
paligraphia paligrafia
palikinesia palicinesia
palilalia palilalia
palilexia palilexia
palilogia palilogia
palindrome palíndromo
palindromic palindrómico
palindromic encephalopathy encefalopatía
   palindrómica
palingraphia palingrafia
palinlexia palinlexia
palinopia palinopia
palinopsia palinopsia
palinphrasia palinfrasia
paliopsy paliopsia
paliphrasia palifrasia
pallanesthesia palanestesia
pallesthesia palestesia
pallesthetic palestético
pallesthetic sensibility sensibilidad palestética
palliative paliativo
pallidal palidal
pallidal syndrome síndrome palidal
pallidectomy palidectomía
pallidoamygdalotomy palidoamigdalotomía
pallidoansotomy palidoansotomía
pallidohypothalamic palidohipotalámico
pallidohypothalamic tract tracto
   palidohipotalámico
pallidotomy palidotomía
pallidum pálido
pallium palio

palm-chin reflex reflejo palma-barbilla
palmaesthesia palmestesia
palmar palmar
palmar conductance conductancia palmar
palmar grasp reflex reflejo de agarre palmar
palmar reflex reflejo palmar
palmar resistance resistencia palmar
palmar response respuesta palmar
palmesthesia palmestesia
palmesthesis palmestesis
palmic pálmico
palmistry quiromancia
palmodic palmódico
palmomandibular palmomandibular
palmomandibular reflex reflejo
     palmomandibular
palmomental palmomentoniano
palmomental reflex reflejo palmomentoniano
palmus palmo
palpebral palpebral
palpebral fissure fisura palpebral
palpitation palpitación
palsy parálisis
pamoate pamoato
pananxiety panansiedad
panarteritis panarteritis
panchreston pancrestón
Pancoast syndrome síndrome de Pancoast
Pancoast tumor tumor de Pancoast
pancreatic pancreático
pancreatic encephalopathy encefalopatía
     pancreática
pancreatitis pancreatitis
pandemic pandémico
pandiculation pandiculación
Pandy's reaction reacción de Pandy
panel panel
panencephalitis panencefalitis
panesthesia panestesia
pang punzada
panglossia panglosia
panic pánico
panic attack ataque de pánico
panic disorder trastorno de pánico
panic disorder with agoraphobia trastorno de
     pánico con agorafobia
panic disorder without agoraphobia
     trastorno de pánico sin agorafobia
panic in fires pánico en fuegos
panmixia panmixia
panneuritis panneuritis
panneuritis endemica panneuritis endémica
panneurosis panneurosis
panodic panódico
panophobia panofobia
panoramic memory memoria panorámica
panphobia panfobia
panplegia panplejía
panpsychism panpsiquismo
pansexualism pansexualismo
pantalgia pantalgia
pantanencephalia pantanencefalia
pantanencephaly pantanencefalia
pantaphobia pantafobia
panthodic pantódico

pantomime pantomima
pantophobia pantofobia
pantry-check technique técnica de inspección
     de despensa
Panum phenomenon fenómeno de Panum
paper and pencil test prueba de papel y lápiz
paper-folding test prueba de doblar papel
paper pica pica de papel
Papez circle círculo de Papez
Papez circuit circuito de Papez
Papez theory of emotion teoría de emoción
     de Papez
papilla papila
papilledema papiledema
papilloma papiloma
papilloma neuropathicum papiloma
     neuropático
papilloma neuroticum papiloma neurótico
paraballism parabalismo
parabiosis parabiosis
parabiotic parabiótico
parabiotic preparation preparación
     parabiótica
parablepsia parablepsia
parabulia parabulia
paracarcinomatous paracarcinomatoso
paracarcinomatous encephalomyelopathy
     encefalomielopatía paracarcinomatosa
paracarcinomatous myelopathy mielopatía
     paracarcinomatosa
paracenesthesia paracenestesia
paracentral paracentral
paracentral lobule lóbulo paracentral
paracentral sulcus surco paracentral
paracentral vision visión paracentral
parachromatopsia paracromatopsia
parachromopsia paracromopsia
parachute reflex reflejo de paracaidas
paracinesia paracinesia
paracinesis paracinesis
paracontrast paracontraste
paracousia paracusia
paracousis paracusis
paracusia paracusia
paracusis paracusis
paracyclic ovulation ovulación paracíclica
paracyesis paraciesis
paradigm paradigma
paradigm clash choque de paradigmas
paradigm of associative inhibition paradigma
     de inhibición asociativa
paradigmatic paradigmático
paradigmatic association asociación
     paradigmática
paradipsia paradipsia
paradox paradoja
paradoxical paradójico
paradoxical cold frío paradójico
paradoxical extensor reflex reflejo extensor
     paradójico
paradoxical flexor reflex reflejo flexor
     paradójico
paradoxical incontinence incontinencia
     paradójica
paradoxical injunction mandato paradójico

paradoxical intention intención paradójica
paradoxical intervention intervención
     paradójica
paradoxical orgasm orgasmo paradójico
paradoxical patellar reflex reflejo rotuliano
     paradójico
paradoxical pupil pupila paradójica
paradoxical pupillary phenomenon
     fenómeno pupilar paradójico
paradoxical pupillary reflex reflejo pupilar
     paradójico
paradoxical reaction reacción paradójica
paradoxical reflex reflejo paradójico
paradoxical response respuesta paradójica
paradoxical sleep sueño paradójico
paradoxical technique técnica paradójica
paradoxical therapy terapia paradójica
paradoxical triceps reflex reflejo del tríceps
     paradójico
paradoxical warmth calor moderado
     paradójico
paraequilibrium paraequilibrio
paraerotism paraerotismo
paraesthesia paraestesia
parafovea parafovea
paraganglioma paraganglioma
paragenital paragenital
parageusia parageusia
parageusic parageúsico
paragnomen paragnomen
paragnosia paragnosia
paragrammatism paragramatismo
paragraph-meaning test prueba de
     significado de párrafo
paragraphia paragrafía
parahypnosis parahipnosis
parahypophysis parahipófisis
parakinesia paracinesia
parakinesis paracinesis
paralalia paralalia
paralalia literalis paralalia literal
paralanguage paralenguaje
paraldehyde paraldehído
paraleprosis paraleprosis
paralepsy paralepsia
paralexia paralexia
paralgesia paralgesia
paralgia paralgia
paralinguistic paralingüístico
paralinguistic feature característica
     paralingüística
paralinguistics paralingüística
paralipophobia paralipofobia
parallax paralaje
parallel paralelo
parallel distributed processing procesamiento
     distribuido paralelo
parallel dream sueño paralelo
parallel forms formas paralelas
parallel law ley paralela
parallel play juego paralelo
parallel processing procesamiento paralelo
parallel search búsqueda paralela
parallel visual computation cómputo visual
     paralelo

parallelism paralelismo
paralog parálogo
paralogia paralogía
paralogism paralogismo
paralogy paralogía
paralysis parálisis
paralysis agitans parálisis agitante
paralytic paralítico
paralytic chorea corea paralítica
paralytic dementia demencia paralítica
paralytic ileus íleo paralítico
paralytic micosis micosis paralítica
paralytic miosis miosis paralítica
paralytic mydriasis midriasis paralítica
paralytic scoliosis escoliosis paralítica
paralyzant paralizante
paralyze paralizar
paralyzing paralizante
paralyzing vertigo vértigo paralizante
parameter parámetro
parameter dragging arrastramiento de
     parámetro
parameter-estimation technique técnica de
     estimación de parámetros
paramethadione parametadiona
parametric paramétrico
parametric statistics estadística paramétrica
parametric test of significance prueba
     paramétrica de significación
parametrismus parametrismo
paramimia paramimia
paramimism paramimismo
paramnesia paramnesia
paramusia paramusia
paramyoclonus paramioclono
paramyotonia paramiotonía
paramyotonia congenita paramiotonía
     congénita
paramyotonus paramiotono
paranalgesia paranalgesia
paraneoplastic paraneoplásico
paraneoplastic limbic encephalitis encefalitis
     límbica paraneoplásica
paraneural paraneural
paraneural infiltration infiltración paraneural
paranoia paranoia
paranoia originaria paranoia originaria
paranoia querulans paranoia quejumbrosa
paranoia scale escala de paranoia
paranoia senilis paranoia senil
paranoiac paranoico
paranoid paranoide
paranoid anxiety ansiedad paranoide
paranoid character carácter paranoide
paranoid condition condición paranoide
paranoid delusion delusión paranoide
paranoid dementia demencia paranoide
paranoid disorder trastorno paranoide
paranoid erotism erotismo paranoide
paranoid hostility hostilidad paranoide
paranoid ideation ideación paranoide
paranoid litigious state estado litigioso
     paranoide
paranoid melancholia melancolía paranoide
paranoid personality personalidad paranoide

paranoid personality disorder trastorno de personalidad paranoide
paranoid psychosis psicosis paranoide
paranoid scale escala paranoide
paranoid-schizoid position posición paranoide-esquizoide
paranoid schizophrenia esquizofrenia paranoide
paranoid-schizotypal personality disorder trastorno de personalidad paranoide-esquizotípico
paranoid state estado paranoide
paranoid trend tendencia paranoide
paranoid type tipo paranoide
paranoid type schizophrenia esquizofrenia tipo paranoide
paranoidal paranoide
paranomasia paranomasia
paranomia paranomia
paranormal paranormal
paranormal cognition cognición paranormal
paranormal phenomenon fenómeno paranormal
paranosic paranósico
paranosic gain ganancia paranósica
paranosis paranosis
paraparesis paraparesia
paraparetic paraparético
parapathia parapatía
parapathy parapatía
paraperitoneal paraperitoneal
paraperitoneal nephrectomy nefrectomía paraperitoneal
paraphasia parafasia
paraphasic parafásico
paraphemia parafemia
paraphia parafia
paraphilia parafilia
paraphilic parafílico
paraphilic coercive disorder trastorno coercitivo parafílico
paraphobia parafobia
paraphonia parafonía
paraphora paráfora
paraphrase paráfrasis
paraphrasia parafrasia
paraphrenia parafrenia
paraphysial parafisial
paraphysial cyst quiste parafisial
parapithymia parapitimia
paraplectic parapléctico
paraplegia paraplejía
paraplegia dolorosa paraplejía dolorosa
paraplegia in extension paraplejía en extensión
paraplegia in flexion paraplejía en flexión
paraplegic parapléjico
parapoplexy parapoplejía
parapraxia parapraxia
parapraxis parapraxis
paraprofessional paraprofesional
parapsia parapsia
parapsychology parapsicología
parapsychosis parapsicosis
parareaction pararreacción

parareflexia pararreflexia
parasagittal parasagital
parasexuality parasexualidad
parasite parásito
parasitic parasítico
parasitic superego superego parasítico
parasitism parasitismo
parasitophobia parasitofobia
parasocial parasocial
parasocial speech habla parasocial
parasomnia parasomnia
parasuicide parasuicidio
parasympathetic parasimpático
parasympathetic drug droga parasimpática
parasympathetic nervous system sistema nervioso parasimpático
parasympathicotonia parasimpaticotonía
parasympatholytic parasimpaticolítico
parasympathomimetic parasimpaticomimético
parasympathomimetic drug droga parasimpaticomimética
parataxia parataxia
parataxic paratáxico
parataxic distortion distorsión paratáxica
parataxic mode modo paratáxico
parataxis parataxis
paratheresiomania parateresiomanía
parathormone parathormona
parathymia paratimia
parathyroid paratiroideo
parathyroid glands glándulas paratiroides
parathyroid hormone hormona paratiroidea
parathyroid tetany tetania paratiroidea
parathyroidism paratiroidismo
parathyroprival paratiroprivo
parathyroprival tetany tetania paratiropriva
paratonia paratonía
paratype paratipo
paratypic paratípico
paravariation paravariación
paraventricular nucleus núcleo paraventricular
paraverbal paraverbal
paraverbal therapy terapia paraverbal
paravertebral paravertebral
paravertebral ganglionic chain cadena ganglionar paravertebral
paraxial paraxial
parectropia parectropia
paregoric paregórico
pareidolia pareidolia
parencephalia parencefalia
parencephalitis parencefalitis
parencephalocele parencefalocele
parencephalous parencefaloso
parenchyma parénquima
parenchymatous parenquimatoso
parenchymatous neuritis neuritis parenquimatosa
parenchymatous neurosyphilis neurosífilis parenquimatosa
parens patriae parens patriae
parent padre, madre
parent burnout agotamiento de padre,

agotamiento de madre
parent-child communication comunicación
padre-hijo, comunicación padre-hija,
comunicación madre-hijo, comunicación
madre-hija
parent-child model modelo padre-hijo,
modelo padre-hija, modelo madre-hijo,
modelo madre-hija
parent-child problem problema padre-hijo,
problema padre-hija, problema madre-hijo,
problema madre-hija
parent-child relational problem problema
relacional padre-hijo, problema relacional
padre-hija, problema relacional madre-hijo,
problema relacional madre-hija
parent counseling asesoramiento de padres
parent education educación de padres
parent-effectiveness training entrenamiento
de efectividad de padres
parent image imagen de padre, imagen de
madre
parent-infant bonding vinculación
padre-infante, vinculación madre-infante
parent-infant interaction interacción
padre-infante, interacción madre-infante
parent-infant interactions at birth
interacciones padre-infante en nacimiento,
interacciones madre-infante en nacimiento
parent therapist program programa de
terapeutas padres
parental parental
parental alcoholism alcoholismo parental
parental attitude actitud parental
parental behavior conducta parental
parental conflict conflicto parental
parental death muerte parental
parental discord discordia parental
parental divorce divorcio parental
parental expectations expectaciones
parentales
parental fit ajuste parental
parental inadequacy insuficiencia parental
parental influence influencia parental
parental intercourse relación parental
parental permissiveness permisividad
parental
parental perplexity perplejidad parental
parental rejection rechazo parental
parental separation separación parental
parental speech habla parental
parental style estilo parental
parenteral parenteral
parenteral drug administration
administración de droga parenteral
parenthood paternidad, maternidad
parepithymia parepitimia
parerethisis pareretisis
parergasia parergasia
parerosia parerosia
paresis paresia
paresthesia parestesia
paresthetic parestésico
paretic parético
paretic curve curva parética
paretic impotence impotencia parética

paretic muscles músculos paréticos
paretic psychosis psicosis parética
pargyline pargilina
parietal parietal
parietal bones huesos parietales
parietal cortex corteza parietal
parietal drift tendencia parietal
parietal lobe lóbulo parietal
parietooccipital parietooccipital
parietooccipital sulcus surco parietooccipital
Parinaud's ophthalmoplegia oftalmoplejía de
Parinaud
Parinaud's syndrome síndrome de Parinaud
Parkinson's disease enfermedad de Parkinson
Parkinson's facies facies de Parkinson
parkinsonian parkinsoniano
parkinsonism parkinsonismo
parole libertad condicional
paroneiria paroniria
paroniria paroniria
parophresia parofresia
parorexia parorexia
parosmia parosmia
parosphresia parosfresia
parosphresis parosfresis
parotid gland glándula parótida
parous para
paroxysm paroxismo
paroxysmal paroxístico
paroxysmal cerebral dysrhythmia disritmia
cerebral paroxística
paroxysmal drinking beber paroxístico
paroxysmal dyskinesia discinesia paroxística
paroxysmal sleep sueño paroxístico
parricide parricidio
Parry's disease enfermedad de Parry
Parry-Romberg syndrome síndrome de
Parry-Romberg
pars pro toto pars pro toto
parsimony parsimonia
part instinct instinto parcial
parthenogenesis partenogénesis
parthenophobia partenofobia
partial parcial
partial adjustment ajuste parcial
partial aim fin parcial
partial correlation correlación parcial
partial epilepsy epilepsia parcial
partial hospitalization hospitalización parcial
partial insanity insania parcial
partial instinct instinto parcial
partial lipodystrophy lipodistrofia parcial
partial regression regresión parcial
partial reinforcement refuerzo parcial
partial-reinforcement effect efecto de
refuerzo parcial
partial remission remisión parcial
partial-report method método de informe
parcial
partial seizure acceso parcial
partial sight vista parcial
partial tone tono parcial
partialism parcialismo
partiality parcialidad
partialization parcialización

participant participante
participant observation observación de participante
participant observer observador participante
participation participación
participative participante
participative management administración participante
particular particular
particular complex complejo particular
particularism particularismo
partition partición
partition measure medida de partición
partner relational problem problema relacional de pareja
partner-swapping intercambio de parejas
parturiphobia parturifobia
parturition parto
paruresis paruresis
passing stranger effect efecto de extraño pasajero
passion pasión
passional pasional
passional attitude actitud pasional
passive pasivo
passive aggression agresión pasiva
passive-aggressive pasivo-agresivo
passive-aggressive behavior conducta pasiva-agresiva
passive-aggressive personality personalidad pasiva-agresiva
passive-aggressive personality disorder trastorno de personalidad pasiva-agresiva
passive-aggressive scale escala pasiva-agresiva
passive analysis análisis pasivo
passive avoidance evitación pasiva
passive-avoidance learning aprendizaje pasivo de evitación
passive castration complex complejo de castración pasivo
passive dependency dependencia pasiva
passive-dependent personality personalidad pasiva-dependiente
passive euthanasia eutanasia pasiva
passive immunity inmunidad pasiva
passive incontinence incontinencia pasiva
passive introversion introversión pasiva
passive learning aprendizaje pasivo
passive listening escuchar pasivo
passive mode of consciousness modo pasivo de conciencia
passive-receptive longing añoranza pasiva-receptiva
passive recreation recreación pasiva
passive therapist terapeuta pasivo
passive therapy terapia pasiva
passive tremor temblor pasivo
passive vocabulary vocabulario pasivo
passivism pasivismo
passivity pasividad
pastoral counseling asesoramiento pastoral
patch amnesia amnesia localizada
patella rótula
patellar rotuliano

patellar reflex reflejo rotuliano
patellar tendon reflex reflejo del tendón rotuliano
patelloadductor reflex reflejo rotuloaductor
patellometer rotulómetro
paternal paternal
paternal behavior conducta paternal
paternalism paternalismo
paternity paternidad
paternity blues depresión de paternidad
pathematic patemático
pathematic aphasia afasia patemática
pathergasia patergasia
pathetic patético
pathetic fallacy falacia patética
pathetic nerve nervio patético
pathetism patetismo
pathic pático
pathobiography patobiografía
pathobiology patobiología
pathoclisis patoclisis
pathocure patocura
pathodixia patodixia
pathoformic patofórmico
pathogen patógeno
pathogenesis patogénesis
pathogenic patogénico
pathogenic family pattern patrón familiar patogénico
pathogeny patogenia
pathognomic patognómico
pathognomonic patognomónico
pathognomonic signs signos patognomónicos
pathognomy patognomía
pathognostic patognóstico
pathography patografía
pathohysteria patohisteria
pathokinesis patocinesis
patholesia patolesia
pathologic patológico
pathological patológico
pathological drowsiness modorra patológica
pathological fallacy falacia patológica
pathological gambling jugar patológico
pathological grief reaction reacción de aflicción patológica
pathological guilt culpabilidad patológica
pathological intoxication intoxicación patológica
pathological lying mentir patológico
pathological mendicancy mendicidad patológica
pathological sleepiness somnolencia patológica
pathological trait rasgo patológico
pathology patología
pathomimesis patomimesis
pathomimicry patomímica
pathomiosis patomiosis
pathomorphism patomorfismo
pathoneurosis patoneurosis
pathophobia patofobia
pathophrenesis patofrenesis
pathophysiological patofisiológico
pathophysiological pattern patrón

patofisiológico
pathophysiology patofisiología
pathoplasty patoplastia
pathopsychology patopsicología
pathopsychosis patopsicosis
pathosis patosis
pathway vía
patient paciente
patient-care audit auditoría de cuidado de
 pacientes
patient-centered services servicios centrados
 en pacientes
patient government gobierno de pacientes
patient obligations obligaciones de pacientes
patient-oriented consultation consultación
 orientada a pacientes
patient responsibility responsabilidad del
 paciente
patients' rights derechos de pacientes
patriarchal patriarcal
patriarchal family familia patriarcal
patricide patricidio
Patrick's test prueba de Patrick
patrilineal patrilineal
patrilineal descent descendencia patrilineal
patriophobia patriofobia
patroiophobia patroiofobia
pattern patrón
pattern analysis análisis de patrón
pattern discrimination discriminación de
 patrón
pattern learning aprendizaje de patrón
pattern of emotions patrón de emociones
pattern perception percepción de patrón
pattern recognition reconocimiento de patrón
pattern sensitive epilepsy epilepsia sensitiva a
 patrón
paucity escasez
paucity of speech escasez del habla
pause pausa
Pavlov method método de Pavlov
pavlovian pavloviano
pavlovian conditioning condicionamiento
 pavloviano
pavlovian learning aprendizaje pavloviano
pavlovianism pavlovianismo
pavor diurnus pavor diurno
pavor nocturnus pavor nocturno
peak-clipping recorte de picos
peak experience experiencia cumbre
pearl tumor tumor perlado
Pearson chi square tests pruebas de ji
 cuadrada de Pearson
peccatiphobia pecatifobia
pecking order jerarquía de dominancia
pectoral pectoral
pectoral reflex reflejo pectoral
pectoralgia pectoralgia
pectus carinatum pecho carinado
pedagogy pedagogía
pederast pederasta
pederasty pederastia
pederosis pederosis
pedestrian movement movimiento pedestre
pediatric pediátrico

pediatric psychology psicología pediátrica
pediatric psychopharmacology
 psicofarmacología pediátrica
pediatrics pediatría
pedicatio pedicación
pedication pedicación
pediculophobia pediculofobia
pedionalgia pedionalgia
pedioneuralgia pedioneuralgia
pediophobia pediofobia
pedolalia pedolalia
pedologia pedología
pedologist pedólogo
pedology pedología
pedomorphism pedomorfismo
pedomorphosis pedomorfosis
pedophilia pedofilia
pedophilia and unbelieving parents pedofilia
 y padres incrédulos
pedophilic pedofílico
pedophobia pedofobia
pedotrophy pedotrofia
peduncle pedúnculo
peduncular peduncular
peduncular hallucinosis alucinosis peduncular
pedunculotomy pedunculotomía
peer paritario
peer counseling asesoramiento paritario
peer group grupo paritario
peer-group pressure presión de grupo
 paritario
peer-group therapy terapia de grupo paritario
peer influence influencia paritaria
peer interaction interacción paritaria
peer play juego paritario
peer pressure presión paritaria
peer pressure and drinking presión paritaria
 y beber
peer pressure and drug use presión paritaria
 y uso de drogas
peer pressure and smoking presión paritaria
 y fumar
peer rating clasificación paritaria
peer relations relaciones paritarias
peer relations and anxiety relaciones
 paritarias y ansiedad
peer relationship relación paritaria
peer review revisión paritaria
peer separation separación paritaria
pegboard tablero de clavijas
Pelizaeus-Merzbacher disease enfermedad de
 Pelizaeus-Merzbacher
pellagra pelagra
pellet trozo de comida
pelvifemoral pelvifemoral
pelvifemoral muscular dystrophy distrofia
 muscular pelvifemoral
pemoline pemolina
penalty penalidad
pencil and paper test prueba de lápiz y papel
pendular knee-jerk sacudida de rodilla
 pendular
penetrance penetrancia
penetration penetración
penetration response respuesta de

penetración
penfluridol penfluridol
peniaphobia peniafobia
penile peniano
penile erection erección peniana
penile plethysmograph pletismógrafo peniano
penile tumescence tumescencia peniana
penilingus penilingus
penis pene
penis captivus pene cautivo
penis envy envidia de pene
penis fear temor a penes
penology penología
pension neurosis neurosis de pensión
pentatonic pentatónico
pentazocine pentazocina
pentetrazol pentetrazol
pentobarbital pentobarbital
pentylenetetrazol pentilenotetrazol
peonage peonaje
peotillomania peotilomanía
Pepper syndrome síndrome de Pepper
pepsin pepsina
pepsinogen pepsinógeno
peptic péptico
peptic ulcer úlcera péptica
peptide péptido
peptide bond enlace peptídico
peptidergic peptidérgico
perazine perazina
perceive percibir
perceived percibido
perceived object objeto percibido
perceived pseudohallucination
    seudoalucinación percibida
perceived reality realidad percibida
perceived self yo percibido
percentile percentila
percentile norm norma percentil
percentile rank rango percentil
percentile score puntuación percentil
percept percepto
percept analysis análisis de perceptos
percept image imagen perceptiva
perception percepción
perception deafness sordera de percepción
perception-hallucination
    percepción-alucinación
perception of heat percepción de calor
perception of illness percepción de
    enfermedad
perception of spatial relations percepción de
    relaciones espaciales
perception time tiempo de percepción
perceptive perceptivo
perceptive impairment and nerve loss
    deterioro perceptivo y pérdida nerviosa
perceptivity perceptividad
perceptual perceptivo
perceptual abnormality anormalidad
    perceptiva
perceptual adaptation adaptación perceptiva
perceptual anchoring anclaje perceptivo
perceptual competency competencia
    perceptiva

perceptual consciousness conciencia
    perceptiva
perceptual constancy constancia perceptiva
perceptual cues señales perceptivas
perceptual cycle ciclo perceptivo
perceptual defect defecto perceptivo
perceptual defense defensa perceptiva
perceptual deficit déficit perceptivo
perceptual deficits and brain damage
    déficits perceptivos y daño cerebral
perceptual development desarrollo perceptivo
perceptual disability discapacidad perceptiva
perceptual disorder trastorno perceptivo
perceptual distortion distorsión perceptiva
perceptual disturbance disturbio perceptivo
perceptual expansion expansión perceptiva
perceptual extinction extinción perceptiva
perceptual field campo perceptivo
perceptual filtering filtración perceptiva
perceptual image imagen perceptiva
perceptual induction inducción perceptiva
perceptual learning aprendizaje perceptivo
perceptual localization localización
    perceptiva
perceptual maintenance mantenimiento
    perceptivo
perceptual masking enmascaramiento
    perceptivo
perceptual-motor disability discapacidad
    perceptiva-motora
perceptual-motor dysfunction disfunción
    perceptiva-motora
perceptual-motor learning aprendizaje
    perceptivo-motor
perceptual-motor match apareamiento
    perceptivo-motor
perceptual-motor region región
    perceptiva-motora
perceptual-motor skills destrezas
    perceptiva-motoras
perceptual organization organización
    perceptiva
perceptual processes procesos perceptivos
perceptual processing procesamiento
    perceptivo
perceptual psychology psicología perceptiva
perceptual restructuring reestructuración
    perceptiva
perceptual rivalry rivalidad perceptiva
perceptual schema esquema perceptivo
perceptual segregation segregación
    perceptiva
perceptual sensitization sensibilización
    perceptiva
perceptual set predisposición perceptiva
perceptual sociogram sociograma perceptivo
perceptual speed velocidad perceptiva
perceptual structure estructura perceptiva
perceptual style estilo perceptivo
perceptual synthesis síntesis perceptiva
perceptual task tarea perceptiva
perceptual training entrenamiento perceptivo
perceptual transactionalism
    transaccionalismo perceptivo
perceptual transformation transformación

perceptiva
perceptual vigilance vigilancia perceptiva
perceptualization perceptualización
perceptually handicapped minusválido
perceptivamente
percipient perceptor
percutaneous percutáneo
percutaneous radiofrequency gangliolysis
gangliólisis por radiofrecuencia percutánea
percutaneous stimulation estimulación
percutánea
perencephaly perencefalia
perennial dream sueño perenne
Perez reflex reflejo de Perez
perfect correlation correlación perfecta
perfect negative relationship relación
negativa perfecta
perfect pitch tono perfecto
perfect positive relationship relación positiva
perfecta
perfectionism perfeccionismo
perforator perforador
performance ejecución
performance anxiety ansiedad de ejecución
performance assessment evaluación de
ejecución
performance neurosis neurosis de ejecución
performance requirements requisitos de
ejecución
performance test prueba de ejecución
performative performativo
pergolide pergolida
perhaps neurosis neurosis del quizás
periamygdaloid cortex corteza
periamigdaloide
periarterial periarterial
periarterial sympathectomy simpatectomía
periarterial
periblepsis periblepsia
pericardial pericárdico
pericardial reflex reflejo pericárdico
perichareia pericareia
periciazine periciazina
pericranitis pericranitis
periencephalitis periencefalitis
perikaryon pericarion
periluteal phase dysphoric disorder trastorno
disfórico de fase perilútea
perilymph perilinfa
perimacular perimacular
perimacular vision visión perimacular
perimeningitis perimeningitis
perimeter perímetro
perimetry perimetría
perinatal perinatal
perinatal complications complicaciones
perinatales
perinatal events eventos perinatales
perinatal herpes virus infection infección por
virus de herpes perinatal
perinatal history historial perinatal
perinatal infection infección perinatal
perinatal morbidity morbilidad perinatal
perinatal period periodo perinatal
perinatal stress estrés perinatal

perineural perineural
perineural anesthesia anestesia perineural
perineural infiltration infiltración perineural
perineuritis perineuritis
period periodo
period prevalence prevalencia de periodo
periodic periódico
periodic catatonia catatonía periódica
periodic drinking beber periódico
periodic edema edema periódico
periodic migrainous neuralgia neuralgia
migrañosa periódica
periodic paralysis parálisis periódica
periodic psychosis of puberty psicosis
periódica de pubertad
periodic reinforcement refuerzo periódico
periodicity periodicidad
periodicity theory teoría de periodicidad
periosteal perióstico
periosteal elevator elevador perióstico
periosteal reflex reflejo perióstico
peripachymeningitis peripaquimeningitis
peripathologist peripatólogo
peripheral periférico
peripheral apnea apnea periférica
peripheral dysostosis with nasal hypoplasia
disostosis periférica con hipoplasia nasal
peripheral nervous system sistema nervioso
periférico
peripheral neuropathy neuropatía periférica
peripheral scotoma escotoma periférico
peripheral tabes tabes periférica
peripheral vision visión periférica
peripheralism periferalismo
periphery periferia
periphery of the retina periferia de la rétina
perispondylitis periespondilitis
peristasis perístasis
peritoneal peritoneal
peritoneal dialysis diálisis peritoneal
peritoneal space espacio peritoneal
peritonism peritonismo
peritonitis peritonitis
periventricular periventricular
permanence permanencia
permanence concept concepto de
permanencia
permanent permanente
permanent dominant idea idea dominante
permanente
permanent memory memoria permanente
permanent planning planificación permanente
permeability permeabilidad
permeable permeable
permissive permisivo
permissive doll play juego con muñecas
permisivo
permissive environment ambiente permisivo
permissive hypothesis of affective disorders
hipótesis permisiva de trastornos afectivos
permissive parent padre permisivo, madre
permisiva
permissiveness permisividad
pernicious pernicioso
pernicious anemia anemia perniciosa

pernicious trend tendencia perniciosa
peroneal peroneo
peroneal muscular atrophy atrofia muscular peronea
peroneal phenomenon fenómeno peroneo
perphenazine perfenazina
perplexed perplejo
perplexity perplejidad
perplexity state estado de perplejidad
persecution persecución
persecution complex complejo de persecución
persecution syndrome síndrome de persecución
persecutory persecutorio
persecutory anxiety ansiedad persecutoria
persecutory delusion delusión persecutoria
persecutory delusional disorder trastorno delusorio persecutorio
perseverance perseverancia
perseveration perseveración
perseveration deficit déficit de perseveración
perseveration set predisposición de perseveración
perseverative perseverante
perseverative error error perseverante
perseverative functional autonomy autonomía funcional perseverante
perseverative speech habla perseverante
perseverative trace rastro perseverante
persistence persistencia
persistence of vision persistencia de visión
persistent persistente
persistent puberism puberismo persistente
persistent tremor temblor persistente
person-centered theory teoría centrada en la persona
person in the patient persona en el paciente
person perception percepción de personas
persona persona
personal personal
personal adjustment ajuste personal
personal attribution atribución personal
personal audit auditoría personal
personal care home hogar de cuidado personal
personal constant constante personal
personal construct constructo personal
personal construct theory teoría de constructo personal
personal data sheet hoja de datos personales
personal determinant determinante personal
personal development desarrollo personal
personal disjunction disyunción personal
personal disorganization desorganización personal
personal disposition disposición personal
personal-distance zone zona de distancia personal
personal document documento personal
personal-document analysis análisis de documentos personales
personal-document method método de documentos personales
personal equation ecuación personal
personal fitness aptitud personal

personal growth crecimiento personal
personal-growth group grupo de crecimiento personal
personal-growth laboratory laboratorio de crecimiento personal
personal history historial personal
personal-history questionnaire cuestionario de historial personal
personal identity identidad personal
personal image imagen personal
personal injury lesión personal
personal motivation motivación personal
personal myth mito personal
personal relationship relación personal
personal-social inventory inventario personal-social
personal-social motive motivo personal-social
personal space espacio personal
personal-space invasion invasión de espacio personal
personal unconscious inconsciente personal
personalism personalismo
personalistic personalista
personalistic psychology psicología personalista
personality personalidad
personality assessment evaluación de personalidad
personality change cambio de personalidad
personality characteristics características de personalidad
personality cult culto de personalidad
personality deterioration deterioración de personalidad
personality development desarrollo de personalidad
personality disintegration desintegración de personalidad
personality disorder trastorno de personalidad
personality disorders scale escala de trastornos de personalidad
personality dynamics dinámica de personalidad
personality factors factores de personalidad
personality formation formación de personalidad
personality integration integración de personalidad
personality inventory inventario de personalidad
personality organization organización de personalidad
personality pattern disturbance disturbio de patrón de personalidad
personality problem problema de personalidad
personality profile perfil de personalidad
personality psychology psicología de personalidad
personality research investigación de personalidad
personality sphere esfera de personalidad
personality structure estructura de personalidad

personality syndrome síndrome de
  personalidad
personality test prueba de personalidad
personality theory teoría de personalidad
personality trait rasgo de personalidad
personality-trait disturbance disturbio de
  rasgo de personalidad
personality-trait theory teoría de rasgo de
  personalidad
personality type tipo de personalidad
personalization personalización
personalized personalizado
personalized instruction instrucción
  personalizada
personification personificación
personified personificado
personified self yo personificado
personnel personal
personnel data datos del personal
personnel evaluation evaluación del personal
personnel placement colocación del personal
personnel psychology psicología del personal
personnel selection selección del personal
personnel specifications especificaciones del
  personal
personnel test prueba del personal
personnel training entrenamiento del personal
personology personología
perspective perspectiva
persuasion persuasión
persuasion therapy terapia de persuasión
persuasive persuasivo
persuasive communication comunicación
  persuasiva
persuasive therapy terapia persuasiva
pervasive penetrante
pervasive developmental disorder trastorno
  penetrante del desarrollo
perverse perverso
perversion perversión
pervert pervertido
perverted pervertido
perverted logic lógica pervertida
perverted thinking pensamiento pervertido
pervigilium pervigilium
pessimism pesimismo
pet animal de compañía
petechial hemorrhages hemorragias
  petequiales
petit mal pequeño mal
petit mal epilepsy epilepsia de pequeño mal
petit mal seizure acceso de pequeño mal
petrifaction petrifacción
petrification petrificación
petrositis petrositis
petrousitis petrositis
Pette-Doring disease enfermedad de
  Pette-Doring
peyote peyote
Pfaundler-Hurler syndrome síndrome de
  Pfaundler-Hurler
Pfeiffer's syndrome síndrome de Pfeiffer
Pfuhl's sign signo de Pfuhl
phacoma facoma
phacomatosis facomatosis

phacoscope facoscopio
Phaedra complex complejo de Fedra
phagocytosis fagocitosis
phagomania fagomanía
phagophobia fagofobia
phakoma facoma
phakomatosis facomatosis
phalanx falange
phallic fálico
phallic character carácter fálico
phallic level nivel fálico
phallic love amor fálico
phallic mother madre fálica
phallic-narcissistic character carácter
  fálico-narcisista
phallic-oedipal fálico-edípico
phallic phase fase fálica
phallic pride orgullo fálico
phallic primacy primacía fálica
phallic sadism sadismo fálico
phallic stage etapa fálica
phallic symbol símbolo fálico
phallic woman mujer fálica
phallicism falicismo
phallism falismo
phallocentric falocéntrico
phallocentric culture cultura falocéntrica
phallometry falometría
phallophobia falofobia
phallus falo
phallus envy envidia de falo
phaneromania faneromanía
phantasm fantasma
phantasmagoria fantasmagoría
phantasmatomoria fantasmatomoria
phantasmology fantasmología
phantasmoscopia fantasmoscopia
phantasmoscopy fantasmoscopia
phantom fantasma
phantom breast pecho fantasma
phantom limb miembro fantasma
phantom limb pain dolor de miembro
  fantasma
phantom limb sensation sensación de
  miembro fantasma
phantom-lover syndrome síndrome de
  amante fantasma
phantom reaction reacción fantasma
pharmaceutical farmacéutico
pharmacodynamic farmacodinámico
pharmacodynamic tolerance tolerancia
  farmacodinámica
pharmacogenetics farmacogenética
pharmacogenic farmacogénico
pharmacogenic orgasm orgasmo
  farmacogénico
pharmacogeriatrics farmacogeriatría
pharmacokinetics farmacocinética
pharmacological farmacológico
pharmacological antagonism antagonismo
  farmacológico
pharmacological experiment experimento
  farmacológico
pharmacological experimentation
  experimentación farmacológica

pharmacology farmacología
pharmacomania farmacomanía
pharmacopeia farmacopea
pharmacophilia farmacofilia
pharmacophobia farmacofobia
pharmacopsychoanalysis farmacopsicoanálisis
pharmacopsychosis farmacopsicosis
pharmacotherapy farmacoterapia
pharmacotherapy for affective disorders farmacoterapia para trastornos afectivos
pharmacotherapy for anxiety disorders farmacoterapia para trastornos ansiosos
pharmacotherapy for attention-deficit disorders farmacoterapia para trastornos de déficit de atención
pharmacotherapy for autism farmacoterapia para autismo
pharmacotherapy for depression farmacoterapia para depresión
pharmacotherapy for eating disorders farmacoterapia para trastornos del comer
pharmacothymia farmacotimia
pharyngeal faríngeo
pharyngeal anesthesia anestesia faríngea
pharyngeal keratosis queratosis faríngea
pharyngeal reflex reflejo faríngeo
pharyngismus faringismo
pharyngoplegia faringoplejía
pharyngospasm faringoespasmo
pharynx faringe
phase fase
phase cue señal de fase
phase delay demora de fase
phase difference diferencia de fases
phase of life fase de vida
phase of life problem problema de fase de vida
phase sequence secuencia de fase
phase shift traslado de fase
phasic fásico
phasic activation activación fásica
phasic function función fásica
phasic reflex reflejo fásico
phasmophobia fasmofobia
phasophrenia fasofrenia
phenacemide fenacemida
phenacetin fenacetina
phenadoxone fenadoxona
phenazocine fenazocina
phencyclidine fenciclidina
phencyclidine abuse abuso de fenciclidina
phencyclidine anxiety disorder trastorno de ansiedad de fenciclidina
phencyclidine delirium delirio de fenciclidina
phencyclidine delusional disorder trastorno delusorio de fenciclidina
phencyclidine dependence dependencia de fenciclidina
phencyclidine intoxication intoxicación por fenciclidina
phencyclidine mood disorder trastorno del humor de fenciclidina
phencyclidine psychotic disorder trastorno psicótico de fenciclidina

phencyclidine psychotic disorder with delusions trastorno psicótico de fenciclidina con delusiones
phencyclidine psychotic disorder with hallucinations trastorno psicótico de fenciclidina con alucinaciones
phencyclidine use disorder trastorno de uso de fenciclidina
phendimetrazine fendimetrazina
phenelzine fenelzina
phengophobia fengofobia
phenmetrazine fenmetrazina
phenobarbital fenobarbital
phenocopy fenocopia
phenomenal fenomenal
phenomenal absolutism absolutismo fenomenal
phenomenal field campo fenomenal
phenomenal motion moción fenomenal
phenomenal pattern patrón fenomenal
phenomenal regression regresión fenomenal
phenomenal report informe fenomenal
phenomenal self yo fenomenal
phenomenalism fenomenalismo
phenomenalistic fenomenalista
phenomenalistic introspection introspección fenomenalista
phenomenistic fenomenístico
phenomenistic causality causalidad fenomenística
phenomenistic thought pensamiento fenomenístico
phenomenological fenomenológico
phenomenological analysis análisis fenomenológico
phenomenological field campo fenomenológico
phenomenological method método fenomenológico
phenomenological reality realidad fenomenológica
phenomenology fenomenología
phenomenon fenómeno
phenomenon identification identificación de fenómeno
phenothiazine fenotiazina
phenothiazine death muerte por fenotiazina
phenotype fenotipo
phensuximide fensuximida
phentermine fentermina
phentolamine fentolamina
phenylalanine fenilalanina
phenylalanine disorder trastorno de fenilalanina
phenylbutazone fenilbutazona
phenylethylamine feniletilamina
phenylketonuria fenilcetonuria
phenylpyruvic fenilpirúvico
phenylpyruvic acid ácido fenilpirúvico
phenylpyruvic amentia amencia fenilpirúvica
phenylpyruvic oligophrenia oligofrenia fenilpirúvica
phenyltoloxamine feniltoloxamina
phenytoin fenitoína
pheromone feromona

phi phi
phi coefficient coeficiente phi
phi motion moción phi
phi phenomenon fenómeno phi
Phillipson's reflex reflejo de Phillipson
philogenitive filogenitivo
philology filología
philomimesia filomimesia
philoprogenitive filoprogenitivo
philosophical filosófico
philosophical psychology psicología filosófica
philosophical psychotherapy psicoterapia
   filosófica
philosophy filosofía
phimosis fimosis
phlebitis flebitis
phlebotomy flebotomía
phlegm flema
phlegmatic flemático
phlegmatic temperament temperamento
   flemático
phlegmatic type tipo flemático
phobanthropy fobantropía
phobia fobia
phobic fóbico
phobic anxiety ansiedad fóbica
phobic attitude actitud fóbica
phobic character carácter fóbico
phobic companion compañero fóbico
phobic disorder trastorno fóbico
phobic neurosis neurosis fóbica
phobic reaction reacción fóbica
phobophobia fobofobia
phocomelia focomelia
pholcodine folcodina
phon fonio
phonasthenia fonastenia
phonation fonación
phone fono
phoneme fonema
phoneme-grapheme correspondence
   correspondencia fonema-grafema
phonemic fonémico
phonemic disorder trastorno fonémico
phonemic restoration effect efecto de
   restauración fonémica
phonemics fonémica
phonetic fonético
phonetic alphabet alfabeto fonético
phonetic method método fonético
phonetic segment segmento fonético
phonetics fonética
phonic fónico
phonic method método fónico
phonic spasm espasmo fónico
phonics fónica
phonism fonismo
phonogram fonograma
phonography fonografía
phonological fonológico
phonological development desarrollo
   fonológico
phonological disorder trastorno fonológico
phonology fonología
phonomania fonomanía

phonomyoclonus fonomioclono
phonomyography fonomiografía
phonopathy fonopatía
phonophobia fonofobia
phonopsia fonopsia
phonoscope fonoscopio
phoria foria
phorometry forometría
phosphate fosfato
phosphene fosfeno
phosphodiesterase fosfodiesterasa
phosphorous fósforo
phosphorylation fosforilación
phot fotio
photalgia fotalgia
photaugiaphobia fotaugiafobia
photerythrosity foteritrosidad
photerythrous foteritro
photesthesia fotestesia
photic fótico
photic sensitivity sensibilidad fótica
photic stimulation estimulación fótica
photism fotismo
photobiology fotobiología
photochemistry fotoquímica
photochromatic fotocromático
photochromatic interval intervalo
   fotocromático
photocoagulation fotocoagulación
photodynia fotodinia
photodysphoria fotodisforia
photoesthetic fotoestético
photogenic fotogénico
photogenic epilepsy epilepsia fotogénica
photographic memory memoria fotográfica
photokinesis fotocinesis
photoma fotoma
photomania fotomanía
photometer fotómetro
photometrazol fotometrazol
photometrazol test prueba de fotometrazol
photometric fotométrico
photometric brightness brillantez fotométrica
photometric measurement medición
   fotométrica
photometry fotometría
photomyoclonus fotomioclono
photon fotón
photoperiodism fotoperiodismo
photophobia fotofobia
photophobic fotofóbico
photopic fotópico
photopic luminosity luminosidad fotópica
photopic-sensitivity curve curva de
   sensibilidad fotópica
photopic vision visión fotópica
photopigment fotopigmento
photopsia fotopsia
photopsin fotopsina
photopsy fotopsia
photoptarmosis fotoptarmosis
photoreceptor fotorreceptor
photosensitivity fotosensibilidad
phototaxis fototaxis
phototherapy fototerapia

phototropism fototropismo
phrase frase
phrase-structure grammar gramática de
  estructura de frases
phren fren
phrenalgia frenalgia
phrenasthenia frenastenia
phrenectomy frenectomía
phrenemphraxis frenenfraxis
phrenetic frenético
phrenic frénico
phrenic nerve nervio frénico
phrenicectomy frenicectomía
phreniclasia freniclasia
phrenicoexeresis frenicoexéresis
phreniconeurectomy freniconeurectomía
phrenicotomy frenicotomía
phrenicotripsy frenicotripsia
phrenitic frenítico
phrenocardia frenocardia
phrenoglottic frenoglótico
phrenologist frenólogo
phrenology frenología
phrenophagia frenofagia
phrenoplegia frenoplejía
phrenoplegy frenoplejía
phrenopraxic frenopráxico
phrenospasm frenoespasmo
phrenotropic frenotrópico
phrictopathia frictopatía
phrictopathic frictopático
phronemophobia fronemofobia
phthinoid ftinoide
phthiriophobia ftiriofobia
phthisiomania tisiomanía
phthisiophobia tisiofobia
phylaxis filaxis
phyloanalysis filoanálisis
phylobiology filobiología
phylogenesis filogénesis
phylogenetic filogenético
phylogenetic memory memoria filogenética
phylogenetic principle principio filogenético
phylogenetic symptom síntoma filogenético
phylogeny filogenia
phylopathology filopatología
phylum filum
physaliphorous fisalíforo
physaliphorous cell célula fisalífora
physiatrics fisiatría
physiatrist fisiatra
physical físico
physical abuse abuso físico
physical abuse and development abuso físico
  y el desarrollo
physical abuse and premature death abuso
  físico y muerte prematura
physical abuse and self-esteem abuso físico y
  autoestima
physical abuse of adult abuso físico de adulto
physical abuse of child abuso físico de niño
physical activity actividad física
physical anthropology antropología física
physical appearance apariencia física
physical assault acometimiento físico

physical attractiveness atractividad física
physical changes cambios físicos
physical changes in adolescence cambios
  físicos en adolescencia
physical condition condición física
physical custody custodia física
physical dependence dependencia física
physical development desarrollo físico
physical disability discapacidad física
physical disorder trastorno físico
physical education educación física
physical exercise ejercicio físico
physical fitness aptitud física
physical fitness of children aptitud física de
  niños
physical handicap minusvalía física
physical illness enfermedad física
physical medicine medicina física
physical punishment castigo físico
physical stimulus estímulo físico
physical teratogen teratógeno físico
physical therapist terapueta físico
physical therapy terapia física
physicalism fisicalismo
physician's assistant asistente de médico
physiodrama fisiodrama
physiodynamic fisiodinámico
physiodynamic therapy terapia fisiodinámica
physiogenesis fisiogénesis
physiogenetic fisiogenético
physiogenic fisiogénico
physiognomic fisionómico
physiognomic perception percepción
  fisionómica
physiognomic thinking pensamiento
  fisionómico
physiognomy fisionomía
physiognosis fisiognosis
physiological fisiológico
physiological age edad fisiológica
physiological antagonism antagonismo
  fisiológico
physiological dependence dependencia
  fisiológica
physiological drive impulso fisiológico
physiological feedback retroalimentación
  fisiológica
physiological limit límite fisiológico
physiological maintenance mantenimiento
  fisiológico
physiological memory memoria fisiológica
physiological motive motivo fisiológico
physiological need necesidad fisiológica
physiological nystagmus nistagmo fisiológico
physiological paradigm paradigma fisiológico
physiological psychology psicología
  fisiológica
physiological response respuesta fisiológica
physiological-response specificity
  especificidad de respuestas fisiológicas
physiological self-regulation autorregulación
  fisiológica
physiological zero cero fisiológico
physiology fisiología
physiology of emotion fisiología de emoción

physioneurosis fisioneurosis
physiopathology fisiopatología
physioplastic fisioplástico
physiopsychic fisiopsíquico
physiotherapy fisioterapia
physique físico
physique type tipo físico
physocephaly fisocefalia
physostigmine fisostigmina
pia mater piamadre
piaarachnitis piaracnitis
pianist's cramp calambre de pianista
piano player's cramp calambre de tocador de piano
piano theory teoría de piano
piano theory of hearing teoría de piano de audición
piblokto piblokto
pica pica
Pick's atrophy atrofia de Pick
Pick's body cuerpo de Pick
Pick's disease enfermedad de Pick
Pick's syndrome síndrome de Pick
pickwickian syndrome síndrome de Pickwick
picrotoxin picrotoxina
pictogram pictograma
pictophilia pictofilia
picture-anomalies test prueba de anomalías de pinturas
picture-arrangement test prueba de ordenación de pinturas
picture-completion test prueba de terminación de pinturas
picture-frustration study estudio de frustración en pinturas
picture-interpretation test prueba de interpretación de pinturas
picture world test prueba de mundo en pintura
Piderit drawings dibujos de Piderit
pidgin lengua franca
Pierre Robin's syndrome síndrome de Pierre Robin
piesesthesia piesestesia
Pigem's question pregunta de Pigem
pigment pigmento
pigment layer capa de pigmento
pill-rolling enrollado de bolitas
pilocarpine pilocarpina
piloerection piloerección
piloid piloide
piloid astrocytoma astrocitoma piloide
piloid gliosis gliosis piloide
pilojection piloyección
pilomotor pilomotor
pilomotor reflex reflejo pilomotor
pilomotor response respuesta pilomotora
pilot study estudio piloto
Piltz reflex reflejo de Piltz
Piltz sign signo de Piltz
piminodine piminodina
pimozide pimozida
pinazepam pinazepam
pineal pineal
pineal body cuerpo pineal

pineal cyst quiste pineal
pineal gland glándula pineal
pineal substance sustancia pineal
pinealectomy pinealectomía
pinealoma pinealoma
pinealopathy pinealopatía
Pinel's system sistema de Pinel
Pinel-Haslam syndrome síndrome de Pinel-Haslam
pineoblastoma pineoblastoma
ping-pong fracture fractura en ping-pong
ping-pong gaze mirada fija de ping-pong
pink disease enfermedad rosada
pink noise ruido rosado
pinna pinna
pinocytosis pinocitosis
pipamperone pipamperona
Piper's law ley de Piper
piperacetazine piperacetazina
piperazine piperazina
piperidine piperidina
pipotiazine pipotiazina
pipradrol pipradrol
piriform area área piriforme
Pisa syndrome síndrome de Pisa
pitch tono
pitch discrimination discriminación de tono
pithiatism pitiatismo
pithiatric pitiátrico
Pitres' rule regla de Pitres
Pitres' sign signo de Pitres
pituicytoma pituicitoma
pituitarism pituitarismo
pituitary pituitaria
pituitary adamantinoma adamantinoma pituitario
pituitary adenoma adenoma pituitario
pituitary apoplexy apoplejía pituitaria
pituitary basophilia basofilia pituitaria
pituitary cachexia caquexia pituitaria
pituitary disorder trastorno pituitario
pituitary gland glándula pituitaria
pituitary stalk section sección del tallo pituitario
pity lástima
place learning aprendizaje de lugar
place theory teoría de lugar
place theory of hearing teoría de lugar de audición
placebo placebo
placebo effect efecto de placebo
placement colocación
placement counseling asesoramiento de colocación
placement test prueba de colocación
placenta placenta
placenta praevia placenta previa
placenta previa placenta previa
placental placentario
placental hormone hormona placentaria
placental immunity inmunidad placentaria
placental infection infección placentario
placentitis placentitis
plane plano
planned planificado

planned comparison comparación planificada
planned learning environment ambiente de aprendizaje planificado
planned parenthood procreación planificada
planned test prueba planificada
planning planificación
planomania planomanía
planophrasia planofrasia
planotopokinesia planotopocinesia
plantalgia plantalgia
plantar plantar
plantar muscle reflex reflejo muscular plantar
plantar reflex reflejo plantar
plantigrade plantígrado
plaque placa
plasma plasma
plasma level nivel plasmático
plasmapheresis plasmaféresis
plasmid plásmido
plastic-arts therapy terapia de artes plásticas
plastic surgery cirugía plástica
plastic tonus tono plástico
plasticity plasticidad
plateau meseta
plateau phase fase de meseta
plateau speech habla de meseta
platelet plaqueta
platelet count cuenta de plaquetas
platonic idea idea platónica
platonic ideal ideal platónico
platonic love amor platónico
platonization platonización
platonize platonizar
platybasia platibasia
platycephalic platicefálico
platycephaly platicefalia
platykurtic platicúrtico
platykurtosis platicurtosis
play juego
play acting actuación de juego
play and language juego y lenguaje
play behavior conducta de juego
play behavior in autism conducta de juego en autismo
play development desarrollo de juego
play group grupo de juego
play-group psychotherapy psicoterapia de grupo de juego
play pattern patrón de juego
play therapy terapia de juego
playful juguetón
playing dead fingirse muerto
pleasant placentero
pleasure placer
pleasure center centro de placer
pleasure ego ego del placer
pleasure-pain principle principio de placer-dolor
pleasure principle principio del placer
pleasure-unpleasure principle principio de placer-dolor
pleiotropic pleiotrópico
pleiotropy pleiotropía
pleniloquence plenilocuencia
pleocytosis pleocitosis

pleonasm pleonasmo
pleonexia pleonexia
plethysmograph pletismógrafo
pleurothotonos pleurotótonos
pleurothotonus pleurotótonos
plexectomy plexectomía
plexiform plexiforme
plexiform neurofibroma neurofibroma plexiforme
plexiform neuroma neuroma plexiforme
plexitis plexitis
plexus plexo
plosive explosivo
plumbism plumbismo
Plummer's disease enfermedad de Plummer
plural marriage matrimonio plural
pluralism pluralismo
pluralistic pluralista
pluralistic ignorance ignorancia pluralista
pluralistic utilitarianism utilitarismo pluralista
plutomania plutomanía
pneumatocele neumatocele
pneumatorrhachis neumatorraquis
pneumocardiograph neumocardiógrafo
pneumocele neumocele
pneumocephalus neumocefalia
pneumococcal meningitis meningitis neumocócica
pneumocranium neumocráneo
pneumoencephalogram neumoencefalograma
pneumoencephalography neumoencefalografía
pneumogastric neumogástrico
pneumogastric nerve nervio neumogástrico
pneumograph neumógrafo
pneumonia neumonía
pneumoorbitography neumoorbitografía
pneumophonia neumofonía
pneumorrhachis neumorraquis
pneumotaxic neumotáxico
pneumotaxic center centro neumotáxico
pneumotaxic localization localización neumotáxica
pneumotherapy neumoterapia
pneumothorax neumotórax
pneumoventricle neumoventrículo
pnigophobia pnigofobia
podismus podismo
podospasm podoespasmo
podospasmus podoespasmo
Poetzl effect efecto de Poetzl
Poggendorf illusion ilusión de Poggendorf
poiesis poiesis
poikilothymia poiquilotimia
poinephobia poinefobia
point punto
point estimate estimado de punto
point-for-point correspondence correspondencia punto por punto
point-localization test prueba de localización de punto
point mutation mutación de punto
point of regard punto de mirada
point of subjective equality punto de igualdad

subjetiva
point prevalence prevalencia de punto
point scale escala de puntos
point-to-point correspondence
  correspondencia de punto a punto
pointing apuntamiento
pointing the bone apuntamiento del hueso
poisoning envenenamiento
Poisson distribution distribución de Poisson
poker back espondilitis deformante
polar body cuerpo polar
polar continuum continuo polar
polar opposites opuestos polares
polarity polaridad
polarization polarización
police power poder de policía
policy política
policy analysis análisis de política
polio polio
polioclastic policlástico
poliodystrophia poliodistrofia
poliodystrophia cerebri progressiva infantilis
  poliodistrofia cerebral progresiva infantil
poliodystrophy poliodistrofia
polioencephalitis polioencefalitis
polioencephalitis infectiva polioencefalitis
  infecciosa
polioencephalomeningomyelitis
  polioencefalomeningomielitis
polioencephalomyelitis polioencefalomielitis
polioencephalopathy polioencefalopatía
poliomyelencephalitis poliomielencefalitis
poliomyelitis poliomielitis
poliomyeloencephalitis poliomieloencefalitis
poliomyelopathy poliomielopatía
political genetics genética política
political psychiatry psiquiatría política
pollakiuria polaquiuria
pollicomental policomental
pollicomental reflex reflejo policomental
pollodic polódico
Pollyanna mechanism mecanismo de Poliana
polyandry poliandria
polychromate policromato
polychromatic policromático
polycinematosomnography
  policinematosomnografía
polyclonia policlonia
Polycrates complex complejo de Polícrates
polycratism policratismo
polycyesis policiesis
polydactyl polidáctilo
polydactylism polidactilismo
polydipsia polidipsia
polydrug abuse abuso polídroga
polydrug addiction adicción polídroga
polydystrophic oligophrenia oligofrenia
  polidistrófica
polyesthesia poliestesia
polyestrous poliestro
polygamy poligamia
polygenic poligénico
polygenic traits rasgos poligénicos
polyglot polígloto
polyglot amnesia amnesia políglota

polyglot neophasia neofasia políglota
polyglot reaction reacción políglota
polygon polígono
polygraph polígrafo
polygraph test prueba de polígrafo
polygyny poliginia
polygyria poligiria
polyhybrid polihíbrido
polyleptic poliléptico
polylogia polilogia
polymatric polimátrico
polymorph polimorfo
polymorphism polimorfismo
polymorphous polimorfo
polymorphous perverse sexuality sexualidad
  perversa polimorfa
polymorphous perversion perversión
  polimorfa
polymyalgia polimialgia
polymyalgia arteritica polimialgia arterítica
polymyalgia rheumatica polimialgia
  reumática
polymyoclonus polimioclono
polymyositis polimiositis
polyneuralgia polineuralgia
polyneuritic polineurítico
polyneuritic psychosis psicosis polineurítica
polyneuritis polineuritis
polyneuronitis polineuronitis
polyneuropathy polineuropatía
polyonomy polionomía
polyopia poliopía
polyopsia poliopsia
polyorchid poliórquido
polyp pólipo
polyparesis poliparesia
polypeptide polipéptido
polyphagia polifagia
polyphallic polifálico
polypharmacy polifarmacia
polyphasic polifásico
polyphasic activity actividad polifásica
polyphasic sleep rhythm ritmo de sueño
  polifásico
polyphobia polifobia
polyphony polifonía
polyphrasia polifrasia
polyplegia poliplejía
polypnea polipnea
polypnoea polipnea
polyposia poliposia
polyposis poliposis
polypsychism polipsiquismo
polyradiculitis polirradiculitis
polyradiculomyopathy polirradiculomiopatía
polyradiculoneuritis polirradiculoneuritis
polyradiculoneuropathy
  polirradiculoneuropatía
polyradiculopathy polirradiculopatía
polysemy polisemia
polysensory polisensorial
polysensory unit unidad polisensorial
polyserositis poliserositis
polysomnogram polisomnograma
polysomnography polisomnografía

polysteraxic polisteráxico
polysurgical addiction adicción poliquirúrgica
polysynaptic polisináptico
polysynaptic arc arco polisináptico
polysynaptic reflex arc arco reflejo
  polisináptico
polytoxicomaniac politoxicomaníaco
polyuria poliuria
polyvitamin therapy terapia polivitamínica
Pompadour fantasy fantasía de Pompadour
Pompe's disease enfermedad de Pompe
ponopathy ponopatía
ponophobia ponofobia
pons pons
pontile pontino
pontile apoplexy apoplejía pontina
pontine pontino
pontine angle tumor tumor del ángulo
  pontino
pontine apoplexy apoplejía pontina
pontine hemorrhage hemorragia pontina
pontine nucleus núcleo pontino
pontine sleep sueño pontino
pontocerebellar pontocerebeloso
pontocerebellar-angle syndrome síndrome
  del ángulo pontocerebeloso
pontocerebellar-angle tumor tumor del
  ángulo pontocerebeloso
Ponzo illusion ilusión de Ponzo
Pool's phenomenon fenómeno de Pool
Pool-Schlesinger sign signo de
  Pool-Schlesinger
pooling combinación
poor mothering cuidados maternales pobres
popular response respuesta popular
popularity popularidad
population población
population density densidad poblacional
population genetics genética poblacional
population research investigación poblacional
porencephalia porencefalia
porencephalic porencefálico
porencephalitis porencefalitis
porencephalous porencéfalo
porencephaly porencefalia
poriomania poriomanía
poriomanic poriomaníaco
poriomanic fugue fuga poriomaníaca
pornerastic pornerástico
pornographomania pornografomanía
pornography pornografía
pornolagnia pornolagnia
porosis porosis
porphobilinogen porfobilinógeno
porphyria porfiria
porphyrinuria porfirinuria
porphyrismus porfirismo
porropsia porropsia
portal-systemic encephalopathy encefalopatía
  portal sistémica
Porter's law ley de Porter
Porteus maze laberinto de Porteus
portmanteau word palabra híbrida
portosystemic encephalopathy encefalopatía
  portosistémica

posiomania posiomanía
position posición
position agnosia agnosia de posición
position factor factor de posición
position habit hábito de posición
position preference preferencia de posición
position sense sentido de posición
positive positivo
positive acceleration aceleración positiva
positive adaptation adaptación positiva
positive afterimage imagen persistente
  positiva
positive attitude actitud positiva
positive attitude change cambio de actitud
  positivo
positive cathexis catexis positiva
positive conditioned reflex reflejo
  condicionado positivo
positive correlation correlación positiva
positive eugenics eugenesia positiva
positive feedback retroalimentación positiva
positive incentive incentivo positivo
positive induction inducción positiva
positive motivation motivación positiva
positive regard estimación positiva
positive reinforcement refuerzo positivo
positive reinforcer reforzador positivo
positive retroaction retroaccíon positiva
positive reward recompensa positiva
positive spike pattern patrón de puntas
  positivas
positive transfer transferencia positiva
positive transference transferencia positiva
positive tropism tropismo positivo
positive valence valencia positiva
positively positivamente
positively bathmotropic positivamente
  batmotrópico
positivism positivismo
positron positrón
positron-emission tomography tomografía de
  emisión de positrones
possession posesión
possessive posesivo
possessive instinct instinto posesivo
possessiveness posesividad
post hoc post hoc
post-test prueba posterior
postadrenalectomy syndrome síndrome
  posadrenalectomía
postambivalence posambivalencia
postambivalent phase fase posambivalente
postapoplectic posapopléctico
postcentral poscentral
postcentral area área poscentral
postcentral gyrus circunvolución poscentral
postconcussion posconcusión
postconcussion neurosis neurosis
  posconcusión
postconcussion syndrome síndrome
  posconcusión
postconventional level nivel posconvencional
postconventional level of moral development
  nivel posconvencional del desarrollo moral
postconventional stage of moral development

etapa posconvencional del desarrollo moral
postdiphtheritic posdiftérico
postdiphtheritic paralysis parálisis
  posdiftérica
postdisaster posdesastre
postdisaster adaptation adaptación
  posdesastre
postdivorce posdivorcio
postdivorce adjustment ajuste posdivorcio
postdormital posdormital
postdormital chalastic fit ataque calástico
  posdormital
postdormitum posdormitum
postemotive schizophrenia esquizofrenia
  posemotiva
postemployment posempleo
postemployment services servicios posempleo
postencephalitic posencefalítico
postencephalitic amnesia amnesia
  posencefalítica
postencephalitis posencefalitis
postencephalitis syndrome síndrome
  posencefalitis
postepileptic posepiléptico
postepileptic twilight state estado crepuscular
  posepiléptico
posterior posterior
posterior cerebral artery arteria cerebral
  posterior
posterior column cordotomy cordotomía de
  columna posterior
posterior commissure comisura posterior
posterior communicating artery arteria
  comunicante posterior
posterior diencephalon diencéfalo posterior
posterior forceps fórceps posterior
posterior fossa fosa posterior
posterior inferior cerebellar artery
  syndrome síndrome arterial cerebeloso
  inferior posterior
posterior nephrectomy nefrectomía posterior
posterior nucleus núcleo posterior
posterior orbital gyrus circunvolución orbital
  posterior
posterior parietal area área parietal posterior
posterior parietal lobe lóbulo parietal
  posterior
posterior rachischisis raquisquisis posterior
posterior rhizotomy rizotomía posterior
posterior root raíz posterior
posterior sclerosis esclerosis posterior
posterior spinal sclerosis esclerosis espinal
  posterior
posterior subarachnoidean space espacio
  subaracnoideo posterior
posterior thalamus tálamo posterior
posterolateral posterolateral
posterolateral sclerosis esclerosis
  posterolateral
postexperimental posexperimental
postexperimental inquiry pregunta
  posexperimental
postganglionic posganglionar
postganglionic autonomic neuron neurona
  autonómica posganglionar

posthallucinogen posalucinógeno
posthallucinogen perception disorder
  trastorno de percepción posalucinógena
posthemiplegic poshemipléjico
posthemiplegic athetosis atetosis
  poshemipléjica
posthemiplegic chorea corea poshemipléjica
posthion postión
posthypnotic poshipnótico
posthypnotic amnesia amnesia poshipnótica
posthypnotic psychosis psicosis poshipnótica
posthypnotic suggestion sugestión
  poshipnótica
postictal posictal
postictal depression depresión posictal
postictal state estado posictal
posticus póstico
posticus palsy parálisis póstica
posticus paralysis parálisis póstica
postinfectious posinfeccioso
postinfectious psychosis psicosis
  posinfecciosa
postmature posmaduro
postmaturity posmadurez
postmeningitic posmeningítico
postmeningitic hydrocephalus hidrocefalia
  posmeningítica
postmortem posmortem
postmortem examination examinación
  posmortem
postnatal posnatal
postnatal sensorineural lesion lesión
  sensorineural posnatal
postneuritic posneurítico
postoedipal posedípico
postoperative posoperatorio
postoperative delirium delirio posoperatorio
postoperative disorder trastorno
  posoperatorio
postoperative tetany tetania posoperatoria
postparalytic posparalítico
postpartal pospartal
postpartal eclamptic symptom síntoma
  eclámptico pospartal
postpartal period periodo pospartal
postpartum posparto
postpartum blues depresión posparto
postpartum depression depresión posparto
postpartum emotional disturbances
  disturbios emocionales posparto
postpartum mania manía posparto
postpartum pituitary necrosis syndrome
  síndrome de necrosis pituitaria posparto
postpartum psychosis psicosis posparto
postreconstructive surgery cirugía
  posreconstructiva
postremity postremidad
postremity principle principio de postremidad
postrotational nystagmus nistagmo
  posrotacional
postschizophrenic posesquizofrénico
postschizophrenic depression depresión
  posesquizofrénica
postseparation postseparación
postsynaptic postsináptico

postsynaptic potential potencial postsináptico
posttetanic potentiation potenciación
    postetánica
posttraumatic postraumático
posttraumatic amnesia amnesia
    postraumática
posttraumatic communicating hydrocephalus
    hidrocefalia comunicante postraumática
posttraumatic constitution constitución
    postraumática
posttraumatic delirium delirio postraumático
posttraumatic dementia demencia
    postraumática
posttraumatic disorder trastorno
    postraumático
posttraumatic epilepsy epilepsia
    postraumática
posttraumatic headache dolor de cabeza
    postraumática
posttraumatic hydrocephalus hidrocefalia
    postraumática
posttraumatic leptomeningeal cyst quiste
    leptomeníngeo postraumático
posttraumatic neurosis neurosis
    postraumática
posttraumatic osteoporosis osteoporosis
    postraumática
posttraumatic personality disorder trastorno
    de personalidad postraumática
posttraumatic psychosis psicosis
    postraumática
posttraumatic stress disorder trastorno de
    estrés postraumático
posttraumatic stress syndrome síndrome de
    estrés postraumático
posttraumatic syndrome síndrome
    postraumático
postulate postulado
postulational method método postulacional
postural postural
postural control control postural
postural myoneuralgia mioneuralgia postural
postural reflex reflejo postural
postural set predisposición postural
postural syncope síncope postural
postural tremor temblor postural
postural vertigo vértigo postural
posture postura
posture sense sentido de postura
posturing posturación
posturology posturología
postvaccinal posvacunal
postvaccinal encephalitis encefalitis
    posvacunal
postventral nucleus núcleo posventral
potamophobia potamofobia
potassium potasio
potassium bromide bromuro de potasio
potassium cyanate cianato de potasio
potassium deprivation privación de potasio
potassium nitrate nitrato de potasio
potence potencia
potency potencia
potent potente
potential potencial

potentiality potencialidad
Pott's abscess absceso de Pott
Pott's disease enfermedad de Pott
Pott's paralysis parálisis de Pott
Pott's paraplegia paraplejía de Pott
Pott's puffy tumor tumor edematoso de Pott
Potzl phenomenon fenómeno de Potzl
Potzl syndrome síndrome de Potzl
poverty pobreza
poverty of content of speech pobreza de
    contenido del habla
poverty of ideas pobreza de ideas
poverty of speech pobreza del habla
Powassan encephalitis encefalitis por
    Powassan
power poder
power-coercive strategy estrategia
    poder-coercitiva
power complex complejo de poder
power factor factor de poder
power field campo de poder
power figure figura de poder
power function función de poder
power test prueba de poder
powerless impotente
powerlessness impotencia
practice práctica
practice curve curva de práctica
practice effect efecto de práctica
practice limit límite de práctica
practice material material de práctica
practice period periodo de práctica
practice theory of play teoría de práctica del
    juego
practice trial ensayo de práctica
Prader-Labhart-Willi syndrome síndrome de
    Prader-Labhart-Willi
Prader-Willi syndrome síndrome de
    Prader-Willi
pragmatagnosia pragmatagnosia
pragmatamnesia pragmatamnesia
pragmatic pragmático
pragmatics pragmática
pragmatism pragmatismo
praise elogio
prandial prandial
prandial drinking beber prandial
praxiology praxiología
praxis praxis
praxitherapeutics praxiterapéutica
prazepam prazepam
preadaptive preadaptivo
preadolescence preadolescencia
preambivalence preambivalencia
preataxic preatáxico
precenter precentro
precentral area área precentral
precentral gyrus circunvolución precentral
precipitant precipitante
precipitating precipitante
precipitating cause causa precipitante
precision precisión
precision law ley de precisión
precision of process precisión de proceso
preclinical preclínico

preclinical psychopharmacology
  psicofarmacología preclínica
precocious precoz
precocious aging envejecimiento precoz
precocious development desarrollo precoz
precocious puberty pubertad precoz
precocity precocidad
precoding precodificación
precognition precognición
preconcept preconcepto
preconception preconcepción
preconceptual stage etapa preconceptual
preconditioning precondicionamiento
preconscious preconsciente
preconscious thinking pensamiento
  preconsciente
preconventional preconvencional
preconventional level nivel preconvencional
preconventional level of moral development
  nivel preconvencional del desarrollo moral
preconvulsive preconvulsivo
precuneus precúneo
precursor precursor
precursor load strategy estrategia de carga
  precursora
predation predatismo
predatory predatorio
predatory aggression agresión predatoria
predatory attack ataque predatorio
predatory behavior conducta predatoria
predelay reinforcement refuerzo predemora
predementia predemencia
predementia praecox predemencia precoz
predestination predestinación
predeterminism predeterminismo
predication predicación
predicative thinking pensamiento predicativo
prediction predicción
prediction of behavior predicción de
  conducta
prediction of mortality predicción de
  mortalidad
prediction study estudio de predicción
predictive predictivo
predictive efficiency eficiencia predictiva
predictive index índice predictivo
predictive validity validez predictiva
predictive value valor predictivo
predictor predictor
predictor variable variable predictora
predisaster predesastre
predisaster adaptation adaptación predesastre
predisposition predisposición
predivorce predivorcio
predivorce counseling asesoramiento
  predivorcio
predormital predormital
predormitum predormitum
preeclampsia preeclampsia
preference preferencia
preference behavior conducta de preferencia
preference method método de preferencias
preference test prueba de preferencia
preferential preferencial
preferential perception percepción

preferencial
preferred provider organization
  organización de proveedores preferidos
prefigurative culture cultura prefigurativa
preformism preformismo
prefrontal prefrontal
prefrontal area área prefrontal
prefrontal leukotomy leucotomía prefrontal
prefrontal lobotomy lobotomía prefrontal
preganglionic preganglionar
preganglionic autonomic neuron neurona
  autonómica preganglionar
pregenital pregenital
pregenital factor factor pregenital
pregenital level nivel pregenital
pregenital love amor pregenital
pregenital organization organización
  pregenital
pregenital phase fase pregenital
pregenital stage etapa pregenital
pregnancy embarazo
pregnancy fantasy fantasía de embarazo
pregnancy loss pérdida de embarazo
prehemiplegic prehemipléjico
prehensile prensil
prehension prensión
preictal preictal
prejudice prejuicio
prelinguistic prelingüístico
prelinguistic period periodo prelingüístico
prelogical prelógico
prelogical mind mente prelógica
prelogical thinking pensamiento prelógico
Premack's principle principio de Premack
premaniacal premaníaco
premarital premarital
premarital counseling asesoramiento
  premarital
premature prematuro
premature birth nacimiento prematuro
premature ejaculation eyaculación prematura
premature infant infante prematuro
premature infants and affective development
  infantes prematuros y desarrollo afectivo
prematurity premadurez
premeditation premeditación
premenstrual premenstrual
premenstrual disorder trastorno premenstrual
premenstrual dysphoric disorder trastorno
  disfórico premenstrual
premenstrual-stress syndrome síndrome de
  estrés premenstrual
premenstrual syndrome síndrome
  premenstrual
premenstrual tension tensión premenstrual
premenstrual-tension state estado de tensión
  premenstrual
premenstrual-tension syndrome síndrome de
  tensión premenstrual
premise premisa
premoral stage etapa premoral
premorality premoralidad
premorbid premórbido
premorbid adjustment ajuste premórbido
premorbid personality personalidad

premórbida
premotor premotor
premotor area área premotora
premotor cortex corteza premotora
premotor syndrome síndrome premotor
prenatal prenatal
prenatal care cuidado prenatal
prenatal development desarrollo prenatal
prenatal development and alcohol abuse
     desarrollo prenatal y abuso de alcohol
prenatal development and drug abuse
     desarrollo prenatal y abuso de drogas
prenatal developmental anomaly anomalía
     del desarrollo prenatal
prenatal diagnosis diagnóstico prenatal
prenatal effects of alcohol efectos prenatales
     del alcohol
prenatal history historial prenatal
prenatal influences influencias prenatales
prenatal period periodo prenatal
prenatal sensorineural lesion lesión
     sensorineural prenatal
preoccupation preocupación
preoedipal preedípico
preoedipal factor factor preedípico
preoedipal level nivel preedípico
preoedipal phase fase preedípica
preoedipal stage etapa preedípica
preoperational preoperacional
preoperational phase fase preoperacional
preoperational stage etapa preoperacional
preoperational thinking pensamiento
     preoperacional
preoperational thought pensamiento
     preoperacional
preoperational thought stage etapa de
     pensamiento preoperacional
preoperatory preoperatorio
preoperatory level nivel preoperatorio
preoperatory period periodo preoperatorio
preoperatory stage etapa preoperatoria
preoperatory thought pensamiento
     preoperatorio
preoptic preóptico
preoptic area área preóptica
preorgasmic preorgásmico
preparalytic preparalítico
preparation preparación
preparation for hospitalization preparación
     para hospitalización
preparatory preparatorio
preparatory interval intervalo preparatorio
preparatory response respuesta preparatoria
preparatory set predisposición preparatoria
prepared preparado
prepared childbirth parto preparado
prepartal prepartal
prepartal eclamptic symptom síntoma
     eclámptico prepartal
preperception prepercepción
prephallic prefálico
prephallic masturbation equivalent
     equivalente de masturbación prefálico
prepotent prepotente
prepotent reflex reflejo prepotente

prepotent response respuesta prepotente
prepotent stimulus estímulo prepotente
preprogramming preprogramación
prepsychotic prepsicótico
prepsychotic panic pánico prepsicótico
prepsychotic personality personalidad
     prepsicótica
prepsychotic psychosis psicosis prepsicótica
prepuberal prepuberal
prepuberal stage etapa prepuberal
prepubertal prepubertal
prepuberty prepubertad
prepubescence prepubescencia
prepuce prepucio
prepuce of clitoris prepucio del clítoris
prepuce of penis prepucio del pene
preputium prepucio
preputium clitoridis prepucio del clítoris
preputium penis prepucio del pene
prepyriform area área prepiriforme
prerecognition hypothesis hipótesis de
     prerreconocimiento
presacral presacro
presacral neurectomy neurecotmía presacra
presacral sympathectomy simpatectomía
     presacra
presbyacusis presbiacusis
presbycusis presbicusis
presbyophrenia presbiofrenia
presbyopia presbiopía
preschizophrenic preesquizofrénico
preschizophrenic ego ego preesquizofrénico
preschool preescolar
preschool children niños preescolares
preschool program programa preescolar
presenile presenil
presenile degeneration degeneración presenil
presenile dementia demencia presenil
presenile gangrene gangrena presenil
presenility presenilidad
presenium presenium
presentation presentación
presolution presolución
presolution variability variabilidad
     presolución
prespeech prehabla
prespeech development desarrollo prehabla
prespeech stage etapa prehabla
press factores ambientales apremiantes
press-need pattern patrón de factores
     ambientales apremiantes y necesidades
pressoreceptor presorreceptor
pressoreceptor reflex reflejo presorreceptor
pressure presión
pressure anesthesia anestesia a presión
pressure gradient gradiente de presión
pressure of activity presión de actividad
pressure of ideas presión de ideas
pressure of speech presión del habla
pressure palsy parálisis por presión
pressure paralysis parálisis por presión
pressure point punto de presión
pressure receptor receptor de presión
pressure sensation sensación de presión
pressure sense sentido de presión

pressure-sensitive spot punto sensitivo a presión
pressure sore llaga por presión
pressure spot punto de presión
pressure testicular atrophy atrofia testicular de presión
pressure-threshold test prueba de umbral de presión
pressure-volume index índice de presión-volumen
pressured speech habla apresurada
prestige prestigio
prestige motive motivo de prestigio
prestige suggestion sugestión de prestigio
prestriate area área preestriada
presuperego presuperego
presuperego phase fase presuperego
presupposition presuposición
presynaptic presináptico
presynaptic inhibition inhibición presináptica
pretend fingir
pretest prepueba
pretraumatic pretraumático
pretraumatic personality personalidad pretraumática
prevalence prevalencia
prevalence of behavior problems prevalencia de problemas de conducta
prevalence of eating disorders prevalencia de trastornos del comer
prevention prevención
prevention of anxiety prevención de ansiedad
prevention of child abuse prevención de abuso de niños
prevention of child sexual abuse prevención de abuso sexual de niños
prevention of eating disorders prevención de trastornos del comer
preventive preventivo
preventive intervention intervención preventiva
preventive medicine medicina preventiva
preventive psychiatry psiquiatría preventiva
preventive therapy terapia preventiva
preverbal preverbal
preverbal construct constructo preverbal
prevocational prevocacional
prevocational training entrenamiento prevocacional
priapism priapismo
pride orgullo
prima facie prima facie
primacy primacía
primacy effect efecto de primacía
primal primal
primal anxiety ansiedad primal
primal depression depresión primal
primal fantasy fantasía primal
primal ictal automatism automatismo ictal primal
primal pain dolor primal
primal repression represión primal
primal scene escena primal
primal scream grito primal
primal therapy terapia primal

primal trauma trauma primal
primary primario
primary abilities habilidades primarias
primary aging envejecimiento primario
primary amebic meningoencephalitis meningoencefalitis amebiana primaria
primary amenorrhea amenorrea primaria
primary amentia amencia primaria
primary amyloidosis amiloidosis primario
primary anxiety ansiedad primaria
primary area área primaria
primary attention atención primaria
primary autonomous function función autónoma primaria
primary behavior disorder trastorno de conducta primario
primary care physician médico de cuidado primario
primary caretaker custodio primario
primary cause causa primaria
primary circular reaction reacción circular primaria
primary cognition cognición primaria
primary color color primario
primary cortex corteza primaria
primary cortical zone zona cortical primaria
primary data datos primarios
primary degenerative dementia demencia degenerativa primaria
primary degenerative dementia of Alzheimer type demencia degenerativa primaria de tipo Alzheimer
primary dementia demencia primaria
primary diagnosis diagnóstico primario
primary drive impulso primario
primary dysmenorrhea dismenorrea primaria
primary empathy empatía primaria
primary environment ambiente primario
primary erectile dysfunction disfunción eréctil primaria
primary factor factor primario
primary familial xanthomatosis xantomatosis familiar primario
primary gain ganancia primaria
primary generalized epilepsy epilepsia generalizada primaria
primary group grupo primario
primary health care cuidado de salud primario
primary hue matiz primario
primary hydrocephalus hidrocefalia primaria
primary hypersomnia hipersomnia primaria
primary hypersomnia disorder trastorno de hipersomnia primaria
primary ictal automatism automatismo ictal primario
primary identification identificación primaria
primary impotence impotencia primaria
primary insomnia insomnio primario
primary integration integración primaria
primary masochism masoquismo primario
primary memory memoria primaria
primary mental abilities habilidades mentales primarias
primary mental deficiency deficiencia mental

primaria
primary mental image imagen mental
primaria
primary microcephaly microcefalia primaria
primary microorchidism microorquidismo
primario
primary motivation motivación primaria
primary narcissism narcisismo primario
primary narcissistic identification
identificación narcisista primaria
primary need necesidad primaria
primary neurasthenia neurastenia primaria
primary neuronal degeneration degeneración
neuronal primaria
primary object objeto primario
primary object-love amor de objeto primario
primary orgasmic dysfunction disfunción
orgásmica primaria
primary parkinsonism parkinsonismo
primario
primary personality personalidad primaria
primary physician médico primario
primary prevention prevención primaria
primary prevention of psychopathology
prevención primaria de psicopatología
primary process proceso primario
primary progressive cerebellar degeneration
degeneración cerebelosa progresiva
primaria
primary psychic process proceso psíquico
primario
primary quality cualidad primaria
primary reaction reacción primaria
primary reinforcement refuerzo primario
primary reinforcer reforzador primario
primary repression represión primaria
primary retarded ejaculation eyaculación
retardada primaria
primary reward conditioning
condicionamiento de recompensa primaria
primary senile dementia demencia senil
primaria
primary sensation sensación primaria
primary sex characteristics características
sexuales primarias
primary sexual characteristics características
sexuales primarias
primary shock choque primario
primary signal system sistema de primera
señal
primary signaling system sistema de primera
señal
primary social unit unidad social primaria
primary sociopath sociópata primario
primary stuttering tartamudez primaria
primary symptoms síntomas primarios
primary task tarea primaria
primary territory territorio primario
primary thinking pensamiento primario
primary thought disorder trastorno de
pensamiento primario
primary tumor tumor primario
primary zone zona primaria
primate primate
primate behavior conducta de primates

primate studies estudios de primates
prime of life flor de la vida
primidone primidona
priming preparación
primipara primípara
primitivation primitivación
primitive primitivo
primitive idealization idealización primitiva
primitive mentality mentalidad primitiva
primitive narcissism narcisismo primitivo
primitive superego superego primitivo
primitive thinking pensamiento primitivo
primitivization primitivización
primordial primordial
primordial image imagen primordial
primordial impulse impulso primordial
primordial nanosmia nanosmia primordial
primordial panic pánico primordial
principal principal
principal-component method método de
componente principal
principal diagnosis diagnóstico principal
principal factors factores principales
principle principio
principle learning aprendizaje de principios
principle of anticipatory maturation
principio de maduración anticipatoria
principle of belongingness principio de
pertenencia
principle of constancy principio de constancia
principle of economy principio de economía
principle of equipotentiality principio de
equipotencialidad
principle of inertia principio de inercia
principle of maximum contrast principio de
contraste máximo
principle of optimal stimulation principio de
estimulación óptima
principle of Pragnanz principio de Pragnanz
principle of primacy principio de primacía
principle of recency principio de lo más
reciente
principle of the irresistible impulse principio
del impulso irresistible
prior-entry law ley de entrada previa
prior history historial previo
prism prisma
prison prisión
prison neurosis neurosis de prisión
prison psychologist psicólogo de prisión
prison psychosis psicosis de prisión
prisoner's dilemma dilema del prisionero
privacy privacidad
private privado
private acceptance aceptación privada
private mental hospital hospital mental
privado
private opinion opinión privada
privation privación
privilege privilegio
privileged communication comunicación
privilegiada
proactive proactivo
proactive inhibition inhibición proactiva
proactive interference interferencia proactiva

probabilism probabilismo
probabilistic probabilístico
probabilistic functionalism funcionalismo
    probabilístico
probability probabilidad
probability curve curva de probabilidades
probability density densidad de
    probabilidades
probability distribution distribución de
    probabilidades
probability function función de
    probabilidades
probability learning aprendizaje de
    probabilidades
probability matching pareo de probabilidades
probability of response probabilidad de
    respuesta
probability ratio razón de probabilidades
probability sampling muestreo de
    probabilidades
probability space espacio de probabilidades
probability table tabla de probabilidades
probability theory teoría de probabilidades
probable probable
probable error error probable
proband probando
probarbital probarbital
probe sonda, investigación
probenecid probenecid
probing exploración
problem problema
problem behavior conducta problema
problem box caja problema
problem checklist lista de comprobación de
    problemas
problem child niño problema
problem drinker bebedor problema
problem drinking beber problema
problem-oriented record registro orientado a
    problemas
problem related to abuse problema
    relacionado con abuso
problem related to neglect problema
    relacionado con negligencia
problem solving resolución de problemas
problem-solving behavior conducta de
    resolución de problemas
problem-solving interview entrevista de
    resolución de problemas
problematic problemático
problems with hearing problemas con la
    audición
procaine procaína
procedure procedimiento
procedure for establishing competency
    procedimiento para establecer competencia
process proceso
process analysis análisis de proceso
process attitude actitud de proceso
process evaluation evaluación de proceso
process observer observador de proceso
process psychosis psicosis de proceso
process research investigación de proceso
process schizophrenia esquizofrenia de
    proceso

processing procesamiento
processing error error de procesamiento
processor procesador
prochlorperazine proclorperazina
procrastination procrastinación
proctalgia proctalgia
proctalgia fugax proctalgia fugaz
proctoparalysis proctoparálisis
proctophobia proctofobia
proctoplegia proctoplejía
proctospasm proctoespasmo
procursive procursivo
procursive chorea corea procursiva
procursive epilepsy epilepsia procursiva
procyclidine prociclidina
prodigy prodigio
prodromal prodromal
prodromal myopia miopía prodromal
prodromal symptom síntoma prodromal
prodrome pródromo
prodromic prodrómico
prodromic dream sueño prodrómico
prodromic phase fase prodrómica
product producto
product appeal atractivo de producto
product image imagen de producto
product scale escala de productos
production producción
production method método de producción
productive productivo
productive love amor productivo
productive memory memoria productiva
productive orientation orientación productiva
productive personality personalidad
    productiva
productive symptom síntoma productivo
productive thinking pensamiento productivo
productiveness productividad
productiveness in language productividad en
    lenguaje
productivity productividad
proestrus proestro
profession profesión
professional profesional
professional aptitude test prueba de aptitud
    profesional
professional code código profesional
professional consultation consultación
    profesional
professional ethics ética profesional
professional manager administrador
    profesional
professional neurasthenia neurastenia
    profesional
professional neurosis neurosis profesional
professional spasm espasmo profesional
profile perfil
profile analysis análisis de perfil
profile chart esquema de perfil
profile-matching system sistema de pareo de
    perfiles
profound mental retardation retardo mental
    profundo
progeria progeria
progesterone progesterona

progestin progestina
progestogen progestógeno
prognosis pronóstico
prognostic pronosticador
prognostic test prueba pronosticadora
program programa
program evaluation evaluación de programa
program impact impacto de programa
program-impact evaluation evaluación de
impacto de programa
programmed programado
programmed instruction instrucción
programada
programmed learning aprendizaje
programado
programmed practice práctica programada
programmed text texto programado
programming programación
progression progresión
progression law ley de progresión
progressive progresivo
progressive bulbar palsy parálisis bulbar
progresiva
progressive bulbar paralysis parálisis bulbar
progresiva
progressive cerebral poliodystrophy
poliodistrofia cerebral progresiva
progressive cerebral tremor temblor cerebral
progresivo
progressive degenerative subcortical
encephalopathy encefalopatía subcortical
degenerativa progresiva
progressive diaphyseal dysplasia displasia
diafisaria progresiva
progressive education educación progresiva
progressive infantile cerebral poliodystrophy
poliodistrofia cerebral infantil progresiva
progressive lingual hemiatrophy hemiatrofia
lingual progresiva
progressive lipodystrophy lipodistrofia
progresiva
progressive multifocal leukoencephalopathy
leucoencefalopatía multifocal progresiva
progressive muscular atrophy atrofia
muscular progresiva
progressive muscular dystrophy distrofia
muscular progresiva
progressive myopia miopía progresiva
progressive relaxation relajación progresiva
progressive-relaxation therapy terapia de
relajación progresiva
progressive spinal amyotrophy amiotrofia
espinal progresiva
progressive spinal-muscular atrophy atrofia
espinomuscular progresiva
progressive subcortical encephalopathy
encefalopatía subcortical progresiva
progressive supranuclear palsy parálisis
supranuclear progresiva
progressive teleological regression regresión
teleológica progresiva
progressive teleological-regression hypothesis
hipótesis de regresión teleológica
progresiva
progressive torsion spasm espasmo de torsión

progresivo
progressive total total progresivo
prohibited prohibido
prohibited behavior conducta prohibida
prohormone prohormona
project proyecto
project method método de proyecto
projected jealousy celos proyectados
projection proyección
projection area área de proyección
projection fiber fibra de proyección
projection therapy terapia de proyección
projective proyectivo
projective device aparato proyectivo
projective doll play juego con muñecas
proyectivo
projective identification identificación
proyectiva
projective method método proyectivo
projective personality assessment evaluación
de personalidad proyectiva
projective play juego proyectivo
projective psychotherapy psicoterapia
proyectiva
projective technique técnica proyectiva
projective test prueba proyectiva
prolactin prolactina
prolactin-producing adenoma adenoma
productor de prolactina
prolactinoma prolactinoma
prolapse prolapso
proliferation proliferación
proliferative proliferativo
proliferative phase fase proliferativa
prolonged-sleep therapy terapia de sueño
prolongado
prolonged-sleep treatment tratamiento de
sueño prolongado
promazine promazina
promethazine prometazina
promiscuity promiscuidad
promiscuous promiscuo
promotion neurosis neurosis de promoción
prompt apunte
pronation pronación
pronator reflex reflejo pronador
prone prono
pronoun reversal inversión de pronombres
proof prueba
proofreader's illusion ilusión de corrector
propaedeutic propedéutico
propaedeutic task tarea propedéutica
propaganda propaganda
propaganda analysis análisis de propaganda
propagation propagación
propanolol propranolol
propensity propensión
prophase profase
prophetic profético
prophetic dream sueño profético
prophylactic profiláctico
prophylactic maintenance mantenimiento
profiláctico
prophylaxis profilaxis
propinquity propincuidad

propiomazine propiomazina
proportion proporción
proposition proposición
propositus propositus
propoxyphene propoxifeno
propoxyphene dependence dependencia de
  propoxifeno
propranolol propranolol
proprietary drug droga propietaria
proprioception propiocepción
proprioceptive propioceptivo
proprioceptive reflex reflejo propioceptivo
proprioceptive sensibility sensibilidad
  propioceptiva
proprioceptor propioceptor
propulsion propulsión
propulsion gait marcha de propulsión
prosencephalon prosencéfalo
prosocial prosocial
prosocial aggression agresión prosocial
prosocial behavior conducta prosocial
prosodic prosódico
prosodic features características prosódicas
prosody prosodia
prosopagnosia prosopagnosia
prosopalgia prosopalgia
prosopalgic prosopálgico
prosoplegia prosoplejía
prosopodiplegia prosopodiplejía
prosoponeuralgia prosoponeuralgia
prosopoplegia prosoplejía
prosopoplegic prosopopléjico
prosopospasm prosopoespasmo
prospective prospectivo
prospective research investigación
  prospectiva
prospective study estudio prospectivo
prospermia proespermia
prostaglandin prostaglandina
prostate gland glándula prostática
prostatectomy prostatectomía
prosternation prosternación
prosthesis prótesis
prosthetist prosteta
prostitution prostitución
prostration postración
protanomaly protanomalía
protanopia protanopía
protease proteasa
protection protección
protection factor factor de protección
protective laryngeal reflex reflejo laríngeo
  protector
protein proteína
protein deficiency deficiencia de proteína
protein synthesis síntesis de proteína
protein-synthesis inhibitors inhibidores de
  síntesis de proteína
protension protensión
protensity protensidad
protest protesta
protest psychosis psicosis de protesta
prothetic protético
prothipendyl protipendilo
prothrombin protrombina

prothrombin time tiempo de protrombina
prothymia protimia
protocol protocolo
protomasochism protomasoquismo
protopathic protopático
protopathic sensibility sensibilidad
  protopática
protopathic system sistema protopático
protophallic protofálico
protophallic phase fase protofálica
protoplasm protoplasma
protoplasmic protoplásmico
protoplasmic astrocyte astrocito
  protoplásmico
protoplasmic astrocytoma astrocitoma
  protoplásmico
protospasm protoespasmo
prototaxic prototáxico
prototaxic mode modo prototáxico
prototaxis prototaxis
prototheory prototeoría
prototype prototipo
protracted withdrawal syndrome síndrome
  de retiro prolongado
protriptyline protriptilina
protruded disk disco protruido
proverbs test prueba de proverbios
provisional provisional
provisional diagnosis diagnóstico provisional
provisional try intento provisional
proxemics proxémica
proxibarbal proxibarbal
proximal proximal
proximal receptor receptor proximal
proximal response respuesta proximal
proximal stimulus estímulo proximal
proximity proximidad
proximity principle principio de proximidad
proximoataxia proximoataxia
proximodistal proximodistal
proximodistal development desarrollo
  proximodistal
prudery gazmoñería
pruritus prurito
psammocarcinoma psamocarcinoma
psammoma psamoma
psammoma body cuerpo de psamoma
psammomatous psamomatoso
psammomatous meningioma meningioma
  psamomatoso
psammous psamoso
pselaphesia pselafesia
pselaphesis pselafesia
psellism pselismo
pseudagraphia seudoagrafia
pseudaphia seudoafia
pseudesthesia seudoestesia
pseudo-Graefe sign signo seudo-Graefe
pseudoaffective seudoafectivo
pseudoaffective behavior conducta
  seudoafectiva
pseudoaggression seudoagresión
pseudoagrammatism seudoagramatismo
pseudoagraphia seudoagrafia
pseudoamnesia seudoamnesia

pseudoangina seudoangina
pseudoanhedonia seudoanhedonia
pseudoapoplexy seudoapoplejía
pseudoapraxia seudoapraxia
pseudoataxia seudoataxia
pseudoathetosis seudoatetosis
pseudoauthenticity seudoautenticidad
pseudoblepsia seudoblepsia
pseudoblepsis seudoblepsis
pseudobulbar seudobulbar
pseudobulbar paralysis parálisis seudobulbar
pseudocatatonia seudocatatonía
pseudocephalocele seudocefalocele
pseudocholinesterase seudocolinesterasa
pseudochondroplasia seudocondroplasia
pseudochorea seudocorea
pseudochromesthesia seudocromestesia
pseudochromesthesis seudocromestesia
pseudoclonus seudoclono
pseudocollusion seudocolusión
pseudocoma seudocoma
pseudocommunication seudocomunicación
pseudocommunity seudocomunidad
pseudoconditioning seudocondicionamiento
pseudoconversation seudoconversación
pseudoconvulsion seudoconvulsión
pseudocopulation seudocopulación
pseudocyesis seudociesis
pseudodementia seudodemencia
pseudoepilepsy seudoepilepsia
pseudoesthesia seudoestesia
pseudofamily seudofamilia
pseudofeedback seudorretroalimentación
pseudoflexibilitas seudoflexibilitas
pseudoganglion seudoganglio
pseudogeusesthesia seudogeusestesia
pseudogeusia seudogeusia
pseudographia seudografia
pseudohallucination seudoalucinación
pseudohermaphrodism seudohermafrodismo
pseudohermaphrodite seudohermafrodita
pseudohomosexual seudohomosexual
pseudohomosexuality seudohomosexualidad
pseudohydrocephalus seudohidrocefalia
pseudohydrocephaly seudohidrocefalia
pseudohydrophobia seudohidrofobia
pseudohypersexuality seudohipersexualidad
pseudohypertrophic seudohipertrófico
pseudohypertrophic muscular atrophy
　　atrofia muscular seudohipertrófica
pseudohypertrophic muscular dystrophy
　　distrofia muscular seudohipertrófica
pseudohypertrophic muscular paralysis
　　parálisis muscular seudohipertrófica
pseudohypnosis seudohipnosis
pseudohypoparathyroidsm
　　seudohipoparatiroidismo
pseudoidentification seudoidentificación
pseudoindependent seudoindependiente
pseudoindependent personality personalidad
　　seudoindependiente
pseudoinsomnia seudoinsomnio
pseudoisochromatic seudoisocromático
pseudoisochromatic chart esquema
　　seudoisocromático

pseudolalia seudolalia
pseudologia seudología
pseudologia fantastica seudología fantástica
pseudologia phantastica seudología fantástica
pseudomalignancy seudomalignidad
pseudomania seudomanía
pseudomasturbation seudomasturbación
pseudomature seudomaduro
pseudomature syndrome síndrome
　　seudomaduro
pseudomemory seudomemoria
pseudomeningitis seudomeningitis
pseudomnesia seudomnesia
pseudomotivation seudomotivación
pseudomuscular seudomuscular
pseudomuscular hypertrophy hipertrofia
　　seudomuscular
pseudomutuality seudomutualidad
pseudonarcotism seudonarcotismo
pseudonecrophilia seudonecrofilia
pseudoneoplasm seudoneoplasma
pseudoneurogenic seudoneurogénico
pseudoneurogenic bladder vejiga
　　seudoneurogénica
pseudoneuroma seudoneuroma
pseudoneurotic seudoneurótico
pseudoneurotic schizophrenia esquizofrenia
　　seudoneurótica
pseudonomania seudonomanía
pseudoparalysis seudoparálisis
pseudoparameter seudoparámetro
pseudoparanoia seudoparanoia
pseudoparaplegia seudoparaplejía
pseudoparesis seudoparesia
pseudoparkinsonism seudoparkinsonismo
pseudoperitonitis seudoperitonitis
pseudopersonality seudopersonalidad
pseudophone seudófono
pseudophotesthesia seudofotestesia
pseudoplegia seudoplejía
pseudoprecocious seudoprecoz
pseudoprecocious puberty pubertad
　　seudoprecoz
pseudoprodigy seudoprodigio
pseudopsia seudopsia
pseudopsychology seudopsicología
pseudopsychopathic seudopsicopático
pseudopsychopathic schizophrenia
　　esquizofrenia seudopsicopática
pseudopsychosis seudopsicosis
pseudoretardation seudorretardo
pseudorosette seudorroseta
pseudoschizophrenia seudoesquizofrenia
pseudoschizophrenic seudoesquizofrénico
pseudoschizophrenic neurosis neurosis
　　seudoesquizofrénica
pseudoscience seudociencia
pseudosclerosis seudoesclerosis
pseudoscope seudoscopio
pseudoseizure seudoacceso
pseudosenility seudosenilidad
pseudosexuality seudosexualidad
pseudosmia seudosmia
pseudotabes seudotabes
pseudotransference seudotransferencia

pseudotumor seudotumor
pseudotumor cerebri seudotumor cerebral
pseudoventricle seudoventrículo
psi psi
psi phenomenon fenómeno psi
psi process proceso psi
psilocin psilocina
psilocybin psilocibina
psittacism psitacismo
psopholalia psofolalia
psoriasis psoriasis
psychagogy psicagogía
psychalgalia psicalgalia
psychalgia psicalgia
psychalia psicalia
psychanopsia psicanopsia
psychasthenia psicastenia
psychataxia psicataxia
psychauditory psicauditivo
psyche psiquis
psychedelic psicodélico
psychedelic drug droga psicodélica
psychedelic experience experiencia
    psicodélica
psychedelic therapy terapia psicodélica
psychehormic psiquehórmico
psycheism psiqueismo
psychelytic psiquelítico
psychentonia psiquentonía
psychephoric psiquefórico
psycheplastic psiqueplástico
psychiatric psiquiátrico
psychiatric aide ayudante psiquiátrico
psychiatric anaphylaxis anafilaxis psiquiátrica
psychiatric case register registro de casos
    psiquiátricos
psychiatric classification clasificación
    psiquiátrica
psychiatric clinic clínica psiquiátrica
psychiatric consultation consultación
    psiquiátrica
psychiatric diagnosis diagnóstico psiquiátrico
psychiatric disability discapacidad
    psiquiátrica
psychiatric disorder trastorno psiquiátrico
psychiatric emergency emergencia
    psiquiátrica
psychiatric epidemic epidemia psiquiátrica
psychiatric epidemiology epidemiología
    psiquiátrica
psychiatric examination examinación
    psiquiátrica
psychiatric history historial psiquiátrico
psychiatric hospital hospital psiquiátrico
psychiatric illness enfermedad psiquiátrica
psychiatric interview entrevista psiquiátrica
psychiatric-medical history historial
    psiquiátrico-médico
psychiatric nosology nosología psiquiátrica
psychiatric rehabilitation rehabilitación
    psiquiátrica
psychiatric screening cribado psiquiátrico
psychiatric services servicios psiquiátricos
psychiatric social treatment tratamiento
    social psiquiátrico

psychiatric social work trabajo social
    psiquiátrico
psychiatric social worker trabajador social
    psiquiátrico
psychiatric team equipo psiquiátrico
psychiatric trend tendencia psiquiátrica
psychiatric unit unidad psiquiátrica
psychiatrics psiquiatría
psychiatrism psiquiatrismo
psychiatrist psiquiatra
psychiatry psiquiatría
psychic psíquico
psychic anaphylaxis anafilaxis psíquica
psychic apparatus aparato psíquico
psychic ataxia ataxia psíquica
psychic blindness ceguera psíquica
psychic contagion contagio psíquico
psychic determinism determinismo psíquico
psychic divorce divorcio psíquico
psychic energizer energizador psíquico
psychic energy energía psíquica
psychic equivalent equivalente psíquico
psychic force fuerza psíquica
psychic helplessness impotencia psíquica
psychic impotence impotencia psíquica
psychic inertia inercia psíquica
psychic isolation aislamiento psíquico
psychic masochism masoquismo psíquico
psychic masturbation masturbación psíquica
psychic mobility movilidad psíquica
psychic norm norma psíquica
psychic pain dolor psíquico
psychic paralysis parálisis psíquica
psychic reality realidad psíquica
psychic reflex arc arco reflejo psíquico
psychic research investigación psíquica
psychic scar cicatriz psíquica
psychic secretion secreción psíquica
psychic seizure acceso psíquico
psychic suicide suicidio psíquico
psychic tension tensión psíquica
psychic tic tic psíquico
psychic tone tono psíquico
psychic trauma trauma psíquico
psychic vaginismus vaginismo psíquico
psychical psíquico
psychicism psiquicismo
psychinosis psiquinosis
psychism psiquismo
psychoacoustic psicoacústico
psychoacoustic test prueba psicoacústica
psychoacoustics psicoacústica
psychoactive psicoactivo
psychoactive drug droga psicoactiva
psychoactive drug abuse abuso de droga
    psicoactiva
psychoactive substance sustancia psicoactiva
psychoactive substance abuse abuso de
    sustancia psicoactiva
psychoactive substance amnestic disorder
    trastorno amnésico de sustancia psicoactiva
psychoactive substance anxiety disorder
    trastorno de ansiedad de sustancia
    psicoactiva
psychoactive substance delirium delirio por

sustancia psicoactiva
psychoactive substance delusional disorder
trastorno delusorio por sustancia
psicoactiva
psychoactive substance dementia　demencia
por sustancia psicoactiva
psychoactive substance dependence
dependencia de sustancia psicoactiva
psychoactive substance hallucinosis
alucinosis de sustancia psicoactiva
**psychoactive substance-induced organic
mental disorder**　trastorno mental orgánico
inducido por sustancia psicoactiva
psychoactive substance intoxication
intoxicación por sustancia psicoactiva
psychoactive substance mood disorder
trastorno del humor por sustancia
psicoactiva
**psychoactive substance organic mental
disorder**　trastorno mental orgánico por
sustancia psicoactiva
psychoactive substance personality disorder
trastorno de personalidad por sustancia
psicoactiva
psychoactive substance use disorder
trastorno de uso de sustancia psicoactiva
psychoactive substance withdrawal　retiro de
sustancia psicoactiva
psychoallergy　psicoalergia
psychoanaleptic　psicoanaléptico
psychoanaleptica　psicoanaléptica
psychoanalysis　psicoanálisis
psychoanalyst　psicoanalista
psychoanalytic　psicoanalítico
psychoanalytic anthropology　antropología
psicoanalítica
psychoanalytic development psychology
psicología del desarrollo psicoanalítico
psychoanalytic group psychotherapy
psicoterapia de grupo psicoanalítica
psychoanalytic psychiatry　psiquiatría
psicoanalítica
psychoanalytic psychotherapy　psicoterapia
psicoanalítica
psychoanalytic setting　ambiente psicoanalítico
psychoanalytic situation　situación
psicoanalítica
psychoanalytic stage　etapa psicoanalítica
psychoanalytic theory　teoría psicoanalítica
psychoanalytic theory of attachment　teoría
psicoanalítica del apego
psychoanalytic therapy　terapia psicoanalítica
psychoanalytic treatment　tratamiento
psicoanalítico
psychoasthenia　psicoastenia
psychoasthenics　psicoasténica
psychoataxia　psicoataxia
psychoauditory　psicoauditivo
psychobioanalysis　psicobioanálisis
psychobiogram　psicobiograma
psychobiological　piscobiológico
psychobiological factor　factor piscobiológico
psychobiology　psicobiología
psychocardiac　psicocardíaco
psychocardiac reflex　reflejo psicocardíaco

psychocatharsis　psicocatarsis
psychochemistry　psicoquímica
psychochemistry intelligence　inteligencia
psicoquímica
psychochrome　psicocromo
psychochromesthesia　psicocromestesia
psychocortical　psicocortical
psychocultural　psicocultural
psychocultural stress　estrés psicocultural
psychodiagnosis　psicodiagnóstico
psychodiagnostics　psicodiagnóstica
psychodietetics　psicodietética
psychodometer　psicodómetro
psychodometry　psicodometría
psychodrama　psicodrama
psychodrama form　forma de psicodrama
psychodrama group therapy　terapia de grupo
de psicodrama
psychodramatic shock　choque psicodramático
psychodynamic　psicodinámico
psychodynamic cerebral system　sistema
cerebral psicodinámico
psychodynamic psychotherapy　psicoterapia
psicodinámica
psychodynamic theory　teoría psicodinámica
psychodynamics　psicodinámica
psychoeducation　psicoeducación
psychoeducational　psicoeducativo
psychoeducational diagnostician
diagnosticador psicoeducativo
psychoeducational model　modelo
psicoeducativo
psychoeducational problem　problema
psicoeducativo
psychoeducational program　programa
psicoeducativo
psychoendocrinology　psicoendocrinología
psychoexploration　psicoexploración
psychogalvanic　psicogalvánico
psychogalvanic reaction　reacción
psicogalvánica
psychogalvanic reflex　reflejo psicogalvánico
psychogalvanic response　respuesta
psicogalvánica
psychogalvanic skin reaction　reacción de piel
psicogalvánica
psychogalvanic skin reflex　reflejo de piel
psicogalvánico
psychogalvanic skin response　respuesta de
piel psicogalvánica
psychogalvanometer　psicogalvanómetro
psychogender　psicogénero
psychogenesis　psicogénesis
psychogenetic　psicogenético
psychogenetics　psicogenética
psychogenic　psicogénico
psychogenic amnesia　amnesia psicogénica
psychogenic aspermia　aspermia psicogénica
psychogenic constipation　constipación
psicogénica
psychogenic deafness　sordera psicogénica
psychogenic disorder　trastorno psicogénico
psychogenic drug　droga psicogénica
psychogenic fugue　fuga psicogénica
psychogenic hallucination　alucinación

psicogénica
psychogenic hypersomnia hipersomnia
  psicogénica
psychogenic megacolon megacolon
  psicogénico
psychogenic motive motivo psicogénico
psychogenic mutism mutismo psicogénico
psychogenic need necesidad psicogénica
psychogenic nocturnal polydipsia polidipsia
  nocturna psicogénica
psychogenic nocturnal polydipsia syndrome
  síndrome de polidipsia nocturna
  psicogénica
psychogenic pain dolor psicogénico
psychogenic pain disorder trastorno de dolor
  psicogénico
psychogenic polydipsia polidipsia psicogénica
psychogenic pruritus prurito psicogénico
psychogenic psychosis psicosis psicogénica
psychogenic stupor estupor psicogénico
psychogenic syndrome síndrome psicogénico
psychogenic torticollis tortícolis psicogénico
psychogenic vomiting vómitos psicogénicos
psychogeny psicogenia
psychogeriatrics psicogeriatría
psychogerontology psicogerontología
psychogeusic psicogéusico
psychognosia psicognosia
psychogogic psicogógico
psychogonical psicogónico
psychogony psicogonia
psychogram psicograma
psychograph psicógrafo
psychographic psicográfico
psychographic disturbance disturbio
  psicográfico
psychographics psicográfica
psychography psicografía
psychohistory psicohistoria
psychoimmunology psicoinmunología
psychoinfantilism psicoinfantilismo
psychokinesia psicocinesia
psychokinesis psicocinesia
psychokym psicoquimo
psycholagny psicolagnia
psycholegal psicolegal
psycholepsis psicolepsis
psycholepsy psicolepsia
psycholeptica psicoléptica
psycholinguistic psicolingüístico
psycholinguistic abilities habilidades
  psicolingüísticas
psycholinguistics psicolingüística
psychologic psicológico
psychologic abuse abuso psicológico
psychological psicológico
psychological abuse abuso psicológico
psychological anaphylaxis anafilaxis
  psicológica
psychological aphrodisiac afrodisiaco
  psicológico
psychological autopsy autopsia psicológica
psychological capacity capacidad psicológica
psychological contract contrato psicológico
psychological counseling asesoramiento

psicológico
psychological defense system sistema de
  defensa psicológico
psychological deficit déficit psicológico
psychological dependence dependencia
  psicológica
psychological distance distancia psicológica
psychological effects efectos psicológicos
psychological effects of exercise efectos
  psicológicos del ejercicio
psychological effects of hospitalization
  efectos psicológicos de hospitalización
psychological environment ambiente
  psicológico
psychological esthetics estética psicológica
psychological examination examinación
  psicológica
**psychological factor affecting medical
  condition** factor psicológico afectando una
  condición médica
**psychological factor affecting physical
  condition** factor psicológico afectando una
  condición física
psychological factors factores psicológicos
psychological field campo psicológico
psychological freedom libertad psicológica
psychological game juego psicológico
psychological geography geografía
  psicológica
psychological health salud psicológica
psychological invalidism invalidismo
  psicológico
psychological laboratory laboratorio
  psicológico
psychological linguistics lingüística
  psicológica
psychological maltreatment maltrato
  psicológico
psychological me yo psicológico
psychological measure medida psicológica
psychological moment momento psicológico
psychological motive motivo psicológico
psychological need necesidad psicológica
psychological need for dreaming necesidad
  psicológica para soñar
psychological network red psicológica
psychological programming therapy terapia
  de programación psicológica
psychological rapport rapport psicológico
psychological rating scale escala de
  clasificación psicológica
psychological reactance reactancia
  psicológica
psychological refractory period periodo
  refractario psicológico
psychological rehabilitation rehabilitación
  psicológica
psychological scale escala psicológica
psychological science ciencia psicológica
psychological space espacio psicológico
psychological statistics estadística psicológica
psychological stress estrés psicológico
psychological teratogen teratógeno
  psicológico
psychological test prueba psicológica

psychological time tiempo psicológico
psychological tremor temblor psicológico
psychological type tipo psicológico
psychological warfare guerra psicológica
psychological weaning destete psicológico
psychological zero cero psicológico
psychologism psicologismo
psychologist psicólogo
psychologist's fallacy falacia de psicólogo
psychology psicología
psycholytic psicolítico
psycholytic therapy terapia psicolítica
psychometric psicométrico
psychometric examination examinación
　　psicométrica
psychometric function función psicométrica
psychometrician psicometrista
psychometrics psicométrica
psychometrist psicometrista
psychometry psicometría
psychomimetic psicomimético
psychomimic psicomímico
psychomimic syndrome síndrome
　　psicomímico
psychomotility psicomovilidad
psychomotor psicomotor
psychomotor action acción psicomotora
psychomotor agitation agitación psicomotora
psychomotor attack ataque psicomotor
psychomotor disorder trastorno psicomotor
psychomotor epilepsy epilepsia psicomotora
psychomotor excitement excitación
　　psicomotora
psychomotor hallucination alucinación
　　psicomotora
psychomotor retardation retardo psicomotor
psychomotor seizure acceso psicomotor
psychomotor stimulant estimulante
　　psicomotor
psychomotor stimulus estímulo psicomotor
psychomotor test prueba psicomotora
psychomusic psicomúsica
psychoneural psiconeural
psychoneural parallelism paralelismo
　　psiconeural
psychoneuroid psiconeuroide
psychoneuroimmunology
　　psiconeuroinmunología
psychoneurosis psiconeurosis
psychoneurosis maidica psiconeurosis
　　maídica
psychoneurotic psiconeurótico
psychoneurotic depressive reaction reacción
　　depresiva psiconeurótica
psychoneurotic inventory inventario
　　psiconeurótico
psychonomic psiconómico
psychonomics psiconómica
psychonomy psiconomía
psychonosology psiconosología
psychonoxious psiconocivo
psychooncology psicooncología
psychoparesis psicoparesia
psychopath psicópata
psychopathia psicopatía

psychopathic psicopático
psychopathic deviance desviación psicopática
psychopathic deviance scale escala de
　　desviación psicopática
psychopathic personality personalidad
　　psicopática
psychopathist psicopatista
psychopathological psicopatológico
psychopathologist psicopatólogo
psychopathology psicopatología
psychopathology in adolescence
　　psicopatología en adolescencia
psychopathy psicopatía
psychopedagogy psicopedagogía
psychopedics psicopedia
psychopenetration psicopenetración
psychopenetration test prueba de
　　psicopenetración
psychopharmaceutical psicofarmacéutico
psychopharmacological psicofarmacológico
psychopharmacological drug droga
　　psicofarmacológica
psychopharmacology psicofarmacología
psychopharmacotherapy psicofarmacoterapia
psychophobia psicofobia
psychophysical psicofísico
psychophysical dualism dualismo psicofísico
psychophysical function función psicofísica
psychophysical law ley psicofísica
psychophysical methods métodos psicofísicos
psychophysical parallelism paralelismo
　　psicofísico
psychophysical relationship relación
　　psicofísica
psychophysics psicofísica
psychophysiologic psicofisiológico
psychophysiologic cardiovascular reaction
　　reacción cardiovascular psicofisiológica
psychophysiologic disorder trastorno
　　psicofisiológico
psychophysiologic effects of exercise efectos
　　psicofisiológicos del ejercicio
psychophysiologic endocrine reaction
　　reacción endocrina psicofisiológica
psychophysiologic gastrointestinal reaction
　　reacción gastrointestinal psicofisiológica
psychophysiologic genitourinary reaction
　　reacción genitourinaria psicofisiológica
psychophysiologic hemic and lymphatic
　　reaction reacción hémica y linfática
　　psicofisiológica
psychophysiologic manifestation
　　manifestación psicofisiológica
psychophysiologic musculoskeletal reaction
　　reacción musculoesquelética
　　psicofisiológica
psychophysiologic nervous system reaction
　　reacción del sistema nervioso
　　psicofisiológica
psychophysiologic respiratory reaction
　　reacción respiratoria psicofisiológica
psychophysiologic skin reaction reacción de
　　piel psicofisiológica
psychophysiologic special sense reaction
　　reacción de sentido especial psicofisiológica

psychophysiological psicofisiológico
psychophysiology psicofisiología
psychoplegia psicoplejía
psychopneumatology psiconeumatología
psychopolitics psicopolítica
psychoprophylaxis psicoprofilaxis
psychoreaction psicorreacción
psychorelaxation psicorrelajación
psychorhythmia psicorritmia
psychormic psicórmico
psychorrhea psicorrea
psychorrhythmia psicorritmia
psychoscience psicociencia
psychosensorial psicosensorial
psychosensory psicosensorial
psychosensory aphasia afasia psicosensorial
psychosexual psicosexual
psychosexual development desarrollo
psicosexual
psychosexual development in adolescence
desarrollo psicosexual en adolescencia
psychosexual disorder trastorno psicosexual
psychosexual dysfunction disfunción
psicosexual
psychosexual history historial psicosexual
psychosexual moratorium moratoria
psicosexual
psychosexual pain disorder trastorno de
dolor psicosexual
psychosexual stage etapa psicosexual
psychosexual stages of development etapas
psicosexuales del desarrollo
psychosexual therapy terapia psicosexual
psychosexual trauma trauma psicosexual
psychosexuality psicosexualidad
psychosis psicosis
psychosis in sleep deprivation psicosis en
privación de sueño
psychosis of association psicosis de
asociación
psychosis of syphilis psicosis de sífilis
psychosis with cardiorenal disease psicosis
con enfermedad cardiorrenal
psychosis with cerebral arteriosclerosis
psicosis con arterioesclerosis cerebral
psychosis with mental retardation psicosis
con retardo mental
psychosocial psicosocial
psychosocial deprivation privación
psicosocial
psychosocial development desarrollo
psicosocial
psychosocial dwarfism enanismo psicosocial
psychosocial factors factores psicosociales
psychosocial model modelo psicosocial
psychosocial model of development modelo
psicosocial del desarrollo
psychosocial moratorium moratoria
psicosocial
psychosocial retardation retardo psicosocial
psychosocial stage etapa psicosocial
psychosocial stages of development etapas
psicosociales del desarrollo
psychosocial stressor estresante psicosocial
psychosocial system sistema psicosocial

psychosocial theory teoría psicosocial
psychosocial therapy terapia psicosocial
psychosocially psicosocialmente
psychosocially determined short stature
estatura corta determinada psicosocialmente
psychosoma psicosoma
psychosomatic psicosomático
psychosomatic disorder trastorno
psicosomático
psychosomatic disorder and chronic illness
trastorno psicosomático y enfermedad
crónica
psychosomatic medicine medicina
psicosomática
psychosomatic suicide suicidio psicosomático
psychosomimetic psicosomimético
psychostimulant psicoestimulante
psychostimulant drug droga psicoestimulante
psychosurgery psicocirugía
psychosynthesis psicosíntesis
psychotechnician psicotécnico
psychotechnics psicotécnica
psychotechnology psicotecnología
psychotherapeutic psicoterapéutico
psychotherapeutic drug droga
psicoterapéutica
psychotherapeutics psicoterapéutica
psychotherapist psicoterapeuta
psychotherapy psicoterapia
psychotherapy by reciprocal inhibitions
psicoterapia por inhibiciones recíprocas
psychotherapy for children psicoterapia para
niños
psychotherapy technique técnica de
psicoterapia
psychotic psicótico
psychotic character carácter psicótico
psychotic delusion delusión psicótica
psychotic delusions scale escala de delusiones
psicóticas
psychotic depression depresión psicótica
psychotic depression scale escala de
depresión psicótica
psychotic depressive reaction reacción
depresiva psicótica
psychotic disorder trastorno psicótico
**psychotic disorder due to general medical
condition** trastorno psicótico debido a
condición médica general
psychotic episode episodio psicótico
psychotic manifestation manifestación
psicótica
psychotic surrender rendición psicótica
psychotic thinking pensamiento psicótico
psychotic thinking scale escala de
pensamiento psicótico
psychoticism psicoticismo
psychotogen psicotógeno
psychotogenic psicotogénico
psychotomimetic psicotomimético
psychotomimetic drug droga psicotomimética
psychotoxicomania psicotoxicomanía
psychotropic psicotrópico
psychotropic drug droga psicotrópica
psychroalgia psicroalgia

psychroesthesia psicroestesia
psychrophobia psicrofobia
pteronophobia pteronofobia
ptosis ptosis
ptosis sympathetica ptosis simpática
ptyalism ptialismo
puberal puberal
puberism puberismo
pubertal pubertal
pubertal sexual recapitulation recapitulación
   sexual pubertal
pubertal stage etapa pubertal
pubertas praecox pubertad precoz
puberty pubertad
puberty rites ritos de pubertad
puberum dysphonia disfonía de pubertad
pubes pubes
pubescence pubescencia
pubescency pubescencia
pubescent pubescente
pubic púbico
pubic rites ritos púbicos
pubis pubis
public público
public-distance zone zona de distancia pública
public health salud pública
public health model modelo de salud pública
public mental hospital hospital mental
   público
public opinion opinión pública
public-opinion poll encuesta de opinión
   pública
public-service psychology psicología de
   servicio público
public territory territorio público
pudenda pudenda
pudendal pudendo
pudendal nerve nervio pudendo
puerile pueril
puerilism puerilismo
puerperal puerperal
puerperal convulsion convulsión puerperal
puerperal disorder trastorno puerperal
puerperal eclampsia eclampsia puerperal
puerperal osteomalacia osteomalacia
   puerperal
puerperal psychosis psicosis puerperal
puerperium puerperio
Pulfrich phenomenon fenómeno de Pulfrich
pulmonary pulmonar
pulmonary disorder trastorno pulmonar
pulmonic pulmónico
pulmonic stenosis estenosis pulmónica
pulmonocoronary pulmonocoronario
pulmonocoronary reflex reflejo
   pulmonocoronario
pulsating neurasthenia neurastenia pulsátil
pulse pulso
pulvinar pulvinar
pun equívoco
punctate punteado
punctum punto
punctum dolorosum punto doloroso
punctum vasculosum punto vascular
puncture punción

punding acicaladura sin propósito por
   anfetaminas
punishment castigo
punishment and aggression castigo y
   agresión
punishment by reciprocity castigo por
   reciprocidad
punishment dream sueño de castigo
punishment fear temor al castigo
punitive punitivo
pupil pupila
pupil-teacher fit ajuste alumno-maestro
pupillary pupilar
pupillary reflex reflejo pupilar
pupillary-skin reflex reflejo pupilar-cutáneo
pupillomotor pupilomotor
pupilloplegia pupiloplejía
pupillotonia pupilotonía
pupillotonic pupilotónico
pupillotonic pseudotabes seudotabes
   pupilotónica
pure puro
pure absence ausencia pura
pure aphasia afasia pura
pure erotomania erotomanía pura
pure hue matiz puro
pure meaning significado puro
pure microcephaly microcefalia pura
pure obsession obsesión pura
pure phi phenomenon fenómeno phi puro
pure research investigación pura
pure-stimulus act acto de estímulo puro
pure tone tono puro
pure-tone audiometry audiometría de tono
   puro
puritan puritano
puritan complex complejo puritano
Purkinje afterimage imagen persistente de
   Purkinje
Purkinje cells células de Purkinje
Purkinje effect efecto de Purkinje
Purkinje figure figura de Purkinje
Purkinje network red de Purkinje
Purkinje phenomenon fenómeno de Purkinje
Purkinje-Sanson images imágenes de
   Purkinje-Sanson
Purkinje shift cambio de Purkinje
Purmann's method método de Purmann
puromycin puromicina
purple púrpura
purpose propósito
purposeful accident accidente intencionado
purposeless sin propósito
purposeless hyperactivity hiperactividad sin
   propósito
purposive intencionado
purposive accident accidente intencionado
purposive psychology psicología intencionada
pursuit eye movements movimientos de ojos
   de rastreo
pursuit reaction reacción de rastreo
purulent encephalitis encefalitis purulenta
putamen putamen
Putnam-Dana syndrome síndrome de
   Putnam-Dana

putrid pútrido
puzzle box caja rompecabeza
pycnic pícnico
pycnodysostosis picnodisostosis
pycnoepilepsy picnoepilepsia
pycnolepsy picnolepsia
pyelonephritis pielonefritis
pyencephalus piencéfalo
Pygmalion effect efecto de Pigmalión
pygmalionism pigmalionismo
pyknic pícnico
pyknic type tipo pícnico
pyknodysostosis picnodisostosis
pyknoepilepsy picnoepilepsia
pyknolepsy picnolepsia
pyknophrasia picnofrasia
pyloric stenosis estenosis pilórica
pyocephalus piocefalia
pyogenic piógeno
pyogenic pachymeningitis paquimeningitis
  piógena
pyramid pirámide
pyramid sign signo piramidal
pyramidal piramidal
pyramidal cells células piramidales
pyramidal motor system sistema motor
  piramidal
pyramidal system sistema piramidal
pyramidal tract tracto piramidal
pyramidal tractotomy tractotomía piramidal
pyramidotomy piramidotomía
pyrazolone pirazolona
pyrexeophobia pirexeofobia
pyrexiophobia pirexiofobia
pyridostigmine piridostigmina
pyridoxine piridoxina
pyriform area área piriforme
pyriform cortex corteza piriforme
pyriform lobe lóbulo piriforme
pyrogen pirógeno
pyrolagnia pirolagnia
pyromania piromanía
pyromaniac piromaníaco
pyrophobia pirofobia
pyroptothymia piroptotimia
pyrosis pirosis

Q

Q data datos Q
Q method método Q
Q methodology metodología Q
Q sort clasificación Q
Q technique técnica Q
Q test prueba Q
quadrangular therapy terapia cuadrangular
quadrant cuadrante
quadrantanopia cuadrantanopía
quadrantanopsia cuadrantanopsia
quadrantic hemianopsia hemianopsia
  cuadrántica
quadrate lobule lóbulo cuadrado
quadriceps reflex reflejo del cuadríceps
quadrigemina cuadrigémino
quadriparesis cuadriparesia
quadripedal extensor reflex reflejo extensor
  cuadripedal
quadriplegia cuadriplejía
quadriplegic cuadripléjico
qualitative cualitativo
qualitative approach acercamiento cualitativo
qualitative aspects aspectos cualitativos
qualitative judgment juicio cualitativo
quality calidad, cualidad
quality assessment evaluación de calidad
quality assurance evaluación de calidad
quality of life calidad de vida
quality of mood calidad del humor
quality of speech calidad del habla
quanta cuantos
quantal cuantal
quantal hypothesis hipótesis cuantal
quantitative cuantitativo
quantitative approach acercamiento
  cuantitativo
quantitative electrophysiological battery
  batería electrofisiológica cuantitativa
quantitative genetics genética cuantitativa
quantitative judgment juicio cuantitativo
quantitative score puntuación cuantitativa
quantitative semantics semántica cuantitativa
quantitative variable variable cuantitativa
quantity cantidad
quantity of speech cantidad del habla
quantum cuanto
quantum theory teoría cuántica
quartile cuartil
quartile deviation desviación cuartílica
quasi-experimental cuasiexperimental
quasi-experimental design diseño
  cuasiexperimental
quasi-experimental research investigación
  cuasiexperimental

quasi-experimental study estudio
   cuasiexperimental
quasi-group cuasigrupo
quasi-need cuasinecesidad
Quasimodo complex complejo de Cuasimodo
quaternity cuaternidad
quazepam cuazepam
Queckenstedt-Stookey test prueba de
   Queckenstedt-Stookey
querulent quejumbroso
querulous quejumbroso
question pregunta
question stage etapa de preguntas
questionary cuestionario
questionnaire cuestionario
quick rápido
quickening primeros movimientos fetales
   percibidos
Quincke's disease enfermedad de Quincke
Quincke's edema edema de Quincke
Quincke's puncture punción de Quincke
Quincke tubes tubos de Quincke
quota control control de cuotas
quota sampling muestreo por cuotas
quotidian cotidiano
quotidian variability variabilidad cotidiana
quotient cociente

R correlation correlación R
rabbit syndrome síndrome de conejo
rabies rabia
raccoon eye ojo de mapache
race raza
race differences diferencias raciales
race prejudice prejuicio racial
rachicentesis raquicentesis
rachigraph raquígrafo
rachilysis raquílisis
rachiocentesis raquiocentesis
rachiochysis raquioquisis
rachiometer raquiómetro
rachiopathy raquiopatía
rachioplegia raquioplejía
rachioscoliosis raquioescoliosis
rachiotome raquiótomo
rachiotomy raquiotomía
rachischisis raquisquisis
rachischisis partialis raquisquisis parcial
rachischisis posterior raquisquisis posterior
rachischisis totalis raquisquisis total
rachitome raquítomo
rachitomy raquitomía
racialism racismo
racism racismo
radial radial
radial phenomenon fenómeno radial
radial reflex reflejo radial
radiance radiancia
radiant energy energía radiante
radiant flux flujo radiante
radiation radiación
radiation myelopathy mielopatía por
   radiación
radiation sickness enfermedad por radiación
radiation somnolence syndrome síndrome de
   somnolencia por radiación
radiation therapy terapia de radiación
radical radical
radical behaviorism conductismo radical
radical hysterectomy histerectomía radical
radical mastectomy mastectomía radical
radical therapy terapia radical
radicalism radicalismo
radicotomy radicotomía
radiculalgia radiculalgia
radicular radicular
radicular syndrome síndrome radicular
radiculectomy radiculectomía
radiculitis radiculitis
radiculoganglionitis radiculoganglionitis
radiculomeningomyelitis
   radiculomeningomielitis

radiculomyelopathy radiculomielopatía
radiculoneuropathy radiculoneuropatía
radiculopathy radiculopatía
radioactive radiactivo
radioactive isotope isótopo radiactivo
radioactive tracer trazador radiactivo
radioautography radioautografía
radiobicipital radiobicipital
radiobicipital reflex reflejo radiobicipital
radiogram radiograma
radiograph radiografía
radioimmunoassay radioinmunoanálisis
radioisotope radioisótopo
radioisotope cisternography cisternografía
  con radioisótopos
radiologic radiológico
radiologic technologist tecnólogo radiológico
radiometer radiómetro
radiomimetic radiomimético
radiomimetic drug droga radiomimética
radioneuritis radioneuritis
radionuclide radionúclido
radionuclide cisternography cisternografía
  con radionúclidos
radioperiosteal radioperióstico
radioperiosteal reflex reflejo radioperióstico
radiophobia radiofobia
radioreceptor radiorreceptor
radiotherapy radioterapia
radix radix
Raeder's paratrigeminal syndrome síndrome
  paratrigeminal de Raeder
rage rabia
rage reflex reflejo de rabia
railway illusion ilusión de ferrocarril
Raman effect efecto de Raman
Raman shift cambio de Raman
rami communicantes rami communicantes
ramicotomy ramicotomía
ramisection ramisección
ramitis ramitis
Ramsay Hunt's syndrome síndrome de
  Ramsay Hunt
ramus ramus
random aleatorio
random activity actividad aleatoria
random assignment asignación aleatoria
random error error aleatorio
random factor factor aleatorio
random group grupo aleatorio
random mating apareamiento aleatorio
random model modelo aleatorio
random movement movimiento aleatorio
random noise ruido aleatorio
random number número aleatorio
random-number table tabla de números
  aleatorios
random observation observación aleatoria
random sample muestra aleatoria
random variable variable aleatoria
random waves ondas aleatorias
randomization aleatorización
randomization test prueba de aleatorización
randomize aleatorizar
randomized aleatorizado

randomized clinical trial ensayo clínico
  aleatorizado
randomized-group design diseño de grupo
  aleatorizado
range intervalo
range effect efecto de intervalo
range of audibility intervalo de audibilidad
range-of-motion exercises ejercicios de
  intervalo de moción
range restriction restricción de intervalo
rank rango
rank-difference correlation correlación por
  diferencias de rangos
rank order orden de rango
rank-order correlation correlación por orden
  de rangos
ranked distribution distribución de rangos
Rankian therapy terapia de Rankian
Ranschburg effect efecto de Ranschburg
Ranvier's node nódulo de Ranvier
rape violación
rape and violent pornography violación y
  pornografía violenta
rape counseling asesoramiento tras violación
rape fantasy fantasía de violación
rape trauma syndrome síndrome de trauma
  de violación
raphe rafe
rapid-change theory teoría de cambios
  rápidos
rapid eye movement movimientos oculares
  rápidos
rapid eye movement behavior disorder
  trastorno de conducta de movimientos
  oculares rápidos
rapid eye movement density densidad de
  movimientos oculares rápidos
rapid eye movement deprivation privación
  de movimientos oculares rápidos
rapid eye movement deprivation and
  schizophrenia privación de movimientos
  oculares rápidos y esquizofrenia
rapid eye movement latency latencia de
  movimientos oculares rápidos
rapid eye movement sleep sueño de
  movimientos oculares rápidos
rapid eye movement sleep efficiency
  eficiencia de sueño de movimientos
  oculares rápidos
rapid eye movement sleep in infants sueño
  de movimientos oculares rápidos en
  infantes
rapid eye movement sleep in newborns
  sueño de movimientos oculares rápidos en
  recién nacidos
rapid eye movement storm tormenta de
  movimientos oculares rápidos
rapid speech habla rápida
rapport rapport
rapture rapto
rapture-of-the-deep syndrome síndrome de
  rapto de la profundidad
raptus raptus
raptus action acción por rapto
raptus melancholicus raptus melancholicus

rate tasa, ritmo, índice
rate of change tasa de cambio
rate of first admission tasa de primeras admisiones
rate of occurrence tasa de ocurrencia
rate of production of speech velocidad de producción del habla
Rathke's cleft cyst quiste hendido de Rathke
Rathke's cyst quiste de Rathke
Rathke's pouch tumor tumor de bolsa de Rathke
ratification theory teoría de ratificación
rating clasificación
rating scale escala de clasificación
ratio razón
ratio estimation estimación de proporciones
ratio production producción de proporciones
ratio reinforcement refuerzo de proporciones
ratio scale escala de proporciones
rational racional
rational authority autoridad racional
rational-emotive therapy terapia racional-emotiva
rational equation ecuación racional
rational group therapy terapia de grupo racional
rational learning aprendizaje racional
rational-legal authority autoridad racional-legal
rational problem-solving resolución de problemas racional
rational psychology psicología racional
rational psychotherapy psicoterapia racional
rational therapy terapia racional
rational type tipo racional
rational uniformity uniformidad racional
rationale razón fundamental
rationalism racionalismo
rationality racionalidad
rationalization racionalización
rationalize racionalizar
Rauwolfia Rauwolfia
raw data datos en bruto
raw score puntuación en bruto
Rayleigh equation ecuación de Rayleigh
Raymond type of apoplexy apoplejía de tipo Raymond
Raynaud's disease enfermedad de Raynaud
Raynaud's phenomenon fenómeno de Raynaud
reactance reactancia
reactance theory teoría de reactancia
reaction reacción
reaction chain cadena de reacción
reaction formation formación reactiva
reaction of degeneration reacción de degeneración
reaction pattern patrón de reacción
reaction potential potencial de reacción
reaction process proceso de reacción
reaction product producto de reacción
reaction range intervalo de reacción
reaction-specific energy energía específica de reacción
reaction time tiempo de reacción

reaction to disaster reacción a desastre
reaction type tipo de reacción
reactional reaccional
reactional biography biografía reaccional
reactivation reactivación
reactivation of memory reactivación de memoria
reactivation process proceso de reactivación
reactive reactivo
reactive alcoholism alcoholismo reactivo
reactive astrocyte astrocito reactivo
reactive attachment disorder trastorno de apego reactivo
reactive attachment disorder of early childhood trastorno de apego reactivo de niñez temprana
reactive attachment disorder of infancy trastorno de apego reactivo de infancia
reactive cell célula reactiva
reactive confusion confusión reactiva
reactive depression depresión reactiva
reactive disorder trastorno reactivo
reactive ego alteration alteración del ego reactiva
reactive excitation excitación reactiva
reactive inhibition inhibición reactiva
reactive mania manía reactiva
reactive measure medida reactiva
reactive paranoid psychosis psicosis paranoide reactiva
reactive psychosis psicosis reactiva
reactive reinforcement refuerzo reactivo
reactive schizophrenia esquizofrenia reactiva
reactive type tipo reactivo
reactivity reactividad
readiness disposición, preparación
readiness law ley de preparación
readiness test prueba de preparación
reading lectura
reading age edad de lectura
reading comprehension comprensión de lectura
reading disability discapacidad de lectura
reading-disabled incapacitado de lectura
reading disorder trastorno de lectura
reading epilepsy epilepsia de lectura
reading quotient cociente de lectura
reading readiness disposición de lectura
reading retardation retardo de lectura
reading skills destrezas de lectura
reading skills acquisition adquisición de destrezas de lectura
reading span lapso de lectura
reading test prueba de lectura
readmission readmisión
reafference reaferencia
real real
real anxiety ansiedad real
real definition definición real
real loss pérdida real
real love amor real
real motion moción real
real pride orgullo real
real self yo real
real time tiempo real

realism realismo
realism factor factor de realismo
realistic realista
realistic stage etapa realista
realistic thinking pensamiento realista
reality realidad
reality adaptation adaptación a la realidad
reality-adaptive supportive psychotherapy
   psicoterapia de apoyo adaptiva de realidad
reality anxiety ansiedad de realidad
reality assumption asunción de realidad
reality awareness conciencia de realidad
reality confrontation confrontación de
   realidad
reality denial negación de realidad
reality ego ego de realidad
reality group therapy terapia de grupo de
   realidad
reality life of ego vida del ego de realidad
reality orientation orientación de realidad
reality principle principio de realidad
reality system sistema de realidad
reality test prueba de realidad
reality therapy terapia de realidad
reason razón
reasoning razonamiento
reasoning mania manía de razonamiento
reassociation reasociación
reassurance aquietamiento
reattachment readhesión
reattribution technique técnica de
   reatribución
rebellious rebelde
rebelliousness rebeldía
rebirth renacimiento
rebirth fantasy fantasía de renacimiento
rebound eating comer de rebote
rebound effect efecto de rebote
rebound insomnia insomnio de rebote
rebound phenomenon fenómeno de rebote
rebound phenomenon of Gordon Holmes
   fenómeno de rebote de Gordon Holmes
rebus jeroglífico
recall recordación
recall method método de recordación
recall test prueba de recordación
recapitulation recapitulación
recapitulation theory teoría de recapitulación
recathexis recatexis
receiver recibidor
receiver operating characteristic
   característica operatorio de recibidor
receiving hospital hospital receptor
recency effect efecto de lo más reciente
recent memory memoria reciente
recent past memory memoria del pasado
   reciente
receptive receptivo
receptive amimia amimia receptiva
receptive aphasia afasia receptiva
receptive character carácter receptivo
receptive dysphasia disfasia receptiva
receptive-expressive aphasia afasia
   receptiva-expresiva
receptive field campo receptivo

receptive language lenguaje receptivo
receptive language disorder trastorno del
   lenguaje receptivo
receptive orientation orientación receptiva
receptive personality personalidad receptiva
receptivity receptividad
receptoma receptoma
receptor receptor
receptor complex complejo de receptores
receptor field campo de receptor
receptor potential potencial de receptor
receptor site sitio de receptor
recess receso
recessive recesivo
recessive gene gen recesivo
recessive inheritance herencia recesiva
recessive trait rasgo recesivo
recidivation recidiva
recidivism recidivismo
recidivism rate tasa de recidivismo
recidivist recidivista
recipiomotor recipiomotor
reciprocal recíproco
reciprocal altruism altruismo recíproco
reciprocal assimilation asimilación recíproca
reciprocal determinism determinismo
   recíproco
reciprocal inhibition inhibición recíproca
reciprocal inhibition and desensitization
   inhibición recíproca y desensibilización
reciprocal-inhibition psychotherapy
   psicoterapia de inhibición recíproca
reciprocal-inhibition therapy terapia de
   inhibición recíproca
reciprocal innervation inervación recíproca
reciprocal overlap solapo recíproco
reciprocal punishment castigo recíproco
reciprocal regulation regulación recíproca
reciprocal roles papeles recíprocos
reciprocal translocation traslocación
   recíproca
reciprocity reciprocidad
reciprocity norm norma de reciprocidad
recitation method método de recitación
Recklinghausen's disease enfermedad de
   Recklinghausen
recognition reconocimiento
recognition memory memoria de
   reconocimiento
recognition method método de
   reconocimiento
recognition procedure procedimiento de
   reconocimiento
recognition site sitio de reconocimiento
recognition span lapso de reconocimiento
recognition technique técnica de
   reconocimiento
recognition test prueba de reconocimiento
recognition time tiempo de reconocimiento
recognition vocabulary vocabulario de
   reconocimiento
recollection recordación
recombinant deoxyribonucleic acid ácido
   desoxirribonucleico recombinante
recombination recombinación

recommencement mania manía de
   recomenzar
recompensation recompensación
reconciliation reconciliación
reconditioning recondicionamiento
reconditioning therapy terapia de
   recondicionamiento
reconstituted family familia reconstituida
reconstitution reconstitución
reconstruction reconstrucción
reconstruction method método de
   reconstrucción
reconstructive reconstructivo
reconstructive memory memoria
   reconstructiva
reconstructive psychotherapy psicoterapia
   reconstructiva
reconstructive surgery cirugía reconstructiva
record registro
recording registro
recovery recuperación
recovery and reorganization recuperación y
   reorganización
recovery of function recuperación de función
recovery ratio razón de recuperación
recovery stage etapa de recuperación
recovery time tiempo de recuperación
recovery wish deseo de recuperación
recreation recreación
recreation specialist especialista de
   recreación
recreational recreativo
recreational therapy terapia recreativa
recreational use of drugs uso de drogas
   recreativo
recruiting response respuesta de
   reclutamiento
recruiting system sistema de reclutamiento
recruitment reclutamiento
recruitment by cults reclutamiento por cultos
rectal rectal
rectal disease enfermedad rectal
rectangular distribution distribución
   rectangular
rectilinear rectilíneo
rectilinear distribution distribución rectilínea
rectoanal reflex reflejo rectoanal
rectocardiac rectocardíaco
rectocardiac reflex reflejo rectocardíaco
rectolaryngeal rectolaríngeo
rectolaryngeal reflex reflejo rectolaríngeo
rectophobia rectofobia
recumbent recumbente
recurrent recurrente
recurrent circuit circuito recurrente
recurrent collateral inhibition inhibición
   colateral recurrente
recurrent depression depresión recurrente
recurrent dream sueño recurrente
recurrent encephalopathy encefalopatía
   recurrente
recurrent inhibition inhibición recurrente
red-green blindness ceguera rojo-verde
red-green color blindness ceguera al color
   rojo-verde

red-green response respuesta rojo-verde
red neuralgia neuralgia roja
red nucleus núcleo rojo
redintegration redintegración
redintegrative redintegrativo
redintegrative memory memoria
   redintegrativa
reduced reducido
reduced cue señal reducida
reduced score puntación reducida
reduction division división de reducción
reduction screen pantalla de reducción
reductionism reduccionismo
reductive reductivo
reductive approach acercamiento reductivo
reductive interpretation interpretación
   reductiva
redundancy redundancia
reduplicated babbling balbuceo reduplicado
reduplicative memory deception decepción
   de memoria reduplicativa
reduplicative paramnesia paramnesia
   reduplicativa
reeducation reeducación
reeducative reeducativo
reeducative therapy terapia reeducativa
reenactment reconstrucción
reentry reentrada
reevaluation reevaluación
reevaluation counseling asesoramiento de
   reevaluación
reference referencia
reference axes ejes de referencia
reference group grupo de referencia
reference-group theory teoría de grupo de
   referencia
reference memory memoria de referencia
reference vector vector de referencia
referent referente
referral referido
referred referido
referred pain dolor referido
referred sensation sensación referida
reflect reflejar
reflected reflejado
reflected color color reflejado
reflection reflexión
reflection of feeling reflexión de sensación
reflection spectrum espectro de reflexión
reflectivity-impulsivity
   reflectividad-impulsividad
reflex reflejo
reflex act acto reflejo
reflex anosmia anosmia refleja
reflex arc arco reflejo
reflex association asociación refleja
reflex circle círculo reflejo
reflex circuit circuito reflejo
reflex control control reflejo
reflex epilepsy epilepsia refleja
reflex excitability excitabilidad refleja
reflex facilitation facilitación refleja
reflex figure figura refleja
reflex headache dolor de cabeza reflejo
reflex incontinence incontinencia refleja

reflex inhibition inhibición refleja
reflex iridoplegia iridoplejía refleja
reflex latency latencia refleja
reflex movement movimiento reflejo
reflex neurogenic bladder vejiga neurogénica refleja
reflex psychology psicología refleja
reflex reserve reserva refleja
reflex sensation sensación refleja
reflex sensitization sensibilización refleja
reflex sensitization theory teoría de sensibilización refleja
reflex therapy terapia refleja
reflex time tiempo reflejo
reflexogenic reflexogénico
reflexogenic zone zona reflexogénica
reflexogenous reflexógeno
reflexograph reflexógrafo
reflexology reflexología
reflexometer reflexómetro
reflexophil reflexófilo
reflexophile reflexófilo
reflexotherapy reflexoterapia
reflux reflujo
reflux management administración de reflujo
reformist delusion delusión reformista
refraction refracción
refraction index índice de refracción
refractory refractario
refractory mental illness enfermedad mental refractaria
refractory period periodo refractario
refractory state estado refractario
Refsum's disease enfermedad de Refsum
Refsum's syndrome síndrome de Refsum
regeneration regeneración
regeneration of nerves regeneración de nervios
regimen régimen
region región
region of rejection región de rechazo
regional regional
regional anesthetic anestésico regional
regional cerebral blood flow flujo sanguíneo cerebral regional
regional hypothermia hipotermia regional
registration registro
regnancy predominio
regnant predominante
regnant process proceso predominante
regression regresión
regression analysis análisis de regresión
regression coefficient coeficiente de regresión
regression curve curva de regresión
regression equation ecuación de regresión
regression line línea de regresión
regression neurosis neurosis de regresión
regression time tiempo de regresión
regression toward the mean regresión hacia la media
regression weight peso de regresión
regressive regresivo
regressive alcoholism alcoholismo regresivo
regressive electroshock therapy terapia de electrochoques regresiva

regressive-reconstructive approach acercamiento regresivo-reconstructivo
regressive schizophrenia esquizofrenia regresiva
regressive transference neurosis neurosis de transferencia regresiva
regret remordimiento
regularity regularidad
regulation regulación
regulation of breathing during sleep regulación de respiración durante sueño
regulation of emotion regulación de emoción
regulation of hunger regulación de hambre
regulatory regulador
regulatory behavior conducta reguladora
regulatory system sistema regulador
regurgitation regurgitación
rehabilitate rehabilitar
rehabilitation rehabilitación
rehabilitation center centro de rehabilitación
rehabilitation counselor asesor de rehabilitación
rehabilitation medicine medicina de rehabilitación
rehabilitation program programa de rehabilitación
rehabilitation psychologist psicólogo de rehabilitación
rehabilitation stage etapa de rehabilitación
rehabilitation team equipo de rehabilitación
rehearsal ensayo
rehospitalization rehospitalización
reification cosificación
reification fallacy falacia de cosificación
reinforce reforzar
reinforcement refuerzo
reinforcement analysis análisis de refuerzo
reinforcement counseling asesoramiento de refuerzo
reinforcement effect efecto de refuerzo
reinforcement gradient gradiente de refuerzo
reinforcement schedule programa de refuerzo
reinforcement theory teoría de refuerzo
reinforcer reforzador
reinforcing reforzante
reinforcing cause causa reforzante
reinforcing stimulus estímulo reforzante
reinnervation reinervación
reintegration reintegración
Reissner's membrane membrana de Reissner
Reiter's syndrome síndrome de Reiter
rejecting-neglecting parent padre rechazador-negligente, madre rechazadora-negligente
rejection rechazo
rejuvenation rejuvenecimiento
rejuvenation fantasy fantasía de rejuvenecimiento
relapse recaída
relapse prevention prevención de recaída
relapse rate tasa de recaídas
relation relación
relational relacional
relational learning aprendizaje relacional
relational problem problema relacional

relational problem related to general medical condition problema relacional relacionado a condición médica general
relational problem related to mental disorder problema relacional relacionado a trastorno mental
relational threshold umbral relacional
relational word palabra relacional
relationship relación
relationship history historial de relaciones
relationship therapy terapia de relación
relative (adj) relativo
relative (n) pariente
relative deprivation-gratification privación-gratificación relativa
relative frequency frecuencia relativa
relative infertility infertilidad relativa
relative motion moción relativa
relative pitch tono relativo
relative position posición relativa
relative refractory period periodo refractario relativo
relative risk riesgo relativo
relative risk in epidemology riesgo relativo en epidemología
relative size tamaño relativo
relativism relativismo
relativity relatividad
relativity of reality relatividad de realidad
relaxation relajación
relaxation-induced anxiety ansiedad inducida por relajación
relaxation principle principio de relajación
relaxation response respuesta de relajación
relaxation therapy terapia de relajación
relaxation training entrenamiento de relajación
relearning reaprendizaje
relearning method método de reaprendizaje
release inhibitor inhibidor de liberación
release phenomenon fenómeno de liberación
release therapy terapia de liberación
releaser disparador
releasing mechanism mecanismo liberador
releasing stimulus estímulo liberador
relevant relevante
relevant other otro relevante
reliability confiabilidad
reliability coefficient coeficiente de confiabilidad
reliability of test confiabilidad de prueba
reliability sampling muestreo de confiabilidad
reliable confiable
reliance confianza
relief alivio
relief-discomfort quotient cociente de alivio-incomodidad
relief-distress quotient cociente de alivio-angustia
relieve aliviar
religious delusion delusión religiosa
religious mania manía religiosa
religious problem problema religioso
relocation reubicación
Remak's reflex reflejo de Remak

Remak's sign signo de Remak
remarry volver a contraer matrimonio
remedial remediador
remedial reading lectura remediadora
remedial therapy terapia remediadora
remembrance remembranza
reminiscence reminiscencia
reminiscent reminiscente
reminiscent aura aura reminiscente
reminiscent neuralgia neuralgia reminiscente
remission remisión
remitting remitente
remitting schizophrenia esquizofrenia remitente
remorse remordimiento
remote remoto
remote association asociación remota
remote-association test prueba de asociación remota
remote conditioning condicionamiento remoto
remote dependency dependencia remota
remote masking enmascaramiento remoto
remote memory memoria remota
remote perception percepción remota
remotivation remotivación
removal protection protección por remoción
renal renal
Renpenning's syndrome síndrome de Renpenning
Renshaw cell célula de Renshaw
renunciation renunciación
reorganization reorganización
reorganization principle principio de reorganización
reorganization theory teoría de reorganización
repair mechanism mecanismo de reparación
reparation reparación
repertoire repertorio
repetition repetición
repetition compulsion compulsión de repetición
repetition-compulsion principle principio de repetición-compulsión
repetition law ley de repetición
repetition reaction reacción de repetición
repetitive repetitivo
repetitive pattern patrón repetitivo
replacement reemplazo
replacement formation formación de reemplazo
replacement memory memoria de reemplazo
replacement sampling muestreo con reemplazo
replacement therapy terapia de reemplazo
replicate replicar
replication replicación
replication therapy terapia de replicación
reporting child abuse reportando abuso de niños
represent representar
representation representación
representative representativo
representative design diseño representativo
representative factors factores

representativos
representative intelligence inteligencia
   representativa
representative measure medida
   representativa
representative sample muestra representativa
representative sampling muestreo
   representativo
representative score puntuación
   representativa
representative value valor representativo
repress reprimir
repressed reprimido
repressed complex complejo reprimido
repression represión
repression-resistance represión-resistencia
repression scale escala de represión
repression-sensitization scale escala de
   represión-sensibilización
repressive represivo
repressive approach acercamiento represivo
repressive personality personalidad represiva
repressor represor
reproduction reproducción
reproduction method método de
   reproducción
reproduction procedure procedimiento de
   reproducción
reproduction theory teoría de reproducción
reproductive reproductivo
reproductive assimilation asimilación
   reproductiva
reproductive behavior conducta reproductiva
reproductive facilitation facilitación
   reproductiva
reproductive failure fracaso reproductivo
reproductive function función reproductiva
reproductive instinct instinto reproductivo
reproductive interference interferencia
   reproductiva
reproductive isolation aislamiento
   reproductivo
reproductive memory memoria reproductiva
reproductive mortality mortalidad
   reproductiva
reproductive ritual ritual reproductivo
reproductive strength fuerza reproductiva
reproductive thinking pensamiento
   reproductivo
reproductive type tipo reproductivo
repulsion repulsión
required requerido
required behavior conducta requerida
required relationship relación requerida
rescue fantasy fantasía de rescate
research investigación
reserpine reserpina
reserve reserva
reservoir reservorio
residence rate tasa de residencia
resident residente
resident treatment facility instalación de
   tratamiento de residentes
residential residencial
residential care cuidado residencial

residential school escuela residencial
residential treatment tratamiento residencial
residential treatment facility instalación de
   tratamiento residencial
residual residual
residual amnesia amnesia residual
residual schizophrenia esquizofrenia residual
residual type schizophrenia esquizofrenia de
   tipo residual
residue residuo
resignation resignación
resinous resinoso
resistance resistencia
resistance phase fase de resistencia
resistance stage etapa de resistencia
resistance to extinction resistencia a extinción
resistance to stress resistencia al estrés
resistance to temptation resistencia a
   tentación
resistant resistente
resistant attachment apego resistente
resocialization resocialización
resolution resolución
resolution of crisis resolución de crisis
resolution phase fase de resolución
resolving power poder de resolución
resonance theory teoría de resonancia
resonance theory of hearing teoría de
   resonancia de audición
resonator resonador
resource recurso
resource person persona de recursos
resource teacher maestro de recursos
respiration respiración
respiration rate ritmo de respiración
respirator respirador
respiratory respiratorio
respiratory anosmia anosmia respiratoria
respiratory depression depresión respiratoria
respiratory disorder trastorno respiratorio
respiratory-distress syndrome síndrome de
   dificultad respiratoria
respiratory eroticism erotismo respiratorio
respiratory impairment sleep disorder
   trastorno del sueño de deterioro respiratorio
respiratory pattern patrón respiratorio
respiratory pause pausa respiratoria
respiratory therapy terapia respiratoria
respirograph respirógrafo
respondent respondiente
respondent behavior conducta respondiente
respondent conditioning condicionamiento
   respondiente
response respuesta
response acquiescence aquiescencia de
   respuesta
response amplitude amplitud de respuesta
response attitude actitud de respuesta
response bias sesgo de respuestas
response circuit circuito de respuestas
response class clase de respuestas
response cost costo de respuesta
response deviation desviación de respuestas
response differentiation diferenciación de
   respuestas

response dispersion dispersión de respuestas
response equivalence equivalencia de
  respuestas
response generalization generalización de
  respuestas
response-generalization principle principio
  de generalización de respuestas
response hierarchy jerarquía de respuestas
response intensity intensidad de respuestas
response latency latencia de respuesta
response learning aprendizaje de respuesta
response magnitude magnitud de respuesta
response oriented orientado a respuestas
response prevention prevención de respuestas
response-produced cues señales producidas
  por respuestas
response rate tasa de respuestas
response set predisposición de respuesta
response-shock interval intervalo de
  respuesta-choque
response specificity especificidad de respuesta
response strength fuerza de respuesta
response system sistema de respuestas
response threshold umbral de respuesta
response time tiempo de respuesta
response variable variable de respuesta
responsibility responsabilidad
responsive responsivo
rest home hogar de descanso
rest period periodo de descanso
restatement repetición
resting potential potencial de reposo
restitution restitución
restitutional restitucional
restitutional schizophrenia esquizofrenia
  restitucional
restless inquieto
restless leg pierna inquieta
restless leg syndrome síndrome de piernas
  inquietas
restlessness inquietud
restoration therapy terapia de restauración
Restorff effect efecto de Restorff
restraint control
restricted restringido
restricted affect afecto restringido
restricted code código restringido
restricted learning aprendizaje restringido
restriction restricción
restriction endonuclease endonucleasa de
  restricción
restructure reestructurar
resymbolization resimbolización
retaliation represalia
retardation retardo
retarded depression depresión retardada
retarded ejaculation eyaculación retardada
retarded maturation maduración retardada
retarded schizophrenia esquizofrenia
  retardada
retention retención
retention control training entrenamiento de
  control de retención
retention curve curva de retención
retention hysteria histeria de retención

retention of affect retención de afecto
retentive memory memoria retentiva
retest reprueba
retest consistency consistencia de reprueba
reticular reticular
reticular activating system sistema activante
  reticular
reticular formation formación reticular
reticular membrane membrana reticular
reticular nucleus núcleo reticular
reticulotomy reticulotomía
retifism retifismo
retina retina
retinal retinal
retinal bipolar cells células bipolares retinales
retinal cone cono retinal
retinal densitometry densitometría retinal
retinal disparity disparidad retinal
retinal element elemento retinal
retinal field campo retinal
retinal fusion fusión retinal
retinal ganglion cell célula ganglionar retinal
retinal hemorrhage hemorragia retinal
retinal horizontal cells células horizontales
  retinales
retinal image imagen retinal
retinal light luz retinal
retinal macula mácula retinal
retinal mixture mezcla retinal
retinal oscillation oscilación retinal
retinal rivalry rivalidad retinal
retinal rods bastoncillos retinales
retinal size tamaño retinal
retinal zone zona retinal
retinene retineno
retinitis retinitis
retinoblastoma retinoblastoma
retinocerebral retinocerebral
retinocerebral angiomatosis angiomatosis
  retinocerebral
retinodiencephalic retinodiencefálico
retinodiencephalic degeneration
  degeneración retinodiencefálica
retinoscope retinoscopio
retirement retiro
retirement counseling asesoramiento de retiro
retirement neurosis neurosis de retiro
retraction retracción
retraction nystagmus nistagmo de retracción
retreat retiro
retreat from reality retiro de la realidad
retrieval recuperación
retroactive retroactivo
retroactive association asociación retroactiva
retroactive facilitation facilitación retroactiva
retroactive inhibition inhibición retroactiva
retroactive interference interferencia
  retroactiva
retroactive therapy terapia retroactiva
retrobulbar retrobulbar
retrobulbar neuritis neuritis retrobulbar
retrocochlear retrococlear
retrocochlear deafness sordera retrococlear
retrocollic retrocólico
retrocollic spasm espasmo retrocólico

retrocollis retrocolis
retrocursive retrocursivo
retrocursive absence ausencia retrocursiva
retroflexion retroflexión
retrogasserian retrogasseriano
retrogasserian neurectomy neurecotmía
retrogasseriana
retrogasserian neurotomy neurotomía
retrogasseriana
retrogenesis retrogénesis
retrograde retrógrado
retrograde amnesia amnesia retrógrada
retrograde chromatolysis cromatólisis
retrógrada
retrograde degeneration degeneración
retrógrada
retrograde ejaculation eyaculación retrógrada
retrograde memory memoria retrógrada
retrography retrografía
retrogression retrogresión
retrolental fibroplasia fibroplasia retrolental
retropulsion retropulsión
retropulsive retropulsivo
retropulsive epilepsy epilepsia retropulsiva
retrospection retrospección
retrospective retrospectivo
retrospective falsification falsificación
retrospectiva
retrospective medical audit auditoría médica
retrospectiva
retrospective report informe retrospectivo
retrospective research investigación
retrospectiva
retrospective study estudio retrospectivo
Rett's disorder trastorno de Rett
Rett's syndrome síndrome de Rett
revenge venganza
revenge rape violación por venganza
reverberating circuit circuito reverberante
reverberatory circuit circuito reverberatorio
reverie ensueño
reversal inversión
reversal learning aprendizaje inverso
reversal of affect inversión de afecto
reverse tolerance tolerancia inversa
reversibility reversibilidad
reversible reversible
reversible decortication descorticación
reversible
reversible figure figura reversible
reversible perspective perspectiva reversible
reversible shock choque reversible
reversion reversión
review revisión
Revilliod's sign signo de Revilliod
revolving-door phenomenon fenómeno de
puerta giratoria
revolving-door policy política de puerta
giratoria
reward recompensa
reward by the superego recompensa por el
superego
reward delay demora de recompensa
reward expectancy expectación de
recompensa

reward system sistema de recompensa
Rexed lamina lámina de Rexed
Reye's syndrome síndrome de Reye
Rh blood group grupo sanguíneo Rh
Rh blood group incompatibility
incompatibilidad de grupo sanguíneo Rh
Rh factor factor Rh
Rh reaction reacción Rh
rhabdophobia rabdofobia
rhathymia ratimia
rheobase reobase
rheoencephalogram reoencefalograma
rheoencephalography reoencefalografía
rheotaxis reotaxis
rheotropism reotropismo
rheumatic reumático
rheumatic chorea corea reumática
rheumatic tetany tetania reumática
rheumatic torticollis tortícolis reumático
rheumatism reumatismo
rheumatoid reumatoide
rheumatoid arthritis artritis reumatoide
rheumatoid spondylitis espondilitis
reumatoide
rhigosis rigosis
rhigotic rigótico
rhinencephalon rinencéfalo
rhinolalia rinolalia
rhinorrhea rinorrea
rhizomelic rizomélico
rhizomeningomyelitis rizomeningomielitis
rhizotomy rizotomía
rhodopsin rodopsina
rhombencephalic sleep sueño rombencefálico
rhombencephalon rombencéfalo
rhombocele rombocele
rhomboidal romboidal
rhomboidal sinus seno romboidal
rhypophagy ripofagia
rhypophobia ripofobia
rhythm ritmo
rhythm and periodicity ritmo y periodicidad
rhythm disorder trastorno de ritmo
rhythm method método de ritmo
rhythm method of contraception método de
ritmo de contracepción
rhythm test prueba de ritmo
rhythmic rítmico
rhythmic chorea corea rítmica
rhythmic sensory-bombardment therapy
terapia de bombardeo sensorial rítmica
rhythmic stimulation estimulación rítmica
rhythmicity ritmicidad
ribonuclease ribonucleasa
ribonucleic acid ácido ribonucleico
ribosome ribosoma
Ribot's law ley de Ribot
Ricco's law ley de Ricco
rich interpretation interpretación rica
Richards-Rundel syndrome síndrome de
Richards-Rundel
rickets raquitismo
Ridgway color system sistema de colores de
Ridgway
Rieger's syndrome síndrome de Rieger

Riese hearing audición de Riese
right-and-wrong test prueba de lo correcto e incorrecto
right-footed dextropedal
right-handed diestro
right-left discrimination discriminación derecha-izquierda
right-left disorientation desorientación derecha-izquierda
right-left orientation orientación derecha-izquierda
right-or-wrong test prueba de lo correcto o incorrecto
right to refuse treatment derecho de rehusar tratamiento
right to treatment derecho a tratamiento
righting enderezamiento
righting reaction reacción de enderezamiento
righting reflex reflejo de enderezamiento
rights of patients derechos de pacientes
rights of the disabled derechos de los incapacitados
rigid rígido
rigid-akinetic syndrome síndrome rígido-acinético
rigid control control rígido
rigid family familia rígida
rigid pupil pupila rígida
rigidity rigidez
Riley-Day syndrome síndrome de Riley-Day
ring chromosome cromosoma anular
ring-finger dermatitis dermatitis de dedo anular
ring-wall lesion lesión anular de pared
risk riesgo
risk factor factor de riesgo
risk hypothesis hipótesis de riesgo
risk level nivel de riesgo
risk management administración de riesgo
risk-taking behavior conducta arriesgada
rite rito
Ritter's law ley de Ritter
Ritter's tetanus tétanos de Ritter
Ritter-Rollet phenomenon fenómeno de Ritter-Rollet
ritual ritual
ritualistic ritualista
ritualistic behavior conducta ritualista
rivalry rivalidad
Robert's syndrome síndrome de Robert
Robertson pupil pupila de Robertson
robotics robótica
rocking balanceo
rod bastoncillo
rod of Corti bastoncillo de Corti
rod vision visión de bastoncillos
rodonalgia rodonalgia
Roger's reflex reflejo de Roger
rolandic epilepsy epilepsia rolándica
role papel
role behavior conducta de papel
role category categoría de papel
role conflict conflicto de papel
role confusion confusión de papel
role deprivation privación de papel

role diffusion difusión de papel
role discontinuity discontinuidad de papel
role distancing distanciamiento de papel
role distortion distorsión de papel
role expectation expectación de papel
role experimentation experimentación de papel
role fixation fijación de papel
role model modelo de papel
role obsolescence obsolescencia de papel
role of physical attractiveness in interpersonal attraction papel de atractividad física en atracción interpersonal
role-playing desempeño de papeles
role rehearsal ensayo de papel
role reversal inversión de papeles
role shift cambio de papel
role specialization especialización de papel
role theory of personality teoría de papeles de personalidad
Romano-Ward syndrome síndrome de Romano-Ward
romantic love amor romántico
Romberg's disease enfermedad de Romberg
Romberg's sign signo de Romberg
Romberg's symptom síntoma de Romberg
Romberg's syndrome síndrome de Romberg
Romberg's trophoneurosis trofoneurosis de Romberg
Romberg-Howship symptom síntoma de Romberg-Howship
Romberg test prueba de Romberg
rombergism rombergismo
Romeo and Juliet effect efecto de Romeo y Julieta
root raíz
root conflict conflicto raíz
root problem problema raíz
rooting reflex reflejo de hociquear
Rorschach test prueba de Rorschach
Rosanoff list lista de Rosanoff
Rosanoff test prueba de Rosanoff
Rose's cephalic tetanus tétanos cefálico de Rose
Rosenbach's law ley de Rosenbach
Rosenbach's sign signo de Rosenbach
Rosenbach-Gmelin test prueba de Rosenbach-Gmelin
Rosenthal effect efecto de Rosenthal
Rosenthal fiber fibra de Rosenthal
rosette roseta
Rossolimo's reflex reflejo de Rossolimo
Rossolimo's sign signo de Rossolimo
rostral rostral
rostral transentorial herniation herniación transtentorial rostral
rotary-pursuit procedure procedimiento de rastreo rotatorio
rotary-pursuit test prueba de rastreo rotatorio
rotation rotación
rotation perception percepción de rotación
rotation system sistema de rotación
rotatory rotatorio
rotatory spasm espasmo rotatorio

rotatory tic tic rotatorio
rotatory vertigo vértigo rotatorio
rote learning aprendizaje mecánico
rote recall recordación mecánica
Roth's disease enfermedad de Roth
Roth-Berhardt disease enfermedad de
    Roth-Berhardt
Rothmund-Thomson syndrome síndrome de
    Rothmund-Thomson
roughness discrimination discriminación de
    aspereza
round window ventana redonda
Roussy-Levy disease enfermedad de
    Roussy-Levy
Roussy-Levy syndrome síndrome de
    Roussy-Levy
routine rutina
rubella rubéola
Rubin's figure figura de Rubin
Rubinstein-Taybi syndrome síndrome de
    Rubinstein-Taybi
rubrospinal tract tracto rubroespinal
rudiment rudimento
Ruffini corpuscle corpúsculo de Ruffini
Ruffini end organ órgano terminal de Ruffini
Ruffini ending terminación de Ruffini
Ruffini papillary ending terminación papilar
    de Ruffini
rule learning aprendizaje de reglas
rule of abstinence regla de abstinencia
rule of thumb regla práctica
rules of the game reglas del juego
rumination rumiación
rumination disorder of infancy trastorno de
    rumiación de infancia
ruminative ruminativo
rumor rumor
Rumpf's sign signo de Rumpf
run away fugarse
runway corredor
rupophobia rupofobia
ruptured disk disco rupturado
rural environment ambiente rural
Russell's sign signo de Russell
Russell's syndrome síndrome de Russell
Rust's disease enfermedad de Rust
Rust's phenomenon fenómeno de Rust
rut celo
rypophobia ripofobia

S

S-curve curva en S
sabulous sabuloso
saccadic sacádico
saccadic eye movement movimiento ocular
    sacádico
saccadic movement movimiento sacádico
saccule sáculo
sacral sacral
sacral division división sacral
sacral nerve nervio sacral
sacrifice (n) sacrificio
sacrifice (v) sacrificar
sacrolisthesis sacrolistesis
sacrum sacro
sadism sadismo
sadist sadista
sadistic sádico
sadistic personality personalidad sádica
sadistic personality disorder trastorno de
    personalidad sádica
sadistic rape violación sádica
sadness tristeza
sadomasochism sadomasoquismo
sadomasochistic sadomasoquista
sadomasochistic relationship relación
    sadomasoquista
Saenger's sign signo de Saenger
safety and health education educación de
    seguridad y salud
safety device aparato de seguridad
safety motive motivo de seguridad
safety need necesidad de seguridad
safety psychology psicología de seguridad
sagittal sagital
sagittal axis eje sagital
sagittal fissure fisura sagital
sagittal section sección sagital
Saint Anthony's dance danza de San Antonio
Saint John's dance danza de San Juan
Saint Vitus dance danza de San Vito
salaam convulsion convulsión en zalema
salbutamol salbutamol
sales psychology psicología de ventas
sales-survey technique técnica de encuesta de
    ventas
salicylate salicilato
salience prominencia
salivary glands glándulas salivales
salivation salivación
Salpetriere school escuela de Salpetriere
salpingectomy salpingectomía
salt balance balance de sal
saltation saltación
saltatory saltatorio

saltatory chorea corea saltatoria
saltatory conduction conducción saltatoria
saltatory spasm espasmo saltatorio
sample muestra
sample bias sesgo de muestra
sample space espacio de muestra
sample standard deviation desviación estándar de muestra
sampling muestreo
sampling distribution distribución de muestreo
sampling error error de muestreo
sampling population población de muestreo
sampling reliability confiabilidad de muestreo
sampling stability estabilidad de muestreo
sampling theory teoría de muestreo
sampling validity validez de muestreo
sampling variability variabilidad de muestreo
sampling with replacement muestreo con reemplazo
sampling without replacement muestreo sin reemplazo
sanable sanable
sanatorium sanatorio
sanction sanción
sand body cuerpo de arena
sand tumor tumor de arena
sandbox marriage matrimonio de cajón de arena
Sandhoff's disease enfermedad de Sandhoff
Sandifer's syndrome síndrome de Sandifer
Sandler's triad tríada de Sandler
sane cuerdo
Sanfilippo's syndrome síndrome de Sanfilippo
sanguine sanguíneo
sanguine type tipo sanguíneo
sanguineous sanguíneo
sanitarium sanatorio
sanity cordura
Sanson images imágenes de Sanson
Sapir-Whorf hypothesis hipótesis de Sapir-Whorf
sapphism safismo
sarcasm sarcasmo
sarcoma sarcoma
sarmassation sarmasación
satanophobia satanofobia
satellite satélite
satellite clinic clínica satélite
satellite housing vivienda satélite
satellitosis satelitosis
satiation saciedad
satiety saciedad
satiety center centro de saciedad
satisfaction satisfacción
satisfaction of instincts satisfacción de instintos
saturated test prueba saturada
saturation saturación
saturnine saturnino
saturnine encephalopathy encefalopatía saturnina
saturnine pseudogeneral paralysis parálisis seudogeneral saturnina

saturnine tremor temblor saturnino
satyriasis satiriasis
satyrism satirismo
sauce Bearnaise effect efecto de salsa bearnesa
Saunders-Sutton syndrome síndrome de Saunders-Sutton
savage salvaje
sawtooth waves onda de dientes de sierra
scabiophobia escabiofobia
scala media scala media
scala tympani scala tympani
scala vestibuli scala vestibuli
scalability escalabilidad
scalar analysis análisis escalar
scale escala
scale of measurement escala de medición
scale value valor escalar
scalenectomy escalenectomía
scalenotomy escalenotomía
scalenus anterior syndrome síndrome del escaleno anterior
scaling escalamiento
scalloping festoneado
scalogram escalograma
scalogram analysis análisis de escalograma
scalp cuero cabelludo
scalp contusion contusión del cuero cabelludo
scalp infection infección del cuero cabelludo
scalp laceration laceración del cuero cabelludo
Scanlon plan plan de Scanlon
scanning exploración
scapegoat chivo expiatorio
scapegoat mechanism mecanismo de chivo expiatorio
scaphohydrocephalus escafohidrocefalia
scaphohydrocephaly escafohidrocefalia
scapular reflex reflejo escapular
scapulohumeral escapulohumeral
scapulohumeral atrophy atrofia escapulohumeral
scapulohumeral reflex reflejo escapulohumeral
scapuloperiosteal reflex reflejo escapuloperióstico
Scarpa's ganglion ganglio de Scarpa
Scarpa's method método de Scarpa
scatologia escatología
scatologic escatológico
scatological escatológico
scatology escatología
scatophagy escatofagia
scatophobia escatofobia
scatter dispersión
scatter analysis análisis de dispersión
scatter diagram diagrama de dispersión
scattering desparramamiento
scavenging behavior conducta carroñera
scelalgia escelalgia
scelerophobia escelerofobia
scelotyrbe escelotirbe
Schaffer's reflex reflejo de Schaffer
Schaumberg's disease enfermedad de Schaumberg

schedule programa, horario, lista
schedule of reinforcement programa de
   refuerzo
Scheffe test prueba de Scheffe
Scheid cyanotic syndrome síndrome cianótico
   de Scheid
Scheie's syndrome síndrome de Scheie
schema esquema
schematic esquemático
schematic image imagen esquemática
scheme esquema, ardid
Schiff-Sherrington phenomenon fenómeno
   de Schiff-Sherrington
Schilder's disease enfermedad de Schilder
Schirmer's syndrome síndrome de Schirmer
schism cisma
schistorrhachis esquistorraquis
schistosomiasis esquistosomiasis
schizencephalic esquizencefálico
schizencephalic microcephaly microcefalia
   esquizencefálica
schizencephaly esquizencefalia
schizoaffective esquizoafectivo
schizoaffective disorder trastorno
   esquizoafectivo
schizoaffective psychosis psicosis
   esquizoafectiva
schizobipolar esquizobipolar
schizocaria esquizocaria
schizogen esquizógeno
schizogyria esquizogiria
schizoid esquizoide
schizoid character carácter esquizoide
schizoid disorder trastorno esquizoide
schizoid disorder of adolescence trastorno
   esquizoide de adolescencia
schizoid disorder of childhood trastorno
   esquizoide de niñez
schizoid fantasy fantasía esquizoide
schizoid-manic state estado
   esquizoide-maníaco
schizoid personality personalidad esquizoide
schizoid personality disorder trastorno de
   personalidad esquizoide
schizoid personality scale escala de
   personalidad esquizoide
schizoid position posición esquizoide
schizoid scale escala esquizoide
schizoidia esquizoidia
schizoidism esquizoidismo
schizokinesis esquizocinesis
schizomania esquizomanía
schizomanic esquizomaníaco
schizomimetic esquizomimético
schizophasia esquizofasia
schizophrasia esquizofrasia
schizophrenia esquizofrenia
schizophrenia in remission esquizofrenia en
   remisión
schizophrenia scale escala de esquizofrenia
schizophrenic esquizofrénico
schizophrenic disorder trastorno
   esquizofrénico
schizophrenic episode episodio esquizofrénico
schizophrenic excitement excitación

esquizofrénica
schizophrenic personality personalidad
   esquizofrénica
schizophrenic psychosis psicosis
   esquizofrénica
schizophrenic reaction reacción
   esquizofrénica
schizophrenic spectrum espectro
   esquizofrénico
schizophrenic state estado esquizofrénico
schizophrenic surrender rendición
   esquizofrénica
schizophrenic thought disorder trastorno de
   pensamiento esquizofrénico
schizophreniform esquizofreniforme
schizophreniform disorder trastorno
   esquizofreniforme
schizophreniform psychosis psicosis
   esquizofreniforme
schizophrenogenic esquizofrenogénico
schizophrenogenic parent padre
   esquizofrenogénico, madre
   esquizofrenogénica
schizotaxia esquizotaxia
schizothemia esquizotemia
schizothymia esquizotimia
schizothymic esquizotímico
schizothymic personality personalidad
   esquizotímica
schizotonia esquizotonía
schizotypal esquizotípico
schizotypal disorder trastorno esquizotípico
schizotypal personality personalidad
   esquizotípica
schizotypal personality disorder trastorno de
   personalidad esquizotípica
schizotypal scale escala esquizotípica
Schlesinger's sign signo de Schlesinger
Schmidt's disorder trastorno de Schmidt
Schmidt's syndrome síndrome de Schmidt
Schmorl's nodule nódulo de Schmorl
Schneider's first-rank symptoms síntomas de
   primer rango de Schneider
schneiderian criteria for depressive
   personality criterios de Schneider para
   personalidad depresiva
schneiderian first-rank symptoms síntomas
   de primer rango de Schneider
schneiderian symptom síntoma de Schneider
scholastic escolástico
scholastic acceleration aceleración escolástica
scholastic achievement test prueba de
   aprovechamiento escolástico
Scholz' disease enfermedad de Scholz
school adjustment ajuste escolar
school gang pandilla escolar
school history historial escolar
school phobia fobia escolar
school problem problema escolar
school psychology psicología escolar
school refusal denegación escolar
school refusal syndrome síndrome de
   denegación escolar
Schuller's phenomenon fenómeno de
   Schuller

Schultze's sign signo de Schultze
Schwann cells células de Schwann
Schwann sheath vaina de Schwann
schwannoma schwannoma
schwannosis schwannosis
Schwartz tractotomy tractotomía de Schwartz
sciatic ciático
sciatic neuralgia neuralgia ciática
sciatic neuritis neuritis ciática
sciatic scoliosis escoliosis ciática
sciatica ciática
scientific approach acercamiento científico
scientific attitude actitud científica
scientific illiteracy analfabetismo científico
scientific law ley científica
scientific management administración
    científica
scientific method método científico
scientific psychology psicología científica
scintillating scotoma escotoma centelleante
scintillator centelleador
scissor gait marcha en tijeras
sclera esclerótica
sclerencephalia esclerencefalia
sclerencephaly esclerencefalia
sclerosis esclerosis
sclerosis of white matter esclerosis de la
    sustancia blanca
sclerotic esclerótico
sclerotic layer capa esclerótica
scoliosis escoliosis
scoliotic escoliótico
scope alcance
scopolamine escopolamina
scopophilia escopofilia
scopophobia escopofobia
scoptophilia escoptofilia
score puntuación
scoring tanteo
scotoma escotoma
scotomatization escotomatización
scotomization escotomización
scotophilia escotofilia
scotophobia escotofobia
scotopic escotópico
scotopic adaptation adaptación escotópica
scotopic vision visión escotópica
scotopsin escotopsina
scratch reflex reflejo de rascarse
screen pantalla
screen defense defensa cubriente
screen fantasy fantasía cubriente
screen memory memoria cubriente
screening cribado
screening program programa cribador
screening test prueba cribadora
script analysis análisis de libreto
scrivener's palsy parálisis de escritor
scrotum escroto
scrupulosity escrupulosidad
scrupulous escrupuloso
Scull's dilemma dilema de Scull
seance sesión espiritista
search búsqueda
Seashore tests pruebas de Seashore

seasickness mareo
seasonal affective disorder trastorno afectivo
    temporal
seasonal cycle ciclo temporal
seasonal depression depresión temporal
seasonal energy syndrome síndrome de
    energía temporal
seasonal mood disorder trastorno del humor
    temporal
seasonal pattern patrón temporal
seclusion reclusión
seclusion need necesidad de reclusión
secobarbital secobarbital
second cranial nerve segundo nervio craneal
second negative phase segunda fase negativa
second-order conditioning condicionamiento
    de segundo orden
second-order factor factor de segundo orden
second-order language lenguaje de segundo
    orden
second signal system sistema de segundas
    señales
second signaling system sistema de segundas
    señales
secondary secundario
secondary advantage ventaja secundaria
secondary aging envejecimiento secundario
secondary amenorrhea amenorrea secundaria
secondary amyloidosis amiloidosis secundaria
secondary area área secundaria
secondary attention atención secundaria
secondary autoerotism autoerotismo
    secundario
secondary cause causa secundaria
secondary circular reaction reacción circular
    secundaria
secondary conditioning condicionamiento
    secundario
secondary cortical zone zona cortical
    secundaria
secondary defense symptoms síntomas de
    defensas secundarias
secondary degeneration degeneración
    secundaria
secondary dementia demencia secundaria
secondary depression depresión secundaria
secondary deviance desviación secundaria
secondary drive impulso secundario
secondary-drive theory teoría de impulso
    secundario
secondary elaboration elaboración secundaria
secondary encephalitis encefalitis secundaria
secondary environment ambiente secundario
secondary erectile dysfunction disfunción
    eréctil secundaria
secondary evaluation evaluación secundaria
secondary extinction extinción secundaria
secondary gain ganancia secundaria
secondary generalized epilepsy epilepsia
    generalizada secundaria
secondary group grupo secundario
secondary hydrocephalus hidrocefalia
    secundaria
secondary identification identificación
    secundaria

secondary impotence impotencia secundaria
secondary integration integración secundaria
secondary mania manía secundaria
secondary memory memoria secundaria
secondary mental deficiency deficiencia
  mental secundaria
secondary motivation motivación secundaria
secondary narcissism narcisismo secundario
secondary oocyte oocito secundario
secondary personality personalidad
  secundaria
secondary prevention prevención secundaria
secondary process proceso secundario
secondary quality calidad secundaria
secondary reinforcement refuerzo secundario
secondary reinforcer reforzador secundario
secondary relationship relación secundaria
secondary repression represión secundaria
secondary retarded ejaculation eyaculación
  retardada secundaria
secondary revision revisión secundaria
secondary reward recompensa secundaria
secondary reward conditioning
  condicionamiento de recompensa
  secundaria
secondary sensation sensación secundaria
secondary sex characteristics características
  sexuales secundarias
secondary signaling system sistema de
  señales secundario
secondary sleep disorder trastorno del sueño
  secundario
secondary stuttering tartamudez secundaria
secondary symptoms síntomas secundarios
secondary territory territorio secundario
secondary tumor tumor secundario
secret control control secreto
secretin secretina
sect secta
section sección
secular secular
secure seguro
secure attachment apego seguro
secure base effect efecto de base segura
security seguridad
security blanket manta de seguridad
security operations operaciones de seguridad
sedation sedación
sedation threshold umbral de sedación
sedative sedante
sedative abuse abuso de sedante
sedative anxiety disorder trastorno de
  ansiedad de sedante
sedative delirium delirio de sedante
sedative dependence dependencia de sedante
sedative drug droga sedante
sedative-hypnotic sedante-hipnótico
sedative-hypnotic drug droga
  sedante-hipnótica
sedative intoxication intoxicación por sedante
sedative mood disorder trastorno del humor
  de sedante
sedative occupation ocupación sedante
sedative persisting amnestic disorder
  trastorno amnésico persistente de sedante

sedative persisting dementia demencia
  persistente de sedante
sedative psychotic disorder trastorno
  psicótico de sedante
sedative psychotic disorder with delusions
  trastorno psicótico de sedante con
  delusiones
**sedative psychotic disorder with
  hallucinations** trastorno psicótico de
  sedante con alucinaciones
sedative sexual dysfunction disfunción sexual
  de sedante
sedative sleep disorder trastorno del sueño de
  sedante
sedative use disorder trastorno de uso de
  sedante
sedative withdrawal retiro de sedante
sedativism sedativismo
sedimentation sedimentación
seduction seducción
seductive seductivo
Seeligmuller's sign signo de Seeligmuller
segmental segmentario
segmental anesthesia anestesia segmentaria
segmental neuritis neuritis segmentaria
segmental neuropathy neuropatía segmentaria
segmentation segmentación
segregation segregación
Seitelberger's disease enfermedad de
  Seitelberger
seizure acceso
seizure dyscontrol descontrol por acceso
sejunction sejunción
selaphobia selafobia
selected group grupo seleccionado
selection selección
selection bias sesgo de selección
selection index índice de selección
selection test prueba de selección
selectionism seleccionismo
selective selectivo
selective adaptation adaptación selectiva
selective amnesia amnesia selectiva
selective analysis análisis selectivo
selective attachment apego selectivo
selective attention atención selectiva
selective inattention inatención selectiva
selective learning aprendizaje selectivo
selective listening audición selectiva
selective memory memoria selectiva
selective perception percepción selectiva
selective response respuesta selectiva
selective retention retención selectiva
selective use of hypnosis uso selectivo de
  hipnosis
self yo, identidad propia, personalidad
self-abasement autoabatimiento
self-absorption absorción propia
self-abuse autoabuso
self-acceptance autoaceptación
self-accusation autoacusación
self-actualization actualización propia
self-administered test prueba
  autoadministrada
self-alienation autoalienación

self-analysis autoanálisis
self-appraisal autoevaluación
self-assessment autoevaluación
self-attack autoataque
self-awareness conciencia propia
self-blaming autoculpación
self-blaming depression depresión de autoculpación
self-care autocuidado
self-censure autocensura
self-centered egocéntrico
self-certainty autocertidumbre
self-commitment autoconfinamiento
self-concept autoconcepto
self-concept test prueba de autoconcepto
self-confidence confianza propia
self-consciousness conciencia propia, cohibición
self-consistency autoconsistencia
self-contempt autodesprecio
self-contemptuous autodespreciativo
self-control autodominio
self-control techniques técnicas de autodominio
self-control therapy terapia de autodominio
self-correlation autocorrelación
self-criticism autocrítica
self-deception autodecepción
self-defeating autoderrotante
self-defeating behavior conducta autoderrotante
self-defeating personality disorder trastorno de personalidad autoderrotante
self-demand feeding alimentación por demanda propia
self-demand schedule programa de demanda propia
self-demand schedule of feeding programa de alimentación por demanda propia
self-denial autonegación
self-deprecatory remark comentario autodespreciativo
self-derogation autoderogación
self-desensitization autodesensibilización
self-destructive behavior conducta autodestructiva
self-destructiveness autodestructividad
self-determination autodeterminación
self-development autodesarrollo
self-differentiation autodiferenciación
self-directed autodirigido
self-direction autodirección
self-discipline autodisciplina
self-disclosure autodivulgación
self-discovery autodescubrimiento
self-dynamism autodinamismo
self-effacement modestia
self-efficacy autoeficacia
self-employment empleo por cuenta propia
self-esteem autoestima
self-evaluation autoevaluación
self-evident evidente
self-examination autoexaminación
self-expression autoexpresión
self-extension autoextensión

self-extinction autoextinción
self-feeding autoalimentación
self-fellator autofelator
self-fulfilling prophecy profecía autorrealizante
self-fulfillment autorrealización
self-gratification autogratificación
self-hate odio propio
self-help autoayuda
self-help group grupo de autoayuda
self-hypnorelaxation autohipnorrelajación
self-hypnosis autohipnosis
self ideal yo ideal
self-identification autoidentificación
self-image autoimagen
self-image of abused children autoimagen de niños abusados
self-injurious autoperjudicial
self-injurious behavior conducta autoperjudicial
self-instruction autoinstrucción
self-instructional autoinstruccional
self-inventory autoinventario
self-irrumation autoirrumación
self-knowledge autoconocimiento
self-love amor propio
self-managed autoadministrado
self-managed reinforcement refuerzo autoadministrado
self-management autoadministración
self-maximation automaximación
self-monitoring automonitorización
self-mutilation automutilación
self-observation autoobservación
self-perception autopercepción
self-perception theory teoría de autopercepción
self-preservation autopreservación
self-preservation instinct instinto de autopreservación
self-psychology autopsicología
self-punishment autocastigo
self-rating autoclasificación
self-rating scale escala de autoclasificación
self-rating test prueba de autoclasificación
self-realization autorrealización
self-recitation recitación propia
self-reference autorreferencia
self-regard autoestimación
self-regulation autorregulación
self-reinforcement autorrefuerzo
self-reliance confianza propia
self-report inventory inventario de autoinforme
self-reporting autoinformante
self-respect respeto propio
self-revelation autorrevelación
self-selection autoselección
self-sentiment sentimiento propio
self-serving de beneficio propio
self-serving bias sesgo de beneficio propio
self-stimulation autoestimulación
self-stimulation mechanism mecanismo de autoestimulación
self-system sistema del yo

self-terminating search búsqueda
   autoterminante
self-theory autoteoría
self-understanding entendimiento propio
self-worth valor propio
selfish gene gen egoísta
Selter's disease enfermedad de Selter
semantene semantena
semantic semántico
semantic aphasia afasia semántica
semantic code código semántico
semantic component componente semántico
semantic conditioning condicionamiento
   semántico
semantic confusion confusión semántica
semantic counseling asesoramiento semántico
semantic dementia demencia semántica
semantic differential diferencial semántico
semantic dissociation disociación semántica
semantic feature característica semántica
semantic generalization generalización
   semántica
semantic jargon jerga semántica
semantic memory memoria semántica
semantic network red semántica
semantic paraphrasia parafrasia semántica
semantic psychosis psicosis semántica
semantic satiation saciedad semántica
semantic space espacio semántico
semantic therapy terapia semántica
semanticity semanticidad
semantics semántica
semantogenic semantogénico
semantogenic disorder trastorno
   semantogénico
semasiography semasiografía
semeiology semiología
semeiopathic semiopático
semeiosis semiosis
semeiotic semiótico
semeiotic function función semiótica
semeiotics semiótica
semen semen
semenuria semenuria
semicircular canal canal semicircular
semicoma semicoma
semicomatose semicomatoso
semiconscious semiconsciente
semiconsonant semiconsonante
semimembranosus semimembranoso
semimembranosus reflex reflejo
   semimembranoso
seminal seminal
seminal discharge descarga seminal
seminal duct conducto seminal
seminal vesicles vesículas seminales
semination seminación
seminiferous tubules túbulos seminíferos
semiology semiología
semiopathic semiopático
semiosis semiosis
semiotic semiótico
semiotic movement movimiento semiótico
semiotics semiótica
semitendinosus semitendinoso

semitendinosus reflex reflejo semitendinoso
semitendinous semitendinoso
semitone semitono
semivowel semivocal
Semon's law ley de Semon
Semon-Hering theory teoría de
   Semon-Hering
senescence senescencia
senescent senescente
senescent pedophilia pedofilia senescente
senile senil
senile artiopathic psychosis psicosis
   artiopática senil
senile brain disease enfermedad cerebral senil
senile chorea corea senil
senile delirium delirio senil
senile dementia demencia senil
senile dementia of Alzheimer type demencia
   senil de tipo Alzheimer
senile deterioration deterioración senil
senile involution involución senil
senile keratosis queratosis senil
senile memory memoria senil
senile osteomalacia osteomalacia senil
senile paraplegia paraplejía senil
senile plaque placa senil
senile psychosis psicosis senil
senile tremor temblor senil
senilism senilismo
senility senilidad
senium senium
senium praecox senium praecox
sensate focus enfoque en sensaciones
sensate focus learning aprendizaje de enfoque
   en sensaciones
sensation sensación
sensation increment incremento de sensación
sensation level nivel de sensación
sensation-seeking buscante de sensaciones
sensation threshold umbral de sensación
sensation type tipo de sensación
sensation unit unidad de sensación
sensationalism sensacionalismo
sense sentido
sense datum dato sensorial
sense distance distancia sensorial
sense experience experiencia sensorial
sense feeling sensación sensorial
sense illusion ilusión sensorial
sense impression impresión sensorial
sense limen limen sensorial
sense modality modalidad sensorial
sense of equilibrium sentido de equilibrio
sense of guilt sentido de culpabilidad
sense of humor sentido del humor
sense of identity sentido de identidad
sense of self sentido de identidad propia
sense organ órgano sensorial
sense perception percepción sensorial
sense quality cualidad sensorial
sensed difference diferencia percibida
sensibility sensibilidad
sensible sensible, sensato
sensiferous sensífero
sensigenous sensígeno

sensimeter sensímetro
sensitive sensitivo
sensitive period periodo sensitivo
sensitive zone zona sensitiva
sensitivity sensibilidad
sensitivity training entrenamiento de sensibilidad
sensitivity training group grupo de entrenamiento de sensibilidad
sensitization sensibilización
sensitization-repression scale escala de sensibilización-represión
sensitizer sensibilizador
sensomobile sensomóvil
sensomobility sensomovilidad
sensor sensor
sensorial sensorial
sensoriglandular sensoriglandular
sensorimotor sensorimotor
sensorimotor aphasia afasia sensorimotora
sensorimotor development desarrollo sensorimotor
sensorimotor intelligence inteligencia sensorimotora
sensorimotor level nivel sensorimotor
sensorimotor period periodo sensorimotor
sensorimotor phase fase sensorimotora
sensorimotor process proceso sensorimotor
sensorimotor rhythm ritmo sensorimotor
sensorimotor stage etapa sensorimotora
sensorimotor theory teoría sensorimotora
sensorimuscular sensorimuscular
sensorineural sensorineural
sensorineural deafness sordera sensorineural
sensorineural hearing loss pérdida de audición sensorineural
sensorineural impairment deterioro sensorineural
sensorium sensorio
sensorivascular sensorivascular
sensorivasomotor sensorivasomotor
sensory sensorial
sensory acuity agudeza sensorial
sensory adaptation adaptación sensorial
sensory alexia alexia sensorial
sensory amimia amimia sensorial
sensory amusia amusia sensorial
sensory aphasia afasia sensorial
sensory apraxia apraxia sensorial
sensory area área sensorial
sensory ataxia ataxia sensorial
sensory automatism automatismo sensorial
sensory awareness conciencia sensorial
sensory-awareness group grupo de conciencia sensorial
sensory-awareness procedure procedimiento de conciencia sensorial
sensory capacity capacidad sensorial
sensory conditioning condicionamiento sensorial
sensory-conditioning system sistema de condicionamiento sensorial
sensory conformance conformidad sensorial
sensory conversion symptom síntoma de conversión sensorial

sensory cortex corteza sensorial
sensory cue señal sensorial
sensory defect defecto sensorial
sensory deficit déficit sensorial
sensory deprivation privación sensorial
sensory discrimination discriminación sensorial
sensory disorder trastorno sensorial
sensory disturbance disturbio sensorial
sensory drive impulso sensorial
sensory epilepsy epilepsia sensorial
sensory-evoked potential potencial evocado sensorial
sensory experience experiencia sensorial
sensory exploration exploración sensorial
sensory extinction extinción sensorial
sensory feedback retroalimentación sensorial
sensory field campo sensorial
sensory gating desconexión periódica sensorial
sensory habit hábito sensorial
sensory homunculus homúnculo sensorial
sensory image imagen sensorial
sensory impairment deterioro sensorial
sensory inattention inatención sensorial
sensory-information store almacén de información sensorial
sensory input entrada sensorial
sensory-integrative functioning funcionamiento integrativo sensorial
sensory interaction interacción sensorial
sensory isolation aislamiento sensorial
sensory memory memoria sensorial
sensory modality modalidad sensorial
sensory-motor sensorimotor
sensory-motor intelligence inteligencia sensorimotora
sensory-motor level nivel sensorimotor
sensory-motor period periodo sensorimotor
sensory-motor stage etapa sensorimotora
sensory neglect negligencia sensorial
sensory nerve nervio sensorial
sensory neuron neurona sensorial
sensory neuronopathy neuronopatía sensorial
sensory organization organización sensorial
sensory paralysis parálisis sensorial
sensory pathway vía sensorial
sensory-perceptual test prueba sensorial-perceptiva
sensory polyneuropathy polineuropatía sensorial
sensory precipitated epilepsy epilepsia precipitada sensorial
sensory preconditioning precondicionamiento sensorial
sensory process proceso sensorial
sensory processing procesamiento sensorial
sensory projection area área de proyección sensorial
sensory psychophysiology psicofisiología sensorial
sensory quality cualidad sensorial
sensory-reaction type tipo de reacción sensorial
sensory register registro sensorial

sensory root raíz sensorial
sensory self-stimulation autoestimulación
  sensorial
sensory stimulation estimulación sensorial
sensory stimulus estímulo sensorial
sensory system sistema sensorial
sensory test prueba sensorial
sensory transduction transducción sensorial
sensual sensual
sensualism sensualismo
sensuality sensualidad
sensum sentido
sensuous sensual
sentence-completion method método de
  terminación de oraciones
sentence-completion test prueba de
  terminación de oraciones
sentence-repetition test prueba de repetición
  de oraciones
sentience percepción básica
sentient consciente
sentiment sentimiento
sentimentality sentimentalismo
separation separación
separation anxiety ansiedad de separación
separation anxiety disorder trastorno de
  ansiedad de separación
separation anxiety disorder of childhood
  trastorno de ansiedad de separación de
  niñez
separation distress angustia de separación
separation-individuation
  separación-individuación
sepsis sepsis
septal septal
septal area área septal
septic séptico
septicemia septicemia
septicemia psychosis psicosis de septicemia
septooptic dysplasia displasia septoóptica
septum septum
septum pellucidum septum pellucidum
sequela secuela
sequence secuencia
sequence preference preferencia de secuencia
sequential secuencial
sequential analysis análisis secuencial
sequential design diseño secuencial
sequential marriages matrimonios
  secuenciales
sequential memory memoria secuencial
sequential test prueba secuencial
sequestration separación, secuestro
serendipity serendipismo
serial serial
serial-anticipation method método de
  anticipación serial
serial association asociación serial
serial behavior conducta serial
serial discriminator discriminador serial
serial exploration exploración serial
serial-exploration method método de
  exploración serial
serial interpretation interpretación serial
serial learning aprendizaje serial

serial memory memoria serial
serial-memory search búsqueda de memoria
  serial
serial monogamy monogamia serial
serial-order learning aprendizaje de orden
  serial
serial polygamy poligamia serial
serial-position curve curva de posición serial
serial-position effect efecto de posición serial
serial processing procesamiento serial
serial recall recordación serial
serial response respuesta serial
serial search búsqueda serial
serialization serialización
seriation seriación
series serie
serotonergic serotonérgico
serotonergic neuron neurona serotonérgica
serotonergic receptor receptor serotonérgico
serotonergic synapse sinapsis serotonérgica
serotonergic tract tracto serotonérgico
serotonin serotonina
serotonin inhibitor inhibidor de serotonina
serotonin receptor receptor de serotonina
serous seroso
serous apoplexy apoplejía serosa
serous meningitis meningitis serosa
serous otitis media otitis media serosa
serpentine aneurysm aneurisma serpentino
Sertoli cells células de Sertoli
serum suero
serum albumin albúmina sérica
serum amylase amilasa sérica
serum bicarbonate bicarbonato sérico
serum bromide bromuro sérico
serum caffeine level nivel de cafeína sérico
serum calcium calcio sérico
serum ceruloplasmin ceruloplasmina sérica
serum chloride cloruro sérico
serum copper cobre sérico
serum ferritin ferritina sérica
serum folate folato sérico
serum folic acid ácido fólico sérico
serum glutamic-pyruvic transaminase
  transaminasa glutámica-pirúvica sérica
serum glutamyl transaminase transaminasa
  glutamil sérica
serum heavy metal intoxication intoxicación
  por metal pesado sérico
serum iron hierro sérico
serum level nivel sérico
serum magnesium magnesio sérico
serum phosphorous fósforo sérico
serum potassium potasio sérico
serum prolactin prolactina sérica
serum protein proteína sérica
serum salicylate salicilato sérico
serum sodium sodio sérico
serum testosterone testosterona sérica
serum vitamin A vitamina A sérica
serum vitamin B-12 vitamina B-12 sérica
servomechanism servomecanismo
set conjunto, predisposición
set point punto fijo
seventh cranial nerve séptimo nervio craneal

seventh sense séptimo sentido
severe mental retardation retardo metal severo
severity severidad
sewing spasm espasmo de costurero
sex anomaly anomalía sexual
sex-appropriate behavior conducta apropiada de sexo
sex assignment asignación sexual
sex change cambio de sexo
sex characteristics características sexuales
sex chromatin cromatina sexual
sex-chromosomal aberration aberración cromosómica sexual
sex chromosome cromosoma sexual
sex chromosome disorder trastorno de cromosoma sexual
sex counseling asesoramiento sexual
sex determination determinación de sexo
sex differences diferencias sexuales
sex differentiation diferenciación sexual
sex discrimination discriminación sexual
sex distribution distribución sexual
sex drive impulso sexual
sex education educación sexual
sex fear temor al sexo
sex feeling sensación sexual
sex hormone hormona sexual
sex hygiene higiene sexual
sex identification identificación sexual
sex identity identidad sexual
sex-influenced character caracter influenciado por sexo
sex-influenced gene gen influenciado por sexo
sex instinct instinto sexual
sex interest interés sexual
sex-limited limitado por sexo
sex linkage enlace al sexo
sex-linked ligado al sexo
sex-linked character carácter ligado al sexo
sex-linked gene gen ligado al sexo
sex object objeto sexual
sex offender ofensor sexual
sex offense ofensa sexual
sex organs órganos sexuales
sex perversion perversión sexual
sex preselection preselección de sexo
sex ratio razón sexual
sex reassignment reasignación sexual
sex rehabilitation rehabilitación sexual
sex reversal inversión de sexo
sex rivalry rivalidad sexual
sex role papel sexual
sex-role development desarrollo de papel sexual
sex-role inversion inversión de papeles sexuales
sex-role stereotype estereotipo de papel sexual
sex selection selección sexual
sex sensations sensaciones sexuales
sex service servicio sexual
sex therapy terapia sexual
sex trauma trauma sexual
sex-typed categorizado por sexo

sex-typing tipificación sexual
sexism sexismo
sexological sexológico
sexological examination examinación sexológica
sexology sexología
sexopathy sexopatía
sexual aberration aberración sexual
sexual abstinence abstinencia sexual
sexual abuse abuso sexual
sexual abuse and day care abuso sexual y cuidado diurno
sexual abuse of adult abuso sexual de adulto
sexual abuse of child abuso sexual de niño
sexual adjustment ajuste sexual
sexual aggression agresión sexual
sexual aim fin sexual
sexual anesthesia anestesia sexual
sexual anomaly anomalía sexual
sexual anorexia anorexia sexual
sexual anxiety ansiedad sexual
sexual apathy apatía sexual
sexual arousal despertamiento sexual
sexual arousal disorder trastorno del despertamiento sexual
sexual assault acometimiento sexual
sexual attitude restructuring program programa de reestructuración de actitudes sexuales
sexual attitudes actitudes sexuales
sexual aversion aversión sexual
sexual aversion disorder trastorno del aversión sexual
sexual behavior conducta sexual
sexual behavioral problems problemas conductuales sexuales
sexual change cambio sexual
sexual characteristics características sexuales
sexual concern preocupación sexual
sexual contact contacto sexual
sexual counseling asesoramiento sexual
sexual curiosity curiosidad sexual
sexual delusion delusión sexual
sexual desire deseo sexual
sexual desire disorder trastorno del deseo sexual
sexual development desarrollo sexual
sexual deviancy desviación sexual
sexual deviation desviación sexual
sexual differentiation diferenciación sexual
sexual dimorphism dimorfismo sexual
sexual discrimination discriminación sexual
sexual disorder trastorno sexual
sexual domination dominación sexual
sexual drive impulso sexual
sexual dysfunction disfunción sexual
sexual dysfunction due to general medical condition disfunción sexual debido a condición médica general
sexual education educación sexual
sexual energy energía sexual
sexual exhibition exhibición sexual
sexual expectations expectativas sexuales
sexual exploration exploración sexual
sexual fantasy fantasía sexual

sexual feeling sensación sexual
sexual functioning funcionamiento sexual
sexual guilt culpabilidad sexual
sexual harassment hostigamiento sexual
sexual health salud sexual
sexual history historial sexual
sexual hygiene higiene sexual
sexual identification identificación sexual
sexual identity identidad sexual
sexual infantilism infantilismo sexual
sexual inhibition inhibición sexual
sexual instinct instinto sexual
sexual intercourse relación sexual
sexual interest interés sexual
sexual inversion inversión sexual
sexual involution involución sexual
sexual latency latencia sexual
sexual life vida sexual
sexual lifestyle estilo de vida sexual
sexual love amor sexual
sexual masochism masoquismo sexual
sexual maturation maduración sexual
sexual maturity madurez sexual
sexual molestation acoso sexual
sexual motivation motivación sexual
sexual negativism negativismo sexual
sexual neurasthenia neurastenia sexual
sexual object objeto sexual
sexual offender ofensor sexual
sexual offense ofensa sexual
sexual orgasm orgasmo sexual
sexual orientation orientación sexual
sexual-orientation distress angustia por
    orientación sexual
sexual-orientation disturbance disturbio de
    orientación sexual
sexual pain dolor sexual
sexual pain disorder trastorno de dolor sexual
sexual partner pareja sexual
sexual perversion perversión sexual
sexual polarization polarización sexual
sexual potency potencia sexual
sexual preference preferencia sexual
sexual problem problema sexual
sexual provocation provocación sexual
sexual readiness disposición sexual
sexual reassignment reasignación sexual
sexual reflex reflejo sexual
sexual regulation regulación sexual
sexual rehabilitation rehabilitación sexual
sexual reproduction reproducción sexual
sexual response respuesta sexual
sexual response cycle ciclo de respuestas
    sexuales
sexual rivalry rivalidad sexual
sexual role papel sexual
sexual sadism sadismo sexual
sexual sadomasochism sadomasoquismo
    sexual
sexual script libreto sexual
sexual selection selección sexual
sexual self-esteem autoestima sexual
sexual sensation sensación sexual
sexual stimulation estimulación sexual
sexual surrogate sustituto sexual

sexual synergism sinergismo sexual
sexual tension tensión sexual
sexual trauma trauma sexual
sexual value system sistema de valores sexual
sexual vandalism vandalismo sexual
sexualism sexualismo
sexuality sexualidad
sexuality in adolescence sexualidad en
    adolescencia
sexuality index índice de sexualidad
sexuality of dream content sexualidad del
    contenido de sueños
sexualization sexualización
sexualize sexualizar
sexually sexualmente
sexually transmitted disease enfermedad
    transmitida sexualmente
shadowing repetición inmediata
shaking palsy parálisis temblorosa
shallowness of affect superficialidad de afecto
sham disorder trastorno simulado
sham feeding alimentación simulada
sham feeding procedure procedimiento de
    alimentación simulada
sham-movement vertigo vértigo de
    movimientos falsos
sham operation operación simulada
sham rage rabia simulada
sham surgery cirugía simulada
shaman chamán
shame vergüenza
shamelessness desvergüenza
shape constancy constancia de forma
shaping modelamiento
shared paranoid disorder trastorno paranoide
    compartido
shared psychotic disorder trastorno psicótico
    compartido
shared reality realidad compartida
shaving cramp calambre de afeitar
Sheehan's syndrome síndrome de Sheehan
Sheldon's constitutional theory teoría
    constitucional de Sheldon
Sheldon's constitutional theory of personality
    teoría constitucional de Sheldon de
    personalidad
shell shock choque por casquillos
shelter care cuidado en refugio
sheltered workshop taller refugiado
Sherrington's law ley de Sherrington
Sherrington phenomenon fenómeno de
    Sherrington
Shipley-Hartford scale escala de
    Shipley-Hartford
shiver tiritar
shock choque
shock phase fase de choque
shock-shock interval intervalo choque-choque
shock therapy terapia de choques
shock treatment tratamiento de choques
short-answer test prueba de respuestas cortas
short-circuit appeal atractivo de corto
    circuito
short-circuiting cortocircuitado
short-stare epilepsy epilepsia de mirada fija

corta
short-term a corto plazo
short-term anxiety-provoking psychotherapy psicoterapia provocante de ansiedad a corto plazo
short-term memory memoria a corto plazo
short-term psychotherapy psicoterapia a corto plazo
short-term therapy terapia a corto plazo
shoulder-girdle syndrome síndrome hombro-cinturón
shoulder-hand syndrome síndrome hombro-mano
shudder estremecimiento
shut-in personality personalidad encerrada
shuttle box caja dividida en dos
Shy-Drager syndrome síndrome de Shy-Drager
shyness timidez
shyness disorder trastorno de timidez
sialidosis sialidosis
sialoaerophagy sialoaerofagia
sialorrhea sialorrea
Siamese twins gemelos siameses
sibilant sibilante
sibling hermano, hermana
sibling relational problem problema relacional de hermanos
sibling relationship relación de hermanos
sibling rivalry rivalidad de hermanos
sicchasia sicasia
sick enfermo
sick headache migraña
sick role papel de enfermo
sickness enfermedad
side effect efecto secundario
side impulse impulso secundario
sideration sideración
siderodromophobia siderodromofobia
siderophobia siderofobia
Sidman avoidance evitación de Sidman
Sidman avoidance schedule programa de evitación de Sidman
Siegert's sign signo de Siegert
Siemerling-Creutzfeldt disease enfermedad de Siemerling-Creutzfeldt
sigh suspiro
sight vista
sight method método de vista
sight vocabulary vocabulario de vista
sight word palabra de vista
sigma sigma
sigma score puntuación sigma
sigmation sigmación
sigmatism sigmatismo
sign signo
sign blindness ceguera de signos
sign language lenguaje de signos
sign learning aprendizaje por signos
sign of the orbicularis signo del orbicular
sign-significance relation relación de significación de signos
sign stimulus estímulo por signo
sign system sistema de signos
sign test prueba de signos

signal señal
signal anxiety ansiedad de señal
signal-detection task tarea de detección de señales
signal-detection theory teoría de detección de señales
signal-to-noise ratio razón de señal a ruido
signaled señalado
signaling system sistema de señalamiento
significance significación
significance level nivel de significación
significant significante
significant difference diferencia significativa
significant other otro significante
signify significar
Signorelli's sign signo de Signorelli
silence silencio
silent silencioso
silent area área silenciosa
silent pause pausa silenciosa
silent period periodo silencioso
silent speech habla silenciosa
Silver's syndrome síndrome de Silver
Silver-Russell syndrome síndrome de Silver-Russell
similarities test prueba de similitudes
similarity similitud
similarity paradox paradoja de similitud
Simmonds' disease enfermedad de Simmonds
Simon's sign signo de Simon
simple absence ausencia simple
simple causation causalidad simple
simple correlation correlación simple
simple depression depresión simple
simple mastectomy mastectomía simple
simple phobia fobia simple
simple schizophrenia esquizofrenia simple
simple skull fracture fractura de cráneo simple
simple structure estructura simple
simple tone tono simple
simple type tipo simple
simulant simulador
simulate simular
simulated simulado
simulated environment ambiente simulado
simulated family familia simulada
simulation simulación
simulator simulador
simultagnosia simultagnosia
simultanagnosia simultanagnosia
simultaneity simultaneidad
simultaneous simultáneo
simultaneous conditioning condicionamiento simultáneo
simultaneous contrast contraste simultáneo
simultaneous fertilization fertilización simultánea
simultaneous tactile sensation sensación táctil simultánea
sine wave onda senoidal
single-blind study estudio ciego
single-case experimental design diseño experimental de caso único
single-channel model modelo de canal único

single custody custodia única
single-episode depression depresión de
  episodio único
single-gene defect defecto de gen único
single-parent family familia de padre solo,
  familia de madre sola
single photon emission tomography
  tomografía de emisión de fotón único
single-subject design diseño de sujeto único
single-unit recording registro de unidad única
single-variable technique técnica de variable
  única
single word stage etapa de palabra única
singultus singulto
sinistral sinistral
sinistrality sinistralidad
sinistropedal sinistropedal
sinography sinografía
sinus seno
sinus phlebitis flebitis sinusal
sinus reflex reflejo sinusal
sinus rhomboidalis seno romboidal
sinusoidal sinusoidal
sitiophobia sitofobia
sitophobia sitofobia
situated identities identidades situadas
situation situación
situation anxiety ansiedad de situación
situation neurosis neurosis de situación
situation set predisposición para una situación
situation test prueba de situación
situational situacional
situational analysis análisis situacional
situational anxiety ansiedad situacional
situational approach acercamiento situacional
situational crisis crisis situacional
situational depression depresión situacional
situational determinant determinante
  situacional
situational homosexuality homosexualidad
  situacional
situational hypoactive sexual desire deseo
  sexual hipoactivo situacional
situational neurosis neurosis situacional
situational orgasmic dysfunction disfunción
  orgásmica situacional
situational psychosis psicosis situacional
situational reaction reacción situacional
situational sampling muestreo situacional
situational-stress test prueba de estrés
  situacional
situational test prueba situacional
situational therapy terapia situacional
situationalism situacionalismo
sixth cranial nerve sexto nervio craneal
sixth sense sexto sentido
size-age confusion confusión de tamaño-edad
size constancy constancia de tamaño
size discrimination discriminación de tamaños
size perception percepción de tamaño
size-weight illusion ilusión de tamaño-peso
Sjogren-Larsson syndrome síndrome de
  Sjogren-Larsson
Sjoqvist tractotomy tractotomía de Sjoqvist
Skaggs-Robinson hypothesis hipótesis de

Skaggs-Robinson
skeletal esqueletal
skeletal age edad esqueletal
skeletal muscle músculo esqueletal
skeletal-system deformity deformidad del
  sistema esqueletal
Skene's glands glándulas de Skene
skewness asimetría
skiascope esquiascopio
skill destreza
skill learning aprendizaje de destreza
skin conductance response respuesta de
  conductancia cutánea
skin disease enfermedad cutánea
skin disorder trastorno cutáneo
skin eroticism erotismo cutáneo
skin-muscle reflex reflejo cutáneo-muscular
skin potential potencial cutáneo
skin-pupillary reflex reflejo cutáneo-pupilar
skin receptor receptor cutáneo
skin reflex reflejo cutáneo
skin sense sentido cutáneo
skin stimulation estimulación cutánea
Skinner box caja de Skinner
skinnerian conditioning condicionamiento de
  Skinner
skull cráneo
skull fracture fractura de cráneo
sleep sueño
sleep apnea apnea del sueño
sleep architecture arquitectura del sueño
sleep center centro del sueño
sleep characteristics características del sueño
sleep deprivation privación del sueño
sleep disorder trastorno del sueño
sleep disorder due to general medical
  condition trastorno del sueño debido a
  condición médica general
sleep dissociation disociación del sueño
sleep disturbance disturbio del sueño
sleep drive impulso de sueño
sleep drunkenness embriaguez del sueño
sleep efficiency eficiencia del sueño
sleep epilepsy epilepsia del sueño
sleep fear temor al sueño
sleep history historial del sueño
sleep-induced apnea apnea inducida por el
  sueño
sleep-induced respiratory ailment dolencia
  respiratoria inducida por el sueño
sleep-inducing peptide péptido inducidor de
  sueño
sleep latency latencia del sueño
sleep learning aprendizaje en sueño
sleep mentation mentación del sueño
sleep numbness entumecimiento del sueño
sleep paralysis parálisis del sueño
sleep patterns patrones del sueño
sleep patterns in autism patrones del sueño
  en autismo
sleep patterns in depression patrones del
  sueño en depresión
sleep reports informes del sueño
sleep research investigación del sueño
sleep restriction therapy terapia de

restricción del sueño
sleep rhythm ritmo del sueño
sleep spindle huso del sueño
sleep stages etapas del sueño
sleep state estado de sueño
sleep terror disorder trastorno de terror del
  sueño
sleep time tiempo de sueño
sleep treatment tratamiento de sueño
sleep-wake cycle ciclo de dormir-despertar
sleep-wake schedule disorder trastorno del
  horario de dormir-despertar
sleepiness somnolencia
sleeping sickness enfermedad del dormir
sleeptalker somniloquista
sleeptalking somnilocuencia
sleepwalking sonambulismo
sleepwalking disorder trastorno de
  sonambulismo
sleeve graft injerto en manga
slip of the pen error de la pluma
slip of the tongue error de la lengua
slope pendiente
slow speech habla lenta
slow virus virus lento
slow-wave sleep sueño de ondas lentas
Sluder's syndrome síndrome de Sluder
slurred speech habla indistinta
small group grupo pequeño
small-penis complex complejo de pene
  pequeño
small-sample statistics estadística de muestras
  pequeñas
small-sample theory teoría de muestras
  pequeñas
smegma esmegma
smell olfato
smell blindness ceguera olfativa
smell mechanism mecanismo olfativo
smell prism prisma olfativa
Smellie's scissors tijeras de Smellie
Smith-Lemli-Opitz syndrome síndrome de
  Smith-Lemli-Opitz
Smith-Robinson operation operación de
  Smith-Robinson
smoking fumar
smoking behavior conducta de fumar
snapping reflex reflejo de castañeteo
Sneddon's syndrome síndrome de Sneddon
Snellen chart esquema de Snellen
Snellen test prueba de Snellen
snow blindness ceguera por nieve
sociability sociabilidad
sociability index índice de sociabilidad
sociability rating clasificación de sociabilidad
sociable sociable
sociable type tipo sociable
social social
social accommodation acomodación social
social action acción social
social-action program programa de acción
  social
social activity actividad social
social adaptation adaptación social
social-adequacy index índice de suficiencia

social
social adjustment ajuste social
social-adjustment theory teoría de ajuste
  social
social age edad social
social agency agencia social
social aggregate agregado social
social anchoring anclaje social
social animal animal social
social animism animismo social
social anorexia anorexia social
social anthropology antropología social
social anxiety ansiedad social
social assimilation asimilación social
social atmosphere atmósfera social
social atom átomo social
social attitude actitud social
social behavior conducta social
social being ser social
social bond vínculo social
social breakdown syndrome síndrome de
  colapso social
social case work trabajo de casos sociales
social category categoría social
social change cambio social
social class clase social
social climate clima social
social code código social
social cognition cognición social
social cohesion cohesión social
social comparison comparación social
social-comparison theory teoría de
  comparación social
social competence competencia social
social compliance acatamiento social
social consciousness conciencia social
social constructionism construccionismo
  social
social contact contacto social
social contagion contagio social
social context contexto social
social control control social
social cue señal social
social darwinism darwinismo social
social decrement decremento social
social density densidad social
social deprivation privación social
social deprivation syndrome síndrome de
  privación social
social desirability deseabilidad social
social-desirability bias sesgo de deseabilidad
  social
social determinism determinismo social
social development desarrollo social
social diagnosis diagnóstico social
social differentiation diferenciación social
social dilemma dilema social
social disability syndrome síndrome de
  discapacidad social
social disintegration desintegración social
social distance distancia social
social-distance scale escala de distancia social
social drive impulso social
social dyad díada social
social dynamics dinámica social

social ecology ecología social
social engineer ingeniero social
social equality igualdad social
social equilibrium equilibrio social
social exchange theory teoría de intercambio social
social facilitation facilitación social
social factor factor social
social feedback retroalimentación social
social fission fisión social
social fixity fijeza social
social flexibility flexibilidad social
social gerontology gerontología social
social group grupo social
social habit hábito social
social heritage herencia social
social hunger hambre social
social imitation imitación social
social immobility inmovilidad social
social impact impacto social
social-impact assessment evaluación de impacto social
social imperception impercepción social
social impulse impulso social
social increment incremento social
social indicator indicador social
social influence influencia social
social inhibition inhibición social
social-inquiry model modelo de indagación social
social insect insecto social
social instinct instinto social
social institution institución social
social integration integración social
social integration-disintegration model modelo de integración-desintegración social
social intelligence inteligencia social
social interaction interacción social
social interaction therapy terapia de interacción social
social interest interés social
social intervention intervención social
social introversion introversión social
social introversion scale escala de introversión social
social island isla social
social isolate aislado social
social isolation aislamiento social
social-isolation syndrome síndrome de aislamiento social
social lag atraso social
social learning aprendizaje social
social learning group therapy terapia de grupo de aprendizaje social
social learning theory teoría de aprendizaje social
social maladjustment inadaptación social
social masochism masoquismo social
social maturity madurez social
social meaning significado social
social mind mente social
social mobility movilidad social
social mores costumbres sociales
social motive motivo social
social movement movimiento social

social need necesidad social
social network red social
social network therapy terapia de red social
social norm norma social
social object objeto social
social order orden social
social organism organismo social
social organization organización social
social pathology patología social
social perception percepción social
social phenomenon fenómeno social
social phobia fobia social
social play juego social
social policy planning planificación de política social
social pressure presión social
social problem problema social
social process proceso social
social psychiatry psiquiatría social
social psychology psicología social
social psychophysiology psicofisiología social
social pyramid pirámide social
social quotient cociente social
social readjustment rating scale escala de clasificación de reajuste social
social reality realidad social
social recognition reconocimiento social
social recovery recuperación social
social reform reforma social
social rehabilitation rehabilitación social
social reinforcement refuerzo social
social rejection rechazo social
social relations test prueba de relaciones sociales
social resistance resistencia social
social responsibility responsabilidad social
social-responsibility norm norma de responsabilidad social
social role papel social
social sanction sanción social
social scale escala social
social selection selección social
social self yo social
social sensitivity sensibilidad social
social services servicios sociales
social-sexual relationship relación social-sexual
social situation situación social
social skills destrezas sociales
social skills deficit déficit de destrezas sociales
social skills training entrenamiento de destrezas sociales
social space espacio social
social status estado social
social stimulus estímulo social
social stratification estratificación social
social stress estrés social
social-stress theory teoría del estrés social
social stressor estresante social
social structure estructura social
social support apoyo social
social technology tecnología social
social tension tensión social
social therapy terapia social

social time tiempo social
social transmission transmisión social
social trap trampa social
social type tipo social
social value valor social
social welfare bienestar social
social welfare program programa de
   bienestar social
social withdrawal retirada social
social work trabajo social
social-work aide ayudante de trabajo social
social worker trabajador social
social zone zona social
socialization socialización
socialization of individuals socialización de
   individuos
socialization process proceso de socialización
socialize socializar
socialized socializado
socialized-aggressive conduct disorder
   trastorno de conducta agresiva socializada
socialized drive impulso socializado
socialized-nonaggressive conduct disorder
   trastorno de conducta no agresiva
   socializada
socialized speech habla socializada
socially socialmente
socially intimate model modelo socialmente
   íntimo
societal societal
societal-reaction theory teoría de reacción
   societal
society sociedad
sociobiology sociobiología
sociocenter sociocentro
sociocentric sociocéntrico
sociocentrism sociocentrismo
sociocognitive sociocognitivo
sociocosm sociocosmo
sociocultural sociocultural
sociocultural factors factores socioculturales
sociocultural milieu ambiente sociocultural
sociocultural psychiatry psiquiatría
   sociocultural
sociocusis sociocusis
sociodrama sociodrama
socioeconomic socioeconómico
socioeconomic factors factores
   socioeconómicos
socioeconomic status estado socioeconómico
socioempathy socioempatía
sociofugal space espacio sociófugo
sociogenesis sociogénesis
sociogenetics sociogenética
sociogenic sociogénico
sociogram sociograma
sociolinguistics sociolingüística
sociological sociológico
sociological determinism determinismo
   sociológico
sociological factors factores sociológicos
sociological measures medidas sociológicas
sociology sociología
sociomedical sociomédico
sociometric sociométrico

sociometric analysis análisis sociométrico
sociometric clique peña sociométrica
sociometric distance distancia sociométrica
sociometric test prueba sociométrica
sociometrics sociométrica
sociometry sociometría
socionomics socionomía
sociopath sociópata
sociopathic sociopático
sociopathic behavior conducta sociopática
sociopathic personality personalidad
   sociopática
sociopathic personality disorder trastorno de
   personalidad sociopática
sociopathic personality disturbance disturbio
   de personalidad sociopática
sociopathology sociopatología
sociopathy sociopatía
sociopetal space espacio sociópeto
sociosexual sociosexual
sociotaxis sociotaxis
sociotechnical sociotécnico
sociotechnical model modelo sociotécnico
sociotherapy socioterapia
sodium bicarbonate bicarbonato de sodio
sodium bromide bromuro de sodio
sodium-responsive periodic paralysis
   parálisis periódica responsiva al sodio
sodomist sodomista
sodomite sodomita
sodomy sodomía
soft palate paladar blando
softness suavidad
software programa
Sohval-Soffer syndrome síndrome de
   Sohval-Soffer
sole reflex reflejo plantar
sole tap reflex reflejo de golpecito plantar
solidarity solidaridad
solipsism solipsismo
solitary solitario
solitary aggressive type tipo agresivo solitario
solitary play juego solitario
solitude soledad
solution solución
solution learning aprendizaje por soluciones
solvent inhalation inhalación de solventes
soma soma
somaesthesia somestesia
somatagnosia somatagnosia
somatalgia somatalgia
somatesthesia somatestesia
somatesthetic somatestético
somatic somático
somatic cell célula somática
somatic compliance acatamiento somático
somatic concern preocupación somática
somatic delusion delusión somática
somatic disorder trastorno somático
somatic hallucination alucinación somática
somatic nervous system sistema nervioso
   somático
somatic obsession obsesión somática
somatic paranoid disorder trastorno
   paranoide somático

somatic receptor receptor somático
somatic sense sentido somático
somatic sensory area área sensorial somática
somatic therapy terapia somática
somatic weakness debilidad somática
somatist somatista
somatization somatización
somatization disorder trastorno de
  somatización
somatization reaction reacción de
  somatización
somatobiology somatobiología
somatoform somatoforme
somatoform disorder trastorno somatoforme
somatoform pain disorder trastorno de dolor
  somatoforme
somatoform scale escala somatoforme
somatogenesis somatogénesis
somatogenic somatogénico
somatogenic need necesidad somatogénica
somatognosia somatognosia
somatometry somatometría
somatopathic somatopático
somatopathic drinking beber somatopático
somatophrenia somatofrenia
somatoplasm somatoplasma
somatopsychic somatopsíquico
somatopsychic delusion delusión
  somatopsíquica
somatopsychic disorder trastorno
  somatopsíquico
somatopsychology somatopsicología
somatopsychosis somatopsicosis
somatosense somatosentido
somatosensory somatosensorial
somatosensory cortex corteza somatosensorial
somatosensory evoked potential potencial
  evocado somatosensorial
somatosensory evoked response respuesta
  evocada somatosensorial
somatosensory system sistema
  somatosensorial
somatosexual somatosexual
somatosexuality somatosexualidad
somatostatin somatostatina
somatotherapy somatoterapia
somatotonia somatotonía
somatotonic somatotónico
somatotonic temperament temperamento
  somatotónico
somatotopagnosia somatotopagnosia
somatotopagnosis somatotopagnosis
somatotopic somatotópico
somatotopic organization organización
  somatotópica
somatotopy somatotopia
somatotrophic somatotrófico
somatotrophic hormone hormona
  somatotrófica
somatotropin somatotropina
somatotype somatotipo
somatotypology somatotipología
somesthesia somestesia
somesthesis somestesis
somesthetic somestésico

somesthetic area área somestésica
somesthetic disorder trastorno somestésico
somesthetic stimulation estimulación
  somestésica
somesthetic system sistema somestésico
somite somita
somnambulance sonambulancia
somnambulic epilepsy epilepsia sonámbula
somnambulism sonambulismo
somnambulist sonámbulo
somnambulistic sonambulístico
somnambulistic state estado sonambulístico
somnambulistic trance trance sonambulístico
somnial somnial
somnifacient somnifaciente
somniferous somnífero
somnific somnífico
somnifugous somnífugo
somniloquence somnilocuencia
somniloquism somniloquismo
somniloquist somniquista
somniloquy somniloquia
somnipathist somnípata
somnipathy somnipatía
somnocinematograph somnocinematógrafo
somnocinematography somnocinematografía
somnolence somnolencia
somnolency somnolencia
somnolent somnoliento
somnolent detachment desprendimiento
  somnoliento
somnolentia somnolencia
somnolescent somnolescente
somnolism somnolismo
sonant sonante
sone sonio
sonic boom estampido sónico
sonoencephalogram sonoencefalograma
sonogram sonograma
sonography sonografía
sonometer sonómetro
sonomotor sonomotor
sonomotor response respuesta sonomotora
sophism sofisma
sophistry sofistería
sophomania sofomanía
sopor sopor
soporiferous soporífero
soporific soporífico
soporose soporoso
soporous soporoso
sororate sororato
sorting test prueba de clasificación
sotalol sotalol
Sotos syndrome síndrome de Sotos
sound sonido
sound frequency frecuencia de sonido
sound intensity intensidad de sonido
sound-level meter medidor de intensidad de
  sonido
sound localization localización de sonido
sound-pattern theory teoría de patrón de
  sonido
sound-pattern theory of hearing teoría de
  audición de patrón de sonido

sound perimetry perimetría de sonido
sound-pressure level nivel de presión de sonido
sound shadow sombra de sonido
sound spectrogram espectrograma de sonido
sound spectrograph espectrógrafo de sonido
sound spectrum espectro de sonido
sound wave onda de sonido
sour agrio
sour grapes uvas verdes
sour grapes mechanism mecanismo de uvas verdes
source fuente
source language lenguaje fuente
source trait rasgo fuente
space error error espacial
space factor factor espacial
space orientation orientación espacial
space perception percepción espacial
space psychology psicología espacial
space sense sentido espacial
spacing espaciamiento
span lapso
span of apprehension lapso de aprehensión
span of attention lapso de atención
span of consciousness lapso de conciencia
spasm espasmo
spasmodic espasmódico
spasmodic apoplexy apoplejía espasmódica
spasmodic diathesis diátesis espasmódica
spasmodic ergotism ergotismo espasmódico
spasmodic mydriasis midriasis espasmódica
spasmodic tic tic espasmódico
spasmodic torticollis tortícolis espasmódico
spasmogenic espasmogénico
spasmology espasmología
spasmolygmus espasmoligmo
spasmolysis espasmólisis
spasmolytic espasmolítico
spasmophemia espasmofemia
spasmophilia espasmofilia
spasmophilic espasmofílico
spasmophilic diathesis diátesis espasmofílica
spasmus spasmus
spasmus agitans spasmus agitans
spasmus caninus spasmus caninus
spasmus coordinatus spasmus coordinatus
spasmus nictitans spasmus nictitans
spasmus nutans spasmus nutans
spastic espástico
spastic abasia abasia espástica
spastic aphonia afonía espástica
spastic colitis colitis espástica
spastic diplegia diplejía espástica
spastic dysphonia disfonía espástica
spastic gait marcha espástica
spastic hemiparesis hemiparesia espástica
spastic hemiplegia hemiplejía espástica
spastic miosis miosis espástica
spastic mydriasis midriasis espástica
spastic paralysis parálisis espástica
spastic paraplegia paraplejía espástica
spastic speech habla espástica
spastic spinal paralysis parálisis espinal espástica

spasticity espasticidad
spasticity of conjugate gaze espasticidad de mirada fija conjugada
spatial espacial
spatial ability habilidad espacial
spatial agnosia agnosia espacial
spatial apractagnosia apractagnosia espacial
spatial conformance conformidad espacial
spatial contiguity contigüidad espacial
spatial density densidad espacial
spatial discrimination discriminación espacial
spatial disorder trastorno espacial
spatial orientation orientación espacial
spatial relationship relación espacial
spatial-reversal learning aprendizaje de inversión espacial
spatial summation sumación espacial
spatial threshold umbral espacial
spatial vision visión espacial
Spearman-Brown formula fórmula de Spearman-Brown
Spearman rank correlation correlación de rangos de Spearman
special aptitude aptitud especial
special-aptitude test prueba de aptitudes especiales
special case caso especial
special child niño especial
special class clase especial
special education educación especial
special factor factor especial
special scale escala especial
special school escuela especial
special sensation sensación especial
special sense sentido especial
special-symptom reaction reacción de síntoma especial
special vulnerability vulnerabilidad especial
species especie
species-specific específico de especie
species-specific behavior conducta específica de especie
species-typical típico de especie
specific específico
specific ability habilidad específica
specific aptitude aptitud específica
specific attitude theory teoría de actitud específica
specific developmental disorder trastorno del desarrollo específico
specific developmental dyslexia dislexia del desarrollo específica
specific dynamic pattern patrón dinámico específico
specific energies doctrine doctrina de energías específicas
specific excitant excitante específico
specific hunger hambre específica
specific inhibition inhibición específica
specific language disability discapacidad del lenguaje específica
specific learning disability discapacidad del aprendizaje específica
specific nerve energies energías nerviosas específicas

specific phobia fobia específica
specific-reaction theory teoría de reacción
  específica
specific reading disability discapacidad de
  lectura específica
specific transfer transferencia específica
specificity especificidad
specimen espécimen
specimen record registro de espécimen
specious present presente especioso
spectator espectador
spectator role papel de espectador
spectator therapy terapia de espectador
spectral espectral
spectral absorption absorción espectral
spectral-absorption curve curva de absorción
  espectral
spectral color color espectral
spectral-emission curve curva de emisiones
  espectrales
spectral hue matiz espectral
spectral sensitivity sensibilidad espectral
spectral-sensitivity curve curva de
  sensibilidad espectral
spectrograph espectrógrafo
spectrographic espectrográfico
spectrographic evidence prueba
  espectrográfica
spectrometer espectrómetro
spectrophobia espectrofobia
spectrophotometer espectrofotómetro
spectrophotometry espectrofotometría
spectroscope espectroscopio
spectrum espectro
speculation especulación
speculative especulativo
speculative psychology psicología
  especulativa
speech habla
speech act acto del habla
speech and hearing center centro del habla y
  audición
speech area área del habla
speech audiometry audiometría del habla
speech block bloqueo del habla
speech center centro del habla
speech correction corrección del habla
speech derailment descarrilamiento del habla
speech development desarrollo del habla
speech disorder trastorno del habla
speech disturbance disturbio del habla
speech function función del habla
speech impairment deterioro del habla
speech impediment impedimento del habla
speech in autism habla en autismo
speech lateralization lateralización del habla
speech origin origen del habla
speech pathology patología del habla
speech perception percepción del habla
speech production producción del habla
speech-reading lectura del habla
speech-reception threshold umbral de
  recepción del habla
speech rehabilitation rehabilitación del habla
speech-retarded child niño retardado del

habla
speech synthesizer sintetizador del habla
speech theory teoría del habla
speech therapy terapia del habla
speed velocidad
speed-accuracy tradeoff canje
  velocidad-precisión
speed reading lectura de velocidad
speed test prueba de velocidad
spelencephaly espelencefalia
Spens' syndrome síndrome de Spens
sperm esperma
sperm analysis análisis de esperma
spermatic espermático
spermatid espermátide
spermatocyte espermatocito
spermatogenesis espermatogénesis
spermatogonium espermatogonio
spermatophobia espermatofobia
spermatorrhea espermatorrea
spermatozoid espermatozoide
spermatozoon espermatozoo
spermaturia espermaturia
spermicide espermicida
sphenoidal esfenoidal
sphenoidal herniation herniación esfenoidal
sphenoiditis esfenoiditis
sphenoidostomy esfenoidostomía
sphenoidotomy esfenoidotomía
spheresthesia esferestesia
spherical aberration aberración esférica
sphincter esfínter
sphincter control control esfintérico
sphincter morality moralidad esfintérica
sphincteral achalasia acalasia esfinteral
sphingolipid esfingolípido
sphingolipidosis esfingolipidosis
sphygmograph esfigmógrafo
sphygmomanometer esfigmomanómetro
sphygmometer esfigmómetro
spider fantasy fantasía de arañas
Spielmeyer's acute swelling tumefacción
  aguda de Spielmeyer
Spielmeyer-Sjogren disease enfermedad de
  Spielmeyer-Sjogren
Spielmeyer-Vogt disease enfermedad de
  Spielmeyer-Vogt
spike punta
spike and wave complex complejo de punta y
  onda
spike potential potencial de punta
spike-wave activity actividad de punta-onda
spina espina
spina bifida espina bífida
spina bifida aperta espina bífida abierta
spina bifida cystica espina bífida quística
spina bifida manifesta espina bífida
  manifiesta
spina bifida occulta espina bífida oculta
spinal espinal
spinal accessory nerve nervio accesorio
  espinal
spinal anesthesia anestesia espinal
spinal angiography angiografía espinal
spinal animal animal espinal

spinal apoplexy   apoplejía espinal
spinal arteriography   arteriografía espinal
spinal ataxia   ataxia espinal
spinal atrophy   atrofia espinal
spinal block   bloqueo espinal
spinal canal   canal espinal
spinal column   columna espinal
spinal concussion   concusión espinal
spinal conditioning   condicionamiento espinal
spinal cord   médula espinal
spinal-cord disease   enfermedad de médula
   espinal
spinal-cord injury   lesión de médula espinal
spinal curvature   curvatura espinal
spinal decompression   descompresión espinal
spinal fluid   fluido espinal
spinal fusion   fusión espinal
spinal ganglion   ganglio espinal
spinal gate   puerta espinal
spinal headache   dolor de cabeza espinal
spinal meningitis   meningitis espinal
spinal nerves   nervios espinales
spinal paralysis   parálisis espinal
spinal pia mater   piamadre espinal
spinal poliomyelitis   poliomielitis espinal
spinal puncture   punción espinal
spinal pyramidotomy   piramidotomía espinal
spinal reflex   reflejo espinal
spinal root   raíz espinal
spinal shock   choque espinal
spinal stenosis   estenosis espinal
spinal tap   punción espinal
spinal tonus   tono espinal
spinal tractotomy   tractotomía espinal
spinal transection   transección espinal
spinal trigeminal nucleus   núcleo trigeminal
   espinal
spinal tumor   tumor espinal
spinant   espinante
spindle   huso
spindle wave   onda en huso
spine   espina
spine fusion   fusión espinal
spine sign   signo espinal
spinifungal   espinífugo
spinipetal   espinípeto
spinoadductor reflex   reflejo espinoaductor
spinocerebellar   espinocerebeloso
spinocerebellar tract   tracto espinocerebeloso
spinogalvanization   espinogalvanización
spinothalamic   espinotalámico
spinothalamic cordotomy   cordotomía
   espinotalámica
spinothalamic tract   tracto espinotalámico
spinothalamic tractotomy   tractotomía
   espinotalámica
spiperone   espiperona
spiral aftereffect   efecto posterior espiral
spiral ganglion   ganglio espiral
spiral test   prueba espiral
spiritual problem   problema espiritual
spirograph   espirógrafo
spirometer   espirómetro
splanchnesthesia   esplacnestesia
splanchnesthetic   esplacnestésico

splanchnesthetic sensibility   sensibilidad
   esplacnestésica
splanchnic   esplácnico
splanchnic anesthesia   anestesia esplácnica
splanchnicectomy   esplacnicectomía
splanchnicotomy   esplacnicotomía
splenetic   esplenético
splenium   esplenio
split   dividido
split brain   cerebro dividido
split-brain technique   técnica de cerebro
   dividido
split custody   custodia dividida
split-litter method   método de camada dividida
split personality   personalidad dividida
splitting   división
spoiled   consentido
spoiled child   niño consentido
spoiled-child reaction   reacción de niño
   consentido
spondylalgia   espondilalgia
spondylarthritis   espondilartritis
spondylarthrocace   espondilartrocace
spondylitic   espondilítico
spondylitis   espondilitis
spondylitis deformans   espondilitis deformante
spondylocace   espondilocace
spondylolisthesis   espondilolistesis
spondylolisthetic   espondilolistético
spondylolysis   espondilólisis
spondylomalacia   espondilomalacia
spondylopathy   espondilopatía
spondyloptosis   espondiloptosis
spondylopyosis   espondilopiosis
spondyloschisis   espondilosquisis
spondylosis   espondilosis
spondylosyndesis   espondilosindesis
spondylotomy   espondilotomía
spongiform   espongiforme
spongiform encephalopathy   encefalopatía
   espongiforme
spongioblast   espongioblasto
spongioblastoma   espongioblastoma
spongiocyte   espongiocito
spongy degeneration   degeneración esponjosa
spontaneity   espontaneidad
spontaneity test   prueba de espontaneidad
spontaneity therapy   terapia de espontaneidad
spontaneity training   entrenamiento de
   espontaneidad
spontaneous   espontaneo
spontaneous abortion   aborto espontaneo
spontaneous behavior   conducta espontanea
spontaneous discharge   descarga espontanea
spontaneous hypnosis   hipnosis espontanea
spontaneous imagery   imaginería espontanea
spontaneous movement   movimiento
   espontaneo
spontaneous neural activity   actividad neural
   espontanea
spontaneous recovery   recuperación
   espontanea
spontaneous regression   regresión espontanea
spontaneous remission   remisión espontanea
spontaneous thought   pensamiento espontaneo

spoonerism transposición de sonidos iniciales
sports psychology psicología de deportes
spouse cónyuge
spouse abuse abuso de cónyuge
spouse selection seleccíon de cónyuge
spread of effect propagación del efecto
spreading activation activación propagante
spreading depression depresión propagante
spring finger dedo en resorte
spurious espurio
spurious correlation correlación espuria
spurious meningocele meningocele espurio
spurious torticollis tortícolis espurio
spurt arranque
squeeze technique técnica de presión
squint estrabismo
stabilimeter estabilímetro
stability estabilidad
stability coefficient coeficiente de estabilidad
stability-lability estabilidad-labilidad
stabilized estabilizado
stabilized image imagen estabilizada
stabilized retinal image imagen retinal
    estabilizada
stable estable
staccato speech habla en staccato
stage etapa
stage of exhaustion etapa de agotamiento
stage of resistance etapa de resistencia
stage theory teoría de etapas
stages of sleep etapas del sueño
stagger tambalear
staggers torneo
stagnation estancación
stain colorante
staircase illusion ilusión de escalera
staircase method método de escalera
stalking behavior conducta acechante
stammer (n) tartamudeo
stammer (v) tartamudear
stammering tartamudeo
stance reflex reflejo postural
standard estándar
standard deviation desviación estándar
standard difference diferencia estándar
standard error error estándar
standard error of difference error estándar
    de diferencia
standard error of estimate error estándar del
    estimado
standard error of measurement error
    estándar de medición
standard error of the mean error estándar de
    la media
standard measure medida estándar
standard observer observador estándar
standard ratio razón estándar
standard score puntuación estándar
standard stimulus estímulo estándar
standardization estandarización
standardization group grupo de
    estandarización
standardization of a test estandarización de
    una prueba
standardization sample muestra de

estandarización
standardize estandarizar
standardized estandarizado
standardized interview schedule programa
    de entrevistas estandarizada
standardized measuring device dispositivo de
    medición estandarizada
standardized score puntuación estandarizada
standardized test prueba estandarizada
stapedectomy estapedectomía
stapedius estapedio
stapes estribo
staphyloplegia stafiloplejía
stare mirada fija
Starling's reflex reflejo de Starling
startle sobresalto
startle epilepsy epilepsia por sobresalto
startle reaction reacción de sobresalto
startle reflex reflejo de sobresalto
startle response respuesta de sobresalto
starvation reactions reacciones de hambre
stasibasiphobia estasibasifobia
stasiphobia estasifobia
stasis estasis
stasobasophobia estasobasofobia
stasophobia estasofobia
state estado
state dependence dependencia del estado
state-dependent dependiente del estado
state-dependent learning aprendizaje
    dependiente del estado
state-dependent memory memoria
    dependiente del estado
state of arousal estado de despertamiento
static estático
static ataxia ataxia estática
static convulsion convulsión estática
static equilibrium equilibrio estático
static infantilism infantilismo estático
static reflex reflejo estático
static response respuesta estática
static sense sentido estático
static tremor temblor estático
station test prueba de estación
statistic estadística
statistical estadístico
statistical artifact artefacto estadístico
statistical association asociación estadística
statistical attenuation atenuación estadística
statistical control control estadístico
statistical dependence dependencia estadística
statistical error error estadístico
statistical inference inferencia estadística
statistical interaction interacción estadística
statistical law ley estadística
statistical-learning theory teoría de
    aprendizaje estadística
statistical paradigm paradigma estadística
statistical psychology psicología estadística
statistical regression regresión estadística
statistical significance significación estadística
statistical stability estabilidad estadística
statistical test prueba estadística
statistical trend tendencia estadística
statistics estadística

statoacoustic estatoacústico
statoacoustic nerve nervio estatoacústico
statoconia estatoconía
statocyst estatocisto
statokinetic estatocinético
statokinetic reflex reflejo estatocinético
statokinetic response respuesta estatocinética
statotonic reflex reflejo estatotónico
statue of Condillac estatua de Condillac
status estado
status choreicus estado coreico
status comparison comparación de estado
status convulsivus estado convulsivo
status cribrosus estado criboso
status criticus estado crítico
status dysmyelinisatus estado desmielinizado
status dysraphicus estado disráfico
status epilepticus estado epiléptico
status group grupo de estado
status grouping agrupamiento por estado
status hemicranicus estado hemicraneal
status hypnoticus estado hipnótico
status lacunaris estado lacunar
status marmoratus estado marmóreo
status need necesidad de estado alto
status nervosus estado nervioso
status raptus estado de rapto
status role papel de estado
status sequence secuencia de estados
status spongiosus estado esponjoso
status symbol símbolo de estado
status typhosus estado tifoso
status validity validez de estado
status vertiginosus estado vertiginoso
statutory rape violación estatutaria
statuvolence estatuvolencia
statuvolent estatuvolente
Stauder's lethal catatonia catatonía letal de
  Stauder
stauroplegia estauroplejía
steady estable
steady state estado estable
stealing hurto
Stearns' alcoholic amentia amencia
  alcohólica de Stearns
steatopygia esteatopigia
steatopygy esteatopigia
Steele-Richardson-Olszewski disease
  enfermedad de
  Steele-Richardson-Olszewski
Steele-Richardson-Olszewski syndrome
  síndrome de Steele-Richardson-Olszewski
Steinert's disease enfermedad de Steinert
stellate cell célula estrellada
stellate skull fracture fractura de cráneo
  estrellada
stellectomy estelectomía
sten estén
stenosis estenosis
stenostenosis estenoestenosis
step function función de pasos
step interval intervalo de pasos
stepbrother hermanastro
stepchild alnado, alnada
steppage estepaje

steppage gait marcha de estepaje
stepparent padrastro, madrastra
stepsister hermanastra
stepwise phenomenon fenómeno escalonado
stereoagnosis estereoagnosis
stereoanesthesia estereoanestesia
stereochemical estereoquímico
stereochemical theory teoría estereoquímica
stereochemical theory of smell teoría
  estereoquímica del olfato
stereocilium estereocilio
stereoelectroencephalography
  estereoelectroencefalografía
stereoencephalometry estereoencefalometría
stereoencephalotomy estereoencefalotomía
stereognosis estereognosia
stereognostic estereognóstico
stereogram estereograma
stereopathy estereopatía
stereopsis estereopsis
stereopsyche esteropsiquis
stereoscope estereoscopio
stereoscopic estereoscópico
stereoscopic acuity agudeza estereoscópica
stereoscopic vision visión estereoscópica
stereotactic estereotáctico
stereotactic cordotomy cordotomía
  estereotáctica
stereotactic instrument instrumento
  estereotáctico
stereotactic localization localización
  estereotáctica
stereotactic surgery cirugía estereotáctica
stereotactic tractotomy tractotomía
  estereotáctica
stereotaxic estereotáxico
stereotaxic cordotomy cordotomía
  estereotáxica
stereotaxic instrument instrumento
  estereotáxico
stereotaxic localization localización
  estereotáxica
stereotaxic surgery cirugía estereotáxica
stereotaxic technique técnica estereotáxica
stereotaxis estereotaxis
stereotaxy estereotaxia
stereotropism estereotropismo
stereotype estereotipo
stereotype accuracy precisión de estereotipo
stereotyped estereotipado
stereotyped behavior conducta estereotipada
stereotyped movement movimiento
  estereotipado
stereotyped-movement disorder trastorno de
  movimientos estereotipados
stereotypic estereotípico
stereotypic-movement disorder trastorno de
  movimientos estereotípicos
stereotypical estereotípico
stereotypical role papel estereotípico
stereotypy estereotipia
stereotypy and habit disorder trastorno de
  estereotipia y hábito
stereotypy disorder tratorno de estereotipia
steric estérico

steric theory of odor teoría estérica de olores
sterile estéril
sterility esterilidad
sterilization esterilización
Stern's disease enfermedad de Stern
sternal puncture punción esternal
Sternberg task tarea de Sternberg
sternobrachial reflex reflejo esternobraquial
sternocleidomastoid esternocleidomastoideo
sternutatory absence ausencia estornutatoria
steroid esteroide
steroid withdrawal syndrome síndrome del
   retiro de esteroides
stethoparalysis estetoparálisis
Stevens' law ley de Stevens
Stevens' power law ley de potencia de
   Stevens
Stevens-Johnson syndrome síndrome de
   Stevens-Johnson
Stewart-Holmes sign signo de
   Stewart-Holmes
Stewart-Morel syndrome síndrome de
   Stewart-Morel
sthenia estenia
sthenic esténico
sthenic type tipo esténico
sthenometer estenómetro
sthenoplastic estenoplástico
stiff neck cuello tieso
stigma estigma
stigmatic estigmático
stigmatism estigmatismo
stigmatization estigmatización
Stiles-Crawford effect efecto de
   Stiles-Crawford
Stiller's sign signo de Stiller
Stilling test prueba de Stilling
stilted speech habla tiesa
stimulant estimulante
stimulant abuse abuso de estimulantes
stimulating estimulante
stimulating occupation ocupación estimulante
stimulation estimulación
stimulation effects efectos de estimulación
stimulation method método de estimulación
stimulator estimulador
stimuli estímulos
stimulus estímulo
stimulus attitude actitud de estímulo
stimulus barrier barrera de estímulo
stimulus-bound ligado a estímulo
stimulus continuum continuo de estímulo
stimulus control control de estímulo
stimulus differentiation diferenciación de
   estímulos
stimulus discrimination discriminación de
   estímulos
stimulus element elemento de estímulo
stimulus equivalence equivalencia de
   estímulos
stimulus error error de estímulo
stimulus fading desvanecimiento de estímulo
stimulus field campo de estímulo
stimulus generalization generalización de
   estímulo

stimulus hunger hambre de estímulo
stimulus object objeto de estímulo
stimulus overload sobrecarga de estímulo
stimulus pattern patrón de estímulo
stimulus population población de estímulo
stimulus-processing function función de
   procesamiento de estímulos
stimulus-response estímulo-respuesta
stimulus-response learning aprendizaje por
   estímulo-respuesta
stimulus-response psychology psicología de
   estímulo-respuesta
stimulus-response theory teoría de
   estímulo-respuesta
stimulus-sampling theory teoría de muestreo
   de estímulos
stimulus sensitive myoclonus mioclono
   sensitivo a estímulos
stimulus set predisposición de estímulo
stimulus situation situación de estímulo
stimulus specificity especificidad de estímulo
stimulus-stimulus learning aprendizaje por
   estímulo-estímulo
stimulus substitution sustitución de estímulo
stimulus tension tensión de estímulo
stimulus threshold umbral de estímulo
stimulus trace rastro de estímulo
stimulus value valor de estímulo
stimulus variable variable de estímulo
stimulus word palabra de estímulo
stinginess tacañería
stochastic estocástico
Stockholm syndrome síndrome de Estocolmo
stocking anesthesia anestesia en media
Stoffel's operation operación de Stoffel
stoker's cramps calambres de fogoneros
Stokes' law ley de Stokes
Stokes-Adams disease enfermedad de
   Stokes-Adams
Stokes-Adams syndrome síndrome de
   Stokes-Adams
stoma estoma
stomach activity actividad estomacal
Stookey-Scarff operation operación de
   Stookey-Scarff
stopped image imagen detenida
storage almacenamiento
store almacén
stormy personality personalidad tormentosa
story-recall test prueba de recordación de
   cuento
strabismus estrabismo
strain esfuerzo, raza
straitjacket chaleco de fuerza
strangalesthesia estrangalestesia
strange-hand sign signo de mano extraña
stranger anxiety ansiedad ante extraños
strangulated affect afecto estrangulado
strategic estratégico
strategic compliance acatamiento estratégico
strategic family therapy terapia familiar
   estratégica
strategic intervention intervención estratégica
strategic planning planificación estratégica
strategy estrategia

stratification estratificación
stratified estratificado
stratified sample muestra estratificada
stratified sampling muestreo estratificado
Stratton's experiment experimento de
   Stratton
Straus' sign signo de Straus
Strauss' syndrome síndrome de Strauss
stream of action corriente de acción
stream of consciousness corriente de
   conciencia
stream of thought corriente de pensamiento
street drugs drogas callejeras
strephosymbolia estrefosimbolia
stress estrés
stress-decompensation model modelo de
   estrés-descompensación
stress disorder trastorno de estrés
stress immunity inmunidad de estrés
stress in adolescence estrés en adolescencia
stress in infancy estrés en infancia
stress inoculation inoculación para estrés
stress inoculation training entrenamiento de
   inoculación para estrés
stress interview entrevista bajo estrés
stress management administración de estrés
stress reaction reacción de estrés
stress reduction reducción de estrés
stress related disorder trastorno relacionado
   al estrés
stress response syndrome síndrome de
   respuesta al estrés
stress situation situación de estrés
stress test prueba de estrés
stress theory teoría de estrés
stress tolerance tolerancia de estrés
stressor estresante
stretch receptor receptor de estiramiento
stretch reflex reflejo de estiramiento
stria atrophicae estrías atróficas
stria terminalis estría terminal
striate estriado
striate body cuerpo estriado
striate cortex corteza estriada
striate muscle músculo estriado
striated estriado
striatum estriado
strident estridente
string hilera
stripe of Gennari banda de Gennari
stroboscope estroboscopio
stroboscopic estroboscópico
stroboscopic effect efecto estroboscópico
stroboscopic illusion ilusión estroboscópica
stroboscopic motion moción estroboscópica
stroke ataque, golpe
strong law of effect ley de efecto fuerte
Stroop test prueba de Stroop
structural estructural
structural analysis análisis estructural
structural approach acercamiento estructural
structural family therapy terapia familiar
   estructural
structural hypothesis hipótesis estructural
structural imbalance desequilibrio estructural

structural integration integración estructural
structural matrix matriz estructural
structural model modelo estructural
structural profile perfil estructural
structural psychology psicología estructural
structural scoliosis escoliosis estructural
structural-strategic therapy terapia
   estructural-estratégica
structural therapy terapia estructural
structuralism estructuralismo
structure estructura
structure-of-intellect model modelo de
   estructura de intelecto
structured estructurado
structured family therapy terapia familiar
   estructurada
structured group grupo estructurado
structured interactional group
   psychotherapy psicoterapia de grupo
   interaccional estructurada
structured interview entrevista estructurada
structured stimulus estímulo estructurado
Strumpell's disease enfermedad de Strumpell
Strumpell's phenomenon fenómeno de
   Strumpell
Strumpell's reflex reflejo de Strumpell
Strumpell-Marie disease enfermedad de
   Strumpell-Marie
Strumpell-Westphal disease enfermedad de
   Strumpell-Westphal
strychnine estricnina
strychninism estricninismo
student's disease enfermedad del estudiante
Student's distribution distribución de Student
Student's test prueba de Student
study estudio
stump muñón
stump hallucination alucinación de muñón
stump neuralgia neuralgia de muñón
stun aturdir
stupefacient estupefaciente
stupefactive estupefactivo
stupor estupor
stuporous estuporoso
stuporous catatonia catatonía estuporosa
stuporous depression depresión estuporosa
stuporous mania manía estuporosa
Sturge's disease enfermedad de Sturge
Sturge-Kalischer-Weber syndrome síndrome
   de Sturge-Kalischer-Weber
Sturge-Weber-Dimitri disease enfermedad de
   Sturge-Weber-Dimitri
Sturge-Weber disease enfermedad de
   Sturge-Weber
Sturge-Weber syndrome síndrome de
   Sturge-Weber
stutter (n) tartamudeo
stutter (v) tartamudear
stuttering tartamudez
stygiophobia estigiofobia
style of life estilo de vida
styloradial reflex reflejo estilorradial
subacute subagudo
subacute cerebellar degeneration
   degeneración cerebelosa subaguda

subacute combined degeneration of the spinal cord degeneración combinada subaguda de la médula espinal

subacute delirious state estado delirante subagudo

subacute inclusion body encephalitis encefalitis de cuerpos de inclusión subaguda

subacute necrotizing encephalomyelopathy encefalomielopatía necrotizante subaguda

subacute necrotizing myelitis mielitis necrotizante subaguda

subacute sclerosing leukoencephalitis leucoencefalitis esclerosante subaguda

subacute sclerosing panencephalitis panencefalitis esclerosante subaguda

subacute spongiform encephalopathy encefalopatía espongiforme subaguda

subaffective subafectivo

subaffective dysthymia distimia subafectiva

subaffective spectrum espectro subafectivo

subarachnoid subaracnoideo

subarachnoid hemorrhage hemorragia subaracnoidea

subarachnoid space espacio subaracnoideo

subaverage intellectual functioning funcionamiento intelectual bajo promedio

subcallosal subcalloso

subcallosal gyrus circunvolución subcallosa

subception subcepción

subclavian subclavio

subclavian steal secuestro subclavio

subclavian steal syndrome síndrome de secuestro subclavio

subclinical subclínico

subclinical absence ausencia subclínica

subcoma subcoma

subcoma insulin treatment tratamiento de insulina subcoma

subconscious subconsciente

subconscious memory memoria subconsciente

subconscious mind mente subconsciente

subconscious personality personalidad subconsciente

subconsciousness subconsciencia

subcortical subcortical

subcortical arteriosclerotic encephalopathy encefalopatía arterioesclerótica subcortical

subcortical dementia demencia subcortical

subcortical encephalopathy encefalopatía subcortical

subcortical learning aprendizaje subcortical

subculture subcultura

subcutaneous subcutáneo

subcutaneous injection inyección subcutánea

subcutaneous sensibility sensibilidad subcutánea

subdelirious subdelirante

subdelirious state estado subdelirante

subdelirium subdelirio

subdural subdural

subdural hematoma hematoma subdural

subdural hematorrhachis hematorraquis subdural

subdural hemorrhage hemorragia subdural

subdural hygroma higroma subdural

subependymoma subependimoma

subfalcial subfalcial

subfalcial herniation herniación subfalcial

subfecundity subfecundidad

subgaleal subgaleal

subgaleal emphysema enfisema subgaleal

subgaleal hemorrhage hemorragia subgaleal

subgoal subfin

subgrundation subgrundación

subictal epilepsy epilepsia subictal

subject sujeto

subject-object differentiation diferenciación sujeto-objeto

subject variable variable de sujeto

subjection sujeción

subjective subjetivo

subjective attribute atributo subjetivo

subjective color color subjetivo

subjective contour contorno subjetivo

subjective equality igualdad subjetiva

subjective error error subjetivo

subjective examination examinación subjetiva

subjective expected utility utilidad esperada subjetiva

subjective frequency frecuencia subjetiva

subjective idealism idealismo subjetivo

subjective mentation mentación subjetiva

subjective organization organización subjetiva

subjective orientation orientación subjetiva

subjective-outcome value valor de resultados subjetivos

subjective probability probabilidad subjetiva

subjective psychology psicología subjetiva

subjective scoring tanteo subjetivo

subjective sensation sensación subjetiva

subjective test prueba subjetiva

subjective tone tono subjetivo

subjective vertigo vértigo subjetivo

subjective vision visión subjetiva

subjectivism subjetivismo

subjectivism factor factor de subjetivismo

subjectivity subjetividad

sublimate sublimar

sublimation sublimación

sublimation difficulty dificultad de sublimación

subliminal subliminal

subliminal consciousness conciencia subliminal

subliminal learning aprendizaje subliminal

subliminal perception percepción subliminal

subliminal self yo subliminal

subliminal stimulation estimulación subliminal

subliminal stimulus estímulo subliminal

submania submanía

submission sumisión

submissiveness sumisión

subnormal subnormal

subnormal period of neuron periodo de neurona subnormal

suboccipital suboccipital

suboccipital decompression descompresión

suboccipital
suboccipital neuralgia neuralgia suboccipital
suboccipital neuritis neuritis suboccipital
suboccipital puncture punción suboccipital
subordination subordinación
subpsyche subpsiquis
subshock subchoque
subshock insulin treatment tratamiento de insulina subchoque
subshock therapy terapia de subchoques
substance sustancia
substance abuse abuso de sustancia
substance abuse and child abuse abuso de sustancia y abuso de niños
substance abuse disorder trastorno de abuso de sustancia
substance abuse program programa de abuso de sustancias
substance addiction adicción a sustancia
substance dependence dependencia de sustancia
substance dependence disorder trastorno de dependencia de sustancia
substance-induced chronic psychosis psicosis crónica inducida por sustancia
substance-induced disorder trastorno inducido por sustancia
substance-induced mood disorder trastorno del humor inducido por sustancia
substance-induced organic mental disorder trastorno mental orgánico inducido por sustancia
substance-induced persisting dementia demencia persistente inducida por sustancia
substance-induced sexual dysfunction disfunción sexual inducida por sustancia
substance-induced sleep disorder trastorno del sueño inducido por sustancia
substance-induced syndrome síndrome inducido por sustancia
substance K sustancia K
substance P sustancia P
substance-related delirium delirio relacionado con sustancia
substance-related disorder trastorno relacionado con sustancia
substance-use disorder trastorno de uso de sustancia
substance withdrawal retiro de sustancia
substantia gelatinosa sustancia gelatinosa
substantia nigra sustancia negra
substitute sustituto
substitute formation formación de sustituto
substitute valence valencia sustituta
substitution sustitución
substitution hypothesis hipótesis de sustitución
substitution test prueba de sustitución
substrate sustrato
subsultus subsultus
subsultus clonus subsultus clonus
subsultus tendinum subsultus tendinum
subtemporal subtemporal
subtemporal decompression descompresión subtemporal

subtest subprueba
subtetanic subtetánico
subthalamic subtalámico
subthalamic nucleus núcleo subtalámico
subthalamus subtálamo
subthreshold subumbral
subthreshold potential potencial subumbral
subthreshold stimulus estímulo subumbral
subtraction method método de substracción
subvocal subvocal
subvocal speech habla subvocal
subvocalization subvocalización
success neurosis neurosis del éxito
successive sucesivo
successive approximations aproximaciones sucesivas
successive-approximations method método de aproximaciones sucesivas
successive conditioning condicionamiento sucesivo
successive contrast contraste sucesivo
successive induction inducción sucesiva
successive-intervals method método de intervalos sucesivos
successive-practice method método de práctica sucesiva
successive reproductions reproducciones sucesivas
succinylcholine succinilcolina
succorance need necesidad de socorro
succubus súcubo
sucking reflex reflejo de succión
sudden súbito
sudden infant death syndrome síndrome de muerte de infante súbita
sudden insight penetración súbita
Sudeck's atrophy atrofia de Sudeck
Sudeck's syndrome síndrome de Sudeck
sudoriferous sudorífero
sudoriferous glands glándulas sudoríferas
suffer sufrir
suffering sufrimiento
suffix effect efecto de sufijo
sugar self-selection autoselección de azúcar
suggestibility sugestibilidad
suggestible sugestionable
suggestible stage etapa sugestionable
suggestion sugestión
suggestion therapy terapia de sugestión
suggestive sugestivo
suggestive psychotherapy psicoterapia sugestiva
suggestive therapeutics terapéutica sugestiva
sui generis sui generis
suicidal suicida
suicidal crisis crisis suicida
suicidal ideation ideación suicida
suicide suicidio
suicide attempt intento de suicidio
suicide gesture gesto de suicidio
suicide in adolescence suicidio en adolescencia
suicide prevention prevención de suicidios
suicide-prevention center centro de prevención de suicidios

suicide tendency tendencia suicida
suicidogenic suicidogénico
suicidology suicidología
suigenderism suigenerismo
sulcus surco
sulfate sulfato
sulfatide lipidosis lipidosis sulfátida
sulfatidosis sulfatidosis
sulpiride sulpirida
sum of squares suma de cuadrados
summation sumación, resumen
summation curve curva de sumación
summation effect efecto de sumación
summation tone tono de sumación
Sunday neurosis neurosis de domingo
superego superego
superego anxiety ansiedad del superego
superego lacuna laguna del superego
superego resistance resistencia del superego
superego sadism sadismo del superego
superexcitation superexcitación
superfecundation superfecundación
superfetation superfetación
superficial superficial
superficial reflex reflejo superficial
supergene supergen
superior superior
superior cerebellar artery syndrome
    síndrome arterial cerebeloso superior
superior colliculus colículo superior
superior function función superior
superior hemorrhagic polioencephalitis
    polioencefalitis hemorrágica superior
superior intelligence inteligencia superior
superior longitudinal fasciculus fascículo
    longitudinal superior
superior olivary complex complejo olivar
    superior
superior olivary nucleus núcleo olivar
    superior
superior paraplegia paraplejía superior
superior polioencephalitis polioencefalitis
    superior
superior pulmonary sulcus tumor tumor de
    surco pulmonar superior
superior sagittal sinus seno sagital superior
superiority complex complejo de superioridad
superiority feelings sensaciones de
    superioridad
supermotility supermovilidad
supernatural sobrenatural
supernormal supernormal
supernormal period periodo supernormal
supersonic supersónico
superstition superstición
superstitious supersticioso
superstitious behavior conducta supersticiosa
superstitious control control supersticioso
supervision supervisión
supination supinación
supination reflex reflejo de supinación
supinator jerk sacudida del supinador
supinator longus reflex reflejo del supinador
    largo
supinator reflex reflejo del supinador

supplementary motor area área motora
    suplemental
support apoyo
support group grupo de apoyo
supportive apoyador
supportive ego ego apoyador
supportive-expressive apoyador-expresivo
supportive-expressive psychotherapy
    psicoterapia apoyadora-expresiva
supportive group therapy terapia de grupo
    apoyador
supportive personnel personal apoyador
supportive psychotherapy psicoterapia
    apoyadora
supportive therapy terapia apoyadora
supposition suposición
suppression supresión
suppressive supresor
suppressive therapy terapia supresora
suppressor supresor
suppressor area área supresora
suppressor variable variable supresora
suppurative supurativo
suppurative cerebritis cerebritis supurativa
suppurative encephalitis encefalitis
    supurativa
suprachiasmatic nucleus núcleo
    supraquiasmático
supraclinoid supraclinoideo
supraclinoid aneurysm aneurisma
    supraclinoideo
supraliminal supraliminal
supraliminal stimulus estímulo supraliminal
supramarginal gyrus circunvolución
    supramarginal
supramaximal stimulus estímulo
    supramáximo
supranuclear supranuclear
supranuclear lesion lesión supranuclear
supranuclear palsy parálisis supranuclear
supranuclear paralysis parálisis supranuclear
supraorbital supraorbitario
supraorbital neuralgia neuralgia
    supraorbitaria
supraorbital reflex reflejo supraorbitario
suprapatellar suprarrotuliano
suprapatellar reflex reflejo suprarrotuliano
suprarenal suprarrenal
suprarenal gland glándula suprarrenal
suprarenalectomy suprarrenalectomía
suprasegmental suprasegmentario
suprasegmental reflex reflejo
    suprasegmentario
suprasellar supraselar
suprasellar cyst quiste supraselar
supratentorial supratentorial
supraumbilical supraumbilical
supraumbilical reflex reflejo supraumbilical
surd sordo
surdimutism sordomudez
surdity sordera
surface color color superficial
surface imaging producción de imagen
    superficial
surface pain dolor superficial

surface structure estructura superficial
surface therapy terapia superficial
surface trait rasgo superficial
surgency surgencia
surgery cirugía
surgical microscope microscopio quirúrgico
surrender rendición
surrogate sustituto
surrogate father padre sustituto
surrogate mother madre sustituta
surrogate partner pareja sustituta
surrogate sexual partner pareja sexual
  sustituta
sursumversion sursunversión
survey encuesta
survey research investigación por encuestas
survey test prueba de encuesta
survival guilt culpabilidad de supervivencia
survival of the fittest supervivencia del más
  apto
survival value valor de supervivencia
survivor guilt culpabilidad de supervivientes
survivor syndrome síndrome de superviviente
suspicion sospecha
suspicious sospechoso
suspiciousness recelo
sustentacular cell célula sustentacular
Sutton's law ley de Sutton
suture sutura
suturectomy suturectomía
swallowing reflex reflejo de tragar
sweating test prueba de sudación
sweet dulce
swelled head cabeza hinchada
swelling tumefacción
swimming reflex reflejo de natación
Swindle's ghost fantasma de Swindle
switch process proceso de cambio
Sydenham's chorea corea de Sydenham
Sydenham's disease enfermedad de
  Sydenham
syllabary silabario
syllabic speech habla silábica
syllabic synthesis síntesis silábica
syllable sílaba
syllogism silogismo
syllogistic reasoning razonamiento silogístico
symbiont simbionte
symbiosis simbiosis
symbiotic simbiótico
symbiotic infantile psychosis psicosis infantil
  simbiótica
symbiotic infantile psychotic syndrome
  síndrome psicótico infantil simbiótico
symbiotic marriage matrimonio simbiótico
symbiotic phase fase simbiótica
symbiotic psychosis psicosis simbiótica
symbiotic relationship relación simbiótica
symbiotic stage etapa simbiótica
symbol símbolo
symbol-digit test prueba de símbolos-dígitos
symbol-substitution test prueba de sustitución
  de símbolos
symbolia simbolia
symbolic simbólico

symbolic action acción simbólica
symbolic categorization categorización
  simbólica
symbolic displacement desplazamiento
  simbólico
symbolic function función simbólica
symbolic loss pérdida simbólica
symbolic masturbation masturbación
  simbólica
symbolic mode modo simbólico
symbolic parricide parricidio simbólico
symbolic play juego simbólico
symbolic process proceso simbólico
symbolic realization realización simbólica
symbolic representation representación
  simbólica
symbolic stage etapa simbólica
symbolic synthesis síntesis simbólica
symbolic thinking pensamiento simbólico
symbolic thought pensamiento simbólico
symbolism simbolismo
symbolization simbolización
symbolophobia simbolofobia
symmetric simétrico
symmetric distal neuropathy neuropatía
  distal simétrica
symmetrical simétrico
symmetrical distribution distribución
  simétrica
symmetry simetría
sympathectomy simpatectomía
sympathetectomy simpatetectomía
sympathetic simpático
sympathetic chain cadena simpática
sympathetic division división simpática
sympathetic dyspraxia dispraxia simpática
sympathetic ganglion ganglio simpático
sympathetic hypertonia hipertonía simpática
sympathetic imbalance desequilibrio
  simpático
sympathetic induction inducción simpática
sympathetic iridoplegia iridoplejía simpática
sympathetic nervous system sistema nervioso
  simpático
sympathetic reflex dystrophy distrofia refleja
  simpática
sympathetic vibration vibración simpática
sympathetoblastoma simpatetoblastoma
sympathic simpático
sympathicectomy simpaticectomía
sympathicoblastoma simpaticoblastoma
sympathicogonioma simpaticogonioma
sympathiconeuritis simpaticoneuritis
sympathicopathy simpaticopatía
sympathicotonia simpaticotonía
sympathicotonic simpaticotónico
sympathicotripsy simpaticotripsia
sympathin simpatina
sympathism simpatismo
sympathist simpatista
sympathize simpatizar
sympathizer simpatizante
sympathoblastoma simpatoblastoma
sympathogonioma simpatogonioma
sympatholytic simpatolítico

sympatholytic drug droga simpatolítica
sympathomimetic simpatomimético
sympathomimetic delirium delirio simpatomimético
sympathomimetic delusional disorder trastorno delusorio simpatomimético
sympathomimetic drug droga simpatomimética
sympathomimetic intoxication intoxicación simpatomimética
sympathomimetic withdrawal retiro simpatomimético
sympathy simpatía
sympathy seeking buscante de simpatía
sympatric species especies simpátricas
symptom síntoma
symptom bearer portador de síntomas
symptom choice selección de síntoma
symptom cluster grupo de síntomas
symptom complex complejo de síntomas
symptom experience stage etapa de experimentar un síntoma
symptom formation formación de síntomas
symptom group grupo de síntomas
symptom localization localización de síntomas
symptom neurosis neurosis de síntomas
symptom specificity especificidad de síntomas
symptom substitution sustitución de síntoma
symptom substitution hypothesis hipótesis de sustitución de síntoma
symptom-symbol hypothesis hipótesis de síntoma-símbolo
symptomatic sintomático
symptomatic act acto sintomático
symptomatic alcoholism alcoholismo sintomático
symptomatic autoscopy autoscopia sintomática
symptomatic epilepsy epilepsia sintomática
symptomatic headache dolor de cabeza sintomático
symptomatic impotence impotencia sintomática
symptomatic neuralgia neuralgia sintomática
symptomatic paramyotonia paramiotonía sintomática
symptomatic psychosis psicosis sintomática
symptomatic torticollis tortícolis sintomático
symptomatic treatment tratamiento sintomático
symptoms of depression síntomas de depresión
synalgia sinalgia
synalgic sinálgico
synaphoceptors sinafoceptores
synapse sinapsis
synaptic sináptico
synaptic button botón sináptico
synaptic delay demora sináptica
synaptic knob botón sináptico
synaptic resistance resistencia sináptica
synaptic transmission transmisión sináptica
syncheiria sinqueiria
synchiria sinquiria

synchronic sincrónico
synchronic study estudio sincrónico
synchronism sincronismo
synchronization sincronización
synchronized sincronizado
synchronized sleep sueño sincronizado
synchronous sincrónico
synchronous reflex reflejo sincrónico
synchrony sincronía
synclonic sinclónico
synclonic spasm espasmo sinclónico
synclonus sinclono
syncopal sincopal
syncope síncope
syncopic sincópico
syncretic sincrético
syncretic thought pensamiento sincrético
syncretism sincretismo
syndrome síndrome
syndrome of approximate answers síndrome de respuestas aproximadas
syndrome of approximate relevant answers síndrome de respuestas relevantes aproximadas
syndrome of deviously relevant answers síndrome de respuestas relevantes tortuosas
syndrome of inappropriate secretion of antidiuretic hormone síndrome de secreción inapropiada de hormona antidiurética
syneidesis sineidesis
synencephalocele sinencefalocele
synergic sinérgico
synergic control control sinérgico
synergic drug droga sinérgica
synergism sinergismo
synergistic sinérgico
synergy sinergía
synesthesia sinestesia
synesthesia algica sinestesia álgica
synesthesialgia sinestesialgia
syngamy singamia
synkinesia sincinesia
synkinesis sincinesis
synonym sinónimo
synonym-antonym test prueba de sinónimos-antónimos
synoptic sinóptico
synorchidism sinorquidismo
synorchism sinorquismo
synostosis sinostosis
syntactic sintáctico
syntactic aphasia afasia sintáctica
syntactic component componente sintáctico
syntactical sintáctico
syntactical aphasia afasia sintáctica
syntactics sintáctica
syntality sintalidad
syntax sintaxis
syntaxic mode modo sintáxico
syntaxic thought pensamiento sintáxico
synthesis síntesis
synthetic sintético
synthetic approach acercamiento sintético
synthetic function función sintética

synthetic language lenguaje sintético
synthetic narcotic narcótico sintético
synthetic speech habla sintética
synthetic trainer entrenador sintético
synthetic validity validez sintética
synthetical sintético
syntone síntono
syntonia sintonía
syntonic sintónico
syntonic personality personalidad sintónica
syntropic sintrópico
syntropy sintropía
syphilis sífilis
syphilitic sifilítico
syphilitic meningoencephalitis
    meningoencefalitis sifilítica
syphiloma sifiloma
syphilophobia sifilofobia
syringobulbia siringobulbia
syringocele siringocele
syringoencephalomyelia siringoencefalomielia
syringoid siringoide
syringomeningocele siringomeningocele
syringomyelia siringomielia
syringomyelic siringomiélico
syringomyelic dissociation disociación
    siringomiélica
syringomyelic hemorrhage hemorragia
    siringomiélica
syringomyelocele siringomielocele
syringomyelus siringomielo
syringopontia siringopontia
systaltic sistáltico
system sistema
system analysis análisis de sistemas
systematic sistemático
systematic abstraction abstracción sistemática
systematic approach acercamiento
    sistemático
systematic desensitization desensibilización
    sistemática
systematic distortion distorsión sistemática
systematic error error sistemático
systematic family therapy terapia familiar
    sistemática
systematic observations observaciones
    sistemáticas
systematic rational restructuring
    reestructuración racional sistemática
systematic reinforcement refuerzo
    sistemático
systematic sampling muestreo sistemático
systematic schizophrenia esquizofrenia
    sistemática
systematic vertigo vértigo sistemático
systematization sistematización
systematized delusion delusión sistematizada
systemic sistémico
systemic lupus erythematosus lupus
    eritematoso sistémico
systemic myelitis mielitis sistémica
systemic sense sentido sistémico
systems analysis análisis de sistemas
systems theory teoría de sistemas
systole sístole

systolic blood pressure presión sanguínea
    sistólica

T

T group grupo T
T-maze laberinto en T
T myelotomy mielotomía en T
tabes tabes
tabes diabetica tabes diabética
tabes dorsalis tabes dorsal
tabes ergotica tabes ergótica
tabes spasmodica tabes espasmódica
tabes spinalis tabes espinal
tabetic tabético
tabetic arthropathy artropatía tabética
tabetic crisis crisis tabética
tabetic cuirass coraza tabética
tabetic curve curva tabética
tabetic dissociation disociación tabética
tabetic psychosis psicosis tabética
tabetiform tabetiforme
tabic tábico
tabid tábido
taboo tabú
taboparesis taboparesia
tabula rasa tabla rasa
tabula rasa concept concepto de tabla rasa
tache mancha
tache cerebrale mancha cerebral
tache meningeale mancha meníngea
tache spinale mancha espinal
tachistoscope taquistoscopio
tachyathetosis taquiatetosis
tachycardia taquicardia
tachylalia taquilalia
tachylogia taquilogia
tachyphagia taquifagia
tachyphasia taquifasia
tachyphemia taquifemia
tachyphrasia taquifrasia
tachyphrenia taquifrenia
tachyphylaxis taquifilaxis
tachypnea taquipnea
tachypragia taquipragia
tachytrophism taquitrofismo
tacit tácito
tactic táctico
tactile táctil
tactile agnosia agnosia táctil
tactile amnesia amnesia táctil
tactile anesthesia anestesia táctil
tactile circle círculo táctil
tactile corpuscle corpúsculo táctil
tactile disk disco táctil
tactile hallucination alucinación táctil
tactile hyperesthesia hiperestesia táctil
tactile image imagen táctil
tactile perception percepción táctil

tactile-perceptual disorder trastorno
    táctil-perceptivo
tactile receptor receptor táctil
tactile sensation sensación táctil
tactile sense sentido táctil
tactile stimulation estimulación táctil
taction tacción
tactoagnosia tactoagnosia
tactometer tactómetro
tactual táctil
tactual hallucination alucinación táctil
tactual shape discrimination discriminación
    de forma táctil
tactual size discrimination discriminación de
    tamaño táctil
Tadoma method método de Tadoma
taeniophobia teniofobia
taenophobia tenofobia
tag question pregunta con cola
tailor's cramp calambre de sastre
tailor's spasm espasmo de sastre
Takayasu's disease enfermedad de Takayasu
Talbot brightness brillantez de Talbot
Talbot-Plateau law ley de Talbot-Plateau
talbutal talbutal
talent talento
talion talión
talion principle principio del talión
talipes talipes
talipes spasmodicus talipes espasmódico
talking book libro sonoro
talking typewriter máquina de escribir sonora
Talma's disease enfermedad de Talma
tambour tambor
tandem tándem
tandem reinforcement refuerzo en tándem
tangent screen pantalla tangente
tangential tangencial
tangential speech habla tangencial
tangential thinking pensamiento tangencial
tangentiality tangencialidad
tantrum rabieta
tanyphonia tanifonía
tap golpecito, punción
tapetum tapetum
taphephobia tafefobia
taphophilia tafofilia
taphophobia tafofobia
Tapia's syndrome síndrome de Tapia
tapir mouth boca de tapir
tarantism tarantismo
taraxein taraxeína
Tarchanoff phenomenon fenómeno de
    Tarchanoff
tardive tardío
tardive dyskinesia discinesia tardía
tardive dysmentia dismencia tardía
tardive oral dyskinesia discinesia oral tardía
tardy epilepsy epilepsia tardía
target objetivo
target behavior conducta objetivo
target cell célula objetivo
target language lenguaje objetivo
target organ órgano objetivo
target patient paciente objetivo

target response respuesta objetivo
target set conjunto objetivo
target stimulus estímulo objetivo
Tarlov's cyst quiste de Tarlov
tarsal tunnel syndrome síndrome del túnel tarsiano
tarsophalangeal tarsofalángico
tarsophalangeal reflex reflejo tarsofalángico
Tartini's tone tono de Tartini
tartrate tartrato
Tarui's disease enfermedad de Tarui
task tarea
task analysis análisis de tarea
task demands exigencias de tarea
task design diseño de tarea
task inventory inventario de tareas
task-oriented orientado hacia tarea
task-oriented approach acercamiento orientado hacia tarea
task-oriented group grupo orientado hacia tarea
task-oriented reaction reacción orientada hacia tarea
taste gusto
taste aversion aversión del gusto
taste blindness ceguera al gusto
taste buds papilas del gusto
taste cell célula del gusto
taste perception percepción del gusto
taste tetrahedron tetraedro del gusto
taurine taurina
tautology tautología
tautophone tautófono
taxis taxis
taxonomic taxonómico
taxonomy taxonomía
Tay-Sachs disease enfermedad de Tay-Sachs
teacher-student model modelo maestro-estudiante
teacher-student relationship relación maestro-estudiante
teaching enseñanza
teaching game juego de enseñanza
teaching machine máquina de enseñanza
teaching model modelo de enseñanza
teaching style estilo de enseñanza
team approach acercamiento de equipo
teamwork trabajo en equipo
tears lágrimas
technique técnica
technological illiteracy analfabetismo tecnológico
technopsychology tecnopsicología
tectal tectal
tectal nucleus núcleo tectal
tectorial tectorial
tectorial membrane membrana tectorial
tectum tectum
tegmental tegmental
tegmental syndrome síndrome tegmental
tegmentotomy tegmentotomía
tegmentum tegmentum
teichopsia teicopsia
teknonymy tecnonimia
telalgia telalgia

telangiectasia telangiectasia
telangiectasis telangiectasis
telangiectatic telangiectásico
telangiectatic angiomatosis angiomatosis telangiectásico
telangiectatic glioma glioma telangiectásico
telebinocular telebinocular
teleceptor teleceptor
telegnosis telegnosis
telegraphic speech habla telegráfica
telekinesis telecinesia
telencephalic telencefálico
telencephalic sleep sueño telencefálico
telencephalization telencefalización
telencephalon telencéfalo
teleologic teleológico
teleological teleológico
teleological hallucination alucinación teleológica
teleological regression regresión teleológica
teleology teleología
teleonomic teleonómico
teleonomy teleonomía
teleopsia teleopsia
teleoreceptor teleorreceptor
teleotherapeutics teleoterapéutica
telepathic telepático
telepathic dream sueño telepático
telepathy telepatía
telephone counseling asesoramiento telefónico
telephone scatologia escatología telefónica
telephone support service servicio de apoyo telefónico
telephone theory of hearing teoría de audición de teléfono
telereceptor telerreceptor
telergy telergía
telesis telesis
telestereoscope telestereoscopio
telesthesia telestesia
teletactor teletactor
teletractor teletractor
television and aggression televisión y agresión
telic télico
telic change cambio télico
telodendria telodendria
telodendron telodendrón
telophase telofase
temazepam temazepam
temper genio
temperament temperamento
temperament and suicidal behavior temperamento y conducta suicida
temperance temperancia
temperate temperado
temperature temperatura
temperature effects efectos de temperatura
temperature eroticism erotismo de temperatura
temperature sense sentido de temperatura
temperature spot mancha de temperatura
temporal temporal
temporal arteritis arteritis temporal
temporal avoidance conditioning

condicionamiento de evitación temporal
temporal conditioning condicionamiento
temporal
temporal contiguity contigüidad temporal
temporal discrimination discriminación
temporal
temporal hallucination alucinación temporal
temporal lobe lóbulo temporal
temporal-lobe epilepsy epilepsia de lóbulo
temporal
temporal-lobe illusion ilusión de lóbulo
temporal
temporal-lobe seizure acceso de lóbulo
temporal
temporal-lobe syndrome síndrome de lóbulo
temporal
temporal lobectomy lobectomía temporal
temporal maze laberinto temporal
temporal orientation orientación temporal
temporal-perceptual disorder trastorno
temporal-perceptivo
temporal perspective perspectiva temporal
temporal summation sumación temporal
temporal vision visión temporal
temporary admission admisión temporal
temporary commitment confinamiento
temporal
temporary threshold shift cambio de umbral
temporal
temporomandibular joint syndrome
síndrome de la articulación
temporomandibular
temptation tentación
tendency tendencia
tendency of action tendencia de acción
tender line línea sensible
tender point punto sensible
tender zone zona sensible
tendo Achillis reflex reflejo del tendón de
Aquiles
tendon reflex reflejo tendinoso
tenesmus tenesmo
tenet dogma
tense tenso
tension tensión
tension headache dolor de cabeza por tensión
tension reduction reducción de tensión
tension-reduction theory teoría de reducción
de tensión
tensor tympani tensor timpánico
tenth cranial nerve décimo nervio craneal
tentorium tentorium
tentorium cerebelli tentorium cerebelli
tephromalacia tefromalacia
tephrylometer tefrilómetro
teratogen teratógeno
teratogenesis teratogénesis
teratogenic teratogénico
teratogenic syndrome síndrome teratogénico
teratological teratológico
teratological defect defecto teratológico
teratology teratología
teratophobia teratofobia
terebrant terebrante
terebrating terebrante

terebration terebración
terminal terminal
terminal behavior conducta terminal
terminal button botón terminal
terminal care cuidado terminal
terminal factor factor terminal
terminal illness enfermedad terminal
terminal insomnia insomnio terminal
terminal reinforcement refuerzo terminal
terminal stimulus estímulo terminal
terminal threshold umbral terminal
territorial aggression agresión territorial
territorial dominance dominancia territorial
territoriality territorialidad
territory territorio
terror terror
terror dream sueño de terror
tertiary terciario
tertiary circular reaction reacción circular
terciaria
tertiary cortex corteza terciaria
tertiary cortical zone zona cortical terciaria
tertiary gain ganancia terciaria
tertiary prevention prevención terciaria
test prueba
test accuracy precisión de prueba
test administration adminstración de pruebas
test age edad de prueba
test anxiety ansiedad de pruebas
test battery batería de pruebas
test bias sesgo de prueba
test item artículo de prueba
test of criminal responsibility prueba de
responsabilidad criminal
test of hypothesis prueba de hipótesis
test of significance prueba de significación
test profile perfil de prueba
test-retest prueba-reprueba
test-retest coefficient coeficiente de
prueba-reprueba
test-retest method método de
prueba-reprueba
test-retest reliability confiabilidad de
prueba-reprueba
test scaling escalamiento de prueba
test score puntuación de prueba
test selection selección de prueba
test sophistication sofisticación de prueba
test standardization estandarización de
prueba
test-study-test method método de
prueba-estudio-prueba
testamentary capacity capacidad
testamentaria
testes testes
testicle testículo
testicular testicular
testicular atrophy atrofia testicular
testicular feminization syndrome síndrome
de feminización testicular
testis testis
testitis testitis
testosterone testosterona
tetania tetania
tetania epidemica tetania epidémica

tetania gastrica tetania gástrica
tetania neonatorium tetania neonatal
tetania parathyreopriva tetania paratiropriva
tetania rheumatica tetania reumática
tetanic tetánico
tetanic contraction contracción tetánica
tetanic convulsion convulsión tetánica
tetaniform tetaniforme
tetanigenous tetanígeno
tetanilla tetanilla
tetanism tetanismo
tetanization tetanización
tetanize tetanizar
tetanizing tetanizante
tetanizing shock choque tetanizante
tetanode tetánodo
tetanoid tetanoide
tetanoid chorea corea tetanoide
tetanoid paraplegia paraplejía tetanoide
tetanometer tetanómetro
tetanomotor tetanomotor
tetanus tétanos
tetanus anticus tétanos anticus
tetanus completus tétanos completo
tetanus dorsalis tétanos dorsal
tetanus neonatorum tétanos neonatal
tetanus posticus tétanos posticus
tetany tetania
tetany of alkalosis tetania por alcalosis
tetartanopia tetartanopía
tetrabenazine tetrabenazina
tetrachromatic tetracromático
tetrachromatic theory teoría tetracromática
tetrachromatism tetracromatismo
tetracyclic antidepressant antidepresivo
    tetracíclico
tetrad tétrada
tetrahydrocannabinol tetrahidrocannabinol
tetraparesis tetraparesia
tetraplegia tetraplejía
tetraplegic tetrapléjico
tetrasomy tetrasomia
text blindness ceguera textual
textual textual
texture textura
texture gradient gradiente de textura
thalamectomy talamectomía
thalamic talámico
thalamic lesion lesión talámica
thalamic nucleus núcleo talámico
thalamic pacemaker marcapasos talámico
thalamic syndrome síndrome talámico
thalamic theory of Cannon teoría de Cannon
    talámica
thalamic theory of emotion teoría de emoción
    talámica
thalamotomy talamotomía
thalamus tálamo
thalassophobia talasofobia
thalectomy talectomía
thalidomide talidomida
thanatography tanatografía
thanatology tanatología
thanatomania tanatomanía
thanatophobia tanatofobia

thanatopsy tanatopsia
thanatos tanatos
thanatotic tanatótico
thebaine tebaína
theft hurto
thelarche telarca
thematic temático
thematic paralogia paralogía temática
thematic paraphasia parafasia temática
theme interference interferencia de temas
theomania teomanía
theophobia teofobia
theorem teorema
theoretical teorético
theoretical construct constructo teorético
theoretical equation ecuación teorética
theoretical psychology psicología teorética
theory teoría
theory of aggression teoría de agresión
theory of aging teoría de envejecimiento
theory of anxiety teoría de ansiedad
theory of autism teoría de autismo
theory of cognition teoría de cognición
theory of color vision teoría de visión de
    colores
theory of delinquency teoría de delincuencia
theory of development teoría del desarrollo
theory of emotion teoría de emociones
theotherapy teoterapia
therapeusis terapeusis
therapeutic terapéutico
therapeutic abortion aborto terapéutico
therapeutic agent agente terapéutico
therapeutic alliance alianza terapéutica
therapeutic atmosphere atmósfera terapéutica
therapeutic communication comunicación
    terapéutica
therapeutic community comunidad
    terapéutica
therapeutic crisis crisis terapéutica
therapeutic dose dosis terapéutica
therapeutic dose dependency dependencia de
    dosis terapéutica
therapeutic environment ambiente
    terapéutico
therapeutic group grupo terapéutico
therapeutic-group analysis análisis de grupo
    terapéutico
therapeutic impasse atolladero terapéutico
therapeutic malaria malaria terapéutica
therapeutic matrix matriz terapéutica
therapeutic nihilism nihilismo terapéutico
therapeutic optimism optimismo terapéutico
therapeutic pessimism pesimismo terapéutico
therapeutic reaction reacción terapéutica
therapeutic recreation recreación terapéutica
therapeutic relationship relación terapéutica
therapeutic relaxation relajamiento
    terapéutico
therapeutic role papel terapéutico
therapeutic use uso terapéutico
therapeutic window ventana terapéutica
therapeutics terapéutica
therapeutist terapeuta
therapist terapeuta

therapist obligations obligaciones de terapeuta
therapy terapia
therapy in groups terapia en grupos
therapy puppet muñeco de terapia
theriomorphism teriomorfismo
thermal térmico
thermal anesthesia anestesia térmica
thermal discrimination discriminación térmica
thermal sense sentido térmico
thermal sensitivity sensibilidad térmica
thermalgesia termalgesia
thermalgia termalgia
thermanalgesia termanalgesia
thermanesthesia termanestesia
thermesthesia termestesia
thermesthesiometer termestesiómetro
thermic térmico
thermic anesthesia anestesia térmica
thermic fever fiebre térmica
thermic sense sentido térmico
thermistor termistor
thermoalgesia termoalgesia
thermoanalgesia termoanalgesia
thermoanesthesia termoanestesia
thermocoagulation termocoagulación
thermoesthesia termoestesia
thermoesthesiometer termoestesiómetro
thermography termografía
thermohyperalgesia termohiperalgesia
thermohyperesthesia termohiperestesia
thermohypesthesia termohipestesia
thermohypoesthesia termohipoestesia
thermoneurosis termoneurosis
thermophobia termofobia
thermoreceptor termorreceptor
thermoregulation termorregulación
thermotaxis termotaxis
thermotropism termotropismo
theroid teroide
thesis tesis
theta theta
theta rhythm ritmo theta
theta wave onda theta
thiamine tiamina
thiamine deficiency deficiencia de tiamina
thiazide tiazida
thigmesthesia tigmestesia
thinking pensamiento
thinking compulsion compulsión de pensamiento
thinking disorder trastorno de pensamiento
thinking type tipo de pensamiento
thiopental tiopental
thiopropazate tiopropazato
thioproperazine tioproperazina
thioridazine tioridazina
thiothixene tiotixeno
thiouracil tiouracilo
thioxanthene tioxanteno
third cranial nerve tercer nervio craneal
third dimension tercera dimensión
third ear tercera oreja
third-force therapy terapia de tercera fuerza

third party payer tercero pagador
third-variable problem problema de tercera variable
third ventricle tercer ventrículo
thirst sed
Thomsen's disease enfermedad de Thomsen
thoracic torácico
thoracic nerve nervio torácico
thoracolumbar toracolumbar
thoracolumbar system sistema toracolumbar
thorax tórax
thought pensamiento
thought broadcasting emisión de pensamientos
thought constraint constreñimiento de pensamientos
thought content contenido de pensamientos
thought control control de pensamientos
thought deprivation privación de pensamientos
thought derailment descarrilamiento de pensamientos
thought disorder trastorno de pensamientos
thought disorganization desorganización de pensamientos
thought disturbance disturbio de pensamientos
thought experiment experimento de pensamientos
thought hearing audición de pensamientos
thought impulses impulsos de pensamientos
thought insertion inserción de pensamientos
thought obstruction obstrucción de pensamientos
thought pressure presión de pensamientos
thought process proceso de pensamiento
thought-process disorder trastorno del proceso de pensamientos
thought rehearsal ensayo de pensamientos
thought transference transferencia de pensamientos
thought withdrawal retirada de pensamientos
Thouless ratio razón de Thouless
threat amenaza
three-color theory teoría de tres colores
three-component theory teoría de tres componentes
three-cornered therapy terapia de tres esquinas
three-day schizophrenia esquizofrenia de tres días
threshold umbral
threshold differential diferencial de umbral
threshold of consciousness umbral de conciencia
threshold shift cambio de umbral
threshold stimulus estímulo umbral
thrombosis trombosis
thrombotic trombótico
thrombotic apoplexy apoplejía trombótica
thrombotic hydrocephalus hidrocefalia trombótica
thrombus trombo
thumb opposition oposición de pulgar
thumb reflex reflejo del pulgar

thumb-sucking chuparse el pulgar
Thurstone scale escala de Thurstone
thwart frustrar
thymectomy timectomía
thymine timina
thymogenic timogénico
thymogenic drinking beber timogénico
thymoleptic timoléptico
thymopathic timopático
thymopathy timopatía
thymopsyche timopsiquis
thymus timo
thyrohypophysial tirohipofisario
thyrohypophysial syndrome síndrome
    tirohipofisario
thyroid tiroides
thyroid function test prueba de
    funcionamiento tiroide
thyroid gland glándula tiroides
thyroid hormone hormona tiroide
thyroid-stimulating hormone hormona
    estimulante del tiroides
thyroidectomy tiroidectomía
thyroidism tiroidismo
thyrotoxic tirotóxico
thyrotoxic coma coma tirotóxico
thyrotoxic encephalopathy encefalopatía
    tirotóxica
thyrotoxic myopathy miopatía tirotóxica
thyrotoxicosis tirotoxicosis
thyrotropic tirotrópico
thyrotropic hormone hormona tirotrópica
thyrotropin tirotropina
thyrotropin-releasing hormone hormona
    liberadora de tirotropina
thyroxine tiroxina
tibial phenomenon fenómeno tibial
tic tic
tic de pensee tic de pensamiento
tic disorder trastorno de tic
tic douloureux tic doloroso
tick-borne encephalitis encefalitis transmitida
    por garrapatas
tick paralysis parálisis por garrapata
tickling cosquillas
tigretier tigretier
tigrolysis tigrólisis
timbre timbre
time tiempo
time agnosia agnosia del tiempo
time and motion analysis análisis de tiempo y
    moción
time and rhythm disorder trastorno del
    tiempo y ritmo
time confusion confusión de tiempo
time consciousness conciencia del tiempo
time disorientation desorientación del tiempo
time distortion distorsión del tiempo
time error error del tiempo
time-extended therapy terapia de tiempo
    extendido
time-limited dynamic psychotherapy
    psicoterapia dinámica limitada por tiempo
time-limited psychotherapy psicoterapia
    limitada por tiempo

time-motion study estudio de tiempo y
    moción
time out tiempo fuera
time-out from reinforcement tiempo fuera de
    refuerzo
time-out procedure procedimiento de tiempo
    fuera
time-out technique técnica de tiempo fuera
time perception percepción del tiempo
time perspective perspectiva del tiempo
time sample muestra del tiempo
time score puntuación del tiempo
time sense sentido del tiempo
time sense test prueba del sentido del tiempo
time series serie del tiempo
time study estudio del tiempo
timidity timidez
timiperone timiperona
Tinel's sign signo de Tinel
tinnitus tinnitus
tip-of-the-tongue punta de la lengua
tip-of-the-tongue phenomenon fenómeno de
    punta de la lengua
tissue tejido
tissue rejection rechazo de tejido
tissue respiration respiración de tejidos
titillation titilación
titubation titubeo
tobacco tabaco
tobacco abuse abuso de tabaco
tobacco dependence dependencia de tabaco
tobacco use uso de tabaco
tobacco withdrawal retiro de tabaco
tocomania tocomanía
tocophobia tocofobia
Todd's paralysis parálisis de Todd
Todd's postepileptic paralysis parálisis
    posepiléptica de Todd
toe clonus clono del dedo del pie
toe drop caída de los dedos del pie
toe phenomenon fenómeno de los dedos del
    pie
toe reflex reflejo del dedo del pie
toilet training entrenamiento de inodoro
token economy economía de fichas
token reward recompensa de fichas
tolerance tolerancia
tolerance level nivel de tolerancia
tolerance of ambiguity tolerancia de
    ambigüedad
tolerance of anxiety tolerancia de ansiedad
tolerance test prueba de tolerancia
Tolosa-Hunt syndrome síndrome de
    Tolosa-Hunt
tomography tomografía
tomomania tomomanía
tonal tonal
tonal attribute atributo tonal
tonal bell campana tonal
tonal brightness brillantez tonal
tonal character carácter tonal
tonal color color tonal
tonal density densidad tonal
tonal dimension dimensión tonal
tonal fusion fusión tonal

tonal gap brecha tonal
tonal interaction interacción tonal
tonal intermittence intermitencia tonal
tonal island isla tonal
tonal pattern patrón tonal
tonal range intervalo tonal
tonal scale escala tonal
tonal spectrum espectro tonal
tonal variator variador tonal
tonal volume volumen tonal
tonality tonalidad
tonaphasia tonafasia
tone tono
tone color color de tono
tone deafness sordera de tono
tongue phenomenon fenómeno lingual
tonic tónico
tonic activation activación tónica
tonic-clonic seizure acceso tónico-clónico
tonic conduction conducción tónica
tonic contraction contracción tónica
tonic control control tónico
tonic convulsion convulsión tónica
tonic epilepsy epilepsia tónica
tonic immobility inmovilidad tónica
tonic neck reflex reflejo del cuello tónico
tonic pupil pupila tónica
tonic pupil of Adie pupila tónica de Adie
tonic reflex reflejo tónico
tonic spasm espasmo tónico
tonicity tonicidad
tonicoclonic tonicoclónico
tonitophobia tonitofobia
tonitrophobia tonitrofobia
tonoclonic tonoclónico
tonoclonic spasm espasmo tonoclónico
tonogenic tonogénico
tonogeny tonogenia
tonometer tonómetro
tonometry tonometría
tonotopic tonotópico
tonotopic organization organización
   tonotópica
tonotopic representation representación
   tonotópica
tonotopy tonotopia
tonsillar herniation herniación tonsilar
tonus tono
tool-using behavior conducta de uso de
   herramientas
tooth grinding rechinamiento
tooth spasm espasmo dental
top-down processing procesamiento del tope
   hacia abajo
topagnosis topagnosis
topalgia topalgia
topectomy topectomía
topesthesia topestesia
topical tópico
topoanesthesia topoanestesia
topognosia topognosia
topognosis topognosis
topographagnosia topografagnosia
topographic topográfico
topographical topográfico

topographical disorientation desorientación
   topográfica
topographical hypothesis hipótesis
   topográfica
topographical model modelo topográfico
topographical organization organización
   topográfica
topographical psychology psicología
   topográfica
topographical theory teoría topográfica
topography topografía
topological topológico
topological psychology psicología topológica
topology topología
toponarcosis toponarcosis
toponeurosis toponeurosis
topophobia topofobia
toposcope toposcopio
topothermesthesiometer
   topotermestesiómetro
tornado epilepsy epilepsia de tornado
torpor torpor
torsion torsión
torsion dystonia distonía de torsión
torsion neurosis neurosis de torsión
torsion spasm espasmo de torsión
torsionometer torsionómetro
Torsten Sjogren's syndrome síndrome de
   Torsten Sjogren
torticollar torticolar
torticollis tortícolis
torticollis spastica tortícolis espástico
toruloma toruloma
total aphasia afasia total
total color blindness ceguera al color total
total push therapy terapia de empuje total
totem tótem
totemism totemismo
totemistic totémico
touch sense sentido del tacto
Tourette's disease enfermedad de Tourette
Tourette's disorder trastorno de Tourette
Tourette's syndrome síndrome de Tourette
towers skull cráneo en torre
toxemia toxemia
toxemia of pregnancy toxemia del embarazo
toxic tóxico
toxic delirium delirio tóxico
toxic dementia demencia tóxica
toxic disorder trastorno tóxico
toxic hydrocephalus hidrocefalia tóxica
toxic neuritis neuritis tóxica
toxic psychosis psicosis tóxica
toxic tetanus tétanos tóxico
toxicity toxicidad
toxicomania toxicomanía
toxicophobia toxicofobia
toxin toxina
toxiphobia toxifobia
toxophobia toxofobia
toxoplasmosis toxoplasmosis
trace traza
trace conditioning condicionamiento de traza
trachelagra traquelagra
trachelism traquelismo

trachelismus traquelismo
trachelocyrtosis traquelocirtosis
trachelodynia traquelodinia
trachelokyphosis traquelocifosis
trachelology traquelología
trachoma tracoma
trachyphonia traquifonía
tracking rastreo
tract tracto
tractotomy tractotomía
tradition-directed dirigido hacia tradiciones
traditional marriage matrimonio tradicional
train entrenar
trained reflex reflejo entrenado
training entrenamiento
training aid ayuda para entrenamiento
training analysis análisis de entrenamiento
training evaluation evaluación de entrenamiento
training group grupo de entrenamiento
training school escuela de entrenamiento
training transfer transferencia de entrenamiento
training trial ensayo de entrenamiento
trait rasgo
trait carrier portador de rasgo
trait organization organización de rasgos
trait profile perfil de rasgos
trait theory teoría de rasgo
trait validity validez de rasgo
trait variability variabilidad de rasgo
trance trance
trance coma coma de trance
trance state estado de trance
tranquilizer tranquilizante
tranquilizer abuse abuso de tranquilizante
transaction transacción
transactional transaccional
transactional analysis análisis transaccional
transactional evaluation evaluación transaccional
transactional psychology psicología transaccional
transactional psychotherapy psicoterapia transaccional
transactional theory teoría transaccional
transactional theory of perception teoría de percepción transaccional
transcendental transcendental
transcendental meditation meditación transcendental
transcendental state estado transcendental
transcortical transcortical
transcortical aphasia afasia transcortical
transcortical apraxia apraxia transcortical
transcortical motor aphasia afasia motora transcortical
transcortical sensory aphasia afasia sensorial transcortical
transcription transcripción
transcultural transcultural
transcultural psychiatry psiquiatría transcultural
transcutaneous electrical stimulation estimulación eléctrica transcutánea

transducer transductor
transduction transducción
transductive transductivo
transductive logic lógica transductiva
transductive reasoning razonamiento transductivo
transection transección
transfer transferencia
transfer by generalization transferencia por generalización
transfer function función de transferencia
transfer of learning transferencia de aprendizaje
transfer of principles transferencia de principios
transfer of training transferencia de entrenamiento
transfer ribonucleic acid ácido ribonucleico de transferencia
transferase transferasa
transference transferencia
transference cure cura de transferencia
transference improvement mejora de transferencia
transference neurosis neurosis de transferencia
transference reaction reacción de transferencia
transference remission remisión de transferencia
transference resistance resistencia de transferencia
transferred sensation sensación transferida
transformation transformación
transformation of affect transformación de afecto
transformation rule regla de transformación
transformation theory of anxiety teoría de transformación de ansiedad
transformational transformacional
transformational grammar gramática transformacional
transformed transformado
transformed score puntuación transformada
transformism transformismo
transient transitorio
transient ego ideal ego ideal transitorio
transient global amnesia amnesia global transitoria
transient group grupo transitorio
transient ischemic attack ataque isquémico transitorio
transient situational disturbance disturbio situacional transitorio
transient situational personality disorder trastorno de personalidad situacional transitoria
transient tic disorder trastorno de tic transitorio
transient tremor temblor transitorio
transinstitutionalization transinstitucionalización
transition transición
transitional transicional
transitional cortex corteza transicional

transitional object objeto transicional
transitional probability probabilidad transicional
transitional program programa transicional
transitivism transitivismo
transitivity transitividad
transketolase transcetolasa
translation traducción
translocation translocación
translocation Down's syndrome síndrome de Down de translocación
transmissible transmisible
transmission transmisión
transmission of information transmisión de información
transmitter transmisor
transmitter substance sustancia transmisora
transneuronal transneuronal
transneuronal atrophy atrofia transneuronal
transneuronal degeneration degeneración transneuronal
transorbital transorbitario
transorbital leukotomy leucotomía transorbitaria
transorbital lobotomy lobotomía transorbitaria
transosseous venography venografía transósea
transparency transparencia
transpersonal transpersonal
transpersonal psychology psicología transpersonal
transpersonality transpersonalidad
transplantation trasplante
transposition transposición
transposition behavior conducta de transposición
transposition error error de transposición
transposition of affect transposición de afecto
transposon transposón
transsexual transexual
transsexualism transexualismo
transsituational transituacional
transsynaptic transináptico
transsynaptic chromatolysis cromatólisis transináptica
transsynaptic degeneration degeneración transináptica
transsynaptic filament filamento transináptico
transtentorial transtentorial
transtentorial herniation herniación transtentorial
transverse transversal
transverse myelitis mielitis transversal
transverse section sección transversal
transversectomy transversectomía
transvestic transvéstico
transvestic fetishism fetichismo transvéstico
transvestism transvestismo
transvestite transvestista
transvestitism transvestismo
Transylvania effect efecto de Transilvania
tranylcypromine tranilcipromina
trapezoid body cuerpo trapezoide
trauma trauma

traumasthenia traumastenia
traumatic traumático
traumatic anesthesia anestesia traumática
traumatic anxiety ansiedad traumática
traumatic aphasia afasia traumática
traumatic cervical discopathy discopatía cervical traumática
traumatic delirium delirio traumático
traumatic encephalopathy encefalopatía traumática
traumatic event evento traumático
traumatic experience experiencia traumática
traumatic hemorrhage hemorragia traumática
traumatic meningocele meningocele traumático
traumatic neurasthenia neurastenia traumática
traumatic neuritis neuritis traumática
traumatic neuroma neuroma traumático
traumatic neurosis neurosis traumática
traumatic progressive encephalopathy encefalopatía progresiva traumática
traumatic pseudocatatonia seudocatatonía traumática
traumatic psychosis psicosis traumática
traumatic shock choque traumático
traumatic tetanus tétanos traumático
traumatism traumatismo
traumatization traumatización
traumatize traumatizar
traumatophilia traumatofilia
traumatophilic traumatofílico
traumatophilic diathesis diátesis traumatofílica
traumatophobia traumatofobia
trazodone trazodona
Treacher Collins' syndrome síndrome de Treacher Collins
treated prevalence prevalencia tratada
treatment tratamiento
treatment-evaluation strategy estrategia de evaluación de tratamiento
treatment of alcoholism tratamiento de alcoholismo
treatment of anxiety tratamiento de ansiedad
treatment of autism tratamiento de autismo
treatment of behavior disorders tratamiento de trastornos de conducta
treatment of delinquency tratamiento de delincuencia
treatment of depression tratamiento de depresión
treatment of domestic violence tratamiento de violencia doméstica
treatment of eating disorders tratamiento de trastornos del comer
treatment of learning disabilities tratamiento de discapacidades del aprendizaje
treatment of psychological maltreatment tratamiento de maltrato psicológico
treatment outcome resultados de tratamiento
treatment plan plan de tratamiento
treatment variable variable de tratamiento
trembling tembloroso
trembling abasia abasia temblorosa

trembling palsy parálisis temblorosa
tremogram tremograma
tremograph tremógrafo
tremophobia tremofobia
tremor temblor
tremor artuum tremor artuum
tremor opiophagorum tremor opiophagorum
tremor potatorum tremor potatorum
tremor tendinum tremor tendinum
tremulous trémulo
trend tendencia
trend analysis análisis de tendencia
trend of thought tendencia del pensamiento
trend test prueba de tendencia
Trendelenburg's symptom síntoma de
  Trendelenburg
trepan trépano
trepanation trepanación
trephination trefinación
trephine trefina
trepidant trepidante
trepidation trepidación
triad tríada
triadic triádico
triadic symbiosis simbiosis triádica
triadic therapy terapia triádica
triage triage
trial ensayo
trial analysis análisis de ensayo
trial and error learning aprendizaje por
  tanteo
trial lesson lección de ensayo
trial marriage matrimonio de ensayo
triangular therapy terapia triangular
triangulation triangulación
triazolam triazolam
triazolopyridine antidepressant antidepresivo
  triazolopiridínico
tribade tríbada
tribadism tribadismo
tribady tribadismo
tribasilar synostosis sinostosis tribasilar
triceps reflex reflejo del tríceps
triceps surae reflex reflejo del tríceps sural
trichalgia tricalgia
trichodynia tricodinia
trichoesthesia tricoestesia
trichologia tricología
trichology tricología
Trichomonas vaginalis Trichomonas vaginalis
trichopathophobia tricopatofobia
trichophagy tricofagia
trichophobia tricofobia
trichosis tricosis
trichosis sensitiva tricosis sensitiva
trichotillomania tricotilomanía
trichotomy tricotomía
trichromacy tricromacia
trichromasy tricromacia
trichromat tricrómata
trichromatic tricromático
trichromatic theory teoría tricromática
trichromatism tricromatismo
trichromatopsia tricromatopsia
trichromia tricromia

tricyclic tricíclico
tricyclic antidepressant antidepresivo
  tricíclico
tricyclic drug droga tricíclica
trifacial trifacial
trifacial neuralgia neuralgia trifacial
trigeminal trigeminal
trigeminal cerebral angiomatosis
  angiomatosis cerebral trigeminal
trigeminal decompression descompresión
  trigeminal
trigeminal lemniscus lemnisco trigeminal
trigeminal nerve nervio trigeminal
trigeminal neuralgia neuralgia trigeminal
trigeminal nucleus núcleo trigeminal
trigeminal rhizotomy rizotomía trigeminal
trigeminal tractotomy tractotomía trigeminal
trigeminofacial trigeminofacial
trigeminofacial reflex reflejo trigeminofacial
trigger area área de disparo
trigger finger dedo en gatillo
trigger point punto de gatillo
trigger zone zona de gatillo
trigram trigrama
trigraph trígrafo
trihybrid trihíbrido
trilogy trilogía
trimethadione trimetadiona
trimipramine trimipramina
triolist triolista
triorchid triórquido
triple-X condition condición de triple X
triple-X syndrome síndrome de triple X
triplegia triplejía
triploid triploide
triploid karyotype cariotipo triploide
trisexuality trisexualidad
triskaidekaphobia triscaidecafobia
trismic trísmico
trismoid trismoide
trismus trismo
trismus dolorificus trismo doloroso
trismus neonatorum trismo neonatal
trismus sardonicus trismo sardónico
trisomy trisomia
trisomy 21 trisomia 21
trisomy 21 syndrome síndrome de trisomia
  21
trisomy syndrome síndrome de trisomia
tritanopia tritanopía
trochanter trocánter
trochanter reflex reflejo del trocánter
trochlear troclear
trochlear nerve nervio troclear
trocular nerve nervio trocular
troilism troilismo
Tromner's reflex reflejo de Tromner
trophesic trofésico
trophesy trofesía
trophic trófico
trophic change cambio trófico
trophic function función trófica
trophic gangrene gangrena trófica
trophic hormone hormona trófica
trophicity troficidad

trophism trofismo
trophodermatoneurosis trofodermatoneurosis
trophoneurosis trofoneurosis
trophoneurotic trofoneurótico
trophoneurotic atrophy atrofia trofoneurótica
trophoneurotic leprosy lepra trofoneurótica
trophotropic trofotrópico
trophotropic zone of Hess zona trofotrópica
    de Hess
tropism tropismo
tropotaxis tropotaxis
Trousseau's point punto de Trousseau
Trousseau's sign signo de Trousseau
Trousseau's spot punto de Trousseau
Trousseau's syndrome síndrome de
    Trousseau
Troxler's effect efecto de Troxler
truancy ausencia sin permiso
true anosmia anosmia verdadera
true anxiety ansiedad verdadera
true communication stage etapa de
    comunicación verdadera
true insight penetración verdadera
true value valor verdadero
true zero cero verdadero
truncated distribution distribución truncada
trust confianza
trust versus mistrust confianza contra
    desconfianza
truth serum suero de la verdad
trypanosome tripanosoma
trypanosome fever fiebre por tripanosomas
trypanosomiasis tripanosomiasis
tryptamine triptamina
tryptophan triptófano
tubal ligation ligación tubaria
tubectomy tubectomía
tuberculoma tuberculoma
tuberculomania tuberculomanía
tuberculophobia tuberculofobia
tuberculosis tuberculosis
tuberculous tuberculoso
tuberculous meningitis meningitis tuberculosa
tuberculous spondylitis espondilitis
    tuberculosa
tuberous tuberoso
tuberous sclerosis esclerosis tuberosa
tubulization tubulización
tumefacient tumefaciente
tumefaction tumefacción
tumescence tumescencia
tumor tumor
tunica dartos tunica dartos
tunnel vision visión de túnel
Tuohy needle aguja de Tuohy
turban tumor tumor en turbante
turbid túrbido
Turck's degeneration degeneración de Turck
Turcot syndrome síndrome de Turcot
Turing's test prueba de Turing
Turing machine máquina de Turing
turmoil tumulto
Turner's syndrome síndrome de Turner
turricephaly turricefalia
tussive tusivo

tussive absence ausencia tusiva
twilight attack ataque crepuscular
twilight sleep sueño crepuscular
twilight state estado crepuscular
twilight vision visión crepuscular
twin gemelo
twin study estudio de gemelos
twinge punzada
twitch sacudida
two-factor design diseño de dos factores
two-factor design theory teoría de diseño de
    dos factores
two-neuron arc arco de dos neuronas
two-point discrimination discriminación de
    dos puntos
two-point threshold umbral de dos puntos
two-sided message mensaje de dos lados
two-tailed probability probabilidad de dos
    colas
two-tailed test prueba de dos colas
two-word messages stage etapa de mensajes
    de dos palabras
two-word stage of language development
    etapa de dos palabras del desarrollo del
    lenguaje
tybamate tibamato
tympanic timpánico
tympanic canal canal timpánico
tympanic cavity cavidad timpánica
tympanic membrane membrana timpánica
tympanic reflex reflejo timpánico
tympanometry timpanometría
tympanoplasty timpanoplastia
tympanum tímpano
type tipo
type A behavior conducta tipo A
type A personality personalidad tipo A
type B behavior conducta tipo B
type B personality personalidad tipo B
type fallacy falacia de tipos
type I error error tipo I
type II error error tipo II
type-identity theory teoría de identidad de
    tipo
type of personality tipo de personalidad
typhomania tifomanía
typical típico
typical absence ausencia típica
typicality tipicalidad
typist's cramp calambre de mecanógrafo
typography tipografía
typology tipología
tyramine tiramina
tyrannical behavior conducta tiránica
tyrannism tiranismo
tyrosine tirosina
Tyson's glands glándulas de Tyson

U

Uhthoff sign signo de Uhthoff
ulcer úlcera
ulcer personality personalidad ulcerosa
ulegyria ulegiria
Ullmann's line línea de Ullmann
ulnar ulnar
ulnar reflex reflejo ulnar
ultradian ultradiano
ultradian rhythm ritmo ultradiano
ultrasonic ultrasónico
ultrasonic irradiation irradiación ultrasónica
ultrasonic therapy terapia ultrasónica
ultrasonic waves ondas ultrasónicas
ultrasonosurgery ultrasonocirugía
ultraviolet ultravioleta
ultromotivity ultromotividad
ululation ululación
umbilical cord cordón umbilical
unanticipated crisis crisis no anticipada
unbalanced bilingual bilingüe no balanceado
unbiased insesgado
unbiased error error insesgado
unbiased estimate estimado insesgado
unbiased estimator estimador insesgado
uncal uncal
uncal herniation herniación uncal
uncertainty incertidumbre
uncertainty factor factor de incertidumbre
uncertainty level nivel de incertidumbre
uncinate uncinado
uncinate attack ataque uncinado
uncinate epilepsy epilepsia uncinada
uncinate fasciculus fascículo uncinado
uncinate fit ajuste uncinado
uncinate seizure acceso uncinado
uncomplicated alcohol withdrawal retiro de
    alcohol no complicado
uncomplicated bereavement duelo no
    complicado
unconditional incondicional
unconditional reflex reflejo incondicional
unconditional response respuesta
    incondicional
unconditioned incondicionado
unconditioned reflex reflejo incondicionado
unconditioned response respuesta
    incondicionada
unconditioned stimulus estímulo
    incondicionado
unconscious inconsciente
unconscious cerebration cerebración
    inconsciente
unconscious cognitive process proceso
    cognitivo inconsciente

unconscious drive impulso inconsciente
unconscious factor factor inconsciente
unconscious fantasy fantasía inconsciente
unconscious guilt culpabilidad inconsciente
unconscious homosexuality homosexualidad
    inconsciente
unconscious ideation ideación inconsciente
unconscious impulse impulso inconsciente
unconscious inference inferencia inconsciente
unconscious knowledge conocimiento
    inconsciente
unconscious memory memoria inconsciente
unconscious motivation motivación
    inconsciente
unconscious process proceso inconsciente
unconscious resistance resistencia
    inconsciente
unconsciousness inconsciencia
uncontrolled incontrolado
uncovertebral uncovertebral
underachievement subrendimiento
underachiever quien rinde bajo su potencial
underarousal subdespertamiento
undercontrolled subcontrolado
underdetermined subdeterminado
undergeneralization subgeneralización
undersocialized subsocializado
undersocialized-aggressive-conduct disorder
    trastorno de conducta agresiva
    subsocializada
undersocialized conduct disorder trastorno
    de conducta subsocializada
undersocialized-nonaggressive-conduct
    disorder trastorno de conducta no agresiva
    subsocializada
understand entender
understanding entendimiento
understimulation subestimulación
understimulation theory teoría de
    subestimulación
underweight falto de peso
undifferentiated indiferenciado
undifferentiated cell adenoma adenoma de
    células indiferenciadas
undifferentiated schizophrenia esquizofrenia
    indiferenciada
undifferentiated somatoform disorder
    trastorno somatoforme indiferenciado
undifferentiated type schizophrenia
    esquizofrenia de tipo indiferenciada
undoing revocación
unemployment desempleo
unformed visual hallucination alucinación
    visual sin formar
uniaural uniaural
unidextrous unidextro
unidimensional unidimensional
uniform distribution distribución uniforme
uniformism uniformismo
uniformity uniformidad
unilateral unilateral
unilateral anesthesia anestesia unilateral
unilateral lesion lesión unilateral
unilateral neglect negligencia unilateral
unilateral sensorimotor cortex lesion lesión

de corteza sensorimotora unilateral
unimodal unimodal
uninhibited desinhibido
uninhibited behavior conducta desinhibida
uninhibited neurogenic bladder vejiga
   neurogénica desinhibida
unintentional death muerte no intencionada
uniocular uniocular
uniocular dichromat dicrómata uniocular
uniovular uniovular
uniovular twins gemelos uniovulares
unipolar unipolar
unipolar cell célula unipolar
unipolar depression depresión unipolar
unipolar mania manía unipolar
unipolar manic-depressive psychosis psicosis
   maniacodepresiva unipolar
unipolar neuron neurona unipolar
unipolar psychosis psicosis unipolar
unique único
unique factor factor único
unique hue matiz único
unique trait rasgo único
unisex unisex
unisexual unisexual
unit unidad
universal complex complejo universal
universal grammar gramática universal
universal phobia fobia universal
universal symbol símbolo universal
universalism universalismo
universality universalidad
unknown substance abuse abuso de sustancia
   desconocida
unknown substance anxiety disorder
   trastorno de ansiedad de sustancia
   desconocida
unknown substance delirium delirio de
   sustancia desconocida
unknown substance dependence dependencia
   de sustancia desconocida
unknown substance intoxication intoxicación
   por sustancia desconocida
unknown substance mood disorder trastorno
   del humor de sustancia desconocida
unknown substance persisting amnestic
   disorder trastorno amnésico persistente de
   sustancia desconocida
unknown substance persisting dementia
   demencia persistente de sustancia
   desconocida
unknown substance psychotic disorder
   trastorno psicótico de sustancia desconocida
unknown substance psychotic disorder with
   delusions trastorno psicótico de sustancia
   desconocida con delusiones
unknown substance psychotic disorder with
   hallucinations trastorno psicótico de
   sustancia desconocida con alucinaciones
unknown substance sexual dysfunction
   disfunción sexual de sustancia desconocida
unknown substance sleep disorder trastorno
   del sueño de sustancia desconocida
unknown substance use disorder trastorno de
   uso de sustancia desconocida

unknown substance withdrawal retiro de
   sustancia desconocida
unlearned no aprendido
unpleasant desagradable
unreliability desconfiabilidad
unreliable desconfiable
unresolved no resuelto
unsociable insociable
unsocialized insocializado
unspecified no especificado
unspecified mental disorder trastorno mental
   no especificado
unspecified mental retardation retardo
   mental no especificado
unspecified substance dependence
   dependencia de sustancia no especificada
unstable inestable
unstructured no estructurado
unstructured interview entrevista no
   estructurada
unstructured stimulus estímulo no
   estructurado
unstructured therapy group grupo de terapia
   no estructurada
unsystematized delusion delusión no
   sistematizada
Unverricht's disease enfermedad de
   Unverricht
unweighted no ponderado
upper superior
upper abdominal periosteal reflex reflejo
   perióstico abdominal superior
upper motor neuron neurona motora superior
upper motor neuron lesion lesión de neurona
   motora superior
upper threshold umbral superior
upsilon upsilón
uracil uracilo
uraniscolalia uraniscolalia
uranism uranismo
uranophobia uranofobia
Urbach-Wiethe disease enfermedad de
   Urbach-Wiethe
uremic urémico
uremic polyneuropathy polineuropatía
   urémica
uresis uresis
ureterolysis ureterólisis
urethra uretra
urethral uretral
urethral anxiety ansiedad uretral
urethral character carácter uretral
urethral complex complejo uretral
urethral eroticism erotismo uretral
urethral phase fase uretral
urethral stage etapa uretral
urethrism uretrismo
urethrismus uretrismo
urethritis uretritis
urethrospasm uretroespasmo
urge urgencia
urge incontinence incontinencia de urgencia
urgency urgencia
urgency incontinence incontinencia de
   urgencia

urinalysis urinálisis
urinary urinario
urinary creatinine creatinina urinaria
urinary reflex reflejo urinario
urinary stuttering tartamudez urinaria
urinary tract infection infección del tracto
    urinario
urine orina
uriposia uriposia
urocrisia urocrisia
urocrisis urocrisis
urolagnia urolagnia
urophilia urofilia
urorrhea urorrea
urticaria urticaria
urticaria gigans urticaria gigante
urticaria gigantea urticaria gigante
urticaria tuberosa urticaria tuberosa
urticate urticado
urtication urticación
uterine uterino
uterine fantasy fantasía uterina
uteroplacental uteroplacentario
uteroplacental environment ambiente
    uteroplacentario
uteroplacental insufficiency insuficiencia
    uteroplacentaria
uterus útero
utilitarian utilitario
utilitarian principle principio utilitario
utility utilidad
utilization utilización
utilization review revisión de utilización
utilization review committee comité de
    revisión de utilización
utopia utopía
utricle utrículo
utricular utricular
utricular reflex reflejo utricular
uxoricide uxoricidio

vaccination vacunación
vaccine vacuna
vaccinophobia vacunofobia
vacuum activity actividad en el vacío
vacuum headache dolor de cabeza por vacío
vacuum response respuesta en el vacío
vagal vagal
vagal attack ataque vagal
vagina vagina
vagina dentata vagina dentada
vaginal vaginal
vaginal canal canal vaginal
vaginal envy envidia vaginal
vaginal hypoesthesia hipoestesia vaginal
vaginal orgasm orgasmo vaginal
vaginalplasty vaginalplastía
vaginate vaginar
vaginism vaginismo
vaginismus vaginismo
vaginitis vaginitis
vagolysis vagólisis
vagolytic vagolítico
vagomimetic vagomimético
vagotomy vagotomía
vagotonia vagotonía
vagotonic vagotónico
vagotropic vagotrópico
vagovagal vagovagal
vagus nerve nervio vago
valence valencia
valerian valeriana
valgus valgus
valid válido
valid consent consentimiento válido
validation validación
validity validez
validity and experimental method validez y
    método experimental
validity criterion criterio de validez
validity of lie detection validez de detección
    de mentiras
validity of test validez de prueba
validity scale escala de validez
Valleix's point punto de Valleix
valnoctamide valnoctamida
valproate valproato
valproic acid ácido valproico
value valor
value judgment juicio de valores
value system sistema de valores
valve válvula
van Bogaert's disease enfermedad de van
    Bogaert
van Buchem's syndrome síndrome de van

Buchem
van der Kolk's law ley de van der Kolk
vandalism vandalismo
variability variabilidad
variable variable
variable chorea of Brissaud corea variable de
    Brissaud
variable error error variable
variable-interval reinforcement refuerzo de
    intervalo variable
variable-interval reinforcement schedule
    programa de refuerzo de intervalo variable
variable-interval schedule programa de
    intervalo variable
variable-ratio reinforcement refuerzo de
    razón variable
variable-ratio reinforcement schedule
    programa de refuerzo de razón variable
variable-ratio schedule programa de razón
    variable
variable reinforcement refuerzo variable
variable stimulus estímulo variable
variance varianza
variant variante
variate variable
variation variación
varicella varicela
varicella encephalitis encefalitis de varicela
varus varus
vas deferens vas deferens
vascular vascular
vascular accident accidente vascular
vascular dementia demencia vascular
vascular headache dolor de cabeza vascular
vascular insufficiency insuficiencia vascular
vasculomyelinopathy vasculomielinopatía
vasectomy vasectomía
vasoactive vasoactivo
vasoactive intestinal peptide péptido
    intestinal vasoactivo
vasoconstriction vasoconstricción
vasoconstrictor vasoconstrictor
vasodepression vasodepresión
vasodilatation vasodilatación
vasogenic vasogénico
vasogenic shock choque vasogénico
vasomotor vasomotor
vasomotor absence ausencia vasomotora
vasomotor ataxia ataxia vasomotora
vasomotor epilepsy epilepsia vasomotora
vasomotor imbalance desequilibrio vasomotor
vasomotor instability inestabilidad
    vasomotora
vasomotor spasm espasmo vasomotor
vasoneuropathy vasoneuropatía
vasoneurosis vasoneurosis
vasopressin vasopresina
vasopressor vasopresor
vasopressor reflex reflejo vasopresor
vasoreflex vasorreflejo
vasospasm vasoespasmo
vasostimulant vasoestimulante
vasovagal vasovagal
vasovagal attack ataque vasovagal
vasovagal attack of Gowers ataque vasovagal

de Gowers
vasovagal epilepsy epilepsia vasovagal
vasovagal syncope síncope vasovagal
vasovagal syndrome síndrome vasovagal
vector vector
vegetative vegetativo
vegetative level nivel vegetativo
vegetative nervous system sistema nervioso
    vegetativo
vegetative neurosis neurosis vegetativa
vegetative retreat retiro vegetativo
vegetative state estado vegetativo
vegetative symptom síntoma vegetativo
velar velar
vellicate velicar
vellication velicación
venereal venéreo
venereal disease enfermedad venérea
venereal-disease phobia fobia de enfermedad
    venérea
venereal disease research laboratory test
    prueba del laboratorio de investigación de
    enfermedades venéreas
venereophobia venereofobia
Venn diagram diagrama de Venn
venography venografía
venorespiratory venorrespiratorio
venorespiratory reflex reflejo
    venorrespiratorio
ventilation ventilación
ventral ventral
ventral anterior nucleus núcleo anterior
    ventral
ventral lateral nucleus núcleo lateral ventral
ventral posterior nucleus núcleo posterior
    ventral
ventral root raíz ventral
ventricle ventrículo
ventricle puncture punción de ventrículo
ventricular ventricular
ventricular system sistema ventricular
ventriculitis ventriculitis
ventriculocisternostomy
    ventriculocisternostomía
ventriculogram ventriculograma
ventriculography ventriculografía
ventriculomastoidostomy
    ventriculomastoidostomía
ventriculopuncture ventriculopunción
ventriculoscopy ventriculoscopia
ventriculostomy ventriculostomía
ventriculotomy ventriculotomía
ventromedial ventromedial
ventromedial hypothalamic syndrome
    síndrome hipotalámico ventromedial
ventromedial hypothalamus hipotálamo
    ventromedial
ventromedial nucleus núcleo ventromedial
verapamil verapamil
verbal verbal
verbal ability habilidad verbal
verbal abuse abuso verbal
verbal agraphia agrafia verbal
verbal alexia alexia verbal
verbal amnesia amnesia verbal

verbal aphasia afasia verbal
verbal assault acometimiento verbal
verbal assaults on children acometimientos verbales en niños
verbal automatism automatismo verbal
verbal aversion therapy terapia de aversión verbal
verbal behavior conducta verbal
verbal comprehension comprensión verbal
verbal conditioning condicionamiento verbal
verbal encoding codificación verbal
verbal factor factor verbal
verbal generalization generalización verbal
verbal image imagen verbal
verbal intelligence inteligencia verbal
verbal learning aprendizaje verbal
verbal masochism masoquismo verbal
verbal memory memoria verbal
verbal paraphasia parafasia verbal
verbal rehearsal ensayo verbal
verbal scale escala verbal
verbal search búsqueda verbal
verbal space espacio verbal
verbal stimulation estimulación verbal
verbal stimulus estímulo verbal
verbal test prueba verbal
verbal thought pensamiento verbal
verbalism verbalismo
verbalization verbalización
verbigerate verbigerar
verbigeration verbigeración
verbochromia verbocromia
verbomania verbomanía
verbose verboso
vergence vergencia
veridical verídico
verification verificación
verification time tiempo de verificación
vermis vermis
vernacular vernáculo
vernal encephalitis encefalitis vernal
Vernet's syndrome síndrome de Vernet
Verneuil's neuroma neuroma de Verneuil
vernier vernier
Verocay body cuerpo de Verocay
vertebral vertebral
vertebral artery arteria vertebral
vertebral cervical instability inestabilidad cervical vertebral
vertebral fusion fusión vertebral
vertebral venography venografía vertebral
vertebrectomy vertebrectomía
vertebrobasilar vertebrobasilar
vertebrobasilar system sistema vertebrobasilar
vertex vértice
vertex potential potencial de vértice
vertical axis eje vertical
vertical group grupo vertical
vertical mobility movilidad vertical
vertical sampling muestreo vertical
vertical transmission transmisión vertical
vertical vertigo vértigo vertical
vertiginous vertiginoso
vertigo vértigo

very important person syndrome síndrome de persona muy importante
vesical vesical
vesical reflex reflejo vesical
vestibular vestibular
vestibular adaptation adaptación vestibular
vestibular apparatus aparato vestibular
vestibular canal canal vestibular
vestibular hallucination alucinación vestibular
vestibular membrane membrana vestibular
vestibular nerve nervio vestibular
vestibular receptor receptor vestibular
vestibular sense sentido vestibular
vestibular system sistema vestibular
vestibule vestíbulo
vestibulocerebellar vestibulocerebeloso
vestibulocerebellar ataxia ataxia vestibulocerebelosa
vestibulocochlear vestibulococlear
vestibulocochlear nerve nervio vestibulococlear
vestibuloequilibratory vestibuloequilibratorio
vestibuloequilibratory control control vestibuloequilibratorio
vestibulospinal vestibuloespinal
vestibulospinal reflex reflejo vestibuloespinal
vestibulospinal system sistema vestibuloespinal
vestige vestigio
viable viable
vibration experience experiencia de vibraciones
vibration rate tasa de vibraciones
vibration receptor receptor de vibraciones
vibration sense sentido de vibraciones
vibration syndrome síndrome por vibraciones
vibrator vibrador
vibratory sense sentido vibratorio
vibratory sensibility sensibilidad vibratoria
vicarious vicario
vicarious brain process proceso cerebral vicario
vicarious conditioning condicionamiento vicario
vicarious function función vicaria
vicarious functioning funcionamiento vicario
vicarious learning aprendizaje vicario
vicarious living vivir vicario
vicarious pleasure placer vicario
vicarious satisfaction satisfacción vicaria
vicious circle círculo vicioso
victim víctima
victim psychology psicología de víctima
victim recidivism recidivismo de víctima
victimization victimización
victimology victimología
video techniques técnicas de video
videotape method método de videocinta
Vierordt's law ley de Vierordt
vigil vigilia
vigilambulism vigilambulismo
vigilance vigilancia
viloxazine viloxazina
vinbarbital vinbarbital

Vincent curve curva de Vincent
Vincent method método de Vincent
violence violencia
violence on television violencia en televisión
violence prediction predicción de violencia
violent violento
violent behavior conducta violenta
violent behavior of abused children conducta
    violenta de niños abusados
violinist's cramp calambre de violinista
viraginity viraginidad
viral viral
viral cerebral infection infección cerebral
    viral
Virchow's disease enfermedad de Virchow
Virchow's psammoma psamoma de Virchow
virgophrenia virgofrenia
virilescence virilescencia
virilism virilismo
virulent virulento
virus virus
virus encephalomyelitis encefalomielitis viral
virus infection infección viral
viscera vísceras
visceral visceral
visceral anesthesia anestesia visceral
visceral disorder trastorno visceral
visceral drive impulso visceral
visceral epilepsy epilepsia visceral
visceral learning aprendizaje visceral
visceral neurosis neurosis visceral
visceral sensation sensación visceral
visceral sense sentido visceral
visceroceptor visceroceptor
viscerogenic viscerogénico
viscerogenic reflex reflejo viscerogénico
visceromotor visceromotor
visceromotor reflex reflejo visceromotor
visceroreceptor viscerorreceptor
viscerosensory viscerosensorial
viscerosensory reflex reflejo viscerosensorial
viscerotonia viscerotonía
viscerotonic viscerotónico
viscerotonic temperament temperamento
    viscerotónico
viscosity of libido viscosidad de libido
viscus víscera
visibility visibilidad
visibility coefficient coeficiente de visibilidad
visibility curve curva de visibilidad
visible spectrum espectro visible
visible speech habla visible
vision visión
visual visual
visual accommodation acomodación visual
visual acuity agudeza visual
visual adaptation adaptación visual
visual agnosia agnosia visual
visual agraphia agrafia visual
visual alexia alexia visual
visual allachesthesia alaquestesia visual
visual amnesia amnesia visual
visual angle ángulo visual
visual aphasia afasia visual
visual attention atención visual

visual aura aura visual
visual axis eje visual
visual capture captura visual
visual cliff precipicio visual
visual closure cierre visual
visual cortex corteza visual
visual cycle ciclo visual
visual discrimination discriminación visual
visual disparity disparidad visual
visual-distortion test prueba de distorsión
    visual
visual dominance dominancia visual
visual evoked potential potencial evocado
    visual
visual evoked response respuesta evocada
    visual
visual field campo visual
visual-field defect defecto de campo visual
visual fixation fijación visual
visual hallucination alucinación visual
visual illusion ilusión visual
visual image imagen visual
visual imagery imaginería visual
visual impairment deterioro visual
visual inattention inatención visual
visual induction inducción visual
visual learning aprendizaje visual
visual memory memoria visual
visual memory span lapso de memoria visual
visual-motor visual-motor
visual-motor coordination coordinación
    visual-motora
visual-motor skill destreza visual-motora
visual noise ruido visual
visual orbicularis reflex reflejo orbicular
    visual
visual organization organización visual
visual perception percepción visual
visual projection proyección visual
visual righting reflex reflejo de
    enderezamiento visual
visual search búsqueda visual
visual-search perceptual disorder trastorno
    perceptivo de búsqueda visual
visual space espacio visual
visual span lapso visual
visual-spatial ability habilidad visual-espacial
visual-spatial agnosia agnosia visual-espacial
visual stimulation estimulación visual
visual system sistema visual
visual tracking rastreo visual
visual type tipo visual
visualization visualización
visualization technique técnica de
    visualización
visualize visualizar
visuoauditory visuoauditivo
visuoconstruction defect defecto de
    visuoconstrucción
visuognosis visuognosis
visuomotor visuomotor
visuomotor theory teoría visuomotora
visuopsychic visuopsíquico
visuosensory visuosensorial
visuospatial visuoespacial

visuospatial agnosia agnosia visuoespacial
vital vital
vital capacity capacidad vital
vital signs signos vitales
vital statistics estadística vital
vitalism vitalismo
vitality vitalidad
vitamin vitamina
vitamin B-12 neuropathy neuropatía por vitamina B-12
vitamin deficiency deficiencia de vitamina
vitamin therapy terapia vitamínica
vitrectomy vitrectomía
vitreous vítreo
vitreous hemorrhage hemorragia vítrea
vitreous humor humor vítreo
vivisection vivisección
vocabulary vocabulario
vocabulary growth crecimiento de vocabulario
vocabulary test prueba de vocabulario
vocal vocal
vocal amusia amusia vocal
vocal cord cuerda vocal
vocal tract tracto vocal
vocality vocalidad
vocalization vocalización
vocation vocación
vocational vocacional
vocational adjustment ajuste vocacional
vocational appraisal evaluación vocacional
vocational aptitude aptitud vocacional
vocational-aptitude test prueba de aptitud vocacional
vocational assessment evaluación vocacional
vocational choice selección vocacional
vocational counseling asesoramiento vocacional
vocational development desarrollo vocacional
vocational education educación vocacional
vocational evaluation evaluación vocacional
vocational guidance asesoramiento vocacional
vocational identity identidad vocacional
vocational maladjustment inadaptación vocacional
vocational rehabilitation rehabilitación vocacional
vocational selection selección vocacional
vocational services servicios vocacionales
vocational training entrenamiento vocacional
Vogt-Spielmeyer disease enfermedad de Vogt-Spielmeyer
Vogt syndrome síndrome de Vogt
voice voz
voice disorder trastorno de voz
voice onset time tiempo de comienzo de voz
voice quality calidad de voz
voice sound sonido de voz
voice therapist terapeuta de voz
voiceless sordo
voiceprint espectrograma de voz
Voigt's line línea de Voigt
volar volar
volatile volátil
volatile chemical inhalation inhalación de

sustancia química volátil
volatile solvent dependence dependencia de solvente volátil
volition volición
volitional volitivo
volitional ability habilidad volitiva
volitional tremor temblor volitivo
Volkmann's contracture contractura de Volkmann
voltaic vertigo vértigo voltaico
volubility volubilidad
volume volumen
voluntarism voluntarismo
voluntary voluntario
voluntary admission admisión voluntaria
voluntary ataxia ataxia voluntaria
voluntary commitment confinamiento voluntario
voluntary control control voluntario
voluntary euthanasia eutanasia voluntaria
voluntary hospitalization hospitalización voluntaria
voluntary movement movimiento voluntario
voluntary muscle músculo voluntario
voluntary mutism mutismo voluntario
voluntary nervous system sistema nervioso voluntario
voluntary process proceso voluntario
voluntary response respuesta voluntaria
volunteer bias sesgo de voluntarios
vomiting vómito
vomiting reflex reflejo de vómito
von Domarus principle principio de von Domarus
von Economo's disease enfermedad de von Economo
von Gierke's disease enfermedad de von Gierke
von Gierke's syndrome síndrome de von Gierke
von Graefe's sign signo de von Graefe
von Hippel-Lindau disease enfermedad de von Hippel-Lindau
von Hippel-Lindau syndrome síndrome de von Hippel-Lindau
von Recklinghausen's disease enfermedad de von Recklinghausen
von Restorff effect efecto de von Restorff
voodoo vudú
voyeur voyeur
voyeurism voyeurismo
vulnerability vulnerabilidad
vulnerability factor factor de vulnerabilidad
vulnerability theory teoría de vulnerabilidad
vulnerable vulnerable
vulnerable child niño vulnerable
vulnerable-child syndrome síndrome de niño vulnerable
Vulpian's atrophy atrofia de Vulpian
Vulpian's effect efecto de Vulpian
vulva vulva
vulvectomy vulvectomía
vulvismus vulvismo
Vygotsky blocks bloques de Vygotsky
Vygotsky test prueba de Vygotsky

Waardenburg's syndrome síndrome de
 Waardenburg
Wada dominance test prueba de dominancia
 de Wada
Wada test prueba de Wada
waiter's cramp calambre de camarero
waking center centro del despertar
waking hypnosis hipnosis despierta
waking numbness entumecimiento al
 despertar
Walker tractotomy tractotomía de Walker
Wallenberg's syndrome síndrome de
 Wallenberg
wallerian degeneration degeneración
 walleriana
wallerian law ley de Waller
wandering errante
wandering attention atención errante
wandering cell célula errante
wandering uterus útero errante
wanderlust impulso mórbido de viajar
ward pabellón
Wardrop's method método de Wardrop
warfarin warfarina
warm-up period periodo de calentamiento
warming-up period periodo de calentamiento
Wartenberg's symptom síntoma de
 Wartenberg
wasting palsy parálisis degenerante
wasting paralysis parálisis degenerante
watch test prueba de reloj
watchmaker's cramp calambre de relojero
water intoxication intoxicación por agua
waterfall illusion ilusión de cascada
wave onda
wave amplitude amplitud de onda
wave analyzer analizador de ondas
wave frequency frecuencia de onda
wave of excitation onda de excitación
wavelength longitud de onda
waxy flexibility flexibilidad cerea
weak ego ego débil
weaning destete
Weber's law ley de Weber
Weber's sign signo de Weber
Weber's syndrome síndrome de Weber
Weber-Fechner law ley de Weber-Fechner
Weber test prueba de Weber
wedding night noche de boda
Wedensky facilitation facilitación de
 Wedensky
weekend hospital hospital de fin de semana
weekend neurosis neurosis de fin de semana
weekend parents padres de fin de semana

Weigert stain colorante de Weigert
weight peso
weight control control de peso
weight discrimination discriminación de peso
weight loss therapy terapia de pérdida de
 peso
weight regulation regulación de peso
weighted ponderado
weighting ponderación
Weingrow's reflex reflejo de Weingrow
Weir Mitchell treatment tratamiento de Weir
 Mitchell
Weiss' sign signo de Weiss
well-adjusted bien ajustado
Werdnig-Hoffmann disease enfermedad de
 Werdnig-Hoffmann
Werner's disease enfermedad de Werner
Werner's syndrome síndrome de Werner
Wernicke's aphasia afasia de Wernicke
Wernicke's area área de Wernicke
Wernicke's cramp calambre de Wernicke
Wernicke's dementia demencia de Wernicke
Wernicke's disease enfermedad de Wernicke
Wernicke's encephalopathy encefalopatía de
 Wernicke
Wernicke's fluent encephalopathy
 encefalopatía fluente de Wernicke
Wernicke's reaction reacción de Wernicke
Wernicke's sign signo de Wernicke
Wernicke's syndrome síndrome de Wernicke
Wernicke-Korsakoff encephalopathy
 encefalopatía de Wernicke-Korsakoff
Wernicke-Korsakoff syndrome síndrome de
 Wernicke-Korsakoff
Wernicke-Mann hemiplegia hemiplejía de
 Wernicke-Mann
West's syndrome síndrome de West
western equine encephalomyelitis
 encefalomielitis equina del oeste
Westphal's disease enfermedad de Westphal
Westphal's phenomenon fenómeno de
 Westphal
Westphal's pseudosclerosis seudoesclerosis
 de Westphal
Westphal's pupillary reflex reflejo pupilar de
 Westphal
Westphal's sign signo de Westphal
Westphal-Erb sign signo de Westphal-Erb
Westphal-Leyden syndrome síndrome de
 Westphal-Leyden
Westphal-Piltz phenomenon fenómeno de
 Westphal-Piltz
Westphal-Strumpell pseudosclerosis
 seudoesclerosis de Westphal-Strumpell
wet beriberi beriberi húmedo
wet dream sueño con emisión
Wever-Bray effect efecto de Wever-Bray
Wever-Bray phenomenon fenómeno de
 Wever-Bray
wheelchair silla de ruedas
wheelchair sports deportes con sillas de
 ruedas
whiplash injury lesión en látigo
whipping azotamiento
whispered speech habla susurrada

white commissure comisura blanca
white matter materia blanca
white noise ruido blanco
whole-word method método de palabra completa
Whorf's hypothesis hipótesis de Whorf
wife battering golpeo de esposa
Wilcoxon test prueba de Wilcoxon
Wilder's law of initial value ley de Wilder de valor inicial
Wildervanck's syndrome síndrome de Wildervanck
will voluntad
will disturbance disturbio de voluntad
will factor factor de voluntad
will power fuerza de voluntad
will therapy terapia de voluntad
will to live voluntad de vivir
will to survive voluntad de sobrevivir
Williams syndrome síndrome de Williams
Wilson's disease enfermedad de Wilson
Wilson's syndrome síndrome de Wilson
wink reflex reflejo de guiño
Winkelman's disease enfermedad de Winkelman
winking spasm espasmo de guiños
wisdom sabiduría
wish deseo
wish fulfillment realización de sueño
wishful thinking pensamiento deseoso
witchcraft brujería
withdrawal retiro, retirada
withdrawal delirium delirio de retiro
withdrawal dyskinesia discinesia de retiro
withdrawal method of contraception método de contracepción de retirada
withdrawal reaction reacción de retiro
withdrawal reflex reflejo de retiro
withdrawal symptoms síntomas de retiro
withdrawal syndrome síndrome de retiro
Wohlfart-Kugelberg-Welander disease enfermedad de Wohlfart-Kugelberg-Welander
Wolf-Orton body cuerpo de Wolf-Orton
Wollaston's theory teoría de Wollaston
Wolman's disease enfermedad de Wolman
womb fantasy fantasía de útero
woodcutter's encephalitis encefalitis de leñador
word approximation aproximación de palabras
word association asociación de palabras
word-association technique técnica de asociación de palabras
word-association test prueba de asociación de palabras
word blindness ceguera de palabras
word configuration configuración de palabra
word count cuenta de palabras
word deafness sordera de palabras
word fluency fluencia de palabras
word method método de palabras
word recognition reconocimiento de palabras
word-recognition skills destrezas de reconocimiento de palabras

word salad ensalada de palabras
work addiction adicción al trabajo
work decrement decremento de trabajo
work evaluation evaluación de trabajo
work inhibition inhibición de trabajo
work motivation motivación de trabajo
work paralysis parálisis de trabajo
work rehabilitation center centro de rehabilitación de trabajo
work sample muestra de trabajo
work-space design diseño de espacio de trabajo
work therapy terapia de trabajo
working conditions condiciones de trabajo
working memory memoria trabajadora
working mother madre trabajadora
working through aumento de penetración
worry preocupación
wound herida
wrist clonus clono de muñeca
wrist clonus reflex reflejo del clono de muñeca
wrist drop caída de muñeca
writer's cramp calambre de escritor
writing escritura
writing disorder trastorno de escritura
writing hand mano de escritor
wryneck cuello torcido
wryneck syndrome síndrome de cuello torcido
Wyburn-Mason syndrome síndrome de Wyburn-Mason

X axis eje X
X chromosome cromosoma X
X-linked ligado al X
xanthine xantina
xanthocyanopsia xantocianopsia
xanthomatosis xantomatosis
xanthopsia xantopsia
xenogenous xenógeno
xenoglossia xenoglosia
xenoglossophilia xenoglosofilia
xenoglossophobia xenoglosofobia
xenophobia xenofobia
xenorexia xenorexia
xerostomia xerostomía
xiphodynia xifodinia
xiphoidalgia xifoidalgia
xyrospasm xiroespasmo

Y axis eje Y
Y chromosome cromosoma Y
Yates correction corrección de Yates
yes-no question pregunta de sí-no
yoga yoga
yohimbine yohimbina
Young-Helmholtz theory teoría de
    Young-Helmholtz
Young-Helmholtz theory of color vision
    teoría de Young-Helmholtz de visión de
    color
youth juventud

Z

Zange-Kindler syndrome síndrome de
   Zange-Kindler
Zanoli-Vecchi syndrome síndrome de
   Zanoli-Vecchi
Zappert's syndrome síndrome de Zappert
Zeigarnik effect efecto de Zeigarnik
Zeigarnik phenomenon fenómeno de
   Zeigarnik
zeitgeist zeitgeist
zelophobia celofobia
zelotypia celotipia
Zenker's paralysis parálisis de Zenker
zero-order correlation correlación de orden
   cero
zeta zeta
Ziehen-Oppenheim disease enfermedad de
   Ziehen-Oppenheim
Zipf's law ley de Zipf
Zipf curve curva de Zipf
zoanthropic zoantrópico
zoanthropy zoantropía
Zollner illusion ilusión de Zollner
zona dermatica zona dermática
zona epithelioserosa zona epitelioserosa
zonesthesia zonestesia
zonifugal zonífugo
zonipetal zonípeto
zooerastia zooerastia
zooerasty zooerastia
zoolagnia zoolagnia
zoomania zoomanía
zoomorphism zoomorfismo
zoophile zoófilo
zoophilia zoofilia
zoophilic zoofílico
zoophilism zoofilismo
zoophobia zoofobia
zoopsia zoopsia
zoosadism zoosadismo
zoster encephalomyelitis encefalomielitis
   zoster
Zwaardemaker olfactometer olfatómetro de
   Zwaardemaker
Zwaardemaker smell system sistema de
   olfato de Zwaardemaker
zygomaticus cigomático
zygosis cigosis
zygosity cigosidad
zygote cigoto
zygotic cigótico

ESPAÑOL-INGLÉS
SPANISH-ENGLISH

a corto plazo short-term
a largo plazo long-term
a posteriori a posteriori
a priori a priori
a riesgo at risk
abalienación abalienation
abandonando el campo leaving the field
abandono abandonment
abarognosis abarognosis
abasia abasia
abasia-astasia abasia-astasia
abasia atáxica ataxic abasia
abasia coreica choreic abasia
abasia espástica spastic abasia
abasia temblorosa trembling abasia
abásico abasic
abático abatic
abatimiento abasement
abatir abate
abclusión abclution
abdominal abdominal
abducción abduction
abducente abducens
abducente abducent
abducir abduct
abductor abductor
aberración aberration
aberración cromática chromatic aberration
aberración cromosómica chromosomal
    aberration
aberración cromosómica sexual
    sex-chromosomal aberration
aberración dióptrica dioptric aberration
aberración esférica spherical aberration
aberración mental mental aberration
aberración sexual sexual aberration
aberraciones autosómicas autosomal
    aberrations
aberrante aberrant
abertura aperture
abiatrofia abiatrophy
abiencia abience
abiente abient
abiogenético abiogenetic
abionergia abionergy
abiosis abiosis
abiótico abiotic
abiotrofia abiotrophy
abirritante abirritant
ablación ablatio
ablación del pene ablatio penis
ablactación ablactation
ablepsia ablepsy
ablución ablution

ablutomanía ablutomania
abnerval abnerval
abneural abneural
abominación abomination
aboral aboral
abortivo abortifacient
aborto abortion
aborto espontaneo spontaneous abortion
aborto inducido induced abortion
aborto terapéutico therapeutic abortion
abrasión abrasion
abrasivo abrasive
abrazadera brace
abrazante embracing
abrazo embrace
abreacción abreaction
abreacción motora motor abreaction
abrosia abrosia
absceso abscess
absceso cerebral cerebral abscess
absceso de Pott Pott's abscess
absceso ótico otic abscess
abscisa abscissa
absintio absinthe
absintismo absinthism
absolutismo cultural cultural absolutism
absolutismo fenomenal phenomenal
    absolutism
absoluto absolute
absoluto cultural cultural absolute
absorber absorb, engross
absorción absorption, engrossment
absorción espectral spectral absorption
absorción propia self-absorption
abstinencia abstinence
abstinencia sexual sexual abstinence
abstracción abstraction
abstracción sistemática systematic abstraction
abstracto abstract
absurdidad absurdity
abterminal abterminal
abulia abulia
abúlico abulic
abulomanía abulomania
abultamiento bloating
aburrimiento boredom
abusabilidad abusability
abuso abuse
abuso de adultos adult abuse
abuso de alcohol alcohol abuse
abuso de alcohol crónico chronic alcohol
    abuse
abuso de alcohol y dependencia alcohol
    abuse and dependence
abuso de alucinógenos hallucinogen abuse
abuso de ancianos elderly abuse
abuso de anfetaminas amphetamine abuse
abuso de ansiolítico anxiolytic abuse
abuso de barbituratos barbiturate abuse
abuso de cafeína caffeine abuse
abuso de cannabis cannabis abuse
abuso de cocaína cocaine abuse
abuso de cónyuge spouse abuse
abuso de droga psicoactiva psychoactive
    drug abuse

abuso de drogas drug abuse
abuso de drogas en adolescencia drug abuse in adolescence
abuso de estimulantes stimulant abuse
abuso de fenciclidina phencyclidine abuse
abuso de hipnótico hypnotic abuse
abuso de inhalante inhalant abuse
abuso de laxantes laxative abuse
abuso de mayores elder abuse
abuso de mentanfetaminas methamphetamine abuse
abuso de niños child abuse
abuso de niños y suicidio child abuse and suicide
abuso de niños y uso de alcohol child abuse and alcohol use
abuso de opioide opioid abuse
abuso de otra sustancia other substance abuse
abuso de sedante sedative abuse
abuso de sustancia substance abuse
abuso de sustancia desconocida unknown substance abuse
abuso de sustancia psicoactiva psychoactive substance abuse
abuso de sustancia y abuso de niños substance abuse and child abuse
abuso de sustancias maternal maternal substance abuse
abuso de sustancias químicas chemical abuse
abuso de tabaco tobacco abuse
abuso de tranquilizante tranquilizer abuse
abuso emocional emotional abuse
abuso físico physical abuse
abuso físico de adulto physical abuse of adult
abuso físico de niño physical abuse of child
abuso físico e hiperactividad physical abuse and hyperactivity
abuso físico e inteligencia physical abuse and intelligence
abuso físico y autoestima physical abuse and self-esteem
abuso físico y el desarrollo physical abuse and development
abuso físico y muerte prematura physical abuse and premature death
abuso mental mental abuse
abuso polídroga polydrug abuse
abuso psicológico psychologic abuse
abuso sexual sexual abuse
abuso sexual de adulto sexual abuse of adult
abuso sexual de niño sexual abuse of child
abuso sexual y cuidado diurno sexual abuse and day care
abuso verbal verbal abuse
académico academic
acalasia achalasia
acalasia esfinteral sphincteral achalasia
acalasia esofagal esophageal achalasia
acalculia acalculia
acampsia acampsia
acantamebiasis acanthamebiasis
acantestesia acanthesthesia
acaparamiento hoarding
acarofobia acarophobia

acatafasia acataphasia
acatalepsia acatalepsia
acatama akatama
acatamatesia acatamathesia
acatamatesia akatamathesia
acatamiento compliance
acatamiento estratégico strategic compliance
acatamiento inducido induced compliance
acatamiento motor motor compliance
acatamiento neurótico neurotic compliance
acatamiento normativo normative compliance
acatamiento social social compliance
acatamiento somático somatic compliance
acatexia acathexis
acatisia acathisia
acatisia aguda inducida por neuroléptico neuroleptic-induced acute akathisia
acatisia paraestética acathisia paraesthetica
accesibilidad accessibility
accesible accessible
acceso access, seizure
acceso acinético akinetic seizure
acceso anosognósico anosognosic seizure
acceso audiogénico audiogenic seizure
acceso automático automatic seizure
acceso autónomo autonomic seizure
acceso centrencefálico centrencephalic seizure
acceso de ausencia absence seizure
acceso de conversión conversion seizure
acceso de lóbulo temporal temporal-lobe seizure
acceso de pequeño mal petit mal seizure
acceso epileptiforme epileptiform seizure
acceso erótico erotic seizure
acceso generalizado generalized seizure
acceso gustatorio gustatory seizure
acceso histérico hysterical seizure
acceso masivo massive seizure
acceso mioclónico myoclonic seizure
acceso motor mayor major motor seizure
acceso parcial partial seizure
acceso parcial complejo complex partial seizure
acceso parcial elemental elementary partial seizure
acceso psicomotor psychomotor seizure
acceso psíquico psychic seizure
acceso tónico-clónico tonic-clonic seizure
acceso tónico-clónico generalizado generalized tonic-clonic seizure
acceso uncinado uncinate seizure
accesorio accessory
accesos fragmentados fragmentary seizures
accidental accidental
accidente accident
accidente cerebrovascular cerebrovascular accident
accidente fatal fatal accident
accidente intencionado purposeful accident
accidente intencional intentional accident
accidente vascular vascular accident
acción action
acción afirmativa affirmative action
acción antigonadal antigonadal action

acción automática automatic action
acción casual chance action
acción cognitiva cognitive action
acción en masa mass action
acción-instrumento action-instrument
acción irracional irrational action
acción por rapto raptus action
acción psicomotora psychomotor action
acción-recipiente action-recipient
acción simbólica symbolic action
acción social social action
acción-ubicación action-location
acedia acedia
aceleración acceleration
aceleración del desarrollo developmental
    acceleration
aceleración educacional educational
    acceleration
aceleración escolástica scholastic acceleration
aceleración negativa negative acceleration
aceleración positiva positive acceleration
acenestesia acenesthesia
acento accent
acento extranjero foreign accent
acentuación de interfase interface
    accentuation
aceptación acceptance
aceptación de grupo group acceptance
aceptación privada private acceptance
acercamiento approach
acercamiento a la lectura de experiencias del
    lenguaje language-experience approach to
    reading
acercamiento adaptacional adaptational
    approach
acercamiento adaptivo adaptive approach
acercamiento ambiental environmental
    approach
acercamiento bioquímico biochemical
    approach
acercamiento centrado en la comunidad
    community-centered approach
acercamiento científico scientific approach
acercamiento cognitivo cognitive approach
acercamiento conductual behavioral
    approach
acercamiento conductual para conducta
    anormal behavioral approach to abnormal
    behavior
acercamiento conductual para esquizofrenia
    behavioral approach to schizophrenia
acercamiento constructivo constructive
    approach
acercamiento cualitativo qualitative approach
acercamiento cuantitativo quantitative
    approach
acercamiento de alto riesgo high-risk
    approach
acercamiento de aquí y ahora here-and-now
    approach
acercamiento de Bayes Bayesian approach
acercamiento de caja negra black-box
    approach
acercamiento de equipo team approach
acercamiento de Fechner Fechner's approach

acercamiento de grupos cluster approach
acercamiento de libros de lectura básicos
    basal reader approach
acercamiento de sentido común crítico
    critical common-sense approach
acercamiento descriptivo descriptive
    approach
acercamiento dinámico dynamic approach
acercamiento ecléctico eclectic approach
acercamiento ecológico ecological approach
acercamiento económico economic approach
acercamiento educacional educational
    approach
acercamiento educativo
    diagnóstico-prescriptivo
    diagnostic-prescriptive educational
    approach
acercamiento estructural structural approach
acercamiento ético ethical approach
acercamiento etnográfico ethnographic
    approach
acercamiento freudiano freudian approach
acercamiento idiográfico idiographic
    approach
acercamiento interdisciplinario
    interdisciplinary approach
acercamiento lingüístico linguistic approach
acercamiento lingüístico-cinésico
    linguistic-kinesic approach
acercamiento mecanístico mechanistic
    approach
acercamiento molar molar approach
acercamiento molecular molecular approach
acercamiento multidisciplinario
    multidisciplinary approach
acercamiento naturalista naturalistic
    approach
acercamiento no directivo nondirective
    approach
acercamiento nomotético nomothetic
    approach
acercamiento nosológico nosological
    approach
acercamiento o retirada approach or
    withdrawal
acercamiento orgánico organic approach
acercamiento orientado hacia tarea
    task-oriented approach
acercamiento reductivo reductive approach
acercamiento regresivo-reconstructivo
    regressive-reconstructive approach
acercamiento represivo repressive approach
acercamiento sintético synthetic approach
acercamiento sistemático systematic approach
acercamiento situacional situational approach
acercamiento transcultural cross-cultural
    approach
acerofobia acerophobia
acérvula acervulus
acervulino acervuline
acetaminofeno acetaminophen
acetanilida acetanilide
acetato de ciproterona cyproterone acetate
acetazolamida acetazolamide
acetilasa de colina choline acetylase

acetilcolina acetylcholine
acetilcolinesterasa acetylcholinesterase
acetilfosfato acetylphosphate
acetiltransferasa de colina choline
   acetyltransferase
acetilureas acetylureas
acetofenazina acetophenazine
acetofenetidina acetophenetidine
acetona acetone
acicaladura grooming
acidez acidity
acidificación acidification
ácido acid
ácido acetilsalicílico acetylsalicylic acid
ácido adenílico adenylic acid
ácido aminohidroxibutírico
   aminohydroxybutyric acid
ácido aspártico aspartic acid
ácido barbitúrico barbituric acid
ácido clorazépico clorazepic acid
ácido desoxirribonucleico deoxyribonucleic
   acid
ácido desoxirribonucleico recombinante
   recombinant deoxyribonucleic acid
ácido fenilpirúvico phenylpyruvic acid
ácido fólico folic acid
ácido fólico sérico serum folic acid
ácido gama-aminobutírico
   gamma-aminobutyric acid
ácido glutámico glutamic acid
ácido homovanílico homovanillic acid
ácido lisérgico lysergic acid
ácido malónico malonic acid
ácido nicotínico nicotinic acid
ácido nucleico nucleic acid
ácido ribonucleico ribonucleic acid
ácido ribonucleico de transferencia transfer
   ribonucleic acid
ácido ribonucleico mensajero messenger
   ribonucleic acid
ácido valproico valproic acid
acidosis acidosis
acidosis diabética diabetic acidosis
aciduria argininosuccínica argininosuccinic
   aciduria
ácigos azygous
acinesia akinesia
acinesia álgera akinesia algera
acinesia amnésica akinesia amnestica
acinesis akinesis
acinestesia akinesthesia
acinético akinetic
aclimatación acclimatization
acluofobia achluophobia
acmé acme
acmestesia acmesthesia
acné acne
acolasia acolasia
acometimiento assault
acometimiento físico physical assault
acometimiento sexual sexual assault
acometimiento verbal verbal assault
acometimientos verbales en niños verbal
   assaults on children
acomodación accommodation

acomodación absoluta absolute
   accommodation
acomodación binocular binocular
   accommodation
acomodación de nervio accommodation of
   nerve
acomodación interpersonal interpersonal
   accommodation
acomodación social social accommodation
acomodación visual visual accommodation
acomodativo accommodative
aconativo aconative
acondroplasia achondroplasia
acónito aconite
aconuresis acqnuresis
acoplamiento coupling
acoria acoria
acosado por instintos instinct-ridden
acoso sexual sexual molestation
acrai acrai
acrasia acrasy
acrecentamiento accretion
acreditación accreditation
acroagnosis acroagnosis
acroanestesia acroanesthesia
acroataxia acroataxia
acrobraquicefalia acrobrachycephaly
acrocefalia acrocephaly
acrocefálico acrocephalic
acrocéfalo acrocephalous
acrocianosis acrocyanosis
acrocinesia acrocinesia
acrocinesis acrocinesis
acrodinia acrodynia
acrodisestesia acrodysesthesia
acroedema acroedema
acroestesia acroesthesia
acrofobia acrophobia
acrognosis acrognosis
acrohipotermia acrohypothermia
acromático achromatic
acromatismo achromatism
acromatopsia achromatopsia
acromegalia acromegaly
acromegaloide acromegaloid
acromelalgia acromelalgia
acromial acromial
acromicria acromicria
acromicria congénita congenital acromicria
acroneurosis acroneurosis
acrónimo acronym
acroparestesia acroparesthesia
acrosoma acrosome
acrotrofodinia acrotrophodynia
acrotrofoneurosis acrotrophoneurosis
actina actin
actinoneuritis actinoneuritis
actitud attitude
actitud abstracta abstract attitude
actitud catatonoide catatonoid attitude
actitud categórica categorical attitude
actitud científica scientific attitude
actitud concreta concrete attitude
actitud concretante concretizing attitude
actitud de escuchar listening attitude

actitud de estímulo stimulus attitude
actitud de exposición exposition attitude
actitud de momia mummy attitude
actitud de objeto object attitude
actitud de proceso process attitude
actitud de respuesta response attitude
actitud dionisiaca Dionysian attitude
actitud emocional emotional attitude
actitud fóbica phobic attitude
actitud imperativa imperative attitude
actitud negativa negative attitude
actitud parental parental attitude
actitud pasional passional attitude
actitud positiva positive attitude
actitud social social attitude
actitudes maternales maternal attitudes
actitudes sexuales sexual attitudes
activación activation
activación automática automatic activation
activación fásica phasic activation
activación propagante spreading activation
activación tónica tonic activation
activador activator
actividad activity
actividad aleatoria random activity
actividad antisocial antisocial activity
actividad antisocial oculta concealed
  antisocial activity
actividad autóctona autochthonous activity
actividad autónoma autonomous activity
actividad de bloqueo blocking activity
actividad de compromiso compromise
  activity
actividad de desplazamiento displacement
  activity
actividad de ejercicio exercise activity
actividad de ligadura de libido libido-binding
  activity
actividad de motor fino fine motor activity
actividad de motor grueso gross motor
  activity
actividad de punta-onda spike-wave activity
actividad de rebosamiento overflow activity
actividad dopaminérgica dopaminergic
  activity
actividad eléctrica del cerebro electrical
  activity of the brain
actividad electrodérmica electrodermal
  activity
actividad electrodérmica durante el sueño
  electrodermal activity in sleep
actividad en el vacío vacuum activity
actividad estomacal stomach activity
actividad fetal fetal activity
actividad física physical activity
actividad graduada graded activity
actividad inmovilizante immobilizing activity
actividad locomotora locomotor activity
actividad lúdica ludic activity
actividad neural neural activity
actividad neural espontanea spontaneous
  neural activity
actividad opioide cerebral brain opioid
  activity
actividad orogenital orogenital activity

actividad polifásica polyphasic activity
actividad sexual sexual activity
actividad sexual compulsiva compulsive
  sexual activity
actividad social social activity
actividades autoagresivas autoaggressive
  activities
actividades del diario vivir activities of daily
  living
actividades funcionales functional activities
activismo activism
activo active
activo y pasivo active and passive
acto act
acto adaptivo adaptive act
acto consumatorio consummatory act
acto de estímulo puro pure-stimulus act
acto del habla speech act
acto del habla indirecta indirect speech act
acto-hábito act-habit
acto ideomotor ideomotor act
acto instrumental instrumental act
acto interviniente intervening act
acto reflejo reflex act
acto sintomático symptomatic act
actógrafo actograph
actomiosina actomyosin
actuación de juego play acting
actual actual
actualización actualization
actualización propia self-actualization
actuarial actuarial
acuafobia aquaphobia
acueducto cerebral cerebral aqueduct
acueducto de Silvio aqueduct of Sylvius
acuestesia acuesthesia
aculalia aculalia
aculturación acculturation
aculturar acculturate
acúmetro acoumeter
acumulación accumulation
acumulador de orgón orgone accumulator
acupuntura acupuncture
acusma acousma
acusmatagnosia acousmatagnosis
acusmatamnesia acousmatamnesia
acústica acoustics
acústico acoustic
acusticofobia acousticophobia
achaque infirmity
ad hoc ad hoc
ad lib ad lib
adamantinoma pituitario pituitary
  adamantinoma
adaptabilidad adaptability
adaptabilidad cultural cultural adaptability
adaptación adaptation
adaptación a brillantez brightness adaptation
adaptación a contaminación del aire air
  pollution adaptation
adaptación a la muerte adaptation to death
adaptación a la obscuridad dark adaptation
adaptación a la realidad reality adaptation
adaptación a luz light adaptation
adaptación a sonoridad loudness adaptation

adaptación al color color adaptation
adaptación biológica biological adaptation
adaptación cromática chromatic adaptation
adaptación cruzada cross-adaptation
adaptación cultural cultural adaptation
adaptación de desastre disaster adaptation
adaptación de migración migration
   adaptation
adaptación de percepción de espacio
   adaptation of space perception
adaptación escotópica scotopic adaptation
adaptación negativa negative adaptation
adaptación perceptiva perceptual adaptation
adaptación posdesastre postdisaster
   adaptation
adaptación positiva positive adaptation
adaptación predesastre predisaster adaptation
adaptación selectiva selective adaptation
adaptación sensorial sensory adaptation
adaptación social social adaptation
adaptación vestibular vestibular adaptation
adaptación visual visual adaptation
adaptacional adaptational
adaptivo adaptive
adefagia adephagia
adelanto breakthrough
adelanto cultural culture lead
adelanto neurótico neurotic breakthrough
ademoma de células nulas null-cell adenoma
ademonia ademonia
ademosina ademosyne
adenilciclasa adenyl cyclase
adenina adenine
adenohipófisis adenohypophysis
adenohipofisitis linfocítica lymphocytic
   adenohypophysitis
adenoma adenoma
adenoma acidófilo acidophilic adenoma
adenoma basofílico basophilic adenoma
adenoma basófilo basophil adenoma
adenoma cromófilo chromophil adenoma
adenoma cromófobo chromophobe adenoma
adenoma de células indiferenciadas
   undifferentiated cell adenoma
adenoma eosinófilo eosinophil adenoma
adenoma fetal fetal adenoma
adenoma pituitario pituitary adenoma
adenoma productor de gonadotropinas
   gonadotropin-producing adenoma
adenoma productor de hormona del
   crecimiento growth hormone producing
   adenoma
adenoma productor de prolactina
   prolactin-producing adenoma
adenomatoide adenomatoid
adenoneural adenoneural
adenopatía inguinal inguinal adenopathy
adenosina adenosine
adherencia adherence
adherencia a tratamiento médico adherence
   to medical treatment
adhesiones intertalámicas interthalamic
   adhesions
adiadococinesia adiadochocinesia
adiadococinesis adiadochocinesis

adiaforia adiaphoria
adicción addiction
adicción a laxantes laxative addiction
adicción a objetos object addiction
adicción a opiáceos opiate addiction
adicción a opio opium addiction
adicción a sustancia substance addiction
adicción al trabajo work addiction
adicción alcohólica alcoholic addiction
adicción contra abuso addiction versus abuse
adicción cruzada cross-addiction
adicción de analgésico narcótico narcotic
   analgesic addiction
adicción de barbituratos barbiturate addiction
adicción de heroína heroin addiction
adicción narcótica narcotic addiction
adicción polídroga polydrug addiction
adicción poliquirúrgica polysurgical addiction
adicción a enemas enema addiction
adictivo addictive
adicto addict
adicto al alcohol alcohol-addicted
adiencia adience
adiente adient
adinamia adynamia
adinámico adynamic
adipocito adipocyte
adiposalgia adiposalgia
adiposis cerebral adiposis cerebralis
adiposo adipose
adiposogenital adiposogenital
adipsia adipsia
aditivo additive
aditivos de comida food additives
adivinación divination
adleriano adlerian
administración management, administration
administración científica scientific
   management
administración conductual behavioral
   management
administración conductual y control
   behavioral management and control
administración de aflicción grief
   management
administración de contingencias contingency
   management
administración de crisis crisis management
administración de crisis de conducta
   autodestructiva crisis management of
   self-destructive behavior
administración de crisis de conducta violenta
   crisis management of violent behavior
administración de dolor pain management
administración de dolor multidimensional
   multidimensional pain management
administración de droga parenteral
   parenteral drug administration
administración de drogas por enema enema
   drug administration
administración de estrés stress management
administración de impresiones impression
   management
administración de inyección injection
   administration

administración de reflujo reflux management
administración de riesgo risk management
administración oral oral administration
administración participante participative
  management
administración por objetivos management by
  objectives
administrador profesional professional
  manager
administrando emociones managing emotions
administrando estrés managing stress
administrativo managerial
adminstración de pruebas test administration
admisión admission, intake
admisión informal informal admission
admisión involuntaria involuntary admission
admisión temporal temporary admission
admisión voluntaria voluntary admission
adnerval adnerval
adneural adneural
adoctrinamiento indoctrination
adolescencia adolescence
adolescencia mediana middle adolescence
adolescencia normal normal adolescence
adolescencia tardía late adolescence
adolescencia temprana early adolescence
adolescente adolescent
adolescente autista-presimbiótico
  autistic-presymbiotic adolescent
adopción adoption
adoptados control control adoptees
adoptados índice index adoptees
adoptivo adoptive
adquirido acquired
adquisición acquisition
adquisición de concepto concept acquisition
adquisición de destrezas de lectura reading
  skills acquisition
adquisición de información information
  acquisition
adquisición del lenguaje language acquisition
adquisitividad acquisitiveness
adrenal adrenal
adrenalina adrenaline
adrenérgico adrenergic
adrenocromo adrenochrome
adrenoceptor adrenoceptor
adrenoceptor alfa alpha adrenoceptor
adrenoleucodistrofia adrenoleukodystrophy
adrenomieloneuropatía
  adrenomyeloneuropathy
adrenosterona adrenosterone
adromia adromia
aducción adduction
aductor adductor
adulterio adultery
adultez adulthood
adultez mediana middle adulthood
adultez tardía late adulthood
adultez temprana early adulthood
adulto adult
adultomorfismo adultomorphism
adventicio adventitious
adverso adverse
adyuvante adjuvant

aelurofobia aelurophobia
aerastenia aerasthenia
aeroacrofobia aeroacrophobia
aeroastenia aeroasthenia
aeróbico aerobic
aerofagia aerophagy
aerofobia aerophobia
aeroneurosis aeroneurosis
aerosialofagia aerosialophagy
afagia aphagia
afanisis aphanisis
afaquia aphakia
afasia aphasia
afasia acústica acoustic aphasia
afasia acusticoamnésica acoustico-amnestic
  aphasia
afasia amnésica amnesic aphasia
afasia anómica anomic aphasia
afasia asociativa associative aphasia
afasia atáxica ataxic aphasia
afasia auditiva auditory aphasia
afasia central central aphasia
afasia coclear cochlear aphasia
afasia congénita congenital aphasia
afasia de Broca Broca's aphasia
afasia de conducción conduction aphasia
afasia de jerga jargon aphasia
afasia de Kussmaul Kussmaul's aphasia
afasia de Wernicke Wernicke's aphasia
afasia del desarrollo developmental aphasia
afasia epiléptica adquirida acquired epileptic
  aphasia
afasia expresiva expressive aphasia
afasia fluente fluent aphasia
afasia funcional functional aphasia
afasia global global aphasia
afasia gráfica graphic aphasia
afasia grafomotora graphomotor aphasia
afasia impresiva impressive aphasia
afasia mixta mixed aphasia
afasia motora motor aphasia
afasia motora aferente afferent motor aphasia
afasia motora cortical cortical motor aphasia
afasia motora eferente efferent motor aphasia
afasia motora transcortical transcortical
  motor aphasia
afasia no fluente nonfluent aphasia
afasia nominal nominal aphasia
afasia patemática pathematic aphasia
afasia psicosensorial psychosensory aphasia
afasia pura pure aphasia
afasia receptiva receptive aphasia
afasia receptiva-expresiva
  receptive-expressive aphasia
afasia semántica semantic aphasia
afasia sensorial sensory aphasia
afasia sensorial cortical cortical sensory
  aphasia
afasia sensorial transcortical transcortical
  sensory aphasia
afasia sensorimotora sensorimotor aphasia
afasia sintáctica syntactic aphasia
afasia total total aphasia
afasia transcortical transcortical aphasia
afasia transcortical combinada combined

transcortical aphasia
afasia transcortical mixta mixed transcortical aphasia
afasia traumática traumatic aphasia
afasia verbal verbal aphasia
afasia visual visual aphasia
afásico aphasic
afasiología aphasiology
afasiólogo aphasiologist
afección affection
afección enmascarada masked affection
afectación affectation
afectado affected
afectado germinalmente germinally affected
afectar affect
afectividad affectivity
afectivo affective
afecto affect
afecto amplio broad affect
afecto aplanado flattened affect
afecto apropiado appropriate affect
afecto corporal body affect
afecto dentro del intervalo normal affect within normal range
afecto desprendido detached affect
afecto estrangulado strangulated affect
afecto flotante floating affect
afecto inapropiado inappropriate affect
afecto insulso flat affect
afecto lábil labile affect
afecto restringido restricted affect
afecto rudo blunted affect
afectomotor affectomotor
afectosimbólico affectosymbolic
afectualización affectualization
afectuoso affectionate
afefobia aphephobia
afelxia aphelxia
afemestesia aphemesthesia
afemia aphemia
afémico aphemic
afeminado effeminate
aferencia afference
aferente afferent
afiliación affiliation
afiloponia aphilopony
afinidad affinity
afirmación affirmation
aflicción grief, affliction
aflicción anticipatoria anticipatory grief
aflicción demorada delayed grief
aflicción inhibida inhibited grief
aflicción negada denied grief
aflojamiento loosening
aflojamiento de asociación loosening of association
afonía aphonia
afonía aducida adducted aphonia
afonía espástica spastic aphonia
afonía funcional functional aphonia
afonía histérica hysterical aphonia
afonía paralítica aphonia paralytica
afónico aphonic
afonogelia aphonogelia
aforesis aphoresis

aforia aphoria
afrasia aphrasia
afrenia aphrenia
africada affricate
afrodisia aphrodisia
afrodisiaco aphrodisiac
afrodisiaco psicológico psychological aphrodisiac
afrodisiomanía aphrodisiomania
aftenxia aphthenxia
aftongia aphthongia
agamogénesis agamogenesis
agapaxia agapaxia
agapismo agapism
agarre grasp
agastroneuria agastroneuria
ageismo ageism
agencia agency
agencia de servicios en el hogar home-service agency
agencia social social agency
agenesia agenesia
agenético agenetic
agente agent
agente antiandrogénico antiandrogenic agent
agente antiansiedad antianxiety agent
agente antipsicótico antipsychotic agent
agente bloqueador narcótico narcotic blocking agent
agente catalítico catalytic agent
agente de bloqueo adrenérgico alfa alpha adrenergic blocking agent
agente de bloqueo adrenérgico beta beta adrenergic blocking agent
agente de bloqueo de receptores alfa alpha receptor blocking agent
agente de bloqueo de receptores beta beta receptor blocking agent
agente de cambio change agent
agente excitatorio excitatory agent
agente neuropsicotrópico neuropsychotropic agent
agente provocador agent provocateur
agente quimioterapéutico chemotherapeutic agent
agente terapéutico therapeutic agent
agentes bloqueadores adrenérgicos adrenergic blocking agents
agentes bloqueadores ganglionares ganglionic blocking agents
agerasia agerasia
ageusia ageusia
ageustia ageustia
agiofobia agyiophobia
agiria agyria
agitación agitation
agitación adolescente adolescent turmoil
agitación psicomotora psychomotor agitation
agitado agitated
agitofasia agitophasia
agitografía agitographia
agitolalia agitolalia
aglosia aglossia
aglutinación agglutination
aglutinaciones de imágenes image

agglutinations
agnea agnea
agnosia agnosia
agnosia auditiva auditory agnosia
agnosia de color color agnosia
agnosia de dolor pain agnosia
agnosia de localización localization agnosia
agnosia de posición position agnosia
agnosia del tiempo time agnosia
agnosia digital finger agnosia
agnosia espacial spatial agnosia
agnosia ideacional ideational agnosia
agnosia óptica optic agnosia
agnosia táctil tactile agnosia
agnosia visual visual agnosia
agnosia visual-espacial visual-spatial agnosia
agnosia visuoespacial visuospatial agnosia
agonía agony
agonista agonist
agonista inverso inverse agonist
agorafobia agoraphobia
agorafobia con ataques de pánico
    agoraphobia with panic attacks
agorafobia sin ataques de pánico
    agoraphobia without panic attacks
agorafóbico agoraphobic
agotamiento exhaustion, burnout
agotamiento nervioso nervous exhaustion
agotamiento por calor heat exhaustion
agrafia agraphia
agrafia absoluta absolute agraphia
agrafia acústica acoustic agraphia
agrafia adquirida acquired agraphia
agrafia amnemónica amnemonic agraphia
agrafia atáxica ataxic agraphia
agrafia cerebral cerebral agraphia
agrafia literal literal agraphia
agrafia mental mental agraphia
agrafia motora motor agraphia
agrafia musical musical agraphia
agrafia verbal verbal agraphia
agrafia visual visual agraphia
agráfico agraphic
agrafognosia agraphognosia
agramafasia agrammaphasia
agramatismo agrammatism
agramatología agrammatologia
agranulocitosis agranulocytosis
agregación aggregation
agregado social social aggregate
agresión aggression
agresión airada angry aggression
agresión altruista altruistic aggression
agresión animal animal aggression
agresión anticipatoria anticipatory aggression
agresión antisocial antisocial aggression
agresión autoritaria authoritarian aggression
agresión de dominancia dominance
    aggression
agresión desplazada displaced aggression
agresión directa direct aggression
agresión en juego aggression in play
agresión en trastorno de déficit de atención
    aggression in attention-deficit disorder
agresión hostil hostile aggression

agresión inducida induced aggression
agresión inducida por temor fear-induced
    aggression
agresión instintiva instinctual aggression
agresión instrumental instrumental
    aggression
agresión maternal maternal aggression
agresión no destructiva nondestructive
    aggression
agresión operante operant aggression
agresión pasiva passive aggression
agresión predatoria predatory aggression
agresión prosocial prosocial aggression
agresión sexual sexual aggression
agresión territorial territorial aggression
agresión y abuso de alcohol aggression and
    alcohol abuse
agresión y conducta suicida aggression and
    suicidal behavior
agresividad aggressivity
agresivo aggressive
agrio sour
agriotimia agriothymia
agripnia agrypnia
agripnocoma agrypnocoma
agripnótico agrypnotic
agromania agromania
agrupamiento grouping, clustering
agrupamiento clínico clinical grouping
agrupamiento de pensamientos chunking
agrupamiento heterogéneo heterogeneous
    grouping
agrupamiento homogéneo homogeneous
    grouping
agrupamiento por estado status grouping
agrupamiento por habilidades ability
    grouping
agrupamiento por habilidades académicas
    academic abilities grouping
agudeza acuity
agudeza auditiva auditory acuity
agudeza de audición hearing acuity
agudeza estereoscópica stereoscopic acuity
agudeza mental alertness
agudeza sensorial sensory acuity
agudeza visual visual acuity
agudo acute
aguja needle
aguja de Frazier Frazier's needle
aguja de punción lumbar lumbar puncture
    needle
aguja de Tuohy Tuohy needle
ahedonia ahedonia
ahilognosia ahylognosia
ahipnia ahypnia
ahipnosia ahypnosia
ahistórico ahistorical
ahorcadura erotizada erotized hanging
aicmofobia aichmophobia
aidoiomanía aidoiomania
ailurofobia ailurophobia
aipnia aypnia
airado angry
aislado isolated
aislado social social isolate

aislamiento isolation
aislamiento autista autistic isolation
aislamiento de afecto isolation of affect
aislamiento emocional emotional insulation
aislamiento psíquico psychic isolation
aislamiento reproductivo reproductive
　isolation
aislamiento sensorial sensory isolation
aislamiento social social isolation
aislar isolate
ajeno al ego ego-alien
ajuste adjustment, fit
ajuste alumno-maestro pupil-teacher fit
ajuste de curvas curve fitting
ajuste de divorcio divorce adjustment
ajuste de nacimiento birth adjustment
ajuste de observaciones adjustment of
　observations
ajuste emocional emotional adjustment
ajuste escolar school adjustment
ajuste marital marital adjustment
ajuste ocupacional occupational adjustment
ajuste parcial partial adjustment
ajuste parental parental fit
ajuste personal personal adjustment
ajuste posdivorcio postdivorce adjustment
ajuste premórbido premorbid adjustment
ajuste sexual sexual adjustment
ajuste social social adjustment
ajuste uncinado uncinate fit
ajuste vocacional vocational adjustment
alalia alalia
alálico alalic
alaquestesia allachesthesia
alaquestesia visual visual allachesthesia
alarma alarm
albedo albedo
albinismo albinism
albinismo cutáneo cutaneous albinism
albinismo ocular ocular albinism
albino albino
albúmina albumin
albúmina sérica serum albumin
alcalinidad alkalinity
alcaloide alkaloid
alcaloide de opio opium alkaloid
alcalosis alkalosis
alcance scope
alcaptonuria alcaptonuria
alcohol alcohol
alcohol etílico ethyl alcohol
alcohólico alcoholic
alcoholismo alcoholism
alcoholismo adictivo addictive alcoholism
alcoholismo agudo acute alcoholism
alcoholismo alfa alpha alcoholism
alcoholismo beta beta alcoholism
alcoholismo crónico chronic alcoholism
alcoholismo delta delta alcoholism
alcoholismo épsilon epsilon alcoholism
alcoholismo esencial essential alcoholism
alcoholismo gama gamma alcoholism
alcoholismo maligno malignant alcoholism
alcoholismo parental parental alcoholism
alcoholismo reactivo reactive alcoholism

alcoholismo regresivo regressive alcoholism
alcoholismo sintomático symptomatic
　alcoholism
alcoholofilia alcoholophilia
alcoholofobia alcoholophobia
alcoholomanía alcoholomania
aldosterona aldosterone
aldosteronismo aldosteronism
aleatorio random
aleatorización randomization
aleatorizado randomized
aleatorizar randomize
alector alector
alegación de incompetencia incompetence
　plea
alélico allelic
alelo allele
alelomórfico allelomorphic
alelomorfo allelomorph
alergeno allergen
alergia allergy
alergia de comida food allergy
alérgico allergic
alestesia allesthesia
aleteo flutter
aleteo ocular ocular flutter
aletia alethia
alexia alexia
alexia agnósica agnosic alexia
alexia congénita congenital alexia
alexia incompleta incomplete alexia
alexia literal literal alexia
alexia motora motor alexia
alexia musical musical alexia
alexia óptica optical alexia
alexia sensorial sensory alexia
alexia verbal verbal alexia
alexia visual visual alexia
aléxico alexic
alexitimia alexithymia
alfa alpha
alfabetismo literacy
alfabeto alphabet
alfabeto fonético phonetic alphabet
alfabeto manual manual alphabet
alfaprodina alphaprodine
álgebra de Boole Boolean algebra
algedónico algedonic
algesia algesia
algésico algesic
algesicronómetro algesichronometer
algesímetro algesimeter
algesiogénico algesiogenic
algesiómetro algesiometer
algestesia algesthesia
algestesis algesthesis
algético algetic
algoespasmo algospasm
algofilia algophilia
algofobia algophobia
algogenesia algogenesia
algogénesis algogenesis
algogénico algogenic
algolagnia algolagnia
algometría algometry

algómetro algometer
algopsicalia algopsychalia
algoritmo algorithm
algoritmo clínico clinical algorithm
aliáceo alliaceous
aliado allied
alianza alliance
alianza terapéutica therapeutic alliance
alianza y rompimiento alliance and splitting
alienación alienation, estrangement
alienación interna inner estrangement
alienista alienist
aliento encouragement
aliestesia alliesthesia
alimentación feeding
alimentación a petición demand feeding
alimentación estilo cafetería cafeteria feeding
alimentación ficticia fictitious feeding
alimentación forzada forced feeding
alimentación por biberón bottle-feeding
alimentación por demanda propia
    self-demand feeding
alimentación por pecho breast-feeding
alimentación simulada sham feeding
alimento aliment
alisosis alysosis
aliteración alliteration
aliviar relieve
alivio relief
alma popular folk soul
almacén store
almacén acústico acoustic store
almacén articulatorio articulatory store
almacén de contenido direccionable
    content-addressable store
almacén de información sensorial
    sensory-information store
almacenamiento storage
almacenamiento de memoria memory
    storage
almacenamiento genético genetic storage
almacenamiento icónico iconic storage
alnada stepdaughter
alnado stepson
alobarbital allobarbital
alocéntrico allocentric
alocinesia allokinesis
alocorteza allocortex
alodinia allodynia
aloerótico alloerotic
aloerotismo alloerotism
aloestesia alloesthesia
alofasis allophasis
alófono allophone
alogia alogia
alolalia allolalia
alometría allometry
alomórfico allomorphic
alomorfo allomorph
alónomo allonomous
alopatía allopathy
alopecia alopecia
aloplastia alloplasty
aloplasticidad alloplasticity
alopsicosis allopsychosis

alopsíquico allopsychic
alopsiquis allopsyche
aloquestesia allochesthesia
aloquiria allochiria
alotriofagia allotriophagy
alotriogeusia allotriogeusia
alotriogeustia allotriogeustia
alotriorhexia allotriorhexia
alotriosmia allotriosmia
alotropía allotropy
alotrópico allotropic
aloxana alloxan
alpinismo alpinism
alprazolam alprazolam
alter alter
alter ego alter ego
alteración alteration
alteración cromosómica chromosomal
    alteration
alteración del ego ego alteration
alteración del ego reactiva reactive ego
    alteration
alteregoísmo alteregoism
alternación alternation
alternación demorada delayed alternation
alternante alternating
alternativa alternative
alternativa fija fixed alternative
alternativa menos restrictiva least restrictive
    alternative
altricial altricial
altruismo altruism
altruismo recíproco reciprocal altruism
altruista altruistic
alucinación hallucination
alucinación afectiva affective hallucination
alucinación auditiva auditory hallucination
alucinación cenestésica cenesthesic
    hallucination
alucinación cinestésica kinesthetic
    hallucination
alucinación de concepción hallucination of
    conception
alucinación de muñón stump hallucination
alucinación de percepción hallucination of
    perception
alucinación del humor congruente
    mood-congruent hallucination
alucinación del humor incongruente
    mood-incongruent hallucination
alucinación elemental elementary
    hallucination
alucinación en blanco blank hallucination
alucinación gustatoria gustatory hallucination
alucinación háptica haptic hallucination
alucinación hipnagógica hypnagogic
    hallucination
alucinación hipnopómpica hypnopompic
    hallucination
alucinación inducida induced hallucination
alucinación liliputiense Lilliputian
    hallucination
alucinación micróptica microptic
    hallucination
alucinación negativa negative hallucination

alucinación no afectiva nonaffective
hallucination
alucinación olfatoria olfactory hallucination
alucinación orgánica organic hallucination
alucinación psicogénica psychogenic
hallucination
alucinación psicomotora psychomotor
hallucination
alucinación somática somatic hallucination
alucinación táctil tactile hallucination
alucinación teleológica teleological
hallucination
alucinación temporal temporal hallucination
alucinación vestibular vestibular hallucination
alucinación visual visual hallucination
alucinación visual diminutiva diminutive
visual hallucination
alucinación visual formada formed visual
hallucination
alucinación visual sin formar unformed
visual hallucination
alucinaciones de imagen corporal body
image hallucinations
alucinar hallucinate
alucinatorio hallucinatory
alucinogénico hallucinogenic
alucinógeno hallucinogen
alucinosis hallucinosis
alucinosis aguda acute hallucinosis
alucinosis alcohólica alcoholic hallucinosis
alucinosis de alcohol alcohol hallucinosis
alucinosis de alucinógeno hallucinogen
hallucinosis
alucinosis de bromuro bromide hallucinosis
alucinosis de cannabis cannabis hallucinosis
alucinosis de escena retrospectiva flashback
hallucinosis
alucinosis de sustancia psicoactiva
psychoactive substance hallucinosis
alucinosis orgánica organic hallucinosis
alucinosis peduncular peduncular hallucinosis
alveolar alveolar
amamantamiento eterno eternal suckling
amargo bitter
amartelamiento infatuation
amatividad amativeness
amatofobia amathophobia
amaurosis amaurosis
amaurosis histérica hysterical amaurosis
amaxofobia amaxophobia
ambageusia ambageusia
ambenonio ambenonium
ambición ambition
ambición negativa negative ambition
ambidextrismo ambidextrism
ambidextro ambidextrous
ambiental environmental
ambientalismo environmentalism
ambientalista environmentalist
ambiente environment
ambiente académico academic setting
ambiente aislado isolated environment
ambiente de aprendizaje planificado planned
learning environment
ambiente de conducta behavior setting

ambiente de decisiones decision environment
ambiente de libre acceso free-access
environment
ambiente del hogar home environment
ambiente enriquecido enriched environment
ambiente familiar family environment
ambiente interno internal environment
ambiente libre de barreras barrier-free
environment
ambiente menos restrictivo least restrictive
environment
ambiente neutral neutral environment
ambiente permisivo permissive environment
ambiente primario primary environment
ambiente psicoanalítico psychoanalytic setting
ambiente psicológico psychological
environment
ambiente rural rural environment
ambiente secundario secondary environment
ambiente simulado simulated environment
ambiente sociocultural sociocultural milieu
ambiente terapéutico therapeutic environment
ambiente uteroplacentario uteroplacental
environment
ambigüedad ambiguity
ambigüedad de señal cue ambiguity
ambiguo ambiguous
ambilevo ambilevous
ambisexual ambisexual
ambisexualidad ambisexuality
ambisinistro ambisinister
ambitendencia ambitendency
ambivalencia ambivalence
ambivalencia afectiva affective ambivalence
ambivalencia de la voluntad ambivalence of
the will
ambivalencia del intelecto ambivalence of the
intellect
ambivalencia doble dual ambivalence
ambivalente ambivalent
ambiversión ambiversion
ambivertido ambivert
ambliacusia amblyacousia
ambliafia amblyaphia
ambligeustia amblygeustia
ambliopía amblyopia
amblioscopio amblyoscope
ambrosiaco ambrosiac
ambulación ambulation
ambulatorio ambulatory
ameléctico amelectic
ameleia ameleia
ameliorar ameliorate
amenaza threat
amenaza al ego ego threat
amenaza de abandono abandonment threat
amencia amentia
amencia alcohólica de Stearns Stearns'
alcoholic amentia
amencia del desarrollo developmental
amentia
amencia fenilpirúvica phenylpyruvic amentia
amencia nevoide nevoid amentia
amencia por aislamiento isolation amentia
amencia primaria primary amentia

amencial amential
amenomanía amenomania
amenorrea amenorrhea
amenorrea emocional emotional amenorrhea
amenorrea primaria primary amenorrhea
amenorrea secundaria secondary amenorrhea
ametístico amethystic
ametopterina amethopterin
ametrofia ametrophia
ametropía ametropia
amicofobia amychophobia
amida de ácido lisérgico lysergic acid amide
amígdala amygdala
amigdaloide amygdaloid
amilasa amylase
amilasa sérica serum amylase
amilofagia amylophagia
amiloide amyloid
amiloidosis amyloidosis
amiloidosis familiar familial amyloidosis
amiloidosis primario primary amyloidosis
amiloidosis secundaria secondary amyloidosis
amimia amimia
amimia expresiva expressive amimia
amimia motora motor amimia
amimia receptiva receptive amimia
amimia sensorial sensory amimia
amina amine
aminas biógenas biogenic amines
aminoácido amino acid
aminofilina aminophylline
aminopirina aminopyrine
aminopterina aminopterin
amioestesia amyoesthesia
amiostasia amyostasia
amiostenia amyosthenia
amiotonía amyotonia
amiotonía congénita amyotonia congenita
amiotrofia amyotrophy
amiotrofia espinal progresiva progressive
  spinal amyotrophy
amiotrofia hemipléjica hemiplegic
  amyotrophy
amiotrofia neurálgica neuralgic amyotrophy
amistad friendship
amistades familiares family friends
amistoso friendly
amitriptilina amitriptyline
amnemónico amnemonic
amnesia amnesia
amnesia afectiva affective amnesia
amnesia anterógrada anterograde amnesia
amnesia audioverbal audioverbal amnesia
amnesia auditiva auditory amnesia
amnesia autohipnótica autohypnotic amnesia
amnesia axial axial amnesia
amnesia catatímica catathymic amnesia
amnesia circunscrita circumscribed amnesia
amnesia continua continuous amnesia
amnesia cortical cortical amnesia
amnesia de época epochal amnesia
amnesia disociativa dissociative amnesia
amnesia en la enfermedad de Alzheimer
  amnesia in Alzheimer's disease
amnesia episódica episodic amnesia

amnesia generalizada generalized amnesia
amnesia global global amnesia
amnesia global transitoria transient global
  amnesia
amnesia histérica hysterical amnesia
amnesia infantil infantile amnesia
amnesia lagunar lacunar amnesia
amnesia localizada localized amnesia
amnesia neurológica neurological amnesia
amnesia orgánica organic amnesia
amnesia políglota polyglot amnesia
amnesia posencefalítica postencephalitic
  amnesia
amnesia poshipnótica posthypnotic amnesia
amnesia postraumática posttraumatic
  amnesia
amnesia psicogénica psychogenic amnesia
amnesia residual residual amnesia
amnesia retrógrada retrograde amnesia
amnesia selectiva selective amnesia
amnesia táctil tactile amnesia
amnesia tras lesiones amnesia after lesions
amnesia tras lobectomías amnesia after
  lobectomies
amnesia tras terapia electroconvulsiva
  amnesia after electroconvulsive therapy
amnesia verbal verbal amnesia
amnesia visual visual amnesia
amnésico amnestic
amniocentesis amniocentesis
amniografía amniography
amnios amnion
amniótico amniotic
amobarbital amobarbital
amok amok
amor condicional conditional love
amor de mono monkey love
amor de objeto object love
amor de objeto primario primary object-love
amor del ser being love
amor delusorio delusional loving
amor dorio Dorian love
amor fálico phallic love
amor genital genital love
amor griego Greek love
amor helénico Hellenic love
amor homogénico homogenic love
amor juvenil calf love
amor platónico platonic love
amor por deficiencia deficiency love
amor pregenital pregenital love
amor productivo productive love
amor propio self-love
amor real real love
amor romántico romantic love
amor sexual sexual love
amorfagnosia amorphagnosia
amorfosíntesis amorphosynthesis
amortiguamiento damping
amotivacional amotivational
amoxapina amoxapine
amplificación amplification
amplificador diferencial differential amplifier
amplitud amplitude
amplitud de onda wave amplitude

amplitud de respuesta amplitude of response
ampollita ampulla
amputación amputation
amusia amusia
amusia expresiva expressive amusia
amusia motora motor amusia
amusia sensorial sensory amusia
amusia vocal vocal amusia
anabólico anabolic
anabolismo anabolism
anacamptómetro anacamptometer
anacatestesia anacatesthesia
anaclisis anaclisis
anaclítico anaclitic
anacusia anacusia
anacusis anacusis
anaeróbico anaerobic
anafase anaphase
anafia anaphia
anafilaxis anaphylaxis
anafilaxis psicológica psychological
    anaphylaxis
anafilaxis psiquiátrica psychiatric anaphylaxis
anafilaxis psíquica psychic anaphylaxis
anáfora anaphora
anafrodisia anaphrodisia
anafrodisiaco anaphrodisiac
anaglifo anaglyph
anagliptoscopio anaglyptoscope
anagogia anagogy
anagógico anagogic
anagrama anagram
anal anal
anal-expulsivo anal-expulsive
anal-retentivo anal-retentive
anal-sádico anal-sadistic
analepsis analepsis
analéptico analeptic
analfabetismo illiteracy
analfabetismo científico scientific illiteracy
analfabetismo de computadoras computer
    illiteracy
analfabetismo tecnológico technological
    illiteracy
analgesia analgesia
analgesia álgera analgesia algera
analgesia dolorosa analgesia dolorosa
analgesia hipnótica hypnotic analgesia
analgésico analgesic
analgésico narcótico narcotic analgesic
analgesímetro analgesimeter
analgético analgetic
analgia analgia
analidad anality
análisis analysis
análisis a ciegas blind analysis
análisis a fondo analysis in depth
análisis activo active analysis
análisis anamnésico anamnestic analysis
análisis armónico harmonic analysis
análisis clásico classical analysis
análisis control control analysis
análisis controlado controlled analysis
análisis de actividad activity analysis
análisis de artículos item analysis

análisis de carácter character analysis
análisis de características feature analysis
análisis de componentes componential
    analysis
análisis de conducta behavior analysis
análisis de conducta experimental
    experimental analysis of behavior
análisis de contenido content analysis
análisis de contingencias contingency analysis
análisis de costo-beneficio cost-benefit
    analysis
análisis de costo-efectividad
    cost-effectiveness analysis
análisis de costo-recompensa cost-reward
    analysis
análisis de covarianza analysis of covariance
análisis de decisiones decision analysis
análisis de desastre disaster analysis
análisis de destino fate analysis
análisis de discurso discourse analysis
análisis de dispersión scatter analysis
análisis de documentos personales
    personal-document analysis
análisis de ensayo trial analysis
análisis de entrenamiento training analysis
análisis de errores error analysis
análisis de escalograma scalogram analysis
análisis de escritura handwriting analysis
análisis de esperma sperm analysis
análisis de Fourier Fourier analysis
análisis de grupo group analysis
análisis de grupo terapéutico
    therapeutic-group analysis
análisis de impacto impact analysis
análisis de ji cuadrada chi square analysis
análisis de la resistencia analysis of the
    resistance
análisis de libreto script analysis
análisis de marco frame analysis
análisis de métodos methods analysis
análisis de niños child analysis
análisis de patrón pattern analysis
análisis de perceptos percept analysis
análisis de perfil profile analysis
análisis de política policy analysis
análisis de proceso process analysis
análisis de propaganda propaganda analysis
análisis de refuerzo reinforcement analysis
análisis de regresión regression analysis
análisis de sentimientos feelings analysis
análisis de sistemas systems analysis
análisis de sueños analysis of dreams
análisis de tarea task analysis
análisis de tendencia trend analysis
análisis de tiempo y moción time and motion
    analysis
análisis de trabajo job analysis
análisis de transferencia analysis of
    transference
análisis de varianza analysis of variance
análisis de vecino más lejano furthest
    neighbor analysis
análisis del ego ego analysis
análisis del proceso de interacción
    interaction process analysis

análisis demográfico demographic analysis
análisis didáctico didactic analysis
análisis directo direct analysis
análisis dirigido directed analysis
análisis discriminante discriminant analysis
análisis distributivo distributive analysis
análisis distributivo y síntesis distributive
  analysis and synthesis
análisis escalar scalar analysis
análisis estructural structural analysis
análisis etológico causal causal ethological
  analysis
análisis existencial existential analysis
análisis experimental experimental analysis
análisis factorial factor analysis
análisis factorial inverso inverse factor
  analysis
análisis factorial invertido inverted factor
  analysis
análisis fenomenológico phenomenological
  analysis
análisis fraccional fractional analysis
análisis funcional functional analysis
análisis funcional de ambientes functional
  analysis of environments
análisis gráfico graphic analysis
análisis jerárquico hierarchical analysis
análisis menor minor analysis
análisis multidimensional multidimensional
  analysis
análisis multivariado multivariate analysis
análisis multivariado de variancia
  multivariate analysis of variance
análisis ocupacional occupational analysis
análisis pasivo passive analysis
análisis por síntesis analysis by synthesis
análisis profundo depth analysis
análisis secuencial sequential analysis
análisis selectivo selective analysis
análisis situacional situational analysis
análisis sociométrico sociometric analysis
análisis transaccional transactional analysis
análisis enfocado focused analysis
analista analyst
analítico analytical
analizador analyzer
analizador de ondas wave analyzer
analizando analysand
analogía analogy
análogo analogous
análogo de libido libido analog
anamnesia anamnesia
anamnésico anamnestic
anamnesis anamnesis
anamnesis asociativa associative anamnesis
ananastasia ananastasia
anancasmo anancasm
anancastia anancastia
anancástico anancastic
anandria anandria
anapeirático anapeiratic
anáptico anaptic
anarritmia anarithmia
anartria anarthria
anastasis anastasis

anastomosis anastomosis
anastomosis microneurovascular
  microneurovascular anastomosis
anastomosis microvascular microvascular
  anastomosis
anatomía anatomy
anatopismo anatopism
anaudia anaudia
anciano elderly
ancilostoma ankylostoma
ancla anchor
anclaje anchoring
anclaje del ego anchoring of ego
anclaje perceptivo perceptual anchoring
anclaje social social anchoring
ancho de banda bandwidth
ancho de banda crítico critical bandwidth
andar walking
andar demorado delayed walking
androfilia androphilia
andrófilo androphile
androfobia androphobia
androgénico androgenic
androgenización androgenization
andrógeno androgen
androginia androgyny
androginidad androgyneity
androginismo androgynism
androide android
andromanía andromania
androstenediona androstenedione
androsterona androsterone
anecoico anechoic
anelectrónico anelectronic
anelectrotono anelectrotonus
anemia anemia
anemia cerebral cerebral anemia
anemia de Cooley Cooley's anemia
anemia de Fanconi Fanconi's anemia
anemia esplénica familiar familial splenic
  anemia
anemia perniciosa pernicious anemia
anémico anemic
anemofobia anemophobia
anemotropismo anemotropism
anencefalia anencephaly
anencefálico anencephalic
anencéfalo anencephalous
anepia anepia
anergasia anergasia
anergástico anergastic
anergia anergy
anérgico anergic
anerotismo anerotism
anestecinesia anesthecinesia
anestesia anesthesia
anestesia a presión pressure anesthesia
anestesia cruzada crossed anesthesia
anestesia cutánea cutaneous anesthesia
anestesia de pie foot anesthesia
anestesia diagnóstica diagnostic anesthesia
anestesia disociada dissociated anesthesia
anestesia disociativa dissociative anesthesia
anestesia dolorosa painful anesthesia
anestesia emocional emotional anesthesia

anestesia en cinturón girdle anesthesia
anestesia en guante glove anesthesia
anestesia en media stocking anesthesia
anestesia espinal spinal anesthesia
anestesia esplácnica splanchnic anesthesia
anestesia faríngea pharyngeal anesthesia
anestesia gustatoria gustatory anesthesia
anestesia histérica hysterical anesthesia
anestesia muscular muscular anesthesia
anestesia olfatoria olfactory anesthesia
anestesia perineural perineural anesthesia
anestesia por compresión compression
  anesthesia
anestesia segmentaria segmental anesthesia
anestesia sexual sexual anesthesia
anestesia táctil tactile anesthesia
anestesia térmica thermal anesthesia
anestesia traumática traumatic anesthesia
anestesia unilateral unilateral anesthesia
anestesia visceral visceral anesthesia
anestésico anesthetic
anestésico general general anesthetic
anestésico regional regional anesthetic
anetópata anethopath
anetopatía anethopathy
aneuploidia aneuploidy
aneurisma aneurysm
aneurisma carotídeo cavernoso
  cavernous-carotid aneurysm
aneurisma cerebral congénito congenital
  cerebral aneurysm
aneurisma de Charcot-Bouchard
  Charcot-Bouchard aneurysm
aneurisma en baya berry aneurysm
aneurisma infraclinoideo infraclinoid
  aneurysm
aneurisma intracraneal intracranial aneurysm
aneurisma miliar miliary aneurysm
aneurisma serpentino serpentine aneurysm
aneurisma supraclinoideo supraclinoid
  aneurysm
aneurismectomía aneurysmectomy
aneutanasia aneuthanasia
aneyaculatorio anejaculatory
anfetamina amphetamine
anficrania amphicrania
anfierotismo amphierotism
anfigénesis amphigenesis
anfimixis amphimixis
anfitimia amphithymia
anfotonía amphotony
angina angina
angina de pecho angina pectoris
anginofobia anginophobia
angioblastoma angioblastoma
angioedema angioedema
angiofacomatosis angiophacomatosis
angioglioma angioglioma
angiografía angiography
angiografía cerebral cerebral angiography
angiografía digital digital angiography
angiografía espinal spinal angiography
angiograma angiogram
angioma angioma
angioma encefálico encephalic angioma

angiomatosis angiomatosis
angiomatosis cefalotrigeminal
  cephalotrigeminal angiomatosis
angiomatosis cerebral cerebral angiomatosis
angiomatosis cerebral trigeminal trigeminal
  cerebral angiomatosis
angiomatosis cutaneomeningoespinal
  cutaneomeningospinal angiomatosis
angiomatosis displástica congénita congenital
  dysplastic angiomatosis
angiomatosis encefalofacial encephalofacial
  angiomatosis
angiomatosis encefalotrigeminal
  encephalotrigeminal angiomatosis
angiomatosis oculoencefálica oculoencephalic
  angiomatosis
angiomatosis retinocerebral retinocerebral
  angiomatosis
angiomatosis telangiectásico telangiectatic
  angiomatosis
angioneurectomía angioneurectomy
angioneuredema angioneuredema
angioneurosis angioneurosis
angioneurótico angioneurotic
angioneurotomía angioneurotomy
angiopatía angiopathy
angiopatía amiloide cerebral cerebral
  amyloid angiopathy
angiopatía displástica congénita congenital
  dysplastic angiopathy
angiopático angiopathic
angioscotoma angioscotoma
angiotensina angiotensin
angiotensinógeno angiotensinogen
angor angor
angor animi angor animi
angor pectoris angor pectoris
angstrom angstrom
ángulo de convergencia convergence angle
ángulo visual visual angle
angustia distress
angustia de separación separation distress
angustia fetal fetal distress
angustia por orientación sexual
  sexual-orientation distress
anhedonia anhedonia
anhidrasa carbónica carbonic anhydrase
anhidrosis anhidrosis
anhipnia anhypnia
anhipnosis anhypnosis
aniconia aniconia
anilerdina anilerdine
anilición anilinction
anilidad anility
anilingus anilingus
anillo de Kayser-Fleischer Kayser-Fleischer
  ring
anillo de Landolt Landolt ring
anima anima
animación animation
animación de computadora computer
  animation
animal de compañía pet
animal espinal spinal animal
animal social social animal

animástico animastic
animatismo animatism
animismo animism
animismo social social animism
animosidad animosity
animus animus
aniseiconía aniseikonia
anisocoria anisocoria
anisofrenia anisophrenia
anisoiconia anisoiconia
anisometropía anisometropia
anisopía anisopia
anisotropía anisotropia
anlaje anlage
ano anus
anociasociación anociassociation
anoclesia anochlesia
anodino anodyne
anodontia anodontia
anoesia anoesia
anoesis anoesis
anoético anoetic
anoftalmía anophthalmia
anogenital anogenital
anoia anoia
anomalía anomaly
anomalía congénita congenital anomaly
anomalía craneal cranial anomaly
anomalía cromosómica chromosomal anomaly
anomalía del desarrollo prenatal prenatal developmental anomaly
anomalía metabólica metabolic anomaly
anomalía sexual sexual anomaly
anomalías autosómicas autosomal anomalies
anomalías craneofaciales craniofacial anomalies
anómalo anomalous
anomalopía anomalopia
anomaloscopio anomaloscope
anomia anomia
anómico anomic
anonimato anonymity
anopía anopia
anopsia anopsia
anorético anoretic
anorexia anorexia
anorexia electiva elective anorexia
anorexia nerviosa anorexia nervosa
anorexia sexual sexual anorexia
anorexia social social anorexia
anoréxico anorexic
anorexígeno anorexiant
anorgasmia anorgasmy
anorgásmico anorgasmic
anormal abnormal
anormalidad abnormality
anormalidad cromosómica chromosomal abnormality
anormalidad insulínica insulin abnormality
anormalidad perceptiva perceptual abnormality
anorrectal anorectal
anortografía anorthography
anortopía anorthopia

anortoscópico anorthoscopic
anortosis anorthosis
anosfresia anosphresia
anosmia anosmia
anosmia esencial essential anosmia
anosmia funcional functional anosmia
anosmia mecánica mechanical anosmia
anosmia refleja reflex anosmia
anosmia respiratoria respiratory anosmia
anosmia verdadera true anosmia
anósmico anosmic
anosodiaforia anosodiaphoria
anosognosia anosognosia
anosognósico anosognosic
anovulatorio anovulatory
anoxemia anoxemia
anoxia anoxia
anoxia anémica anemic anoxia
anoxia metabólica metabolic anoxia
anquiloglosia ankyloglossia
anquilosis ankylosis
ansiedad anxiety
ansiedad aguda acute anxiety
ansiedad ante extraños stranger anxiety
ansiedad anticipatoria anticipatory anxiety
ansiedad automática automatic anxiety
ansiedad básica basic anxiety
ansiedad catastrófica catastrophic anxiety
ansiedad competitiva competitive anxiety
ansiedad condicionada conditioned anxiety
ansiedad contra temor anxiety versus fear
ansiedad crónica chronic anxiety
ansiedad de ancianos elderly anxiety
ansiedad de aniquilación annihilation anxiety
ansiedad de aprendizaje learning anxiety
ansiedad de castración castration anxiety
ansiedad de castración anal anal castration anxiety
ansiedad de computadoras computer anxiety
ansiedad de ejecución performance anxiety
ansiedad de examinación examination anxiety
ansiedad de muerte death anxiety
ansiedad de pruebas test anxiety
ansiedad de realidad reality anxiety
ansiedad de señal signal anxiety
ansiedad de separación separation anxiety
ansiedad de situación situation anxiety
ansiedad del ego ego anxiety
ansiedad del id id anxiety
ansiedad del superego superego anxiety
ansiedad depresiva depressive anxiety
ansiedad elemental elemental anxiety
ansiedad en adolescencia anxiety in adolescence
ansiedad erotizada erotized anxiety
ansiedad existencial existential anxiety
ansiedad flotante free-floating anxiety
ansiedad fóbica phobic anxiety
ansiedad generalizada generalized anxiety
ansiedad heterosexual heterosexual anxiety
ansiedad inducida por relajación relaxation-induced anxiety
ansiedad instintiva instinctual anxiety
ansiedad manifiesta manifest anxiety
ansiedad matemática mathematical anxiety

ansiedad moral moral anxiety
ansiedad neurótica neurotic anxiety
ansiedad noética noetic anxiety
ansiedad objetiva objective anxiety
ansiedad oral oral anxiety
ansiedad orgánica organic anxiety
ansiedad paranoide paranoid anxiety
ansiedad persecutoria persecutory anxiety
ansiedad primal primal anxiety
ansiedad primaria primary anxiety
ansiedad real real anxiety
ansiedad sexual sexual anxiety
ansiedad situacional situational anxiety
ansiedad social social anxiety
ansiedad traumática traumatic anxiety
ansiedad uretral urethral anxiety
ansiedad verdadera true anxiety
ansiedad y delincuencia anxiety and
     delinquency
ansiedad y problemas de sueño anxiety and
     sleep problems
ansiolítico anxiolytic
ansioso anxious
antafrodisiaco antaphrodisiac
antagónico antagonistic
antagonismo antagonism
antagonismo bioquímico biochemical
     antagonism
antagonismo de colores color antagonism
antagonismo de drogas drug antagonism
antagonismo farmacológico pharmacological
     antagonism
antagonismo fisiológico physiological
     antagonism
antagonismo funcional functional antagonism
antagonismo químico chemical antagonism
antagonista antagonist
antagonista narcótico narcotic antagonist
antagonista opiáceo opiate antagonist
ante partum ante partum
antecedente antecedent
antefiáltico antephialtic
anterior anterior
anterógrado anterograde
anterolateral anterolateral
antiácido antacid
antiadrenérgico antiadrenergic
antiandrógeno antiandrogen
antiansiedad antianxiety
antibiótico antibiotic
anticatexis anticathexis
anticefalágico anticephalagic
anticipación anticipation
anticipación del papel anticipation of role
anticipatorio anticipatory
anticolinérgico anticholinergic
anticolinesterasa anticholinesterase
anticonformismo anticonformity
anticonvulsivo anticonvulsant
anticuerpo antibody
anticuerpo anticerebro antibrain antibody
antidepresivo antidepressant
antidepresivo atípico atypical antidepressant
antidepresivo tetracíclico tetracyclic
     antidepressant

antidepresivo triazolopiridínico
     triazolopyridine antidepressant
antidepresivo tricíclico tricyclic
     antidepressant
antidepresivos de ancianos elderly
     antidepressants
antidiurético antidiuretic
antidrómico antidromic
antiepiléptico antiepileptic
antierótico anterotic
antiespasmódico antispasmodic
antiestrogénico antiestrogenic
antifetichismo antifetishism
antifóbico antiphobic
antígeno antigen
antihipnótico antihypnotic
antihistamina antihistamine
antiintoxicante antiintoxicant
antiintracepción antiintraception
antimanía antimania
antimaníaco antimaniacal
antimetabolita antimetabolite
antimetropía antimetropia
antimiasténico antimyasthenic
antimicrobiano antimicrobial
antineurálgico antineuralgic
antineurítico antineuritic
antinomía antinomy
antiobsesivo antiobsessive
antiparkinsoniano antiparkinsonian
antipirético antipyretic
antipirina antipyrine
antipraxia antipraxia
antipsicótico antipsychotic
antipsiquiatría antipsychiatry
antirrumiante antiruminant
antisocial antisocial
antitetánico antitetanic
antitónico antitonic
antitrismo antitrismus
antitusivo antitussive
antiviral antiviral
antivitamina antivitamin
antlofobia antlophobia
antojo craving
antojo de comidas food craving
ántrax anthrax
ántrax cerebral cerebral anthrax
antrofosia antrophose
antropocéntrico anthropocentric
antropocentrismo anthropocentrism
antropofagia anthropophagy
antropofobia anthropophobia
antropoide anthropoid
antropología anthropology
antropología aplicada applied anthropology
antropología cognitiva cognitive anthropology
antropología criminal criminal anthropology
antropología cultural cultural anthropology
antropología física physical anthropology
antropología médica medical anthropology
antropología psicoanalítica psychoanalytic
     anthropology
antropología social social anthropology
antropometría anthropometry

antropomorfismo anthropomorphism
antropomorfo anthropomorph
antroponomía anthroponomy
antropopatía anthropopathy
antroposcopia anthroposcopy
antrotipo anthrotype
anulación annulment
añoranza longing, homesickness
añoranza pasiva-receptiva passive-receptive
    longing
apaciguar appease
apalancamiento leverage
apalestesia apallesthesia
apálico apallic
apandria apandria
apantropía apanthropy
aparalítico aparalytic
aparato device
aparato autoinstructivo autoinstructional
    device
aparato autónomo autonomic apparatus
aparato de adquisición del lenguaje language
    acquisition device
aparato de Golgi Golgi apparatus
aparato de seguridad safety device
aparato mental mental apparatus
aparato mnemónico mnemonic device
aparato para desensibilización automática
    device for automatic desensitization
aparato proyectivo projective device
aparato psíquico psychic apparatus
aparato vestibular vestibular apparatus
apareamiento mating
apareamiento aleatorio random mating
apareamiento metamérico metameric match
apareamiento perceptivo-motor
    perceptual-motor match
apareamiento selectivo assortative mating
apareamientos consanguíneos
    consanguineous matings
aparente apparent
apareunia apareunia
aparición apparition
apariencia appearance
apariencia de color color appearance
apariencia física physical appearance
apastia apastia
apatía apathy
apatía erótica erotic apathy
apatía eufórica euphoric apathy
apatía sexual sexual apathy
apático apathetic
apatismo apathism
apego attachment
apego afectivo affectional attachment
apego evitante avoidant attachment
apego fetal fetal attachment
apego inseguro insecure attachment
apego maternal maternal attachment
apego resistente resistant attachment
apego seguro secure attachment
apego selectivo selective attachment
apeirofobia apeirophobia
apelación emocional emotional appeal
apelaciones emocionales en anuncios

emotional appeals in advertising
apercepción apperception
apercepción de sentimiento feeling
    apperception
apercepción sesgada biased apperception
aperceptivo apperceptive
apersonificación appersonification
apestato appestat
apetitivo appetitive
apetito appetite
apifobia apiphobia
apiñamiento crowding
aplanamiento flattening
aplanamiento de afecto flattening of affect
aplasia aplasia
aplástico aplastic
aplestia aplestia
aplicación clínica clinical application
apnea apnea
apnea central central apnea
apnea del sueño sleep apnea
apnea del sueño central central sleep apnea
apnea del sueño obstructiva obstructive sleep
    apnea
apnea inducida por el sueño sleep-induced
    apnea
apnea obstructiva obstructive apnea
apnea periférica peripheral apnea
apneico apneic
apneusis apneusis
apocamnósico apokamnosic
apocamnosis apokamnosis
apocarteresis apocarteresis
apoclesia apoclesis
apodemialgia apodemialgia
apofisario apophysary
apolepsis apolepsis
apomorfina apomorphine
apopatético apopathetic
apopléctico apoplectic
apoplectiforme apoplectiform
apoplectoide apoplectoid
apoplejía apoplexy
apoplejía bulbar bulbar apoplexy
apoplejía de Broadbent Broadbent's apoplexy
apoplejía de tipo Raymond Raymond type of
    apoplexy
apoplejía embólica embolic apoplexy
apoplejía espasmódica spasmodic apoplexy
apoplejía espinal spinal apoplexy
apoplejía funcional functional apoplexy
apoplejía ingravescente ingravescent
    apoplexy
apoplejía neonatal neonatal apoplexy
apoplejía pituitaria pituitary apoplexy
apoplejía pontina pontine apoplexy
apoplejía serosa serous apoplexy
apoplejía trombótica thrombotic apoplexy
apopnixia apopnixis
aporía aporia
aporioneurosis aporioneurosis
apoyador supportive
apoyador-expresivo supportive-expressive
apoyo support
apoyo del ego ego support

apoyo del ego de amigos ego support from friends
apoyo del ego de familia ego support from family
apoyo del ego de grupos ego support from groups
apoyo emocional emotional support
apoyo social social support
apractagnosia apractagnosia
apractagnosia espacial spatial apractagnosia
apráctico apractic
apragmatismo apragmatism
apraxia apraxia
apraxia acinética akinetic apraxia
apraxia álgera apraxia algera
apraxia amnésica amnesic apraxia
apraxia cinestésica kinesthetic apraxia
apraxia constructiva constructive apraxia
apraxia cortical cortical apraxia
apraxia de construcción constructional apraxia
apraxia de inervación innervation apraxia
apraxia de marcha apraxia of gait
apraxia del vestir dressing apraxia
apraxia dinámica dynamic apraxia
apraxia ideacional ideational apraxia
apraxia ideatoria ideatory apraxia
apraxia ideocinética ideokinetic apraxia
apraxia ideomotora ideomotor apraxia
apraxia limbocinética limb-kinetic apraxia
apraxia magnética magnetic apraxia
apraxia motora motor apraxia
apraxia motora ocular ocular motor apraxia
apraxia oculomotora oculomotor apraxia
apraxia sensorial sensory apraxia
apraxia transcortical transcortical apraxia
apráxico apraxic
aprehensión apprehension
aprehensión de evaluación evaluation apprehension
aprehensión directa direct apprehension
aprehensión irresistible irresistible apprehension
aprender learn
aprendido learned
aprendiendo a aprender learning to learn
aprendizaje learning
aprendizaje animal animal learning
aprendizaje apetitivo appetitive learning
aprendizaje asimilativo assimilative learning
aprendizaje asociativo associative learning
aprendizaje aversivo aversive learning
aprendizaje complejo complex learning
aprendizaje conceptual conceptual learning
aprendizaje continuado continued learning
aprendizaje de alternación doble double-alternation learning
aprendizaje de apego attachment learning
aprendizaje de aversión aversion learning
aprendizaje de categorización categorization learning
aprendizaje de conceptos concept learning
aprendizaje de conceptos animal animal concept learning
aprendizaje de descubrimiento discovery learning

aprendizaje de destreza skill learning
aprendizaje de destrezas de motor grueso gross motor skills learning
aprendizaje de discriminación discrimination learning
aprendizaje de enfoque en sensaciones sensate focus learning
aprendizaje de escape escape learning
aprendizaje de escape-evitación escape-avoidance learning
aprendizaje de evitación avoidance learning
aprendizaje de experiencias learning from experience
aprendizaje de infantes infant learning
aprendizaje de inversión espacial spatial-reversal learning
aprendizaje de laberinto maze learning
aprendizaje de lugar place learning
aprendizaje de movimiento movement learning
aprendizaje de orden serial serial-order learning
aprendizaje de pares asociados paired-associates learning
aprendizaje de patrón pattern learning
aprendizaje de principios principle learning
aprendizaje de probabilidades probability learning
aprendizaje de reglas rule learning
aprendizaje de respuesta response learning
aprendizaje de respuesta condicionada conditioned response learning
aprendizaje de todo o nada all-or-none learning
aprendizaje de un ensayo one trial learning
aprendizaje del fondo hacia arriba bottom-up learning
aprendizaje del lenguaje learning of language
aprendizaje dependiente del estado state-dependent learning
aprendizaje discriminativo discriminative learning
aprendizaje disociado dissociated learning
aprendizaje durante sueño learning during sleep
aprendizaje en sueño sleep learning
aprendizaje escondido hidden learning
aprendizaje fetal fetal learning
aprendizaje ideacional ideational learning
aprendizaje imitativo imitative learning
aprendizaje implícito implicit learning
aprendizaje incidental incidental learning
aprendizaje integrante integrative learning
aprendizaje intencional intentional learning
aprendizaje intraneurosensorial intraneurosensory learning
aprendizaje intraserial intraserial learning
aprendizaje inverso reversal learning
aprendizaje latente latent learning
aprendizaje mecánico rote learning
aprendizaje motor motor learning
aprendizaje observacional observational learning
aprendizaje observacional en niños

observational learning in children
aprendizaje observacional y agresión
   observational learning and aggression
aprendizaje operante operant learning
aprendizaje pasivo passive learning
aprendizaje pasivo de evitación
   passive-avoidance learning
aprendizaje pavloviano pavlovian learning
aprendizaje perceptivo perceptual learning
aprendizaje perceptivo-motor
   perceptual-motor learning
aprendizaje por estímulo-estímulo
   stimulus-stimulus learning
aprendizaje por estímulo-respuesta
   stimulus-response learning
aprendizaje por exposición exposure learning
aprendizaje por signos sign learning
aprendizaje por soluciones solution learning
aprendizaje por tanteo trial and error
   learning
aprendizaje programado programmed
   learning
aprendizaje racional rational learning
aprendizaje relacional relational learning
aprendizaje restringido restricted learning
aprendizaje selectivo selective learning
aprendizaje serial serial learning
aprendizaje significativo meaningful learning
aprendizaje sin conciencia learning without
   awareness
aprendizaje social social learning
aprendizaje subcortical subcortical learning
aprendizaje subliminal subliminal learning
aprendizaje temprano early learning
aprendizaje verbal verbal learning
aprendizaje vicario vicarious learning
aprendizaje visceral visceral learning
aprendizaje visual visual learning
aprendizaje y abuso de niños learning and
   child abuse
aprendizaje y desarrollo cognitivo learning
   and cognitive development
aprendizaje y memoria learning and memory
aprendizaje y recompensas learning and
   rewards
aprendizaje y retención learning and
   retention
aprendizaje y señales learning and cues
apriorismo apriorism
aprobación approval
aprobarbital aprobarbital
aproforia aprophoria
apropiado appropriate
aprosexia aprosexia
aprosodia aprosody
aprovechamiento contra aptitud achievement
   versus aptitude
aprovechamiento educacional educational
   achievement
aproximación approximation
aproximación de palabras word
   approximation
aproximaciones sucesivas successive
   approximations
apsicognosia apsychognosia

apsicosis apsychosis
apsiquia apsychia
aptitud aptitude, fitness
aptitud aeróbica aerobic fitness
aptitud cardiovascular cardiovascular fitness
aptitud darwiniana darwinian fitness
aptitud especial special aptitude
aptitud específica specific aptitude
aptitud física physical fitness
aptitud física de niños physical fitness of
   children
aptitud general general aptitude
aptitud genética genetic fitness
aptitud inclusiva inclusive fitness
aptitud mecánica mechanical aptitude
aptitud natural natural aptitude
aptitud para juicio fitness for trial
aptitud personal personal fitness
aptitud vocacional vocational aptitude
apuntamiento pointing
apuntamiento de hueso bone-pointing
apunte prompt
apuro doble double bind
apuro doble bipolar bipolar double bind
aqueiria acheiria
aquiescencia acquiescence
aquiescencia de respuesta response
   acquiescence
aquietamiento reassurance
aquiria achiria
aracnofobia arachnophobia
aracnoideo arachnoid
aracnoiditis arachnoiditis
aracnoiditis adhesiva adhesive arachnoiditis
aracnoiditis neoplásica neoplastic
   arachnoiditis
aracnoiditis obliterativa obliterative
   arachnoiditis
arafia araphia
arbitraje arbitration
arbitrario arbitrary
árbol de decisiones decision tree
árbol vital arbor vitae
arborización arborization
arcaico archaic
arcaísmo archaism
arco arc
arco alfa alpha arc
arco beta beta arc
arco de dos neuronas two-neuron arc
arco de reflejo multisináptico multisynaptic
   reflex arc
arco monosináptico monosynaptic arc
arco multisináptico multisynaptic arc
arco neural neural arc
arco polisináptico polysynaptic arc
arco reflejo reflex arc
arco reflejo monosináptico monosynaptic
   reflex arc
arco reflejo polisináptico polysynaptic reflex
   arc
arco reflejo psíquico psychic reflex arc
ardanestesia ardanesthesia
área area
área bajo la curva area under the curve

área calcarina calcarine area
área crítica critical area
área cultural cultural area
área de asociación association area
área de Broca Broca's area
área de Brodmann Brodmann's area
área de disparo trigger area
área de proyección projection area
área de proyección motora motor projection
   area
área de proyección sensorial sensory
   projection area
área de Wernicke Wernicke's area
área del habla speech area
área del habla de Broca Broca's speech area
área ejecutiva executive area
área estriada area striata
área libre de conflictos conflict-free area
área motora motor area
área motora suplemental supplementary
   motor area
área parietal posterior posterior parietal area
área piriforme piriform area
área poscentral postcentral area
área postrema area postrema
área precentral precentral area
área preestriada prestriate area
área prefrontal prefrontal area
área premotora premotor area
área preóptica preoptic area
área preóptica lateral lateral preoptic area
área prepiriforme prepyriform area
área primaria primary area
área secundaria secondary area
área sensorial sensory area
área sensorial somática somatic sensory area
área septal septal area
área silenciosa silent area
área somestésica somesthetic area
área supresora suppressor area
área precentral intermedia intermediate
   precentral area
áreas de proyección auditiva auditory
   projection areas
áreas olfatorias olfactory areas
arecolina arecoline
arena cerebral brain sand
areola areola
argot argot
argumentatividad argumentativeness
ariepiglótico aryepiglottic
aristogénica aristogenics
aristotélico Aristotelian
aritmética arithmetic
aritmética mental mental arithmetic
aritmomanía arithmomania
armadura del carácter character armor
armonía harmony
armónico harmonic
armónico aural aural harmonic
armonista harmonizer
arquetipo archetype
arquetipo materno mother archetype
arquicerebelo archicerebellum
arquicorteza archicortex

arquitectónico architectonic
arquitectura del sueño sleep architecture
arranque spurt
arranque de crecimiento growth spurt
arranque final end spurt
arranque inicial initial spurt
arrastramiento dragging
arrastramiento de parámetro parameter
   dragging
arrastramiento de pie foot-dragging
arreflexia areflexia
arreglo arrangement
arreglo jerárquico hierarchical arrangement
arreglo neurótico neurotic arrangement
arriesgado hazardous
arrigosis arrhigosis
arrimo cuddling
arrinencefalia arrhinencephaly
arritmia arrhythmia
arritmocinesis arrhythmokinesis
arrobamiento bliss
arrobamiento absoluto absolute bliss
artefacto artifact
artefacto cultural cultural artifact
artefacto estadístico statistical artifact
arteria artery
arteria basilar basilar artery
arteria carótida interna internal carotid
   artery
arteria cerebral anterior anterior cerebral
   artery
arteria cerebral media middle cerebral artery
arteria cerebral posterior posterior cerebral
   artery
arteria comunicante posterior posterior
   communicating artery
arteria dolicoectática dolichoectatic artery
arteria helicina helicine artery
arteria oftálmica ophthalmic artery
arteria vertebral vertebral artery
arterioesclerosis arteriosclerosis
arterioesclerosis cerebral cerebral
   arteriosclerosis
arterioesclerótico arteriosclerotic
arteriografía arteriography
arteriografía cerebral cerebral arteriography
arteriografía espinal spinal arteriography
arteriograma arteriogram
arteriopalmo arteriopalmus
arteritis arteritis
arteritis craneal cranial arteritis
arteritis de células gigantes giant cell arteritis
arteritis de Horton Horton's arteritis
arteritis granulomatoso granulomatous
   arteritis
arteritis temporal temporal arteritis
artes del lenguaje language arts
artes expresivas expressive arts
artes y oficios arts and crafts
articulación articulation
articulación de Charcot Charcot's joint
articulación histérica hysterical joint
articulación infantil infantile articulation
articulación neuropática neuropathic joint
articular articular

artículo item
artículo de prueba test item
artículos amortiguadores buffer items
artículos culturales cultural items
artificialismo artificialism
artrestesia arthresthesia
artritis arthritis
artritis neuropática neuropathic arthritis
artritis reumatoide rheumatoid arthritis
artritismo arthritism
artrodesis arthrodesis
artrogriposis arthrogryposis
artropatía arthropathy
artropatía diabética diabetic arthropathy
artropatía neuropática neuropathic
  arthropathy
artropatía tabética tabetic arthropathy
asa de Meyer-Archambault
  Meyer-Archambault loop
asafolalia asapholalia
asalto assault
ascendencia ascendance
ascendencia-sumisión ascendance-submission
ascendente ascending
ascetismo asceticism
asemasia asemasia
asemia asemia
aséptico aseptic
asertivo assertive
asesinato murder
asesor counselor
asesor de drogas drug counselor
asesor de rehabilitación rehabilitation
  counselor
asesor de rehabilitación industrial industrial
  rehabilitation counselor
asesor de salud mental mental-health
  counselor
asesor genético genetic counselor
asesoramiento counseling, guidance
asesoramiento anticipatorio anticipatory
  guidance
asesoramiento clínico clinical counseling
asesoramiento conjunto conjoint counseling
asesoramiento de adolescentes adolescent
  counseling
asesoramiento de carrera career counseling
asesoramiento de carrera de grupo group
  career counseling
asesoramiento de colocación placement
  counseling
asesoramiento de divorcio divorce counseling
asesoramiento de grupo group counseling
asesoramiento de niños child guidance
asesoramiento de reevaluación reevaluation
  counseling
asesoramiento de refuerzo reinforcement
  counseling
asesoramiento de retiro retirement counseling
asesoramiento de seguimiento follow-up
  counseling
asesoramiento de sobrevivientes counseling
  of survivors
asesoramiento de víctimas counseling of
  victims

asesoramiento del desarrollo developmental
  counseling
asesoramiento directivo directive counseling
asesoramiento ecléctico eclectic counseling
asesoramiento educacional educational
  counseling
asesoramiento en la colocación de niños
  child-placement counseling
asesoramiento familiar family counseling
asesoramiento genético genetic counseling
asesoramiento marital marital counseling
asesoramiento matrimonial marriage
  counseling
asesoramiento matrimonial en grupos
  marriage counseling in groups
asesoramiento multicultural multicultural
  counseling
asesoramiento ocupacional occupational
  counseling
asesoramiento paritario peer counseling
asesoramiento pastoral pastoral counseling
asesoramiento predivorcio predivorce
  counseling
asesoramiento premarital premarital
  counseling
asesoramiento psicológico psychological
  counseling
asesoramiento semántico semantic counseling
asesoramiento sexual sexual counseling
asesoramiento telefónico telephone
  counseling
asesoramiento transcultural cross-cultural
  counseling
asesoramiento tras violación rape counseling
asesoramiento vocacional vocational
  counseling
asesoramiento de padres parent counseling
asexual asexual
asfalgesia asphalgesia
asfixia asphyxia
asfixia neonatal neonatal asphyxia
asignación assignment
asignación aleatoria random assignment
asignación condicional conditional assignment
asignación sexual sex assignment
asilabia asyllabia
asilo asylum
asilo de insanos insane asylum
asilo para adultos adult foster home
asimbolia asymbolia
asimetría asymmetry
asimetría funcional functional asymmetry
asimetría mental mental asymmetry
asimetrías en orientación asymmetries in
  orientation
asimetrías hemisféricas hemispheric
  asymmetries
asimétrico asymmetric
asimilable assimilable
asimilación assimilation
asimilación cultural cultural assimilation
asimilación de objeto object assimilation
asimilación generalizante generalizing
  assimilation
asimilación recíproca reciprocal assimilation

asimilación reproductiva reproductive
  assimilation
asimilación social social assimilation
asimilar assimilate
asíncrono asynchronous
asindesis asyndesis
asinergia asynergia
asinergia mayor de Babinski major asynergia
  of Babinski
asinesia asynesia
asinesis asynesis
asinodia asynodia
asintomático asymptomatic
asíntota asymptote
asintótico asymptotic
asistencia de aula classroom attendance
asistencia posterior aftercare
asistencia postoperatoria aftercare
asistente de médico physician's assistant
asistido por computadora computer-assisted
asitia asitia
asma asthma
asma bronquial bronchial asthma
asma extrínseca extrinsic asthma
asma nerviosa nervous asthma
asociación association
asociación constreñida constrained
  association
asociación contextual contextual association
asociación controlada controlled association
asociación cruzada cross-association
asociación de ideas association of ideas
asociación de palabras word association
asociación de sueños dream association
asociación directa direct association
asociación estadística statistical association
asociación falsa false association
asociación hacia adelante forward association
asociación hacia atrás backward association
asociación indirecta indirect association
asociación inmediata immediate association
asociación libre free association
asociación libre en hipnosis free-association
  in hypnosis
asociación mediata mediate association
asociación paradigmática paradigmatic
  association
asociación por contigüidad association by
  contiguity
asociación refleja reflex association
asociación remota remote association
asociación retroactiva retroactive association
asociación serial serial association
asociación sonora clang association
asociacionismo associationism
asociado associate
asocial asocial
asocialidad asociality
asociativo associative
asonancia assonance
asonia asonia
asoticamanía asoticamania
aspartama aspartame
aspartilglucosaminuria
  aspartylglycosaminuria

aspecto aspect
aspectos cualitativos qualitative aspects
aspectos del desarrollo de ansiedad
  developmental aspects of anxiety
aspermatismo aspermatism
aspermia aspermia
aspermia psicogénica psychogenic aspermia
aspiración aspiration
astasia astasia
astasia-abasia astasia-abasia
astático astatic
astenia asthenia
astenia inducida por calor heat-induced
  asthenia
astenia mental mental asthenia
astenia neurocirculatoria neurocirculatory
  asthenia
asténico asthenic
astenofobia asthenophobia
astenología asthenology
astenopía asthenopia
astereognosia astereognosia
astereognosis astereognosis
asterixis asterixis
astigmatismo astigmatism
astrafobia astraphobia
astrapofobia astrapophobia
astroblastoma astroblastoma
astrocito astrocyte
astrocito ameboide ameboid astrocyte
astrocito fibrilar fibrillary astrocyte
astrocito fibroso fibrous astrocyte
astrocito gemistocítico gemistocytic astrocyte
astrocito protoplásmico protoplasmic
  astrocyte
astrocito reactivo reactive astrocyte
astrocitoma astrocytoma
astrocitoma anaplástico anaplastic
  astrocytoma
astrocitoma gemistocítico gemistocytic
  astrocytoma
astrocitoma grado I grade I astrocytoma
astrocitoma grado II grade II astrocytoma
astrocitoma grado III grade III astrocytoma
astrocitoma grado IV grade IV astrocytoma
astrocitoma piloide piloid astrocytoma
astrocitoma protoplásmico protoplasmic
  astrocytoma
astrocitosis astrocytosis
astrocitosis cerebri astrocytosis cerebri
astroependimoma astroependymoma
astroglia astroglia
astrología astrology
asunción assumption
asunción de pelea-fuga fight-flight
  assumption
asunción de realidad reality assumption
atactilia atactilia
ataque attack
ataque afectivo affective attack
ataque calástico chalastic fit
ataque calástico posdormital postdormital
  chalastic fit
ataque cardíaco heart attack
ataque catapléctico cataplectic attack

ataque cerebeloso cerebellar fit
ataque crepuscular twilight attack
ataque de ansiedad anxiety attack
ataque de ansiedad aguda acute anxiety attack
ataque de ansiedad de sueños dream anxiety attack
ataque de arañazos clawing attack
ataque de caída drop attack
ataque de morder biting attack
ataque de pánico panic attack
ataque de síntomas limitados limited-symptom attack
ataque de sueño neurótico neurotic-sleep attack
ataque isquémico transitorio transient ischemic attack
ataque obsesivo obsessive attack
ataque predatorio predatory attack
ataque psicomotor psychomotor attack
ataque uncinado uncinate attack
ataque vagal vagal attack
ataque vasovagal vasovagal attack
ataque vasovagal de Gowers vasovagal attack of Gowers
ataques de tentación horrenda fits of horrendous temptation
ataráctico ataractic
ataraxia ataraxy
ataráxico ataraxic
atavismo atavism
ataxia ataxia
ataxia aguda acute ataxia
ataxia cerebelosa cerebellar ataxia
ataxia cerebelosa aguda acute cerebellar ataxia
ataxia cerebelosa hereditaria hereditary cerebellar ataxia
ataxia cerebelosa hereditaria de Marie hereditary cerebellar ataxia of Marie
ataxia cinética kinetic ataxia
ataxia de Biemond Biemond's ataxia
ataxia de Briquet Briquet's ataxia
ataxia de Bruns Bruns' ataxia
ataxia de Friedreich Friedreich's ataxia
ataxia de Leyden Leyden's ataxia
ataxia de Marie Marie's ataxia
ataxia espinal spinal ataxia
ataxia espinal hereditaria hereditary spinal ataxia
ataxia estática static ataxia
ataxia hereditaria hereditary ataxia
ataxia histérica hysterical ataxia
ataxia intrapsíquica intrapsychic ataxia
ataxia locomotora locomotor ataxia
ataxia mental mental ataxia
ataxia moral moral ataxia
ataxia motora motor ataxia
ataxia psíquica psychic ataxia
ataxia sensorial sensory ataxia
ataxia telangiectasia ataxia telangiectasia
ataxia vasomotora vasomotor ataxia
ataxia vestibulocerebelosa vestibulocerebellar ataxia
ataxia voluntaria voluntary ataxia

ataxiadinamia ataxiadynamia
ataxiafasia ataxiaphasia
ataxiágrafo ataxiagraph
ataxiagrama ataxiagram
ataxiámetro ataxiameter
atáxico ataxic
ataxiofemia ataxiophemia
ataxiofobia ataxiophobia
ataxofemia ataxophemia
atefobia atephobia
atelesis atelesis
atelia atelia
ateliosis ateliosis
atención attention
atención auditiva auditory attention
atención controlada controlled attention
atención dirigida directed attention
atención e interferencia attention and interference
atención en funcionamiento cognitivo attention in cognitive functioning
atención en hipnosis attention in hypnosis
atención errante wandering attention
atención flotante free-floating attention
atención focal focal attention
atención primaria primary attention
atención secundaria secondary attention
atención selectiva selective attention
atención visual visual attention
atender attend
atenolol atenolol
atensidad attensity
atento attentive
atenuación attenuation
atenuación dimming
atenuación estadística statistical attenuation
atenuador attenuator
ateroesclerosis atherosclerosis
ateromatosis atheromatosis
atetoide athetoid
atetósico athetosic
atetosis athetosis
atetosis congénita doble double congenital athetosis
atetosis doble double athetosis
atetosis poshemipléjica posthemiplegic athetosis
atetótico athetotic
atimia athymia
atípico atypical
atlas cerebral brain atlas
atmósfera atmosphere
atmósfera autoritaria authoritarian atmosphere
atmósfera de grupo group atmosphere
atmósfera democrática democratic atmosphere
atmósfera laissez-faire laissez-faire atmosphere
atmósfera social social atmosphere
atmósfera terapéutica therapeutic atmosphere
atolladero bottleneck, impasse
atolladero de atención bottleneck of attention
atolladero terapéutico therapeutic impasse
atomismo atomism

atomístico atomistic
átomo social social atom
atonía atony
atonicidad attonity
atónico atonic
atopognosia atopognosia
atopognosis atopognosis
atrabiliario atrabiliary
atracción attraction
atracción interpersonal interpersonal attraction
atracción por temor fear appeal
atractividad attractiveness
atractividad física physical attractiveness
atractivo appeal
atractivo de corto circuito short-circuit appeal
atractivo de producto product appeal
atraso lag
atraso cultural cultural lag
atraso del desarrollo developmental lag
atraso maduracional maturational lag
atraso social social lag
atrayente de atención attention-getting
atresia atresia
atribución attribution
atribución ambiental environmental attribution
atribución causal causal attribution
atribución de causalidad attribution of causality
atribución de emoción attribution of emotion
atribución de error error attribution
atribución de responsabilidad attribution of responsibility
atribución disposicional dispositional attribution
atribución personal personal attribution
atributo attribute
atributo de color color attribute
atributo subjetivo subjective attribute
atributo tonal tonal attribute
atributos abstractos abstract attributes
atributos auditivos auditory attributes
atributos comunes common attributes
atributos irrelevantes irrelevant attributes
atrigenerismo altrigenderism
atriopeptina atriopeptin
atrofedema atrophedema
atrofia atrophy
atrofia cerebelosa cerebellar atrophy
atrofia cerebelosa tipo nutricional nutritional type cerebellar atrophy
atrofia cerebral brain atrophy
atrofia de Erb Erb's atrophy
atrofia de Hunt Hunt's atrophy
atrofia de Pick Pick's atrophy
atrofia de Sudeck Sudeck's atrophy
atrofia de Vulpian Vulpian's atrophy
atrofia escapulohumeral scapulohumeral atrophy
atrofia espinal spinal atrophy
atrofia espinomuscular progresiva progressive spinal-muscular atrophy
atrofia facioescapulohumeral

facioscapulohumeral atrophy
atrofia infantil infantile atrophy
atrofia miopática myopathic atrophy
atrofia muscular muscular atrophy
atrofia muscular de Hoffmann Hoffmann's muscular atrophy
atrofia muscular espinal familiar familial spinal muscular atrophy
atrofia muscular espinal progresiva infantil infantile progressive spinal muscular atrophy
atrofia muscular idiopática idiopathic muscular atrophy
atrofia muscular infantil infantile muscular atrophy
atrofia muscular isquémica ischemic muscular atrophy
atrofia muscular juvenil juvenile muscular atrophy
atrofia muscular peronea peroneal muscular atrophy
atrofia muscular progresiva progressive muscular atrophy
atrofia muscular seudohipertrófica pseudohypertrophic muscular atrophy
atrofia neurítica neuritic atrophy
atrofia neurogénica neurogenic atrophy
atrofia neurotrófica neurotrophic atrophy
atrofia olivopontocerebelosa olivopontocerebellar atrophy
atrofia óptica optic atrophy
atrofia testicular testicular atrophy
atrofia testicular de presión pressure testicular atrophy
atrofia transneuronal transneuronal atrophy
atrofia trofoneurótica trophoneurotic atrophy
atrofoderma atrophoderma
atrofoderma neurítica atrophoderma neuriticum
atropina atropine
aturdir stun
audacia adventurousness
audibilidad audibility
audible audible
audición audition
audición coloreada colored audition
audición cromática chromatic audition
audición de color color hearing
audición de pensamientos thought hearing
audición de Riese Riese hearing
audición dicótica dichotic listening
audición en infantes hearing in infants
audición gustatoria gustatory audition
audición persistente afterhearing
audición selectiva selective listening
audífono hearing aid, earphone
audífono contralateral contralateral hearing aid
audioanalgesia audioanalgesia
audiogénico audiogenic
audiograma audiogram
audiología audiology
audiometría audiometry
audiometría de tono puro pure-tone audiometry

audiometría del habla speech audiometry
audiometría diagnóstica diagnostic audiometry
audiometría electroencefálica electroencephalic audiometry
audiómetro audiometer
auditivo auditive
auditoría audit
auditoría de cuidado de pacientes patient-care audit
auditoría médica medical audit
auditoría médica concurrente concurrent medical audit
auditoría médica retrospectiva retrospective medical audit
auditoría personal personal audit
aula classroom
aula abierta open classroom
aulofobia aulophobia
aumento augmentation
aumento de despertamiento arousal boost
aura aura
aura cinestésica kinesthetic aura
aura epiléptica epileptic aura
aura intelectual intellectual aura
aura reminiscente reminiscent aura
aura visual visual aura
aural aural
aurorafobia auroraphobia
auscultación auscultation
ausencia absence
ausencia atípica atypical absence
ausencia atónica atonic absence
ausencia automática automatic absence
ausencia compleja complex absence
ausencia de fantasía fantasy absence
ausencia del padre father absence
ausencia enurética enuretic absence
ausencia epiléptica epileptic absence
ausencia estornutatoria sternutatory absence
ausencia hipertónica hypertonic absence
ausencia mioclónica myoclonic absence
ausencia pura pure absence
ausencia retrocursiva retrocursive absence
ausencia simple simple absence
ausencia subclínica subclinical absence
ausencia típica typical absence
ausencia tusiva tussive absence
ausencia vasomotora vasomotor absence
ausente absent
ausentismo absenteeism
autarquía autarchy
autemesia autemesia
autenticidad authenticity
autía autia
autismo autism
autismo contra esquizofrenia autism versus schizophrenia
autismo contra retardo mental autism versus mental retardation
autismo contra trastorno de déficit de atención autism versus attention-deficit disorder
autismo infantil infantile autism
autismo infantil temprano early infantile

autism
autismo infantil y esquizofrenia de niñez infantile autism and childhood schizophrenia
autismo normal normal autism
autista autistic
autoabatimiento self-abasement
autoabuso self-abuse
autoaceptación self-acceptance
autoacusación self-accusation
autoadministración self-management
autoadministrado self-managed
autoagresión autoaggression
autoalienación self-alienation
autoalimentación self-feeding
autoanálisis self-analysis
autoataque self-attack
autoayuda self-help
autobiográfico autobiographical
autocastigo self-punishment
autocastración autocastration
autocastración anticipatoria anticipatory autocastration
autocatarsis autocatharsis
autocatártico autocathartic
autocensura self-censure
autocéntrico autocentric
autocertidumbre self-certainty
autocinesia autokinesia
autocinesis autokinesis
autocinético autokinetic
autoclasificación self-rating
autoclítico autoclitic
autoconcepto self-concept
autoconfinamiento self-commitment
autoconocimiento self-knowledge
autoconsistencia self-consistency
autocorrelación autocorrelation
autocrítica self-criticism
autóctono autochthonous
autocuidado self-care
autoculpación self-blaming
autodecepción self-deception
autoderogación self-derogation
autoderrotante self-defeating
autodesarrollo self-development
autodescubrimiento self-discovery
autodesensibilización self-desensitization
autodespreciativo self-contemptuous
autodesprecio self-contempt
autodestructividad self-destructiveness
autodeterminación self-determination
autodiferenciación self-differentiation
autodinamismo self-dynamism
autodirección self-direction
autodirigido self-directed
autodisciplina self-discipline
autodisosmofobia autodysosmophobia
autodivulgación self-disclosure
autodominio self-control
autoecolalia autoecholalia
autoecopraxia autoechopraxia
autoeficacia self-efficacy
autoerótico autoerotic
autoerotismo autoerotism

autoerotismo secundario secondary
  autoerotism
autoestima self-esteem
autoestima sexual sexual self-esteem
autoestimación self-regard
autoestimulación self-stimulation
autoestimulación sensorial sensory
  self-stimulation
autoevaluación self-assessment
autoexaminación self-examination
autoexpresión self-expression
autoextensión self-extension
autoextinción self-extinction
autofagia autophagy
autofágico autophagic
autofelación autofellatio
autofelator self-fellator
autofetichismo autofetishism
autofilia autophilia
autoflagelación autoflagellation
autofobia autophobia
autogénico autogenic
autógeno autogenous
autognosis autognosis
autografismo autographism
autogratificación self-gratification
autohipnorrelajación self-hypnorelaxation
autohipnosis self-hypnosis
autohipnótico autohypnotic
autohipnotismo autohypnotism
autoidentificación self-identification
autoimagen self-image
autoimagen de niños abusados self-image of
  abused children
autoinformante self-reporting
autoinmune autoimmune
autoinmunidad autoimmunity
autoinstrucción self-instruction
autoinstruccional self-instructional
autointoxicación autointoxication
autoinventario self-inventory
autoirrumación self-irrumation
autolibido autolibido
autología autology
automasoquismo automasochism
autómata automaton
automático automatic
automatismo automatism
automatismo ambulatorio ambulatory
  automatism
automatismo ante mandatos command
  automatism
automatismo confusional confusional
  automatism
automatismo gestual gestural automatism
automatismo ictal primal primal ictal
  automatism
automatismo ictal primario primary ictal
  automatism
automatismo postraumático inmediato
  immediate posttraumatic automatism
automatismo sensorial sensory automatism
automatismo verbal verbal automatism
automatización automatization
automatización de atención automatization of

  attention
automatógrafo automatograph
automaximación self-maximation
automisofobia automysophobia
automnesia automnesia
automonitorización self-monitoring
automórfico automorphic
automutilación self-mutilation
autonegación self-denial
autonomasia autonomasia
autonomía autonomy
autonomía contra duda autonomy versus
  doubt
autonomía contra vergüenza y duda
  autonomy versus shame and doubt
autonomía de motivos autonomy of motives
autonomía familiar family autonomy
autonomía funcional functional autonomy
autonomía funcional perseverante
  perseverative functional autonomy
autonomía-heteronomía
  autonomy-heteronomy
autónomo autonomous
autonomotrópico autonomotropic
autoobservación self-observation
autopatía autopathy
autopercepción self-perception
autoperjudicial self-injurious
autoplastia autoplasty
autopreservación self-preservation
autopsia autopsy
autopsia psicológica psychological autopsy
autopsicología self-psychology
autopsicosis autopsychosis
autopsíquico autopsychic
autopsiquis autopsyche
autoridad authority
autoridad carismática charismatic authority
autoridad ilegítima nonlegitimate authority
autoridad legal legal authority
autoridad racional rational authority
autoridad racional-legal rational-legal
  authority
autoritario authoritarian
autoritarismo authoritarianism
autorradiografía autoradiography
autorrealización self-fulfillment
autorreferencia self-reference
autorrefuerzo self-reinforcement
autorrefuerzo cognitivo cognitive
  self-reinforcement
autorregulación self-regulation
autorregulación fisiológica physiological
  self-regulation
autorrevelación self-revelation
autosadismo autosadism
autoscopia autoscopy
autoscopia idiopática idiopathic autoscopy
autoscopia sintomática symptomatic
  autoscopy
autoscópico autoscopic
autoselección self-selection
autoselección de azúcar sugar self-selection
autoselección de comida food self-selection
autosexualidad autosexuality

autosexualismo autosexualism
autosimbolismo autosymbolism
autosinoia autosynnoia
autosmia autosmia
autosoma autosome
autosomatognosis autosomatognosis
autosomatognóstico autosomatognostic
autosómico autosomal
autosómico-dominante autosomal-dominant
autosómico-recesivo autosomal-recessive
autosonambulismo autosomnabulism
autosugestibilidad autosuggestibility
autosugestión autosuggestion
autotélico autotelic
autoteoría self-theory
autotomía autotomy
autotopagnosia autotopagnosia
auxanología auxanology
auxiliar auxiliary
aversión aversion
aversión condicionada conditioned aversion
aversión de aprendizaje learning aversion
aversión de comida food aversion
aversión de gusto condicionada conditioned
    taste aversion
aversión del gusto taste aversion
aversión sexual sexual aversion
aversivo aversive
aviofobia aviophobia
avulsión avulsion
avulsión nerviosa nerve avulsion
axial axial
axila axilla
axiología axiology
axioma axiom
axodendrita axodendrite
axólisis axolysis
axón axon
axón mielinizado myelinated axon
axonopatía axonopathy
axonotmesis axonotmesis
axotomía axotomy
ayuda para entrenamiento training aid
ayudante aide
ayudante de salud en el hogar home health
    aide
ayudante de trabajo social social-work aide
ayudante mágico magic helper
ayudante psiquiátrico psychiatric aide
ayudas de memoria memory aids
ayudas del comer eating aids
ayudas electrónicas electronic aids
ayudas funcionales functional aids
ayudas para beber drinking aids
ayudas para el diario vivir daily living aids
ayudas para gatear creeping and crawling
    aids
ayudas para vivir independiente
    independent-living aids
ayudas puericulturales child-care aids
azaciclonol azacyclonol
azaperona azaperone
azoospermia azoospermia
azotador flogger
azotamiento beating, whipping

azotamiento de niño child beating
azotioprina azathioprine
azúcar sanguínea blood sugar

B

bacilofobia bacillophobia
baclofeno baclofen
bacteremia bacteremia
bacterial bacterial
bahnung bahnung
balance balance
balance autónomo autonomic balance
balance de electrólito electrolyte balance
balance de sal salt balance
balanceo rocking
balanceo corporal body rocking
balbuceo babbling
balbuceo en niños sordos babbling in deaf
children
balbuceo manual en niños sordos manual
babbling in deaf children
balbuceo reduplicado reduplicated babbling
balismo ballism
balístico ballistic
balistofobia ballistophobia
banco de ojos eye bank
banda de Gennari stripe of Gennari
bandas de Charpentier Charpentier's bands
bandas de Mach Mach bands
baragnosis baragnosis
barbaralalia barbaralalia
barbital barbital
barbiturato barbiturate
barbituratos de acción intermedia
intermediate-acting barbiturates
barestesia baresthesia
barestesiómetro baresthesiometer
barestesis baresthesis
bariecoia baryecoia
barifonía baryphony
bariglosia baryglossia
barilalia barylalia
baritimia barythymia
barofobia barophobia
barognosis barognosis
barorreceptor baroreceptor
barorreflejo baroreflex
barotaxis barotaxis
barotitis barotitis
barra de Galton Galton bar
barra de mordisco bite bar
barras de Konig Konig bars
barrera barrier
barrera al incesto incest barrier
barrera de estímulo stimulus barrier
barrera hematocerebral blood-brain barrier
barrera hematoencefálica hematoencephalic
barrier
barreras arquitectónicas architectural

barriers
barruntamiento guessing
barrunto guess
bartolinitis bartholinitis
basado en datos data-based
basal basal
base de datos data base
básico basic
basifobia basiphobia
basilar basilar
basistasifobia basistasiphobia
basofilia basophilia
basofilia pituitaria pituitary basophilia
basofilismo basophilism
basofilismo de Cushing Cushing's
basophilism
basofobia basophobia
basostasofobia basostasophobia
baston cane
bastoncillo rod
bastoncillo de Corti rod of Corti
bastoncillos retinales retinal rods
batarismo battarismus
batería battery
batería de logro achievement battery
batería de pruebas battery of tests
batería electrofisiológica cuantitativa
quantitative electrophysiological battery
batianestesia bathyanesthesia
batiestesia bathyesthesia
batihiperestesia bathyhyperesthesia
batihipestesia bathyhypesthia
batmotrópico bathmotropic
batofobia bathophobia
bebedor drinker
bebedor compulsivo compulsive drinker
bebedor problema problem drinker
beber drinking
beber controlado controlled drinking
beber de escape escape drinking
beber disocial dyssocial drinking
beber inveterado inveterate drinking
beber ocupacional occupational drinking
beber paroxístico paroxysmal drinking
beber periódico periodic drinking
beber prandial prandial drinking
beber problema problem drinking
beber somatopático somatopathic drinking
beber timogénico thymogenic drinking
bedlamismo bedlamism
bel bel
belonefobia belonephobia
belladona belladonna
bemegrida bemegride
benactizina benactyzine
benceno benzene
beneceptor beneceptor
beneficiencia beneficence
beneficio básico basic benefit
benigno benign
benperidol benperidol
bentazepam bentazepam
benzaldehído benzaldehyde
benzoctamina benzoctamine
benzodiazepina benzodiazepine

benzofetamina benzphetamine
benzotropina benztropine
beriberi beriberi
beriberi húmedo wet beriberi
beriberi seco dry beriberi
besilato de mesoridazina mesoridazine
   besylate
bestialidad bestiality
beta beta
betahistina betahistine
betanecol bethanechol
bhang bhang
biblioclasta biblioclast
biblioclepto biblioklept
bibliocleptomanía bibliokleptomania
bibliofobia bibliophobia
bibliomanía bibliomania
biblioterapia bibliotherapy
bicarbonato bicarbonate
bicarbonato de sodio sodium bicarbonate
bicarbonato sérico serum bicarbonate
bicultural bicultural
biculturalismo biculturalism
bidé bidet
bidireccionalidad de influencia
   bidirectionality of influence
bien ajustado well-adjusted
bienestar social social welfare
bigamia bigamy
bilabial bilabial
bilateral bilateral
bilharziasis bilharziasis
biliar biliary
bilingüe bilingual
bilingüe balanceado balanced bilingual
bilingüe compuesto compound bilingual
bilingüe coordinado coordinate bilingual
bilingüe no balanceado unbalanced bilingual
bilingüismo bilingualism
bilioso bilious
bilirraquia bilirachia
bilirrubina bilirubin
bimodal bimodal
bimodalidad bimodality
binaural binaural
binocular binocular
binocularidad binocularity
binomial binomial
bioacústica bioacoustics
bioanálisis bioanalysis
biocibernética biocybernetics
biodinámica biodynamics
biodisponibilidad bioavailability
bioenergética bioenergetics
bioestadística biostatistics
bioética bioethics
biofidelidad biofidelity
biofilia biophilia
biofísica biophysics
biogénesis biogenesis
biogenética biogenetics
biógeno biogenic
biografía a fondo biography in depth
biografía reaccional reactional biography
biograma biogram

bioingeniería bioengineering
biología matemática mathematical biology
biológico biological
biologismo biologism
biomecánica biomechanics
biomédico biomedical
biometría biometrics
bionegatividad bionegativity
biónica bionics
biónico bionic
bionómica bionomics
biopsia biopsy
biopsia del corion chorion biopsy
biopsicología biopsychology
biopsicosocial biopsychosocial
biopsíquico biopsychic
bioquímica biochemistry
biorretroalimentación biofeedback
biorretroalimentación para enuresis
   biofeedback for enuresis
biorritmo biorhythm
biosfera biosphere
biosocial biosocial
biotaxis biotaxis
biotaxis de red network biotaxis
biotecnología biotechnology
biotipo biotype
biotipograma biotypogram
biotipología biotypology
biotopo biotope
biotransformación biotransformation
biotransporte biotransport
biperidina biperiden
bipolar bipolar
bipolar I bipolar I
bipolar II bipolar II
bipolaridad bipolarity
bisensorial bisensory
bisexual bisexual
bisexualidad bisexuality
bit bit
bivalencia bivalence
bivariado bivariate
blastoftoria blastophthoria
blastómero blastomere
blástula blastula
blefaroespasmo blepharospasm
bloque block
bloqueador blocker
bloqueador adrenérgico beta beta adrenergic
   blocker
bloqueador beta beta blocker
bloqueador del ego ego block
bloqueo blocking, blockade, block
bloqueo alfa alpha blocking
bloqueo cardíaco heart block
bloqueo de afecto affect block
bloqueo del habla speech block
bloqueo emocional emotional blocking
bloqueo epidural epidural block
bloqueo espinal spinal block
bloqueo genético genetic block
bloqueo narcótico narcotic blockade
bloqueo nervioso nerve block
bloques de Vygotsky Vygotsky blocks

boca de tapir tapir mouth
boca seca dry mouth
bomba de iones ion pump
bombesina bombesin
botón button
botón sináptico synaptic button
botón terminal terminal button
bovarismo bovarism
bradiacusia bradyacusia
bradiartria bradyarthria
bradicardia bradycardia
bradicardia central central bradycardia
bradicinesia bradykinesia
bradicinesia funcional functional
    bradykinesia
bradicinesis bradykinesis
bradiestesia bradyesthesia
bradifagia bradyphagia
bradifasia bradyphasia
bradifemia bradyphemia
bradifrasia bradyphrasia
bradifrenia bradyphrenia
bradiglosia bradyglossia
bradilalia bradylalia
bradilexia bradylexia
bradilogía bradylogia
bradipnea bradypnea
bradipragia bradypragia
bradipsiquia bradypsychia
bradiquinina bradykinin
braditeleocinesia bradyteleocinesia
braditeleocinesis bradyteleokinesis
braditrofia bradytrophia
braidismo braidsm
braille braille
braquial brachial
braquibasia brachybasia
braquicefalia brachycephaly
braquicefálico brachycephalic
braquilineal brachylineal
braquimetropía brachymetropy
braquimórfico brachymorphic
braquisquélico brachyskelic
bratracofobia batrachophobia
brazo mioeléctrico myoelectric arm
brecha gap
brecha aire-hueso air-bone gap
brecha generacional generation gap
brecha tonal tonal gap
bredouillement bredouillement
bregar cope
bregma bregma
breve brief
brevilineal brevilineal
bril bril
brillantez brightness
brillantez de Talbot Talbot brightness
brillantez fotométrica photometric brightness
brillantez tonal tonal brightness
bromazepam bromazepam
bromhidrosis bromhidrosis
bromidrosifobia bromidrosiphobia
bromidrosis bromidrosis
brominismo brominism
bromisovalum bromisovalum

bromocriptina bromocriptine
bromoglutamato bromoglutamate
bromoperidol bromperidol
bromuro bromide
bromuro de calcio calcium bromide
bromuro de potasio potassium bromide
bromuro de sodio sodium bromide
bromuro sérico serum bromide
broncodilación bronchodilation
broncodilatación bronchodilatation
broncodilatador bronchodilator
bronquitis crónica chronic bronchitis
brontofobia brontophobia
brujería witchcraft
bruxismo bruxism
bruxomanía bruxomania
bucal buccal
bucolingual buccolingual
bufotenina bufotenin
bujía internacional international candle
bujía-pie foot-candle
bulbar bulbar
bulbo bulb
bulbo olfatorio accesorio accessory olfactory
    bulb
bulbo terminal de Krause Krause end bulb
bulbocapnina bulbocapnine
bulboespinal bulbospinal
bulbos olfatorios olfactory bulbs
bulesis bulesis
bulimia bulimia
bulimia nerviosa bulimia nervosa
bulímico bulimic
bulmorexia bulmorexia
buprenorfina buprenorphine
bupropiona bupropion
buscador de datos fact-seeker
buscante de sensaciones sensation seeking
buscante de simpatía sympathy seeking
buspirona buspirone
búsqueda search
búsqueda autoterminante self-terminating
    search
búsqueda de memoria serial serial-memory
    search
búsqueda exhaustiva exhaustive search
búsqueda paralela parallel search
búsqueda serial serial search
búsqueda verbal verbal search
búsqueda visual visual search
butabarbital butabarbital
butaperazina butaperazine
butetal butethal
butirofenona butyrophenone
butorfanol butorphanol
butriptilina butriptyline
byte byte

C

caapi caapi
cabeceo nodding
cabeza hinchada swelled head
cacergasia cacergasia
cacodemonia cacodemonia
cacodemonomanía cacodemonomania
cacoetes cacoethes
cacoforia cacophoria
cacogénico cacogenic
cacogeusia cacogeusia
cacolalia cacolalia
cacorrafiofobia kakorrhaphiophobia
cacosmia cacosmia
cacosomnia cacosomnia
cacotimia cacothymia
cadena chain
cadena de conducta behavior chain
cadena de Markoff Markoff chain
cadena de Markov Markov chain
cadena de reacción reaction chain
cadena ganglionar paraverterbral paravertebral ganglionic chain
cadena simpática sympathetic chain
cafard cafard
cafeína caffeine
cafeinismo caffeinism
caída drop
caída de los dedos del pie toe drop
caída de muñeca wrist drop
caída de pie foot drop
cainofobia cainophobia
cainotofobia cainotophobia
caja de obstrucción obstruction box
caja de orgón orgone box
caja de Skinner Skinner box
caja dividida en dos shuttle box
caja negra black box
caja problema problem box
caja rompecabeza puzzle box
calambre cramp
calambre accesorio accessory cramp
calambre de afeitar shaving cramp
calambre de artesano artisan's cramp
calambre de camarero waiter's cramp
calambre de escritor writer's cramp
calambre de mecanógrafo typist's cramp
calambre de memoria memory cramp
calambre de minero miner's cramp
calambre de músico musician's cramp
calambre de pianista pianist's cramp
calambre de relojero watchmaker's cramp
calambre de sastre tailor's cramp
calambre de tocador de piano piano player's cramp

calambre de violinista violinist's cramp
calambre de Wernicke Wernicke's cramp
calambre intermitente intermittent cramp
calambre ocupacional occupational cramp
calambres de fogoneros stoker's cramps
calasis chalasis
calcio sérico serum calcium
calcitonina calcitonin
calculador relámpago lightning calculator
calculi calculi
cálculo calculus
cálculo cerebral cerebral calculus
calibración calibration
calidad quality
calidad de voz voice quality
calidad de vida quality of life
calidad del habla quality of speech
calidad del humor quality of mood
calidad secundaria secondary quality
calificación grading
calificación en educación grading in education
calipedia callipedia
cáliz calyx
calmante calmative
calomanía callomania
calor moderado paradójico paradoxical warmth
caloría calorie
callejón sin salida blind alley
cámara camera
cámara anecoica anechoic chamber
cámara escondida hidden camera
camazepam camazepam
cambio change
cambio ambiental environmental change
cambio asociativo associative shifting
cambio binaural binaural shift
cambio bioconductual biobehavioral shift
cambio cauteloso cautious shift
cambio compulsivo compulsive changing
cambio de actitud congruente congruent attitude change
cambio de actitud negativo negative attitude change
cambio de actitud positivo positive attitude change
cambio de actitudes attitude change
cambio de ambiente change of environment
cambio de atención attention switching
cambio de cinco a siete five-to-seven shift
cambio de códigos code switching
cambio de conducta change of behavior
cambio de papel role shift
cambio de personalidad personality change
cambio de Purkinje Purkinje shift
cambio de Raman Raman shift
cambio de selección choice shift
cambio de sexo sex change
cambio de umbral threshold shift
cambio de umbral temporal temporary threshold shift
cambio de vida change of life
cambio del contexto context shifting
cambio extradimensional extradimensional

shift
cambio geográfico geographical change
cambio sexual sexual change
cambio social social change
cambio télico telic change
cambio trófico trophic change
cambios cognitivos en adultez cognitive changes in adulthood
cambios de audición hearing changes
cambios de audición en adultez hearing changes in adulthood
cambios físicos physical changes
cambios físicos en adolescencia physical changes in adolescence
cambios sexuales de adolescencia adolescent sex changes
camisola camisole
campamento diurno day camp
campana tonal tonal bell
campana y almohadilla bell and pad
campimetría campimetry
campímetro campimeter
campo field
campo audible mínimo minimum audible field
campo conceptual conceptual field
campo de conciencia field of consciousness
campo de conducta behavior field
campo de estímulo stimulus field
campo de fuerza force field
campo de mirada field of regard
campo de ojo eye field
campo de poder power field
campo de receptor receptor field
campo excitatorio excitatory field
campo fenomenal phenomenal field
campo fenomenológico phenomenological field
campo neural binocular binocular neural field
campo perceptivo perceptual field
campo psicológico psychological field
campo receptivo receptive field
campo retinal retinal field
campo sensorial sensory field
campo tegmental gigantocelular gigantocellular tegmental field
campo visual visual field
campos de Forel fields of Forel
camptocormia camptocormia
camptoespasmo camptospasm
camuflaje camouflage
canal canal
canal alimenticio alimentary canal
canal auditivo auditory canal
canal central central canal
canal espinal spinal canal
canal semicircular semicircular canal
canal timpánico tympanic canal
canal vaginal vaginal canal
canal vestibular vestibular canal
canales de comunicación channels of communication
canalización canalization
cancasmo canchasmus

cancelación cancellation
cancelación doble double cancellation
cáncer cancer
cáncer laríngeo laryngeal cancer
cancerofobia cancerophobia
candela candela
candidiasis candidiasis
canibalismo cannibalism
canje velocidad-precisión speed-accuracy tradeoff
cannabis cannabis
cannabismo cannabism
canon de Lloyd Morgan Lloyd Morgan's canon
canon de Morgan Morgan's canon
cantárida cantharides
cantidad quantity
cantidad del habla quantity of speech
cánula cannula
caótico chaotic
capa layer
capa aracnoidea arachnoid layer
capa de pigmento pigment layer
capa del manto mantle layer
capa esclerótica sclerotic layer
capa ganglionar ganglionic layer
capa granular granular layer
capa granular externa external granular layer
capa granular interna internal granular layer
capacidad capacity
capacidad aeróbica aerobic capacity
capacidad cognitiva cognitive capacity
capacidad craneal cranial capacity
capacidad de canal channel capacity
capacidad de códigos code capacity
capacidad de memoria memory capacity
capacidad de memoria general general memory capacity
capacidad disminuida diminished capacity
capacidad legal legal capacity
capacidad medios-fin means-end capacity
capacidad psicológica psychological capacity
capacidad sensorial sensory capacity
capacidad testamentaria testamentary capacity
capacidad vital vital capacity
capacidades integrantes integrative capacities
capas celulares de la corteza cellular layers of cortex
capilar capillary
capitium capitium
cápsula interna internal capsule
cápsula externa external capsule
captodiam captodiam
captodiamina captodiamine
captopril captopril
captura visual visual capture
caput caput
caput succedaneum caput succedaneum
caquectico cachectic
caquexia cachexia
caquexia hipofisaria hypophysial cachexia
caquexia hipofisopriva cachexia hypophysiopriva
caquexia pituitaria pituitary cachexia

caquinación cachinnation
cara a cara face-to-face
carácter character
carácter acaparador hoarding character
carácter adquirido acquired character
carácter anal anal character
carácter anal-agresivo anal-aggressive
    character
carácter anal-expulsivo anal-expulsive
    character
carácter anal-retentivo anal-retentive
    character
carácter autoritario authoritarian character
carácter compulsivo compulsive character
carácter contencioso contentiousness
carácter contrafóbico counterphobic
    character
carácter de exigencia demand character
carácter demoníaco demonic character
carácter depresivo depressive character
carácter epiléptico epileptic character
carácter erótico erotic character
carácter esquizoide schizoid character
carácter explotador exploitative character
carácter fálico phallic character
carácter fálico-narcisista phallic-narcissistic
    character
carácter fóbico phobic character
carácter genital genital character
carácter histérico hysterical character
carácter impulsivo impulsive character
caracter influenciado por sexo sex-influenced
    character
carácter masoquista masochistic character
carácter narcisista narcissistic character
carácter neurótico neurotic character
carácter obsesivo obsessional character
carácter oral oral character
carácter oral-agresivo oral-aggressive
    character
carácter oral-receptivo oral-receptive
    character
carácter paranoide paranoid character
carácter psicótico psychotic character
carácter receptivo receptive character
carácter sumiso compliant character
carácter tonal tonal character
carácter uretral urethral character
característica feature
característica adquirida acquired
    characteristic
característica distintiva distinctive feature
característica operatorio de recibidor
    receiver operating characteristic
característica paralingüística paralinguistic
    feature
característica psicótica del humor
    congruente mood-congruent psychotic
    feature
característica psicótica del humor
    incongruente mood-incongruent psychotic
    feature
característica semántica semantic feature
características de exigencia demand
    characteristics

características de fondo background
    characteristics
características de niñez childhood
    characteristics
características de personalidad personality
    characteristics
características del consumidor consumer
    characteristics
características del sueño sleep characteristics
características electrográficas del ciclo de
    sueño electrographic features of the sleep
    cycle
características emocionales mixtas mixed
    emotional features
características prosódicas prosodic features
características sexuales sexual characteristics
características sexuales primarias primary
    sexual characteristics
características sexuales secundarias
    secondary sexual characteristics
característico characteristic
caracterización characterization
carácter ligado al sexo sex-linked character
caracterología characterology
caras de Brunswik Brunswik faces
carbacol carbachol
carbamato carbamate
carbamazepina carbamazepine
carbidopa carbidopa
carbonato de litio lithium carbonate
carbromal carbromal
carcinofobia carcinophobia
carcinogénico carcinogenic
carcinógeno carcinogen
carcinoma carcinoma
carcinoma leptomeníngeo leptomeningeal
    carcinoma
carcinoma meníngeo meningeal carcinoma
carcinomata carcinomata
carcinomatosis carcinomatosis
carcinomatosis leptomeníngea
    leptomeningeal carcinomatosis
carcinomatosis meníngea meningeal
    carcinomatosis
carcinomatoso carcinomatous
cardenal cardinal
cardíaco cardiac
cardioespasmo cardiospasm
cardiofobia cardiophobia
cardiofrenia cardiophrenia
cardiograma cardiogram
cardiomiopatía cardiomyopathy
cardioneural cardioneural
cardioneurosis cardioneurosis
cardiorespiratorio cardiorespiratory
cardiotóxico cardiotoxic
cardiovascular cardiovascular
carebaria carebaria
carezza carezza
carfenazina carphenazine
carfología carphology
carga loading
carga de casos case load
carga factorial factor loading
cargador magazine

caricatura caricature
cariotipo karyotype
cariotipo triploide triploid karyotype
carisma charisma
carismático charismatic
carisoprodol carisoprodol
carnal carnal
carnosina carnosine
caroteno carotene
carótico carotic
carotídeo carotid
carotodinia carotodynia
carpiano carpal
carpopedal carpopedal
carpoptosia carpoptosia
carpoptosis carpoptosis
cartesiano Cartesian
cartografía de actividad eléctrica cerebral
    brain electrical activity mapping
carúncula caruncula
casa de huéspedes boarding house
casa de transición halfway house
casa urbana cooperativa cooperative urban
    house
casco neurasténico neurasthenic helmet
caso case
caso especial special case
caso índice index case
casta caste
castigo punishment
castigo contingente contingent punishment
castigo de Midas Midas punishment
castigo expiatorio expiatory punishment
castigo físico physical punishment
castigo negativo negative punishment
castigo por reciprocidad punishment by
    reciprocity
castigo recíproco reciprocal punishment
castigo y agresión punishment and aggression
castración castration
castración anal anal castration
castrante castrating
castrar castrate
casual chance
catabólico catabolic
catabolismo catabolism
cataclonia cataclonia
cataclono cataclonus
catafasia cataphasia
catáfora cataphora
catafrenia cataphrenia
catagelofobia catagelophobia
catagénesis catagenesis
catalepsia catalepsy
catalepsia accesoria accessory catalepsy
catalepsia epidémica epidemic catalepsy
cataléptico cataleptic
cataleptoide cataleptoid
catalexia catalexia
catalizador catalyst
catalogía catalogia
catamenia catamenia
catamita catamite
catamnesis catamnesis
catapléctico cataplectic

cataplejía cataplexy
cataplejía del despertar cataplexy of
    awakening
cataptosis cataptosis
catarata cataract
catarsis catharsis
catarsis conversacional conversational
    catharsis
catártico cathartic
catasexual katasexual
catasexualidad katasexuality
catástrofe catastrophe
catastrófico catastrophic
catatimia catathymia
catatímico catathymic
catatonía catatonia
catatonía estuporosa stuporous catatonia
catatonía excitada excited catatonia
catatonía letal lethal catatonia
catatonía letal de Stauder Stauder's lethal
    catatonia
catatonía mortal deadly catatonia
catatonía periódica periodic catatonia
catatónico catatonic
catatonoide catatonoid
catecolamina catecholamine
catéctico cathectic
categoría category
categoría básica basic category
categoría de nivel básico basic level category
categoría de papel role category
categoría natural natural category
categoría social social category
categorías de colores color categories
categórico categorical
categorización categorization
categorización de concepto concept
    categorization
categorización de nivel básico basic level
    categorization
categorización simbólica symbolic
    categorization
categorizado por sexo sex-typed
catelectrotono catelectrotonus
catéter catheter
catexis cathexis
catexis afectiva affective cathexis
catexis corporal body cathexis
catexis de fantasía fantasy cathexis
catexis de necesidad need cathexis
catexis de objeto object cathexis
catexis del ego ego cathexis
catexis libidinal libidinal cathexis
catexis negativa negative cathexis
catexis positiva positive cathexis
catisofobia kathisophobia
catochus catochus
catotrofobia catotrophobia
cauda equina cauda equina
caudal caudal
caumestesia caumesthesia
causa cause
causa eficiente efficient cause
causa mantenedora maintaining cause
causa precipitante precipitating cause

causa primaria primary cause
causa reforzante reinforcing cause
causa secundaria secondary cause
causal causal
causalgia causalgia
causalidad causality
causalidad fenomenística phenomenistic causality
causalidad mecánica mechanical causality
causalidad múltiple multiple causation
causalidad simple simple causation
causas de abuso de niños causes of child abuse
cautela caution
cauteloso guarded
cautivación captivation
cavidad oral oral cavity
cavidad timpánica tympanic cavity
cebocefalia cebocephaly
cecear lisp
ceceo lisping
cefalagia cephalagia
cefalagia de Horton Horton's cephalagia
cefalagia histamínica histaminic cephalagia
cefalagra cephalagra
cefalalgia cephalalgia
cefalea cephalea
cefalea atónita cephalea attonita
cefalea epiléptica epileptic cephalea
cefaledema cephaledema
cefalemia cephalemia
cefalgia cephalgia
cefalgia orgásmica orgasmic cephalgia
cefalhematocele cephalhematocele
cefalhematoma cephalhematoma
cefálico cephalic
cefalitis cephalitis
cefalocaudal cephalocaudal
cefalocele cephalocele
cefalocentesis cephalocentesis
cefalodinia cephalodynia
cefalogénesis cephalogenesis
cefalógiro cephalogyric
cefalohematocele cephalohematocele
cefalohematoma cephalohematoma
cefalohemómetro cephalohemometer
cefalohidrocele cephalhydrocele
cefalomeningitis cephalomeningitis
cefalometría cephalometry
cefalometría fetal fetal cephalometry
cefalomotor cephalomotor
cefalopatía cephalopathy
ceguera blindness
ceguera al azul blue blindness
ceguera al color color blindness
ceguera al color rojo-verde red-green color blindness
ceguera al color total total color blindness
ceguera al gusto taste blindness
ceguera azul-amarilla blue-yellow blindness
ceguera cerebral cerebral blindness
ceguera cortical cortical blindness
ceguera cultural cultural blindness
ceguera de música music blindness
ceguera de objetos object blindness

ceguera de palabras word blindness
ceguera de palabras congénita congenital word blindness
ceguera de palabras del desarrollo developmental word blindness
ceguera de signos sign blindness
ceguera duirna day blindness
ceguera funcional functional blindness
ceguera histérica hysterical blindness
ceguera literal letter blindness
ceguera mental mind blindness
ceguera nocturna night blindness
ceguera olfativa smell blindness
ceguera para las notas note blindness
ceguera por nieve snow blindness
ceguera psíquica psychic blindness
ceguera rojo-verde red-green blindness
ceguera textual text blindness
celda acolchada padded cell
celibato celibacy
celo rut
celofobia zelophobia
celoma celoma
celos jealousy
celos alcohólicos alcoholic jealousy
celos delusorios delusional jealousy
celos mórbidos morbid jealousy
celos proyectados projected jealousy
celoso jealous
celotipia zelotypia
célula cell
célula ameboide ameboid cell
célula bipolar bipolar cell
célula de Opalski Opalski cell
célula de Renshaw Renshaw cell
célula del gusto taste cell
célula en cesta basket cell
célula errante wandering cell
célula estrellada stellate cell
célula fisalífora physaliphorous cell
célula ganglionar ganglion cell
célula ganglionar retinal retinal ganglion cell
célula gemastete gemastete cell
célula gemistocítica gemistocytic cell
célula germinativa germ cell
célula globoide globoid cell
célula granular granular cell
célula haploide haploid cell
célula glial glial cell
célula mitral mitral cell
célula multipolar multipolar cell
célula nerviosa nerve cell
célula neurosecretoria neurosecretory cell
célula objetivo target cell
célula pilosa hair cell
célula reactiva reactive cell
célula somática somatic cell
célula sustentacular sustentacular cell
célula unipolar unipolar cell
celular cellular
células adventicias adventitial cells
células alfa alpha cells
células amacrinas amacrine cells
células beta beta cells
células bipolares retinales retinal bipolar cells

células de Betz Betz cells
células de color color cells
células de Deiters Deiters' cells
células de Martinotti Martinotti cells
células de Purkinje Purkinje cells
células de Sertoli Sertoli cells
células H H cells
células horizontales horizontal cells
células horizontales retinales retinal
    horizontal cells
células intersticiales interstitial cells
células pilosas externas outer hair cells
células pilosas externas del oído external hair
    cells of ear
células pilosas internas internal hair cells
células piramidales pyramidal cells
células retinales sentitivas al movimiento
    movement-sensitive retinal cells
células de Schwann Schwann cells
cenestesia cenesthesia
cenestésico cenesthesic
cenestesis cenesthesis
cenestopatía cenesthopathy
cenofobia cenophobia
cenogamia cenogamy
cenotofobia cenotophobia
cenotropo cenotrope
censor censor
censor endopsíquico endopsychic censor
censura censorship
censura de sueños dream censorship
censura intrapsíquica intrapsychic censorship
centavo cent
centelleador scintillator
centelleo flicker
centelleo auditivo auditory flicker
centelleo cromático chromatic flicker
centesis centesis
centila centile
centimorgan centimorgan
centrado en el niño child-centered
centraje centering
central central
centralismo centralism
centrencefálico centrencephalic
centrífugo centrifugal
centrípeto centripetal
centro center
centro cerebral brain center
centro cortical cortical center
centro de alimentación feeding center
centro de convalecientes convalescent center
centro de crecimiento growth center
centro de crecimiento de potencial humano
    human-potential growth center
centro de crisis crisis center
centro de destoxificación detoxification
    center
centro de diagnóstico y tratamiento de
    adultos adult diagnostic and treatment
    center
centro de evaluación assessment center
centro de evaluación y cribado geriátrico
    geriatric screening and evaluation center
centro de metadona methadone center

centro de placer pleasure center
centro de prevención de suicidios
    suicide-prevention center
centro de quemaduras burn center
centro de rehabilitación rehabilitation center
centro de rehabilitación de trabajo work
    rehabilitation center
centro de saciedad satiety center
centro de salud mental mental health center
centro de salud mental comprensiva
    comprehensive mental health center
centro de salud mental comunitario
    community mental health center
centro del despertar waking center
centro del ego ego center
centro del habla speech center
centro del habla y audición speech and
    hearing center
centro del sueño sleep center
centro diagnóstico diagnostic center
centro diurno day center
centro nervioso nerve center
centro neumotáxico pneumotaxic center
centro transaccional central central
    transactional core
centrocinesia centrokinesia
centrocinético centrokinetic
centrofenoxina centrophenoxine
centroide centroid
centrómero centromere
centros cerebrales superiores higher brain
    centers
centros del habla y audición comunitarios
    community speech and hearing centers
centros del lenguaje language centers
centrosoma centrosome
cepillo terminal end brush
ceptor ceptor
ceptor a distancia distance ceptor
ceptor de contacto contact ceptor
ceptor químico chemical ceptor
cera ósea bone wax
ceramida ceramide
ceraunofobia ceraunophobia
cerebelitis cerebellitis
cerebelo cerebellum
cerebelopontino cerebellopontine
cerebeloso cerebellar
cerebración cerebration
cerebración inconsciente unconscious
    cerebration
cerebral cerebral
cerebralgia cerebralgia
cerebria cerebria
cerebritis cerebritis
cerebritis supurativa suppurative cerebritis
cerebro brain
cerebro aislado isolated brain
cerebro anterior forebrain
cerebro arcaico archaic brain
cerebro dividido divided brain
cerebro intermedio interbrain
cerebro olfatorio olfactory brain
cerebro posterior hindbrain
cerebroesclerosis cerebrosclerosis

cerebroespinal cerebrospinal
cerebroma cerebroma
cerebromacular cerebromacular
cerebromalacia cerebromalacia
cerebromeningitis cerebromeningitis
cerebropatía cerebropathy
cerebrósido cerebroside
cerebrosidosis cerebrosidosis
cerebrosis cerebrosis
cerebrospinante cerebrospinant
cerebrotendinoso cerebrotendinous
cerebrotomía cerebrotomy
cerebrotonía cerebrotonia
cerebrovascular cerebrovascular
ceremonia ceremony
ceremonial ceremonial
ceremonial compulsivo compulsive
    ceremonial
cero absoluto absolute zero
cero audiométrico audiometric zero
cero del desarrollo developmental zero
cero fisiológico physiological zero
cero psicológico psychological zero
cero verdadero true zero
certidumbre certainty
certificable certifiable
certificación certification
certificación de admisión admission
    certification
certificado por junta board certified
certificar certify
ceruloplasmina sérica serum ceruloplasmin
cerumen cerumen
cervical cervical
cervicodinia cervicodynia
cervicotorácico cervicothoracic
cérvix cervix
cesta de compras market basket
cetoesteriode ketosteroid
ciamemazina cyamemazine
cianato de potasio potassium cyanate
cianosis cyanosis
ciática sciatica
ciático sciatic
ciberfobia cyberphobia
cibernética cybernetics
cibofobia cibophobia
cicatriz cicatrix
cicatriz cerebral brain cicatrix
cicatriz meningocerebral meningocerebral
    cicatrix
cicatriz narcisista narcissistic scar
cicatriz psíquica psychic scar
cicatrización cicatrization
ciclandelato cyclandelate
ciclazocina cyclazocine
ciclencefalia cyclencephaly
cíclico cyclic
ciclo cycle
ciclo de actividad activity cycle
ciclo de diseños design cycle
ciclo de dormir-despertar sleep-wake cycle
ciclo de ejercicio exercise cycle
ciclo de ondas cerebrales brain wave cycle
ciclo de respuestas sexuales sexual response

    cycle
ciclo de retroalimentación feedback loop
ciclo de vida life cycle
ciclo diurno diurnal cycle
ciclo de descanso-actividad básico basic
    rest-activity cycle
ciclo endometrial endometrial cycle
ciclo estrual estrus cycle
ciclo gonadal gonadal cycle
ciclo menstrual menstrual cycle
ciclo menstrual anovulatorio anovulatory
    menstrual cycle
ciclo ovárico ovarian cycle
ciclo perceptivo perceptual cycle
ciclo por segundo cycle per second
ciclo temporal seasonal cycle
ciclo visual visual cycle
ciclobarbital cyclobarbital
cicloforia cyclophoria
ciclofosfamida cyclophosphamide
ciclofrenia cyclophrenia
cicloide cycloid
ciclopentolato cyclopentolate
cicloplejía cycloplegia
ciclopléjico cycloplegic
ciclopropano cyclopropane
cicloserina cycloserine
ciclotimia cyclothymia
ciclotímico cyclothymic
ciclotimosis cyclothymosis
cicuta hemlock
ciego blind
ciencia cognitiva cognitive science
ciencia conductual behavioral science
ciencia de la información information science
ciencia normativa normative science
ciencia psicológica psychological science
cierre closure
cierre auditivo auditory closure
cierre visual visual closure
ciesis cyesis
cifoescoliosis kyphoscoliosis
cifosis kyphosis
cifra de riesgo empírico empiric-risk figure
cigomático zygomaticus
cigosidad zygosity
cigosis zygosis
cigótico zygotic
cigoto zygote
ciliar ciliary
cilindro de memoria memory drum
cilindros de Koenig Koenig cylinders
cilio cilium
cilios cilia
ciliotomía ciliotomy
cimatismo kymatism
cimógrafo kymograph
cinaedi cinaedi
cinanestesia cinanesthesia
cinantropía cynanthropy
cinarizina cinnarizine
cinclisis cinclisis
cinconismo cinchonism
cinefantasma kinephantom
cinemática kinematics

cinemorfo kinemorph
cineplastia cineplasty
cinesalgia kinesalgia
cineseismografía cineseismography
cinesia kinesia
cinésica kinesics
cinesiología kinesiology
cinesioneurosis kinesioneurosis
cinesipatía kinesipathy
cinesiterapia kinesitherapy
cinesofobia kinesophobia
cinestesia kinesthesia
cinestésico kinesthetic
cinestesiómetro kinesthesiometer
cinético kinetic
cingulado cingulate
cingulectomía cingulectomy
cingulotomía cingulotomy
cínico cynic
cinismo cynicism
cinofobia cynophobia
cinohapto kinohapt
cinorexia cynorexia
cinturón de Hitzig Hitzig's girdle
cipridofobia cypridophobia
ciprifobia cypriphobia
ciproheptadina cyproheptadine
circadiano circadian
circanual circannual
circuito circuit
circuito de Papez Papez circuit
circuito de respuestas response circuit
circuito recurrente recurrent circuit
circuito reflejo reflex circuit
circuito reverberante reverberating circuit
circuito reverberatorio reverberatory circuit
circuitos neurales neural circuitry
circular circular
circulatorio circulatory
círculo arterial arterial circle
círculo de color color circle
círculo de dispersión dispersion circle
círculo de Landolt Landolt circle
círculo de Papez Papez circle
círculo de Willis circle of Willis
círculo reflejo reflex circle
círculo táctil tactile circle
círculo vicioso vicious circle
circuncisión femenina female circumcision
circunlocución circumlocution
circunscripción circumscription
circunscripción monosintomática
    monosymptomatic circumscription
circunscrito circumscribed
circunstancialidad circumstantiality
circunstancias familiares family
    circumstances
circunvolución gyrus
circunvolución angular angular gyrus
circunvolución callosa callosal gyrus
circunvolución cingulada cingulate gyrus
circunvolución de Heschl Heschl gyrus
circunvolución dentada dentate gyrus
circunvolución fasciolar fasciolar gyrus
circunvolución fusiforme fusiform gyrus

circunvolución lateral lateral gyrus
circunvolución lingual lingual gyrus
circunvolución orbital lateral lateral orbital
    gyrus
circunvolución orbital medial medial orbital
    gyrus
circunvolución orbital posterior posterior
    orbital gyrus
circunvolución poscentral postcentral gyrus
circunvolución precentral precentral gyrus
circunvolución subcallosa subcallosal gyrus
circunvolución supramarginal supramarginal
    gyrus
cirrosis cirrhosis
cirugía surgery
cirugía cardiovascular cardiovascular surgery
cirugía cerebral brain surgery
cirugía craneofacial craniofacial surgery
cirugía criogénica cryogenic surgery
cirugía estereotáctica stereotactic surgery
cirugía estereotáxica stereotaxic surgery
cirugía plástica plastic surgery
cirugía posreconstructiva postreconstructive
    surgery
cirugía reconstructiva reconstructive surgery
cirugía simulada sham surgery
cisa cissa
cisma schism
cisma marital marital schism
cistationinuria cystathioninuria
cisteína cysteine
cisterna cerebellomedularis cisterna
    cerebellomedullaris
cisterna magna cisterna magna
cisternografía cisternography
cisternografía cerebelopontina
    cerebellopontine cisternography
cisternografía con radioisótopos radioisotope
    cisternography
cisternografía con radionúclidos radionuclide
    cisternography
cisvestismo cisvestism
cisvestitismo cisvestitism
citeromanía cytheromania
citoarquitectura cytoarchitecture
citogenética cytogenetics
citogénico cytogenic
citología cytology
citomegalovirus cytomegalovirus
citoplasma cytoplasm
citosina cytosine
citosis cittosis
citotóxico cytotoxic
citrato citrate
civilización civilization
cladosporiosis cladosporiosis
cladosporiosis cerebral cerebral
    cladosporiosis
clan clan
clariaudición clairaudience
claridad clearness, lightness
clarificación clarification
clarividencia clairvoyance
clase class
clase corporativa corporate class

clase de respuestas response class
clase especial special class
clase media middle class
clase social social class
clásico classical
clasificación classification, rating
clasificación de ansiedad classification of
    anxiety
clasificación de cartas card sorting
clasificación de conducta behavior rating
clasificación de conducta anormal
    classification of abnormal behavior
clasificación de delincuencia classification of
    delinquency
clasificación de madurez maturity rating
clasificación de sociabilidad sociability rating
clasificación global global rating
clasificación hedónica hedonic rating
clasificación jerárquica hierarchical
    classification
clasificación multiaxial multiaxial
    classification
clasificación paritaria peer rating
clasificación por mérito merit rating
clasificación psiquiátrica psychiatric
    classification
clasificación Q Q sort
clasificaciones evaluativas evaluative ratings
claudicación claudication
claudicación cerebral cerebral claudication
claudicación intermitente cerebral cerebral
    intermittent claudication
claudicación mental mental claudication
claustrofilia claustrophilia
claustrofobia claustrophobia
claustrofóbico claustrophobic
clava clava
clavo clavus
clazomanía klazomania
cleptofobia kleptophobia
cleptolagnia kleptolagnia
cleptomanía kleptomania
cleptomaníaco kleptomaniac
cliché cliché
cliente client
clima de grupo group climate
clima organizativo organizational climate
clima social social climate
climacofobia climacophobia
climatérico climacteric
climaterio climacterium
climaterio femenino female climacterium
climaterio masculino male climacterium
clímax climax
clínica clinic
clínica conductual behavioral clinic
clínica de asesoramiento de niños
    child-guidance clinic
clínica de dolor pain clinic
clínica de pacientes externos outpatient clinic
clínica de salud mental mental-health clinic
clínica móvil mobile clinic
clínica psiquiátrica psychiatric clinic
clínica satélite satellite clinic
clínico clinical

clinodactilia clinodactyly
clinotaxis klinotaxis
clismafilia klismaphilia
clitoral clitoral
clitoridectomía clitoridectomy
clítoris clitoris
clitrofobia clithrophobia
cloaca cloaca
clobazam clobazam
clomipramina clomipramine
clona clone
clonazepam clonazepam
clonicidad clonicity
clónico clonic
clonicotónico clonicotonic
clonidina clonidine
clonismo clonism
clono clonus
clono de muñeca wrist clonus
clono del dedo del pie toe clonus
clono del tobillo ankle clonus
clonoespasmo clonospasm
cloramfenicol chloramphenicol
clordiazepóxido chlordiazepoxide
clorhidrato hydrochloride
clorhidrato de amantadina amantadine
    hydrochloride
clorhidrato de amilorida amiloride
    hydrochloride
clorhidrato de amitriptilina amitriptyline
    hydrochloride
clorhidrato de cicrimina cycrimine
    hydrochloride
clorhidrato de clorpromazina
    chlorpromazine hydrochloride
clorhidrato de doxepina doxepin
    hydrochloride
clorhidrato de mentanfetamina
    methamphetamine hydrochloride
clorhidrato de meperidina meperidine
    hydrochloride
clorhidrato de metadona methadone
    hydrochloride
clorhidrato de nortriptilina nortriptyline
    hydrochloride
clorimipramina chlorimipramine
clormezanona chlormezanone
cloroquina chloroquine
clorpromazina chlorpromazine
cloruro chloride
cloruro sérico serum chloride
clotiapina clothiapine
clotiazepam clotiazepam
clounismo clownism
cloxazolam cloxazolam
clozapina clozapine
club de ex pacientes ex-patient club
coartado coarctate
coarticulación coarticulation
cobre sérico serum copper
coca coca
cocaína cocaine
cocainismo cocainism
cocainomanía cocainomania
cociente quotient

cociente de actividad activity quotient
cociente de alivio-angustia relief-distress quotient
cociente de alivio-incomodidad relief-discomfort quotient
cociente de custodia custody quotient
cociente de desarrollo developmental quotient
cociente de deterioración deterioration quotient
cociente de edad cerebral brain age quotient
cociente de inteligencia intelligence quotient
cociente de inteligencia de desviación deviation intelligence quotient
cociente de lateralidad cognitiva cognitive laterality quotient
cociente de lectura reading quotient
cociente de logro achievement quotient
cociente educacional educational quotient
cociente social social quotient
cóclea cochlea
cocleagrama cochleagram
coconciencia coconsciousness
cocontracción cocontraction
cóctel cocktail
cóctel lítico lytic cocktail
codeína codeine
codificación encoding
codificación automática automatic encoding
codificación doble dual encoding
codificación perceptiva automática automatic perceptual encoding
codificación verbal verbal encoding
codificar encode
código code
código aferente afferent code
código complicado elaborated code
código de ética code of ethics
código de imaginería imagery code
código genético genetic code
código moral moral code
código profesional professional code
código restringido restricted code
código semántico semantic code
código social social code
codominancia codominance
coeficiente coefficient
coeficiente de alienación coefficient of alienation
coeficiente de asociación association coefficient
coeficiente de concordancia coefficient of concordance
coeficiente de confiabilidad reliability coefficient
coeficiente de contingencia contingency coefficient
coeficiente de correlación coefficient of correlation
coeficiente de determinación coefficient of determination
coeficiente de equivalencia equivalence coefficient
coeficiente de estabilidad coefficient of stability
coeficiente de luminosidad luminosity coefficient

coeficiente de prueba-reprueba test-retest coefficient
coeficiente de regresión regression coefficient
coeficiente de variación coefficient of variation
coeficiente de visibilidad visibility coefficient
coeficiente factorial factor coefficient
coeficiente J J coefficient
coeficiente phi phi coefficient
coenestesia coenesthesia
coercible coercible
coerción coercion
coerción compulsiva compulsive coercion
coercitivo coercive
coexistencia coexistence
coexistencia de neurotransmisores coexistence of neurotransmitters
coexistente coexistent
coexperimentador coexperimenter
cognición cognition
cognición animal animal cognition
cognición del ser being cognition
cognición paranormal paranormal cognition
cognición primaria primary cognition
cognición social social cognition
cognición y lenguaje cognition and language
cognitivista cognitivist
cognitivo cognitive
cognización cognization
cohabitación cohabitation
cohesión cohesion
cohesión de grupo group cohesion
cohesión figural figural cohesion
cohesión social social cohesion
cohesividad cohesiveness
cohorte cohort
coinotropia koinotropy
coital coital
coito coitus
coito interrumpido coitus interruptus
coito oral oral coitus
coito reservado coitus reservatus
coitofobia coitophobia
colaboración collaboration
colapso breakdown
colapso nervioso nervous breakdown
colateral collateral
colchicina colchicine
coleccionismo collecting
colecistoquinina cholecystokinin
colectivo collective
colegio invisible invisible college
cólera cholera
colérico choleric
colesteatoma cholesteatoma
colesterinosis cholesterinosis
colesterinosis cerebrotendinosa cerebrotendinous cholesterinosis
colesterol cholesterol
colgajo flap
colgajo neurovascular neurovascular flap
colgajo óseo bone flap
colgajo óseo libre free bone flap
cólico colic

colículo colliculus
colículo inferior inferior colliculus
colículo superior superior colliculus
colifrenia kolyphrenia
coligación colligation
colina choline
colinérgico cholinergic
colinesterasa cholinesterase
colítico kolytic
colitis colitis
colitis espástica spastic colitis
collum distortum collum distortum
coloboma coloboma
colocación placement
colocación adoptiva foster placement
colocación de electrodo electrode placement
colocación de trabajo job placement
colocación del personal personnel placement
colocación educacional educational placement
colonia colony
colonia de Gheel Gheel colony
color acromático achromatic color
color complementario complementary color
color cromático chromatic color
color de memoria memory color
color de objeto object color
color de película film color
color de tono tone color
color espectral spectral color
color familiar familiar color
color fundamental fundamental color
color inducido induced color
color neutral neutral color
color primario primary color
color reflejado reflected color
color subjetivo subjective color
color superficial surface color
color tonal tonal color
colorante stain
colorante de Golgi Golgi stain
colorante de Marchi Marchi stain
colorante de Nissl Nissl stain
colorante de Weigert Weigert stain
colores antagónicos antagonistic colors
colores de Fechner Fechner's colors
colores en sueños color in dreams
colorimetría colorimetry
colorímetro colorimeter
columna column
columna de Clarke Clarke's column
columna dorsal dorsal column
columna espinal spinal column
coma coma
coma carcinomatoso coma carcinomatosum
coma de Kussmaul Kussmaul's coma
coma de trance trance coma
coma diabético diabetic coma
coma hepático hepatic coma
coma hipoglucémico hypoglycemic coma
coma insulínico insulin coma
coma metabólico metabolic coma
coma no cetónico hiperglucémico
    hiperosmolar hyperosmolar
    hyperglycemic nonketonic coma
coma tirotóxico thyrotoxic coma

comando command
comatoso comatose
combativo combative
combinación combination
comención comention
comensalismo commensalism
comentario autodespreciativo
    self-deprecatory remark
comer compulsivo compulsive eating
comer de rebote rebound eating
comer de uñas nail-biting
comer nocturno night-eating
comer sin saturación eating without
    saturation
comer tierra earth-eating
cometofobia cometophobia
comezón itch
cómico comical
comienzo onset
comisura commissure
comisura anterior anterior commissure
comisura blanca white commissure
comisura cerebral cerebral commissure
comisura del hipocampo hippocampal
    commissure
comisura gris gray commissure
comisura media middle commissure
comisura posterior posterior commissure
comisurotomía commissurotomy
comité de revisión de utilización utilization
    review committee
como si as if
comodidad de contacto contact comfort
comorbilidad comorbidity
compañero companion
compañero de juego invisible invisible
    playmate
compañero fóbico phobic companion
compañero imaginario imaginary companion
compañía humana human companionship
comparable comparable
comparación comparison
comparación de características feature
    comparison
comparación de estado status comparison
comparación emparejada paired comparison
comparación planificada planned comparison
comparación social social comparison
comparación transcultural cross-cultural
    comparison
comparativo comparative
compartimentación compartmentalization
compasión compassion
compatibilidad compatibility
compatible compatible
compensación compensation
compensatorio compensatory
competencia competence
competencia cognitiva cognitive competence
competencia comunitaria community
    competence
competencia de jurado juror competence
competencia de menores para consentir a
    tratamiento competency of minors to
    consent to treatment

competencia de niños testigos competency of
child witnesses
competencia de profesionales competency of
professionals
competencia de testigo competency of witness
competencia en psicología competency in
psychology
competencia para hacer un testamento
competency to make a will
competencia para someterse a juicio
competency to stand trial
competencia para someterse a juicio e
insania competency to stand trial and
insanity
competencia perceptiva perceptual
competency
competencia social social competence
competencia y consentimiento informado
competency and informed consent
competente competent
competitivo competitive
complacencia complacency
complejidad complexity
complejidad cognitiva cognitive complexity
complejo complex
complejo autónomo autonomous complex
complejo claustral claustral complex
complejo cultural culture complex
complejo de abuela grandmother complex
complejo de abuelo grandfather complex
complejo de animación animation complex
complejo de aprendiz apprentice complex
complejo de autoridad authority complex
complejo de Caín Cain complex
complejo de castración castration complex
complejo de castración activo active
castration complex
complejo de castración pasivo passive
castration complex
complejo de Clytemnestra Clytemnestra
complex
complejo de Cuasimodo Quasimodo complex
complejo de demencia de SIDA AIDS
dementia complex
complejo de Demóstenes Demosthenes
complex
complejo de desmembración dismemberment
complex
complejo de Diana Diana complex
complejo de Edipo Oedipus complex
complejo de Edipo invertido inverted
Oedipus complex
complejo de Edipo negativo negative Oedipus
complex
complejo de Electra Electra complex
complejo de Fedra Phaedra complex
complejo de feminidad femininity complex
complejo de Friedmann Friedmann's
complex
complejo de funciones function complex
complejo de Griselda Griselda complex
complejo de Icaro Icarus complex
complejo de ideas complex of ideas
complejo de inferioridad inferiority complex
complejo de Kandinsky-Clerambault

Kandinsky-Clerambault complex
complejo de la Cenicienta Cinderella
complex
complejo de Lear Lear complex
complejo de Madona Madonna complex
complejo de Madona-prostituta
Madonna-prostitute complex
complejo de madre superiora mother
superior complex
complejo de Medea Medea complex
complejo de obscenidad-pureza
obscenity-purity complex
complejo de ondas cerebrales brain wave
complex
complejo de Orestes Orestes complex
complejo de pecho breast complex
complejo de pene pequeño small-penis
complex
complejo de persecución persecution complex
complejo de poder power complex
complejo de Polícrates Polycrates complex
complejo de punta y onda spike and wave
complex
complejo de receptores receptor complex
complejo de síntomas symptom complex
complejo de superioridad superiority
complex
complejo de Yocasta Jocasta complex
complejo del ego ego complex
complejo edípico oedipal complex
complejo fraternal brother complex
complejo K K complex
complejo materno mother complex
complejo nuclear nuclear complex
complejo olivar superior superior olivary
complex
complejo particular particular complex
complejo paterno father complex
complejo puritano puritan complex
complejo reprimido repressed complex
complejo universal universal complex
complejo uretral urethral complex
complementaridad complementarity
complementaridad de interacción
complementarity of interaction
complementario complementary
complemento complement
completamente aleatorizado completely
randomized
completo complete
complicación complication
complicaciones de nacimiento birth
complications
complicaciones perinatales perinatal
complications
componente component
componente semántico semantic component
componente sintáctico syntactic component
componentes de emoción components of
emotion
compos mentis compos mentis
composición de movimiento composition of
movement
comprender comprehend
comprensión comprehension

comprensión comunicativa communicative
comprehension
comprensión de lectura reading
comprehension
comprensión del lenguaje language
comprehension
comprensión léxica lexical comprehension
comprensión verbal verbal comprehension
compresión compression
compresión cerebral cerebral compression
comprobación checking
comprobación de hipótesis hypothesis testing
comprometedor compromiser
compromiso commitment
compromiso ideológico ideological
commitment
compuesto compound
compulsión compulsion
compulsión antisocial antisocial compulsion
compulsión de meditar ansiosamente
brooding compulsion
compulsión de pensamiento thinking
compulsion
compulsión de precisión accuracy compulsion
compulsión de repetición repetition
compulsion
compulsión del comer eating compulsion
compulsiones contra tics compulsions versus
tics
compulsivo compulsive
computadora computer
computar compute
computerizado computerized
cómputo computation
cómputo de calendario calendar calculation
cómputo visual paralelo parallel visual
computation
común common
comuna commune
comunicación communication
comunicación animal animal communication
comunicación consumatoria consummatory
communication
comunicación en infantes ciegos
communication in blind infants
comunicación en niños sordos
communication in deaf children
comunicación gestual gestural communication
comunicación indicativa indexical
communication
comunicación interpersonal interpersonal
communication
comunicación no verbal nonverbal
communication
comunicación no verbal en infantes
nonverbal communication in infants
comunicación persuasiva persuasive
communication
comunicación privilegiada privileged
communication
comunicación terapéutica therapeutic
communication
comunicación y conducta disruptiva
communication and disruptive behavior
comunicativo communicative

comunicología communicology
comunidad community
comunidad de Oneida Oneida community
comunidad homosexual homosexual
community
comunidad terapéutica therapeutic
community
comunidades para personas con minusvalía
mental communities for mentally
handicapped persons
comunión communion
comuniscopio communiscope
conación conation
conario conarium
conativo conative
conato conatus
concatenación concatenation
concebir conceive
concentración concentration
concentración de alcohol sanguínea blood
alcohol concentration
concepción conception
concepción imperativa imperative conception
concepto concept
concepto categórico categorical concept
concepto clave key concept
concepto conjuntivo conjunctive concept
concepto corporal body concept
concepto de aprender a aprender
learn-to-learn concept
concepto de burbuja del espacio personal
bubble concept of personal space
concepto de heces-niño-pene
feces-child-penis concept
concepto de objeto object concept
concepto de permanencia permanence
concept
concepto de tabla rasa tabula rasa concept
concepto del ego corporal body ego concept
concepto demonológico de enfermedad
demonologic concept of illness
concepto disyuntivo disjunctive concept
conceptual conceptual
conceptualización conceptualization
conceptualización abstracta abstract
conceptualization
conciencia conscience, awareness
conciencia alterada altered awareness
conciencia alterada durante
biorretroalimentación altered awareness
during biofeedback
conciencia autoritaria authoritarian
conscience
conciencia colectiva collective consciousness
conciencia cósmica cosmic consciousness
conciencia de cabeza head consciousness
conciencia de contingencias contingency
awareness
conciencia de grupo group consciousness
conciencia de hambre hunger awareness
conciencia de multitud crowd consciousness
conciencia de realidad reality awareness
conciencia del cuerpo body awareness
conciencia del tiempo time consciousness
conciencia dividida divided consciousness

conciencia doble double consciousness
conciencia e hipnosis consciousness and hypnosis
conciencia expandida expanded consciousness
conciencia humanística humanistic conscience
conciencia marginal marginal consciousness
conciencia perceptiva perceptual consciousness
conciencia propia self-awareness
conciencia propia objetiva objective self-awareness
conciencia sensorial sensory awareness
conciencia social social consciousness
conciencia subliminal subliminal consciousness
concomitante concomitant
concordancia concordance
concordancia interpersonal interpersonal concordance
concretar concretize
concreticidad concreteness
concretismo concretism
concretización concretization
concretización activa active concretization
concreto concrete
concurrente concurrent
concusión concussion
concusión cerebral brain concussion
concusión espinal spinal concussion
condenación condemnation
condensación condensation
condición condition
condición control control condition
condición de triple X triple-X condition
condición de Y doble double-Y condition
condición experimental experimental condition
condición física physical condition
condición médica medical condition
condición médica general general medical condition
condición no atribuible a un trastorno mental condition not attributable to a mental disorder
condición ortopédica congénita congenital orthopedic condition
condición paranoide paranoid condition
condicionabilidad conditionability
condicionado conditioned
condicionalismo conditionalism
condicionamiento conditioning
condicionamiento alfa alpha conditioning
condicionamiento apetitivo appetitive conditioning
condicionamiento apetitivo clásico classical appetitive conditioning
condicionamiento asertivo assertive conditioning
condicionamiento asociativo associative conditioning
condicionamiento autónomo autonomic conditioning
condicionamiento autónomo-involuntario autonomic-involuntary conditioning
condicionamiento aversivo aversive conditioning
condicionamiento aversivo clásico classical aversive conditioning
condicionamiento beta beta conditioning
condicionamiento clásico classical conditioning
condicionamiento cognitivo cognitive conditioning
condicionamiento compuesto compound conditioning
condicionamiento contiguo de Guthrie Guthrie's contiguous conditioning
condicionamiento cruzado cross-conditioning
condicionamiento de aversión aversion conditioning
condicionamiento de demora delay conditioning
condicionamiento de escape escape conditioning
condicionamiento de evitación avoidance conditioning
condicionamiento de evitación temporal temporal avoidance conditioning
condicionamiento de orden superior higher-order conditioning
condicionamiento de párpado eyelid conditioning
condicionamiento de reacciones compensatorias conditioning of compensatory reactions
condicionamiento de recompensa primaria primary reward conditioning
condicionamiento de recompensa secundaria secondary reward conditioning
condicionamiento de segundo orden second-order conditioning
condicionamiento de Skinner skinnerian conditioning
condicionamiento de temor fear conditioning
condicionamiento de traza trace conditioning
condicionamiento demorado delayed conditioning
condicionamiento diferencial differential conditioning
condicionamiento durante el sueño conditioning during sleep
condicionamiento encubierto covert conditioning
condicionamiento espinal spinal conditioning
condicionamiento excitatorio excitatory conditioning
condicionamiento exteroceptivo exteroceptive conditioning
condicionamiento falso false conditioning
condicionamiento hacia atrás backward conditioning
condicionamiento inhibitorio inhibitory conditioning
condicionamiento instrumental instrumental conditioning
condicionamiento interoceptivo interoceptive conditioning
condicionamiento operante operant

conditioning
condicionamiento pavloviano pavlovian conditioning
condicionamiento por aproximación approximation conditioning
condicionamiento por aproximación automático auto shaping
condicionamiento por aproximaciones sucesivas conditioning by successive approximations
condicionamiento remoto remote conditioning
condicionamiento respondiente respondent conditioning
condicionamiento secundario secondary conditioning
condicionamiento semántico semantic conditioning
condicionamiento sensorial sensory conditioning
condicionamiento simultáneo simultaneous conditioning
condicionamiento sucesivo successive conditioning
condicionamiento temporal temporal conditioning
condicionamiento verbal verbal conditioning
condicionamiento vicario vicarious conditioning
condiciones ambientales ambient conditions
condiciones atmosféricas atmospheric conditions
condiciones de aprendizaje learning conditions
condiciones de aprendizaje analíticas analytic learning conditions
condiciones de iluminación illumination conditions
condiciones de mérito conditions of worth
condiciones de ruido noise conditions
condiciones de trabajo working conditions
condón condom
conducción conduction, driving
conducción antidrómica antidromic conduction
conducción de aire air conduction
conducción de dolor pain conduction
conducción de nervio nerve conduction
conducción electrotónica electrotonic conduction
conducción neural neural conduction
conducción ósea bone conduction
conducción saltatoria saltatory conduction
conducción tónica tonic conduction
conducta behavior
conducta abrazante embracing behavior
conducta accionada por el tiempo clock-driven behavior
conducta acechante stalking behavior
conducta adaptiva adaptive behavior
conducta adictiva addictive behavior
conducta adjunta adjunctive behavior
conducta agonística agonistic behavior
conducta agresiva aggressive behavior
conducta agresiva animal animal aggressive

behavior
conducta agresiva durante cuidado de niños aggressive behavior during child care
conducta agresiva explosiva explosive aggressive behavior
conducta altruista altruistic behavior
conducta anárquica anarchic behavior
conducta animal animal behavior
conducta anormal abnormal behavior
conducta antinodal antinodal behavior
conducta antipredadora antipredator behavior
conducta antisocial antisocial behavior
conducta antisocial adolescente adolescent antisocial behavior
conducta antisocial adulta adult antisocial behavior
conducta antisocial de niñez childhood antisocial behavior
conducta apetitiva appetitive behavior
conducta apopatética apopathetic behavior
conducta aprendida learned behavior
conducta apropiada de sexo sex-appropriate behavior
conducta arriesgada risk-taking behavior
conducta asertiva assertive behavior
conducta auditiva auditory behavior
conducta autoderrotante self-defeating behavior
conducta autodestructiva self-destructive behavior
conducta autoperjudicial self-injurious behavior
conducta aversiva aversive behavior
conducta bisexual bisexual behavior
conducta carroñera scavenging behavior
conducta catastrófica catastrophic behavior
conducta circular circular behavior
conducta coercitiva coercive behavior
conducta colateral collateral behavior
conducta compulsiva compulsive behavior
conducta copulatoria copulatory behavior
conducta de acicaladura grooming behavior
conducta de alimentación feeding behavior
conducta de apaciguamiento appeasement behavior
conducta de apareamiento mating behavior
conducta de apego attachment behavior
conducta de apego en autismo attachment behavior in autism
conducta de arrimo cuddling behavior
conducta de asirse clinging behavior
conducta de ataque attack behavior
conducta de ayuda helping behavior
conducta de besar kissing behavior
conducta de conflicto conflict behavior
conducta de congelación freezing behavior
conducta de contacto contact behavior
conducta de copiarse copying behavior
conducta de cortejo courtship behavior
conducta de criterio criterion behavior
conducta de deferencia deference behavior
conducta de desplazamiento displacement behavior
conducta de despliegue display behavior

conducta de dolor pain behavior
conducta de enfermedad illness behavior
conducta de entrada entry behavior
conducta de escape escape behavior
conducta de evitación avoidance behavior
conducta de fumar smoking behavior
conducta de género cruzado cross-gender
  behavior
conducta de grupo group behavior
conducta de hipótesis hypothesis behavior
conducta de infantes infant behavior
conducta de infantes y alimentación por
  pecho infant behavior and breast-feeding
conducta de juego play behavior
conducta de juego de infantes infant play
  behavior
conducta de juego en autismo play behavior
  in autism
conducta de jugar gambling behavior
conducta de laberinto maze behavior
conducta de lactancia nursing behavior
conducta de lamedura licking behavior
conducta de masticación chewing behavior
conducta de migración migration behavior
conducta de muchedumbre mob behavior
conducta de multitud crowd behavior
conducta de pandilla gang behavior
conducta de papel role behavior
conducta de preferencia preference behavior
conducta de primates primate behavior
conducta de proximidad immediacy behavior
conducta de resolución de problemas
  problem-solving behavior
conducta de saludo greeting behavior
conducta de salvamento de apariencias
  face-saving behavior
conducta de seguir following behavior
conducta de transposición transposition
  behavior
conducta de uso de herramientas tool-using
  behavior
conducta defensiva defensive behavior
conducta del beber drinking behavior
conducta del comer eating behavior
conducta del consumidor consumer behavior
conducta del morder de dedos finger-biting
  behavior
conducta del prender fuegos fire-setting
  behavior
conducta del vestir dressing behavior
conducta delincuente delinquent behavior
conducta depresiva ciclotímica
  cyclothymic-depressive behavior
conducta desinhibida uninhibited behavior
conducta desorganizada disorganized
  behavior
conducta destructiva destructive behavior
conducta desviada deviant behavior
conducta dirigida a un fin goal-directed
  behavior
conducta dirigida hacia lo interno
  inner-directed behavior
conducta disocial dyssocial behavior
conducta disruptiva disruptive behavior
conducta ecoica echoic behavior

conducta egodistónica ego-dystonic behavior
conducta emitida emitted behavior
conducta emocional emotional behavior
conducta en ascensores behavior in elevators
conducta en cadena chain behavior
conducta en masa mass behavior
conducta encubierta covert behavior
conducta específica de especie
  species-specific behavior
conducta espontanea spontaneous behavior
conducta estereotipada stereotyped behavior
conducta estrambótica bizarre behavior
conducta estrual estrous behavior
conducta evocada elicited behavior
conducta explícita explicit behavior
conducta exploratoria exploratory behavior
conducta explotadora-manipulativa
  exploitative-manipulative behavior
conducta expresiva expressive behavior
conducta externalizante externalizing
  behavior
conducta extraindividual extraindividual
  behavior
conducta homicida homicidal behavior
conducta homosexual homosexual behavior
conducta humana human behavior
conducta implícita implicit behavior
conducta impulsiva impulsive behavior
conducta inadaptiva maladaptive behavior
conducta inapropiada inappropriate behavior
conducta ingestiva ingestive behavior
conducta innata innate behavior
conducta innata contra aprendida innate
  versus learned behavior
conducta instintiva instinctive behavior
conducta instrumental instrumental behavior
conducta intencional intentional behavior
conducta internalizante internalizing
  behavior
conducta intrínseca intrinsic behavior
conducta intuitiva intuitive behavior
conducta involuntaria intencional intentional
  unvoluntary behavior
conducta manipulativa manipulative behavior
conducta maternal maternal behavior
conducta molar molar behavior
conducta molecular molecular behavior
conducta moral moral behavior
conducta moral en niños moral behavior in
  children
conducta motora motor behavior
conducta multideterminada multidetermined
  behavior
conducta no verbal nonverbal behavior
conducta nodal nodal behavior
conducta objetivo target behavior
conducta obligada compelled behavior
conducta observada observed behavior
conducta obsesiva obsessive behavior
conducta operante operant behavior
conducta operativa operative behavior
conducta oral oral behavior
conducta para bregar coping behavior
conducta parental parental behavior
conducta parental de animales animal

parental behavior
conducta pasiva-agresiva passive-aggressive behavior
conducta paternal paternal behavior
conducta predatoria predatory behavior
conducta problema problem behavior
conducta prohibida prohibited behavior
conducta propensa a accidentes accident-prone behavior
conducta prosocial prosocial behavior
conducta que podría ocasionar accidentes accident behavior
conducta reguladora regulatory behavior
conducta relacionada al alcohol alcohol-related behavior
conducta reproductiva reproductive behavior
conducta requerida required behavior
conducta respondiente respondent behavior
conducta ritualista ritualistic behavior
conducta serial serial behavior
conducta seudoafectiva pseudoaffective behavior
conducta sexual sexual behavior
conducta sexual de animales animal sexual behavior
conducta sexual desviada deviant sexual behavior
conducta sobredependiente overdependent behavior
conducta social social behavior
conducta sociopática sociopathic behavior
conducta supersticiosa superstitious behavior
conducta terminal terminal behavior
conducta territorial territorial behavior
conducta territorial de grupo group territorial behavior
conducta territorial intragrupal intragroup territorial behavior
conducta tipo A type A behavior
conducta tipo adolescente adolescent-type behavior
conducta tipo B type B behavior
conducta tiránica tyrannical behavior
conducta trastornada disordered behavior
conducta verbal verbal behavior
conducta violenta violent behavior
conducta violenta de niños abusados violent behavior of abused children
conductancia conductance
conductancia palmar palmar conductance
conductas de atención attending behaviors
conductismo behaviorism
conductismo descriptivo descriptive behaviorism
conductismo ecléctico eclectic behaviorism
conductismo operante operant behaviorism
conductismo radical radical behaviorism
conductista behaviorist
conductividad conductivity
conducto duct
conducto coclear cochlear duct
conducto eyaculatorio ejaculatory duct
conducto seminal seminal duct
conductos de Muller Mullerian ducts
conductual behavioral

conector connector
conexión connection
conexión causal causal connection
conexionismo connectionism
confabulación confabulation
confabulación amnésica amnestic confabulation
confabulosis confabulosis
confederado confederate
conferencia conference
conferencia de carrera career conference
confesión confession
confesión falsa false confession
confiabilidad reliability
confiabilidad de forma equivalente equivalent form reliability
confiabilidad de interobservador interobserver reliability
confiabilidad de muestreo sampling reliability
confiabilidad de observador observer reliability
confiabilidad de pares-nones odd-even reliability
confiabilidad de prueba reliability of test
confiabilidad de prueba-reprueba test-retest reliability
confiabilidad interjueces interjudge reliability
confiable reliable
confianza confidence, trust
confianza básica basic trust
confianza contra desconfianza trust versus mistrust
confianza diagnóstica diagnostic confidence
confianza interpersonal interpersonal trust
confianza propia self-confidence
confidencialidad confidentiality
confidencialidad y consentimiento a tratamiento confidentiality and consent to treatment
confidencialidad y consentimiento informado confidentiality and informed consent
configuración configuration
configuración de palabra word configuration
configuración factorial factor configuration
configuracional configurational
confinamiento confinement
confinamiento civil civil commitment
confinamiento criminal criminal commitment
confinamiento para observación observation commitment
confinamiento temporal temporary commitment
confinamiento voluntario voluntary commitment
confirmación confirmation
conflicto conflict
conflicto básico basic conflict
conflicto central central conflict
conflicto cultural culture conflict
conflicto de acercamiento-acercamiento approach-approach conflict
conflicto de acercamiento doble double approach conflict
conflicto de acercamiento-evitación

approach-avoidance conflict
conflicto de acercamiento-evitación doble
double approach-avoidance conflict
conflicto de evitación doble double avoidance
conflict
conflicto de evitación-evitación
avoidance-avoidance conflict
conflicto de intereses conflict of interest
conflicto de papel role conflict
conflicto de papel interpersonal interpersonal
role conflict
conflicto edípico oedipal conflict
conflicto emocional emotional conflict
conflicto ético ethical conflict
conflicto extrapsíquico extrapsychic conflict
conflicto familiar family conflict
conflicto intergrupo intergroup conflict
conflicto interno internal conflict
conflicto interpersonal interpersonal conflict
conflicto intrapersonal intrapersonal conflict
conflicto intrapsíquico intrapsychic conflict
conflicto marital marital conflict
conflicto neurótico neurotic conflict
conflicto nuclear nuclear conflict
conflicto parental parental conflict
conflicto raíz root conflict
conflicto real actual conflict
conflictos inducidos experimentalmente
experimentally induced conflicts
confluencia confluence
conformidad conformity
conformidad con papel convencional
conventional role conformity
conformidad de autómata automaton
conformity
conformidad del clima climate conformance
conformidad en cultos conformity in cults
conformidad espacial spatial conformance
conformidad funcional functional
conformance
conformidad sensorial sensory conformance
confrontación confrontation
confrontación de realidad reality
confrontation
confrontante confrontational
confundir confound
confusión confusion
confusión acústica acoustic confusion
confusión bisexual bisexual confusion
confusión de autoridad authority confusion
confusión de identidad identity confusion
confusión de papel role confusion
confusión de tamaño-edad size-age confusion
confusión de tiempo time confusion
confusión de valores confusion of values
confusión delirante deliriant confusion
confusión direccional directional confusion
confusión lateral lateral confusion
confusión mental mental confusion
confusión reactiva reactive confusion
confusión semántica semantic confusion
confusional confusional
confusionismo confusionism
congelación freezing
congénito congenital

congestión congestion
congestión cerebral brain congestion
congófilo congophilic
congraciador ingratiating
congraciamiento ingratiation
congruencia congruence
congruente congruent
conjugación conjugation
conjuntiva conjunctiva
conjuntividad conjunctivity
conjuntivo conjunctive
conjunto set
conjunto de respuestas aquiescentes
acquiescent-response set
conjunto indistinto fuzzy set
conjunto nulo null set
conjunto objetivo target set
conjunto vacío empty set
conjuntos inconexos disjoint sets
conmoción cerebral commotio cerebri
conmoción espinal commotio spinalis
connato connate
connotación connotation
cono de color color cone
cono retinal retinal cone
conocer cognize
conocimiento knowledge, consciousness
conocimiento de competencia competence
knowledge
conocimiento de resultados knowledge of
results
conocimiento declarativo declarative
knowledge
conocimiento figurativo figurative knowledge
conocimiento funcional functional knowledge
conocimiento inconsciente unconscious
knowledge
conocimiento operativo operative knowledge
conocimiento por familiaridad knowledge by
acquaintance
conocimiento verídico factual knowledge
conos cones
consanguíneo consanguine
consanguinidad consanguinity
consciente conscious
consecuencias consequences
consecuente consequent
consejo advice
consenso consensus
consensual consensual
consentido spoiled
consentimiento consent
consentimiento informado informed consent
consentimiento informado en investigación
informed consent in research
consentimiento informado y abuso de niños
informed consent and child abuse
consentimiento informado y competencia
informed consent and competency
**consentimiento informado y comprensión de
información** informed consent and
comprehension of information
consentimiento informado y confidencialidad
informed consent and confidentiality
consentimiento informado y toma de

decisiones de pacientes informed consent and patient decision making
consentimiento informado y tratamiento informed consent and treatment
consentimiento válido valid consent
conserva cultural cultural conserve
conservación conservation
conservación-retirada conservation-withdrawal
conservador conservator
conservatismo conservatism
conservativo conservative
consideración consideration
consideraciones culturales en evaluación cultural considerations in assessment
consistencia consistency
consistencia conductual behavioral consistency
consistencia de reprueba retest consistency
consistencia interna internal consistency
consistencia moral moral consistency
consolación consolation
consolidación consolidation
consolidación de memoria memory consolidation
consonancia consonance
consonante consonant
constancia constancy
constancia de brillantez brightness constancy
constancia de color color constancy
constancia de condiciones constancy of conditions
constancia de forma form constancy
constancia de género gender constancy
constancia de objeto object constancy
constancia de objeto libidinal libidinal object constancy
constancia de tamaño size constancy
constancia de ubicación location constancy
constancia del ambiente interno constancy of internal environment
constancia del cociente de inteligencia constancy of the intelligence quotient
constancia del organismo constancy of the organism
constancia perceptiva perceptual constancy
constante constant
constante central central constant
constante de Heinis Heinis constant
constante personal personal constant
constelación constellation
constelación familiar family constellation
constipación constipation
constipación psicogénica psychogenic constipation
constitución constitution
constitución hiperadrenal hyperadrenal constitution
constitución hiperpituitaria hyperpituitary constitution
constitución hipertiroide hyperthyroid constitution
constitución hipoadrenal hypoadrenal constitution
constitución hipoparatiroidea hypoparathyroid constitution
constitución hipopituitaria hypopituitary constitution
constitución postraumática posttraumatic constitution
constitución psicopática epiléptica epileptic psychopathic constitution
constitucional constitutional
constitutivo constituent
constitutivo inmediato immediate constituent
constreñimiento constraint
constreñimiento de movimiento constraint of movement
constreñimiento de pensamientos constraint of thought
constricción constriction
constrictor de la vagina constrictor vaginae
construcción de nido nest-building
construccionismo constructionism
construccionismo social social constructionism
constructivismo constructivism
constructivo constructive
constructo construct
constructo constelatorio constellatory construct
constructo empírico empirical construct
constructo hipotético hypothetical construct
constructo personal personal construct
constructo preverbal preverbal construct
constructo teorético theoretical construct
constructos de orden superior higher-order constructs
consultación consultation
consultación centrada en los colegas colleague-centered consultation
consultación orientada a pacientes patient-oriented consultation
consultación profesional professional consultation
consultación psiquiátrica psychiatric consultation
consultor consultant
consultor industrial industrial consultant
consumatorio consummatory
consumerismo consumerism
consumidor consumer
consumo calórico caloric intake
consumo de café coffee consumption
contacto contact
contacto con la realidad contact with reality
contacto corporal body contact
contacto corporal y apego body contact and attachment
contacto cultural culture contact
contacto ocular eye contact
contacto oral-genital oral-genital contact
contacto sexual sexual contact
contacto social social contact
contador counter
contagio contagion
contagio de emergencia emergency contagion
contagio de grupo group contagion
contagio emocional emotional contagion
contagio en masa mass contagion

contagio psíquico psychic contagion
contagio social social contagion
contaminación contamination
contaminación de ruido noise pollution
contaminación del aire air pollution
contemplación contemplation
contemplación de cristal crystal gazing
contemporaneidad contemporaneity
contemporáneo contemporaneous
contención de agresión curbing of aggression
contención de costos cost containment
contencioso contentious
contenido content
contenido de alcohol sanguíneo blood alcohol
    content
contenido de entrevista interview content
contenido de pensamientos thought content
contenido de sueños dream content
contenido de sueños latente latent dream
    content
contenido icónico iconic content
contenido latente latent content
contenido manifiesto manifest content
contenido mental mental content
contentivo contentive
contexto context
contexto social social context
contextual contextual
contextualismo contextualism
contigüidad contiguity
contigüidad de las asociaciones contiguity of
    associations
contigüidad espacial spatial contiguity
contigüidad temporal temporal contiguity
continencia continence
continencia masculina male continence
continente continent
contingencia contingency
contingente contingent
continuación continuation
continuación buena good continuation
continuante continuant
continuidad continuity
continuidad del cuidado continuity of care
continuo (adj) continuous
continuo (n) continuum
continuo de estímulo stimulus continuum
continuo introversión-extroversión
    introversion-extroversion continuum
continuo polar polar continuum
contorno contour
contorno anómalo anomalous contour
contorno cognitivo cognitive contour
contorno de entonación intonation contour
contorno ilusorio illusory contour
contorno isofónico isophonic contour
contorno subjetivo subjective contour
contraafecto counteraffect
contrabalanceo counterbalancing
contracatexis countercathexis
contracción contraction
contracción carpopedal carpopedal
    contraction
contracción isométrica isometric contraction
contracción isotónica isotonic contraction

contracción muscular muscle contraction
contracción tetánica tetanic contraction
contracción tónica tonic contraction
contracepción contraception
contraceptivo contraceptive
contracompulsión countercompulsion
contracondicionamiento counterconditioning
contracondicionamiento con hipnotismo
    counterconditioning with hypnotism
contraconformidad counterconformity
contractibilidad contractibility
contractilidad contractility
contractual contractual
contractura contracture
contractura de Volkmann Volkmann's
    contracture
contractura funcional functional contracture
contractura orgánica organic contracture
contractural contractural
contracultura counterculture
contrachoque countershock
contradictorio contradictory
contraego counter ego
contrafisura contrafissura
contrafobia counterphobia
contrafóbico counterphobic
contrafórmula counterformula
contragolpe contrecoup
contrahechos counterfactual
contraidentificación counteridentification
contraindicación contraindication
contrainversión counterinvestment
contrairritante counterirritant
contralateral contralateral
contrario counter
contrarrestar counter
contrasexual contrasexual
contraste contrast
contraste conductual behavioral contrast
contraste cromático chromatic contrast
contraste de brillantez brightness contrast
contraste de color color contrast
contraste negativo negative contrast
contraste simultáneo simultaneous contrast
contraste sucesivo successive contrast
contrasugestibilidad contrasuggestibility
contrasugestión countersuggestion
contratación con contingencias contingency
    contracting
contrato contract
contrato con contingencias contingency
    contract
contrato conductual behavioral contract
contrato de conducta behavior contract
contrato de evaluación evaluation contract
contrato interactivo interactional contract
contrato matrimonial marriage contract
contrato psicológico psychological contract
contratransferencia countertransference
contravolición countervolition
contravoluntad counterwill
contrectación contrectation
control control
control autonómico aprendido learned
    autonomic control

control aversivo aversive control
control cerebral brain control
control cognitivo cognitive control
control compulsivo compulsive restraint
control conductual behavioral control
control cortical cortical control
control de apetito appetite control
control de balance balance control
control de conducta behavior control
control de cuotas quota control
control de estímulo stimulus control
control de gemelo co-twin control
control de grupo group control
control de impulsos impulse control
control de mente mind control
control de movimiento movement control
control de natalidad birth control
control de obesidad control of obesity
control de pensamiento adaptivo adaptive
    control of thought
control de pensamientos thought control
control de peso weight control
control de retroalimentación feedback
    control
control de variables control of variables
control de vejiga bladder control
control del ego ego control
control discriminativo discriminative control
control esfintérico sphincter control
control estadístico statistical control
control experimental experimental control
control guiado conceptualmente conceptually
    guided control
control idiodinámico idiodynamic control
control interpersonal interpersonal control
control intestinal bowel control
control postural postural control
control reflejo reflex control
control rígido rigid control
control secreto secret control
control sinérgico synergic control
control social social control
control supersticioso superstitious control
control tónico tonic control
control vestibuloequilibratorio
    vestibuloequilibratory control
control voluntario voluntary control
controlado controlled
controlador controlling
controles de carro car controls
controles de mano hand controls
controles internos inner controls
controversia controversy
controversia herencia-ambiente
    heredity-environment controversy
controversia naturaleza-crianza
    nature-nurture controversy
contusión contusion
contusión cerebral cerebral contusion
contusión del cuero cabelludo scalp
    contusion
convaleciente convalescent
convención convention
convencional conventional
convencionalismo conventionality

convergencia convergence
convergente convergent
conversacional conversational
conversacionalismo conversationalism
conversacionalismo de cóctel cocktail-party
    conversationalism
conversión conversion
conversión de emoción conversion of emotion
converso converse
convexidad convexity
convexobasia convexobasia
convolución convolution
convulsión convulsion
convulsión clónica clonic convulsion
convulsión coordinada coordinate convulsion
convulsión en zalema salaam convulsion
convulsión febril febrile convulsion
convulsión histérica hysterical convulsion
convulsión histeroide hysteroid convulsion
convulsión infantil infantile convulsion
convulsión mímica mimic convulsion
convulsión por éter ether convulsion
convulsión postraumática inmediata
    immediate posttraumatic convulsion
convulsión puerperal puerperal convulsion
convulsión estática static convulsion
convulsión tetánica tetanic convulsion
convulsión tónica tonic convulsion
convulsivante convulsant
convulsivo convulsive
conyugal conjugal
cónyuge spouse
cónyuge celoso jealous spouse
cooperación cooperation
cooperación antagónica antagonistic
    cooperation
cooperadores cooperators
cooperativo cooperative
coordenada coordinate
coordenadas cartesianas Cartesian
    coordinates
coordinación coordination
coordinación audiovisual audiovisual
    coordination
coordinación de motor fino fine motor
    coordination
coordinación de proyectos secundarios
    coordination of secondary schemes
coordinación motora motor coordination
coordinación ojo-mano eye-hand coordination
coordinación visual-motora visual-motor
    coordination
coordinado coordinated
coordinar coordinate
copión copycat
copofobia kopophobia
coprofagia coprophagy
coprofemia coprophemia
coprofilia coprophilia
coprofílico coprophilic
coprófilo coprophil
coprofobia coprophobia
coprofrasia coprophrasia
coprolagnia coprolagnia
coprolalia coprolalia

coprología coprology
copropraxia copropraxia
copulación copulation
coraza cuirass
coraza analgésica analgesic cuirass
coraza tabética tabetic cuirass
corazón irritable irritable heart
cordectomía cordectomy
corditis tuberosa chorditis tuberosa
cordoma chordoma
cordón umbilical umbilical cord
cordopexia cordopexy
cordotomía cordotomy
cordotomía abierta open cordotomy
cordotomía anterolateral anterolateral
    cordotomy
cordotomía de columna posterior posterior
    column cordotomy
cordotomía espinotalámica spinothalamic
    cordotomy
cordotomía estereotáctica stereotactic
    cordotomy
cordotomía estereotáxica stereotaxic
    cordotomy
cordura sanity
corea chorea
corea-acantocitosis chorea-acanthocytosis
corea automática automatic chorea
corea danzante dancing chorea
corea de Henoch Henoch's chorea
corea de Huntington Huntington's chorea
corea de Huntington de niñez childhood
    Huntington's chorea
corea de Morvan Morvan's chorea
corea de Sydenham Sydenham's chorea
corea degenerativa degenerative chorea
corea dimidiata chorea dimidiata
corea eléctrica electric chorea
corea festinante chorea festinans
corea fibrilar fibrillary chorea
corea gravídea chorea gravidarum
corea habitual habit chorea
corea hemilateral hemilateral chorea
corea hereditaria hereditary chorea
corea histérica hysterical chorea
corea juvenil juvenile chorea
corea laríngea laryngeal chorea
corea mayor chorea major
corea menor chorea minor
corea metódica methodical chorea
corea mimética mimetic chorea
corea nutans chorea nutans
corea paralítica paralytic chorea
corea poshemipléjica posthemiplegic chorea
corea procursiva procursive chorea
corea progresiva crónica chronic progressive
    chorea
corea reumática rheumatic chorea
corea rítmica rhythmic chorea
corea rotatoria chorea rotatoria
corea saltatoria saltatory chorea
corea senil senile chorea
corea tetanoide tetanoid chorea
corea variable de Brissaud variable chorea of
    Brissaud

coreal choreal
coreico choreic
coreiforme choreiform
coreoatetoide choreoathetoid
coreoatetosis choreoathetosis
coreoatetosis hereditaria hereditary
    choreoathetosis
coreofrasia choreophrasia
coreoide choreoid
coreomanía choreomania
coriomeningitis choriomeningitis
coriomeningitis linfocítica lymphocytic
    choriomeningitis
corion chorion
corium corium
córnea cornea
cornezuelo de centeno ergot
coroides choroid
corolario corollary
coronal coronal
coronario coronary
corporal corporal
corpúsculo corpuscle
corpúsculo de Dogiel Dogiel's corpuscle
corpúsculo de Pacini pacinian corpuscle
corpúsculo de Ruffini Ruffini corpuscle
corpúsculo táctil tactile corpuscle
corpúsculos de Golgi Golgi corpuscles
corpúsculos de Golgi-Mazzoni
    Golgi-Mazzoni corpuscles
corpúsculos de Meissner Meissner's
    corpuscles
corpúsculos de Merkel Merkel's corpuscles
corrección correction
corrección de Yates Yates correction
corrección del habla speech correction
corrección para barruntamiento correction
    for guessing
corrección para casualidad correction for
    chance
corrección para continuidad correction for
    continuity
correctivo corrective
corredor runway
correlación correlation
correlación biserial biserial correlation
correlación cruzada cross-correlation
correlación curvilínea curvilinear correlation
correlación de orden cero zero-order
    correlation
correlación de primera orden first-order
    correlation
correlación de rangos de Spearman
    Spearman rank correlation
correlación directa direct correlation
correlación espuria spurious correlation
correlación ilusoria illusory correlation
correlación indirecta indirect correlation
correlación inversa inverse correlation
correlación lineal linear correlation
correlación múltiple multiple correlation
correlación negativa negative correlation
correlación neurológica neurological
    correlation
correlación no lineal nonlinear correlation

correlación parcial partial correlation
correlación perfecta perfect correlation
correlación por diferencias de rangos
    rank-difference correlation
correlación por orden de rangos rank-order
    correlation
correlación positiva positive correlation
correlación R R correlation
correlación simple simple correlation
correlación y regresión correlation and
    regression
correlacionado correlated
correlacional correlational
correlacionar correlate
correlativo correlative
correspondencia correspondence
correspondencia cruzada
    cross-correspondence
correspondencia de punto a punto
    point-to-point correspondence
correspondencia fonema-grafema
    phoneme-grapheme correspondence
correspondencia punto por punto
    point-for-point correspondence
corriente current
corriente de acción stream of action
corriente de conciencia stream of
    consciousness
corriente de demarcación demarcation
    current
corriente de lesión current of injury
corriente de pensamiento stream of thought
corriente nerviosa nerve current
corriente neural neural current
corte cutting
corte de trenzas braid-cutting
corte familiar family court
cortejo courtship
corteza cortex
corteza adrenal adrenal cortex
corteza agranular agranular cortex
corteza auditiva auditory cortex
corteza calcarina calcarine cortex
corteza cerebelosa cerebellar cortex
corteza cerebral cerebral cortex
corteza cingulada cingulate cortex
corteza de asociación association cortex
corteza estriada striate cortex
corteza extrínseca extrinsic cortex
corteza frontal frontal cortex
corteza granular granular cortex
corteza inferotemporal inferotemporal cortex
corteza intrínseca intrinsic cortex
corteza límbica limbic cortex
corteza motora motor cortex
corteza parietal parietal cortex
corteza periamigdaloide periamygdaloid
    cortex
corteza piriforme pyriform cortex
corteza premotora premotor cortex
corteza primaria primary cortex
corteza sensorial sensory cortex
corteza somatosensorial somatosensory
    cortex
corteza terciaria tertiary cortex

corteza transicional transitional cortex
corteza visual visual cortex
corteza visual no estriada nonstriate visual
    cortex
cortical cortical
corticalización corticalization
corticectomía corticectomy
corticobulbar corticobulbar
corticoespinal corticospinal
corticófugo corticofugal
corticoide corticoid
corticonuclear corticonuclear
corticopontino corticopontine
corticosteroide corticosteroid
corticosterona corticosterone
corticotropina corticotropine
cortina cortin
cortisol cortisol
cortisona cortisone
cortocircuitado short-circuiting
coruscación coruscation
cosificación reification
cosmología cosmology
cosquillas tickling
costo de respuesta response cost
costo máximo permisible maximum allowable
    cost
costumbres mores
costumbres sociales social mores
coterapia cotherapy
cotidiano quotidian
covada couvade
covarianza covariance
coyuntura juncture
crack crack
craneal cranial
cráneo skull
cráneo bífido bifid cranium
cráneo en hoja de trébol cloverleaf skull
cráneo en mapa maplike skull
cráneo en torre towers skull
craneoanfitomía craniamphitomy
craneocele craniocele
craneoesclerosis craniosclerosis
craneoestenosis craniostenosis
craneofacial craniofacial
craneofaringioma craniopharyngioma
craneofaringioma papilomatoso quístico
    cystic papillomatous craniopharyngioma
craneognomia craniognomy
craneógrafo craniograph
craneología craniology
craneología de Gall Gall's craniology
craneomalacia craniomalacia
craneomalacia circunscrita circumscribed
    craniomalacia
craneomeningocele craniomeningocele
craneometría craniometry
craneopatía craniopathy
craneoplastia cranioplasty
craneopunción craniopuncture
craneorraquisquisis craniorrhachischisis
craneosacra craniosacral
craneoscopia cranioscopy
craneosinostosis craniosynostosis

craneosquisis cranioschisis
craneotabes craniotabes
craneotomía craniotomy
craneotomía desprendida detached
   craniotomy
craneotomía osteoplástica osteoplastic
   craniotomy
craneotomía unida attached craniotomy
craneotonoscopia craniotonoscopy
craneotripesis craniotrypesis
craniectomía craniectomy
craniectomía lineal linear craniectomy
creatinina creatinine
creatinina urinaria urinary creatinine
creatividad creativity
creativo creative
crecimiento growth
crecimiento cognitivo cognitive growth
crecimiento continuo continuous growth
crecimiento de membrana membrane growth
crecimiento de vocabulario vocabulary
   growth
crecimiento diferencial differential growth
crecimiento horizontal horizontal growth
crecimiento mental mental growth
crecimiento personal personal growth
credibilidad credibility
credulidad credulity
creencia belief
creencia de equivalencia equivalence belief
creencia irracional irrational belief
creencias de la crianza de niños child-rearing
   beliefs
crematofobia chrematophobia
crematomanía chrematomania
crematorrea chrematorrhea
cremnofobia cremnophobia
crepuscular crepuscular
cresta neural neural crest
cretinismo cretinism
crialgesia cryalgesia
crianestesia cryanesthesia
crianza nurture
crianza cruzada cross-fostering
crianza de niños child-rearing
cribado screening
cribado de portadores carrier screening
cribado de recién nacidos newborn screening
cribado fetal fetal screening
cribado genético genetic screening
cribado metabólico metabolic screening
cribado psiquiátrico psychiatric screening
criestesia cryesthesia
crimen por sentimiento de culpabilidad
   crime from sense of guilt
criminal criminal
criminalidad criminality
criminalismo criminalism
criminología criminology
criminosis criminosis
crimodinia crymodynia
criocirugía cryosurgery
crioespasmo cryospasm
criofobia cryophobia
criogénico cryogenic

criohipofisectomía cryohypophysectomy
criopalidectomía cryopallidectomy
criopulvinectomía cryopulvinectomy
criosonda cryoprobe
criotalamectomía cryothalamectomy
criptestesia cryptesthesia
criptococoma cryptococcoma
criptococosis cryptococcosis
criptofasia cryptophasia
criptografía cryptography
criptomnesia cryptomnesia
criptorquidismo cryptorchidism
criptórquido cryptorchid
criptorquismo cryptorchism
criptotia cryptotia
crisis crisis
crisis accidental accidental crisis
crisis adolescente adolescent crisis
crisis catatímica catathymic crisis
crisis de edad mediana midlife crisis
crisis de identidad identity crisis
crisis de vida life crisis
crisis de vida y salud life crisis and health
crisis del desarrollo developmental crisis
crisis existencial existential crisis
crisis familiar family crisis
crisis gástrica gastric crisis
crisis global global crisis
crisis hipertensiva hypertensive crisis
crisis laríngea laryngeal crisis
crisis maduracional maturational crisis
crisis no anticipada unanticipated crisis
crisis normativa normative crisis
crisis oculógira oculogyric crisis
crisis situacional situational crisis
crisis suicida suicidal crisis
crisis tabética tabetic crisis
crisis terapéutica therapeutic crisis
crispación crispation
cristalización crystallization
cristalización en helecho ferning
cristalofobia crystallophobia
criterio criterion
criterio de cuadrados mínimos least-squares
   criterion
criterio de validez validity criterion
criterios criteria
criterios de exclusión exclusion criteria
criterios de inclusión inclusion criteria
criterios de muerte death criteria
criterios de Schneider para personalidad
   depresiva schneiderian criteria for
   depressive personality
crítico critical
crocidismo crocidismus
croma chroma
cromafín chromaffin
cromafinoma chromaffinoma
cromafinopatía chromaffinopathy
cromaticidad chromaticity
cromático chromatic
cromátide chromatid
cromatina chromatin
cromatina-negativo chromatin-negative
cromatina-positivo chromatin-positive

cromatina sexual sex chromatin
cromatinólisis chromatinolysis
cromatofobia chromatophobia
cromatografía chromatography
cromatólisis chromatolysis
cromatólisis central central chromatolysis
cromatólisis retrógrada retrograde chromatolysis
cromatólisis transináptica transsynaptic chromatolysis
cromatolítico chromatolytic
cromatopsia chromatopsia
cromestesia chromesthesia
cromhidrosis chromhidrosis
cromidrosis chromidrosis
cromofobia chromophobia
cromólisis chromolysis
cromómero chromomere
cromopsia chromopsia
cromosoma chromosome
cromosoma acrocéntrico acrocentric chromosome
cromosoma anular ring chromosome
cromosoma sexual sex chromosome
cromosoma X X chromosome
cromosoma X frágil fragile X chromosome
cromosoma Y Y chromosome
cromosómico chromosomal
cromosómico chromosomic
cromoterapia chromotherapy
cromotopsia chromotopsia
cronaxia chronaxy
cronaxis chronaxis
cronicidad chronicity
crónico chronic
cronobiología chronobiology
cronofisiología chronophysiology
cronofobia chronophobia
cronognosis chronognosis
cronógrafo chronograph
cronometría chronometry
cronometría mental mental chronometry
cronométrica mental mental chronometrics
cronométrico chronometric
cronómetro de caída fall chronometer
cronoscopio chronoscope
cronotaraxia chronotaraxia
cronotaraxis chronotaraxis
cronoterapia chronotherapy
crucial crucial
crueldad cruelty
crueldad hacia animales animal cruelty
crusotomía crusotomy
cruzado crossed
Cryptococcus Cryptococcus
ctonofagia chthonophagy
cuadrado latino Latin square
cuadrados mínimos least-squares
cuadrantanopía quadrantanopia
cuadrantanopsia quadrantanopsia
cuadrante quadrant
cuadrigémino quadrigemina
cuadriparesia quadriparesis
cuadriplejía quadriplegia
cuadripléjico quadriplegic

cualidad quality
cualidad abstracta abstract quality
cualidad determinante determining quality
cualidad primaria primary quality
cualidad sensorial sensory quality
cualitativo qualitative
cuantal quantal
cuantitativo quantitative
cuanto quantum
cuantos quanta
cuartil quartile
cuarto de Ames Ames room
cuarto distorsionado distorted room
cuarto momento fourth moment
cuasiexperimental quasi-experimental
cuasigrupo quasi-group
cuasinecesidad quasi-need
cuaternidad quaternity
cuatro fases de la práctica médica four phases of medical practice
cuazepam quazepam
cubo de Necker Necker cube
cuco bogeyman
cuello neck
cuello de búfalo buffalo neck
cuello tieso stiff neck
cuello torcido wryneck
cuenta de palabras word count
cuenta de plaquetas platelet count
cuento de hadas fairy tale
cuerda del tímpano chorda tympani
cuerda vocal vocal cord
cuerdo sane
cuerno anterior anterior horn
cuerno lateral lateral horn
cuero cabelludo scalp
cuerpo body, corpus
cuerpo calloso corpus callosum
cuerpo cavernoso corpora cavernosa
cuerpo celular cell body
cuerpo contra mente body versus mind
cuerpo de arena sand body
cuerpo de Barr Barr body
cuerpo de Lafora Lafora body
cuerpo de Lewy Lewy body
cuerpo de Pick Pick's body
cuerpo de psamoma psammoma body
cuerpo de Verocay Verocay body
cuerpo de Wolf-Orton Wolf-Orton body
cuerpo esponjoso corpus spongiosum
cuerpo estriado corpus striatum
cuerpo estriado striate body
cuerpo F F body
cuerpo geniculado lateral lateral geniculate body
cuerpo geniculado medial medial geniculate body
cuerpo lúteo corpus luteum
cuerpo mamilar mammillary body
cuerpo olivar olivary body
cuerpo pineal pineal body
cuerpo polar polar body
cuerpo trapezoide trapezoid body
cuerpos arenáceos corpora arenacea
cuerpos citoides cytoid bodies

cuerpos cuadrigéminos corpora quadrigemina
cuerpos de Nissl Nissl bodies
cuerpos geniculados geniculate bodies
cuestión issue
cuestión central central issue
cuestión naturaleza-crianza nature-nurture
    issue
cuestionario questionnaire
cuestionario de historial personal
    personal-history questionnaire
cuestionario de Holmes-Rahe Holmes-Rahe
    questionnaire
cuestionario de opiniones opinionaire
cuestiones económicas del divorcio economic
    issues of divorce
cuestiones éticas ethical issues
cuestiones éticas en el derecho a tratamiento
    ethical issues in right to treatment
cuestiones éticas en la clasificación ethical
    issues in classification
cuestiones éticas en la educación ethical
    issues in education
cuestiones éticas en la negligencia profesional
    ethical issues in malpractice
cuestiones éticas en la psicología ethical
    issues in psychology
cuestiones éticas en la psicología correccional
    ethical issues in correctional psychology
cuestiones éticas en la psiquiatría ethical
    issues in psychiatry
cuestiones éticas y consentimiento informado
    ethical issues and informed consent
cuestiones éticas y la confidencialidad ethical
    issues and confidentiality
cuidado care
cuidado a largo plazo long-term care
cuidado administrado managed care
cuidado adoptivo adoptive care
cuidado alterno alternate care
cuidado ambulatorio ambulatory care
cuidado auxiliar ancillary care
cuidado comunitario community care
cuidado custodial custodial care
cuidado de acompañante attendant care
cuidado de ancianos care of elderly
cuidado de familia adoptiva foster-family
    care
cuidado de la cría care of young
cuidado de niños child-care
cuidado de salud health care
cuidado de salud mental administrado
    managed mental health care
cuidado de salud primario primary health
    care
cuidado dental dental care
cuidado diurno day care
cuidado diurno en el hogar del niño day care
    in the child's home
cuidado domiciliario domiciliary care
cuidado en el hogar home care
cuidado en refugio shelter care
cuidado extendido extended care
cuidado familiar family care
cuidado institucional institutional care
cuidado intensivo intensive care

cuidado médico medical care
cuidado prenatal prenatal care
cuidado residencial residential care
cuidado terminal terminal care
cuidado y protección care and protection
cuidados maternales mothering
cuidados maternales pobres poor mothering
cuidados maternales suficientemente buenos
    good-enough mothering
cuidados maternos múltiples multiple
    mothering
cuidante caregiver
cuidante en la red social del niño caregiver
    in child's social network
culmen culmen
culpa blame
culpabilidad guilt
culpabilidad de supervivencia survival guilt
culpabilidad de supervivientes survivor guilt
culpabilidad inconsciente unconscious guilt
culpabilidad neurótica neurotic guilt
culpabilidad patológica pathological guilt
culpabilidad sexual sexual guilt
culpable guilty
culpando a la víctima blaming the victim
culto cult
culto de héroes hero worship
culto de personalidad cult of personality
cultura culture
cultura coexistente coexistent culture
cultura cofigurativa cofigurative culture
cultura de drogas drug culture
cultura de niños children's culture
cultura falocéntrica phallocentric culture
cultura familiar family culture
cultura familiar indígena indigenous family
    culture
cultura popular folkways
cultura prefigurativa prefigurative culture
cultural cultural
culturalistas culturalists
cumarina coumarin
cumulativo cumulative
cuneiforme cuneate
cunilición cunnilinction
cunilingüista cunnilinguist
cunilingus cunnilingus
cunnus cunnus
cura de transferencia transference cure
cura por fe faith cure
curación healing
curación holísitica holistic healing
curación mental mental healing
curación popular folk healing
curación por fe faith healing
curador healer
curandero popular folk healer
curar heal
curare curare
curiosidad curiosity
curiosidad sexual sexual curiosity
currículo curriculum
curso de acción action stream
curso de vida life course
curtosis kurtosis

curva curve
curva de absorción espectral
  spectral-absorption curve
curva de aprendizaje learning curve
curva de crecimiento growth curve
curva de distribución distribution curve
curva de Ebbinghaus Ebbinghaus curve
curva de emisiones espectrales
  spectral-emission curve
curva de frecuencias frequency curve
curva de frecuencias cumulativas cumulative
  frequency curve
curva de Gompertz Gompertz curve
curva de luminosidad luminosity curve
curva de memoria memory curve
curva de moduladores modulator curve
curva de olvido forgetting curve
curva de posición serial serial-position curve
curva de práctica practice curve
curva de probabilidades probability curve
curva de probabilidades normal normal
  probability curve
curva de regresión regression curve
curva de respuestas cumulativas cumulative
  response curve
curva de retención retention curve
curva de retención de Ebbinghaus
  Ebbinghaus curve of retention
curva de sensibilidad espectral
  spectral-sensitivity curve
curva de sensibilidad fotópica
  photopic-sensitivity curve
curva de sumación summation curve
curva de Vincent Vincent curve
curva de visibilidad visibility curve
curva de Zipf Zipf curve
curva en forma de campana bell-shaped
  curve
curva en J J curve
curva en mariposa butterfly curve
curva en S S-curve
curva en U invertida inverted-U curve
curva gauseana gaussian curve
curva logarítmica logarithmic curve
curva logística logistic curve
curva meningítica meningitic curve
curva normal normal curve
curva parética paretic curve
curva tabética tabetic curve
curvatura espinal spinal curvature
curvilíneo curvilinear
cushingoide cushingoid
custodia custody
custodia conjunta joint custody
custodia dividida split custody
custodia física physical custody
custodia legal legal custody
custodia única single custody
custodio caretaker
custodio primario primary caretaker
cutáneo cutaneous

CH

chaleco de fuerza straitjacket
chamán shaman
chancroide chancroid
chica de cita call girl
chico de cita call boy
chivo expiatorio scapegoat
choque shock
choque cultural cultural shock
choque de paradigmas paradigm clash
choque de piel eléctrico electric skin shock
choque del futuro future shock
choque delirante delirious shock
choque demorado delayed shock
choque depresivo depressive crash
choque diferido deferred shock
choque eléctrico electric shock
choque electroconvulsivo electroconvulsive
  shock
choque eretístico erethistic shock
choque espinal spinal shock
choque insulínico insulin shock
choque irreversible irreversible shock
choque por casquillos shell shock
choque por interrupción break shock
choque primario primary shock
choque psicodramático psychodramatic shock
choque reversible reversible shock
choque tetanizante tetanizing shock
choque traumático traumatic shock
choque vasogénico vasogenic shock
chuparse el pulgar thumb-sucking
chupete pacifier

D

dactiloespasmo dactylospasm
dactilología dactylology
dada de alta discharge
dada de alta involuntaria involuntary
   discharge
dador de datos fact-giver
daltonismo daltonism
dantroleno dantrolene
danza de San Antonio Saint Anthony's dance
danza de San Juan Saint John's dance
danza de San Vito Saint Vitus dance
daño cerebral brain damage
daño cerebral mínimo minimal brain damage
daño cerebral y trastornos psiquiátricos
   brain damage and psychiatric disorders
daño propio self-harm
daño propio deliberado deliberate self-harm
dapsona dapsone
dar y tomar give-and-take
dardo y cúpula dart and dome
darwinismo darwinism
darwinismo social social darwinism
Dasein Dasein
dato datum
dato sensorial sense datum
datos data
datos biográficos biographical data
datos de identificación identifying data
datos del personal personnel data
datos en bruto raw data
datos primarios primary data
datos Q Q data
Dauerschlaf Dauerschlaf
deber duty
deber de advertir duty to warn
debilidad debility
debilidad de color color weakness
debilidad del ego ego weakness
debilidad mental feeble-mindedness
debilidad somática somatic weakness
debrisoquina debrisoquin
decadencia decadence
decalaje decalage
decalaje horizontal horizontal decalage
decalaje oblicuo oblique decalage
decanoato decanoate
deceleración deceleration
decepción deception
decepción de memoria reduplicativa
   reduplicative memory deception
decibel decibel
decil decile
décimo nervio craneal tenth cranial nerve
decisión decision

decisión abortiva abortive decision
decisión automática automatic decision
decisión de Brawner Brawner decision
decisión de Gault Gault decision
decisión de grupo group decision
declaración statement
declaración condicional conditional statement
declaración de derechos bill of rights
declarativo declarative
declinación de memoria asociada con la edad
   age-associated memory decline
decremento decrement
decremento cognitivo cognitive decrement
decremento de trabajo work decrement
decremento social social decrement
decúbito decubitus
decusación decussation
dedo en gatillo trigger finger, jerk finger
dedo en resorte spring finger
deducción deduction
deductivo deductive
defectivo defective
defecto defect
defecto bioquímico biochemical defect
defecto cognitivo cognitive defect
defecto congénito congenital defect
defecto de campo field defect
defecto de campo cuadrántico homónimo
   homonymous quadrantic field defect
defecto de campo visual visual-field defect
defecto de conciencia awareness defect
defecto de gen único single-gene defect
defecto de memoria memory defect
defecto de nacimiento birth defect
defecto de tubo neural neural-tube defect
defecto de visuoconstrucción
   visuoconstruction defect
defecto genético genetic defect
defecto metabólico metabolic defect
defecto neurológico neurological defect
defecto óptico optical defect
defecto orgánico organic defect
defecto orgánico del sistema nervioso central
   organic defect of the central nervous
   system
defecto perceptivo perceptual defect
defecto sensorial sensory defect
defecto teratológico teratological defect
defectos de nacimiento de genitales birth
   defects of genitalia
defendencia defendance
defendible defensible
defensa defense
defensa cubriente screen defense
defensa de insania insanity defense
defensa del carácter character defense
defensa del ego ego defense
defensa madura mature defense
defensa neurótica neurotic defense
defensa perceptiva perceptual defense
defensas del ego y conducta violenta ego
   defenses and violent behavior
defensivo defensive
defensor advocate
deferencia deference

deficiencia deficiency
deficiencia de ácido nicotínico nicotinic acid
  deficiency
deficiencia de calcio calcium deficiency
deficiencia de color color deficiency
deficiencia de hemisferio hemisphere
  deficiency
deficiencia de proteína protein deficiency
deficiencia de tiamina thiamine deficiency
deficiencia de vitamina vitamin deficiency
deficiencia dietética dietary deficiency
deficiencia mental mental deficiency
deficiencia mental primaria primary mental
  deficiency
deficiencia mental secundaria secondary
  mental deficiency
deficiencia nutricional nutritional deficiency
déficit deficit
déficit cognitivo cognitive deficit
déficit de atención attention deficit
déficit de destrezas sociales social skills
  deficit
déficit de perseveración perseveration deficit
déficit de relaciones interpersonales
  interpersonal relationship deficit
déficit del desarrollo developmental deficit
déficit del lenguaje language deficit
déficit del lenguaje y abuso de niños
  language deficit and child abuse
déficit del lenguaje y daño cerebral language
  deficit and brain damage
déficit del lenguaje y pruebas de inteligencia
  language deficit and intelligence tests
déficit ipsilateral ipsilateral deficit
déficit perceptivo perceptual deficit
déficit psicológico psychological deficit
déficit sensorial sensory deficit
déficits cognitivos en niños abusados
  cognitive deficits in abused children
déficits cognitivos y daño cerebral cognitive
  deficits and brain damage
**déficits del desarrollo en trastorno de
  personalidad fronteriza** developmental
  deficits in borderline personality disorder
déficits perceptivos y daño cerebral
  perceptual deficits and brain damage
definición definition
definición nominal nominal definition
definición operacional operational definition
definición real real definition
definitivo definitive
deflexión deflection
deformación deformation
deformación del yo deformation of the self
deformidad deformity
deformidad congénita congenital deformity
deformidad de Arnold-Chiari Arnold-Chiari
  deformity
deformidad del sistema esqueletal
  skeletal-system deformity
deformidad selar en J J-sella deformity
degeneración degeneration
degeneración adiposogenital adiposogenital
  degeneration
degeneración anterógrada anterograde

degeneration
degeneración ascendente ascending
  degeneration
degeneración cerebelosa progresiva primaria
  primary progressive cerebellar
  degeneration
degeneración cerebelosa subaguda subacute
  cerebellar degeneration
degeneración cerebromacular
  cerebromacular degeneration
**degeneración combinada subaguda de la
  médula espinal** subacute combined
  degeneration of the spinal cord
degeneración de Turck Turck's degeneration
degeneración descendiente descending
  degeneration
degeneración esponjosa spongy degeneration
degeneración fascicular fascicular
  degeneration
degeneración focal focal degeneration
degeneración granulovacuolar
  granulovacuolar degeneration
degeneración gris gray degeneration
degeneración hepatolenticular
  hepatolenticular degeneration
degeneración neuroaxonal neuroaxonal
  degeneration
degeneración neurofibrilar neurofibrillary
  degeneration
degeneración neuronal neuronal degeneration
degeneración neuronal infantil infantile
  neuronal degeneration
degeneración neuronal primaria primary
  neuronal degeneration
degeneración olivopontocerebelosa
  olivopontocerebellar degeneration
degeneración ortógrada orthograde
  degeneration
degeneración presenil presenile degeneration
degeneración progresiva lenticular lenticular
  progressive degeneration
degeneración retinodiencefálica
  retinodiencephalic degeneration
degeneración retrógrada retrograde
  degeneration
degeneración secundaria secondary
  degeneration
degeneración transináptica transsynaptic
  degeneration
degeneración transneuronal transneuronal
  degeneration
degeneración walleriana wallerian
  degeneration
degenerado degenerate
degenerativo degenerative
degradación degradation
degradado degraded
degustación degustation
dehidroisoandrosterona
  dehydroisoandrosterone
deixis deixis
déjà entendu déjà entendu
déjà eprouvé déjà eprouvé
déjà fait déjà fait
déjà pensé déjà pensé

déjà raconté déjà raconté
déjà vécu déjà vécu
déjà voulu déjà voulu
déjà vu déjà vu
dejo aftertaste
deleción deletion
deletreo con dedos finger spelling
deliberado deliberate
delincuencia delinquency
delincuencia adaptiva adaptive delinquency
delincuencia geriátrica geriatric delinquency
delincuencia juvenil juvenile delinquency
delincuente delinquent
delirante delirious
delirio delirium
delirio agudo acute delirium
delirio anfetamina amphetamine delirium
delirio ansioso anxious delirium
delirio bajo low delirium
delirio de abstinencia abstinence delirium
delirio de agotamiento exhaustion delirium
delirio de alcohol alcohol delirium
delirio de alucinógeno hallucinogen delirium
delirio de ansiolítico anxiolytic delirium
delirio de belladona belladonna delirium
delirio de cannabis cannabis delirium
delirio de cloruro de amonio ammonium
  chloride delirium
delirio de cocaína cocaine delirium
delirio de fenciclidina phencyclidine delirium
delirio de hipnótico hypnotic delirium
delirio de inhalante inhalant delirium
delirio de metamorfosis delirium of
  metamorphosis
delirio de opioide opioid delirium
delirio de otra sustancia other substance
  delirium
delirio de persecución delirium of persecution
delirio de retiro withdrawal delirium
delirio de sedante sedative delirium
delirio de sustancia desconocida unknown
  substance delirium
delirio debido a condición médica general
  delirium due to general medical condition
delirio del retiro de alcohol alcohol
  withdrawal delirium
delirio del retiro de barbituratos barbiturate
  withdrawal delirium
delirio en enfermedad aguda delirium in
  acute illness
delirio enfocado focused delirium
delirio grave delirium grave
delirio murmurante muttering delirium
delirio musitante delirium mussitans
delirio ocupacional occupational delirium
delirio orgánico organic delirium
delirio por colapso collapse delirium
delirio por sustancia psicoactiva
  psychoactive substance delirium
delirio posoperatorio postoperative delirium
delirio postraumático posttraumatic delirium
delirio relacionado con sustancia
  substance-related delirium
delirio senil senile delirium
delirio simpatomimético sympathomimetic

delirium
delirio tóxico toxic delirium
delirio traumático traumatic delirium
delirium tremens delirium tremens
delirium verborum delirium verborum
delorazepam delorazepam
delta delta
delusión delusion
delusión aislada isolated delusion
delusión alopsíquica allopsychic delusion
delusión autóctona autochthonous delusion
delusión autopsíquica autopsychic delusion
delusión de autoacusación delusion of
  self-accusation
delusión de celos delusion of jealousy
delusión de control delusion of control
delusión de empobrecimiento delusion of
  impoverishment
delusión de estar controlado delusion of
  being controlled
delusión de grandeza delusion of grandeur
delusión de grandeza grandiose delusion
delusión de infestación infestation delusion
delusión de infidelidad delusion of infidelity
delusión de influencia delusion of influence
delusión de interpretación interpretation
  delusion
delusión de Mignon Mignon delusion
delusión de negación delusion of negation
delusión de observación delusion of
  observation
delusión de pasividad delusion of passivity
delusión de pecado y culpabilidad delusion
  of sin and guilt
delusión de persecución delusion of
  persecution
delusión de pobreza delusion of poverty
delusión de referencia delusion of reference
delusión del humor congruente
  mood-congruent delusion
delusión del humor incongruente
  mood-incongruent delusion
delusión dismórfica dysmorphic delusion
delusión encapsulada encapsulated delusion
delusión erótica erotic delusion
delusión estrambótica bizarre delusion
delusión expansiva expansive delusion
delusión fragmentado fragmentary delusion
delusión hipocondríaca hypochondriacal
  delusion
delusión nihilística nihilistic delusion
delusión no sistematizada unsystematized
  delusion
delusión paranoide paranoid delusion
delusión persecutoria persecutory delusion
delusión psicótica psychotic delusion
delusión reformista reformist delusion
delusión religiosa religious delusion
delusión sexual sexual delusion
delusión sistematizada systematized delusion
delusión somática somatic delusion
delusión somatopsíquica somatopsychic
  delusion
delusiones múltiples multiple delusions
delusorio delusional

demarcación demarcation
demencia dementia
demencia alcohólica alcoholic dementia
demencia apopléctica dementia apoplectica
demencia arterioesclerótica arteriosclerotic dementia
demencia asociada con alcoholismo dementia associated with alcoholism
demencia atrófica atrophic dementia
demencia atrófica abiotrófica abiotrophic atrophic dementia
demencia catatónica catatonic dementia
demencia de alcohol alcohol dementia
demencia de Alzheimer Alzheimer's dementia
demencia de ancianos elderly dementia
demencia de Binswagner Binswanger's dementia
demencia de boxeador boxer's dementia
demencia de droga nootrópica de tipo de Alzheimer nootropic drug dementia of Alzheimer type
demencia de noradrenalina de tipo de Alzheimer noradrenaline dementia of Alzheimer type
demencia de tipo Alzheimer dementia of Alzheimer type
demencia de Wernicke Wernicke's dementia
demencia degenerativa degenerative dementia
demencia degenerativa primaria primary degenerative dementia
demencia degenerativa primaria de tipo Alzheimer primary degenerative dementia of Alzheimer type
demencia dialítica dementia dialytica
demencia epiléptica epileptic dementia
demencia hebefrénica hebephrenic dementia
demencia mioclónica myoclonic dementia
demencia multiinfarto multiinfarct dementia
demencia orgánica organic dementia
demencia paralítica dementia paralytica
demencia paralítica de Lissauer Lissauer's dementia paralytica
demencia paranoide dementia paranoides
demencia persistente de alcohol alcohol persisting dementia
demencia persistente de ansiolítico anxiolytic persisting dementia
demencia persistente de hipnótico hypnotic persisting dementia
demencia persistente de inhalante inhalant persistent dementia
demencia persistente de otra sustancia other substance persisting dementia
demencia persistente de sedante sedative persisting dementia
demencia persistente de sustancia desconocida unknown substance persisting dementia
demencia persistente inducida por sustancia substance-induced persisting dementia
demencia por diálisis dialysis dementia
demencia por drogas drug dementia
demencia por sustancia psicoactiva psychoactive substance dementia
demencia postraumática posttraumatic dementia
demencia precoz dementia praecox
demencia presenil dementia praesenilis
demencia primaria primary dementia
demencia pugilística dementia pugilistica
demencia secundaria secondary dementia
demencia semántica semantic dementia
demencia senil senile dementia
demencia senil de tipo Alzheimer senile dementia of Alzheimer type
demencia senil primaria primary senile dementia
demencia subcortical subcortical dementia
demencia tóxica toxic dementia
demencia vascular vascular dementia
demente demented
demofobia demophobia
demografía demography
demográfico demographic
demoníaco demonic
demonofobia demonophobia
demonología demonology
demonológico demonologic
demonomanía demonomania
demora delay
demora de fase phase delay
demora de gratificación delay of gratification
demora de recompensa delay of reward
demora de refuerzo delay of reinforcement
demora del desarrollo developmental delay
demora sináptica synaptic delay
demora tras cambio change-over delay
demorado delayed
demostración demonstration
demostración de afecto affect display
demostración facial facial display
demostraciones Ames Ames demonstrations
dendrita dendrite
dendrofilia dendrophily
dendrofilia dendrophilia
denegación escolar school refusal
denotación denotation
denotativo denotative
densidad density
densidad de movimientos oculares rápidos rapid eye movement density
densidad de probabilidades probability density
densidad espacial spatial density
densidad externa outside density
densidad interna inside density
densidad poblacional population density
densidad social social density
densidad tonal tonal density
densitometría retinal retinal densitometry
dental dental
dentatectomía dentatectomy
deontología deontology
dependencia dependency
dependencia anfetamina amphetamine dependence
dependencia cruzada cross-dependence
dependencia cruzada de alucinógenos

cross-dependence of hallucinogens
dependencia de alcohol alcohol dependence
dependencia de alucinógeno hallucinogen dependence
dependencia de ansiolítico anxiolytic dependence
dependencia de campo field dependence
dependencia de cannabis cannabis dependence
dependencia de cocaína cocaine dependence
dependencia de codeína codeine dependence
dependencia de dosis terapéutica therapeutic dose dependency
dependencia de drogas drug dependence
dependencia de fenciclidina phencyclidine dependence
dependencia de hipnótico hypnotic dependence
dependencia de inhalante inhalant dependence
dependencia de morfina morphine dependence
dependencia de nicotina nicotine dependence
dependencia de opio opium dependence
dependencia de opioide opioid dependence
dependencia de otra sustancia other substance dependence
dependencia de propoxifeno propoxyphene dependence
dependencia de sedante sedative dependence
dependencia de solvente volátil volatile solvent dependence
dependencia de sustancia substance dependence
dependencia de sustancia desconocida unknown substance dependence
dependencia de sustancia no especificada unspecified substance dependence
dependencia de sustancia psicoactiva psychoactive substance dependence
dependencia de tabaco tobacco dependence
dependencia de terapia dependence on therapy
dependencia del estado state dependence
dependencia emocional emotional dependence
dependencia estadística statistical dependence
dependencia física physical dependence
dependencia fisiológica physiological dependence
dependencia instrumental instrumental dependence
dependencia mórbida morbid dependency
dependencia narcótica narcotic dependence
dependencia oral oral dependence
dependencia pasiva passive dependency
dependencia psicológica psychological dependence
dependencia química chemical dependence
dependencia remota remote dependency
dependiente dependent
dependiente del estado state-dependent
depletivo depletive
deportes con sillas de ruedas wheelchair sports

depravación depravation
depravado depraved
depresión depression
depresión agitada agitated depression
depresión aguda acute depression
depresión anaclítica anaclitic depression
depresión ansiosa anxious depression
depresión atípica atypical depression
depresión autónoma autonomous depression
depresión causada por separación depression caused by separation
depresión clásica classical depression
depresión con ansiedad anxiety depression
depresión contra esquizofrenia depression versus schizophrenia
depresión contra síndrome mental orgánico depression versus organic mental syndrome
depresión contra trastorno de ansiedad depression versus anxiety disorder
depresión crónica chronic depression
depresión de ancianos elderly depression
depresión de autoculpación self-blaming depression
depresión de episodio único single-episode depression
depresión de maternidad maternity blues
depresión de paternidad paternity blues
depresión del padre father blues
depresión delusoria delusional depression
depresión doble double depression
depresión e impotencia aprendida depression and learned helplessness
depresión en adolescentes depression in adolescents
depresión en adultez depression in adulthood
depresión en niños abusados depression in abused children
depresión en preadolescentes depression in preadolescents
depresión endógena endogenous depression
depresión endogenomórfica endogenomorphic depression
depresión enmascarada masked depression
depresión estuporosa stuporous depression
depresión exógena exogenous depression
depresión leve mild depression
depresión maternal maternal depression
depresión mayor major depression
depresión menopáusica menopausal depression
depresión moderada moderate depression
depresión monopolar monopolar depression
depresión neurótica neurotic depression
depresión no reactiva nonreactive depression
depresión involutiva involutional depression
depresión posictal postictal depression
depresión posesquizofrénica postschizophrenic depression
depresión posparto postpartum depression
depresión primal primal depression
depresión profunda deep depression
depresión propagante spreading depression
depresión psicótica psychotic depression
depresión reactiva reactive depression
depresión recurrente recurrent depression

depresión respiratoria respiratory depression
depresión retardada retarded depression
depresión secundaria secondary depression
depresión simple simple depression
depresión situacional situational depression
depresión temporal seasonal depression
depresión tras muerte parental depression following parental death
depresión unipolar unipolar depression
depresión y ansiedad depression and anxiety
depresión y conducta suicida depression and suicidal behavior
depresión y suicidio depression and suicide
depresión y trastornos de ansiedad depression and anxiety disorders
depresivo depressive
depresivo del sistema nervioso central central nervous system depressant
depresomotor depressomotor
depresor depressor
deprimido depressed
depurar debug
derecho a tratamiento right to treatment
derecho de rehusar tratamiento right to refuse treatment
derecho de salud health law
derecho familiar family law
derecho moral moral right
derechos de los incapacitados rights of the disabled
derechos de niños children's rights
derechos de niños para consentir a tratamiento children's rights to consent to treatment
derechos de niños para rehusar tratamiento children's rights to refuse treatment
derechos de pacientes rights of patients
derechos de personas retardadas mentalmente mentally retarded persons' rights
derechos legales legal rights
dereísmo dereism
dereístico dereistic
derivación derivation, bypass
derivación extraintracraneal extraintracranial bypass
derivación inversa inverse derivation
derivado derivative
derivado del alcohol alcohol derivative
derivado del indol indole derivative
dermatitis dermatitis
dermatitis de dedo anular ring-finger dermatitis
dermatitis por contacto contact dermatitis
dermatofobia dermatophobia
dermatoglifo dermatoglyphics
dermatoma dermatome
dermatoneurosis dermatoneurosis
dermatosiofobia dermatosiophobia
dermatotlasia dermatothlasia
dermatozoico dermatozoic
dermografía dermographia
dermoneurosis dermoneurosis
desaferentación deafferentation
desafío defiance

desagradable unpleasant
desagregación disaggregation
desagresivización deaggressivization
desaliento dejection
desambiguación disambiguation
desanalizar deanalize
desarrollo development
desarrollo adolescente adolescent development
desarrollo adulto adult development
desarrollo afectivo affective development
desarrollo anormal abnormal development
desarrollo atípico atypical development
desarrollo cefalocaudal cephalocaudal development
desarrollo cognitivo cognitive development
desarrollo cognitivo en adultos cognitive development in adults
desarrollo cognitivo y desarrollo del lenguaje cognitive development and language development
desarrollo conceptual conceptual development
desarrollo conductual behavioral development
desarrollo de apoyo del ego development of ego support
desarrollo de atención development of attention
desarrollo de carácter character development
desarrollo de carrera career development
desarrollo de cognición development of cognition
desarrollo de currículo curriculum development
desarrollo de destrezas interpersonales interpersonal skills development
desarrollo de emociones development of emotions
desarrollo de género gender development
desarrollo de identidad identity development
desarrollo de infantes infant development
desarrollo de juego play development
desarrollo de la conducta humana development of human behavior
desarrollo de lapso de vida life-span development
desarrollo de niñez temprana early childhood development
desarrollo de niños child development
desarrollo de papel de género gender-role development
desarrollo de papel sexual sex-role development
desarrollo de percepción development of perception
desarrollo de personalidad personality development
desarrollo de personalidad atípica atypical personality development
desarrollo de temor development of fear
desarrollo del ego ego development
desarrollo del habla speech development
desarrollo del lenguaje development of language

desarrollo del lenguaje en balbuceo language development in babbling
desarrollo emocional emotional development
desarrollo fetal fetal development
desarrollo físico physical development
desarrollo fonológico phonological development
desarrollo genital genital development
desarrollo humano human development
desarrollo intelectual intellectual development
desarrollo intelectual adulto adult intellectual development
desarrollo mental mental development
desarrollo moral moral development
desarrollo motor motor development
desarrollo neonatal neonatal development
desarrollo neurológico neurological development
desarrollo neuropsicológico neuropsychological development
desarrollo normal normal development
desarrollo perceptivo perceptual development
desarrollo personal personal development
desarrollo precoz precocious development
desarrollo prehabla prespeech development
desarrollo prenatal prenatal development
desarrollo prenatal y abuso de alcohol prenatal development and alcohol abuse
desarrollo prenatal y abuso de drogas prenatal development and drug abuse
desarrollo proximodistal proximodistal development
desarrollo psicosexual psychosexual development
desarrollo psicosexual en adolescencia psychosexual development in adolescence
desarrollo psicosocial psychosocial development
desarrollo sensorimotor sensorimotor development
desarrollo sexual sexual development
desarrollo social social development
desarrollo vocacional vocational development
desarrollo y ambiente development and environment
desastre disaster
desastre natural natural disaster
desatención hemiespacial hemispatial neglect
desaventajado disadvantaged
desaventajado culturalmente culturally disadvantaged
descarga discharge
descarga afectiva affective discharge
descarga catéctica cathectic discharge
descarga de afecto discharge of affect
descarga de ansiedad anxiety discharge
descarga de cancelación cancellation discharge
descarga demorada delayed discharge
descarga emocional emotional release
descarga espontanea spontaneous discharge
descarga neural neural discharge
descarga persistente afterdischarge
descarga seminal seminal discharge
descarrilamiento derailment

descarrilamiento cognitivo cognitive derailment
descarrilamiento de pensamientos thought derailment
descarrilamiento de volición derailment of volition
descarrilamiento del habla speech derailment
descatexis decathexis
descendencia matrilineal matrilineal descent
descendencia patrilineal patrilineal descent
descendiente descending
descentración decentration
descentración afectiva affective decentration
descentralización decentralization
descentramiento decentering
descentrar decenter
descerebración decerebration
descerebración sin sangre bloodless decerebration
descerebrardo decerebrate
descerebrizar decerebrize
descodificación decoding
descodificar decode
descompensación decompensation
descomponer decompose
descomposición decomposition
descomposición de movimiento decomposition of movement
descomposición del ego decomposition of ego
descompresión decompression
descompresión cerebral cerebral decompression
descompresión espinal spinal decompression
descompresión interna internal decompression
descompresión nerviosa nerve decompression
descompresión orbital orbital decompression
descompresión suboccipital suboccipital decompression
descompresión subtemporal subtemporal decompression
descompresión trigeminal trigeminal decompression
descondicionamiento deconditioning
desconexión disconnection
desconexión periódica gating
desconexión periódica sensorial sensory gating
desconfiabilidad unreliability
desconfiable unreliable
desconfianza mistrust
desconfianza básica basic mistrust
desconfianza contra confianza mistrust versus trust
descontextualización decontextualization
descontrol dyscontrol
descontrol de emergencia emergency dyscontrol
descontrol episódico episodic dyscontrol
descontrol instintivo instinctual dyscontrol
descontrol por acceso seizure dyscontrol
descorticación decortication
descorticación cerebral cerebral decortication
descorticación reversible reversible decortication

descorticar decorticate
descortización decortization
descripción description
descripción de conducta description of behavior
descriptar decrypt
descriptivo descriptive
descubrimiento discovery
descubrimiento de casos case finding
descubrimiento de concepto concept discovery
desdiferenciación dedifferentiation
deseabilidad social social desirability
desempeño de papeles role-playing
desempeño de papeles múltiples multiple-role playing
desempleo unemployment
desensibilización desensitization
desensibilización automatizada automated desensitization
desensibilización de contacto contact desensitization
desensibilización imaginal imaginal desensitization
desensibilización sistemática systematic desensitization
deseo wish, desire
deseo de incesto incest wish
deseo de libido libido wish
deseo de muerte death wish
deseo de recuperación recovery wish
deseo del id id wish
deseo hijo-pene child-penis wish
deseo incestuoso incestuous desire
deseo irracional irrational desire
deseo sexual sexual desire
deseo sexual deteriorado impaired sexual desire
deseo sexual hiperactivo hyperactive sexual desire
deseo sexual hipoactivo hypoactive sexual desire
deseo sexual hipoactivo situacional situational hypoactive sexual desire
deseo sexual inhibido inhibited sexual desire
deseo-sueño masoquista masochistic wish-dream
desequilibrio imbalance
desequilibrio aminoácido amino acid imbalance
desequilibrio autónomo autonomic imbalance
desequilibrio de electrólito electrolyte imbalance
desequilibrio del desarrollo developmental imbalance
desequilibrio estructural structural imbalance
desequilibrio simpático sympathetic imbalance
desequilibrio vasomotor vasomotor imbalance
deserotizar deerotize
deserpidina deserpidine
desesperación desperation
desesperado despairing
desexualización desexualization

desfeminación defemination
desfiguración disfigurement
desfiguración facial facial disfigurement
desfusión defusion
desganglionar deganglionate
desgaste attrition
desgenitalización degenitalization
deshabituación dishabituation
deshidratación dehydration
deshipnotizar dehypnotize
deshumanización dehumanization
designante allocator
desilusión disillusionment
desimbolización desymbolization
desincentivo disincentive
desincrónico desynchronous
desincronización desynchronization
desincronizado desynchronized
desincronosis desynchronosis
desincronosis circadiano circadian desynchronosis
desindividuación deindividuation
desindividuación en grupos deindividuation in groups
desinhibición disinhibition
desinhibición conductual behavioral disinhibition
desinhibido uninhibited
desinstintualización deinstinctualization
desinstitucionalización deinstitutionalization
desintegración disintegration
desintegración de personalidad disintegration of personality
desintegración social social disintegration
desintegrante disintegrative
desipramina desipramine
deslibidinización delibidinization
desliz freudiano freudian slip
desmayarse faint
desmayo faint
desmayo alcohólico alcoholic blackout
desmayo parcial gray-out
desmembración dismemberment
desmetildiazepam desmethyldiazepam
desmetilimipramina desmethylimipramine
desmielinación demyelination
desmielinización demyelinization
desmielinizante demyelinating
desmodinia desmodynia
desmopresina desmopressin
desmoralización demoralization
desmoralizado demoralized
desmorfinización demorphinization
desnarcisismo denarcissism
desnervación denervation
desnervar denervate
desneutralización deneutralization
desnutrición malnutrition
desnutrición fetal fetal malnutrition
desobediencia disobedience
desobediencia civil civil disobedience
desobediente disobedient
desocialización desocialization
desoralidad deorality
desorganización disorganization

desorganización autónoma autonomic
  disorganization
desorganización cerebral cerebral
  disorganization
desorganización conceptual conceptual
  disorganization
desorganización de pensamientos thought
  disorganization
desorganización personal personal
  disorganization
desorganizado disorganized
desorientación disorientation
desorientación del tiempo time disorientation
desorientación derecha-izquierda right-left
  disorientation
desorientación topográfica topographical
  disorientation
desparramamiento scattering
despeciación despeciation
despersonalización depersonalization
despersonificación depersonification
despertamiento arousal
despertamiento autónomo autonomic arousal
despertamiento de impulso drive arousal
despertamiento de necesidades need arousal
despertamiento emocional emotional arousal
despertamiento general general arousal
despertamiento sexual sexual arousal
despertamiento sexual hiperactivo
  hyperactive sexual arousal
despertamiento sexual hipoactivo hypoactive
  sexual arousal
despertamiento sexual inhibido inhibited
  sexual arousal
despertamiento y emociones arousal and
  emotions
desplacer previo foredispleasure
desplazado displaced
desplazamiento displacement
desplazamiento de afecto affect displacement
desplazamiento de conflicto conflict
  displacement
desplazamiento de costos cost shifting
desplazamiento de Doppler Doppler shift
desplazamiento de impulso drive
  displacement
desplazamiento del afecto displacement of
  affect
desplazamiento en el lenguaje displacement
  in language
desplazamiento forzado forced displacement
desplazamiento relacionado al trabajo
  job-related displacement
desplazamiento simbólico symbolic
  displacement
despoblación depopulation
despolarización depolarization
despreciativo contemptuous
desprecio contempt
desprendido detached
desprendimiento detachment
desprendimiento intelectual intellectual
  detachment
desprendimiento somnoliento somnolent
  detachment

desprogramación deprogramming
desrealización derealization
destete weaning
destete psicológico psychological weaning
destino destination, fate
destino común common fate
destoxicación detoxication
destoxificación detoxification
destoxificación de alcohol alcohol
  detoxification
destreza skill
destreza para bregar del ego ego-coping skill
destreza fundamental fundamental skill
destreza manual manual dexterity
destreza visual-motora visual-motor skill
destrezas adaptivas adaptive skills
destrezas adjuntas adjunctive skills
destrezas auditivas auditory skills
destrezas básicas basic skills
destrezas de comunicación communication
  skills
destrezas de lectura reading skills
destrezas de motor fino fine motor skills
destrezas de motor grueso gross motor skills
destrezas de nivel superior higher-level skills
destrezas de reconocimiento de palabras
  word-recognition skills
destrezas del diario vivir daily living skills
destrezas del lenguaje language skills
destrezas del lenguaje expresivas expressive
  language skills
destrezas funcionales functional skills
destrezas interpersonales interpersonal skills
destrezas motoras motor skills
destrezas para bregar coping skills
destrezas para bregar y niños abusados
  coping skills and abused children
destrezas perceptiva-motoras
  perceptual-motor skills
destrezas sociales social skills
destrezas genéricas generic skills
destronamiento dethroning
destructividad destructiveness
destructividad en conducta de juego
  destructiveness in play behavior
destructivo destructive
destrudo destrudo
desuso disuse
desutilidad disutility
desvanecimiento fading
desvanecimiento de estímulo stimulus fading
desventaja ambiental environmental
  disadvantage
desvergüenza shamelessness
desviación deviation
desviación cuartílica quartile deviation
desviación de comunicación communication
  deviance
desviación de conflicto conflict detouring
desviación de respuestas response deviation
desviación del ego ego deviation
desviación del sistema nervioso central
  central nervous system deviation
desviación estándar standard deviation
desviación estándar de muestra sample

standard deviation
desviación media mean deviation
desviación promedia average deviation
desviación psicopática psychopathic deviance
desviación secundaria secondary deviance
desviación sexual sexual deviation
desviado deviant
detección detection
detección auditiva auditory detection
detección de despertamiento arousal
     detection
detección de mentiras lie detection
detección de moción motion detection
detección y reconocimiento detection and
     recognition
detector de características feature detector
detector de mentiras lie detector
detector ideal ideal detector
detectores de límites boundary detectors
detención detention
deterioración deterioration
deterioración alcohólica alcoholic
     deterioration
deterioración de atención deterioration of
     attention
deterioración de hábito habit deterioration
deterioración de personalidad personality
     deterioration
deterioración emocional emotional
     deterioration
deterioración epiléptica epileptic
     deterioration
deterioración intelectual intellectual
     deterioration
deterioración mental mental deterioration
deterioración neurológica neurological
     deterioration
deterioración senil senile deterioration
deteriorado impaired
deteriorativo deteriorative
deterioro decay
deterioro impairment
deterioro cognitivo cognitive impairment
deterioro de audición hearing impairment
deterioro de funcionamiento académico
     impairment of academic functioning
deterioro de memoria memory impairment
deterioro del habla speech impairment
deterioro del habla no organico nonorganic
     speech impairment
deterioro del habla orgánico organic speech
     impairment
deterioro sensorineural sensorineural
     impairment
deterioro mental mental impairment
deterioro neurológico neurological
     impairment
deterioro neurológico y abuso de niños
     neurological impairment and child abuse
deterioro perceptivo y pérdida nerviosa
     perceptive impairment and nerve loss
deterioro sensorial sensory impairment
deterioro visual visual impairment
determinación determination
determinación ambiental environmental

determination
determinación de sexo sex determination
determinación genética genetic determination
determinador determiner
determinante determinant
determinante ambiental environmental
     determinant
determinante de conducta behavior
     determinant
determinante de sueño dream determinant
determinante dominante dominant
     determinant
determinante organísmico organismic
     determinant
determinante personal personal determinant
determinante situacional situational
     determinant
determinantes cognitivos de emoción
     cognitive determinants of emotion
determinativo determinative
determinismo determinism
determinismo biológico biological
     determinism
determinismo biosocial biosocial determinism
determinismo cultural cultural determinism
determinismo psíquico psychic determinism
determinismo recíproco reciprocal
     determinism
determinismo social social determinism
determinismo sociológico sociological
     determinism
detumescencia detumescence
deuda de oxígeno oxygen debt
deuteranomalía deuteranomaly
deuteranopía deuteranopia
deuteropatía deuteropathy
devaluación devaluation
devolución devolution
dexametasona dexamethasone
dexanfetamina dexamphetamine
dextrado dextrad
dextralidad dextrality
dextralidad-sinistralidad dextrality-sinistrality
dextran dextran
dextroanfetamina dextroamphetamine
dextrocerebral dextrocerebral
dextrofobia dextrophobia
dextromanual dextromanual
dextropedal dextropedal
dextrosinistral dextrosinistral
día libre de droga drug holiday
diabetes diabetes
diabetes de comienzo en madurez
     maturity-onset diabetes
diabetes dependiente de insulina
     insulin-dependent diabetes
diabetes insípida diabetes insipidus
diabetes insípida nefrógena nephrogenic
     diabetes insipidus
diabetes maternal maternal diabetes
diabetes mellitus diabetes mellitus
diabético diabetic
diacetilmorfina diacetylmorphine
diacrónico diachronic
díada dyad

díada social social dyad
diádico dyadic
diadococinesis diadochokinesis
diafemétrico diaphemetric
diaforesis diaphoresis
diagnosticador diagnostician
diagnosticador psicoeducativo
  psychoeducational diagnostician
diagnóstico (adj) diagnostic
diagnóstico (n) diagnosis
diagnóstico clínico clinical diagnosis
diagnóstico computerizado computerized
  diagnosis
diagnóstico conductual behavioral diagnosis
diagnóstico de ansiedad diagnosis of anxiety
diagnóstico de trastorno de personalidad
  fronteriza diagnosis of borderline
  personality disorder
diagnóstico de trastornos de eliminación
  diagnosis of elimination disorders
diagnóstico diferencial differential diagnosis
diagnóstico diferencial de depresión
  differential diagnosis of depression
diagnóstico diferencial de trastornos del
  comer differential diagnosis of eating
  disorders
diagnóstico diferido deferred diagnosis
diagnóstico médico medical diagnosis
diagnóstico negativo negative diagnosis
diagnóstico organizativo organizational
  diagnosis
diagnóstico prenatal prenatal diagnosis
diagnóstico primario primary diagnosis
diagnóstico provisional provisional diagnosis
diagnóstico psiquiátrico psychiatric diagnosis
diagnóstico social social diagnosis
diagnóstico principal principal diagnosis
diagrama diagram
diagrama de área area diagram
diagrama de barras bar diagram
diagrama de bloques block diagram
diagrama de cromaticidad chromaticity
  diagram
diagrama de dispersión scatter diagram
diagrama de Venn Venn diagram
dialéctico dialectical
dialecto dialect
diálisis dialysis
diálisis peritoneal peritoneal dialysis
diálogo dialogue
diamina diamine
dianoético dianoetic
diario log
diario de actividad activity log
diario vivir daily living
diarrea diarrhea
diarrea nocturna nocturnal diarrhea
diasquisis diaschisis
diastematocrania diastematocrania
diastematomielia diastematomyelia
diástole diastole
diataxia diataxia
diataxia cerebral cerebral diataxia
diatermia diathermy
diátesis diathesis

diátesis artrítica arthritic diathesis
diátesis contractural contractural diathesis
diátesis espasmódica spasmodic diathesis
diátesis espasmofílica spasmophilic diathesis
diátesis lítica lithic diathesis
diátesis traumatofílica traumatophilic
  diathesis
diazepam diazepam
diazóxido diazoxide
dibenzepina dibenzepin
dibujo drawing
dibujo automático automatic drawing
dibujo con espejo mirror-drawing
dibujo en hipnosis drawing in hypnosis
dibujos de Piderit Piderit drawings
diccionario de colores de Maerz y Paul
  Maerz and Paul color dictionary
dicloralfenazona dichloralphenazone
dicótico dichotic
dicotomía dichotomy
dicotomía cuerpo-mente body-mind
  dichotomy
dicromacia dichromacy
dicrómata dichromat
dicrómata uniocular uniocular dichromat
dicromatismo dichromatism
dicromatismo anómalo anomalous
  dichromatism
dicromatopsia dichromatopsia
dicromia dichromia
dicrómico dichromic
dicromopsia dichromopsia
dictador dictator
didáctico didactic
diencefálico diencephalic
diencéfalo diencephalon
diencéfalo posterior posterior diencephalon
diencefalosis diencephalosis
diestro dexter
dieta diet
dieta hedónica hedonic diet
dieta macrobiótica macrobiotic diet
dietético dietary
dietilamida de ácido lisérgico lysergic acid
  diethylamide
dietilestilbestrol diethylstilbestrol
dietilpropion diethylpropion
dietiltriptamina diethyltryptamine
difamar malign
difenhidramina diphenhydramine
difenilhidantoína diphenylhydantoin
difenoxilato diphenoxylate
diferencia difference
diferencia de cohortes cohort differences
diferencia de fases phase difference
diferencia del tiempo binaural binaural time
  difference
diferencia escasamente notable just
  noticeable difference
diferencia estándar standard difference
diferencia percibida sensed difference
diferencia significante significant difference
diferenciación differentiation
diferenciación celular cell differentiation
diferenciación de estímulos stimulus

differentiation
diferenciación de respuestas response
differentiation
diferenciación sexual sexual differentiation
diferenciación social social differentiation
diferenciación sujeto-objeto subject-object
differentiation
diferencial differential
diferencial de umbral threshold differential
diferencial semántico semantic differential
diferencias casuales chance differences
diferencias culturales cultural differences
diferencias de edad age differences
diferencias de género gender differences
diferencias de grupos group differences
diferencias entre neonatos neonate
differences
diferencias individuales individual differences
diferencias individuales en el desarrollo del
lenguaje individual differences in language
development
diferencias individuales en percepción
individual differences in perception
diferencias individuales en personalidad
individual differences in personality
diferencias interaurales interaural differences
diferencias interindividuales interindividual
differences
diferencias intraindividuales intraindividual
differences
diferencias laterales lateral differences
diferencias raciales race differences
diferencias sexuales sex differences
diferente culturalmente culturally different
diferido deferred
dificultad difficulty
dificultad de alimentación feeding difficulty
dificultad de artículo item difficulty
dificultad de concentración concentration
difficulty
dificultad de sublimación sublimation
difficulty
difracción diffraction
difteria diphtheria
diftérico diphtheritic
difusión diffusion
difusión de identidad identity diffusion
difusión de identidad maligna malignant
identity diffusion
difusión de papel role diffusion
difusión de responsabilidad diffusion of
responsibility
difuso diffuse
digital digital
digitalgia parestésica digitalgia paresthetica
dígrafo digraph
dihidrocodeína dihydrocodeine
dihidroergotoxina dihydroergotoxine
dihidromorfina dihydromorphine
dihidroxifenilalanina dihydroxyphenylalanine
dilapidación dilapidation
dilatación dilation
dildo dildo
dilema dilemma
dilema de Scull Scull's dilemma

dilema del prisionero prisoner's dilemma
dilema moral moral dilemma
dilema necesidad-temor need-fear dilemma
dilema social social dilemma
diltiazem diltiazem
dimenhidrinato dimenhydrinate
dimensión dimension
dimensión de grupo group dimension
dimensión tonal tonal dimension
dimensiones de criterio criterion dimensions
dimensiones de trabajo job dimensions
dimercaprol dimercaprol
dimetilanfetamina dimethylamphetamine
dimetiltriptamina dimethyltryptamine
dimetoxianfetamina dimethoxyamphetamine
dimorfismo dimorphism
dimorfismo cerebral brain dimorphism
dimorfismo sexual sexual dimorphism
dina dyne
dinámica dynamics
dinámica adaptacional adaptational dynamics
dinámica conductual behavioral dynamics
dinámica de aula classroom dynamics
dinámica de grupo group dynamics
dinámica infantil infantile dynamics
dinámica organizativa organizational
dynamics
dinámica social social dynamics
dinámica de personalidad personality
dynamics
dinámico dynamic
dinamismo dynamism
dinamismo de lujuria lust dynamism
dinamismo mental mental dynamism
dinamismo oral oral dynamism
dinamogénesis dynamogenesis
dinamómetro dynamometer
dinomanía dinomania
dionismo dionism
dioptría diopter
diótico diotic
dióxido de carbono carbon dioxide
dipipanona dipipanone
dipiridamol dipyridamole
diplacusia diplacusis
diplejía diplegia
diplejía atáxica ataxic diplegia
diplejía espástica spastic diplegia
diplejía facial facial diplegia
diplejía facial congénita congenital facial
diplegia
diplejía infantil infantile diplegia
diplejía masticatoria masticatory diplegia
diploide diploid
diploidia diploidy
diplomielia diplomyelia
diplopía diplopia
dippoldismo dippoldism
dipsesis dipsesis
dipsomanía dipsomania
dipsosis dipsosis
diptongo diphthong
diquefobia dikephobia
dirección address
direccional directional

direccionalidad directionality
directivo directive
directivo genético genetic directive
directivo implícito implied directive
directivo indirecto indirect directive
directo direct
dirigación dirigation
dirigido directed
dirigido hacia el exterior outer-directed
dirigido hacia lo interno inner-directed
dirigido hacia otros other-directed
dirigido hacia tradiciones tradition-directed
dirogomotor dirigomotor
dirrínico dirhinic
disacusia dysacusia
disacusis dysacusis
disafia dysaphia
disáfico dysaphic
disantigrafia dysantigraphia
disartria dysarthria
disartria apráxica apraxic dysarthria
disartria atáxica ataxic dysarthria
disartria atetoide athetoid dysarthria
disartria atetótica athetotic dysarthria
disartria literal dysarthria literalis
disartria silábica espasmódica dysarthria
   syllabaris spasmodica
disártrico dysarthric
disartrosis dysarthrosis
disasociación disassociation
disautonomía dysautonomia
disautonomía familiar familial dysautonomia
disbasia dysbasia
disbasia lordótica progresiva dysbasia
   lordotica progressiva
disbulia dysbulia
disbúlico dysbulic
discalculia dyscalculia
discapacidad disability
discapacidad aritmética arithmetic disability
discapacidad de aprendizaje learning
   disability
discapacidad de dibujo drawing disability
discapacidad de lectura reading disability
discapacidad de lectura específica specific
   reading disability
discapacidad del aprendizaje específica
   specific learning disability
discapacidad del desarrollo developmental
   disability
discapacidad del lenguaje language disability
discapacidad del lenguaje específica specific
   language disability
discapacidad del lenguaje general general
   language disability
discapacidad física physical disability
discapacidad motora motor disability
discapacidad perceptiva perceptual disability
discapacidad perceptiva-motora
   perceptual-motor disability
discapacidad psiquiátrica psychiatric
   disability
**discapacidades de aprendizaje en víctimas de
   abuso de niños** learning disabilities in
   child abuse victims

discapacidades en abstraer abstracting
   disabilities
discectomía discectomy
discinesia dyskinesia
discinesia álgera dyskinesia algera
discinesia biliar biliary dyskinesia
discinesia de retiro withdrawal dyskinesia
discinesia extrapiramidal extrapiramidal
   dyskinesia
discinesia oral oral dyskinesia
discinesia oral tardía tardive oral dyskinesia
discinesia orofacial orofacial dyskinesia
discinesia paroxística paroxysmal dyskinesia
discinesia tardía tardive dyskinesia
discinesia tardía inducida por neuroléptico
   neuroleptic-induced tardive dyskinesia
discinesis dyskinesis
discinético dyskinetic
disciplina discipline
disciplina de aula classroom discipline
disciplina formal formal discipline
disciplina mental mental discipline
disco disk
disco de Masson Masson disk
disco herniado herniated disk
disco óptico optic disk
disco protruido protruded disk
disco rupturado ruptured disk
disco táctil tactile disk
disco táctil de Merkel Merkel's tactile disk
discogénico discogenic
discografía discography
discograma discogram
discoimesis dyscoimesis
discontinuación breakoff
discontinuidad discontinuity
discontinuidad de papel role discontinuity
discontinuo discontinuous
discopatía discopathy
discopatía cervical traumática traumatic
   cervical discopathy
discordancia discordance
discordia discord
discordia afectiva affective disharmony
discordia familiar family discord
discordia marital marital discord
discordia parental parental discord
discos de Maxwell Maxwell disks
discotomía discotomy
discrasia dyscrasia
discrepancia discrepancy
discrepante discrepant
discreto discrete
discriminabilidad discriminability
discriminación discrimination
discriminación apariencia-realidad
   appearance-reality discrimination
discriminación aprendida learned
   discrimination
discriminación auditiva auditory
   discrimination
discriminación condicional conditional
   discrimination
discriminación contextual contextual
   discrimination

discriminación cromática chromatic discrimination
discriminación de aspereza roughness discrimination
discriminación de brillantez brightness discrimination
discriminación de centelleo flicker discrimination
discriminación de dos puntos two-point discrimination
discriminación de estímulos stimulus discrimination
discriminación de forma táctil tactual shape discrimination
discriminación de formas form discrimination
discriminación de frecuencias frequency discrimination
discriminación de intensidad intensity discrimination
discriminación de matices hue discrimination
discriminación de objetos object discrimination
discriminación de patrón pattern discrimination
discriminación de peso weight discrimination
discriminación de señales adquirida acquired discrimination of cues
discriminación de tamaño táctil tactual size discrimination
discriminación de tamaños size discrimination
discriminación de tono pitch discrimination
discriminación derecha-izquierda right-left discrimination
discriminación en condicionamiento clásico discrimination in classical conditioning
discriminación en servicios psiquiátricos discrimination in psychiatric services
discriminación espacial spatial discrimination
discriminación sensorial sensory discrimination
discriminación sexual sexual discrimination
discriminación temporal temporal discrimination
discriminación térmica thermal discrimination
discriminación visual visual discrimination
discriminado discriminated
discriminador serial serial discriminator
discriminante discriminating
discriminativo discriminative
discromatopsia dyschromatopsia
discronación dischronation
discronismo dyschronism
discurso discourse
discusión discussion
disdiadococinesia dysdiadochokinesia
disdiadococinesis dysdiadochokinesis
diseminación de evaluación evaluation dissemination
diseminado disseminated
diseneia dyseneia
diseño design
diseño ambiental environmental design

diseño ambiental interdisciplinario interdisciplinary environmental design
diseño antes-después before-after design
diseño cuasiexperimental quasi-experimental design
diseño de aula abierta open-classroom design
diseño de despliegue display design
diseño de dos factores two-factor design
diseño de equipo equipment design
diseño de espacio de trabajo work-space design
diseño de grupo aleatorizado randomized-group design
diseño de grupo apareado matched-group design
diseño de hospital hospital design
diseño de instrumento instrument design
diseño de métodos experimentales design of experimental methods
diseño de placebo balanceado balanced placebo design
diseño de sujeto único single-subject design
diseño de tarea task design
diseño de trabajo job design
diseño en bloque block design
diseño experimental experimental design
diseño experimental de caso único single-case experimental design
diseño factorial factorial design
diseño mixto mixed design
diseño representativo representative design
diseño secuencial sequential design
diseretismo dyserethism
disergasia dysergasia
disergia dysergia
disestesia dysesthesia
disfagia dysphagia
disfagia espástica dysphagia spastica
disfasia dysphasia
disfasia del desarrollo developmental dysphasia
disfasia expresiva expressive dysphasia
disfasia receptiva receptive dysphasia
disfemia dysphemia
disfilaxia dysphylaxia
disfluidez dysfluency
disfonía dysphonia
disfonía de pubertad puberum dysphonia
disfonía espástica spastic dysphonia
disfonía funcional functional dysphonia
disfónico dysphonic
disforia dysphoria
disforia de género gender dysphoria
disforia histeroide hysteroid dysphoria
disforia nerviosa dysphoria nervosa
disfórico dysphoric
disfrasia dysphrasia
disfrenia dysphrenia
disfrute enjoyment
disfunción dysfunction
disfunción cerebral cerebral dysfunction
disfunción cerebral mínima minimal cerebral dysfunction
disfunción de atención attention dysfunction
disfunción de eje hipotalámico-pituitario

hypothalamic-pituitary axis dysfunction
disfunción de lóbulo frontal frontal lobe dysfunction
disfunción de procesamiento central central-processing dysfunction
disfunción emocional emotional dysfunction
disfunción emocional en adolescencia emotional dysfunction in adolescence
disfunción emocional y abuso de niños emotional dysfunction and child abuse
disfunción eréctil erectile dysfunction
disfunción eréctil primaria primary erectile dysfunction
disfunción eréctil secundaria secondary erectile dysfunction
disfunción neuroendocrina neuroendocrine dysfunction
disfunción neuropsicológica neuropsychological dysfunction
disfunción orgásmica orgasmic dysfunction
disfunción orgásmica primaria primary orgasmic dysfunction
disfunción orgásmica situacional situational orgasmic dysfunction
disfunción perceptiva-motora perceptual-motor dysfunction
disfunción psicosexual psychosexual dysfunction
disfunción psicosexual atípica atypical psychosexual dysfunction
disfunción sexual sexual dysfunction
disfunción sexual anfetamina amphetamine sexual dysfunction
disfunción sexual de ansiolítico anxiolytic sexual dysfunction
disfunción sexual de cocaína cocaine sexual dysfunction
disfunción sexual de hipnótico hypnotic sexual dysfunction
disfunción sexual de opioide opioid sexual dysfunction
disfunción sexual de otra sustancia other substance sexual dysfunction
disfunción sexual de sedante sedative sexual dysfunction
disfunción sexual de sustancia desconocida unknown substance sexual dysfunction
disfunción sexual debido a condición médica general sexual dysfunction due to general medical condition
disfunción sexual femenina female sexual dysfunction
disfunción sexual inducida por sustancia substance-induced sexual dysfunction
disfunción sexual masculina male sexual dysfunction
disfuncional dysfunctional
disgenesia dysgenesis
disgenesia gonadal gonadal dysgenesis
disgenesia ovárica ovarian dysgenesis
disgénico dysgenic
disgeusia dysgeusia
disglucosis dysglucosis
disgnosia dysgnosia
disgrafia dysgraphia

disgramatismo dysgrammatism
dishomofilia dyshomophilia
disidentidad dysidentity
disimbiosis dyssymbiosis
disimilación dissimilation
disimulación dissimulation
disimulador dissimulator
disinergia dyssynergia
disinergia cerebelosa dyssynergia cerebellaris
disinergia cerebelosa mioclónica dyssynergia cerebellaris myoclonica
disinergia cerebelosa progresiva dyssynergia cerebellaris progressiva
dislalia dyslalia
dislexia dyslexia
dislexia del desarrollo developmental dyslexia
dislexia del desarrollo específica specific developmental dyslexia
disléxico dyslexic
dislocación de cadera hip dislocation
dislogia dyslogia
dismegalopsia dysmegalopsia
dismencia dysmentia
dismencia tardía tardive dysmentia
dismenorrea dysmenorrhea
dismenorrea esencial essential dysmenorrhea
dismenorrea funcional functional dysmenorrhea
dismenorrea inflamatoria inflammatory dysmenorrhea
dismenorrea membranosa membranous dysmenorrhea
dismenorrea obstructiva obstructive dysmenorrhea
dismenorrea primaria primary dysmenorrhea
dismetría dysmetria
dismetropsia dysmetropsia
dismielinación dysmyelination
dismimia dysmimia
dismiotonía dysmyotonia
dismnesia dysmnesia
dismnésico dysmnesic
dismórfico dysmorphic
dismorfobia dysmorphobia
dismorfofobia dysmorphophobia
dismorfomanía dysmorphomania
disnea dyspnea
disnistaxis dysnystaxis
disociación dissociation
disociación albuminocitológica albuminocytologic dissociation
disociación del sueño sleep dissociation
disociación doble double dissociation
disociación e hipnosis dissociation and hypnosis
disociación semántica semantic dissociation
disociación siringomiélica syringomyelic dissociation
disociación tabética tabetic dissociation
disociado dissociated
disocial dyssocial
disociar dissociate
disociativo dissociative
disomnia dyssomnia
disomnia en niñez dyssomnia in childhood

disonancia dissonance
disonancia cognitiva cognitive dissonance
disorexia dysorexia
disosmia dysosmia
disostosis dysostosis
disostosis craneofacial craniofacial dysostosis
disostosis periférica con hipoplasia nasal
    peripheral dysostosis with nasal hypoplasia
dispalia dyspallia
disparate nonsense
disparates cómicos comical nonsense
dispareunia dyspareunia
dispareunia femenina female dyspareunia
dispareunia femenina debido a condición
    médica general female dyspareunia due to
    general medical condition
dispareunia funcional functional dyspareunia
dispareunia masculina debido a condición
    médica general male dyspareunia due to
    general medical condition
disparidad disparity
disparidad binocular binocular disparity
disparidad retinal retinal disparity
disparidad visual visual disparity
dispercepción dysperception
dispercepción metabólica metabolic
    dysperception
dispermia dysspermia
dispersión dispersion
dispersión de respuestas response dispersion
dispersión discriminal discriminal dispersion
displasia dysplasia
displasia cerebral cerebral dysplasia
displasia de cadera hip dysplasia
displasia diafisaria progresiva progressive
    diaphyseal dysplasia
displasia septoóptica septooptic dysplasia
displástico dysplastic
disponesis dysponesis
disponibilidad availability
disposición disposition, readiness
disposición conductual behavioral disposition
disposición de explosión explosion readiness
disposición de lectura reading readiness
disposición del desarrollo developmental
    readiness
disposición depresiva constitucional
    constitutional depressive disposition
disposición maníaca constitucional
    constitutional manic disposition
disposición medios-fines means-ends
    readiness
disposición personal personal disposition
disposición sexual sexual readiness
disposicional dispositional
dispositivo de medición estandarizada
    standardized measuring device
dispositivo intrauterino intrauterine device
dispraxia dyspraxia
dispraxia simpática sympathetic dyspraxia
disprosodia dysprosody
disputa dispute
disputa de custodia custody dispute
disquecia dyschezia
disquiral dyschiral

disquiria dyschiria
disquirial dyscheiral
disritmia dysrhythmia
disritmia cerebral cerebral dysrhythmia
disritmia cerebral paroxística paroxysmal
    cerebral dysrhythmia
disritmia electroencefalográfica
    electroencephalographic dysrhythmia
disritmia mayor major dysrhythmia
disrupción disruption
disruptivo disruptive
distal distal
distancia distance
distancia entre narices nose distance
distancia funcional functional distance
distancia interocular interocular distance
distancia interpersonal interpersonal distance
distancia interpersonal óptima optimal
    interpersonal distance
distancia psicológica psychological distance
distancia sensorial sense distance
distancia social social distance
distancia sociométrica sociometric distance
distanciamiento de papel role distancing
distasia dysstasia
distaxia dystaxia
distimia dysthymia
distimia subafectiva subaffective dysthymia
distímico dysthymic
distinción dado-nuevo given-new distinction
distinción de forma-función form-function
    distinction
distintivo distinctive
distiquia dystychia
distocia dystocia
distonía dystonia
distonía aguda acute dystonia
distonía aguda inducida por neuroléptico
    neuroleptic-induced acute dystonia
distonía de torsión torsion dystonia
distonía lenticular dystonia lenticularis
distonía muscular deformante dystonia
    musculorum deformans
distónico dystonic
distorsión distortion
distorsión de compromiso compromise
    distortion
distorsionado distorted
distorsión de amplitud amplitude distortion
distorsión de figura-fondo figure-ground
    distortion
distorsión de imagen corporal body image
    distortion
distorsión de memoria memory distortion
distorsión de papel role distortion
distorsión del ego ego distortion
distorsión del tiempo time distortion
distorsión metonímica metonymic distortion
distorsión paratáxica parataxic distortion
distorsión perceptiva perceptual distortion
distorsión por transferencia distortion by
    transference
distorsión sistemática systematic distortion
distracción distraction
distractibilidad distractibility

distractor distractor
distraíble distractible
distribución distribution
distribución asimétrica asymmetric distribution
distribución bimodal bimodal distribution
distribución binomial binomial distribution
distribución de Bernoulli Bernoulli distribution
distribución de frecuencias frequency distribution
distribución de frecuencias agrupadas grouped frequency distribution
distribución de frecuencias cumulativas cumulative frequency distribution
distribución de muestreo sampling distribution
distribución de Poisson Poisson distribution
distribución de práctica distribution of practice
distribución de probabilidades probability distribution
distribución de rangos ranked distribution
distribución de Student Student's distribution
distribución en U invertida inverted-U distribution
distribución F F distribution
distribución gauseana gaussian distribution
distribución hipergeométrica hypergeometric distribution
distribución multimodal multimodal distribution
distribución multinomial multinomial distribution
distribución normal normal distribution
distribución rectangular rectangular distribution
distribución rectilínea rectilinear distribution
distribución sexual sex distribution
distribución simétrica symmetrical distribution
distribución truncada truncated distribution
distribución uniforme uniform distribution
distributivo distributive
distrofia dystrophy
distrofia adiposogenital adiposogenital dystrophy
distrofia de Barnes Barnes' dystrophy
distrofia de Duchenne Duchenne's dystrophy
distrofia de Landouzy-Dejerine Landouzy-Dejerine dystrophy
distrofia distal distal dystrophy
distrofia miotónica myotonic dystrophy
distrofia muscular muscular dystrophy
distrofia muscular de cinturones de miembros limb-girdle muscular dystrophy
distrofia muscular de Leyden-Mobius Leyden-Mobius muscular dystrophy
distrofia muscular de niñez childhood muscular dystrophy
distrofia muscular facioescapulohumeral facioscapulohumeral muscular dystrophy
distrofia muscular pelvifemoral pelvifemoral muscular dystrophy
distrofia muscular progresiva progressive muscular dystrophy

distrofia muscular seudohipertrófica pseudohypertrophic muscular dystrophy
distrofia muscular seudohipertrófica adulta adult pseudohypertrophic muscular dystrophy
distrofia muscular tardía tipo Becker Becker type tardive muscular dystrophy
distrofia neuroaxonal infantil infantile neuroaxonal dystrophy
distrofia oftalmopléjica ophthalmoplegic dystrophy
distrofia refleja simpática sympathetic reflex dystrophy
distrofoneurosis dystrophoneurosis
distropía dystropy
disturbio disturbance
disturbio afásico aphasic disturbance
disturbio asociado con enfermedad mental orgánica disturbance associated with organic mental disease
disturbio asociado con fenómenos de conversión disturbance associated with conversion phenomena
disturbio conceptual conceptual disturbance
disturbio de ansiedad anxiety disturbance
disturbio de apetito appetite disturbance
disturbio de asociación association disturbance
disturbio de asociaciones disturbance of associations
disturbio de atención disturbance of attention
disturbio de conceptualización corporal body conceptualization disturbance
disturbio de conciencia disturbance of consciousness
disturbio de conducta conduct disturbance
disturbio de enfoque focusing disturbance
disturbio de hábito habit disturbance
disturbio de identidad identity disturbance
disturbio de imagen corporal body image disturbance
disturbio de memoria disturbance of memory
disturbio de movimiento movement disturbance
disturbio de orientación sexual sexual-orientation disturbance
disturbio de patrón de personalidad personality pattern disturbance
disturbio de pensamientos thought disturbance
disturbio de personalidad sociopática sociopathic personality disturbance
disturbio de rasgo de personalidad personality-trait disturbance
disturbio de voluntad will disturbance
disturbio del comer eating disturbance
disturbio del habla speech disturbance
disturbio del sueño sleep disturbance
disturbio emocional emotional disturbance
disturbio en contenido de pensamientos disturbance in content of thought
disturbio en el habla disturbance in speech
disturbio en la forma de pensar disturbance in form of thinking

disturbio en sugestibilidad disturbance in suggestibility
disturbio interactivo interactive disturbance
disturbio mental mental disturbance
disturbio mixto mixed disturbance
disturbio motor motor disturbance
disturbio perceptivo perceptual disturbance
disturbio psicográfico psychographic disturbance
disturbio sensorial sensory disturbance
disturbio situacional transitorio transient situational disturbance
disturbios emocionales posparto postpartum emotional disturbances
disuasivo deterrent
disulfiram disulfiram
disulfuro de carbono carbon disulfide
disuria dysuria
disyunción disjunction
disyunción personal personal disjunction
disyuntivo disjunctive
diuresis diuresis
diurético diuretic
diurno diurnal
divagación divagation
divergencia divergence
divergente divergent
diversidad cultural cultural diversity
diversivo diversive
dividido divided
división splitting
división celular cell division
división craneal cranial division
división craneosacra craniosacral division
división de reducción reduction division
división sacral sacral division
división simpática sympathetic division
divorcio divorce
divorcio comunitario community divorce
divorcio coparental coparental divorce
divorcio económico economic divorce
divorcio emocional emotional divorce
divorcio legal legal divorce
divorcio parental parental divorce
divorcio psíquico psychic divorce
divulgación disclosure
divulgación de decepciones disclosure of deceptions
dixirazina dixyrazine
dizigótico dizygotic
doble double
doble ciego double-blind
doble sentido double meaning
dócil docile
docilidad docility
doctor descalzo barefoot doctor
doctrina doctrine
doctrina de energías específicas specific energies doctrine
doctrina del mejor interés best interest doctrine
doctrina del mejor interés del niño best interest of the child doctrine
documentación documentation
documentación de abuso de niños

documentation of child abuse
documento personal personal document
dogma dogma
dol dol
dolencia ailment
dolencia funcional functional ailment
dolencia respiratoria inducida por el sueño sleep-induced respiratory ailment
dolicocefalia dolichocephaly
dolicocefálico dolichocephalic
dolicomórfico dolichomorphic
dolor pain
dolor agudo acute pain
dolor central central pain
dolor clínico clinical pain
dolor crónico chronic pain
dolor cutáneo cutaneous pain
dolor de cabeza headache
dolor de cabeza bilioso bilious headache
dolor de cabeza ciego blind headache
dolor de cabeza coital coital headache
dolor de cabeza de capa de plomo lead-cap headache
dolor de cabeza de Horton Horton's headache
dolor de cabeza de migraña migraine headache
dolor de cabeza espinal spinal headache
dolor de cabeza fibrosítico fibrositic headache
dolor de cabeza histamínico histaminic headache
dolor de cabeza nodular nodular headache
dolor de cabeza orgánico organic headache
dolor de cabeza por tensión tension headache
dolor de cabeza por vacío vacuum headache
dolor de cabeza postraumática posttraumatic headache
dolor de cabeza reflejo reflex headache
dolor de cabeza sintomático symptomatic headache
dolor de cabeza vascular vascular headache
dolor de espalda backache
dolor de mente mind pain
dolor de miembro fantasma phantom limb pain
dolor del cáncer cancer pain
dolor en cinturón girdle pain
dolor en sueños pain in dreams
dolor experimental experimental pain
dolor eyaculatorio ejaculatory pain
dolor funcional functional pain
dolor heterotópico heterotopic pain
dolor homotópico homotopic pain
dolor intratable intractable pain
dolor musculoesquelético musculoskeletal pain
dolor nervioso nerve pain
dolor nocturno night pain
dolor orgánico organic pain
dolor primal primal pain
dolor psicogénico psychogenic pain
dolor psíquico psychic pain
dolor referido referred pain
dolor relampagueante flashing pain

dolor sexual sexual pain
dolor superficial surface pain
dolores de cabeza crónicos chronic headaches
dolores de cabeza en grupo cluster headaches
dolores del crecimiento growing pains
dolorífico dolorific
dolorimetría dolorimetry
dolorología dolorology
doloroso painful
domatofobia domatophobia
domesticado domesticated
doméstico domestic
domiciliario domiciliary
domicilio domicile
dominación sexual sexual domination
dominador dominator
dominancia dominance
dominancia cerebral cerebral dominance
dominancia cerebral mixta mixed cerebral
    dominance
dominancia cortical cortical dominance
dominancia cruzada crossed dominance
dominancia de ojo eye dominance
dominancia genética genetic dominance
dominancia hemisférica hemispheric
    dominance
dominancia lateral lateral dominance
dominancia manual manual dominance
dominancia mixta mixed dominance
dominancia ocular ocular dominance
dominancia-sumisión dominance-submission
dominancia territorial territorial dominance
dominancia visual visual dominance
dominante dominant
dominio mastery
domperidona domperidone
donatismo donatism
dopa dopa
dopamina dopamine
dopamina y depresión dopamine and
    depression
dopamina y estado afectivo dopamine and
    affective state
dopaminérgico dopaminergic
dorafobia doraphobia
doromanía doromania
dorsal dorsal
dorsolateral dorsolateral
dorsomedial dorsomedial
dosis dose
dosis terapéutica therapeutic dose
dotación genética genetic endowment
dotado gifted
doxapram doxapram
doxilamina doxylamine
doxogénico doxogenic
dramático dramatic
dramatismo dramatism
dramatización dramatization
dramatogénico dramatogenic
drapetomanía drapetomania
droga drug
droga alucinogénica hallucinogenic drug
droga antiansiedad antianxiety drug
droga antidepresiva antidepressant drug

droga antidepresiva heterocíclica
    heterocyclic antidepressant drug
droga antiepiléptica antiepileptic drug
droga antimaníaca antimaniac drug
droga antiparkinsoniana antiparkinsonian
    drug
droga antipsicótica antipsychotic drug
droga antiviral antiviral drug
droga ataráctica ataractic drug
droga de bloqueo adrenérgico alfa alpha
    adrenergic blocking drug
droga de bloqueo adrenérgico beta beta
    adrenergic blocking drug
droga de mantenimiento maintenance drug
droga de predilección drug of choice
droga depresiva depressant drug
droga dopaminérgica dopaminergic drug
droga estabilizante del humor
    mood-stabilizing drug
droga estimulante adrenérgico alfa alpha
    adrenergic stimulating drug
droga hipnótica hypnotic drug
droga hipnótica-sedante hypnotic-sedative
    drug
droga huérfana orphan drug
droga inmunosupresiva immunosuppresive
    drug
droga narcótica narcotic drug
droga neuroléptica neuroleptic drug
droga no psicotrópica nonpsychotropic drug
droga parasimpática parasympathetic drug
droga parasimpaticomimética
    parasympathomimetic drug
droga propietaria proprietary drug
droga psicoactiva psychoactive drug
droga psicodélica psychedelic drug
droga psicoestimulante psychostimulant drug
droga psicofarmacológica
    psychopharmacological drug
droga psicogénica psychogenic drug
droga psicoterapéutica psychotherapeutic
    drug
droga psicotomimética psychotomimetic drug
droga psicotrópica psychotropic drug
droga radiomimética radiomimetic drug
droga sedante sedative drug
droga sedante-hipnótica sedative-hypnotic
    drug
droga simpatolítica sympatholytic drug
droga simpatomimética sympathomimetic
    drug
droga sinérgica synergic drug
droga tricíclica tricyclic drug
drogadicción drug addiction
drogas adrenérgicas adrenergic drugs
drogas alterantes de mente mind-altering
    drugs
drogas alterantes del humor mood-altering
    drugs
drogas callejeras street drugs
drogas catiónicas cationic drugs
drogas colinérgicas cholinergic drugs
drogas de entrada gateway drugs
drogas de mostrador over-the-counter drugs
drogas modificadas designer drugs

drogas para el dolor drugs for pain
drogas para tratar enfermedad mental drugs for treating mental illness
drómico dromic
dromofobia dromophobia
dromolepsia dromolepsy
dromomanía dromomania
droperidol droperidol
dualismo dualism
dualismo cartesiano Cartesian dualism
dualismo interactivo interactive dualism
dualismo psicofísico psychophysical dualism
ductus deferens ductus deferens
duda doubt
duda obsesiva obsessive doubt
duelo bereavement, mourning
duelo anticipatorio anticipatory mourning
duelo contra depresión mayor bereavement versus major depression
duelo fingido feigned bereavement
duelo no complicado uncomplicated bereavement
duelo por infantes bereavement by infants
duelo por niños bereavement by children
dulce sweet
duplicación del ego ego duplication
duplicativo duplicative
duplicidad duplicity
duración duration
duración crítica critical duration
duración de alimentación por pecho duration of breast-feeding
duración de ciclo cycle length
duración de coma duration of coma
duración de estadía length of stay
duración de sueños length of dreams
duramadre dura mater
duraplastia duraplasty
dureza hardness
dureza de audición hardness of hearing
durmiente liviano light sleeper
durmiente liviano contra durmiente profundo light sleeper versus deep sleeper

E

ebriecación ebriecation
eccema eczema
ecciesis eccyesis
ecdemomanía ecdemomania
ecdemonomanía ecdemonomania
ecdisiasmo ecdysiasm
ecforia ecphoria
ecforizar ecphorize
eclactisma eclactisma
eclampsia eclampsia
eclampsia nutans eclampsia nutans
eclampsia puerperal puerperal eclampsia
eclámptico eclamptic
eclamptogénico eclamptogenic
eclamptógeno eclamptogenous
eclecticismo eclecticism
ecléctico eclectic
eclimia eclimia
eclipse cerebral cerebral eclipse
eclipse mental mental eclipse
ecmnesia ecmnesia
ecnoia ecnoia
eco echo
ecoacusia echoacousia
ecocardiografía echocardiography
ecocardiograma echocardiogram
ecocinesia echokinesia
ecocinesis echokinesis
ecoencefalografía echoencephalography
ecoencefalógrafo echoencephalograph
ecofarmacología ecopharmacology
ecofobia ecophobia
ecofotonía echophotony
ecofrasia echophrasia
ecografia echographia
ecoico echoic
ecolalia echolalia
ecolalia en autismo echolalia in autism
ecolalia y adquisición del lenguaje echolalia and language acquisition
ecolalia y comprensión echolalia and comprehension
ecolalia y lenguaje echolalia and language
ecolalia y trastornos del lenguaje echolalia and language disorders
ecología ecology
ecología conductual behavioral ecology
ecología humana human ecology
ecología social social ecology
ecológico ecological
ecomanía ecomania
ecomatismo echomatism
ecomimia echomimia
ecomotismo echomotism

econdrosis ecchondrosis
econdrosis fisalífora ecchondrosis
    physaliphora
econdrosis fisaliforme ecchondrosis
    physaliformis
economía cognitiva cognitive economy
economía de fichas token economy
economía de moción motion economy
económico economic
ecopalilalia echopalilalia
ecopatía echopathy
ecopraxia echopraxia
ecopsicología ecopsychology
ecopsiquiatría ecopsychiatry
ecosfera ecosphere
ecosistema ecosystem
ecoubicación echolocation
ecouteur ecouteur
ecouteurismo ecouteurism
ectipo ectype
ectodermo ectoderm
ectógeno ectogenous
ectomorfia ectomorphy
ectomórfico ectomorphic
ectomorfo ectomorph
ectopia pupilar ectopia pupillae
ectópico ectopic
ectoplasma ectoplasm
ecuación equation
ecuación de colores color equation
ecuación de Rayleigh Rayleigh equation
ecuación de regresión regression equation
ecuación empírica empirical equation
ecuación personal personal equation
ecuación racional rational equation
ecuación teorética theoretical equation
edad age
edad anatómica anatomical age
edad basal basal age
edad Binet Binet age
edad calendario calendar age
edad carpiana carpal age
edad crítica age critique
edad cronológica chronological age
edad de concepción conception age
edad de lectura reading age
edad de logro achievement age
edad de prueba test age
edad de retorno age de retour
edad del desarrollo developmental age
edad dental dental age
edad e inteligencia age and intelligence
edad educacional educational age
edad emocional emotional age
edad esqueletal skeletal age
edad fisiológica physiological age
edad gestacional gestational age
edad madura middle age
edad maternal maternal age
edad máxima maximal age
edad mediana midlife
edad menstrual menstrual age
edad mental mental age
edad mental basal basal mental age
edad social social age

edema edema
edema angioneurótico angioneurotic edema
edema angioneurótico hereditario hereditary
    angioneurotic edema
edema azul blue edema
edema cerebral cerebral edema
edema circunscrita circumscribed edema
edema de Quincke Quincke's edema
edema periódico periodic edema
edípico oedipal
edipismo oedipism
Edipo completo complete Oedipus
educabilidad educability
educable educable
educación education
educación abierta open education
educación ambiental environmental education
educación compensatoria compensatory
    education
educación continuada continuing education
educación cooperativa cooperative education
educación de asesor counselor education
educación de conductor driver education
educación de danza dance education
educación de drogas drug education
educación de movimiento movement
    education
educación de niñez temprana early childhood
    education
educación de padres parent education
educación de seguridad y salud safety and
    health education
educación del consumidor consumer
    education
educación especial special education
educación familiar family education
educación física physical education
educación graduada graduate education
educación individual individual education
educación médica continuada continuing
    medical education
educación moral moral education
educación progresiva progressive education
educación sexual sexual education
educación vocacional vocational education
educacional educational
educativo educative
efebiatría ephebiatrics
efectancia effectance
efectividad effectiveness
efectividad de liderazgo leadership
    effectiveness
efectivo effective
efecto effect
efecto adverso adverse effect
efecto anticolinérgico anticholinergic effect
efecto atmosférico atmosphere effect
efecto autocinético autokinetic effect
efecto de Abney Abney's effect
efecto de adhesión bandwagon effect
efecto de aislamiento isolation effect
efecto de amortiguamiento damping effect
efecto de asimilación assimilation effect
efecto de Barnum Barnum effect
efecto de base segura secure base effect

efecto de Bernoulli Bernoulli effect
efecto de Bezold-Brucke Bezold-Brucke effect
efecto de borde edge effect
efecto de bumerán boomerang effect
efecto de certidumbre certainty effect
efecto de circunstantes bystander effect
efecto de cohorte cohort effect
efecto de contraste contrast effect
efecto de contraste de entrevistas interview contrast effect
efecto de Coolidge Coolidge effect
efecto de Crespi Crespi effect
efecto de crisis crisis effect
efecto de cumpleaños birthday effect
efecto de Cushing Cushing effect
efecto de deterioración deterioration effect
efecto de dilución dilution effect
efecto de dique levee effect
efecto de Doppler Doppler effect
efecto de extraño pasajero passing stranger effect
efecto de García García effect
efecto de Glick Glick effect
efecto de Greenspoon Greenspoon effect
efecto de halo halo effect
efecto de Hawthorne Hawthorne effect
efecto de interacción interaction effect
efecto de intervalo range effect
efecto de la puerta en la cara door-in-the-face effect
efecto de las expectaciones del experimentador experimenter-expectancy effect
efecto de lo más reciente recency effect
efecto de McCollough McCollough effect
efecto de navaja clasp-knife effect
efecto de nivelación leveling effect
efecto de Orbeli Orbeli effect
efecto de papagallo chatterbox effect
efecto de Pigmalión Pygmalion effect
efecto de placebo placebo effect
efecto de Poetzl Poetzl effect
efecto de posición serial serial-position effect
efecto de primacía primacy effect
efecto de profundidad cinético kinetic depth effect
efecto de Purkinje Purkinje effect
efecto de práctica practice effect
efecto de Raman Raman effect
efecto de Ranschburg Ranschburg effect
efecto de rebote rebound effect
efecto de refuerzo reinforcement effect
efecto de refuerzo parcial partial-reinforcement effect
efecto de restauración fonémica phonemic restoration effect
efecto de Restorff Restorff effect
efecto de Romeo y Julieta Romeo and Juliet effect
efecto de Rosenthal Rosenthal effect
efecto de salsa bearnesa sauce Bearnaise effect
efecto de sótano basement effect
efecto de Stiles-Crawford Stiles-Crawford effect

efecto de suelo floor effect
efecto de sufijo suffix effect
efecto de sumación summation effect
efecto de tope ceiling effect
efecto de Transilvania Transylvania effect
efecto de Troxler Troxler's effect
efecto de von Restorff von Restorff effect
efecto de Vulpian Vulpian's effect
efecto de Wever-Bray Wever-Bray effect
efecto de Zeigarnik Zeigarnik effect
efecto del alcohol fetal fetal alcohol effect
efecto del orden order effect
efecto del pie en la puerta foot-in-the-door effect
efecto directo direct effect
efecto distal distal effect
efecto electrocardiográfico electrocardiographic effect
efecto estroboscópico stroboscopic effect
efecto extrapiramidal extrapyramidal effect
efecto formativo fashioning effect
efecto no específico nonspecific effect
efecto posterior aftereffect
efecto posterior espiral spiral aftereffect
efecto principal main effect
efecto secundario side effect
efecto secundario autónomo autonomic side effect
efecto de Land Land effect
efector effector
efectos adversos de medicación adverse effects of medication
efectos ambientales en el desarrollo cognitivo environmental effects on cognitive development
efectos configuracionales configurational effects
efectos de abuso de niños effects of child abuse
efectos de abuso sexual de niños effects of child sexual abuse
efectos de anfetaminas amphetamine effects
efectos de cafeína effects of caffeine
efectos de confinamiento confinement effects
efectos de contraste al entrevistar contrast effects in interviewing
efectos de decisiones decision effects
efectos de drogas drug effects
efectos de drogas en detección de mentiras drug effects in lie detection
efectos de edad age effects
efectos de estimulación stimulation effects
efectos de estrés effects of stress
efectos de hospitalización effects of hospitalization
efectos de interferencia interference effects
efectos de irradiación irradiation effects
efectos de la aspirina aspirin effects
efectos de la humedad humidity effects
efectos de presión del aire air pressure effects
efectos de privación deprivation effects
efectos de ruido noise effects
efectos de temperatura temperature effects

efectos del calor heat effects
efectos del contexto context effects
efectos del entrevistador interviewer effects
efectos del éter ether effects
efectos del experimentador experimenter
    effects
efectos del frío cold effects
efectos indirectos indirect effects
efectos neurofisiológicos del ejercicio
    neurophysiological effects of exercise
efectos posteriores de moción motion
    aftereffects
efectos posteriores figurales figural
    aftereffects
efectos prenatales del alcohol prenatal effects
    of alcohol
efectos psicofisiológicos del ejercicio
    psychophysiologic effects of exercise
efectos psicológicos psychological effects
efectos psicológicos de hospitalización
    psychological effects of hospitalization
efectos psicológicos del ejercicio
    psychological effects of exercise
efectos ambientales environmental effects
efedrina ephedrine
eferente efferent
eficacia efficacy
eficiencia de pronosticación forecasting
    efficiency
eficiencia del sueño sleep efficiency
eficiencia del sueño de movimientos oculares
    rápidos rapid eye movement sleep
    efficiency
eficiencia predictiva predictive efficiency
eficiente efficient
efímero ephemeral
egersis egersis
ego ego
ego antilibidinal antilibidinal ego
ego apoyador supportive ego
ego auxiliar auxiliary ego
ego corporal body ego
ego de realidad reality ego
ego de sueños dream ego
ego débil weak ego
ego del placer pleasure ego
ego ideal ego ideal
ego ideal transitorio transient ego ideal
ego preesquizofrénico preschizophrenic ego
egocéntrico egocentric
egocentrismo egocentrism
egocentrismo durante adolescencia
    egocentrism during adolescence
egodistónico ego-dystonic
egointegrativo ego-integrative
egoísmo egoism
egoísta egoistic
egomanía egomania
egomorfismo egomorphism
egopatía egopathy
egosintónico ego-syntonic
egoteísmo egotheism
egótico egotic
egotismo egotism
egotista egotistic

egotista egotistical
egotización egotization
egotropía egotropy
egotrópico egotropic
egregorsis egregorsis
eidético eidetic
eidoptometría eidoptometry
Eigenwelt Eigenwelt
Einstellung Einstellung
eisoptrofobia eisoptrophobia
eje axis
eje cefalocaudal cephalocaudal axis
eje hipotalámico-pituitario
    hypothalamic-pituitary axis
eje óptico optical axis
eje sagital sagittal axis
eje vertical vertical axis
eje visual visual axis
eje X X axis
eje Y Y axis
ejecución performance
ejecución académica academic performance
ejecución de trabajo job performance
ejecutivo executive
ejemplo negativo negative example
ejercicio exercise
ejercicio aeróbico aerobic exercise
ejercicio agudo acute exercise
ejercicio como conducta para bregar
    exercise as coping behavior
ejercicio como distracción exercise as
    distraction
ejercicio crónico chronic exercise
ejercicio de conciencia awareness exercise
ejercicio e imagen corporal exercise and
    body image
ejercicio físico physical exercise
ejercicios de intervalo de moción
    range-of-motion exercises
ejercicios de Kegel Kegel exercises
ejercicios intergrupales intergroup exercises
ejes correlacionados correlated axes
ejes de referencia reference axes
ejes diagnósticos diagnostic axes
ejes factoriales factor axes
elaboración elaboration
elaboración secundaria secondary elaboration
elación elation
electivo elective
electroanalgesia electroanalgesia
electrocardiógrafo electrocardiograph
electrocardiograma electrocardiogram
electrocerebral electrocerebral
electrocontractilidad electrocontractility
electroconvulsivo electroconvulsive
electrocorticografía electrocorticography
electrocorticograma electrocorticogram
electrocutáneo electrocutaneous
electrochoque electroshock
electrodérmico electrodermal
electrodiagnóstico electrodiagnosis
electrodo electrode
electrodo de calomel calomel electrode
electroencefalografía electroencephalography
electroencefalográfico

electroencephalographic
electroencefalógrafo electroencephalograph
electroencefalograma electroencephalogram
electroencefalograma isoeléctrico isoelectric electroencephalogram
electroencefalograma plano flat electroencephalogram
electroespectrografía electrospectrography
electroespinografía electrospinography
electroespinograma electrospinogram
electroestimulación electrostimulation
electrofisiología electrophysiology
electrofobia electrophobia
electroforesis electrophoresis
electrofrénico electrophrenic
electrográfico electrographic
electrólito electrolyte
electrolepsia electrolepsy
electromagnético electromagnetic
electromicturición electromicturition
electromiógrafo electromyograph
electromiograma electromyogram
electromuscular electromuscular
electronarcosis electronarcosis
electroneurografía electroneurography
electroneurólisis electroneurolysis
electroneuromiografía electroneuromyography
electrónico electronic
electronistagmografía electronystagmography
electrooculograma electrooculogram
electroolfatograma electroolfactogram
electropatología electropathology
electroplejía electroplexy
electrorretinograma electroretinogram
electrosueño electrosleep
electroterapéutico electrotherapeutic
electroterapia electrotherapy
electroterapia cerebral cerebral electrotherapy
electrotónico electrotonic
electrotono electrotonus
elefantiasis elephantiasis
elefantiasis neuromatosa elephantiasis neuromatosa
elemental elementary
elementarismo elementarism
elemento element
elemento de estímulo stimulus element
elemento mental mental element
elemento O O element
elemento retinal retinal element
elementos de pensamiento elements of thought
elementos del lenguaje elements of language
eleuteromanía eleutheromania
elevación elevation
elevador levator
elevador perióstico periosteal elevator
eliminación elimination
elipsis ellipsis
elogio praise
elucidación elucidation
emancipación emancipation
emancipado emancipated

emasculación emasculation
embarazo pregnancy
embarazo adolescente adolescent pregnancy
embarazo bigémino bigeminal pregnancy
embarazo de trompa de Falopio Fallopian-tube pregnancy
embarazo ectópico ectopic pregnancy
embarazo extrauterino extrauterine pregnancy
embarazo falso false pregnancy
embarazo histérico hysterical pregnancy
embarazo normal normal pregnancy
emblema emblem
embolalia embolalia
embolismo embolism
embolismo cerebral cerebral embolism
embolización embolization
embolofasia embolophasia
embolofrasia embolophrasia
embololalia embololalia
embriaguez drunkenness
embriaguez del sueño sleep drunkenness
embriaguez sensiblera maudlin drunkenness
embriología embryology
embrión embryo
embriónico embryonic
emenia emmenia
emeniopatía emmeniopathy
emergencia emergency, emergence
emergencia de empatía emergence of empathy
emergencia psiquiátrica psychiatric emergency
emergente emergent
emergentismo emergentism
emesis emesis
emetofobia emetophobia
emetomanía emetomania
emetropía emmetropia
émico emic
emilcamato emylcamate
emisión emission
emisión de pensamientos thought broadcasting
emisión nocturna nocturnal emission
emitir emit
emoción emotion
emoción defensiva defensive emotion
emoción expresada expressed emotion
emoción fría cold emotion
emoción fundamental fundamental emotion
emocional emotional
emocionalidad emotionality
emocionalidad expresada expressed emotionality
emocionalmente emotionally
emociones condicionadas conditioned emotions
emociones discretas discrete emotions
emociones ictales ictal emotions
emotiovascular emotiovascular
emotivo emotive
empalme de genes gene-splicing
empatía empathy
empatía generativa generative empathy

empatía primaria primary empathy
empático empathic
empatizar empathize
empírico empirical
empirismo empiricism
empleado employee
empleo employment
empleo por cuenta propia self-employment
empobrecimiento intelectual intellectual
    impoverishment
emprostótonos emprosthotonos
emulación emulation
enanismo dwarfism
enanismo diastrófico diastrophic dwarfism
enanismo nanocefálico nanocephalic
    dwarfism
enanismo por privación deprivation dwarfism
enanismo psicosocial psychosocial dwarfism
enantato enanthate
enantiobiosis enantiobiosis
enantiodromia enantiodromia
enantiopático enantiopathic
encadenamiento chaining
encadenamiento accidental accidental
    chaining
encadenamiento auditivo auditory sequencing
encadenamiento de conducta behavior
    chaining
encadenamiento de Markoff Markoff
    chaining
encadenamiento de Markov Markov chaining
encadenamiento hacia atrás backward
    chaining
encapsulación encapsulation
encapsulado encapsulated
encatalepsia encatalepsis
encefalalgia encephalalgia
encefalastenia encephalasthenia
encefalatrofía encephalatrophy
encefalatrófico encephalatrophic
encefalauxa encephalauxe
encefalemia encephalemia
encefálico encephalic
encefalina enkephalin
encefalítico encephalitic
encefalitis encephalitis
encefalitis alérgica experimental
    experimental allergic encephalitis
encefalitis de Bickerstaff Bickerstaff's
    encephalitis
encefalitis de cuerpos de inclusión
    inclusion-body encephalitis
encefalitis de cuerpos de inclusión subaguda
    subacute inclusion body encephalitis
encefalitis de Dawson Dawson's encephalitis
encefalitis de leñador woodcutter's
    encephalitis
encefalitis de varicela varicella encephalitis
encefalitis epidémica epidemic encephalitis
encefalitis equina equine encephalitis
encefalitis hemorrágica encephalitis
    hemorrhagica
encefalitis hemorrágica aguda acute
    hemorrhagic encephalitis
encefalitis hemorrágica de arsfenamina

    arsphenamine hemorrhagic encephalitis
encefalitis hiperérgica hyperergic encephalitis
encefalitis hipersómnica hypersomnic
    encephalitis
encefalitis letárgica encephalitis lethargica
encefalitis límbica paraneoplásica
    paraneoplastic limbic encephalitis
encefalitis metabólica metabolic encephalitis
encefalitis mioclónica myoclonic encephalitis
encefalitis necrotizante necrotizing
    encephalitis
encefalitis necrotizante aguda acute
    necrotizing encephalitis
encefalitis neonatal encephalitis neonatorum
encefalitis periaxial concéntrica encephalitis
    periaxialis concentrica
encefalitis periaxial difusa encephalitis
    periaxialis diffusa
encefalitis piogénica encephalitis pyogenica
encefalitis por Bunyavirus Bunyavirus
    encephalitis
encefalitis por Coxsackie Coxsackie
    encephalitis
encefalitis por herpes herpes encephalitis
encefalitis por herpes simple herpes simplex
    encephalitis
encefalitis por Iheus Ilheus encephalitis
encefalitis por Mengo Mengo encephalitis
encefalitis por plomo lead encephalitis
encefalitis por Powassan Powassan
    encephalitis
encefalitis posvacunal postvaccinal
    encephalitis
encefalitis purulenta purulent encephalitis
encefalitis secundaria secondary encephalitis
encefalitis subcortical crónica encephalitis
    subcorticalis chronica
encefalitis supurativa suppurative encephalitis
encefalitis transmitida por garrapatas
    tick-borne encephalitis
encefalitis vernal vernal encephalitis
encefalitogénico encephalitogenic
encefalitógeno encephalitogen
encefalización encephalization
encéfalo encephalon
encefalocele encephalocele
encefalodinia encephalodynia
encefalodisplasia encephalodysplasia
encefaloesclerosis encephalosclerosis
encefalografía encephalography
encefalografía de aire air encephalography
encefalograma encephalogram
encefalograma isoeléctrico isoelectric
    encephalogram
encefaloide encephaloid
encefalolito encephalolith
encefalología encephalology
encefaloma encephaloma
encefalomalacia encephalomalacia
encefalomeningitis encephalomeningitis
encefalomeningocele encephalomeningocele
encefalomeningopatía
    encephalomeningopathy
encefalómetro encephalometer
encefalomielitis encephalomyelitis

encefalomielitis alérgica experimental
experimental allergic encephalomyelitis
encefalomielitis diseminada aguda acute
disseminated encephalomyelitis
encefalomielitis equina del este eastern
equine encephalomyelitis
encefalomielitis equina del oeste western
equine encephalomyelitis
encefalomielitis granulomatosa
granulomatous encephalomyelitis
encefalomielitis miálgica epidémica epidemic
myalgic encephalomyelitis
encefalomielitis miálgica benigna benign
myalgic encephalomyelitis
encefalomielitis viral virus encephalomyelitis
encefalomielitis zoster zoster
encephalomyelitis
encefalomielocele encephalomyelocele
encefalomieloneuropatía
encephalomyeloneuropathy
encefalomieloneuropatía inespecífica
nonspecific encephalomyeloneuropathy
encefalomielopatía encephalomyelopathy
encefalomielopatía carcinomatosa
carcinomatous encephalomyelopathy
encefalomielopatía miálgica epidémica
epidemic myalgic encephalomyelopathy
encefalomielopatía necrotizante necrotizing
encephalomyelopathy
encefalomielopatía necrotizante subaguda
subacute necrotizing encephalomyelopathy
encefalomielopatía paracarcinomatosa
paracarcinomatous encephalomyelopathy
encefalomielorradiculitis
encephalomyeloradiculitis
encefalomielorradiculopatía
encephalomyeloradiculopathy
encefalomiocarditis encephalomyocarditis
encefalonarcosis encephalonarcosis
encefalopatía encephalopathy
encefalopatía arterioesclerótica subcortical
subcortical arteriosclerotic encephalopathy
encefalopatía de Binswanger Binswanger's
encephalopathy
encefalopatía de Gayet-Wernicke
Gayet-Wernicke's encephalopathy
encefalopatía de Wernicke Wernicke's
encephalopathy
encefalopatía de Wernicke-Korsakoff
Wernicke-Korsakoff encephalopathy
encefalopatía desmielinizante demyelinating
encephalopathy
encefalopatía epileptogénica epileptogenic
encephalopathy
encefalopatía espongiforme spongiform
encephalopathy
encefalopatía espongiforme subaguda
subacute spongiform encephalopathy
encefalopatía familiar familial
encephalopathy
encefalopatía fluente de Wernicke
Wernicke's fluent encephalopathy
encefalopatía hepática hepatic
encephalopathy
encefalopatía hipercinética hyperkinetic

encephalopathy
encefalopatía hipernatrémica hypernatremic
encephalopathy
encefalopatía hipertensiva hypertensive
encephalopathy
encefalopatía metabólica metabolic
encephalopathy
encefalopatía palindrómica palindromic
encephalopathy
encefalopatía pancreática pancreatic
encephalopathy
encefalopatía por bilirrubina bilirubin
encephalopathy
encefalopatía por mercurio mercury
encephalopathy
encefalopatía por plomo lead encephalopathy
encefalopatía portal sistémica portal-systemic
encephalopathy
encefalopatía portosistémica portosystemic
encephalopathy
encefalopatía progresiva traumática
traumatic progressive encephalopathy
encefalopatía recurrente recurrent
encephalopathy
encefalopatía saturnina saturnine
encephalopathy
encefalopatía subcortical subcortical
encephalopathy
encefalopatía subcortical degenerativa
progresiva progressive degenerative
subcortical encephalopathy
encefalopatía subcortical progresiva
progressive subcortical encephalopathy
encefalopatía tirotóxica thyrotoxic
encephalopathy
encefalopatía traumática traumatic
encephalopathy
encefalopiosis encephalopyosis
encefalopsia encephalopsy
encefalopsicosis encephalopsychosis
encefalorragia encephalorrhagia
encefaloscopia encephaloscopy
encefaloscopio encephaloscope
encefalosis encephalosis
encefalosquisis encephaloschisis
encefalotlipsis encephalothlipsis
encefalotomía encephalotomy
encefalótomo encephalotome
encefalotrigeminal encephalotrigeminal
encigótico enzygotic
encogimiento de cabezas head-shrinking
encopresis encopresis
encopresis funcional functional encopresis
encripción encryption
encubierto covert
encuentro encounter
encuesta survey
encuesta de actitudes attitude survey
encuesta de actitudes de empleados
employee attitude survey
encuesta de consumidores consumer survey
encuesta de evaluación de necesidades
needs-assessment survey
encuesta de opinión pública public-opinion
poll

encuesta de opiniones opinion poll
encuesta indirecta indirect survey
encuesta normativa normative survey
enculturación enculturation
endarterectomía endarterectomy
endémico endemic
enderezamiento righting
endoaneurismoplastía endoaneurysmoplasty
endoaneurismorrafia endoaneurysmorrhaphy
endocarditis endocarditis
endocarditis bacterial bacterial endocarditis
endocatección endocathection
endocepto endocept
endocrinismo endocrinism
endocrino endocrine
endocrinología endocrinology
endocrinología conductual behavioral
  endocrinology
endocrinológico endocrinological
endocrinopatía endocrinopathy
endodermo endoderm
endofasia endophasia
endogamia endogamy
endogénesis endogenesis
endogenético endogenetic
endogenia endogeny
endogénico endogenic
endógeno endogenous
endogenomórfico endogenomorphic
endolinfa endolymph
endometrio endometrium
endometritis endometritis
endomorfia endomorphy
endomórfico endomorphic
endomorfo endomorph
endomusia endomusia
endoneuritis endoneuritis
endonucleasa endonuclease
endonucleasa de restricción restriction
  endonuclease
endoperineuritis endoperineuritis
endopsíquico endopsychic
endoreactivo endoreactive
endorfina endorphin
endorfina alfa alpha endorphin
endorfina beta beta endorphin
enelicomorfismo enelicomorphism
enema enema
energía energy
energía de acción específica action-specific
  energy
energía de afecto affect energy
energía de vida life energy
energía dirigida bound energy
energía específica de reacción
  reaction-specific energy
energía nerviosa nervous energy
energía psíquica psychic energy
energía radiante radiant energy
energía sexual sexual energy
energías nerviosas específicas specific nerve
  energies
energizador energizer
energizador psíquico psychic energizer
enervación enervation

enfático emphatic
enfermedad disease, sickness, illness
enfermedad aguda acute illness
enfermedad arterial coronaria coronary
  artery disease
enfermedad atípica atypical disease
enfermedad autoinmune autoimmune disease
enfermedad bipolar bipolar illness
enfermedad bipolar atípica atypical bipolar
  disease
enfermedad caison caisson disease
enfermedad cardíaca heart disease
enfermedad cardíaca e ira heart disease and
  anger
enfermedad cardiovascular cardiovascular
  disease
enfermedad catastrófica catastrophic illness
enfermedad cerebral brain disease
enfermedad cerebral senil senile brain
  disease
enfermedad cerebrovascular cerebrovascular
  disease
enfermedad cíclica cyclic illness
enfermedad circular circular illness
enfermedad citomegálica cytomegalic disease
enfermedad como autocastigo illness as
  self-punishment
enfermedad cutánea skin disease
enfermedad danzante dancing disease
enfermedad de Adams-Stokes Adams-Stokes
  disease
enfermedad de adaptación adaptation disease
enfermedad de Addison Addison's disease
enfermedad de administrador manager
  disease
enfermedad de Akureyri Akureyri disease
enfermedad de Alexander Alexander's
  disease
enfermedad de Alpers Alpers' disease
enfermedad de altitud altitude sickness
enfermedad de Alzheimer Alzheimer's
  disease
enfermedad de Aran-Duchenne
  Aran-Duchenne disease
enfermedad de Ballet Ballet's disease
enfermedad de Balo Balo's disease
enfermedad de Bamberger Bamberger's
  disease
enfermedad de Bannister Bannister's disease
enfermedad de Batten Batten's disease
enfermedad de Batten-Mayou Batten-Mayou
  disease
enfermedad de Bayle Bayle's disease
enfermedad de Beard Beard's disease
enfermedad de Bechterew Bechterew's
  disease
enfermedad de Begbie Begbie's disease
enfermedad de Behcet Behcet's disease
enfermedad de Bernhardt Bernhardt's
  disease
enfermedad de Bielschowsky Bielschowsky's
  disease
enfermedad de Binswanger Binswanger's
  disease
enfermedad de Blocq Blocq's disease

enfermedad de Bourneville Bourneville's
disease
enfermedad de Bourneville-Pringle
Bourneville-Pringle disease
enfermedad de Boyle Boyle's disease
enfermedad de Brissaud Brissaud's disease
enfermedad de Brodie Brodie's disease
enfermedad de Brushfield-Wyatt
Brushfield-Wyatt disease
enfermedad de Buerger Buerger's disease
enfermedad de Buschke Buschke's disease
enfermedad de Busse-Buschke
Busse-Buschke disease
enfermedad de cabello ensortijado
kinky-hair disease
enfermedad de caerse falling sickness
enfermedad de Canavan Canavan's disease
enfermedad de células de inclusión
inclusion-cell disease
enfermedad de células I I-cell disease
enfermedad de Charcot Charcot's disease
enfermedad de Charcot-Marie-Tooth
Charcot-Marie-Tooth disease
enfermedad de Cheyne Cheyne's disease
enfermedad de Christensen-Krabbe
Christensen-Krabbe disease
enfermedad de Conradi Conradi's disease
enfermedad de Cottunius Cottunius disease
enfermedad de Creutzfeldt-Jakob
Creutzfeldt-Jakob disease
enfermedad de Crigler-Najjar Crigler-Najjar
disease
enfermedad de Crouzon Crouzon's disease
enfermedad de Cruveilhier Cruveilhier's
disease
enfermedad de cuerpos de Lafora Lafora
body disease
enfermedad de Cushing Cushing's disease
enfermedad de Danielssen Danielssen's
disease
enfermedad de Danielssen-Boeck
Danielssen-Boeck disease
enfermedad de Dejerine Dejerine's disease
enfermedad de Dejerine-Sottas
Dejerine-Sottas disease
enfermedad de descompresión
decompression sickness
enfermedad de Devic Devic's disease
enfermedad de Down Down's disease
enfermedad de Dubini Dubini's disease
enfermedad de Duchenne Duchenne's
disease
enfermedad de Duchenne-Aran
Duchenne-Aran disease
enfermedad de Durante Durante's disease
enfermedad de Economo Economo's disease
enfermedad de Engelmann Engelmann's
disease
enfermedad de Erb Erb's disease
enfermedad de Erb-Charcot Erb-Charcot
disease
enfermedad de Erichsen Erichsen's disease
enfermedad de Eulenburg Eulenburg's
disease
enfermedad de Fabry Fabry's disease

enfermedad de Fahr Fahr's disease
enfermedad de Falret Falret's disease
enfermedad de Feer Feer's disease
enfermedad de Flatau-Schilder
Flatau-Schilder disease
enfermedad de Folling Folling's disease
enfermedad de Fothergill Fothergill's disease
enfermedad de Friedmann Friedmann's
disease
enfermedad de Friedreich Friedreich's
disease
enfermedad de Fuerstner Fuerstner's disease
enfermedad de Gairdner Gairdner's disease
enfermedad de Gaucher Gaucher's disease
enfermedad de Gerhardt Gerhardt's disease
enfermedad de Gerlier Gerlier's disease
enfermedad de Gilles de la Tourette Gilles
de la Tourette's disease
enfermedad de Goldflam Goldflam disease
enfermedad de Goldscheider Goldscheider's
disease
enfermedad de Gowers Gowers disease
enfermedad de Graefe Graefe's disease
enfermedad de Graves Graves' disease
enfermedad de Greenfield Greenfield's
disease
enfermedad de Grieg Grieg's disease
enfermedad de Guinon Guinon's disease
enfermedad de Gunther Gunther's disease
enfermedad de Hakim Hakim's disease
enfermedad de Hallervorden-Spatz
Hallervorden-Spatz disease
enfermedad de Hammond Hammond's
disease
enfermedad de Hansen Hansen's disease
enfermedad de Hartnup Hartnup disease
enfermedad de Heidenheim Heidenheim's
disease
enfermedad de Heine-Medin Heine-Medin
disease
enfermedad de Heller Heller's disease
enfermedad de Herrmann Herrmann's
disease
enfermedad de hígado alcohólica alcoholic
liver disease
enfermedad de Hippel Hippel's disease
enfermedad de Hippel-Landau
Hippel-Landau disease
enfermedad de Hirshsprung Hirshsprung's
disease
enfermedad de Hoppe-Goldflam
Hoppe-Goldflam disease
enfermedad de Huntington Huntington's
disease
enfermedad de Jakob-Creutzfeldt
Jakob-Creutzfeldt disease
enfermedad de Janet Janet's disease
enfermedad de Jansky-Bielschowsky
Jansky-Bielschowsky disease
enfermedad de Kempf Kempf's disease
enfermedad de Klippel Klippel's disease
enfermedad de Krabbe Krabbe's disease
enfermedad de Kraepelin Kraepelin's disease
enfermedad de Kufs Kufs disease
enfermedad de Kugelberg-Welander

Kugelberg-Welander disease
enfermedad de la risa laughing sickness
enfermedad de Lafora Lafora's disease
enfermedad de Langdon Down Langdon
    Down's disease
enfermedad de Lasegue Lasegue's disease
enfermedad de Leber Leber's disease
enfermedad de Leigh Leigh's disease
enfermedad de Leroy Leroy's disease
enfermedad de Lhermitte-Duclos
    Lhermitte-Duclos disease
enfermedad de Lindau Lindau's disease
enfermedad de Little Little's disease
enfermedad de Lou Gehrig Lou Gehrig's
    disease
enfermedad de Luft Luft's disease
enfermedad de Machado-Joseph
    Machado-Joseph disease
enfermedad de Marchiafava-Bignami
    Marchiafava-Bignami disease
enfermedad de Marie-Strumpell
    Marie-Strumpell disease
enfermedad de médula espinal spinal-cord
    disease
enfermedad de membrana hialina
    hyaline-membrane disease
enfermedad de Merzbacher-Pelizaeus
    Merzbacher-Pelizaeus disease
enfermedad de Milton Milton's disease
enfermedad de Minamata Minamata disease
enfermedad de Mitchell Mitchell's disease
enfermedad de Mobius Mobius disease
enfermedad de moción motion sickness
enfermedad de Morgagni Morgagni's disease
enfermedad de Morvan Morvan's disease
enfermedad de Moschowitz Moschowitz's
    disease
enfermedad de Neftel Neftel's disease
enfermedad de neuronas motoras motor
    neuron disease
enfermedad de Nielsen Nielsen's disease
enfermedad de Niemann-Pick Niemann-Pick
    disease
enfermedad de Norrie Norrie's disease
enfermedad de Oppenheim Oppenheim's
    disease
enfermedad de orina de jarabe de arce
    maple syrup urine disease
enfermedad de Paget Paget's disease
enfermedad de Parkinson Parkinson's
    disease
enfermedad de Parry Parry's disease
enfermedad de Pelizaeus-Merzbacher
    Pelizaeus-Merzbacher disease
enfermedad de Pette-Doring Pette-Doring
    disease
enfermedad de Pick Pick's disease
enfermedad de Plummer Plummer's disease
enfermedad de Pompe Pompe's disease
enfermedad de Pott Pott's disease
enfermedad de prisa hurry sickness
enfermedad de Quincke Quincke's disease
enfermedad de Raynaud Raynaud's disease
enfermedad de Recklinghausen
    Recklinghausen's disease

enfermedad de Refsum Refsum's disease
enfermedad de Romberg Romberg's disease
enfermedad de Roth Roth's disease
enfermedad de Roth-Berhardt Roth-Berhardt
    disease
enfermedad de Roussy-Levy Roussy-Levy
    disease
enfermedad de Rust Rust's disease
enfermedad de saltador jumper disease
enfermedad de Sandhoff Sandhoff's disease
enfermedad de Schaumberg Schaumberg's
    disease
enfermedad de Schilder Schilder's disease
enfermedad de Scholz Scholz' disease
enfermedad de Seitelberger Seitelberger's
    disease
enfermedad de Selter Selter's disease
enfermedad de Siemerling-Creutzfeldt
    Siemerling-Creutzfeldt disease
enfermedad de Simmonds Simmonds'
    disease
enfermedad de sistemas combinados
    combined system disease
enfermedad de Spielmeyer-Sjogren
    Spielmeyer-Sjogren disease
enfermedad de Spielmeyer-Vogt
    Spielmeyer-Vogt disease
enfermedad de Steele-Richardson-Olszewski
    Steele-Richardson-Olszewski disease
enfermedad de Steinert Steinert's disease
enfermedad de Stern Stern's disease
enfermedad de Stokes-Adams Stokes-Adams
    disease
enfermedad de Strumpell Strumpell's disease
enfermedad de Strumpell-Marie
    Strumpell-Marie disease
enfermedad de Strumpell-Westphal
    Strumpell-Westphal disease
enfermedad de Sturge Sturge's disease
enfermedad de Sturge-Weber Sturge-Weber
    disease
enfermedad de Sturge-Weber-Dimitri
    Sturge-Weber-Dimitri disease
enfermedad de Sydenham Sydenham's
    disease
enfermedad de Takayasu Takayasu's disease
enfermedad de Talma Talma's disease
enfermedad de Tarui Tarui's disease
enfermedad de Tay-Sachs Tay-Sachs disease
enfermedad de Thomsen Thomsen's disease
enfermedad de Tourette Tourette's disease
enfermedad de Unverricht Unverricht's
    disease
enfermedad de Urbach-Wiethe
    Urbach-Wiethe disease
enfermedad de van Bogaert van Bogaert's
    disease
enfermedad de Virchow Virchow's disease
enfermedad de Vogt-Spielmeyer
    Vogt-Spielmeyer disease
enfermedad de von Economo von Economo's
    disease
enfermedad de von Gierke von Gierke's
    disease
enfermedad de von Hippel-Lindau von

Hippel-Lindau disease
enfermedad de von Recklinghausen von
Recklinghausen's disease
enfermedad de Werdnig-Hoffmann
Werdnig-Hoffmann disease
enfermedad de Werner Werner's disease
enfermedad de Wernicke Wernicke's disease
enfermedad de Westphal Westphal's disease
enfermedad de Wilson Wilson's disease
enfermedad de Winkelman Winkelman's
disease
enfermedad de
Wohlfart-Kugelberg-Welander
Wohlfart-Kugelberg-Welander disease
enfermedad de Wolman Wolman's disease
enfermedad de Ziehen-Oppenheim
Ziehen-Oppenheim disease
enfermedad del dormir sleeping sickness
enfermedad del estudiante student's disease
enfermedad desmielinizante demyelinating
disease
enfermedad dinámica dynamic disease
enfermedad emocional emotional illness
enfermedad extrapiramidal extrapyramidal
disease
enfermedad fatal fatal illness
enfermedad física physical illness
enfermedad funcional functional illness
enfermedad genetotrófica genetotrophic
disease
enfermedad hepatolenticular hepatolenticular
disease
enfermedad iatrogénica iatrogenic illness
enfermedad infecciosa infectious disease
enfermedad maniacodepresivo
manic-depressive illness
enfermedad matutina morning sickness
enfermedad mental mental illness
enfermedad mental refractaria refractory
mental illness
enfermedad neoplásica neoplastic disease
enfermedad nerviosa nervous disease
enfermedad neuromuscular neuromuscular
disease
enfermedad obstructiva obstructive disease
enfermedad ósea bone disease
enfermedad poliquística infantil infantile
polycystic disease
enfermedad por radiación radiation sickness
enfermedad psiquiátrica psychiatric illness
enfermedad pulmonar obstructiva crónica
chronic obstructive pulmonary disease
enfermedad quística medular medullary
cystic disease
enfermedad rectal rectal disease
enfermedad rosada pink disease
enfermedad terminal terminal illness
enfermedad transmitida sexualmente
sexually transmitted disease
enfermedad venérea venereal disease
enfermedad y estrés disease and stress
enfermedades de adaptación diseases of
adaptation
enfermedades y cambios de vida disease and
life changes

enfermería de coordinación liaison nursing
enfermo sick
enfermo mental crónico chronic mentally ill
enfermo simulado malingerer
enfisema emphysema
enfisema subgaleal subgaleal emphysema
enfocado focused
enfoque focusing
enfoque en sensaciones sensate focus
enfriamiento de afecto cooling of affect
engendrado por reproducción consanguínea
inbred
engrafia engraphia
engrama engram
engrama de funciones function engram
engullidor gorger
engullidor-vomitador gorger-vomiter
engullir gorge
enisofobia enissophobia
enlace linkage
enlace al sexo sex linkage
enlace asociativo associative linkage
enlace genético genetic linkage
enlace peptídico peptide bond
enlutar mourn
enmascaramiento masking
enmascaramiento auditivo auditory masking
enmascaramiento hacia atrás backward
masking
enmascaramiento lateral lateral masking
enmascaramiento lateral mutuo mutual
lateral masking
enmascaramiento perceptivo perceptual
masking
enmascaramiento remoto remote masking
enomanía enomania
enosimanía enosimania
enosiofobia enosiophobia
enredamiento enmeshment
enriquecido enriched
enriquecimiento enrichment
enriquecimiento ambiental environmental
enrichment
enriquecimiento de trabajo job enrichment
ensalada de palabras word salad
ensamblaje celular cell assembly
ensayo trial, assay
ensayo abierto open trial
ensayo clínico clinical trial
ensayo clínico aleatorizado randomized
clinical trial
ensayo clínico controlado controlled clinical
trial
ensayo cognitivo cognitive rehearsal
ensayo complicado elaborative rehearsal
ensayo conductual behavioral rehearsal
ensayo de adquisición acquisition trial
ensayo de aprendizaje learning trial
ensayo de captura catch trial
ensayo de entrenamiento training trial
ensayo de extinción extinction trial
ensayo de observación observation trial
ensayo de papel role rehearsal
ensayo de pensamientos thought rehearsal
ensayo de práctica practice trial

ensayo en blanco blank trial
ensayo verbal verbal rehearsal
enseñanza teaching
enseñanza clínica clinical teaching
enseñanza dialéctica dialectical teaching
ensueño daydream
ensueño de héroe hero daydream
ensueño de héroe triunfador conquering-hero
  daydream
ensueño hipnagógico hypnagogic reverie
entasia entasia
entasis entasis
entático entatic
entelequia entelechy
entender understand
entendimiento understanding
entendimiento empático empathic
  understanding
entendimiento propio self-understanding
enteroceptor enteroceptor
entidad entity
entlasis enthlasis
entodermo entoderm
entomofobia entomophobia
entonación intonation
entóptico entoptic
entrada input
entrada-salida input-output
entrada sensorial sensory input
entrampamiento entrapment
entrecruzamiento crossover
entrecruzamiento doble ciego double-blind
  crossover
entrelazado interlocking
entrenador sintético synthetic trainer
entrenamiento training
entrenamiento asertivo assertive training
entrenamiento audiovisual audiovisual
  training
entrenamiento auditivo auditory training
entrenamiento autogénico autogenic training
entrenamiento aversivo aversive training
entrenamiento cooperativo cooperative
  training
**entrenamiento de administración de
  ansiedad** anxiety management training
entrenamiento de biorretroalimentación
  biofeedback training
entrenamiento de cargador magazine
  training
entrenamiento de comunicación
  communication training
entrenamiento de control control training
entrenamiento de control de retención
  retention control training
entrenamiento de destrezas de comunicación
  communication skills training
entrenamiento de destrezas sociales social
  skills training
entrenamiento de dominio mastery training
entrenamiento de efectividad de padres
  parent-effectiveness training
entrenamiento de empatía empathy training
entrenamiento de escape escape training
entrenamiento de espontaneidad spontaneity

training
entrenamiento de evitación avoidance
  training
entrenamiento de hábito habit training
entrenamiento de inoculación para estrés
  stress inoculation training
entrenamiento de inodoro toilet training
entrenamiento de laboratorio laboratory
  training
entrenamiento de liderazgo leadership
  training
entrenamiento de memoria memory training
entrenamiento de ondas alfa alpha wave
  training
entrenamiento de relajación relaxation
  training
entrenamiento de sensibilidad sensitivity
  training
entrenamiento del entrevistador interviewer
  training
entrenamiento del personal personnel
  training
entrenamiento en el trabajo on-the-job
  training
entrenamiento en relaciones humanas
  human-relations training
entrenamiento intestinal bowel training
entrenamiento perceptivo perceptual training
entrenamiento prevocacional prevocational
  training
entrenamiento vocacional vocational training
entrenamiento de vejiga bladder training
entrenar train
entrevista interview
entrevista con amobarbital amobarbital
  interview
entrevista bajo estrés stress interview
entrevista conjunta conjoint interview
entrevista de asesoramiento counseling
  interview
entrevista de empleo employment interview
entrevista de evaluación evaluation interview
entrevista de grupo group interview
entrevista de resolución de problemas
  problem-solving interview
entrevista de salida exit interview
entrevista de sistemas de familia family
  systems interview
entrevista de trabajo job interview
entrevista diagnóstica diagnostic interview
entrevista directa direct interview
entrevista estructurada structured interview
entrevista inicial initial interview
entrevista inicial de grupo familiar family
  group intake
entrevista no directiva nondirective interview
entrevista no estructurada unstructured
  interview
entrevista profunda depth interview
entrevista psiquiátrica psychiatric interview
entrevistador interviewer
entropía entropy
entumecimiento numbness
entumecimiento al despertar waking
  numbness

entumecimiento del sueño sleep numbness
enturbado clouded
enturbiamiento clouding
enturbiamiento de conciencia clouding of consciousness
enuresis enuresis
enuresis funcional functional enuresis
enuresis nocturna nocturnal enuresis
enurético enuretic
envejecimiento aging
envejecimiento biológico biological aging
envejecimiento e inteligencia aging and intelligence
envejecimiento precoz precocious aging
envejecimiento primario primary aging
envejecimiento secundario secondary aging
envenenamiento poisoning
envenenamiento por arsénico arsenic poisoning
envenenamiento por aspirina aspirin poisoning
envenenamiento por gas gas poisoning
envenenamiento por monóxido de carbono carbon monoxide poisoning
envenenamiento por nitrógeno nitrogen poisoning
envenenamiento por plomo lead poisoning
envenenamiento por solano nightshade poisoning
envenenamiento por tetracloruro de carbono carbon tetrachloride poisoning
envidia envy
envidia de falo phallus envy
envidia de pecho breast envy
envidia de pene penis envy
envidia vaginal vaginal envy
envoltura caliente hot pack
envoltura fría cold pack
envolvimiento involvement
envolvimiento de circunstantes bystander involvement
envolvimiento del ego ego involvement
envolvimiento del padre con alimentación por pecho father's involvement with breast-feeding
envolvimiento extrapiramidal extrapyramidal involvement
enzima enzyme
eonismo eonism
eosofobia eosophobia
ependimitis ependymitis
epéndimo ependyma
ependimoblastoma ependymoblastoma
ependimoma ependymoma
ependimoma mixopapilar myxopapillary ependymoma
epicrítico epicritic
epidemia epidemic
epidemia de danza dance epidemic
epidemia psiquiátrica psychiatric epidemic
epidemiología epidemiology
epidemiología de trastornos mentales epidemiology of mental disorders
epidemiología psiquiátrica psychiatric epidemiology

epidermis epidermis
epididimitis epididymitis
epidídimo epididymis
epidural epidural
epidurografía epidurography
epifenomenalismo epiphenomenalism
epifenómeno epiphenomenon
epifisiopatía epiphysiopathy
epífisis epiphysis
epigástrico epigastric
epigénesis epigenesis
epigenético epigenetic
epiglotis epiglottis
epilempsia epilempsis
epilepsia epilepsy
epilepsia abdominal abdominal epilepsy
epilepsia acinética akinetic epilepsy
epilepsia activada activated epilepsy
epilepsia alcohólica alcoholic epilepsy
epilepsia alucinatoria hallucinatory epilepsy
epilepsia anosognósica anosognosic epilepsy
epilepsia astática mioclónica myoclonic astatic epilepsy
epilepsia atónica atonic epilepsy
epilepsia audiogénica audiogenic epilepsy
epilepsia automática automatic epilepsy
epilepsia autónoma autonomic epilepsy
epilepsia centrencefálica centrencephalic epilepsy
epilepsia cortical cortical epilepsy
epilepsia de gran mal grand mal epilepsy
epilepsia de Kojewnikoff Kojewnikoff's epilepsy
epilepsia de lectura reading epilepsy
epilepsia de lóbulo temporal temporal-lobe epilepsy
epilepsia de mirada fija corta short-stare epilepsy
epilepsia de pequeño mal petit mal epilepsy
epilepsia de tornado tornado epilepsy
epilepsia del comer eating epilepsy
epilepsia del sueño sleep epilepsy
epilepsia diencefálica diencephalic epilepsy
epilepsia enmascarada masked epilepsy
epilepsia focal focal epilepsy
epilepsia fotogénica photogenic epilepsy
epilepsia gelástica gelastic epilepsy
epilepsia generalizada primaria primary generalized epilepsy
epilepsia generalizada secundaria secondary generalized epilepsy
epilepsia idiopática idiopathic epilepsy
epilepsia jacksoniana jacksonian epilepsy
epilepsia laríngea laryngeal epilepsy
epilepsia local local epilepsy
epilepsia matutina matutinal epilepsy
epilepsia mayor major epilepsy
epilepsia menor minor epilepsy
epilepsia mioclónica myoclonic epilepsy
epilepsia mioclónica juvenil juvenile myoclonic epilepsy
epilepsia musicogénica musicogenic epilepsy
epilepsia nocturna nocturnal epilepsy
epilepsia nutatoria epilepsia nutans
epilepsia parcial partial epilepsy

epilepsia parcial continua epilepsia partialis
continua
epilepsia por sobresalto startle epilepsy
epilepsia postraumática posttraumatic
epilepsy
epilepsia postraumática temprana early
posttraumatic epilepsy
epilepsia precipitada compleja complex
precipitated epilepsy
epilepsia precipitada sensorial sensory
precipitated epilepsy
epilepsia procursiva procursive epilepsy
epilepsia psicomotora psychomotor epilepsy
epilepsia refleja reflex epilepsy
epilepsia retropulsiva retropulsive epilepsy
epilepsia rolándica rolandic epilepsy
epilepsia sensitiva a patrón pattern sensitive
epilepsy
epilepsia sensorial sensory epilepsy
epilepsia sintomática symptomatic epilepsy
epilepsia sonámbula somnambulic epilepsy
epilepsia subictal subictal epilepsy
epilepsia tardía late epilepsy
epilepsia tónica tonic epilepsy
epilepsia tónica-clónica generalizada
generalized tonic-clonic epilepsy
epilepsia uncinada uncinate epilepsy
epilepsia vasomotora vasomotor epilepsy
epilepsia vasovagal vasovagal epilepsy
epilepsia visceral visceral epilepsy
epiléptico epileptic
epileptiforme epileptiform
epileptogénico epileptogenic
epileptógeno epileptogenous
epileptoide epileptoid
epiloia epiloia
epimenorragia epimenorrhagia
epinefrina epinephrine
epinósico epinosic
epinosis epinosis
episódico episodic
episodio episode
episodio amnésico amnestic episode
episodio de conducta behavior episode
episodio de depresión mayor major
depression episode
episodio depresivo depressive episode
episodio depresivo mayor major depressive
episode
episodio esquizofrénico schizophrenic episode
episodio esquizofrénico agudo acute
schizophrenic episode
episodio hipomaníaco hypomanic episode
episodio maníaco manic episode
episodio psicótico psychotic episode
epispadias epispadias
epistasis epistasis
epistémico epistemic
epistemofilia epistemophilia
epistemología epistemology
epistemología genética genetic epistemology
epitálamo epithalamus
epitelio epithelium
epitelio olfatorio olfactory epithelium
epitelioma epithelioma

época epoch
epónimo eponym
épsilon epsilon
equeosis echeosis
equidad equity
equilibración equilibration
equilibrio equilibrium
equilibrio biológico biological equilibrium
equilibrio dinámico dynamic equilibrium
equilibrio estático static equilibrium
equilibrio narcisista narcissistic equilibrium
equilibrio social social equilibrium
equilibrio homeostático homeostatic
equilibrium
equinofobia equinophobia
equipo equipment, team
equipo de crisis crisis team
equipo de evaluación assessment team
equipo de rehabilitación rehabilitation team
equipo para el modelado de arcilla
clay-modeling equipment
equipo psiquiátrico psychiatric team
equipotencialidad equipotentiality
equipotencialidad de señales equipotentiality
of cues
equivalencia equivalence
equivalencia de estímulos stimulus
equivalence
equivalencia de respuestas response
equivalence
equivalencia de señales equivalence of cues
equivalencia de señales adquirida acquired
equivalence of cues
equivalencia motora motor equivalence
equivalente equivalent
equivalente de ansiedad anxiety equivalent
equivalente de certidumbre certainty
equivalent
equivalente de edad age-equivalent
equivalente de grado grade equivalent
equivalente de masturbación masturbation
equivalent
equivalente de masturbación prefálico
prephallic masturbation equivalent
equivalente epiléptico epileptic equivalent
equivalente psíquico psychic equivalent
equivocación mistake
equivocación básica basic mistake
equivocación de categoría category mistake
equívoco double entendre, pun
era descriptiva descriptive era
era juvenil juvenile era
erección erection
erección peniana penile erection
eréctil erectile
erecto erect
eremiofobia eremiophobia
eremofilia eremophilia
eremofobia eremophobia
eretísmico erethismic
eretismo erethism
eretístico erethistic
eretítico erethitic
eretizofrenia erethizophrenia
eretizofrénico erethizophrenic

ereutofobia ereuthophobia
ergasia ergasia
ergasiofobia ergasiophobia
ergasiomanía ergasiomania
ergástico ergastic
ergastoplasma ergastoplasm
érgico ergic
ergio erg
ergodialepsia ergodialepsis
ergofobia ergophobia
ergógrafo ergograph
ergomanía ergomania
ergonomía ergonomics
ergopsicometría ergopsychometry
ergotamina ergotamine
ergoterapia ergotherapy
ergotismo ergotism
ergotismo espasmódico spasmodic ergotism
ergotrópico ergotropic
eritermalgia erythermalgia
eritralgia erythralgia
eritredema erythredema
eritrismo erythrism
eritrofobia erythrophobia
eritroleucoblastosis erythroleukoblastosis
eritromelalgia erythromelalgia
eritroprosopalgia erythroprosopalgia
eritropsia erythropsia
erogeneidad erogeneity
erógeno erogenous
Eros Eros
erosión erosion
erosión cervical cervical erosion
erótico erotic
erotismo eroticism
erotismo anal anal eroticism
erotismo cutáneo skin eroticism
erotismo de temperatura temperature eroticism
erotismo del ego ego erotism
erotismo genital genital eroticism
erotismo labial lip eroticism
erotismo olfartorio olfactory eroticism
erotismo oral oral eroticism
erotismo orgánico organ eroticism
erotismo paranoide paranoid erotism
erotismo respiratorio respiratory eroticism
erotismo uretral urethral eroticism
erotización erotization
erotizado erotized
erotizar eroticize
erotócrata erotocrat
erotofobia erotophobia
erotogénesis erotogenesis
erotogenético erotogenetic
erotogénico erotogenic
erotografomanía erotographomania
erotolalia erotolalia
erotomanía erotomania
erotomanía pura pure erotomania
erotomaníaco erotomanic
erotopatía erotopathy
erotopático erotopathic
errante wandering
errático erratic

error error
error absoluto absolute error
error accidental accidental error
error aleatorio random error
error alfa alpha error
error anticipatorio anticipatory error
error beta beta error
error casual chance error
error compensatorio compensating error
error constante constant error
error de agrupamiento grouping error
error de anticipación anticipation error
error de articulación articulation error
error de atribución attribution error
error de atribución fundamental fundamental attribution error
error de estimado error of estimate
error de estímulo stimulus error
error de intrusión intrusion error
error de la lengua slip of the tongue
error de la pluma slip of the pen
error de medición error of measurement
error de metabolismo ingénito inborn error of metabolism
error de muestreo sampling error
error de procesamiento processing error
error de transposición transposition error
error de ubicación location error
error de varianza error of variance
error del tiempo time error
error espacial space error
error estadístico statistical error
error estándar standard error
error estándar de diferencia standard error of difference
error estándar de la media standard error of the mean
error estándar de medición standard error of measurement
error estándar del estimado standard error of estimate
error experimental experimental error
error genético genetic error
error insesgado unbiased error
error motivado motivated error
error perseverante perseverative error
error probable probable error
error promedio average error
error sistemático systematic error
error subjetivo subjective error
error tipo I type I error
error tipo II type II error
error variable variable error
errores de confusión confusion errors
eructación eructation
eructo belch
erupción de instinto instinct eruption
escabiofobia scabiophobia
escafohidrocefalia scaphohydrocephaly
escala scale
escala absoluta absolute scale
escala acromática-cromática achromatic-chromatic scale
escala aditiva additive scale
escala agresiva aggressive scale

escala anomia anomie scale
escala antisocial antisocial scale
escala balanceada balanced scale
escala categórica categorical scale
escala compulsiva compulsive scale
escala continua continuous scale
escala cromática chromatic scale
escala de abuso de alcohol alcohol abuse
scale
escala de abuso de drogas drug abuse scale
escala de actitudes attitude scale
escala de amor love scale
escala de androginia androgyny scale
escala de ansiedad anxiety scale
escala de autoclasificación self-rating scale
escala de Bellevue Bellevue scale
escala de Binet Binet scale
escala de Binet-Simon Binet-Simon scale
escala de clasificación rating scale
escala de clasificación absoluta absolute
rating scale
escala de clasificación bipolar bipolar rating
scale
escala de clasificación conductual behavioral
rating scale
escala de clasificación de cambios de vida
life-change rating scale
escala de clasificación de reajuste social
social readjustment rating scale
escala de clasificación detallada itemized
rating scale
escala de clasificación gráfica graphic rating
scale
escala de clasificación molar molar rating
scale
escala de clasificación psicológica
psychological rating scale
escala de colores color scale
escala de coma coma scale
escala de conducta adaptiva adaptive
behavior scale
escala de confianza interpersonal
interpersonal trust scale
escala de decibelios decibel scale
escala de delusiones psicóticas psychotic
delusions scale
escala de depresión depression scale
escala de depresión psicótica psychotic
depression scale
escala de desviación psicopática psychopathic
deviance scale
escala de deterioración deterioration scale
escala de dificultad difficulty scale
escala de distancia social social-distance scale
escala de distimia dysthymia scale
escala de edad age scale
escala de equivalente de edad age-equivalent
scale
escala de esquizofrenia schizophrenia scale
escala de etnocentrismo ethnocentrism scale
escala de fuerza del ego ego strength scale
escala de grado grade scale
escala de hipocondriasis hypochondriasis
scale
escala de hipomanía hypomania scale

escala de histeria hysteria scale
escala de infante infant scale
escala de infrecuencia infrequency scale
escala de inteligencia intelligence scale
escala de intervalos interval scale
escala de intervalos iguales equal-interval
scale
escala de introversión social social
introversion scale
escala de letalidad lethality scale
escala de Likert Likert scale
escala de Mach Mach scale
escala de masculinidad-feminidad
masculinity-femininity scale
escala de medición measurement scale
escala de mentación mentation scale
escala de mentiras lie scale
escala de Ostwald Ostwald scale
escala de paranoia paranoia scale
escala de pensamiento psicótico psychotic
thinking scale
escala de personalidad esquizoide schizoid
personality scale
escala de potencial alérgica allergic potential
scale
escala de preferencia liking scale
escala de productos product scale
escala de proporciones ratio scale
escala de puntos point scale
escala de represión repression scale
escala de represión-sensibilización
repression-sensitization scale
escala de Shipley-Hartford Shipley-Hartford
scale
escala de susceptibilidad hipnótica hypnotic
susceptibility scale
escala de Thurstone Thurstone scale
escala de trastornos de personalidad
personality disorders scale
escala de validez validity scale
escala dependiente dependent scale
escala derivada derived scale
escala e e scale
escala especial special scale
escala esquizoide schizoid scale
escala esquizotípica schizotypal scale
escala evitante avoidant scale
escala F F scale
escala fronteriza borderline scale
escala hipomaníaca hypomanic scale
escala histriónica histrionic scale
escala interna-externa internal-external scale
escala ipsativa ipsative scale
escala K K scale
escala mental mental scale
escala narcisista narcissistic scale
escala nominal nominal scale
escala obstétrica obstetrical scale
escala ordinal ordinal scale
escala paranoide paranoid scale
escala pasiva-agresiva passive-aggressive
scale
escala psicológica psychological scale
escala social social scale
escala somatoforme somatoform scale

escala tonal tonal scale
escala verbal verbal scale
escalabilidad scalability
escalamiento scaling
escalamiento de artículo item scaling
escalamiento de Guttman Guttman scaling
escalamiento de Kruskal-Shepard
   Kruskal-Shepard scaling
escalamiento de prueba test scaling
escalamiento indirecto indirect scaling
escalamiento ipsativo ipsative scaling
escalamiento multidimensional
   multidimensional scaling
escalamiento no métrico nonmetric scaling
escalamiento por edad y grado age-grade
   scaling
escalas de categorías category scales
escalas del desarrollo developmental scales
escalenectomía scalenectomy
escalenotomía scalenotomy
escalera de asesoramiento counseling ladder
escalograma scalogram
escape escape
escape a enfermedad escape into illness
escape condicionado conditioned escape
escape de culpa blame escape
escape de la realidad escape from reality
escape de libertad escape from freedom
escapismo escapism
escapulohumeral scapulohumeral
escasez paucity
escasez del habla paucity of speech
escatofagia scatophagy
escatofobia scatophobia
escatología scatologia
escatología telefónica telephone scatologia
escatológico scatological
escelalgia scelalgia
escelerofobia scelerophobia
escelotirbe scelotyrbe
escena primal primal scene
escena retrospectiva flashback
esclerencefalia sclerencephaly
esclerosis sclerosis
esclerosis combinada combined sclerosis
esclerosis cortical laminar laminar cortical
   sclerosis
esclerosis de Alzheimer Alzheimer's sclerosis
esclerosis de Canavan Canavan's sclerosis
esclerosis de la sustancia blanca sclerosis of
   white matter
esclerosis del manto mantle sclerosis
esclerosis difusa diffuse sclerosis
esclerosis diseminada disseminated sclerosis
esclerosis espinal lateral lateral spinal
   sclerosis
esclerosis espinal posterior posterior spinal
   sclerosis
esclerosis familiar infantil difusa diffuse
   infantile familial sclerosis
esclerosis focal focal sclerosis
esclerosis hipocámpica hippocampal sclerosis
esclerosis insular insular sclerosis
esclerosis lateral amiotrófica amyotrophic
   lateral sclerosis

esclerosis lobar lobar sclerosis
esclerosis múltiple multiple sclerosis
esclerosis neuroglial neuroglial sclerosis
esclerosis posterior posterior sclerosis
esclerosis posterolateral posterolateral
   sclerosis
esclerosis tuberosa tuberous sclerosis
esclerótica sclera
esclerótico sclerotic
escolástico scholastic
escoliosis scoliosis
escoliosis ciática sciatic scoliosis
escoliosis compensatorio compensatory
   scoliosis
escoliosis estructural structural scoliosis
escoliosis osteopática osteopathic scoliosis
escoliosis paralítica paralytic scoliosis
escoliótico scoliotic
escopofilia scopophilia
escopofobia scopophobia
escopolamina scopolamine
escoptofilia scoptophilia
escorzo foreshortening
escotadura notch
escotadura de Kernohan Kernohan's notch
escotofilia scotophilia
escotofobia scotophobia
escotoma scotoma
escotoma absoluto absolute scotoma
escotoma centelleante scintillating scotoma
escotoma de color color scotoma
escotoma mental mental scotoma
escotoma periférico peripheral scotoma
escotomatización scotomatization
escotomización scotomization
escotópico scotopic
escotopsina scotopsin
escritura writing
escritura atáxica ataxic writing
escritura automática automatic writing
escritura en espejo mirror-writing
escroto scrotum
escrupulosidad scrupulosity
escrupuloso scrupulous
escuchar con el tercer oído listening with the
   third ear
escuchar pasivo passive listening
escudo ideacional ideational shield
escuela alternativa alternative school
escuela austríaca Austrian school
escuela de entrenamiento training school
escuela de Nancy Nancy school
escuela de Salpetriere Salpetriere school
escuela del desarrollo developmental school
escuela especial special school
escuela existencial existential school
escuela ginebrina Genevan school
escuela humanística humanistic school
escuela residencial residential school
esencia essence
esencial essential
eserina eserine
esfenoidal sphenoidal
esfenoiditis sphenoiditis
esfenoidostomía sphenoidostomy

esfenoidotomía sphenoidotomy
esfera de personalidad personality sphere
esfera libre de conflictos conflict-free sphere
esferestesia spheresthesia
esfigmógrafo sphygmograph
esfigmomanómetro sphygmomanometer
esfigmómetro sphygmometer
esfingolípido sphingolipid
esfingolipidosis sphingolipidosis
esfingolipidosis cerebral cerebral
    sphingolipidosis
esfínter sphincter
esfínteres anales anal sphincters
esfuerzo effort
esfuerzo distribuido distributed effort
esmegma smegma
esoetmoiditis esoethmoiditis
esoforia esophoria
esotropía esotropia
espacial spatial
espaciamiento spacing
espacio auditivo auditory space
espacio de campo field space
espacio de grupo group space
espacio de muestra sample space
espacio de probabilidades probability space
espacio de vida life space
espacio factorial factor space
espacio hodológico hodological space
espacio peritoneal peritoneal space
espacio personal personal space
espacio psicológico psychological space
espacio semántico semantic space
espacio social social space
espacio sociófugo sociofugal space
espacio sociópeto sociopetal space
espacio subaracnoideo subarachnoid space
espacio subaracnoideo posterior posterior
    subarachnoidean space
espacio verbal verbal space
espacio visual visual space
espantado frightened
espantado a muerte frightened to death
espanto fright
espantoso frightening
espasmo spasm
espasmo anorrectal anorectal spasm
espasmo bronquial bronchial spasm
espasmo canino canine spasm
espasmo carpopedal carpopedal spasm
espasmo cínico cynic spasm
espasmo clónico clonic spasm
espasmo danzante dancing spasm
espasmo de afecto affect spasm
espasmo de Bell Bell's spasm
espasmo de cabeceo nodding spasm
espasmo de costurero sewing spasm
espasmo de guiños winking spasm
espasmo de intención intention spasm
espasmo de sastre tailor's spasm
espasmo de torsión torsion spasm
espasmo de torsión progresivo progressive
    torsion spasm
espasmo dental tooth spasm
espasmo facial facial spasm

espasmo fónico phonic spasm
espasmo funcional functional spasm
espasmo habitual habit spasm
espasmo hemifacial hemifacial spasm
espasmo histriónico histrionic spasm
espasmo infantil infantile spasm
espasmo masticatorio masticatory spasm
espasmo mímico mimic spasm
espasmo móvil mobile spasm
espasmo muscular muscle spasm
espasmo nictitante nictitating spasm
espasmo oculógiro oculogyric spasm
espasmo ocupacional occupational spasm
espasmo profesional professional spasm
espasmo retrocólico retrocollic spasm
espasmo rotatorio rotatory spasm
espasmo saltatorio saltatory spasm
espasmo sinclónico synclonic spasm
espasmo tónico tonic spasm
espasmo tonoclónico tonoclonic spasm
espasmo vasomotor vasomotor spasm
espasmódico spasmodic
espasmofemia spasmophemia
espasmofilia spasmophilia
espasmofílico spasmophilic
espasmogénico spasmogenic
espasmoligmo spasmolygmus
espasmólisis spasmolysis
espasmolítico spasmolytic
espasmología spasmology
espasticidad spasticity
espasticidad de mirada fija conjugada
    spasticity of conjugate gaze
espasticidad de navaja clasp-knife spasticity
espástico spastic
especialista de discapacidades de aprendizaje
    learning disability specialist
especialista de recreación recreation
    specialist
especialista en asesoramiento guidance
    specialist
especialización de hemisferio hemisphere
    specialization
especialización de papel role specialization
especialización hemisférica hemispheric
    specialization
especialización lateral lateral specialization
especie species
especies simpátricas sympatric species
especificaciones del personal personnel
    specifications
especificidad specificity
especificidad de estímulo stimulus specificity
especificidad de impulso drive specificity
especificidad de respuesta response
    specificity
especificidad de respuesta individual
    individual-response specificity
especificidad de respuestas fisiológicas
    physiological-response specificity
especificidad de síntomas symptom
    specificity
específico specific
específico de cultura culture-specific
específico de especie species-specific

espécimen specimen
espectador spectator
espectral spectral
espectro spectrum
espectro acústico acoustic spectrum
espectro auditivo auditory spectrum
espectro de absorción absorption spectrum
espectro de fortificación fortification
    spectrum
espectro de reflexión reflection spectrum
espectro de sonido sound spectrum
espectro depresivo depressive spectrum
espectro electromagnético electromagnetic
    spectrum
espectro esquizofrénico schizophrenic
    spectrum
espectro subafectivo subaffective spectrum
espectro tonal tonal spectrum
espectro visible visible spectrum
espectrofobia spectrophobia
espectrofotometría spectrophotometry
espectrofotómetro spectrophotometer
espectrofotómetro infrarrojo infrared
    spectrophotometer
espectrográfico spectrographic
espectrógrafo spectrograph
espectrógrafo de sonido sound spectrograph
espectrograma de sonido sound spectrogram
espectrograma de voz voiceprint
espectrómetro spectrometer
espectroscopio spectroscope
especulación speculation
especulativo speculative
espejo unidireccional one-way mirror
espejuelos eyeglasses
espelencefalia spelencephaly
esperma sperm
espermático spermatic
espermátide spermatid
espermatocito spermatocyte
espermatofobia spermatophobia
espermatogénesis spermatogenesis
espermatogonio spermatogonium
espermatorrea spermatorrhea
espermatozoide spermatozoid
espermatozoo spermatozoon
espermaturia spermaturia
espermicida spermicide
espina spine
espina bífida spina bifida
espina bífida abierta spina bifida aperta
espina bífida manifiesta spina bifida
    manifesta
espina bífida oculta spina bifida occulta
espina bífida quística spina bifida cystica
espina dendrítica dendritic spine
espina hendida cleft spine
espinal spinal
espinante spinant
espinífugo spinifungal
espinípeto spinipetal
espinocerebeloso spinocerebellar
espinogalvanización spinogalvanization
espinotalámico spinothalamic
espiperona spiperone

espiral de Arquímedes Archimedes spiral
espíritu adquisitivo acquisitive spirit
espíritu comunal communal spirit
espíritu comunitario community spirit
espirógrafo spirograph
espirómetro spirometer
esplacnestesia splanchnesthesia
esplacnestésico splanchnesthetic
esplacnicectomía splanchnicectomy
esplácnico splanchnic
esplacnicotomía splanchnicotomy
esplenético splenetic
esplenio splenium
espondilalgia spondylalgia
espondilartritis spondylarthritis
espondilartrocace spondylarthrocace
espondilítico spondylitic
espondilitis spondylitis
espondilitis anquilosante ankylosing
    spondylitis
espondilitis de Kummell Kummell's
    spondylitis
espondilitis deformante spondylitis
    deformans
espondilitis reumatoide rheumatoid
    spondylitis
espondilitis tuberculosa tuberculous
    spondylitis
espondilocace spondylocace
espondilólisis spondylolysis
espondilolistesis spondylolisthesis
espondilolistético spondylolisthetic
espondilomalacia spondylomalacia
espondilopatía spondylopathy
espondilopiosis spondylopyosis
espondiloptosis spondyloptosis
espondilosindesis spondylosyndesis
espondilosis spondylosis
espondilosis cervical cervical spondylosis
espondilosis hiperostótica hyperostotic
    spondylosis
espondilosquisis spondyloschisis
espondilotomía spondylotomy
espongiforme spongiform
espongioblasto spongioblast
espongioblastoma spongioblastoma
espongiocito spongiocyte
espontaneidad spontaneity
espontaneo spontaneous
esposa golpeada battered wife
espurio spurious
esqueletal skeletal
esquema schema, chart
esquema cognitivo cognitive schema
esquema corporal body schema
esquema de perfil profile chart
esquema de Snellen Snellen chart
esquema perceptivo perceptual schema
esquema seudoisocromático
    pseudoisochromatic chart
esquemático schematic
esquiascopio skiascope
esquistorraquis schistorrhachis
esquistosomiasis schistosomiasis
esquizencefalia schizencephaly

esquizencefálico schizencephalic
esquizoafectivo schizoaffective
esquizobipolar schizobipolar
esquizocaria schizocaria
esquizocinesis schizokinesis
esquizofasia schizophasia
esquizofrasia schizophrasia
esquizofrenia schizophrenia
esquizofrenia aguda acute schizophrenia
esquizofrenia ambulatoria ambulatory
   schizophrenia
esquizofrenia anérgica anergic schizophrenia
esquizofrenia catastrófica catastrophic
   schizophrenia
esquizofrenia catatónica catatonic
   schizophrenia
esquizofrenia crónica chronic schizophrenia
esquizofrenia de comienzo tardío late-onset
   schizophrenia
esquizofrenia de niñez childhood
   schizophrenia
esquizofrenia de proceso process
   schizophrenia
esquizofrenia de síntomas negativos
   negative-symptom schizophrenia
esquizofrenia de tipo desorganizada
   disorganized type schizophrenia
esquizofrenia de tipo indiferenciada
   undifferentiated type schizophrenia
esquizofrenia de tipo residual residual type
   schizophrenia
esquizofrenia de tres días three-day
   schizophrenia
esquizofrenia desorganizada disorganized
   schizophrenia
esquizofrenia en remisión schizophrenia in
   remission
esquizofrenia fronteriza borderline
   schizophrenia
esquizofrenia hebefrénica hebephrenic
   schizophrenia
esquizofrenia indiferenciada undifferentiated
   schizophrenia
esquizofrenia indiferenciada aguda acute
   undifferentiated schizophrenia
esquizofrenia indiferenciada crónica chronic
   undifferentiated schizophrenia
esquizofrenia larval larval schizophrenia
esquizofrenia latente latent schizophrenia
esquizofrenia mixta mixed schizophrenia
esquizofrenia no regresiva nonregressive
   schizophrenia
esquizofrenia no sistemática nonsystematic
   schizophrenia
esquizofrenia nuclear nuclear schizophrenia
esquizofrenia paranoide paranoid
   schizophrenia
esquizofrenia posemotiva postemotive
   schizophrenia
esquizofrenia reactiva reactive schizophrenia
esquizofrenia regresiva regressive
   schizophrenia
esquizofrenia remitente remitting
   schizophrenia
esquizofrenia residual residual schizophrenia

esquizofrenia restitucional restitutional
   schizophrenia
esquizofrenia retardada retarded
   schizophrenia
esquizofrenia seudoneurótica pseudoneurotic
   schizophrenia
esquizofrenia seudopsicopática
   pseudopsychopathic schizophrenia
esquizofrenia simple simple schizophrenia
esquizofrenia sistemática systematic
   schizophrenia
esquizofrenia tipo catatónico catatonic type
   schizophrenia
esquizofrenia tipo I de Crow Crow type I
   schizophrenia
esquizofrenia tipo II de Crow Crow type II
   schizophrenia
esquizofrenia tipo paranoide paranoid type
   schizophrenia
esquizofrénico schizophrenic
esquizofrénico anérgico anergic
   schizophrenic
esquizofrénico quemado burned-out
   schizophrenic
esquizofreniforme schizophreniform
esquizofrenogénico schizophrenogenic
esquizógeno schizogen
esquizogiria schizogyria
esquizoide schizoid
esquizoidia schizoidia
esquizoidismo schizoidism
esquizomanía schizomania
esquizomaníaco schizomanic
esquizomimético schizomimetic
esquizotaxia schizotaxia
esquizotemia schizothemia
esquizotimia schizothymia
esquizotímico schizothymic
esquizotípico schizotypal
esquizotonía schizotonia
estabilidad stability
estabilidad de muestreo sampling stability
estabilidad del ego ego stability
estabilidad emocional emotional stability
estabilidad estadística statistical stability
estabilidad-labilidad stability-lability
estabilidad ocupacional occupational stability
estabilímetro stabilimeter
estabilizado stabilized
estabilizador del humor mood stabilizer
estable stable
establecimiento establishment
establecimiento de fin goal setting
establecimiento de límites limit setting
estadía extendida extended stay
estadística statistic
estadística correlacional correlational
   statistics
estadística de muestras pequeñas
   small-sample statistics
estadística descriptiva descriptive statistics
estadística inferencial inferential statistics
estadística libre de distribuciones
   distribution-free statistics
estadística no paramétrica nonparametric

statistics
estadística paramétrica parametric statistics
estadística psicológica psychological statistics
estadística vital vital statistics
estadístico statistical
estado state
estado afectivo affective state
estado alfa alpha state
estado apálico apallic state
estado ausente absent state
estado catatónico catatonic state
estado circulatorio adrenérgico adrenergic
   circulatory state
estado cognitivo cognitive state
estado comatoso comatose state
estado como de sueño dreamlike state
estado conductual behavioral state
estado confusional confusional state
estado confusional agudo acute confusional
   state
estado consciente conscious state
estado convulsivo convulsive state
estado coreico status choreicus
estado crepuscular twilight state
estado crepuscular alcohólico alcoholic
   twilight state
estado crepuscular claro clear twilight state
estado crepuscular posepiléptico
   postepileptic twilight state
estado criboso status cribrosus
estado crítico status criticus
estado de agotamiento exhaustion state
estado de ansiedad anxiety state
estado de ansiedad contra autismo anxiety
   state versus autism
estado de ansiedad contra esquizofrenia
   anxiety state versus schizophrenia
estado de ansiedad contra trastorno evitante
   anxiety state versus avoidant disorder
estado de conciencia alterado altered state of
   consciousness
estado de conciencia alterno alternate state of
   consciousness
estado de despertamiento state of arousal
estado de fatiga fatigue state
estado de fuga fugue state
estado de fusión fusion state
estado de impulso drive state
estado de necesidad need state
estado de negación delusorio crónico chronic
   delusional state of negation
estado de perplejidad perplexity state
estado de rapto status raptus
estado de respuesta adrenérgica adrenergic
   response state
estado de sueño sleep state, dream state
estado de sueño profundo deep-sleep state
estado de tensión premenstrual
   premenstrual-tension state
estado de trance trance state
estado defensivo defensiveness
estado degenerativo degenerative status
estado del ego ego state
estado del ego adulto adult ego state
estado del ego de niño child ego state

estado delirante delirious state
estado delirante subagudo subacute delirious
   state
estado delusorio erotomaníaca erotomanic
   delusional state
estado delusorio litigioso litigious delusional
   state
estado desmielinizado status dysmyelinisatus
estado disráfico status dysraphicus
estado enturbado clouded state
estado enturbado epiléptico epileptic clouded
   state
estado epiléptico status epilepticus
estado esponjoso status spongiosus
estado esquizofrénico schizophrenic state
estado esquizoide-maníaco schizoid-manic
   state
estado estable steady state
estado excitatorio excitatory state
estado excitatorio central central excitatory
   state
estado excitatorio local local excitatory state
estado extático ecstatic state
estado final end state
estado fronterizo borderline state
estado hemicraneal status hemicranicus
estado hipererídico hypereridic state
estado hipnagógico hypnagogic state
estado hipnogógico hypnogogic state
estado hipnoideo hypnoid state
estado hipnótico hypnotic state
estado hipomaníaco hypomanic state
estado histérico hysterical state
estado intencional intentional state
estado interno internal state
estado lacunar status lacunaris
estado litigioso paranoide paranoid litigious
   state
estado maníaco manic state
estado marásmico marasmic state
estado marital marital status
estado marmóreo status marmoratus
estado mental mental status
estado nervioso status nervosus
estado paranoide paranoid state
estado paranoide alcohólico alcoholic
   paranoid state
estado paranoide involutivo involutional
   paranoid state
estado posictal postictal state
estado refractario refractory state
estado social social status
estado socioeconómico socioeconomic status
estado sonambulístico somnambulistic state
estado soñador dreamy state
estado subdelirante subdelirious state
estado tifoso status typhosus
estado transcendental transcendental state
estado vegetativo vegetative state
estado vertiginoso status vertiginosus
estados del ego fluctuantes fluctuating ego
   states
estados del ego múltiples multiple ego states
estados superiores de conciencia higher
   states of consciousness

estallido burst
estampido sónico sonic boom
estancación stagnation
estancamiento analítico analytic stalemate
estándar standard
estandarización standardization
estandarización de prueba test
  standardization
estandarizado standardized
estandarizar standardize
estapedectomía stapedectomy
estapedio stapedius
estasibasifobia stasibasiphobia
estasifobia stasiphobia
estasis stasis
estasobasofobia stasobasophobia
estasofobia stasophobia
estático static
estatoacústico statoacoustic
estatocinético statokinetic
estatocisto statocyst
estatoconía statoconia
estatua de Condillac statue of Condillac
estatura corta determinada psicosocialmente
  psychosocially determined short stature
estatuvolencia statuvolence
estatuvolente statuvolent
estauroplejía stauroplegia
esteatopigia steatopygy
estelectomía stellectomy
estematología esthematology
estén sten
estenia sthenia
esténico sthenic
estenoestenosis stenostenosis
estenómetro sthenometer
estenoplástico sthenoplastic
estenosis stenosis
estenosis espinal spinal stenosis
estenosis mitral mitral stenosis
estenosis pilórica pyloric stenosis
estenosis pulmónica pulmonic stenosis
estepaje steppage
estereoagnosis stereoagnosis
estereoanestesia stereoanesthesia
estereocilio stereocilium
estereoelectroencefalografía
  stereoelectroencephalography
estereoencefalometría stereoencephalometry
estereoencefalotomía stereoencephalotomy
estereognosia stereognosis
estereognóstico stereognostic
estereograma stereogram
estereograma de Julesz Julesz's stereogram
estereopatía stereopathy
estereopsis stereopsis
estereoquímico stereochemical
estereoscópico stereoscopic
estereoscopio stereoscope
estereotáctico stereotactic
estereotaxia stereotaxy
estereotáxico stereotaxic
estereotaxis stereotaxis
estereotipado stereotyped
estereotipia stereotypy

estereotipia oral oral stereotypy
estereotípico stereotypical
estereotipo stereotype
estereotipo del entrevistador interviewer
  stereotype
estereotipo de papel sexual sex-role
  stereotype
estereotropismo stereotropism
estérico steric
estéril sterile
esterilidad sterility
esterilización sterilization
esternocleidomastoideo sternocleidomastoid
esteroide steroid
esteropsiquis stereopsyche
estesia esthesia
estesiódico esthesiodic
estesiofisiología esthesiophysiology
estesiogénesis esthesiogenesis
estesiogénico esthesiogenic
estesiografía esthesiography
estesiología esthesiology
estesiometría esthesiometry
estesiómetro esthesiometer
estesioneuroblastoma esthesioneuroblastoma
estesioneuroblastoma olfatorio olfactory
  esthesioneuroblastoma
estesioneurocitoma esthesioneurocytoma
estesioneurosis esthesioneurosis
estesionosis esthesionosus
estesioscopia esthesioscopy
estesódico esthesodic
estética esthetics
estética ambiental environmental esthetics
estética experimental experimental aesthetics
estética psicológica psychological esthetics
estético esthetic
estetoparálisis stethoparalysis
estigiofobia stygiophobia
estigma stigma
estigmático stigmatic
estigmatismo stigmatism
estigmatización stigmatization
estilo style
estilo adaptivo adaptive style
estilo cognitivo cognitive style
estilo de aprendizaje learning style
estilo de aprendizaje cognitivo cognitive
  learning style
estilo de comando command style
estilo de enseñanza teaching style
estilo de liderazgo leadership style
estilo de vida lifestyle
estilo de vida sexual sexual lifestyle
estilo para bregar coping style
estilo para bregar y estrés coping style and
  stress
estilo parental parental style
estilo perceptivo perceptual style
estilos de comunicación communication styles
estilos para bregar de niños coping styles of
  children
estima esteem
estima corporal body esteem
estimación estimation

estimación de categoría category estimation
estimación de magnitud magnitude estimation
estimación de proporciones ratio estimation
estimación positiva positive regard
estimación positiva condicional conditional positive regard
estimado estimate
estimado de intervalo interval estimate
estimado de punto point estimate
estimado insesgado unbiased estimate
estimador de probabilidad máxima maximum-likelihood estimator
estimador insesgado unbiased estimator
estimulación stimulation
estimulación ambiental environmental stimulation
estimulación amigdaloide amygdaloid stimulation
estimulación auditiva auditory stimulation
estimulación autogenital autogenital stimulation
estimulación cerebral brain stimulation
estimulación cerebral eléctrica electrical brain stimulation
estimulación cerebral por audio audio brain stimulation
estimulación cerebral química chemical brain stimulation
estimulación cutánea skin stimulation
estimulación de columna dorsal dorsal column stimulation
estimulación del sistema nervioso eléctrico electrical nervous system stimulation
estimulación eléctrica electrical stimulation
estimulación eléctrica de la corteza electrical stimulation of cortex
estimulación eléctrica transcutánea transcutaneous electrical stimulation
estimulación electrocutánea electrocutaneous stimulation
estimulación endógena endogenous stimulation
estimulación exógena exogenous stimulation
estimulación fótica photic stimulation
estimulación genital genital stimulation
estimulación intracraneal intracranial stimulation
estimulación intracraneal eléctrica electrical intracranial stimulation
estimulación lenticular-fascículo lenticular-fasciculus stimulation
estimulación olfatoria olfactory stimulation
estimulación percutánea percutaneous stimulation
estimulación quimérica chimeric stimulation
estimulación química chemical stimulation
estimulación rítmica rhythmic stimulation
estimulación sensorial sensory stimulation
estimulación sexual sexual stimulation
estimulación simultánea doble double simultaneous stimulation
estimulación somestésica somesthetic stimulation
estimulación subliminal subliminal stimulation

estimulación táctil tactile stimulation
estimulación transcraneal eléctrica electrical transcranial stimulation
estimulación verbal verbal stimulation
estimulación visual visual stimulation
estimulador stimulator
estimulante (adj) stimulating
estimulante (n) stimulant
estimulante del sistema nervioso central central nervous system stimulant
estimulante psicomotor psychomotor stimulant
estímulo stimulus
estímulo adecuado adequate stimulus
estímulo anómalo anomalous stimulus
estímulo auditivo auditory stimulus
estímulo aversivo aversive stimulus
estímulo condicionado conditioned stimulus
estímulo consumatorio consummatory stimulus
estímulo de centelleo flicker stimulus
estímulo de comparación comparison stimulus
estímulo de despertamiento de impulso drive-arousal stimulus
estímulo de fin goal stimulus
estímulo de sueño dream stimulus
estímulo degradado degraded stimulus
estímulo diferencial differential stimulus
estímulo discrepante discrepant stimulus
estímulo discriminante discriminant stimulus
estímulo discriminativo discriminative stimulus
estímulo discriminativo negativo negative discriminative stimulus
estímulo distal distal stimulus
estímulo efectivo effective stimulus
estímulo estándar standard stimulus
estímulo estructurado structured stimulus
estímulo físico physical stimulus
estímulo funcional functional stimulus
estímulo heterólogo heterologous stimulus
estímulo homólogo homologous stimulus
estímulo iatrotrópico iatrotropic stimulus
estímulo inadecuado inadequate stimulus
estímulo incidental incidental stimulus
estímulo incondicionado unconditioned stimulus
estímulo indiferente indifferent stimulus
estímulo ineficaz ineffective stimulus
estímulo liberador releasing stimulus
estímulo liminal liminal stimulus
estímulo mantenedor maintaining stimulus
estímulo máximo maximal stimulus
estímulo neutral neutral stimulus
estímulo no estructurado unstructured stimulus
estímulo objetivo target stimulus
estímulo por signo sign stimulus
estímulo prepotente prepotent stimulus
estímulo proximal proximal stimulus
estímulo psicomotor psychomotor stimulus
estímulo reforzante reinforcing stimulus
estímulo-respuesta stimulus-response
estímulo sensorial sensory stimulus

estructura endopsíquica

estímulo social social stimulus
estímulo subliminal subliminal stimulus
estímulo subumbral subthreshold stimulus
estímulo supraliminal supraliminal stimulus
estímulo supramáximo supramaximal
stimulus
estímulo terminal terminal stimulus
estímulo umbral threshold stimulus
estímulo variable variable stimulus
estímulo verbal verbal stimulus
estímulos stimuli
estímulos accidentales accidental stimuli
estímulos antecedentes antecedent stimuli
estímulos compuestos compound stimuli
estímulos constantes constant stimuli
estímulos de color color stimuli
estímulos de impulso drive stimuli
estímulos externos external stimuli
estímulos externos antes del sueño external
stimuli prior to sleep
estímulos externos durante el sueño external
stimuli during sleep
estocástico stochastic
estoma stoma
estrabismo strabismus
estrabismo convergente convergent
strabismus
estrabismo de Braid Braid's strabismus
estrabismo divergente divergent strabismus
estradiol estradiol
estrambótico bizarre
estrangalestesia strangalesthesia
estrategia strategy
estrategia cognitiva cognitive strategy
estrategia de aprendizaje learning strategy
estrategia de carga precursora precursor
load strategy
estrategia de evaluación de tratamiento
treatment-evaluation strategy
estrategia de reto challenge strategy
estrategia defensiva defensive strategy
estrategia empírica-racional
empirical-rational strategy
estrategia K K strategy
estrategia mnemónica mnemonic strategy
estrategia normativa-reeducativa
normative-reeducative strategy
estrategia para bregar coping strategy
estrategia poder-coercitiva power-coercive
strategy
estrategias de codificaciones coding strategies
estrategias de decisiones decision strategies
estrategias de defensa defense strategies
estrategias inferenciales inferential strategies
estratégico strategic
estratificación stratification
estratificación social social stratification
estratificado stratified
estrefosimbolia strephosymbolia
estremecimiento shudder
estrés stress
estrés ambiental environmental stress
estrés biológico biological stress
estrés crónico chronic stress
estrés de eventos de la vida life-event stress

estrés de papel de género gender-role stress
estrés de trabajo job stress
estrés de vida life stress
estrés del ego ego stress
estrés e hipertensión stress and hypertension
estrés económico economic stress
estrés ejecutivo executive stress
estrés emocional emotional stress
estrés en adolescencia stress in adolescence
estrés en infancia stress in infancy
estrés exógeno exogenous stress
estrés focal focal stress
estrés maternal maternal stress
estrés ocupacional occupational stress
estrés perinatal perinatal stress
estrés por calor heat stress
estrés psicocultural psychocultural stress
estrés psicológico psychological stress
estrés social social stress
estresante stressor
estresante agudo acute stressor
estresante del desarrollo developmental
stressor
estresante psicosocial psychosocial stressor
estresante social social stressor
estresantes crónicos chronic stressors
estresantes del desarrollo en adolescencia
developmental stressors in adolescence
estresantes del desarrollo en niños
preescolares developmental stressors in
preschool children
estría meningítica meningitic streak
estría terminal stria terminalis
estriado striated
estrías atróficas stria atrophicae
estrías olfatorias mediales medial olfactory
stria
estribo stapes
estricnina strychnine
estricninismo strychninism
estridente strident
estriol estriol
estro estrus
estroboscópico stroboscopic
estroboscopio stroboscope
estrógeno estrogen
estromanía estromania
estrona estrone
estructura structure
estructura cerebral brain structure
estructura cognitiva cognitive structure
estructura de campo field structure
estructura de clases class structure
estructura de datos data structure
estructura de grupo group structure
estructura de personalidad personality
structure
estructura de recompensa competitiva
competitive reward structure
estructura de recompensa cooperativa
cooperative reward structure
estructura del carácter character structure
estructura del ego ego structure
estructura del ojo eye structure
estructura endopsíquica endopsychic

structure
estructura factorial factor structure
estructura familiar family structure
estructura genética genetic structure
estructura genital genital structure
estructura iniciadora initiating structure
estructura mental mental structure
estructura perceptiva perceptual structure
estructura profunda deep structure
estructura simple simple structure
estructura social social structure
estructura superficial surface structure
estructurado structured
estructural structural
estructuralismo structuralism
estudio study
estudio abierto open study
estudio análogo analogue study
estudio ciego blind study
estudio clínico clinical study
estudio cuasiexperimental quasi-experimental
  study
estudio de adopción adoption study
estudio de caso case study
estudio de cohorte cohort study
estudio de control de casos case control study
estudio de frustración en pinturas
  picture-frustration study
estudio de gemelos twin study
estudio de historiales de casos case history
  study
estudio de moción motion study
estudio de predicción prediction study
estudio de riesgo familiar family risk study
estudio de seguimiento follow-up study
estudio de tiempo y moción time-motion
  study
estudio del tiempo time study
estudio diacrónico diachronic study
estudio doble ciego double-blind study
estudio ecológico ecological study
estudio etnológico ethnological study
estudio exploratorio exploratory study
estudio longitudinal longitudinal study
estudio multivariado multivariate study
estudio natural natural study
estudio piloto pilot study
estudio prospectivo prospective study
estudio retrospectivo retrospective study
estudio sincrónico synchronic study
estudio transversal cross-sectional study
estudios correlacionales correlational studies
estudios de animales animal studies
estudios de audición dicótica dichotic
  listening studies
estudios de familias family studies
estudios de fatiga fatigue studies
estudios de infantes infant studies
estudios de niños adoptados adopted-child
  studies
estudios de primates primate studies
estudios del flujo sanguíneo cerebral
  cerebral blood flow studies
estudios en la obscuridad darkness studies
estupefaciente stupefacient

estupefactivo stupefactive
estupor stupor
estupor acinético akinetic stupor
estupor benigno benign stupor
estupor catatónico catatonic stupor
estupor de Cairns Cairns' stupor
estupor depresivo depressive stupor
estupor diencefálico diencephalic stupor
estupor emocional emotional stupor
estupor exhaustivo exhaustive stupor
estupor histérico hysterical stupor
estupor maligno malignant stupor
estupor maníaco manic stupor
estupor narcótico narcotic stupor
estupor psicogénico psychogenic stupor
estuporoso stuporous
etambutol ethambutol
etanol ethanol
etanolismo ethanolism
etapa stage
etapa anal anal stage
etapa anal-expulsiva anal-expulsive stage
etapa anal-retentiva anal-retentive stage
etapa anal-sádico anal-sadistic stage
etapa autónoma autonomous stage
etapa de agotamiento exhaustion stage
etapa de codificación de reglas codification
  of rules stage
etapa de comunicación verdadera true
  communication stage
etapa de dos palabras del desarrollo del
  lenguaje two-word stage of language
  development
etapa de educación education stage
etapa de equidad equity stage
etapa de erotismo oral oral-eroticism stage
etapa de experimentar un síntoma symptom
  experience stage
etapa de formación de gramática grammar
  formation stage
etapa de vida life stage
etapa de igualdad equality stage
etapa de independencia moral moral
  independence stage
etapa de individuación individuation stage
etapa de latencia latency stage
etapa de latencia del desarrollo psicosexual
  latency stage of psychosexual development
etapa de mensajes de dos palabras two-word
  messages stage
etapa de morder biting stage
etapa de operaciones concretas concrete
  operations stage
etapa de operaciones formales formal
  operations stage
etapa de palabra única single word stage
etapa de pensamiento preoperacional
  preoperational thought stage
etapa de preguntas question stage
etapa de realismo moral moral realism stage
etapa de recuperación recovery stage
etapa de rehabilitación rehabilitation stage
etapa de resistencia resistance stage
etapa del desarrollo developmental stage
etapa del desarrollo de gramática grammar

development stage
etapa deuterofálica deuterophallic stage
etapa edípica oedipal stage
etapa fálica phallic stage
etapa fetal fetal stage
etapa genital genital stage
etapa germinativa germinal stage
etapa heterónoma heteronomous stage
etapa holofrástica holophrastic stage
etapa icónica iconic stage
etapa intuitiva intuitive stage
etapa lingüística linguistic stage
etapa locomotora genital locomotor-genital
  stage
etapa muscular-anal muscular-anal stage
etapa operatoria operatory stage
etapa operatoria formal formal operatory
  stage
etapa oral oral stage
etapa oral-sádica oral-sadistic stage
etapa oral-sensorial oral-sensory stage
etapa posconvencional del desarrollo moral
  postconventional stage of moral
  development
etapa preconceptual preconceptual stage
etapa preedípica preoedipal stage
etapa pregenital pregenital stage
etapa prehabla prespeech stage
etapa premoral premoral stage
etapa preoperacional preoperational stage
etapa preoperatoria preoperatory stage
etapa prepuberal prepuberal stage
etapa psicoanalítica psychoanalytic stage
etapa psicosexual psychosexual stage
etapa psicosocial psychosocial stage
etapa pubertal pubertal stage
etapa realista realistic stage
etapa sensorimotora sensorimotor stage
etapa simbiótica symbiotic stage
etapa simbólica symbolic stage
etapa sugestionable suggestible stage
etapa uretral urethral stage
etapa de reacción de alarma alarm reaction
  stage
etapas cognitivas cognitive stages
etapas conductuales de niños children's
  behavioral stages
etapas del sueño sleep stages
etapas psicosexuales del desarrollo
  psychosexual stages of development
etapas psicosociales del desarrollo
  psychosocial stages of development
état état
état crible état crible
etclorvinol ethchlorvynol
éter ether
eteromanía etheromania
ética ethics
ética aplicada applied ethics
ética biomédica biomedical ethics
ética de logro achievement ethic
ética descriptiva descriptive ethics
ética médica medical ethics
ética normativa normative ethics
ética profesional professional ethics

ético ethical
etilamina ethylamine
etilfenacemida ethylphenacemide
etinamato ethinamate
etiología etiology
etiología de depresión etiology of depression
etiología de trastornos del comer etiology of
  eating disorders
etiología y clasificación etiology and
  classification
etiológico etiological
etiqueta diagnóstica diagnostic label
etiquetaje labeling
etmocefalia ethmocephaly
étnico ethnic
etnocentrismo ethnocentrism
etnociencia ethnoscience
etnografía ethnography
etnográfico ethnographic
etnología ethnology
etnológico ethnological
etnometodología ethnomethodology
etnopsicofarmacología
  ethnopsychopharmacology
etnopsicología ethnopsychology
etnopsiquiatría ethnopsychiatry
etnosemántica ethnosemantics
etofarmacología ethopharmacology
etograma ethogram
etología ethology
etológico ethological
etólogo ethologist
etopropazina ethopropazine
etosuximida ethosuximide
etriptamina etryptamine
eudemonia eudemonia
eudemonia afectiva affective eudemonia
euergasia euergasia
euestrés eustress
euforético euphoretic
euforia euphoria
euforia falsa false euphoria
euforia relacionada a evento event-related
  euphoria
eufórico euphoric
euforígeno euphoriant
euforoalucinógeno euphorohallucinogen
eufunción eufunction
eugenesia eugenics
eugenesia negativa negative eugenics
eugenesia positiva positive eugenics
eugénico eugenic
eugenismo eugenism
eugnosia eugnosia
eumetría eumetria
eumórfico eumorphic
eunoia eunoia
eunuco eunuch
eunucoide eunuchoid
eunucoidismo eunuchoidism
euosmia euosmia
eupraxia eupraxia
eurimorfo eurymorph
euriplástico euryplastic
euritmia eurhythmia

eurotofobia eurotophobia
eusténico eusthenic
eutanasia euthanasia
eutanasia activa active euthanasia
eutanasia pasiva passive euthanasia
eutanasia voluntaria voluntary euthanasia
eutelegenesia eutelegenesis
euténica euthenics
eutimia euthymia
eutímico euthymic
eutiquia eutychia
eutónico eutonic
evaluación assessment, evaluation
evaluación ambiental environmental
  assessment
evaluación asistida por computadora
  computer-assisted assessment
evaluación automatizada automated
  assessment
evaluación cervical cervical evaluation
evaluación clínica clinical assessment
evaluación cognitiva cognitive appraisal
evaluación comunitaria community
  assessment
evaluación conductual behavioral assessment
evaluación de agudeza assessment of acuity
evaluación de análisis de red
  network-analysis evaluation
evaluación de ansiedad assessment of anxiety
evaluación de autismo assessment of autism
evaluación de calidad quality assessment
evaluación de competencia para someterse a
  juicio assessment of competency to stand
  trial
evaluación de comunicación assessment of
  communication
evaluación de conducta behavior assessment
evaluación de coordinación assessment of
  coordination
evaluación de cuidado médico medical care
  evaluation
evaluación de delincuencia assessment of
  delinquency
evaluación de depresión assessment of
  depression
evaluación de destrezas de comunicación
  communication skills assessment
evaluación de destrezas sociales assessment
  of social skills
evaluación de discapacidades de aprendizaje
  assessment of learning disabilities
evaluación de discrepancias discrepancy
  evaluation
evaluación de disfunción emocional
  assessment of emotional dysfunction
evaluación de ejecución performance
  assessment
evaluación de empleado employee evaluation
evaluación de entrenamiento training
  evaluation
evaluación de estilo de vida lifestyle
  assessment
evaluación de impacto de programa
  program-impact evaluation
evaluación de impacto social social-impact

assessment
evaluación de inteligencia intelligence
  assessment
evaluación de investigación evaluation of
  research
evaluación de línea base base line assessment
evaluación de necesidades needs assessment
evaluación de necesidades comunitarias
  community needs assessment
evaluación de niños child assessment
evaluación de organicidad organicity
  assessment
evaluación de personalidad personality
  assessment
evaluación de personalidad proyectiva
  projective personality assessment
evaluación de proceso process evaluation
evaluación de programa program evaluation
evaluación de responsabilidad criminal
  assessment of criminal responsibility
evaluación de resultados outcome evaluation
evaluación de retroalimentación feedback
  evaluation
evaluación de trabajo work evaluation
evaluación de trastornos de conducta
  assessment of behavior disorders
evaluación de trastornos del comer
  assessment of eating disorders
evaluación del desarrollo developmental
  assessment
evaluación del lenguaje assessment of
  language
evaluación del personal personnel evaluation
evaluación educacional educational
  assessment
evaluación familiar family assessment
evaluación forense forensic assessment
evaluación formativa formative evaluation
evaluación funcional functional assessment
evaluación individualizada individualized
  assessment
evaluación intelectual intellectual assessment
evaluación intelectual de trastornos del
  desarrollo intellectual assessment of
  developmental disorders
evaluación interna in-house evaluation
evaluación médica medical assessment
evaluación multiaxial multiaxial assessment
evaluación multimodal multimodal
  assessment
evaluación naturalista naturalistic assessment
evaluación neurológica neurological
  evaluation
evaluación neuropsicológica
  neuropsychological assessment
evaluación nutricional nutritional assessment
evaluación objetiva objective assessment
evaluación operacional operational evaluation
evaluación para educación especial
  assessment for special education
evaluación psicológica transcultural
  cross-cultural psychological assessment
evaluación secundaria secondary evaluation
evaluación transaccional transactional
  evaluation

evaluación transcultural cross-cultural
   assessment
evaluación vocacional vocational assessment
evaluado evaluated
evaluador evaluator
evaluando niños assessing children
evaluando niños para psicoterapia assessing
   children for psychotherapy
evaluativo evaluative
evasión evasion
evasivo evasive
evento event
evento conjunto joint event
evento de salida exit event
evento perturbador disturbing event
evento traumático traumatic event
eventos de la vida life events
eventos independientes independent events
eventos mutuamente exclusivos mutually
   exclusive events
eventos perinatales perinatal events
eversión eversion
evidente evident
eviración eviration
evisceroneurotomía evisceroneurotomy
evitación avoidance
evitación activa active avoidance
evitación condicionada conditioned avoidance
evitación de conflicto conflict avoidance
evitación de culpa blame avoidance
evitación de operante libre free-operant
   avoidance
evitación de Sidman Sidman avoidance
evitación pasiva passive avoidance
evitación y aprendizaje de escape avoidance
   and escape learning
evitante avoidant
evocado evoked
evocador evocative
evocar evoke
evolución evolution
evolución convergente convergent evolution
evolución del cerebro evolution of brain
evolución emergente emergent evolution
evolución mental mental evolution
evolutilidad evolutility
ex paciente ex-patient
ex post facto ex post facto
exacerbar exacerbate
exaferencia exafference
exageración exaggeration
exageración en gracia exaggeration in wit
exaltación exaltation
exaltación maníaca maniacal exaltation
exaltado exalted
examinación examination
examinación de seguimiento follow-up
   examination
examinación del estado mental mental-status
   examination
examinación mental mental examination
examinación neurológica neurological
   examination
examinación objetiva objective examination
examinación posmortem postmortem

examination
examinación psicológica psychological
   examination
examinación psicométrica psychometric
   examination
examinación psiquiátrica psychiatric
   examination
examinación sexológica sexological
   examination
examinación subjetiva subjective examination
excéntrico eccentric
excepción exception
excepcional exceptional
excesivamente excessively
excesivo excessive
excitabilidad excitability
excitabilidad de neurona excitability of
   neuron
excitabilidad refleja reflex excitability
excitable excitable
excitación excitement
excitación-calma excitement-calm
excitación catatónica catatonic excitement
excitación de aniversario anniversary
   excitement
excitación esquizofrénica schizophrenic
   excitement
excitación maníaca manic excitement
excitación neural neural excitation
excitación psicomotora psychomotor
   excitement
excitación reactiva reactive excitation
excitación sexual inhibida inhibited sexual
   excitement
excitación sexual previa foreplay
excitación y conducción excitation and
   conduction
excitado excited
excitante excitant
excitante específico specific excitant
excitatorio excitatory
excitomotor excitomotor
exclamación exclamation
exclusión exclusion
exclusión defensiva defensive exclusion
excoriación excoriation
excoriación neurótica neurotic excoriation
excremento excrement
exencefalia exencephaly
exencefálico exencephalic
exencéfalo exencephalous
exencefalocele exencephalocele
exhaustivo exhaustive
exhibición de cortejo courtship display
exhibición sexual sexual exhibition
exhibicionismo exhibitionism
exhibicionista exhibitionist
exhilarante exhilarant
exigencia ambiental environmental demand
exigencias de tarea task demands
existencia existence
existencial existential
existencialismo existentialism
éxito académico academic success
exocatección exocathection

exocitosis exocytosis
exocrino exocrine
exoforia exophoria
exoftalmía exophthalmia
exoftalmos exophthalmos
exogamia exogamy
exogénesis exogenesis
exogenético exogenetic
exogénico exogenic
exógeno exogenous
exón exon
exonerativo exonerative
exopsíquico exopsychic
exorcismo exorcism
exosomático exosomatic
exótico exotic
exotropía exotropia
expansión expansion
expansión de conciencia consciousness
   expansion
expansión perceptiva perceptual expansion
expansividad expansiveness
expansivo expansive
expectación expectation
expectación ansiosa anxious expectation
expectación catastrófica catastrophic
   expectation
expectación de muerte death expectation
expectación de papel role expectation
expectación de recompensa reward
   expectancy
expectación medios-fines means-ends
   expectation
expectaciones parentales parental
   expectations
expectativa de vida life expectancy
expectativas sexuales sexual expectations
experiencia experience
experiencia ¡ajá! aha experience
experiencia afectiva affective experience
experiencia colectiva collective experience
experiencia cumbre peak experience
experiencia cutánea cutaneous experience
experiencia de grupo group experience
experiencia de nacimiento birth experience
experiencia de vibraciones vibration
   experience
experiencia emocional correctiva corrective
   emotional experience
experiencia espantosa frightening experience
experiencia fuera del cuerpo out-of-body
   experience
experiencia inmediata immediate experience
experiencia psicodélica psychedelic
   experience
experiencia sensorial sensory experience
experiencia terapéutica humana human
   therapeutic experience
experiencia traumática traumatic experience
experiencial experiential
experiencias de vida temprana early life
   experiences
experiencias tempranas early experiences
experimentación experimentation
experimentación ambiental environmental

experimentation
experimentación de campo field
   experimentation
experimentación de papel role
   experimentation
experimentación farmacológica
   pharmacological experimentation
experimentador experimenter
experimental experimental
experimento experiment
experimento análogo analogue experiment
experimento control control experiment
experimento crucial crucial experiment
experimento de aislamiento isolation
   experiment
experimento de asociación association
   experiment
experimento de campo field experiment
experimento de complicación complication
   experiment
experimento de detección detection
   experiment
experimento de grupo group experiment
experimento de memoria memory
   experiment
experimento de pensamientos thought
   experiment
experimento de privación deprivation
   experiment
experimento de reacción demorada delayed
   reaction experiment
experimento de selección choice experiment
experimento de selección múltiple
   multiple-choice experiment
experimento de Stratton Stratton's
   experiment
experimento en blanco blank experiment
experimento factorial factorial experiment
experimento farmacológico pharmacological
   experiment
experimento Gedanken Gedanken experiment
experimento global global experiment
experimento mental mental experiment
experimento miniatura miniature experiment
experimentos de nervios cruzados
   crossed-nerve experiments
expiación expiation
expiatorio expiatory
explicación explanation
explicación de conducta explanation of
   behavior
explícito explicit
exploración exploration
exploración cerebral brain scan
exploración de objetos object exploration
exploración diversiva diversive exploration
exploración sensorial sensory exploration
exploración serial serial exploration
exploración sexual sexual exploration
exploratorio exploratory
explosivo explosive
explotación exploitation
explotación de niños exploitation of children
explotador exploiting
exposición exposure

exposición a agresión e imitación exposure to
　aggression and imitation
exposición a plomo y desarrollo cognitivo
　lead exposure and cognitive development
exposición imaginal imaginal exposure
expresión expression
expresión aberrante de energía aberrant
　energy expression
expresión de afecto expression of affect
expresión de disfrute expression of
　enjoyment
expresión de genes gene expression
expresión de ira expression of anger
expresión de repugnancia expression of
　disgust
expresión de temor expression of fear
expresión emocional emotional expression
expresión emocional en infantes ciegos
　emotional expression in blind infants
expresión emocional en preescolares
　emotional expression in preschoolers
expresión facial facial expression
expresionismo abstracto abstract
　expressionism
expresividad expressivity
expresivo expressive
éxtasis ecstasy
extático ecstatic
extensión extension
extensión de efecto effect spread
extensor extensor
exteriorización exteriorization
exteriorizar exteriorize
externalización externalization
externalización de problemas externalization
　of problems
externalizante externalizing
externalizante-internalizante
　externalizing-internalizing
externo external
exteroceptivo exteroceptive
exteroceptor exteroceptor
exterofectivo exterofective
exteropsíquico exteropsychic
extinción extinction
extinción de conducta extinction of behavior
extinción de conducta con hipnotismo
　extinction of behavior with hypnotism
extinción del ego extinction of ego
extinción diferencial differential extinction
extinción en aprendizaje extinction in
　learning
extinción encubierta covert extinction
extinción experimental experimental
　extinction
extinción latente latent extinction
extinción perceptiva perceptual extinction
extinción secundaria secondary extinction
extinción sensorial sensory extinction
extinguido extinguished
extinguir extinguish
extirpación extirpation
extracepción extraception
extracraneal extracranial
extractivo extractive

extradimensional extradimensional
extradural extradural
extraespectral extraspectral
extraindividual extraindividual
extramarital extramarital
extrapiramidal extrapyramidal
extrapolar extrapolate
extrapsíquico extrapsychic
extrapunitivo extrapunitive
extrasensorial extrasensory
extraspectivo extraspective
extraversión extraversion
extraversión-introversión
　extraversion-introversion
extravertido extravert
extrayección extrajection
extremidad extremity
extremo extreme
extrínseco extrinsic
extropunitivo extropunitive
extrospección extrospection
extroversión extroversion
extrovertido extrovert
eyaculación ejaculation
eyaculación ausente absent ejaculation
eyaculación demorada delayed ejaculation
eyaculación femenina female ejaculation
eyaculación masculina male ejaculation
eyaculación precoz ejaculatio praecox
eyaculación prematura premature ejaculation
eyaculación retardada retarded ejaculation
eyaculación retardada primaria primary
　retarded ejaculation
eyaculación retardada secundaria secondary
　retarded ejaculation
eyaculación retrógrada retrograde ejaculation
eyaculatorio ejaculatory

F

fábula fable
fabulación fabulation
facies facies
facies de duende elfin facies
facies de Hutchinson Hutchinson's facies
facies de Parkinson Parkinson's facies
facies dolorosa facies dolorosa
facies miasténica myasthenic facies
facies miopática myopathic facies
facilitación facilitation
facilitación asociativa associative facilitation
facilitación conductual behavioral facilitation
facilitación de conducta asertiva assertive
    behavior facilitation
facilitación de Wedensky Wedensky
    facilitation
facilitación heterosináptica heterosynaptic
    facilitation
facilitación neural neural facilitation
facilitación refleja reflex facilitation
facilitación reproductiva reproductive
    facilitation
facilitación retroactiva retroactive facilitation
facilitación social social facilitation
facilitador facilitator
faciocefalalgia faciocephalalgia
facioescapulohumeral facioscapulohumeral
faciolingual faciolingual
facioplejía facioplegia
facoma phacoma
facomatosis phacomatosis
facoscopio phacoscope
factibilidad feasibility
facticio factitious
factor factor
factor aleatorio random factor
factor antirriesgo antirisk factor
factor C C factor
factor cognitivo cognitive factor
factor común common factor
factor de complejidad complexity factor
factor de crecimiento neural neural growth
    factor
factor de densidad uniforme factor of
    uniform density
factor de despertamiento cortical cortical
    arousal factor
factor de Frankenstein Frankenstein factor
factor de grupo group factor
factor de incertidumbre uncertainty factor
factor de poder power factor
factor de posición position factor
factor de primer orden first-order factor
factor de protección protection factor

factor de realismo realism factor
factor de riesgo risk factor
factor de segundo orden second-order factor
factor de subjetivismo subjectivism factor
factor de tono hedónico hedonic-tone factor
factor de voluntad will factor
factor de vulnerabilidad vulnerability factor
factor espacial space factor
factor especial special factor
factor experimental experimental factor
factor familiar familial factor
factor fijo fixed factor
factor G G factor
factor general general factor
factor gestalt gestalt factor
factor hereditario hereditary factor
factor inconsciente unconscious factor
factor intrínseco intrinsic factor
factor liberador de corticotropina
    corticotropine-releasing factor
factor liberador de hormona del crecimiento
    growth hormone releasing factor
factor motivacional motivational factor
factor neurotrófico neurotrophic factor
factor numérico number factor
factor nutricional nutritional factor
factor piscobiológico psychobiological factor
factor preedípico preoedipal factor
factor pregenital pregenital factor
factor primario primary factor
factor psicológico afectando una condición
    física psychological factor affecting
    physical condition
factor psicológico afectando una condición
    médica psychological factor affecting
    medical condition
factor Rh Rh factor
factor social social factor
factor solapante overlapping factor
factor terminal terminal factor
factor único unique factor
factor verbal verbal factor
factores afectivos-cognitivos
    affective-cognitive factors
factores anatómicos anatomical factors
factores biógenos biogenic factors
factores biológicos biological factors
factores biológicos en depresión biological
    factors in depression
factores biológicos en el desarrollo biological
    factors in development
factores biológicos en esquizofrenia
    biological factors in schizophrenia
factores biológicos en trastornos del humor
    biological factors in mood disorders
factores biológicos que afectan la sexualidad
    biological factors affecting sexuality
factores constitucionales constitutional factors
factores culturales cultural factors
factores culturales en conducta cultural
    factors in behavior
factores culturales en depresión cultural
    factors in depression
factores culturales en emoción cultural
    factors in emotion

factores de decisiones decision factors
factores de inmunidad immunity factors
factores de inmunidad celular cellular
 immunity factors
factores de inmunidad humoral humoral
 immunity factors
factores de interés interest factors
factores de personalidad personality factors
factores del desarrollo developmental factors
factores endogenéticos endogenetic factors
factores endogénicos endogenic factors
factores endógenos endogenous factors
factores etiológicos etiologic factors
factores etiológicos en accidentes etiologic
 factors in accidents
factores étnicos ethnic factors
factores exógenos exogenous factors
factores externos external factors
factores externos en agresión external factors
 in aggression
factores genéticos genetic factors
factores genéticos en agresión genetic factors
 in aggression
factores genéticos en altruismo genetic
 factors in altruism
factores genéticos en autismo genetic factors
 in autism
factores genéticos en emociones genetic
 factors in emotions
factores genéticos en epilepsia genetic factors
 in epilepsy
factores genéticos en esquizofrenia genetic
 factors in schizophrenia
factores genéticos en hipertensión genetic
 factors in hypertension
factores genéticos en inteligencia genetic
 factors in intelligence
factores genéticos en la enfermedad de
 Alzheimer genetic factors in Alzheimer's
 disease
factores genéticos en memoria genetic
 factors in memory
factores genéticos en personalidad genetic
 factors in personality
factores genéticos en trastornos afectivos
 genetic factors in affective disorders
factores genéticos en trastornos del comer
 genetic factors in eating disorders
factores genéticos en trastornos mentales
 genetic factors in mental disorders
factores humanos human factors
factores internos internal factors
factores internos en agresión internal factors
 in aggression
factores principales principal factors
factores psicológicos psychological factors
factores psicosociales psychosocial factors
factores que influencian el apego factors
 influencing attachment
factores que influencian el desarrollo factors
 influencing development
factores representativos representative
 factors
factores socioculturales sociocultural factors
factores socioeconómicos socioeconomic

factors
factores sociológicos sociological factors
factorización factoring
facultad faculty
facultad de criticar criticizing faculty
facultad mental mental faculty
facultativo facultative
fagocitosis phagocytosis
fagofobia phagophobia
fagomanía phagomania
falacia fallacy
falacia a posteriori a posteriori fallacy
falacia de cosificación reification fallacy
falacia de efectos fijos fixed-effects fallacy
falacia de psicólogo psychologist's fallacy
falacia de tasa base base rate fallacy
falacia de terminación opcional
 optional-stopping fallacy
falacia de tipos type fallacy
falacia del jugador gambler's fallacy
falacia patética pathetic fallacy
falacia patológica pathological fallacy
falange phalanx
falectomía fallectomy
falicismo phallicism
fálico phallic
fálico-edípico phallic-oedipal
falismo phallism
falo phallus
falocéntrico phallocentric
falofobia phallophobia
falometría phallometry
falsa alarma false alarm
falsedad falsehood
falsete falsetto
falsificable falsifiable
falsificación falsification
falsificación de memoria memory falsification
falsificación retrospectiva retrospective
 falsification
falso false
falsonegativo false negative
falsopositivo false positive
falta fault
falta básica basic fault
falta de empatía lack of empathy
falta de energía energy lack
falta de envolvimiento lack of involvement
falta de lógica illogicality
falta de motivación lack of motivation
falta de penetrancia lack of penetrance
faltante defaulter
faltante de drogas drug defaulter
falto de peso underweight
falx cerebelli falx cerebelli
falx cerebri falx cerebri
familia family
familia adoptiva foster family
familia alcohólica alcoholic family
familia caótica chaotic family
familia centrada en el niño child-centered
 family
familia disfuncional dysfunctional family
familia extendida extended family
familia matriarcal matriarchal family

familia mezclada blended family
familia nuclear nuclear family
familia ocupacional occupational family
familia patriarcal patriarchal family
familia reconstituida reconstituted family
familia rígida rigid family
familia simulada simulated family
familia y abuso de sustancias family and substance abuse
familianismo familianism
familiar familiar
familias abusivas abusive families
fanatismo fanaticism
faneromanía phaneromania
fantaseo activo active fantasying
fantasía fantasy
fantasía agresiva aggressive fantasy
fantasía autista autistic fantasy
fantasía canibalística cannibalistic fantasy
fantasía cubriente screen fantasy
fantasía de arañas spider fantasy
fantasía de cortesana courtesan fantasy
fantasía de embarazo pregnancy fantasy
fantasía de felatorismo fellatio fantasy
fantasía de incesto incest fantasy
fantasía de Pompadour Pompadour fantasy
fantasía de rejuvenecimiento rejuvenation fantasy
fantasía de renacimiento rebirth fantasy
fantasía de rescate rescue fantasy
fantasía de útero womb fantasy
fantasía de violación rape fantasy
fantasía de violación anal anal rape fantasy
fantasía erotizada eroticized fantasy
fantasía esquizoide schizoid fantasy
fantasía forzada forced fantasy
fantasía heteral hetaeral fantasy
fantasía inconsciente unconscious fantasy
fantasía masoquista masochistic fantasy
fantasía necrofílica necrophilic fantasy
fantasía nocturna night fantasy
fantasía obsesiva obsessive fantasy
fantasía primal primal fantasy
fantasía sexual sexual fantasy
fantasía uterina uterine fantasy
fantasía de afecto affect fantasy
fantasías anales anal fantasies
fantasias de azotamiento beating fantasies
fantasma phantom
fantasma de Bidwell Bidwell's ghost
fantasma de Swindle Swindle's ghost
fantasmagoría phantasmagoria
fantasmatomoria phantasmatomoria
fantasmología phantasmology
fantasmoscopia phantasmoscopy
faringe pharynx
faríngeo pharyngeal
faringismo pharyngismus
faringoespasmo pharyngospasm
faringoplejía pharyngoplegia
farmacéutico pharmaceutical
farmacocinética pharmacokinetics
farmacodinámico pharmacodynamic
farmacofilia pharmacophilia
farmacofobia pharmacophobia

farmacogenética pharmacogenetics
farmacogenética conductual behavioral pharmacogenetics
farmacogénico pharmacogenic
farmacogeriatría pharmacogeriatrics
farmacología pharmacology
farmacológico pharmacological
farmacomanía pharmacomania
farmacopea pharmacopeia
farmacopsicoanálisis pharmacopsychoanalysis
farmacopsicosis pharmacopsychosis
farmacoterapia pharmacotherapy
farmacoterapia de megadosis megadose pharmacotherapy
farmacoterapia para autismo pharmacotherapy for autism
farmacoterapia para depresión pharmacotherapy for depression
farmacoterapia para trastornos afectivos pharmacotherapy for affective disorders
farmacoterapia para trastornos ansiosos pharmacotherapy for anxiety disorders
farmacoterapia para trastornos de déficit de atención pharmacotherapy for attention-deficit disorders
farmacoterapia para trastornos del comer pharmacotherapy for eating disorders
farmacotimia pharmacothymia
fasciculación fasciculation
fascicular fascicular
fascículo fasciculus
fascículo arqueado arcuate fasciculus
fascículo cuneiforme fasciculus cuneatus
fascículo del cerebro anterior medial medial forebrain bundle
fascículo gracilis fasciculus gracilis
fascículo lateral lateral bundle
fascículo longitudinal inferior inferior longitudinal fasciculus
fascículo longitudinal superior superior longitudinal fasciculus
fascículo medial medial bundle
fascículo olivococlear olivocochlear bundle
fascículo tegmental dorsal dorsal tegmental bundle
fascículo uncinado uncinate fasciculus
fascículos fasciculi
fascículos propios fasciculi proprii
fascinación fascination
fascinante fascinating
fase phase
fase anabólica anabolic phase
fase anal anal phase
fase apetitiva appetitive phase
fase autista autistic phase
fase canibalística cannibalistic phase
fase clónica clonic phase
fase contrachoque countershock phase
fase de agotamiento exhaustion phase
fase de ayuno fasting phase
fase de choque shock phase
fase de excitación excitement phase
fase de excitación de respuesta sexual excitement phase of sexual response
fase de latencia latency phase

fase de meseta plateau phase
fase de resistencia resistance phase
fase de resolución resolution phase
fase de vida phase of life
fase del desarrollo developmental phase
fase edípica oedipal phase
fase fálica phallic phase
fase genital genital phase
fase incorporativa oral oral-incorporative
    phase
fase libidinal libidinal phase
fase lútea luteal phase
fase mágica magic phase
fase oral oral phase
fase orgásmica orgasmic phase
fase posambivalente postambivalent phase
fase preedípica preoedipal phase
fase pregenital pregenital phase
fase preoperacional preoperational phase
fase presuperego presuperego phase
fase prodrómica prodromic phase
fase proliferativa proliferative phase
fase protofálica protophallic phase
fase sensorimotora sensorimotor phase
fase simbiótica symbiotic phase
fase uretral urethral phase
fásico phasic
fasmofobia phasmophobia
fasofrenia phasophrenia
fastidium cibi fastidium cibi
fastidium potus fastidium potus
fatal fatal
fatalismo fatalism
fatiga fatigue
fatiga auditiva auditory fatigue
fatiga de combate combat fatigue
fatuidad fatuity
faucial faucial
fausse reconnaissance fausse reconnaissance
faux de mieux faux de mieux
favoritismo favoritism
favoritismo en grupo exclusivo in-group
    favoritism
febrifobia febriphobia
febril febrile
fecundación fecundation
fecundar fecundate
fecundidad fecundity
felación fellatio
felator fellator
felatorismo fellatorism
felatriz fellatrix
felicidad happiness
femenino feminine
feminidad femininity
feminismo feminism
feminista feminist
feminización feminization
fenacemida phenacemide
fenacetina phenacetin
fenadoxona phenadoxone
fenazocina phenazocine
fenciclidina phencyclidine
fendimetrazina phendimetrazine
fenelzina phenelzine

fenestra ovalis fenestra ovalis
fenestra rotunda fenestra rotunda
fenestración fenestration
fenetilina fenethylline
fenfluramina fenfluramine
fenfluramina en autismo fenfluramine in
    autism
fengofobia phengophobia
fenilalanina phenylalanine
fenilbutazona phenylbutazone
fenilcetonuria phenylketonuria
feniletilamina phenylethylamine
fenilpirúvico phenylpyruvic
feniltoloxamina phenyltoloxamine
fenitoína phenytoin
fenmetrazina phenmetrazine
fenobarbital phenobarbital
fenocopia phenocopy
fenomenal phenomenal
fenomenalismo phenomenalism
fenomenalista phenomenalistic
fenomenístico phenomenistic
fenómeno phenomenon
fenómeno antidrómico antidromic
    phenomenon
fenómeno autoscópico autoscopic
    phenomenon
fenómeno cervicolumbar cervicolumbar
    phenomenon
fenómeno de Arago Arago phenomenon
fenómeno de Aubert Aubert phenomenon
fenómeno de Aubert-Forster Aubert-Forster
    phenomenon
fenómeno de Babinski Babinski's
    phenomenon
fenómeno de Bell Bell's phenomenon
fenómeno de cadera hip phenomenon
fenómeno de Capgras Capgras' phenomenon
fenómeno de cóctel cocktail-party
    phenomenon
fenómeno de constancia constancy
    phenomenon
fenómeno de Cushing Cushing phenomenon
fenómeno de déjà vu déjà vu phenomenon
fenómeno de Dejerine-Lichtheim
    Dejerine-Lichtheim phenomenon
fenómeno de desincronosis circadiano jet-lag
    phenomenon
fenómeno de desprendimiento breakoff
    phenomenon
fenómeno de dirección errada misdirection
    phenomenon
fenómeno de Doppelganger Doppelganger
    phenomenon
fenómeno de Duckworth Duckworth's
    phenomenon
fenómeno de eco echo phenomenon
fenómeno de escape escape phenomenon
fenómeno de Fere Fere phenomenon
fenómeno de flexión de cadera hip-flexion
    phenomenon
fenómeno de Fregoli Fregoli's phenomenon
fenómeno de Grasset Grasset's phenomenon
fenómeno de Grasset-Gaussel
    Grasset-Gaussel phenomenon

fenómeno de guiño mandibular jaw-winking
  phenomenon
fenómeno de Gunn Gunn phenomenon
fenómeno de Hertwig-Magendie
  Hertwig-Magendie phenomenon
fenómeno de Hoffmann Hoffmann's
  phenomenon
fenómeno de Honi Honi phenomenon
fenómeno de identificación identification
  phenomenon
fenómeno de Isakower Isakower phenomenon
fenómeno de jamais jamais phenomenon
fenómeno de Kohler-Restorff
  Kohler-Restorff phenomenon
fenómeno de Kohnstamm Kohnstamm's
  phenomenon
fenómeno de Kuhne Kuhne's phenomenon
fenómeno de la mano de Dejerine Dejerine's
  hand phenomenon
fenómeno de Leichtenstern Leichtenstern's
  phenomenon
fenómeno de liberación release phenomenon
fenómeno de los dedos del pie toe
  phenomenon
fenómeno de Marcus Gunn Marcus Gunn
  phenomenon
fenómeno de Napalkov Napalkov
  phenomenon
fenómeno de navaja clasp-knife phenomenon
fenómeno de Negro Negro's phenomenon
fenómeno de no reflujo no reflow
  phenomenon
fenómeno de Panum Panum phenomenon
fenómeno de pecho fantasma breast-phantom
  phenomenon
fenómeno de pierna leg phenomenon
fenómeno de Pool Pool's phenomenon
fenómeno de Potzl Potzl phenomenon
fenómeno de puerta giratoria revolving-door
  phenomenon
fenómeno de Pulfrich Pulfrich phenomenon
fenómeno de punta de la lengua
  tip-of-the-tongue phenomenon
fenómeno de Purkinje Purkinje phenomenon
fenómeno de Raynaud Raynaud's
  phenomenon
fenómeno de rebote rebound phenomenon
fenómeno de rebote de Gordon Holmes
  rebound phenomenon of Gordon Holmes
fenómeno de Ritter-Rollet Ritter-Rollet
  phenomenon
fenómeno de rodilla knee phenomenon
fenómeno de rompimiento breakaway
  phenomenon
fenómeno de rueda dentada cogwheel
  phenomenon
fenómeno de Rust Rust's phenomenon
fenómeno de Schiff-Sherrington
  Schiff-Sherrington phenomenon
fenómeno de Schuller Schuller's phenomenon
fenómeno de Sherrington Sherrington
  phenomenon
fenómeno de Strumpell Strumpell's
  phenomenon
fenómeno de Tarchanoff Tarchanoff

phenomenon
fenómeno de Westphal Westphal's
  phenomenon
fenómeno de Westphal-Piltz Westphal-Piltz
  phenomenon
fenómeno de Wever-Bray Wever-Bray
  phenomenon
fenómeno de Zeigarnik Zeigarnik
  phenomenon
fenómeno del brazo arm phenomenon
fenómeno del dedo finger phenomenon
fenómeno escalonado stepwise phenomenon
fenómeno facial facialis phenomenon
fenómeno frénico cruzado crossed phrenic
  phenomenon
fenómeno gestalt gestalt phenomenon
fenómeno lingual tongue phenomenon
fenómeno paradójico de Hunt Hunt's
  paradoxical phenomenon
fenómeno paranormal paranormal
  phenomenon
fenómeno peroneo peroneal phenomenon
fenómeno phi phi phenomenon
fenómeno phi puro pure phi phenomenon
fenómeno psi psi phenomenon
fenómeno pupilar de Galassi Galassi's
  pupillary phenomenon
fenómeno pupilar paradójico paradoxical
  pupillary phenomenon
fenómeno radial radial phenomenon
fenómeno social social phenomenon
fenómeno tibial tibial phenomenon
fenomenología phenomenology
fenomenología existencial existential
  phenomenology
fenomenológico phenomenological
fenómenos de extinción extinction phenomena
fenotiazina phenothiazine
fenotiazina alifática aliphatic phenothiazine
fenotipo phenotype
fensuximida phensuximide
fentermina phentermine
fentolamina phentolamine
feral feral
feromona pheromone
ferritina sérica serum ferritin
ferruginación ferrugination
fertilidad fertility
fertilidad diferencial differential fertility
fertilidad neta net fertility
fertilización fertilization
fertilización simultánea simultaneous
  fertilization
festinación festination
festinante festinant
festoneado scalloping
fetación fetation
fetal fetal
fetalismo fetalism
fetiche fetish
fetichismo fetishism
fetichismo bestial beast fetishism
fetichismo de pies foot fetishism
fetichismo transvéstico transvestic fetishism
fetichístico fetishistic

feto fetus
feto a riesgo fetus at risk
fetología fetology
fibra fiber
fibra A A fiber
fibra B B fiber
fibra C C fiber
fibra colateral collateral fiber
fibra de proyección projection fiber
fibra de Rosenthal Rosenthal fiber
fibra muscular muscle fiber
fibra nerviosa nerve fiber
fibras comisurales commissural fibers
fibras corticobulbares corticobulbar fibers
fibras corticonucleares corticonuclear fibers
fibras de asociación association fibers
fibras de Muller Muller's fibers
fibras intercerebrales intercerebral fibers
fibras intrafusales intrafusal fibers
fibras nerviosas corticófugas corticofugal
    nerve fibers
fibrilación fibrillation
fibrilar fibrillary
fibrilla fibril
fibrilla neural neural fibril
fibriofobia fibriophobia
fibrogliosis fibrogliosis
fibroma fibroma
fibroneuroma fibroneuroma
fibroplasia retrolental retrolental fibroplasia
fibropsamoma fibropsammoma
fibrosis fibrosis
fibrosis leptomeníngea leptomeningeal
    fibrosis
fibrosis quística cystic fibrosis
fibrosítico fibrositic
fibrositis fibrositis
fibrositis cervical cervical fibrositis
fibroso fibrous
ficción fiction
ficción directiva directive fiction
ficción neurótica neurotic fiction
ficticio fictitious
fiduciario fiduciary
fiebre fever
fiebre baja low fever
fiebre cerebroespinal cerebrospinal fever
fiebre de leche difásica diphasic milk fever
fiebre de máquina machine fever
fiebre meningotifoidea meningotyphoid fever
fiebre por tripanosomas trypanosome fever
fiebre térmica thermic fever
figura figure
figura ambigua ambiguous figure
figura cerrada closed figure
figura compuesta composite figure
figura de autoridad authority figure
figura de fortificación fortification figure
figura de identificación identification figure
figura de Orbison Orbison figure
figura de poder power figure
figura de Purkinje Purkinje figure
figura de Rubin Rubin's figure
figura disparatada nonsense figure
figura encerrada embedded figure

figura escondida hidden figure
figura-fondo figure-ground
figura imposible impossible figure
figura materna mother figure
figura paterna father figure
figura refleja reflex figure
figura reversible reversible figure
figura socorrante helpful figure
figura y fondo figure and ground
figural figural
figuras de Gottschaldt Gottschaldt figures
figuras de Lissajou Lissajou's figures
figurativo figurative
fijación fixation
fijación afectiva affective fixation
fijación anormal abnormal fixation
fijación binocular binocular fixation
fijación canibalística cannibalistic fixation
fijación de afecto affect fixation
fijación de ansiedad anxiety fixation
fijación de atención fixation of attention
fijación de libido libido fixation
fijación de papel role fixation
fijación en el padre father fixation
fijación en la madre mother fixation
fijación oral oral fixation
fijación oral narcisista narcissistic oral
    fixation
fijación visual visual fixation
fijación freudiana freudian fixation
fijamente fixedly
fijar fixate
fijeza fixity
fijeza funcional functional fixity
fijeza social social fixity
fijo fixed
filamento transináptico transsynaptic filament
filaxis phylaxis
filial filial
filicidio filicide
filioparental filioparental
filoanálisis phyloanalysis
filobiología phylobiology
filogénesis phylogenesis
filogenético phylogenetic
filogenia phylogeny
filogenitivo philogenitive
filología philology
filomimesia philomimesia
filopatología phylopathology
filoprogenitivo philoprogenitive
filosofía philosophy
filosofía coercitiva coercive philosophy
filosofía moral moral philosophy
filosófico philosophical
filtración perceptiva perceptual filtering
filtro filter
filtro acústico acoustic filter
filum phylum
fimbria fimbria
fimosis phimosis
fin goal, aim
fin de la vida life goal
fin externo external aim
fin instintivo instinctual aim

fin interno internal aim
fin latente latent goal
fin manifiesto manifest goal
fin parcial partial aim
fin sexual sexual aim
finalismo finalism
finalismo ficticio fictional finalism
fingido feigned
fingimiento feigning
fingimiento de muerte death feigning
fingir feign
fingirse muerto playing dead
firmeza funcional functional fixedness
fisalíforo physaliphorous
fisiatra physiatrist
fisiatría physiatrics
fisicalismo physicalism
físico (adj) physical
físico (n) physique
fisiodinámico physiodynamic
fisiodrama physiodrama
fisiogénesis physiogenesis
fisiogenético physiogenetic
fisiogénico physiogenic
fisiognosis physiognosis
fisiología physiology
fisiología de emoción physiology of emotion
fisiología de eyaculación ejaculation
    physiology
fisiológico physiological
fisión fission
fisión social social fission
fisioneurosis physioneurosis
fisionomía physiognomy
fisionómico physiognomic
fisiopatología physiopathology
fisioplástico physioplastic
fisiopsíquico physiopsychic
fisioterapia physiotherapy
fisocefalia physocephaly
fisostigmina physostigmine
fístula fistula
fístula craneosinusal craniosinus fistula
fisura fissure
fisura calcarina calcarine fissure
fisura central central fissure
fisura de Rolando fissure of Rolando
fisura de Silvio fissure of Sylvius
fisura lateral lateral fissure
fisura longitudinal longitudinal fissure
fisura palpebral palpebral fissure
fisura sagital sagittal fissure
fláccido flaccid
flagelación flagellation
flagelantismo flagellantism
flagelomanía flagellomania
flavismo flavism
flebitis phlebitis
flebitis sinusal sinus phlebitis
flebotomía phlebotomy
flema phlegm
flemático phlegmatic
flexibilidad cerea waxy flexibility
flexibilidad cognitiva cognitive flexibility
flexibilidad del contexto context flexibility

flexibilidad social social flexibility
flexibilitas cerea flexibilitas cerea
flexible flexible
flexión flexion
flexor flexor
flocilación floccillation
flor de la vida prime of life
floreo de naipes card-stacking
florido flowery
flotante floating
fluanisona fluanisone
fluctuación fluctuation
fluctuación contextual contextual fluctuation
fluctuación de atención fluctuation of
    attention
fluctuaciones del humor fluctuations of mood
fluencia de palabras word fluency
fluente fluent
flufenacina fluphenazine
fluidazepam fluidazepam
fluidez fluency
fluidez asociativa associative fluency
fluidez ideacional ideational fluency
fluidez intermodal intermodal fluency
fluido fluid
fluido amniótico amniotic fluid
fluido espinal spinal fluid
flujo axoplásmico axoplasmic flow
flujo luminoso luminous flux
flujo radiante radiant flux
flujo sanguíneo cerebral regional regional
    cerebral blood flow
flunitrazepam flunitrazepam
fluoxetina fluoxetine
flupentixol flupentixol
flurazepam flurazepam
fluspirileno fluspirilene
flutazolam flutazolam
fobantropía phobanthropy
fobia phobia
fobia a enfermedades disease phobia
fobia a los gatos cat phobia
fobia al cáncer cancer phobia
fobia al dolor pain phobia
fobia de aire air phobia
fobia de animales animal phobia
fobia de enfermedad venérea
    venereal-disease phobia
fobia de morir dying phobia
fobia escolar school phobia
fobia específica specific phobia
fobia simple simple phobia
fobia social social phobia
fobia universal universal phobia
fobias comunes common phobias
fóbico phobic
fóbico mixto mixed phobic
fobofobia phobophobia
focal focal
foco focus
foco de atención focus of attention
focomelia phocomelia
focos epileptogénicos epileptogenic foci
folato folate
folato sérico serum folate

folclor folklore
folcodina pholcodine
folículo follicle
folículo de de Graaf Graafian follicle
folículo ovárico ovarian follicle
folículo piloso hair follicle
folie folie
folie à cinq folie à cinq
folie à deux folie à deux
folie à double forme folie à double forme
folie à famille folie à famille
folie à pleusirs folie à pleusirs
folie à quatre folie à quatre
folie à trois folie à trois
folie circulaire folie circulaire
folie collective folie collective
folie communiquée folie communiquée
folie d'action folie d'action
folie démonomaniaque folie démonomaniaque
folie des grandeurs folie des grandeurs
folie des des persécutions folie des
    persécutions
folie du doute folie du doute
folie du pourquoi folie du pourquoi
folie gémellaire folie gémellaire
folie hypocondriaque folie hypocondriaque
folie imitative folie imitative
folie imposée folie imposée
folie instantanée folie instantanée
folie morale folie morale
folie paralytique folie paralytique
folie pénitentiare folie pénitentiare
folie raisonnante folie raisonnante
folie simulée folie simulée
folie simultanè folie simultanè
folie systématisée folie systématisée
folie utérine folie utérine
folie vaniteuse folie vaniteuse
folium folium
fonación phonation
fonastenia phonasthenia
fondo background, fund
fondo de información fund of information
fondo de inteligencia fund of intelligence
fonema phoneme
fonema medial medial phoneme
fonémica phonemics
fonémico phonemic
fonética phonetics
fonético phonetic
fónica phonics
fónico phonic
fonio phon
fonismo phonism
fono phone
fonofobia phonophobia
fonografía phonography
fonograma phonogram
fonología phonology
fonológico phonological
fonomanía phonomania
fonomioclono phonomyoclonus
fonomiografía phonomyography
fonopatía phonopathy
fonopsia phonopsia

fonoscopio phonoscope
fontanela fontanelle
foramen foramen
foramen interventricular de Monro
    interventricular foramen of Monro
foramen intervertebral intervertebral
    foramen
foramen magno foramen magnum
foraminotomía foraminotomy
forceps anterior anterior forceps
fórceps mayor forceps major
fórceps menor forceps minor
fórceps posterior posterior forceps
forense forensic
foria phoria
forma arquetípica archetypal form
forma buena good shape
forma de psicodrama psychodrama form
forma equivalente equivalent form
formación formation
formación de actitudes formation of attitudes
formación de compromiso compromise
    formation
formación de concepto concept formation
formación de hábitos habit formation
formación de identidad identity formation
formación de identidad adolescente
    adolescent identity formation
formación de identidad de género
    gender-identity formation
formación de identidad en adolescencia
    identity formation in adolescence
formación de impresión impression formation
formación de personalidad personality
    formation
formación de reemplazo replacement
    formation
formación de síntomas symptom formation
formación de sueños dream formation
formación de sustituto substitute formation
formación del ego ego formation
formación hacia atrás back-formation
formación reactiva reaction formation
formación reticular reticular formation
formalismo formalism
formante formant
formas alternas alternate forms
formas comparables comparable forms
formas de compuestos combining forms
formas de depresión relacionadas con la
    edad age-related forms of depression
formas paralelas parallel forms
formativo formative
formato format
formato de tratamiento format of treatment
formicación formication
fórmula formula
fórmula de Flesch Flesch formula
fórmula de Harris Harris' formula
fórmula de Jellinek Jellinek's formula
fórmula de Spearman-Brown
    Spearman-Brown formula
formulación diagnóstica diagnostic
    formulation
formulación dinámica dynamic formulation

fórmulas de Kuder-Richardson
  Kuder-Richardson formulas
fornicación fornication
fornicar fornicate
fórnix fornix
forometría phorometry
fortificación fortification
fortuito haphazard
forzado forced
fosa fossa
fosa hipofisaria hypophysial fossa
fosa media middle fossa
fosa posterior posterior fossa
fosfato phosphate
fosfeno phosphene
fosfocinasa de creatina creatine
  phosphokinase
fosfodiesterasa phosphodiesterase
fosforilación phosphorylation
fósforo phosphorous
fósforo sérico serum phosphorous
fossula fossula
fotalgia photalgia
fotaugiafobia photaugiaphobia
foteritro photerythrous
foteritrosidad photerythrosity
fotestesia photesthesia
fótico photic
fotio phot
fotismo photism
fotobiología photobiology
fotocinesis photokinesis
fotocoagulación photocoagulation
fotocromático photochromatic
fotodinia photodynia
fotodisforia photodysphoria
fotoestético photoesthetic
fotofobia photophobia
fotofóbico photophobic
fotogénico photogenic
fotoma photoma
fotomanía photomania
fotometrazol photometrazol
fotometría photometry
fotométrico photometric
fotómetro photometer
fotomioclono photomyoclonus
fotomioclono hereditario hereditary
  photomyoclonus
fotón photon
fotoperiodismo photoperiodism
fotópico photopic
fotopigmento photopigment
fotopsia photopsy
fotopsina photopsin
fotoptarmosis photoptarmosis
fotoquímica photochemistry
fotorreceptor photoreceptor
fotosensibilidad photosensitivity
fototaxis phototaxis
fototerapia phototherapy
fototropismo phototropism
fovea fovea
fovea centralis fovea centralis
foveal foveal

fracaso failure
fracaso a través del éxito failure through
  success
fracaso del ego ego failure
fracaso en avisar failure to warn
fracaso en enlutar failure to mourn
fracaso en medrar failure to thrive
fracaso en medrar no orgánico nonorganic
  failure to thrive
**fracaso en medrar no orgánico y abuso de
  niños** nonorganic failure to thrive and
  child abuse
fracaso reproductivo reproductive failure
fraccional fractional
fraccionamiento fractionation
fractura fracture
fractura abierta open fracture
fractura capilar capillary fracture
fractura complicada complicated fracture
fractura de Chance Chance fracture
fractura de cráneo skull fracture
fractura de cráneo abierta open skull
  fracture
fractura de cráneo basal basal skull fracture
fractura de cráneo cerrada closed skull
  fracture
fractura de cráneo compuesta compound
  skull fracture
fractura de cráneo conminuta comminuted
  skull fracture
fractura de cráneo deprimida depressed
  skull fracture
fractura de cráneo diastática diastatic skull
  fracture
fractura de cráneo estrellada stellate skull
  fracture
fractura de cráneo lineal linear skull fracture
fractura de cráneo simple simple skull
  fracture
fractura de crecimiento growing fracture
fractura de verdugo hangman's fracture
fractura deprimida depressed fracture
fractura directa direct fracture
fractura en canaleta gutter fracture
fractura en ping-pong ping-pong fracture
fractura indirecta indirect fracture
fractura neurogénica neurogenic fracture
fractura por contragolpe fracture by
  contrecoup
frágil fragile
fragmentación fragmentation
fragmentación de pensamiento fragmentation
  of thinking
fragmentado fragmentary
frase phrase
frecuencia frequency
frecuencia de centelleo flicker frequency
frecuencia de centelleo crítica critical flicker
  frequency
frecuencia de ejercicio exercise frequency
frecuencia de fusión fusion frequency
frecuencia de fusión crítica critical fusion
  frequency
frecuencia de genes gene frequency
frecuencia de onda wave frequency

frecuencia de sonido sound frequency
frecuencia dominante dominant frequency
frecuencia esperada expected frequency
frecuencia marginal marginal frequency
frecuencia obtenida obtained frequency
frecuencia relativa relative frequency
frecuencia subjetiva subjective frequency
fren phren
frenalgia phrenalgia
frenastenia phrenasthenia
frenectomía phrenectomy
frenenfraxis phrenemphraxis
frenesí frenzy
frenético frenetic
frenicectomía phrenicectomy
freniclasia phreniclasia
frénico phrenic
frenicoexéresis phrenicoexeresis
freniconeurectomía phreniconeurectomy
frenicotomía phrenicotomy
frenicotripsia phrenicotripsy
frenillo frenulum
frenítico phrenitic
frenocardia phrenocardia
frenoespasmo phrenospasm
frenofagia phrenophagia
frenoglótico phrenoglottic
frenología phrenology
frenólogo phrenologist
frenoplejía phrenoplegy
frenopráxico phrenopraxic
frenotrópico phrenotropic
freudiano freudian
frialdad coldness
fricativo fricative
frictopatía phrictopathia
frictopático phrictopathic
frigidez frigidity
frígido frigid
frío paradójico paradoxical cold
fronemofobia phronemophobia
frontal frontal
fronterizo borderline
frotación frotteurism
frotador frotteur
fructosuria fructosuria
frustración frustration
frustración de castigo frustration from punishment
frustración y agresión frustration and aggression
frustrar frustrate
frustratorio frustrative
frutal fruity
ftinoide phthinoid
ftiriofobia phthiriophobia
fucosidosis fucosidosis
fuente source
fuente ilegal illegal source
fuente informal informal source
fuerza force
fuerza asociativa associative strength
fuerza bruta brute force
fuerza central central force
fuerza de campo field force

fuerza de hábito habit strength
fuerza de hábito efectiva effective habit strength
fuerza de respuesta response strength
fuerza de voluntad will power
fuerza del ego ego strength
fuerza psíquica psychic force
fuerza reproductiva reproductive strength
fuga flight, fugue, elopement
fuga a enfermedad flight into illness
fuga a fantasía flight into fantasy
fuga a realidad flight into reality
fuga a salud flight into health
fuga de colores flight of colors
fuga de ideas flight of ideas
fuga de la realidad flight from reality
fuga disociativa dissociative fugue
fuga o pelea flight or fight
fuga poriomaníaca poriomanic fugue
fuga psicogénica psychogenic fugue
fugarse run away
fulgurante fulgurant
fulminante fulminant
fumar smoking
fumar cigarrillos cigarette smoking
funcinonamiento bajo promedio intelectual intellectual subaverage functioning
función function
función adaptiva de soñar adaptive function of dreaming
función alomérica allomeric function
función autónoma autonomous function
función autónoma primaria primary autonomous function
función cardiovascular cardiovascular function
función cognitiva cognitive function
función cognitiva del sueño cognitive function of sleep
función de densidad density function
función de despertamiento arousal function
función de pasos step function
función de poder power function
función de probabilidades probability function
función de procesamiento de estímulos stimulus-processing function
función de señal cue function
función de sensibilidad de contraste contrast sensitivity function
función de sueños dream function
función de transferencia transfer function
función de transferencia de modulación modulation transfer function
función del ego ego function
función del ego autónomo autonomous ego function
función del ego ejecutivo executive ego function
función del ego existencial existential ego function
función del habla speech function
función discriminante discriminant function
función en U invertida inverted-U function
función fásica phasic function

función gnóstica gnostic function
función inferior inferior function
función isomérica isomeric function
función libre de conflictos conflict-free
    function
función localizada localized function
función mental mental function
función motora motor function
función psicofísica psychophysical function
función psicométrica psychometric function
función reproductiva reproductive function
función semiótica semeiotic function
función simbólica symbolic function
función sintética synthetic function
función superior superior function
función trófica trophic function
función vicaria vicarious function
funcional functional
funcionalidad affordance
funcionalismo functionalism
funcionalismo conductual behavioral
    functionalism
funcionalismo probabilístico probabilistic
    functionalism
funcionamiento functioning
funcionamiento académico academic
    functioning
funcionamiento cognitivo cognitive
    functioning
funcionamiento del ego en preescolares ego
    functioning in preschoolers
funcionamiento emocional emotional
    functioning
funcionamiento familiar family functioning
funcionamiento inmunológico immunological
    functioning
funcionamiento integrativo sensorial
    sensory-integrative functioning
funcionamiento intelectual intellectual
    functioning
funcionamiento intelectual bajo promedio
    subaverage intellectual functioning
funcionamiento intelectual fronterizo
    borderline intellectual functioning
funcionamiento óptimo optimal functioning
funcionamiento sexual sexual functioning
funcionamiento vicario vicarious functioning
funciones cerebrales brain functions
funciones comunicativas communicative
    functions
funciones de familia functions of family
funciones de mantenimiento maintenance
    functions
funciones intelectuales intellectual functions
fundamental fundamental
funicular funicular
funiculitis funiculitis
furor furor
furor epiléptico epileptic furor
furor epilepticus furor epilepticus
fusión fusion
fusión binaural binaural fusion
fusión binocular binocular fusion
fusión cromática chromatic fusion
fusión de colores color fusion

fusión espinal spinal fusion
fusión instintiva instinctual fusion
fusión retinal retinal fusion
fusión tonal tonal fusion
fusión vertebral vertebral fusion
fútil futile
futurística futuristics

G

galactorrea galactorrhea
galactosemia galactosemia
galea galea
galeantropía galeanthropy
galeatomía galeatomy
galeofobia galeophobia
galimatías gibberish
galvánico galvanic
galvanómetro galvanometer
galvanotropismo galvanotropism
gama gamma
gamacismo gammacism
gameto gamete
gamofobia gamophobia
gamonomanía gamonomania
ganancia gain
ganancia epinósica epinosic gain
ganancia narcisista narcissistic gain
ganancia paranósica paranosic gain
ganancia por enfermedad gain by illness
ganancia primaria primary gain
ganancia secundaria secondary gain
ganancia terciaria tertiary gain
gancho calvárico calvarial hook
gangliectomía gangliectomy
ganglio ganglion
ganglio aberrante aberrant ganglion
ganglio cerebral cerebral ganglion
ganglio de Gasser Gasserian ganglion
ganglio de Scarpa Scarpa's ganglion
ganglio espinal spinal ganglion
ganglio espiral spiral ganglion
ganglio trigeminal ganglion trigeminale
ganglio simpático sympathetic ganglion
gangliocitoma gangliocytoma
ganglioglioma ganglioglioma
gangliólisis gangliolysis
gangliólisis por radiofrecuencia percutánea
  percutaneous radiofrequency gangliolysis
ganglioma ganglioma
ganglión habenular habenular ganglion
ganglionar ganglionic
ganglionectomía ganglionectomy
ganglioneuroma ganglioneuroma
ganglioneuroma central central
  ganglioneuroma
ganglioneuromatosis ganglioneuromatosis
ganglionitis ganglionitis
ganglionostomía ganglionostomy
gangliopléjico ganglioplegic
ganglios ganglia
ganglios basales basal ganglia
gangliosidosis gangliosidosis
gangliosidosis generalizada generalized

gangliosidosis
gangliosidosis GM1 GM1 gangliosidosis
gangliosidosis GM2 GM2 gangliosidosis
gangliosidosis GM3 GM3 gangliosidosis
ganglitis gangliitis
gangrena gangrene
gangrena presenil presenile gangrene
gangrena trófica trophic gangrene
Ganzfeld Ganzfeld
gargalanestesia gargalanesthesia
gargalestesia gargalesthesia
gargolismo gargoylism
gástrico gastric
gastrina gastrin
gastroenteritis gastroenteritis
gastrointestinal gastrointestinal
gastroparálisis gastroparalysis
gastroparesia gastroparesis
gastrulación gastrulation
gateamiento crawling
gatofobia gatophobia
gauseano gaussian
gay gay
gazmoñería prudery
gefirofobia gephyrophobia
Gegenhalten Gegenhalten
gelasmo gelasmus
gelotripsia gelotripsy
gemelo twin
gemelología gemellology
gemelos biovulares biovular twins
gemelos dicigóticos dizygotic twins
gemelos encigóticos enzygotic twins
gemelos fraternos fraternal twins
gemelos idénticos identical twins
gemelos monocigóticos monozygotic twins
gemelos monocoriónicos monochorionic twins
gemelos monoovulares monovular twins
gemelos siameses Siamese twins
gemelos uniovulares uniovular twins
gemistocítico gemistocytic
gemistocito gemistocyte
gemistocitoma gemistocytoma
gen gene
gen dominante dominant gene
gen egoísta selfish gene
gen influenciado por sexo sex-influenced
  gene
gen intermedio intermediate gene
gen ligado al sexo sex-linked gene
gen recesivo recessive gene
genealogía genealogy
generación generation
generación de hipótesis hypothesis generation
generación filial filial generation
generalidad generality
generalización generalization
generalización acústica acoustic
  generalization
generalización de estímulo stimulus
  generalization
generalización de respuestas response
  generalization
generalización en aprendizaje generalization
  in learning

generalización semántica semantic
  generalization
generalización verbal verbal generalization
generalizado generalized
generatividad generativity
generatividad contra absorción propia
  generativity versus self-absorption
generatividad contra estancación
  generativity versus stagnation
generativo generative
genérico generic
género gender
género hormonal hormonal gender
genes de enzimas enzyme genes
genética genetics
genética conductual behavioral genetics
genética cuantitativa quantitative genetics
genética de conducta behavior genetics
genética poblacional population genetics
genética política political genetics
geneticismo geneticism
genético genetic
genetista geneticist
genetofobia genetophobia
genetotrófico genetotrophic
genial genial
génico genic
geniculado geniculate
genidéntico genidentic
genio genius, temper
genital genital
genitales genitalia
genitales ambiguos ambiguous genitalia
genitales externos external genitalia
genitales femeninos female genitalia
genitales masculinos male genitalia
genitalidad genitality
genitalizar genitalize
genitourinario genitourinary
genocopia genocopy
genofobia genophobia
genograma genogram
genoma genome
genotípico genotypical
genotipo genotype
genotipo dominante dominant genotype
gens gens
genu genu
geofagia geophagy
geofagismo geophagism
geografía psicológica psychological
  geography
geotaxis geotaxis
geotropismo geotropism
geriatría geriatrics
geriátrico geriatric
geriopsicosis geriopsychosis
germinativo germinal
germinoma germinoma
gerocomía gerocomy
gerofilia gerophilia
gerofobia gerophobia
geromorfismo geromorphism
gerontofilia gerontophilia
gerontofobia gerontophobia

gerontología gerontology
gerontología social social gerontology
gerontológico gerontological
geropsicología geropsychology
geropsiquiatría geropsychiatry
gestación gestation
gestágeno gestagen
gestalt gestalt
gestalt autóctono autochthonous gestalt
gestalt bueno good gestalt
gestaltismo gestaltism
gesticulación gesticulation
gesto gesture
gesto de suicidio suicide gesture
gestual gestural
geumafobia geumaphobia
geusia geusis
gigantismo gigantism
gigantismo cerebral cerebral gigantism
gimnofobia gymnophobia
ginandria gynandry
ginandro gynander
ginandromorfo gynandromorph
ginecología gynecology
ginecomanía gynecomania
ginecomastia gynecomastia
ginefobia gynephobia
ginofobia gynophobia
ginomonoecismo gynomonoecism
girectomía gyrectomy
girectomía frontal frontal gyrectomy
giroespasmo gyrospasm
gitagismo githagism
glabro glabrous
glande glans
glande del clítoris glans clitoris
glande del pene glans penis
glándula gland
glándula adrenal adrenal gland
glándula de secreción interna internal
  secretion gland
glándula endocrina endocrine gland
glándula exocrina exocrine gland
glándula lagrimal lacrimal gland
glándula parótida parotid gland
glándula pineal pineal gland
glándula pituitaria pituitary gland
glándula prostática prostate gland
glándula suprarrenal suprarenal gland
glándula tiroides thyroid gland
glándulas bulbouretrales bulbourethral
  glands
glándulas de Bartholin Bartholin's glands
glándulas de Littre Littre's glands
glándulas de Skene Skene's glands
glándulas de Tyson Tyson's glands
glándulas mamarias mammary glands
glándulas paratiroides parathyroid glands
glándulas salivales salivary glands
glándulas sudoríferas sudoriferous glands
glaucoma glaucoma
glaucoma de baja tensión low tension
  glaucoma
glia glia
glicina glycine

glicinato glycinate
glioblastoma glioblastoma
glioblastosis cerebral glioblastosis cerebri
glioma glioma
glioma de la médula espinal glioma of the
spinal cord
glioma de quiasma óptico glioma of optic
chiasm
glioma gigantocelular gigantocellular glioma
glioma mixto mixed glioma
glioma nasal nasal glioma
glioma telangiectásico telangiectatic glioma
glioma telangiectodes glioma telangiectodes
gliomatosis gliomatosis
gliomatoso gliomatous
gliomixoma gliomyxoma
glioneuroma glioneuroma
gliosarcoma gliosarcoma
gliosis gliosis
gliosis de Chaslin Chaslin's gliosis
gliosis isomorfa isomorphous gliosis
gliosis piloide piloid gliosis
glisando glissando
global global
globo globus
globo histérico globus hystericus
globo pálido globus pallidus
glomectomía glomectomy
glosal glossal
glosocinestésico glossokinesthetic
glosodinia glossodynia
glosodiniotropismo glossodyniotropism
glosodontotropismo glossodontotropism
glosoespasmo glossospasm
glosofaríngeo glossopharyngeal
glosofobia glossophobia
glosolabiofaríngeo glossolabiopharyngeal
glosolabiolaríngeo glossolabiolaryngeal
glosolalia glossolalia
glosólisis glossolysis
glosoplejía glossoplegia
glososíntesis glossosynthesis
glotal glottal
glotidoespasmo glottidospasm
glotis glottis
glucagón glucagon
glucocorticoide glucocorticoid
glucógeno glycogen
glucogenólisis glycogenolysis
glucogenosis glycogenosis
glucogeusia glycogeusia
glucorraquia glycorrhachia
glucosa glucose
glutamato glutamate
glutamato monosódico monosodium
glutamate
glutamilo glutamyl
glutetimida glutethimide
gnosia gnosia
gnóstico gnostic
gobierno de pacientes patient government
golpe de calor heat stroke
golpeado battered
golpeamiento de cabeza head-banging
golpecito tap

golpecito de talón heel tap
golpeo de esposa wife battering
golpeteo de cabeza head-knocking
goma intracraneal intracranial gumma
gónada gonad
gonadal gonadal
gonadocéntrico gonadocentric
gonadotrófico gonadotrophic
gonadotropina gonadotropin
gonadotropina coriónica humana human
chorionic gonadotropin
gonadotropina menopáusica humana human
menopausal gonadotropin
gonadotropina pituitaria anterior anterior
pituitary gonadotropin
gonococo gonococcus
gonorrea gonorrhea
gradiente gradient
gradiente axial axial gradient
gradiente de acercamiento approach gradient
gradiente de consolidación consolidation
gradient
gradiente de demora de recompensa delay of
reward gradient
gradiente de efecto effect gradient
gradiente de evitación avoidance gradient
gradiente de excitación excitation gradient
gradiente de fin goal gradient
gradiente de generalización generalization
gradient
gradiente de generalización de estímulo
gradient of stimulus generalization
gradiente de generalización de respuestas
gradient of response generalization
gradiente de presión pressure gradient
gradiente de refuerzo reinforcement gradient
gradiente de textura texture gradient
gradiente del desarrollo anterior-posterior
anterior-posterior development gradient
grado degree
grado de libertad degree of freedom
grafanestesia graphanesthesia
grafema grapheme
grafestesia graphesthesia
gráfica graph
gráfica de barras bar graph
gráfica de expectación expectancy chart
gráfico graphic
gráficos de computadora computer graphics
grafodina graphodyne
grafoespasmo graphospasm
grafofobia graphophobia
grafología graphology
grafomanía graphomania
grafometría graphometry
grafomotor graphomotor
grafopatología graphopathology
graforrea graphorrhea
gramática grammar
gramática de estructura de frases
phrase-structure grammar
gramática generativa generative grammar
gramática transformacional transformational
grammar
gramática universal universal grammar

gran crisis grand crisis
gran mal grand mal
grandiosidad grandiosity
grandioso grandiose
granulaciones aracnoideas arachnoid granulations
gránulo granule
granuloma granuloma
granuloma inguinal granuloma inguinale
granulomatoso granulomatous
gránulos de Crooke Crooke's granules
gratificación gratification
gratificación de instintos gratification of instincts
gratificación de necesidades need gratification
gratificación oral oral gratification
gravidez gravidity
gregario gregarious
gregarismo gregariousness
gris central central gray
gris neutral neutral gray
grises de Hering Hering grays
grito cry, scream
grito de nacimiento birth cry
grito epiléptico epileptic cry
grito para socorro cry for help
grito primal primal scream
grupo group
grupo abierto open group
grupo aleatorio random group
grupo apareado matched group
grupo aspiracional aspirational group
grupo carboxilo carboxyl group
grupo cerrado closed group
grupo clínico clinical group
grupo coactuante coacting group
grupo continuo continuous group
grupo control control group
grupo de acción action group
grupo de acción comunitario community-action group
grupo de actitudes attitude cluster
grupo de apoyo support group
grupo de apoyo adolescente adolescent support group
grupo de apoyo familiar family support group
grupo de asistencia posterior aftercare group
grupo de asunciones básicas basic assumptions group
grupo de autoayuda self-help group
grupo de ayuda mutua mutual aid group
grupo de cara a cara face-to-face group
grupo de conciencia sensorial sensory-awareness group
grupo de contacto directo direct-contact group
grupo de correlaciones correlation cluster
grupo de crecimiento personal personal-growth group
grupo de crisis crisis group
grupo de criterio criterion group
grupo de discusión discussion group
grupo de encuentro encounter group

grupo de entrenamiento training group
grupo de entrenamiento de sensibilidad sensitivity training group
grupo de estado status group
grupo de estandarización standardization group
grupo de inducción de cambio change induction group
grupo de integridad integrity group
grupo de intervención de crisis crisis intervention group
grupo de juego play group
grupo de maratón marathon group
grupo de miembros membership group
grupo de norma norm group
grupo de orientación de admisión intake-orientation group
grupo de referencia reference group
grupo de relaciones humanas human-relations group
grupo de síntomas symptom group
grupo de terapia no estructurada unstructured therapy group
grupo disociativo dissociative group
grupo estructurado structured group
grupo étnico ethnic group
grupo excluído out-group
grupo exclusivo in-group
grupo experiencial experiential group
grupo experimental experimental group
grupo familiar family group
grupo general blanket group
grupo horizontal horizontal group
grupo laissez-faire laissez-faire group
grupo marginal marginal group
grupo medio median group
grupo minoritario minority group
grupo natural natural group
grupo ocupacional occupational group
grupo orientado hacia tarea task-oriented group
grupo paritario peer group
grupo paritario homosocial homosocial peer group
grupo pequeño small group
grupo primario primary group
grupo sanguíneo Rh Rh blood group
grupo secundario secondary group
grupo seleccionado selected group
grupo sin líder leaderless group
grupo social social group
grupo T T group
grupo terapéutico therapeutic group
grupo transitorio transient group
grupo vertical vertical group
grupos comparables comparable groups
grupos equivalentes equivalent groups
grupos solapantes overlapping groups
guanina guanine
guerra psicológica psychological warfare
gustación gustation
gustatismo gustatism
gustatorio gustatory
gusto taste
gusto de color color taste

gutural guttural
guturotetania gutturotetany

hábeas corpus habeas corpus
habilidad ability
habilidad abstracta abstract ability
habilidad de aprendizaje learning ability
habilidad de procesamiento de información
  information-processing ability
habilidad espacial spatial ability
habilidad específica specific ability
habilidad general general ability
habilidad mecánica mechanical ability
habilidad mental mental ability
habilidad numérica numerical ability
habilidad ocupacional occupational ability
habilidad para bregar coping ability
habilidad perceptiva de infantes infant
  perceptual ability
habilidad verbal verbal ability
habilidad visual-espacial visual-spatial ability
habilidad volitiva volitional ability
habilidades cognitivas cognitive abilities
habilidades cristalizadas crystallized abilities
habilidades fluidas fluid abilities
habilidades intramodales intramodal abilities
habilidades mentales primarias primary
  mental abilities
habilidades primarias primary abilities
habilidades psicolingüísticas psycholinguistic
  abilities
habilidades transmodales cross-modal
  abilities
habilitación habilitation
hábitat habitat
hábito habit
hábito apopléctico habitus apoplecticus
hábito de accidentes accident habit
hábito de posición position habit
hábito de quejas complaint habit
hábito motor motor habit
hábito nervioso nervous habit
hábito sensorial sensory habit
hábito social social habit
hábito tísico habitus phthisicus
hábitos de alimentación feeding habits
hábitos del comer eating habits
habituación habituation
habituación de cocaína cocaine habituation
habituación eléctrica electrical habituation
habituación en aprendizaje habituation in
  learning
habituación en aprendizaje animal
  habituation in animal learning
habituación y categorización habituation and
  categorization
habituado habituated

habla speech
habla alta loud speech
habla apresurada pressured speech
habla asinérgica asynergic speech
habla atáxica ataxic speech
habla automática automatic speech
habla bilateral bilateral speech
habla bucal buccal speech
habla cerebelosa cerebellar speech
habla clara articulate speech
habla de eco echo speech
habla de meseta plateau speech
habla de paladar hendido cleft-palate speech
habla de sentimientos feeling-talk
habla del cuidante caregiver speech
habla delusoria delusional speech
habla demorada delayed speech
habla distraíble distractible speech
habla dramática dramatic speech
habla egocéntrica egocentric speech
habla emocional emotional speech
habla en autismo speech in autism
habla en staccato staccato speech
habla encubierta covert speech
habla espástica spastic speech
habla excesivamente alta excessively loud
   speech
habla excesivamente suave excessively soft
   speech
habla explosiva explosive speech
habla facial facial talk
habla hesitante hesitant speech
habla imitativa imitative speech
habla implícita implicit speech
habla indirecta indirect speech
habla indistinta slurred speech
habla infantil infantile speech
habla interna inner speech
habla internalizada internalized speech
habla lacónica laconic speech
habla lenta slow speech
habla monótona monotonous speech
habla orgánica organ speech
habla parasocial parasocial speech
habla parental parental speech
habla perseverante perseverative speech
habla rápida rapid speech
habla silábica syllabic speech
habla silenciosa silent speech
habla sintética synthetic speech
habla socializada socialized speech
habla subvocal subvocal speech
habla susurrada whispered speech
habla tangencial tangential speech
habla telegráfica telegraphic speech
habla tiesa stilted speech
habla visible visible speech
habromanía habromania
hachís hashish
hadefobia hadephobia
hafalgesia haphalgesia
hafefobia haphephobia
hagioterapia hagiotherapy
halazepam halazepam
haloperidol haloperidol

haloperidol en autismo haloperidol in autism
haloperidol en síndrome de Tourette
   haloperidol in Tourette's syndrome
haloxazolam haloxazolam
hamartofobia hamartophobia
hamaxofobia hamaxophobia
hambre hunger
hambre de afecto affect hunger
hambre de aire air hunger
hambre de estímulo stimulus hunger
hambre específica specific hunger
hambre infantil baby hunger
hambre narcótica narcotic hunger
hambre nerviosa nervous hunger
hambre social social hunger
hambre y anorexia nerviosa hunger and
   anorexia nervosa
haploide haploid
haploidia haploidy
haplología haplology
haptefobia haptephobia
háptica haptics
háptico haptic
haptodisforia haptodysphoria
haptofonía haptophonia
haptómetro haptometer
harmina harmine
harmonía de grupo group harmony
harpaxofobia harpaxophobia
harria harria
hartazgo binge
hartazgo del beber binge drinking
hartazgo del comer binge eating
hartazgo del comprar binge buying
hartazgo del gastar binge spending
hebefilia hebephilia
hebefrenia hebephrenia
hebefrenia depresiva depressive hebephrenia
hebefrenia maníaca manic hebephrenia
hebefrénico hebephrenic
hebético hebetic
hebetud hebetude
heces feces
hechizo charm
hechos de la vida facts of life
hedónico hedonic
hedonismo hedonism
hedonístico hedonistic
hedonofobia hedonophobia
helenologofobia hellenologophobia
helenologomanía hellenologomania
helenomanía hellenomania
helicopodia helicopodia
helicotrema helicotrema
heliencefalitis heliencephalitis
heliofobia heliophobia
heliotropismo heliotropism
helmintofobia helminthophobia
hemangioblastoma hemangioblastoma
hematencéfalo hematencephalon
hematidrosis hematidrosis
hematocefalia hematocephaly
hematocito hematocyte
hematócrito hematocrit
hematoencefálico hematoencephalic

hematofobia hematophobia
hematoma hematoma
hematoma epidural epidural hematoma
hematoma intracraneal intracranial hematoma
hematoma subdural subdural hematoma
hematorraquis hematorrhachis
hematorraquis extradural extradural hematorrhachis
hematorraquis subdural subdural hematorrhachis
hematuria hematuria
hemerafonía hemeraphonia
hemeralopía hemeralopia
hemiacinesia hemiakinesia
hemiacrosomía hemiacrosomia
hemialgia hemialgia
hemiamiostenia hemiamyosthenia
hemianalgesia hemianalgesia
hemianestesia hemianesthesia
hemianestesia alternada alternate hemianesthesia
hemianestesia cruzada crossed hemianesthesia
hemianopía hemianopia
hemianopía heterónima heteronymous hemianopia
hemianopia homónima homonymous hemianopia
hemianópico hemianopic
hemianopsia hemianopsia
hemianopsia bilateral bilateral hemianopsia
hemianopsia binasal binasal hemianopsia
hemianopsia bitemporal bitemporal hemianopsia
hemianopsia cuadrántica quadrantic hemianopsia
hemiapraxia hemiapraxia
hemiasinergia hemiasynergia
hemiasomatagnosia hemiasomatagnosia
hemiasomatognosia hemiasomatognosia
hemiataxia hemiataxia
hemiatetosis hemiathetosis
hemiatrofia hemiatrophy
hemiatrofia facial facial hemiatrophy
hemiatrofia lingual progresiva progressive lingual hemiatrophy
hemibalismo hemiballism
hemicefalalgia hemicephalalgia
hemicigótico hemizygous
hemicigoto hemizygote
hemicorea hemichorea
hemicrania hemicrania
hemicraniectomía hemicraniectomy
hemicraniosis hemicraniosis
hemicraniotomía hemicraniotomy
hemidescorticación hemidecortication
hemidespersonalización hemidepersonalization
hemidisestesia hemidysesthesia
hemiepilepsia hemiepilepsy
hemiespacial hemispatial
hemiespasmo hemispasm
hemifacial hemifacial
hemihidranencefalia hemihydranencephaly

hemihipalgesia hemihypalgesia
hemihiperestesia hemihyperesthesia
hemihipertonía hemihypertonia
hemihipertrofia hemihypertrophy
hemihipestesia hemihypesthesia
hemihipoestesia hemihypoesthesia
hemihipotonía hemihypotonia
hemilaminectomía hemilaminectomy
hemilateral hemilateral
hemiopalgia hemiopalgia
hemiopía hemiopia
hemiparanestesia hemiparanesthesia
hemiparaplejía hemiparaplegia
hemiparesia hemiparesis
hemiparesia espástica spastic hemiparesis
hemiplejía hemiplegia
hemiplejía alternante alternating hemiplegia
hemiplejía ascendente ascending hemiplegia
hemiplejía contralateral contralateral hemiplegia
hemiplejía cruzada hemiplegia cruciata
hemiplejía de Gubler Gubler's hemiplegia
hemiplejía de Wernicke-Mann Wernicke-Mann hemiplegia
hemiplejía doble double hemiplegia
hemiplejía espástica spastic hemiplegia
hemiplejía facial facial hemiplegia
hemiplejía infantil infantile hemiplegia
hemiplejía nocturna nocturnal hemiplegia
hemipléjico hemiplegic
hemisensorial hemisensory
hemisferectomía hemispherectomy
hemisférico hemispheric
hemisferio hemisphere
hemisferio cerebral cerebral hemisphere
hemisferio dominante dominant hemisphere
hemisferio izquierdo left hemisphere
hemisferio menor minor hemisphere
hemisomatognosis hemisomatognosis
hemitemblor hemitremor
hemitermoanestesia hemithermoanesthesia
hemitonía hemitonia
hemocito hemocyte
hemofilia hemophilia
hemofobia hemophobia
hemoglobina hemoglobin
hemorragia hemorrhage
hemorragia cerebral cerebral hemorrhage
hemorragia del tallo cerebral brainstem hemorrhage
hemorragia intracerebral intracerebral hemorrhage
hemorragia intracraneal intracranial hemorrhage
hemorragia intraventricular intraventricular hemorrhage
hemorragia pontina pontine hemorrhage
hemorragia retinal retinal hemorrhage
hemorragia siringomiélica syringomyelic hemorrhage
hemorragia subaracnoidea subarachnoid hemorrhage
hemorragia subdural subdural hemorrhage
hemorragia subgaleal subgaleal hemorrhage
hemorragia traumática traumatic

hemorrhage
hemorragia vítrea vitreous hemorrhage
hemorragia extradural extradural
  hemorrhage
hemorragias petequiales petechial
  hemorrhages
hemorrágico hemorrhagic
hemorraquis hemorrhachis
hemosiderosis hemosiderosis
hemotimia hemothymia
heparitinuria heparitinuria
hepático hepatic
hepatitis hepatitis
hepatitis infecciosa infectious hepatitis
hepatitis viral aguda acute viral hepatitis
hepatolenticular hepatolenticular
herbartianismo Herbartianism
herbívoro herbivorous
herbolario herbalist
heredabilidad heritability
heredabilidad de personalidad heritability of
  personality
heredabilidad y ambiente heritability and
  environment
heredable inheritable
heredado inherited
heredar inherit
hereditario hereditary
hereditarismo hereditarianism
heredoataxia heredoataxia
heredofamiliar heredofamilial
heredopatía heredopathia
heredopatía atáxica polineuritiforme
  heredopathia atactica polyneuritiformis
herencia inheritance, heredity, heritage
herencia arcaica archaic inheritance
herencia de factores múltiples multiple-factor
  inheritance
herencia dominante dominant inheritance
herencia e inteligencia heredity and
  intelligence
herencia multifactorial multifactorial
  inheritance
herencia recesiva recessive inheritance
herencia social social heritage
herida wound
herida narcisista narcissistic wound
hermafrodismo hermaphrodism
hermafrodita hermaphrodite
hermafroditismo hermaphroditism
hermanastra stepsister
hermanastro stepbrother
hermenéutica hermeneutics
hermético hermetic
hernia hernia
hernia cerebral cerebral hernia
hernia meníngea meningeal hernia
herniación herniation
herniación cingulada cingulate herniation
herniación esfenoidal sphenoidal herniation
herniación foraminal foraminal herniation
herniación subfalcial subfalcial herniation
herniación tonsilar tonsillar herniation
herniación transtentorial transtentorial
  herniation

herniación transtentorial caudal caudal
  transtentorial herniation
herniación transtentorial rostral rostral
  transtentorial herniation
herniación uncal uncal herniation
heroína heroin
heroinomanía heroinomania
herpes herpes
herpes genital genital herpes
herpes simple tipo 1 herpes simplex type 1
herpes simple tipo 2 herpes simplex type 2
herpético herpetic
hersaje hersage
hertz hertz
heterarquía heterarchy
heterestesia heteresthesia
heterocéntrico heterocentric
heterocigosidad heterozygosity
heterocigosis heterozygosis
heterocigótico heterozygous
heterocigoto heterozygote
heterocinesia heterokinesia
heterocinesis heterokinesis
heteroclito heteroclite
heterocronía heterochrony
heteroerótico heteroerotic
heteroerotismo heteroerotism
heterofasia heterophasia
heterofemia heterophemy
heterofonía heterophonia
heteroforia heterophoria
heterógamo heterogamous
heterogeneidad heterogeneity
heterogéneo heterogeneous
heterohipnosis heterohypnosis
heterolalia heterolalia
heteroliteral heteroliteral
heterólogo heterologous
heteromorfo heteromorphous
heterónimo heteronymous
heteronomía heteronomy
heterónomo heteronomous
heteropatía heteropathy
heteropsicológico heteropsychologic
heterorexia heterorexia
heterosedasticidad heteroscedasticity
heterosexual heterosexual
heterosexualidad heterosexuality
heterosis heterosis
heterosociabilidad heterosociality
heterosoma heterosome
heterosugestibilidad heterosuggestibility
heterosugestión heterosuggestion
heterotopia heterotopia
heterotópico heterotopic
heterotropía heterotropia
heurística heuristic
hexametonio hexamethonium
hexobarbital hexobarbital
hexosaminidasa A hexosaminidase A
hialofagia hyalophagy
hialofobia hyalophobia
hibernación hibernation
hibridación hybridization
híbrido hybrid

hidantoína hydantoin
hidración hydration
hidralazina hydralazine
hidranencefalia hydranencephaly
hidrato de cloral chloral hydrate
hidrencéfalo hydrencephalus
hidrencefalocele hydrencephalocele
hidrencefalomeningocele
  hydrencephalomeningocele
hidrocefalia hydrocephalus
hidrocefalia comunicante communicating
  hydrocephalus
hidrocefalia comunicante postraumática
  posttraumatic communicating
  hydrocephalus
hidrocefalia congénita congenital
  hydrocephalus
hidrocefalia de compartimiento doble double
  compartment hydrocephalus
hidrocefalia de presión baja low-pressure
  hydrocephalus
hidrocefalia de presión normal normal
  pressure hydrocephalus
hidrocefalia ex vacuo hydrocephalus ex vacuo
hidrocefalia externa external hydrocephalus
hidrocefalia incomunicante
  noncommunicating hydrocephalus
hidrocefalia interna internal hydrocephalus
hidrocefalia obstructiva obstructive
  hydrocephalus
hidrocefalia oculta occult hydrocephalus
hidrocefalia otítica otitic hydrocephalus
hidrocefalia posmeningítica postmeningitic
  hydrocephalus
hidrocefalia postraumática posttraumatic
  hydrocephalus
hidrocefalia primaria primary hydrocephalus
hidrocefalia secundaria secondary
  hydrocephalus
hidrocefalia tóxica toxic hydrocephalus
hidrocefalia trombótica thrombotic
  hydrocephalus
hidrocefálico hydrocephalic
hidrocefalocele hydrocephalocele
hidrocefaloide hydrocephaloid
hidrocele hydrocele
hidrocele espinal hydrocele spinalis
hidrocodona hydrocodone
hidrocortisona hydrocortisone
hidrodipsomanía hydrodipsomania
hidroencefalocele hydroencephalocele
hidrofobia hydrophobia
hidrofóbico hydrophobic
hidrofobofobia hydrophobophobia
hidroforógrafo hydrophorograph
hidromeningocele hydromeningocele
hidromicrocefalia hydromicrocephaly
hidromielia hydromyelia
hidromielocele hydromyelocele
hidrosiringomielia hydrosyringomyelia
hidrosis hidrosis
hidroterapia hydrotherapy
hidroxicina hydroxyzine
hidróxido hydroxide
hidroxitriptamina hydroxytryptamine

hidroxitriptófano hydroxytryptophan
hielofobia hyelophobia
hierofobia hierophobia
hieromanía hieromania
hieroterapia hierotherapy
hierro sérico serum iron
hifedonia hyphedonia
higieiolatría hygieiolatry
higiene hygiene
higiene criminal criminal hygiene
higiene mental mental hygiene
higiene sexual sexual hygiene
higrofobia hygrophobia
higroma hygroma
higroma subdural subdural hygroma
hijos adultos de alcohólicos adult children of
  alcoholics
hijos de alcohólicos children of alcoholics
hilefobia hylephobia
hilera string
hilofobia hylophobia
himen hymen
hinchazón abdominal abdominal bloating
hiosciamina hyoscyamine
hioscina hyoscine
hipacusia hypacusia
hipalgesia hypalgesia
hipalgésico hypalgesic
hipalgia hypalgia
hipalgia histérica hysterical hypalgia
hipantropía hippanthropy
hipengiofobia hypengyophobia
hiperactividad hyperactivity
hiperactividad autónoma autonomic
  hyperactivity
hiperactividad del desarrollo developmental
  hyperactivity
hiperactividad e historial familiar
  hyperactivity and family history
hiperactividad sin propósito purposeless
  hyperactivity
hiperactivo hyperactive
hiperacusia hyperacusia
hiperadrenocorticismo hyperadrenocorticism
hiperafia hyperaphia
hiperáfico hyperaphic
hiperageusia hyperageusia
hiperagresividad hyperaggressivity
hiperaldosternismo hyperaldosternism
hiperalerto hyperalert
hiperalgesia hyperalgesia
hiperalgesia auditiva auditory hyperalgesia
hiperalgésico hyperalgesic
hiperalgia hyperalgia
hiperamonemia hyperammonemia
hiperamonemia cerebroatrófica
  cerebroatrophic hyperammonemia
hiperamoniemia hyperammoniemia
hiperbólico hyperbolic
hiperbulimia hyperbulimia
hipercalcemia hypercalcemia
hipercapnia hypercapnia
hipercarbia hypercarbia
hipercatexis hypercathexis
hipercenestesia hypercenesthesia

hipercinesia hyperkinesia
hipercinesia axial axial hyperkinesia
hipercinesis hyperkinesis
hipercinesis con demora del desarrollo
hyperkinesis with developmental delay
hipercinestesia hyperkinesthesia
hipercinético hyperkinetic
hipercognización hypercognization
hipercompensatorio hypercompensatory
hipercrialgesia hypercryalgesia
hipercriestesia hypercryesthesia
hiperdinamia hyperdynamia
hiperdinámico hyperdynamic
hiperefidrosis hyperephidrosis
hiperemia hyperemia
hiperepitimia hyperepithymia
hiperequema hyperechema
hiperergasia hyperergasia
hipererídico hypereridic
hiperestesia hyperesthesia
hiperestesia auditiva auditory hyperesthesia
hiperestesia cerebral cerebral hyperesthesia
hiperestesia gustatoria gustatory
hyperesthesia
hiperestesia muscular muscular hyperesthesia
hiperestesia olfatoria olfactory hyperesthesia
hiperestesia óptica hyperesthesia optica
hiperestesia táctil tactile hyperesthesia
hiperestético hyperesthetic
hiperexcitabilidad hyperexcitability
hiperfagia hyperphagia
hiperfasia hyperphasia
hiperfeminidad hyperfemininity
hiperforia hyperphoria
hiperfrasia hyperphrasia
hiperfrenia hyperphrenia
hiperfunción hyperfunction
hipergargalestesia hypergargalesthesia
hipergasia hypergasia
hipergenital hypergenital
hipergenitalismo hypergenitalism
hipergeusia hypergeusia
hiperglucemia hyperglycemia
hiperglucemia no cetónica nonketonic
hyperglycemia
hiperglucémico hyperglycemic
hiperglucorraquia hyperglycorrhachia
hipergnosis hypergnosis
hiperhedonia hyperhedonia
hiperhedonismo hyperhedonism
hiperhidrosis hyperhidrosis
hipericalemia hyperkalemia
hiperindependencia hyperindependence
hiperingestión hyperingestion
hiperinsulinismo hyperinsulinism
hiperinsulinismo funcional functional
hyperinsulinism
hiperlexia hyperlexia
hiperlipidemia hyperlipidemia
hiperlipoproteinemia hyperlipoproteinemia
hiperlisinemia hyperlysinemia
hiperlogia hyperlogia
hiperlordosis hyperlordosis
hipermanía hypermania
hipermaníaco hypermanic

hipermasculinidad hypermasculinity
hipermenorrea hypermenorrhea
hipermensia hypermnesia
hipermetamorfosis hypermetamorphosis
hipermetría hypermetria
hipermetropía hypermetropia
hipermiestesia hypermyesthesia
hipermimia hypermimia
hipermiotonía hypermyotonia
hipermovilidad hypermotility
hipernoia hypernoia
hipernómico hypernomic
hiperobesidad hyperobesity
hiperontomorfo hyperontomorph
hiperopía hyperopia
hiperoralidad hyperorality
hiperorexia hyperorexia
hiperosfresia hyperosphresia
hiperosmia hyperosmia
hiperparatiroidismo hyperparathyroidism
hiperparestesia hyperparesthesia
hiperpatía hyperpathia
hiperpipecolatemia hyperpipecolatemia
hiperpirexia por calor heat hyperpyrexia
hiperpituitario hyperpituitary
hiperplasia hyperplasia
hiperplasia adrenal congénita congenital
adrenal hyperplasia
hiperplasia cerebral cerebral hyperplasia
hiperpnea hyperpnea
hiperpolarización hyperpolarization
hiperponesis hyperponesis
hiperpragia hyperpragia
hiperprágico hyperpragic
hiperpraxia hyperpraxia
hiperprosesis hyperprosessis
hiperprosexia hyperprosexia
hiperpsicosis hyperpsychosis
hiperreflexia hyperreflexia
hipersecreción andrógena androgen
hypersecretion
hipersensibilidad hypersensitivity
hipersensibilidad de desnervación
denervation hypersensitivity
hipersexualidad hypersexuality
hipersomnia hypersomnia
hipersomnia primaria primary hypersomnia
hipersomnia psicogénica psychogenic
hypersomnia
hipersomnolencia hypersomnolence
hipersténico hypersthenic
hipertaraquia hypertarachia
hipertelorismo hypertelorism
hipertelorismo ocular ocular hypertelorism
hipertensión hypertension
hipertensión esencial essential hypertension
hipertensión ortostática orthostatic
hypertension
hipertensión y estrés hypertension and stress
hipertensivo hypertensive
hipertermalgesia hyperthermalgesia
hipertermia hyperthermia
hipertermoestesia hyperthermoesthesia
hipertimia hyperthymia
hipertímico hyperthymic

hipertiquia hypertychia
hipertiroide hyperthyroid
hipertiroidismo hyperthyroidism
hipertiroidismo apático apathetic
   hyperthyroidism
hipertonía hypertonia
hipertonía simpática sympathetic hypertonia
hipertonicidad hypertonicity
hipertónico hypertonic
hipertricofobia hypertrichophobia
hipertrofia hypertrophy
hipertrofia seudomuscular pseudomuscular
   hypertrophy
hipertrófico hypertrophic
hipertropía hypertropia
hiperuricemia hyperuricemia
hiperuricosuria hyperuricosuria
hiperventilación hyperventilation
hipervigilancia hypervigilance
hipervigilante hypervigilant
hipervitaminosis hypervitaminosis
hipervolemia hypervolemia
hipestesia hypesthesia
hipestesia olfatoria olfactory hypesthesia
hipnagógico hypnagogic
hipnagogo hypnagogue
hipnalgia hypnalgia
hipnapagógico hypnapagogic
hipnestesia hypnesthesia
hípnico hypnic
hipnoanálisis hypnoanalysis
hipnóbata hypnobat
hipnocatarsis hypnocatharsis
hipnocinematógrafo hypnocinematograph
hipnodóntica hypnodontics
hipnodrama hypnodrama
hipnofobia hypnophobia
hipnofrenosis hypnophrenosis
hipnogénesis hypnogenesis
hipnogénico hypnogenic
hipnogógico hypnogogic
hipnógrafo hypnograph
hipnoideo hypnoid
hipnoidización hypnoidization
hipnolepsia hypnolepsy
hipnología hypnology
hipnólogo hypnologist
hipnonarcosis hypnonarcosis
hipnopatía hypnopathy
hipnopedia hypnopaedia
hipnoplastia hypnoplasty
hipnopómpico hypnopompic
hipnosedante hypnosedative
hipnosigénesis hypnosigenesis
hipnosis hypnosis
hipnosis animal animal hypnosis
hipnosis como tratamiento para dolor
   crónico hypnosis as treatment for chronic
   pain
hipnosis de carretera highway hypnosis
hipnosis despierta waking hypnosis
hipnosis en investigación hypnosis in research
hipnosis en realzado de memoria hypnosis in
   memory enhancement
hipnosis espontanea spontaneous hypnosis

hipnosis letárgica lethargic hypnosis
hipnosis materna mother hypnosis
hipnosis mayor major hypnosis
hipnosis menor minor hypnosis
hipnosis paterna father hypnosis
hipnosis por temor fear hypnosis
hipnosugestión hypnosuggestion
hipnoterapia hypnotherapy
hipnoterapia de distancia distance
   hypnotherapy
hipnoterapia de grupo group hypnotherapy
hipnoterapia ecléctica eclectic hypnotherapy
hipnótico hypnotic
hipnotismo hypnotism
hipnotismo clínico clinical hypnotism
hipnotismo en educación hypnotism in
   education
hipnotismo en terapia hypnotism in therapy
hipnotismo no tradicional nontraditional
   hypnotism
hipnotista hypnotist
hipnotizabilidad hypnotizability
hipnotización hypnotization
hipnotizar hypnotize
hipnotoide hypnotoid
hipo histérico hysterical hiccough
hipoactividad hypoactivity
hipoactivo hypoactive
hipoacusia hypoacusia
hipoafectivo hypoaffective
hipoageusia hypoageusia
hipoalgesia hypoalgesia
hipobaropatía hypobaropathy
hipobulia hypobulia
hipocalcemia hypocalcemia
hipocampo hippocampus
hipocatexis hypocathexis
hipocinesia hypokinesia
hipocinesis hypokinesis
hipocinestesia hypokinesthesia
hipocinético hypokinetic
hipocognización hypocognization
hipocondria hypochondria
hipocondríaco hypochondriac
hipocondrial hypochondrial
hipocondriasis hypochondriasis
hipocondriasis monosintomática
   monosymptomatic hypochondriasis
hipocoresis hypochoresis
hipocresía hypocrisy
hipodepresión hypodepression
hipodérmico hypodermic
hipodoncia hypodontia
hipoemocionalidad hypoemotionality
hipoendocrinismo hypoendocrinism
hipoergasia hypoergasia
hipoergastia hypoergastia
hipoergia hypoergy
hipoestesia hypoesthesia
hipoestesia vaginal vaginal hypoesthesia
hipoevolutismo hypoevolutism
hipofagia hypophagia
hipofisario hypophysial
hipofisectomía hypophysectomy
hipofisectomizar hypophysectomize

hipófisis hypophysis
hipofisitis linfoide lymphoid hypophysitis
hipofobia hippophobia
hipoforia hypophoria
hipofosfatasia hypophosphatasia
hipofrasia hypophrasia
hipofrenia hypophrenia
hipofrenosis hypophrenosis
hipofunción hypofunction
hipoganglionosis hypoganglionosis
hipogástrico hypogastric
hipogenital hypogenital
hipogenitalismo hypogenitalism
hipogeusia hypogeusia
hipoglucemia hypoglycemia
hipoglucémico hypoglycemic
hipoglucorraquia hypoglycorrhachia
hipogonadismo hypogonadism
hipogonadismo con anosmia hypogonadism
  with anosmia
hipohipnótico hypohypnotic
hipolepsiomanía hypolepsiomania
hipolexia hypolexia
hipolipemia hypolipemia
hipologia hypologia
hipomanía hypomania
hipomaníaco hypomanic
hipomelancolía hypomelancholia
hipomenorrea hypomenorrhea
hipometamorfosis hypometamorphosis
hipometría hypometria
hipometropía hypometropia
hipomielinación hypomyelination
hipomielinogénesis hypomyelinogenesis
hipomnesia hypomnesia
hipomovilidad hypomotility
hiponoia hyponoia
hiponoico hyponoic
hipoparatiroidismo hypoparathyroidism
hipopituitario hypopituitary
hipopituitarismo hypopituitarism
hipoplasia hypoplasia
hipoplasia cerebral cerebral hypoplasia
hipoplasia dermal focal focal dermal
  hypoplasia
hipoplástico hypoplastic
hipopraxia hypopraxia
hipoprosesis hypoprosessis
hipoprosexia hypoprosexia
hipopsicosis hypopsychosis
hiporreflexia hyporeflexia
hiposensibilidad hyposensitivity
hiposexualidad hyposexuality
hiposfresia hyposphresia
hiposmia hyposmia
hiposofobia hyposophobia
hiposomnia hyposomnia
hiposomníaco hyposomniac
hipospadias hypospadias
hipostasis hypostasis
hipostenia hyposthenia
hiposteniante hypostheniant
hiposténico hyposthenic
hipotalámico hypothalamic
hipotálamo hypothalamus

hipotálamo lateral lateral hypothalamus
hipotálamo ventromedial ventromedial
  hypothalamus
hipotalamotomía hypothalamotomy
hipotaxia hypotaxia
hipotaxis hypotaxis
hipotémico hypothemic
hipotensión hypotension
hipotensión intracraneal intracranial
  hypotension
hipotensión ortostática orthostatic
  hypotension
hipotensivo hypotensive
hipotermestesia hypothermesthesia
hipotermia hypothermia
hipotermia accidental accidental hypothermia
hipotermia inducida induced hypothermia
hipotermia regional regional hypothermia
hipótesis hypothesis
hipótesis abertural apertural hypothesis
hipótesis adaptiva adaptive hypothesis
hipótesis alfa alpha hypothesis
hipótesis alternativa alternative hypothesis
hipótesis beta beta hypothesis
hipótesis como sí as if hypothesis
hipótesis cuantal quantal hypothesis
hipótesis de afinidad affinity hypothesis
hipótesis de aminas biógenas biogenic amine
  hypothesis
hipótesis de amortiguamiento buffering
  hypothesis
hipótesis de aniversario anniversary
  hypothesis
hipótesis de carga aditiva additive burden
  hypothesis
hipótesis de código doble dual-code
  hypothesis
hipótesis de consolidación consolidation
  hypothesis
hipótesis de constancia constancy hypothesis
hipótesis de contacto contact hypothesis
hipótesis de contacto de intergrupo
  intergroup-contact hypothesis
hipótesis de continuidad continuity
  hypothesis
hipótesis de continuidad de sueños continuity
  hypothesis of dreams
hipótesis de control de puerta gate-control
  hypothesis
hipótesis de criadero breeder hypothesis
hipótesis de descarga de impulso
  drive-discharge hypothesis
hipótesis de distracción distraction hypothesis
hipótesis de dopamina dopamine hypothesis
hipótesis de dopamina de esquizofrenia
  dopamine hypothesis of schizophrenia
hipótesis de empatía-altruismo
  empathy-altruism hypothesis
hipótesis de endorfinas endorphin hypothesis
hipótesis de Feingold Feingold hypothesis
hipótesis de Fiamberti Fiamberti hypothesis
hipótesis de frustración-agresión
  frustration-aggression hypothesis
hipótesis de frustración-regresión
  frustration-regression hypothesis

hipótesis de hipofrontalidad hypofrontality hypothesis

hipótesis de inoculación inoculation hypothesis

hipótesis de la discontinuidad discontinuity hypothesis

hipótesis de las catecolaminas catecholamine hypothesis

hipótesis de maduración maturation hypothesis

hipótesis de maduración-degeneración maturation-degeneration hypothesis

hipótesis de pareo matching hypothesis

hipótesis de prerreconocimiento prerecognition hypothesis

hipótesis de reducción de impulso drive-reduction hypothesis

hipótesis de regresión teleológica progresiva progressive teleological-regression hypothesis

hipótesis de riesgo risk hypothesis

hipótesis de riesgo ético ethical risk hypothesis

hipótesis de Sapir-Whorf Sapir-Whorf hypothesis

hipótesis de síntoma-símbolo symptom-symbol hypothesis

hipótesis de Skaggs-Robinson Skaggs-Robinson hypothesis

hipótesis de sustitución substitution hypothesis

hipótesis de sustitución de síntoma symptom substitution hypothesis

hipótesis de trauma temprano de trastorno autista early trauma hypothesis of autistic disorder

hipótesis de Whorf Whorf's hypothesis

hipótesis del antagonismo antagonism hypothesis

hipótesis del desuso de olvidar disuse hypothesis of forgetting

hipótesis del montón bundle hypothesis

hipótesis diátesis-estrés diathesis-stress hypothesis

hipótesis estructural structural hypothesis

hipótesis experimental experimental hypothesis

hipótesis falsificable falsifiable hypothesis

hipótesis gama gamma hypothesis

hipótesis inversa inverse hypothesis

hipótesis mediumística mediumistic hypothesis

hipótesis mnémica mnemic hypothesis

hipótesis monoamina monoamine hypothesis

hipótesis nula null hypothesis

hipótesis permisiva de trastornos afectivos permissive hypothesis of affective disorders

hipótesis topográfica topographical hypothesis

hipotético hypothetical

hipotimia hypothymia

hipotímico hypothymic

hipotiroideo hypothyroid

hipotiroidismo hypothyroidism

hipotiroidismo congénito congenital hypothyroidism

hipotonía hypotony

hipotonicidad hypotonicity

hipotónico hypotonic

hipotono hypotonous

hipotrofia hypotrophy

hipotropía hypotropia

hipovegetativo hypovegetative

hipovigilancia hypovigility

hipovolemia hypovolemia

hipoxemia hypoxemia

hipoxia hypoxia

hipóxico hypoxic

hipoxifilia hypoxyphilia

hippus hippus

hipsarritmia hypsarrhythmia

hipsicefalia hypsicephaly

hipsicefálico hypsicephalic

hipsocefalia hypsocephaly

hipsofobia hypsophobia

histamina histamine

histamínico histaminic

histerectomía hysterectomy

histerectomía radical radical hysterectomy

histéresis hysteresis

histeria hysteria

histeria ansiosa anxiety hysteria

histeria ártica Arctic hysteria

histeria de combate combat hysteria

histeria de conversión conversion hysteria

histeria de defensa defense hysteria

histeria de fijación fixation hysteria

histeria de grupo group hysteria

histeria de retención retention hysteria

histeria disociativa dissociative hysteria

histeria en masa mass hysteria

histeria epidémica epidemic hysteria

histeria mayor major hysteria

histeria menor minor hysteria

histérico hysterical

histericoneurálgico hystericoneuralgic

histeriforme hysteriform

histeriosis hysteriosis

histerismo hysterics

histerocatalepsia hysterocatalepsy

histeroepilepsia hysteroepilepsy

histerofilia hysterophilia

histerofrénico hysterofrenic

histerogénico hysterogenic

histerógeno hysterogenous

histeroide hysteroid

histeronarcolepsia hysteronarcolepsy

histeropía hysteropia

histerosalpingografía hysterosalpingography

histeroscopia hysteroscopy

histerosintónico hysterosyntonic

histerotrismo hysterotrismus

histiocitosis histiocytosis

histiocitosis de querasina kerasin histiocytosis

histograma histogram

histología histology

histológico histologic

histonectomía histonectomy

historial history

historial biopsicosocial biopsychosocial history

historial de caso case history
historial de la enfermedad presente history of present illness
historial de relaciones relationship history
historial de seguimiento follow-up history
historial de vida life history
historial del sueño sleep history
historial educacional educational history
historial escolar school history
historial familiar family history
historial familiar y psicosis family history and psychosis
historial marital marital history
historial médico medical history
historial ocupacional occupational history
historial perinatal perinatal history
historial personal personal history
historial prenatal prenatal history
historial previo prior history
historial psicosexual psychosexual history
historial psiquiátrico psychiatric history
historial psiquiátrico-médico psychiatric-medical history
historial sexual sexual history
histriónico histrionic
hito milestone
hito del desarrollo developmental milestone
hito motor motor milestone
hodofobia hodophobia
hogar adoptivo foster home
hogar de cuidado domiciliario domiciliary care home
hogar de cuidado personal personal care home
hogar de cuidados médicos nursing home
hogar de descanso rest home
hogar de grupo group home
hogar de huéspedes boarding home
hogar roto broken home
hoja de balance de decisiones decision balance sheet
hoja de datos personales personal data sheet
holergasia holergasia
holísitco holistic
holismo holism
holocordón holocord
holofrase holophrase
holofrástico holophrastic
holografía holography
holográfico holographic
holoprosencefalia holoprosencephaly
holorraquisquisis holorachischisis
holotelencefalia holotelencephaly
hombre afeminado effeminated man
hombre golpeado battered man
homeopatía homeopathy
homeopático homeopathic
homeostasis homeostasis
homeostasis del desarrollo developmental homeostasis
homeostático homeostatic
homeostenosis homeostenosis
homicida homicidal
homicidio homicide
homicidiomanía homicidomania

homiclofobia homichlophobia
homilofobia homilophobia
homilopatía homilopathy
homocigosidad homozygocity
homocigosis homozygosis
homocigoto homozygous
homocistinuria homocystinuria
homoclito homoclite
homoerótico homoerotic
homoerotismo homoerotism
homófilo homophile
homofobia homophobia
homófono homophone
homogamia homogamy
homogeneidad homogeneity
homogeneidad de varianza homogeneity of variance
homogéneo homogeneous
homogénico homogenic
homogenitalidad homogenitality
homógrafo homograph
homolateral homolateral
homología homology
homología conductual behavioral homology
homólogo homologous
homónimo homonym
homosedasticidad homoscedasticity
homosexual homosexual
homosexual latente latent homosexual
homosexualidad homosexuality
homosexualidad accidental accidental homosexuality
homosexualidad adolescente adolescent homosexuality
homosexualidad afeminada effeminate homosexuality
homosexualidad egodistónica ego-dystonic homosexuality
homosexualidad egosintónica ego-syntonic homosexuality
homosexualidad enmascarada masked homosexuality
homosexualidad iatrogénica iatrogenic homosexuality
homosexualidad inconsciente unconscious homosexuality
homosexualidad latente latent homosexuality
homosexualidad manifiesta overt homosexuality
homosexualidad situacional situational homosexuality
homosocial homosocial
homosocialidad homosociality
homotópico homotopic
homúnculo homunculus
homúnculo motor motor homunculus
homúnculo sensorial sensory homunculus
hongo fungus
hongo cerebral fungus cerebri
honradez honesty
horario flexible flexitime
horas de trabajo flexibles flexible work hours
horizontal horizontal
horizonte horizon
hormefobia hormephobia

hormigueo por cocaína   cocaine bug
hormismo   hormism
hormona   hormone
hormona adrenocorticotrópica
  adrenocorticotrophic hormone
hormona antidiurética   antidiuretic hormone
hormona corticotrópica   corticotrophic
  hormone
hormona del crecimiento   growth hormone
hormona estimulante de células intersticiales
  interstitial cell stimulating hormone
hormona estimulante de folículos
  follicle-stimulating hormone
hormona estimulante del tiroides
  thyroid-stimulating hormone
hormona gonadal   gonadal hormone
hormona gonadotrófica   gonadotrophic
  hormone
hormona hipotalámica   hypothalamic
  hormone
hormona lactogénica   lactogenic hormone
hormona liberadora de corticotropina
  corticotropine-releasing hormone
hormona liberadora de gonadotropinas
  gonadotropin-releasing hormone
hormona liberadora de tirotropina
  thyrotropin-releasing hormone
hormona luteinizante   luteinizing hormone
hormona mamotrópica   mammotropic
  hormone
hormona melanocitoestimulante
  melanocyte-stimulating hormone
hormona paratiroidea   parathyroid hormone
hormona placentaria   placental hormone
hormona sexual   sex hormone
hormona somatotrófica   somatotrophic
  hormone
hormona tiroide   thyroid hormone
hormona tirotrópica   thyrotropic hormone
hormona trófica   trophic hormone
hormonal   hormonal
hormonas andrógenas   androgen hormones
horóptero   horopter
hospicio   hospice
hospital   hospital
hospital abierto   open hospital
hospital con fines de lucro   for-profit hospital
hospital de alto volumen   high-volume
  hospital
hospital de bajo volumen   low-volume
  hospital
hospital de cinco días   five-day hospital
hospital de fin de semana   weekend hospital
hospital de puertas abiertas   open-door
  hospital
hospital diurno   day hospital
hospital mental   mental hospital
hospital mental privado   private mental
  hospital
hospital mental público   public mental
  hospital
hospital nocturno   night hospital
hospital psiquiátrico   psychiatric hospital
hospital receptor   receiving hospital
hospital sin fines de lucro   not-for-profit

  hospital
hospitalismo   hospitalism
hospitalitis   hospitalitis
hospitalización   hospitalization
hospitalización involuntaria   involuntary
  hospitalization
hospitalización para psicosis   hospitalization
  for psychosis
hospitalización parcial   partial hospitalization
hospitalización voluntaria   voluntary
  hospitalization
hostigamiento sexual   sexual harassment
hostil   hostile
hostilidad   hostility
hostilidad en juego   hostility in play
hostilidad paranoide   paranoid hostility
hotentotismo   hottentotism
huelga de hambre   hunger strike
huelga de hambre neurótica   neurotic hunger
  strike
huérfano   orphan
hueso mágico   magic bone
huesos parietales   parietal bones
humanismo   humanism
humanístico   humanistic
humillación   humiliation
humor   mood, humor
humor acuoso   aqueous humor
humor anal   anal humor
humor ansioso   anxious mood
humor caprichoso   moodiness
humor de patíbulo   gallows humor
humor delusorio   delusional mood
humor disfórico   dysphoric mood
humor elevado   elevated mood
humor eufórico   euphoric mood
humor eutímico   euthymic mood
humor expansivo   expansive mood
humor irritable   irritable mood
humor lábil   labile mood
humor maníaco   manic mood
humor melancólico   melancholic mood
humor vítreo   vitreous humor
humoral   humoral
hurto   theft
husmeo de datos   data snooping
huso   spindle
huso de color   color spindle
huso del sueño   sleep spindle
huso muscular   muscle spindle
huso neurotendinal   neurotendinal spindle

I

iátrico iatric
iatrogénesis iatrogenesis
iatrogenia iatrogeny
iatrogénico iatrogenic
iconicidad iconicity
icónico iconic
icono icon
iconofobia iconophobia
iconomanía iconomania
ictal ictal
ictericia jaundice
ictericia alérgica allergic jaundice
ictericia nuclear nuclear jaundice
icterus icterus
icterus grave neonatal icterus gravis
  neonatorum
ictiofobia ichthyophobia
ictus ictus
ictus epilepticus ictus epilepticus
ictus paralyticus ictus paralyticus
id id
id-ego id-ego
idea abstracta abstract idea
idea autóctona autochthonous idea
idea compulsiva compulsive idea
idea de influencia idea of influence
idea de irrealidad idea of unreality
idea de referencia idea of reference
idea determinativa determinative idea
idea dominante dominant idea
idea dominante permanente permanent
  dominant idea
idea fija fixed idea
idea hipercuantivalente hyperquantivalent
  idea
idea intrusa obtrusive idea
idea penetrante súbita brainstorm
idea platónica platonic idea
idea secundaria by-idea
idea sobrevalorada overvalued idea
ideación ideation
ideación inconsciente unconscious ideation
ideación paranoide paranoid ideation
ideación suicida suicidal ideation
ideacional ideational
ideal ideal
ideal corporal body ideal
ideal paterna father ideal
ideal platónico platonic ideal
idealismo idealism
idealismo subjetivo subjective idealism
idealización idealization
idealización primitiva primitive idealization
idealización y desilusión idealization and

disillusionment
idealizado idealized
idealizar idealize
ideas expansivas expansive ideas
ideas innatas innate ideas
ideatorio ideatory
idéntico identical
identidad identity
identidad contra confusión de papel identity
  versus role confusion
identidad corporal body identity
identidad cultural cultural identity
identidad de género gender identity
identidad de género núcleo core gender
  identity
identidad de sexo núcleo core sex identity
identidad del ego ego identity
identidad disociativa dissociative identity
identidad familiar family identity
identidad femenina feminine identity
identidad masculina masculine identity
identidad negativa negative identity
identidad personal personal identity
identidad sexual sexual identity
identidad social latente latent social identity
identidad vocacional vocational identity
identidades situadas situated identities
identificación identification
identificación absoluta absolute identification
identificación anaclítica anaclitic
  identification
identificación con el agresor identification
  with the aggressor
identificación cósmica cosmic identification
identificación de categoría category
  identification
identificación de concepto concept
  identification
identificación de fenómeno phenomenon
  identification
identificación de género cruzado
  cross-gender identification
identificación de grupo group identification
identificación de objeto object identification
identificación de olores odor identification
identificación de patrones espaciales
  identification of spatial patterns
identificación defensiva defensive
  identification
identificación errónea misidentification
identificación errónea amnésica amnesic
  misidentification
identificación errónea delusoria delusional
  misidentification
identificación errónea hiperbólica hyperbolic
  misidentification
identificación femenina feminine
  identification
identificación múltiple multiple identification
identificación narcisista primaria primary
  narcissistic identification
identificación parental cruzada
  cross-parental identification
identificación primaria primary identification
identificación proyectiva projective

identification
identificación saludable healthy identification
identificación secundaria secondary
   identification
identificación sexual sexual identification
identificar identify
ideocinético ideokinetic
ideodinámica ideodynamics
ideofobia ideophobia
ideofrenia ideophrenia
ideogenético ideogenetic
ideoglandular ideoglandular
ideográfico ideographic
ideograma ideogram
ideología ideology
ideológico ideological
ideomoción ideomotion
ideomotor ideomotor
ideoplastia ideoplasty
ideoplástico ideoplastic
ideosensorial ideosensory
idiodinámica idiodynamics
idiodinámico idiodynamic
idioespasmo idiospasm
idiofrenia idiophrenia
idiofrénico idiophrenic
idiogamista idiogamist
idioglosia idioglossia
idiográfico idiographic
idiograma idiogram
idiohipnotismo idiohypnotism
idiolalia idiolalia
idiomuscular idiomuscular
idioneurosis idioneurosis
idiopático idiopathic
idioplasma idioplasm
idiopsicológico idiopsychologic
idiorreflejo idioreflex
idiorretinal idioretinal
idiosincrasia idiosyncrasy
idiosincrasia olfatoria idiosyncrasia olfactoria
idiosincrásico idiosyncratic
idiosoma idiosome
idiotrópico idiotropic
idiovariación idiovariation
idoneidad de afecto appropriateness of affect
idoneidad de respuesta emocional
   appropriateness of emotional response
ignipedites ignipedites
ignorancia pluralista pluralistic ignorance
ignorar ignore
igualación equalization
igualación de excitación equalization of
   excitation
igualdad equality
igualdad social social equality
igualdad subjetiva subjective equality
ikota ikota
íleo adinámico adynamic ileus
íleo paralítico paralytic ileus
ileostomía ileostomy
ilícito illicit
ilógico illogical
iluminación illumination
iluminancia illuminance

iluminismo illuminism
iluminómtero de MacBeth MacBeth
   illuminometer
ilusión illusion
ilusión asimilativa assimilative illusion
ilusión asociativa associative illusion
ilusión audiogiral audiogyral illusion
ilusión autocinética autokinetic illusion
ilusión de Aristóteles Aristotle's illusion
ilusión de cascada waterfall illusion
ilusión de Charpentier Charpentier's illusion
ilusión de corrector proofreader's illusion
ilusión de dobles illusion of doubles
ilusión de dobles negativos illusion of
   negative doubles
ilusión de dobles positivos illusion of positive
   doubles
ilusión de escalera staircase illusion
ilusión de ferrocarril railway illusion
ilusión de Hering Hering illusion
ilusión de la luna moon illusion
ilusión de la punta de flecha arrowhead
   illusion
ilusión de lóbulo temporal temporal-lobe
   illusion
ilusión de memoria memory illusion
ilusión de moción illusion of motion
ilusión de movimiento movement illusion
ilusión de Muller-Lyer Muller-Lyer illusion
ilusión de orientación orientation illusion
ilusión de Poggendorf Poggendorf illusion
ilusión de Ponzo Ponzo illusion
ilusión de sueño dream illusion
ilusión de tamaño illusion of size
ilusión de tamaño-peso size-weight illusion
ilusión de Zollner Zollner illusion
ilusión estroboscópica stroboscopic illusion
ilusión geométrica geometric illusion
ilusión horizontal-vertical horizontal-vertical
   illusion
ilusión oculógira oculogyral illusion
ilusión óptica optical illusion
ilusión sensorial sense illusion
ilusión visual visual illusion
ilusional illusional
ilusorio illusory
ilustrador illustrator
imagen image
imagen accidental accidental image
imagen alucinatoria hallucinatory image
imagen auditiva auditory image
imagen compuesta composite image
imagen concreta concrete image
imagen corporal body image
imagen de fantasma ghost image
imagen de Hess Hess image
imagen de memoria memory image
imagen de producto product image
imagen detenida stopped image
imagen eidética eidetic image
imagen esquemática schematic image
imagen estabilizada stabilized image
imagen fija fixed image
imagen generada por computadora
   computer-generated image

imagen general general image
imagen hipnagógica hypnagogic image
imagen hipnogógica hypnogogic image
imagen hipnopómpica hypnopompic image
imagen idealizada idealized image
imagen incidental incidental image
imagen interna inward picture
imagen materna mother image
imagen mental mental image
imagen mental primaria primary mental
   image
imagen motora motor image
imagen óptica optical image
imagen perceptiva perceptual image
imagen persistente afterimage
imagen persistente de Hering Hering
   afterimage
imagen persistente de McCollough
   McCollough afterimage
imagen persistente de memoria memory
   afterimage
imagen persistente de movimiento movement
   afterimage
imagen persistente de Purkinje Purkinje
   afterimage
imagen persistente negativa negative
   afterimage
imagen persistente positiva positive
   afterimage
imagen personal personal image
imagen primordial primordial image
imagen retinal retinal image
imagen retinal estabilizada stabilized retinal
   image
imagen sensorial sensory image
imagen táctil tactile image
imagen verbal verbal image
imagen visual visual image
imágenes de Purkinje-Sanson
   Purkinje-Sanson images
imágenes de Sanson Sanson images
imágenes dobles double images
imaginación imagination
imaginación creativa creative imagination
imaginal imaginal
imaginar imagine
imaginario imaginary
imaginería imagery
imaginería eidética eidetic imagery
imaginería emotiva emotive imagery
imaginería espontanea spontaneous imagery
imaginería mental mental imagery
imaginería visual visual imagery
imaginería y emociones imagery and
   emotions
imago imago
imago paterno father imago
imidazol imidazole
imipramina imipramine
imitación imitation
imitación en infantes imitation in infants
imitación histérica hysterical imitation
imitación interiorizada interiorized imitation
imitación motora motor imitation
imitación social social imitation

imitación y aprendizaje imitation and
   learning
imitación y desarrollo social imitation and
   social development
imitador de mujeres female impersonator
imitativo imitative
impaciencia impatience
impacto impact
impacto de programa program impact
impacto social social impact
impedancia impedance
impedimento impediment
impedimento del habla speech impediment
imperativo imperative
imperativo categórico categorical imperative
imperativo ético ethical imperative
imperativo hipotético hypothetical imperative
imperativo inmoral immoral imperative
impercepción imperception
impercepción social social imperception
imperceptible imperceptible
impersistencia motora motor impersistence
impersonal impersonal
ímpetu impetus
implantación implantation
implantación de nervio nerve implantation
implante implant
implicación implication
implícito implicit
implosión implosion
implosivo implosive
impostor impostor
impostor juvenil juvenile impostor
impotencia impotence, helplessness
impotencia anal anal impotence
impotencia aprendida learned helplessness
impotencia aprendida y apatía learned
   helplessness and apathy
impotencia atónica atonic impotence
impotencia orgásmica orgasmic impotence
impotencia orgástica orgastic impotence
impotencia parética paretic impotence
impotencia primaria primary impotence
impotencia psíquica psychic helplessness
impotencia secundaria secondary impotence
impotencia sintomática symptomatic
   impotence
impotente impotent, powerless
imprecación cursing
impregnación impregnation
impregnación oral oral impregnation
impresión impression
impresión absoluta absolute impression
impresión basilar basilar impression
impresión de universalidad impression of
   universality
impresión maternal maternal impression
impresión mental mental impression
impresión sensorial sense impression
impronta imprinting
impropiedad inappropriateness
impropiedad de afecto inappropriateness of
   affect
improvisación improvisation
impuberismo impuberism

impubertad impuberty
impulsión impulsion
impulsividad impulsivity
impulsividad y conducta suicida impulsivity and suicidal behavior
impulsividad y trastornos del comer impulsivity and eating disorders
impulsividad y trastornos del lenguaje impulsivity and language disorders
impulsivo impulsive
impulso drive
impulso adquirido acquired drive
impulso afectivo affectional drive
impulso agresivo aggressive drive
impulso anormal de trabajar abnormal impulse to work
impulso aprendido learned drive
impulso biológico biological drive
impulso cinético kinetic drive
impulso de actividad activity drive
impulso de curiosidad curiosity drive
impulso de eliminación elimination drive
impulso de exploración exploration drive
impulso de hambre hunger drive
impulso de homonomía homonomy drive
impulso de logro achievement drive
impulso de sueño sleep drive
impulso de temor fear drive
impulso del ego ego drive
impulso destructivo destructive drive
impulso exploratorio exploratory drive
impulso fisiológico physiological drive
impulso hipóxico hypoxic drive
impulso inconsciente unconscious drive
impulso instintivo instinctual drive
impulso irresistible irresistible impulse
impulso manipulativo manipulatory drive
impulso maternal maternal drive
impulso mórbido morbid impulse
impulso mórbido de viajar wanderlust
impulso nervioso nerve impulse
impulso neural neural impulse
impulso neurogénico neurogenic drive
impulso obsesivo obsessive impulse
impulso oral oral drive
impulso primario primary drive
impulso primordial primordial impulse
impulso secundario secondary drive
impulso sensorial sensory drive
impulso sexual sexual drive
impulso social social drive
impulso socializado socialized drive
impulso visceral visceral drive
impulsos de pensamientos thought impulses
impulsos forzados forced impulses
impunitivo impunitive
in loco parentis in loco parentis
in utero in utero
in vitro in vitro
in vivo in vivo
inaccesibilidad inaccessibility
inaccesible inaccessible
inactividad alerta alert inactivity
inadaptación maladjustment
inadaptación social social maladjustment

inadaptación vocacional vocational maladjustment
inadaptado maladjusted
inadaptivo maladaptive
inadecuado inadequate
inanición inanition
inanimado inanimate
inapetencia inappetence
inapropiado inappropriate
inarticulado inarticulate
inasimilable inassimilable
inatención inattention
inatención selectiva selective inattention
inatención sensorial sensory inattention
inatención visual visual inattention
incapacitado disabled
incapacitado de lectura reading-disabled
incendiarismo incendiarism
incentivo incentive
incentivo negativo negative incentive
incentivo positivo positive incentive
incertidumbre uncertainty
incertidumbre de decisiones decision uncertainty
incertidumbre de eventos event uncertainty
incesto incest
incesto madre-hijo mother-son incest
incesto padre-hija father-daughter incest
incestuoso incestuous
incidencia incidence
incidencia de abuso de niños incidence of child abuse
incidental incidental
incidente incident
incipiente incipient
inclinación de cabeza head-tilt
inclusión inclusion
inclusión de clase class inclusion
inclusivo inclusive
incoercible incoercible
incoherencia incoherence
incoherente incoherent
incomodidad discomfort
incompatibilidad incompatibility
incompatibilidad de grupo sanguíneo Rh Rh blood group incompatibility
incompatible incompatible
incompetencia incompetence
incompetencia eyaculatoria ejaculatory incompetence
incompetente incompetent
incompleto incomplete
incondicionado unconditioned
incondicional unconditional
inconexo disjoint
inconformismo nonconformity
inconformismo de género gender nonconformity
incongruencia incongruity
inconmensurable incommensurable
inconsciencia unconsciousness
inconsciente unconscious
inconsciente colectivo collective unconscious
inconsciente descriptivo descriptive unconscious

inconsciente dinámico dynamic unconscious
inconsciente familiar familial unconscious
inconsciente personal personal unconscious
inconstancia inconstancy
incontinencia incontinence
incontinencia de urgencia urgency
  incontinence
incontinencia paradójica paradoxical
  incontinence
incontinencia pasiva passive incontinence
incontinencia por rebosamiento overflow
  incontinence
incontinencia refleja reflex incontinence
incontinente incontinent
incontrolado uncontrolled
incoordinación incoordination
incorporación incorporation
incrédulo doubting
incremental incremental
incremento increment
incremento de sensación sensation increment
incremento social social increment
incubación incubation
incubación de evitación incubation of
  avoidance
íncubo incubus
íncubo familiar family incubus
incumplimiento noncompliance
incumplimiento con tratamiento
  noncompliance with treatment
incumplimiento con tratamiento médico
  noncompliance with medical treatment
incumplimiento con tratamiento para
  trastorno mental noncompliance with
  treatment for mental disorder
incus incus
indagación inquiry
indecencia indecency
indeloxazina indeloxazine
independencia independence
independencia de campo field independence
independencia-dependencia de campo field
  independence-dependence
independencia moral moral independence
independiente independent
independiente del contexto
  context-independent
indeterminado indeterminate
indeterminismo indeterminism
indicador indicator
indicador de características feature indicator
indicador de complejos complex indicator
indicador emocional emotional indicator
indicador social social indicator
indicante indicant
índice index
índice alfa alpha index
índice cefálico cephalic index
índice cefalorraquídeo cephalorrhachidian
  index
índice cerebroespinal cerebrospinal index
índice craneal cranial index
índice de articulación articulation index
índice de confiabilidad index of reliability
índice de deterioración deterioration index

índice de deterioro impairment index
índice de dificultad index of difficulty
índice de discriminación index of
  discrimination
índice de eficiencia de pronóstico index of
  forecasting efficiency
índice de Flesch Flesch index
índice de metabolismo basal basal
  metabolism rate
índice de presión-volumen pressure-volume
  index
índice de privación deprivation index
índice de refracción refraction index
índice de selección selection index
índice de sexualidad sexuality index
índice de sociabilidad sociability index
índice de suficiencia social social-adequacy
  index
índice de tipo corporal index of body build
índice de variabilidad index of variability
índice empático empathic index
índice hiperglucémico hyperglycemic index
índice morfológico morphological index
índice predictivo predictive index
indicio clue
indicios del contexto context clues
indiferencia indifference
indiferenciado undifferentiated
indiferente indifferent
indígena indigenous
indigestión indigestion
indigestión nerviosa nervous indigestion
indirecto indirect
indisociación indissociation
individuación individuation
individual individual
individualidad individuality
individualidad gráfica graphic individuality
individualismo individualism
individualizado individualized
individuo marginal marginal individual
individuo normotenso normotensive
  individual
indol indole
indolamina indolamine
inducción induction
inducción cortical cortical induction
inducción cromática chromatic induction
inducción de concepto concept induction
inducción de enzimas enzyme induction
inducción de luz light induction
inducción de sueño dream induction
inducción de temor fear induction
inducción del humor mood induction
inducción hipnótica hypnotic induction
inducción negativa negative induction
inducción neural neural induction
inducción perceptiva perceptual induction
inducción positiva positive induction
inducción simpática sympathetic induction
inducción sucesiva successive induction
inducción visual visual induction
inducido induced
inducido por drogas drug-induced
inducido por temor fear-induced

inductivo inductive
indulgencia indulgence
indusium griseum indusium griseum
industria industry
industria contra inferioridad industry versus
    inferiority
industrial industrial
inebriación inebriation
inebriedad inebriety
inefabilidad ineffability
inefable ineffable
ineficaz ineffective
inercia inertia
inercia afectiva affective slumber
inercia psíquica psychic inertia
inervación innervation
inervación recíproca reciprocal innervation
inestabilidad instability
inestabilidad ambiental environmental
    instability
inestabilidad cervical vertebral vertebral
    cervical instability
inestabilidad emocional emotional instability
inestabilidad familiar family instability
inestabilidad familiar y conducta suicida
    family instability and suicidal behavior
inestabilidad vasomotora vasomotor
    instability
inestable unstable
inestable emocionalmente emotionally
    unstable
inexistencia non-existence
infancia infancy
infante infant
infante a riesgo infant at risk
infante de alto riesgo high-risk infant
infante prematuro premature infant
infantes prematuros y desarrollo afectivo
    premature infants and affective
    development
infanticidio infanticide
infantil infantile
infantilismo infantilism
infantilismo de Brissaud Brissaud's
    infantilism
infantilismo estático static infantilism
infantilismo sexual sexual infantilism
infantilístico infantilistic
infantilización infantilization
infarto infarct
infarto cerebral cerebral infarct
infección infection
infección bacterial bacterial infection
infección cerebral cerebral infection
infección cerebral bacterial bacterial cerebral
    infection
infección cerebral viral viral cerebral
    infection
infección con citomegalovirus congénita
    congenital cytomegalovirus infection
infección congénita congenital infection
infección del cuero cabelludo scalp infection
infección del tracto urinario urinary tract
    infection
infección fetal fetal infection

infección perinatal perinatal infection
infección placentario placental infection
infección por herpes herpes infection
infección por virus de herpes perinatal
    perinatal herpes virus infection
infección por virus entérico enteric virus
    infection
infección viral virus infection
infeccioso infectious
infecundidad infecundity
inferencia inference
inferencia causal causal inference
inferencia estadística statistical inference
inferencia inconsciente unconscious inference
inferencia lógica logical inference
inferencial inferential
inferior inferior
inferioridad inferiority
inferioridad funcional functional inferiority
inferioridad orgánica organ inferiority
inferotemporal inferotemporal
infertilidad infertility
infertilidad relativa relative infertility
infestación infestation
infibulación infibulation
infidelidad infidelity
infidelidad marital marital infidelity
infiltración infiltration
infiltración paraneural paraneural infiltration
infiltración perineural perineural infiltration
inflamación inflammation
inflamatorio inflammatory
inflexión inflection
influencia influence
influencia de grupo group influence
influencia de grupo en agresión group
    influence on aggression
influencia de grupo en conducta agresiva
    group influence on aggressive behavior
influencia genética genetic influence
influencia genética en autismo genetic
    influence in autism
influencia genética en conducta genetic
    influence in behavior
influencia genética en depresión genetic
    influence in depression
influencia genética en el desarrollo genetic
    influence in development
influencia genética en trastornos mentales
    genetic influence in mental disorders
influencia parental parental influence
influencia paritaria peer influence
influencias prenatales prenatal influences
influenza influenza
influencia social social influence
influyente influencing
información information
información binocular binocular information
información cinética kinetic information
información contextual contextual
    information
información de tasa base base rate
    information
información de trabajo job information
información del fondo hacia arriba

bottom-up information
informado informed
informal informal
informe report
informe fenomenal phenomenal report
informe retrospectivo retrospective report
informes del sueño sleep reports
infradiano infradian
infrahumano infrahuman
infrapsíquico infrapsychic
infrarrojo infrared
infrecuencia infrequency
infundibuloma infundibuloma
infundibulum infundibulum
infusión infusion
ingeniería biogenética biogenetic engineering
ingeniería biomédica biomedical engineering
ingeniería de comunicación communication
  engineering
ingeniería genética genetic engineering
ingeniería humana human engineering
ingeniería microsocial microsocial
  engineering
ingeniero social social engineer
ingénito inborn
ingenuo naive
ingestivo ingestive
ingravescente ingravescent
inguinal inguinal
inhabilidad inability
inhalación inhalation
inhalación de dióxido de carbono carbon
  dioxide inhalation
inhalación de drogas inhalation of drugs
inhalación de pega glue-sniffing
inhalación de solventes solvent inhalation
inhalación de sustancia química volátil
  volatile chemical inhalation
inhalante inhalant
inherente inherent
inhibición inhibition
inhibición académica academic inhibition
inhibición asociativa associative inhibition
inhibición central central inhibition
inhibición colateral recurrente recurrent
  collateral inhibition
inhibición competitiva competitive inhibition
inhibición con refuerzo inhibition with
  reinforcement
inhibición condicionada conditioned
  inhibition
inhibición conductual behavioral inhibition
inhibición cortical cortical inhibition
inhibición de demora inhibition of delay
inhibición de extinción extinction inhibition
inhibición de inhibición inhibition of
  inhibition
inhibición de refuerzo inhibition of
  reinforcement
inhibición de trabajo work inhibition
inhibición del fin aim inhibition
inhibición diferencial differential inhibition
inhibición específica specific inhibition
inhibición externa external inhibition
inhibición interna internal inhibition

inhibición latente latent inhibition
inhibición lateral lateral inhibition
inhibición motora motor inhibition
inhibición ocupacional occupational inhibition
inhibición presináptica presynaptic inhibition
inhibición proactiva proactive inhibition
inhibición reactiva reactive inhibition
inhibición recíproca reciprocal inhibition
inhibición recíproca y desensibilización
  reciprocal inhibition and desensitization
inhibición recurrente recurrent inhibition
inhibición refleja reflex inhibition
inhibición retroactiva retroactive inhibition
inhibición sexual sexual inhibition
inhibición social social inhibition
inhibido inhibited
inhibido del fin aim-inhibited
inhibidor inhibitor
inhibidor de liberación release inhibitor
inhibidor de monoamina oxidasa monoamine
  oxidase inhibitor
inhibidor de serotonina serotonin inhibitor
inhibidores de anhidrasa carbónica carbonic
  anhydrase inhibitors
inhibidores de síntesis de proteína
  protein-synthesis inhibitors
inhibir inhibit
inhibitorio inhibitory
iniciación initiation
iniciador initiator
inicial initial
iniciativa initiative
iniciativa contra culpabilidad initiative
  versus guilt
iniencefalia iniencephaly
injerto graft
injerto en cable cable graft
injerto en manga sleeve graft
injerto fascicular fascicular graft
injerto funicular funicular graft
injerto nervioso nerve graft
inmadurez immaturity
inmadurez del desarrollo developmental
  immaturity
inmadurez emocional emotional immaturity
inmaduro immature
inmanente immanent
inmediación immediacy
inmediato immediate
inminente looming
inmoral immoral
inmoralidad immorality
inmovilidad immobility
inmovilidad social social immobility
inmovilidad tónica tonic immobility
inmovilización immobilization
inmovilizante immobilizing
inmunidad immunity
inmunidad activa active immunity
inmunidad de estrés stress immunity
inmunidad pasiva passive immunity
inmunidad placentaria placental immunity
inmunización immunization
inmunógeno immunogen
inmunógeno conductual behavioral

immunogen
inmunoglobulina immunoglobulin
inmunología immunology
inmunología conductual behavioral
   immunology
inmunológico immunological
inmunosupresión immunosuppression
inmunosupresivo immunosuppresive
innato innate
innato contra aprendido innate versus
   learned
innovación innovation
innovador innovative
inocente innocent
inoculación inoculation
inoculación emocional emotional inoculation
inoculación para estrés stress inoculation
inocular inoculate
inquietarse fidget
inquieto restless
inquietud restlessness
insania insanity
insania cíclica cyclic insanity
insania circular circular insanity
insania constitucional constitutional insanity
insania criminal criminal insanity
insania de Basedow Basedowian insanity
insania de negación negation insanity
insania doble double insanity
insania parcial partial insanity
insano insane
insano criminalmente criminally insane
insecticidas como teratógenos conductuales
   insecticides as behavioral teratogens
insecto social social insect
inseguridad insecurity
inseguro insecure
inseminación insemination
inseminación artificial artificial insemination
inseminación artificial heteróloga
   heterologous artificial insemination
inseminación artificial homóloga homologous
   artificial insemination
insensibilidad insensitivity
insensible insensible
inserción insertion
inserción de pensamientos thought insertion
insesgado unbiased
insociable unsociable
insocializado unsocialized
insolación insolation
insomne insomniac
insomnio insomnia
insomnio de ancianos elderly insomnia
insomnio de comienzo de sueño demorado
   delayed sleep-onset insomnia
insomnio de rebote rebound insomnia
insomnio inducido por hospital
   hospital-induced insomnia
insomnio inicial initial insomnia
insomnio intermitente intermittent insomnia
insomnio mediano middle insomnia
insomnio primario primary insomnia
insomnio terminal terminal insomnia
insomnio y ansiedad insomnia and anxiety

inspección inspection
inspeccionalismo inspectionalism
inspeccionismo inspectionism
inspiración inspiration
inspiración-expiración inspiration-expiration
instalación de cuidado intermedio
   intermediate-care facility
instalación de cuidado y comida board and
   care facility
instalación de tratamiento de residentes
   resident treatment facility
instalación de tratamiento residencial
   residential treatment facility
instalación para el cuidado de niños
   child-care facility
instante instant
instigación instigation
instigador instigator
instigador de sueño dream instigator
instintivo instinctual
instinto instinct
instinto abierto open instinct
instinto agresivo aggressive instinct
instinto cerrado closed instinct
instinto componente component instinct
instinto de autopreservación
   self-preservation instinct
instinto de curiosidad curiosity instinct
instinto de dominio mastery instinct
instinto de manada herd instinct
instinto de muerte death instinct
instinto de vida life instinct
instinto del ego ego instinct
instinto demorado delayed instinct
instinto destructivo destructive instinct
instinto erótico erotic instinct
instinto parcial partial instinct
instinto posesivo possessive instinct
instinto reproductivo reproductive instinct
instinto sexual sexual instinct
instinto social social instinct
instintos complementarios complementary
   instincts
instintualización instinctualization
instintualización del olfato instinctualization
   of smell
institución institution
institución correccional correctional
   institution
institución mental mental institution
institución social social institution
institucional institutional
institucionalismo institutionalism
institucionalización institutionalization
institucionalización y derechos legales
   institutionalization and legal rights
institucionalización y familias
   institutionalization and families
institucionalizar institutionalize
instrucción instruction
instrucción administrada por computadora
   computer-managed instruction
instrucción asistida por computadora
   computer-assisted instruction
instrucción basada en la competencia

competency-based instruction
instrucción directa direct instruction
instrucción en el hogar home instruction
instrucción individualizada individualized instruction
instrucción personalizada personalized instruction
instrucción programada programmed instruction
instruccional instructional
instrumental instrumental
instrumentalismo instrumentalism
instrumento instrument
instrumento de evaluación assessment instrument
instrumento estereotáctico stereotactic instrument
instrumento estereotáxico stereotaxic instrument
insuficiencia insufficiency
insuficiencia adrenocortical adrenocortical insufficiency
insuficiencia cerebrovascular cerebrovascular insufficiency
insuficiencia de párpados insufficiency of eyelids
insuficiencia intelectual intellectual inadequacy
insuficiencia glial glial insufficiency
insuficiencia muscular muscular insufficiency
insuficiencia parental parental inadequacy
insuficiencia uteroplacentaria uteroplacental insufficiency
insuficiencia vascular vascular insufficiency
ínsula insula
insular insular
insularidad insularity
insulina insulin
insulto insult
integración integration
integración cerebral cerebral integration
integración conductual behavioral integration
integración cultural cultural integration
integración de características feature integration
integración de grupo group integration
integración de identidad identity integration
integración de personalidad personality integration
integración del ego ego integration
integración estructural structural integration
integración funcional functional integration
integración intermodal intermodal integration
integración intersensorial intersensory integration
integración primaria primary integration
integración secundaria secondary integration
integración social social integration
integrado integrated
integrante integrative
integrar integrate
integridad integrity
integridad contra desesperación integrity versus despair
integridad del ego ego integrity

integridad del ego contra desesperación ego integrity versus despair
intelecto intellect
intelectual intellectual
intelectualismo intellectualism
intelectualización intellectualization
inteligencia intelligence
inteligencia abstracta abstract intelligence
inteligencia adaptiva adaptive intelligence
inteligencia adulta adult intelligence
inteligencia animal animal intelligence
inteligencia artificial artificial intelligence
inteligencia biológica biological intelligence
inteligencia concreta concrete intelligence
inteligencia cristalizada crystallized intelligence
inteligencia de máquina machine intelligence
inteligencia fluida fluid intelligence
inteligencia fronteriza borderline intelligence
inteligencia humana human intelligence
inteligencia marginal marginal intelligence
inteligencia mecánica mechanical intelligence
inteligencia medida measured intelligence
inteligencia no verbal nonverbal intelligence
inteligencia psicoquímica psychochemistry intelligence
inteligencia representativa representative intelligence
inteligencia sensorimotora sensorimotor intelligence
inteligencia social social intelligence
inteligencia superior superior intelligence
inteligencia verbal verbal intelligence
inteligencia y ambiente intelligence and environment
inteligencia y herencia intelligence and heredity
inteligencia y traslación a la corriente principal intelligence and mainstreaming
intemperancia intemperance
intención intention
intención criminal criminal intent
intención paradójica paradoxical intention
intencionado purposive
intencional intentional
intencionalidad intentionality
intensidad intensity
intensidad de afecto intensity of affect
intensidad de ejercicio exercise intensity
intensidad de fondo background intensity
intensidad de reacción intensity of reaction
intensidad de respuestas response intensity
intensidad de sonido sound intensity
intensidad del humor intensity of mood
intensidad luminosa luminous intensity
intensivo intensive
intento de suicidio suicide attempt
intento provisional provisional try
interacción interaction
interacción acelerada accelerated interaction
interacción afectiva affective interaction
interacción alcohol-metadona alcohol-methadone interaction
interacción de drogas drug interaction
interacción de orden superior higher-order

interaction
interacción de padre-infante father-infant
   interaction
interacción didáctica didactic interaction
interacción estadística statistical interaction
interacción marital marital interaction
interacción paritaria peer interaction
interacción sensorial sensory interaction
interacción social social interaction
interacción tonal tonal interaction
interacciones intersensoriales intersensory
   interactions
interacciones madre-infante mother-infant
   interactions
interacciones y hábitos interactions and habits
interaccionismo interactionism
interactivo interactive
interaural interaural
intercalación intercalation
intercalado intercalated
intercambio de parejas partner-swapping
intercambio fetal-maternal fetal-maternal
   exchange
intercerebral intercerebral
interconductual interbehavioral
intercorrelación intercorrelation
intercortical intercortical
intercuerpo interbody
interdisciplinario interdisciplinary
interego interego
interés interest
interés extrínseco extrinsic interest
interés intrínseco intrinsic interest
interés sexual sexual interest
interés social social interest
interesado interested
intereses ocupacionales occupational interests
interestimulación interstimulation
interestímulo interstimulus
interfase interface
interferencia interference
interferencia asociativa associative
   interference
interferencia de hábito habit interference
interferencia de temas theme interference
interferencia proactiva proactive interference
interferencia reproductiva reproductive
   interference
interferencia retroactiva retroactive
   interference
intergeneracional intergenerational
intergrupo intergroup
interhemisférico interhemispheric
interictal interictal
interindividual interindividual
intermedio intermediate
intermetamorfosis intermetamorphosis
intermisión intermission
intermitencia intermittence
intermitencia tonal tonal intermittence
intermitente intermittent
intermodal intermodal
internado internship
internalización internalization
internalizado internalized

internalizante internalizing
interneurona interneuron
interneurosensorial interneurosensory
interno internal
internuncial internuncial
interobservador interobserver
interocepción interoception
interoceptivo interoceptive
interoceptor interoceptor
interocular interocular
interosistema interosystem
interpelación mand
interpenetración interpenetration
interpersonal interpersonal
interpolado interpolated
interpolar interpolate
interposición interposition
interpretación interpretation
interpretación analítica analytic interpretation
interpretación cognitiva cognitive
   interpretation
interpretación de acción action interpretation
interpretación de defensa defense
   interpretation
interpretación de impulsos impulse
   interpretation
interpretación de sueños dream interpretation
interpretación del id id interpretation
interpretación profunda deep interpretation
interpretación reductiva reductive
   interpretation
interpretación rica rich interpretation
interpretación serial serial interpretation
interpretativo interpretative
interpsicología interpsychology
interrogativo interrogative
interrumpido interrupted
interrupción interruption
intersegmentario intersegmental
intersensorial intersensory
intersexo intersex
intersexualidad intersexuality
intersticial interstitial
intersticio interstice
intersubjetivo intersubjective
intertalámico interthalamic
intervalo interval, range
intervalo acromático achromatic interval
intervalo crítico critical interval
intervalo choque-choque shock-shock interval
intervalo de audibilidad audibility range
intervalo de clase class interval
intervalo de confianza confidence interval
intervalo de demora delay interval
intervalo de discriminación discrimination
   range
intervalo de incertidumbre interval of
   uncertainty
intervalo de interestímulo interstimulus
   interval
intervalo de pasos step interval
intervalo de reacción reaction range
intervalo de respuesta-choque
   response-shock interval
intervalo discriminante discriminating range

intervalo entre ensayos intertrial interval
intervalo fijo fixed interval
intervalo fotocromático photochromatic interval
intervalo intercuartil interquartile range
intervalo lúcido lucid interval
intervalo medio median interval
intervalo metaestético metaesthetic range
intervalo preparatorio preparatory interval
intervalo tonal tonal range
intervención intervention
intervención cognitiva cognitive intervention
intervención comunitaria community intervention
intervención conductual behavioral intervention
intervención de crisis crisis intervention
intervención de emergencia emergency intervention
intervención educacional educational intervention
intervención educativa educative intervention
intervención estratégica strategic intervention
intervención familiar family intervention
intervención para delincuencia intervention for delinquency
intervención paradójica paradoxical intervention
intervención preventiva preventive intervention
intervención social social intervention
intervención temprana early intervention
interviniente intervening
intestinal intestinal
intimidación intimidation
intimidad intimacy
intimidad contra absorción propia intimacy versus self-absorption
intimidad contra aislamiento intimacy versus isolation
intimidar intimidate
íntimo intimate
intolerancia intolerance
intolerancia de ambigüedad intolerance of ambiguity
intolerancia de comida food intolerance
intoxicación intoxication
intoxicación hipnagógica hypnagogic intoxication
intoxicación idiosincrásica idiosyncratic intoxication
intoxicación idiosincrásica por alcohol alcohol idiosyncratic intoxication
intoxicación patológica pathological intoxication
intoxicación por agua water intoxication
intoxicación por alcohol alcohol intoxication
intoxicación por alucinógeno hallucinogen intoxication
intoxicación por anfetaminas amphetamine intoxication
intoxicación por ansiolítico anxiolytic intoxication
intoxicación por barbituratos barbiturate intoxication

intoxicación por bromuro bromide intoxication
intoxicación por cafeína caffeine intoxication
intoxicación por cannabis cannabis intoxication
intoxicación por cocaína cocaine intoxication
intoxicación por disulfuro de carbono carbon disulfide intoxication
intoxicación por etanol ethanol intoxication
intoxicación por fenciclidina phencyclidine intoxication
intoxicación por gasolina gasoline intoxication
intoxicación por hipnótico hypnotic intoxication
intoxicación por inhalante inhalant intoxication
intoxicación por metal metal intoxication
intoxicación por metal pesado heavy metal intoxication
intoxicación por metal pesado sérico serum heavy metal intoxication
intoxicación por opioide opioid intoxication
intoxicación por otra sustancia other substance intoxication
intoxicación por sedante sedative intoxication
intoxicación por sustancia desconocida unknown substance intoxication
intoxicación por sustancia psicoactiva psychoactive substance intoxication
intoxicación simpatomimética sympathomimetic intoxication
intracepción intraception
intraceptivo intraceptive
intracerebral intracerebral
intracisternal intracisternal
intraconsciente intraconscious
intracraneal intracranial
intrafusal intrafusal
intragrupo intragroup
intraindividual intraindividual
intramodal intramodal
intramural intramural
intramuscular intramuscular
intraneurosensorial intraneurosensory
intransitividad intransitivity
intraocular intraocular
intrapersonal intrapersonal
intrapsíquico intrapsychic
intraserial intraserial
intrasujeto intrasubject
intratable intractable
intrauterino intrauterine
intravascular intravascular
intravenoso intravenous
intraventricular intraventricular
intraverbal intraverbal
intrínseco intrinsic
introito introitus
intromisión intromission
intrón intron
intropunitivo intropunitive
introspección introspection
introspección fenomenalista phenomenalistic introspection

introspeccionismo introspectionism
introspectivo introspective
introversión introversion
introversión activa active introversion
introversión-extraversión
    introversion-extraversion
introversión-extroversión
    introversion-extroversion
introversión pasiva passive introversion
introversión social social introversion
introvertido introverted
introyección introjection
intrusión intrusion
intrusivo intrusive
intruso obtrusive
intubación intubation
intubación acueductal aqueductal intubation
intuición intuition
intuitivo intuitive
inundación flooding
inundación emocional emotional flooding
inundación imaginal imaginal flooding
invalidar invalidate
invalidismo invalidism
invalidismo psicológico psychological
    invalidism
inválido invalid
invariable invariable
invariante funcional functional invariant
invarianza invariance
invarianza factorial factorial invariance
invasión de espacio personal personal-space
    invasion
invasión de privacidad invasion of privacy
invasor invasive
invención fabrication
inventario inventory
inventario biográfico biographical inventory
inventario de actividad activity inventory
inventario de ajuste adjustment inventory
inventario de autoinforme self-report
    inventory
inventario de intereses interest inventory
inventario de intereses ocupacionales
    occupational interest inventory
inventario de personalidad personality
    inventory
inventario de tareas task inventory
inventario ecológico ecological inventory
inventario neurótico neurotic inventory
inventario personal-social personal-social
    inventory
inventario psiconeurótico psychoneurotic
    inventory
inventarios de Catell Cattell inventories
inversión inversion, investment
inversión absoluta absolute inversion
inversión anfígena amphigenous inversion
inversión auxiliar auxiliary inversion
inversión de afecto inversion of affect
inversión de conducta behavior reversal
inversión de hábito habit reversal
inversión de letras letter reversal
inversión de papeles role reversal
inversión de papeles sexuales sex-role

reversal
inversión de pronombres pronoun reversal
inversión de señal cue reversal
inversión de sexo sex reversal
inversión ocasional occasional inversion
inversión sexual sexual inversion
inverso inverse
invertido inverted
investigación research, investigation
investigación aplicada applied research
investigación básica basic research
investigación cerebral brain research
investigación conductual behavioral research
investigación cuasiexperimental
    quasi-experimental research
investigación de abuso de niños investigation
    of child abuse
investigación de acción action research
investigación de anuncios advertising
    research
investigación de aparatos de control
    control-devices research
investigación de apoyo advocacy research
investigación de archivos archival research
investigación de campo field research
investigación de evaluación evaluation
    research
investigación de infancia infancy research
investigación de intervención intervention
    research
investigación de laboratorio laboratory
    investigation
investigación de mercado market research
investigación de motivación motivation
    research
investigación de operaciones operations
    research
investigación de personalidad personality
    research
investigación de proceso process research
investigación de resultados outcome research
investigación del consumidor consumer
    research
investigación del sueño sleep research
investigación doble ciego double-blind
    research
investigación empírica empirical research
investigación ex post facto ex post facto
    research
investigación no específica nonspecific
    research
investigación operacional operational
    research
investigación poblacional population research
investigación por encuestas survey research
investigación prospectiva prospective
    research
investigación psíquica psychic research
investigación pura pure research
investigación retrospectiva retrospective
    research
investigación transversal cross-sectional
    research
investigador investigatory
inveterado inveterate

involución involution
involución senil senile involution
involución sexual sexual involution
involuntario involuntary
involutivo involutional
inyección injection
inyección cerebral cerebral injection
inyección hipodérmica hypodermic injection
inyección intramuscular intramuscular injection
inyección intravenosa intravenous injection
inyección intraventricular intraventricular injection
inyección subcutánea subcutaneous injection
iofobia iophobia
iontoforesis iontophoresis
iota iota
iproniazida iproniazid
ipsación ipsation
ipsativo ipsative
ipsilateral ipsilateral
ipsolateral ipsolateral
ira anger
iridociclitis iridocyclitis
iridoparálisis iridoparalysis
iridoplejía iridoplegia
iridoplejía completa complete iridoplegia
iridoplejía refleja reflex iridoplegia
iridoplejía simpática sympathetic iridoplegia
iris iris
irítico iritic
irracional irrational
irracionalidad irrationality
irradiación irradiation
irradiación excitatoria excitatory irradiation
irradiación ultrasónica ultrasonic irradiation
irrealidad irreality
irrelevante irrelevant
irresistible irresistible
irresponsabilidad irresponsibility
irresponsabilidad criminal criminal irresponsibility
irreversible irreversible
irritabilidad irritability
irritabilidad acústica acoustic irritability
irritabilidad de célula irritability of cell
irritabilidad neural neural irritability
irritable irritable
irritación irritation
irrumación irrumation
iscnofonía ischnophonia
iscofonía ischophonia
isla cultural culture island
isla de Reil island of Reil
isla social social island
isla tonal tonal island
islas de Langerhans islands of Langerhans
isocarboxazida isocarboxazid
isocoria isocoria
isocorteza isocortex
isocromosoma isochromosome
isocronal isochronal
isoeléctrico isoelectric
isofilia isophilia
isofílico isophilic

isofónico isophonic
isógamo isogamous
isomorfismo isomorphism
isomorfo isomorphous
isoniazida isoniazid
isopropanol isopropanol
isoproterenol isoproterenol
isosexual isosexual
isotónico isotonic
isótopo radiactivo radioactive isotope
isozima isozyme
isquemia ischemia
isquemia cerebral cerebral ischemia
isquémico ischemic
isquialgia ischialgia
isquiodinia ischiodynia
isquioneuralgia ischioneuralgia
istmoparálisis isthmoparalysis
istmoplejía isthmoplegia
iticifosis ithykyphosis
itilordosis ithylordosis
itinerante itinerant
ixomielitis ixomielitis

J

jactación jactation
jactación de cabeza nocturna jactatio capitis
　nocturna
jactitación jactitation
jamais vu jamais vu
jaula de actividad activity cage
jaula de Bogen Bogen cage
jerarquía hierarchy
jerarquía de ansiedad anxiety hierarchy
jerarquía de dominancia dominance
　hierarchy
jerarquía de familia de hábitos habit family
　hierarchy
jerarquía de hábitos habit hierarchy
jerarquía de Maslow Maslow's hierarchy
jerarquía de motivos motive hierarchy
jerarquía de necesidades need hierarchy
jerarquía de respuestas response hierarchy
jerarquía motivacional motivational
　hierarchy
jerarquía motivacional de Maslow Maslow's
　motivational hierarchy
jerarquía ocupacional occupational hierarchy
jerárquico hierarchical
jerga jargon
jerga neologística neologistic jargon
jerga semántica semantic jargon
ji cuadrada chi square
juego play, game
juego alucinatorio hallucinatory game
juego asociativo associative play
juego con muñecas doll play
juego con muñecas permisivo permissive doll
　play
juego con muñecas proyectivo projective doll
　play
juego conjunto joint play
juego cooperativo cooperative play
juego de enseñanza teaching game
juego de espectador onlooker play
juego de infantes infant play
juego de motivos mixtos mixed-motive game
juego del doctor doctor game
juego del gallina chicken game
juego dramático dramatic play
juego genital genital play
juego imaginativo imaginative play
juego independiente independent play
juego libre free play
juego lingüístico language game
juego modelo model game
juego organizado organized play
juego paralelo parallel play
juego paritario peer play

juego proyectivo projective play
juego psicológico psychological game
juego simbólico symbolic play
juego social social play
juego solitario solitary play
juego y lenguaje play and language
juegos que juega la gente games people play
jugador gambler, player
jugar gambling
jugar compulsivo compulsive gambling
jugar patológico pathological gambling
juguetón playful
juicio judgment
juicio automático automatic judgment
juicio clínico clinical judgment
juicio comparativo comparative judgment
juicio crítico critical judgment
juicio cualitativo qualitative judgment
juicio cuantitativo quantitative judgment
juicio de frecuencias frequency judgment
juicio de valores value judgment
juicio deteriorado impaired judgment
juicio egocéntrico egocentric judgment
juicio moral moral judgment
jungiano jungian
junta board
junta de revisión institucional institutional
　review board
jurisprudencia médica medical jurisprudence
justicia justice
justicia criminal criminal justice
justicia distributiva distributive justice
justicia inmanente immanent justice
justificación justification
juvenil juvenile
juvenilismo juvenilism
juventud youth

K

L

kappa kappa
kernicterus kernicterus
kilobitofobia kilobytophobia
kindling kindling
Klebedenken Klebedenken
Klebenbleiben Klebenbleiben
koro koro
kubisagari kubisagari
kubisagaru kubisagaru
kwashiorkor kwashiorkor

la belle indifference la belle indifference
laberíntico labyrinthine
laberinto maze
laberinto de Elithorn Elithorn maze
laberinto de Porteus Porteus maze
laberinto en T T-maze
laberinto locomotor locomotor maze
laberinto temporal temporal maze
labial labial
lábil labile
labilidad lability
labilidad autónoma autonomic lability
labilidad emocional emotional lability
labilidad-estabilidad lability-stability
labio hendido cleft lip
labio leporino harelip
labio mayor labium majus
labio menor labium minus
labiocorea labiochorea
labiodental labiodental
labioglosofaríngeo labioglossopharyngeal
labioglosolaríngeo labioglossolaryngeal
labiolabial labiolabial
labios mayores labia majora
labios menores labia minora
laboratorio laboratory
laboratorio de crecimiento personal
  personal-growth laboratory
laboratorio psicológico psychological
  laboratory
laceración laceration
laceración cerebral cerebral laceration
laceración del cuero cabelludo scalp
  laceration
lacónico laconic
lacrimación lacrimation
lactación lactation
lactar lactate
lactato lactate
ladrido bark
lagoftalmos lagophthalmos
lagrimal lachrymal
lágrimas tears
lágrimas de cocodrilo crocodile tears
laguna lacuna
laguna cerebral lacuna cerebri
laguna del superego superego lacuna
lagunar lacunar
laissez-faire laissez-faire
lalación lallation
laleo lalling
laliofobia laliophobia
lalofobia lalophobia
lalognosis lalognosis

laloneurosis laloneurosis
lalopatía lalopathy
laloplejía laloplegia
laloquezia lalochezia
lalorrea lalorrhea
lambda lambda
lambert lambert
lambert-pie foot-lambert
lambitus lambitus
lámina lamina
lámina de Rexed Rexed lamina
laminar laminar
laminectomía laminectomy
laminotomía laminotomy
lancinante lancinating
lanugo lanugo
laparoscopia laparoscopy
lapso lapse, span
lapso auditivo auditory span
lapso de aprehensión span of apprehension
lapso de atención attention span
lapso de concentración concentration span
lapso de conciencia span of consciousness
lapso de lectura reading span
lapso de memoria memory span
lapso de memoria auditiva auditory memory
   span
lapso de memoria visual visual memory span
lapso de ojo eye span
lapso de reconocimiento recognition span
lapso de vida life span
lapso ojo-voz eye-voice span
lapso visual visual span
lapsus lapsus
lapsus calami lapsus calami
lapsus linguae lapsus linguae
lapsus memoriae lapsus memoriae
laringe larynx
laringectomía laryngectomy
laringoespasmo laryngospasm
laringoespástico laryngospastic
laringofaringe laryngopharynx
laringoparálisis laryngoparalysis
laringoplejía laryngoplegia
lascivia lasciviousness
lascivo lascivious
lasitud lassitude
lástima pity
lata latah
latencia latency
latencia de movimientos oculares rápidos
   rapid eye movement latency
latencia de respuesta response latency
latencia del sueño sleep latency
latencia refleja reflex latency
latencia sexual sexual latency
latente latent
lateral lateral
lateralidad laterality
lateralidad cerebral cerebral laterality
lateralidad cruzada crossed laterality
lateralidad mixta mixed laterality
lateralización lateralization
lateralización cerebral cerebral lateralization
lateralización del habla speech lateralization

lateropulsión lateropulsion
latirismo lathyrism
latitud latitude
laúdano laudanum
lavado de cerebro brainwashing
laxante laxative
laxo lax
lealtad de marca brand loyalty
lecanomancia lecanomancy
lección de ensayo trial lesson
lectura reading
lectura de pensamientos mind-reading
lectura de velocidad speed reading
lectura del desarrollo developmental reading
lectura del habla speech-reading
lectura en espejo mirror-reading
lectura hacia atrás backward reading
lectura individualizada individualized reading
lectura labial lip-reading
lectura muscular muscle-reading
lectura oral oral reading
lectura remediadora remedial reading
lecheur lecheur
legado de características adquiridas
   inheritance of acquired characteristics
legal legal
legastenia legasthenia
leipolalia leipolalia
lema lemma
lemniscal lemniscal
lemnisco lemniscus
lemnisco lateral lateral lemniscus
lemnisco medial medial lemniscus
lemnisco trigeminal trigeminal lemniscus
lengua franca pidgin
lenguaje language
lenguaje analítico analytic language
lenguaje artificial artificial language
lenguaje corporal body language
lenguaje de conducta behavior language
lenguaje de segundo orden second-order
   language
lenguaje de signos sign language
lenguaje en animales language in animals
lenguaje en autismo language in autism
lenguaje en juego language in play
lenguaje extranjero foreign language
lenguaje figurativo figurative language
lenguaje fuente source language
lenguaje gestual gestural language
lenguaje gestual-postural gestural-postural
   language
lenguaje gráfico graphic language
lenguaje hipocondríaco hypochondriac
   language
lenguaje interno inner language
lenguaje irrelevante irrelevant language
lenguaje manual manual language
lenguaje metafórico metaphoric language
lenguaje natural natural language
lenguaje no verbal nonverbal language
lenguaje objetivo target language
lenguaje orgánico organ language
lenguaje receptivo receptive language
lenguaje sintético synthetic language

lenguaje y percepción language and perception
lente lens
lente del ojo lens of eye
lentes de contacto contact lenses
lenticular lenticular
lepra leprosy
lepra anestésica anesthetic leprosy
lepra articular articular leprosy
lepra mutilante mutilating leprosy
lepra seca dry leprosy
lepra trofoneurótica trophoneurotic leprosy
leprecaunismo leprechaunism
leproso leprous
leptocúrtico leptokurtic
leptocurtosis leptokurtosis
leptomeníngeo leptomeningeal
leptomeninges leptomeninges
leptomeningitis leptomeningitis
leptomeningitis basilar basilar leptomeningitis
leptomorfo leptomorph
leptoprosofia leptoprosophia
leptosoma leptosome
leptosomal leptosomal
leptosómico leptosomic
lerdo normal dull normal
lesbiana lesbian
lesbianismo lesbianism
lesión injury, lesion
lesión anular de pared ring-wall lesion
lesión bilateral bilateral lesion
lesión cerebral brain injury
lesión cerebral por contragolpe contrecoup injury of brain
lesión cortical cortical lesion
lesión de cabeza head injury
lesión de cabeza abierta open head injury
lesión de cabeza cerrada closed head injury
lesión de campo de ojo frontal frontal eye-field lesion
lesión de corteza sensorimotora unilateral unilateral sensorimotor cortex lesion
lesión de disco intervertebral injury of intervertebral disk
lesión de Duret Duret's lesion
lesión de golpe del cerebro coup injury of brain
lesión de hiperextensión-hiperflexión hyperextension-hyperflexion injury
lesión de lóbulo frontal frontal lobe injury
lesión de médula espinal spinal-cord injury
lesión de nacimiento birth injury
lesión de neurona motora superior upper motor neuron lesion
lesión de neuronas motoras motor neuron lesion
lesión del desarrollo developmental injury
lesión en látigo whiplash injury
lesión epileptogénica epileptogenic lesion
lesión personal personal injury
lesión por fórceps forceps injury
lesión sensorineural adulta adult sensorineural lesion
lesión sensorineural posnatal postnatal sensorineural lesion

lesión sensorineural prenatal prenatal sensorineural lesion
lesión supranuclear supranuclear lesion
lesión talámica thalamic lesion
lesión unilateral unilateral lesion
lesiones de quemaduras burn injuries
lesiones sensorineurales de niñez childhood sensorineural lesions
letal lethal
letalidad lethality
letargia lethargy
letárgico lethargic
leteomanía letheomania
letológica lethologica
leucemia leukemia
leucocítico leukocytic
leucocito leukocyte
leucocitosis leukocytosis
leucocitosis emocional emotional leukocytosis
leucodistrofia leukodystrophy
leucodistrofia cerebral progresiva leukodystrophia cerebri progressiva
leucodistrofia de célula globiode globoid cell leukodystrophy
leucodistrofia metacromática metachromatic leukodystrophy
leucoencefalitis leukoencephalitis
leucoencefalitis epidémica aguda acute epidemic leukoencephalitis
leucoencefalitis esclerosante subaguda subacute sclerosing leukoencephalitis
leucoencefalopatía leukoencephalopathy
leucoencefalopatía multifocal progresiva progressive multifocal leukoencephalopathy
leucomielopatía leukomyelopathy
leucotomía leukotomy
leucotomía prefrontal prefrontal leukotomy
leucotomía transorbitaria transorbital leukotomy
leucotomo leukotome
leuencefalina leuenkephalin
levantamiento de conciencia consciousness raising
levirato levirate
levitación levitation
levoanfetamina levoamphetamine
levodopa levodopa
levofobia levophobia
levomepromazina levomepromazine
levopromazina levopromazine
levorfanol levorphanol
léxico lexical
lexicoestadística lexicostatistics
lexicología lexicology
lexicón lexicon
ley law
ley autónoma-afectiva autonomic-affective law
ley biogenética biogenetic law
ley biogenética de Haeckel Haeckel's biogenetic law
ley científica scientific law
ley de Abney Abney's law
ley de acción en masa law of mass action
ley de acción mínima law of least action

ley de asimilación law of assimilation
ley de asociación law of association
ley de avalancha law of avalanche
ley de Bastian Bastian's law
ley de Bell Bell's law
ley de Bell-Magendie Bell-Magendie law
ley de Bichat law of Bichat
ley de Briggs Briggs' law
ley de Broadbent Broadbent's law
ley de Bunsen-Roscoe Bunsen-Roscoe law
ley de Charpentier Charpentier's law
ley de cohesión law of cohesion
ley de combinación law of combination
ley de conducción hacia adelante law of forward conduction
ley de constancia law of constancy
ley de contigüidad law of contiguity
ley de contraste law of contrast
ley de cosenos de Lambert Lambert cosine law
ley de Dale Dale's law
ley de desnervación law of denervation
ley de destino común law of common fate
ley de dirección idéntica law of identical direction
ley de disposición law of readiness
ley de dolor referido law of referred pain
ley de Donders Donders' law
ley de efecto law of effect
ley de efecto empírica empirical law of effect
ley de efecto fuerte strong law of effect
ley de efecto negativo negative law of effect
ley de ejercicio law of exercise
ley de Emmert Emmert's law
ley de entrada previa law of prior entry
ley de equipotencialidad law of equipotentiality
ley de Fechner Fechner's law
ley de Ferry-Porter Ferry-Porter law
ley de Fitt Fitt's law
ley de Flatau Flatau's law
ley de Fourier Fourier's law
ley de frecuencia law of frequency
ley de Fullerton-Cattell Fullerton-Cattell law
ley de Gerhardt-Semon Gerhardt-Semon law
ley de Grasset Grasset's law
ley de Hardy-Weinberg Hardy-Weinberg law
ley de Heymans Heymans' law
ley de Hick Hick's law
ley de Hick-Hyman Hick-Hyman law
ley de Hilton Hilton's law
ley de Hooke Hooke's law
ley de Horner Horner's law
ley de igualdad law of equality
ley de isocronismo law of isochronism
ley de Jackson Jackson's law
ley de Jost Jost's law
ley de Kjersted-Robinson Kjersted-Robinson law
ley de Lambert Lambert's law
ley de Landouzy-Grasset Landouzy-Grasset law
ley de lo más reciente law of recency
ley de localización promedia law of average localization

ley de logaritmo log law
ley de Magendie Magendie's law
ley de Maier Maier's law
ley de Marbe Marbe's law
ley de Merkel Merkel's law
ley de Muller Muller's law
ley de Muller-Schumann Muller-Schumann law
ley de números grandes law of large numbers
ley de Ohm Ohm's law
ley de pareo matching law
ley de parsimonia law of parsimony
ley de Piper Piper's law
ley de Porter Porter's law
ley de potencia de Stevens Stevens' power law
ley de Pragnanz law of Pragnanz
ley de precisión law of precision
ley de preparación readiness law
ley de primacía law of primacy
ley de progresión law of progression
ley de proximidad law of proximity
ley de regresión filial law of filial regression
ley de repetición law of repetition
ley de retrogénesis law of retrogenesis
ley de Ribot Ribot's law
ley de Ricco Ricco's law
ley de Ritter Ritter's law
ley de Rosenbach Rosenbach's law
ley de Semon Semon's law
ley de Sherrington Sherrington's law
ley de Stevens Stevens' law
ley de Stokes Stokes' law
ley de Sutton Sutton's law
ley de Talbot-Plateau Talbot-Plateau law
ley de todo o nada all-or-none law
ley de utilidad decreciente law of diminishing returns
ley de valor inicial law of initial value
ley de van der Kolk van der Kolk's law
ley de ventaja law of advantage
ley de Vierordt Vierordt's law
ley de Waller wallerian law
ley de Weber Weber's law
ley de Weber-Fechner Weber-Fechner law
ley de Wilder de valor inicial Wilder's law of initial value
ley de Zipf Zipf's law
ley del talión lex talionis
ley empírica empirical law
ley estadística statistical law
ley inversa de cuadrados inverse-square law
ley paralela parallel law
ley psicofísica psychophysical law
leyes asociativas associative laws
leyes de certificación certification laws
leyes de confinamiento commitment laws
leyes de Grassmann Grassmann's laws
leyes de Korte Korte's laws
leyes de organización laws of organization
leyes de organización gestalt gestalt laws of organization
leyes de preferencias de colores laws of color preference
leyes del aprendizaje laws of learning

leyes mendelianas mendelian laws
libertad freedom
libertad condicional conditional release,
   parole
libertad de seleccionar freedom to choose
libertad de voluntad freedom of will
libertad psicológica psychological freedom
libidinal libidinal
libidinización libidinization
libidinizar libidinize
libidinoso libidinous
libido libido
libido de objetos object libido
libido del ego ego libido
libido disminuido diminished libido
libido narcisista narcissistic libido
libido orgánico organ libido
libido represado damned-up libido
libre albedrío free will
libre de distribuciones distribution-free
libreto de vida life script
libreto sexual sexual script
libro sonoro talking book
libros para los ciegos books for the blind
licantropía lycanthropy
licomanía lycomania
licorexia lycorexia
líder leader
líder autoritario authoritarian leader
líder burocrático bureaucratic leader
líder centrado en el grupo group-centered
   leader
líder de discusión discussion leader
líder laissez-faire laissez-faire leader
liderazgo leadership
liderazgo doble dual leadership
liderazgo funcional functional leadership
lidocaína lidocaine
ligación tubaria tubal ligation
ligado a estímulo stimulus-bound
ligado al sexo sex-linked
ligado al X X-linked
ligadura ligature
ligadura intravascular intravascular ligature
ligando ligand
ligereza flippancy
ligero flippant
ligofilia lygophilia
límbico limbic
limen limen
limen absoluto absolute limen
limen de diferencia difference limen
limen diferencial differential limen
limen sensorial sense limen
liminal liminal
liminómetro liminometer
limitación limitation
limitación de datos data limitation
limitaciones de pruebas de inteligencia
   limitations of intelligence tests
limitado limited
limitado a la casa housebound
limitado a una cultura culture-bound
limitado al hogar homebound
limitado por sexo sex-limited

límite limit, boundary
límite de audibilidad audibility limit
límite de grupo group boundary
límite de práctica practice limit
límite del ego ego boundary
límite exterior outer boundary
límite externo external boundary
límite fisiológico physiological limit
límite interno internal boundary
límites corporales body boundaries
límites de categorías category boundaries
límites de clase class limits
límites de confianza confidence limits
límites fiduciarios fiducial limits
limofoitas limophoitas
limosis limosis
limotisis limophthisis
límulo limulus
línea line
línea axial axial line
línea base base line
línea base conductual behavioral base line
línea de emergencia hot-line
línea de fijación fixation line
línea de Gubler Gubler's line
línea de regresión regression line
línea de Ullmann Ullmann's line
línea de Voigt Voigt's line
línea sensible tender line
lineal linear
líneas de confusión confusion lines
líneas de Head Head's lines
linfa lymph
linfadenopatía folicular gigante giant
   follicular lymphadenopathy
linfocítico lymphocytic
linfocito lymphocyte
linfoide lymphoid
lingam lingam
linguadental linguadental
lingual lingual
lingüística linguistics
lingüística psicológica psychological
   linguistics
lingüístico linguistic
lingula lingula
linonofobia linonophobia
lipidosis lipidosis
lipidosis cerebral cerebral lipidosis
lipidosis cerebrósida cerebroside lipidosis
lipidosis gangliósida ganglioside lipidosis
lipidosis neuronal neuronal lipidosis
lipidosis sistémica infantil tardía late
   infantile systemic lipidosis
lipidosis sulfátida sulfatide lipidosis
lipocondistrofia lipochondystrophy
lipocondrodistrofia lipochondrodystrophia
lipodistrofia lipodystrophy
lipodistrofia insulínica insulin lipodystrophy
lipodistrofia intestinal intestinal lipodystrophy
lipodistrofia parcial partial lipodystrophy
lipodistrofia progresiva progressive
   lipodystrophy
lipofuscina lipofuscin
lipofuscinosis lipofuscinosis

lipofuscinosis ceroide ceroid lipofuscinosis
lipogranulomatosis de Farber Farber's
    lipogranulomatosis
lipoide lipoid
lipomeningocele lipomeningocele
liquidación de apego liquidation of attachment
líquido cerebroespinal cerebrospinal fluid
lisa lyssa
lisatoterapia lysatotherapy
lisencefalia lissencephaly
lisencefálico lissencephalic
lisinuria lysinuria
lisofobia lyssophobia
lista de comprobación checklist
lista de comprobación de adjetivos adjective
    checklist
lista de comprobación de conducta behavior
    checklist
lista de comprobación de problemas problem
    checklist
lista de Rosanoff Rosanoff list
literal literal
literalismo literalism
litiasis lithiasis
lítico lithic
litigioso litigious
litio lithium
lobar lobar
lobectomía lobectomy
lobectomía temporal temporal lobectomy
lobotomía lobotomy
lobotomía frontal frontal lobotomy
lobotomía prefrontal prefrontal lobotomy
lobotomía transorbitaria transorbital
    lobotomy
lóbulo lobe
lóbulo cuadrado quadrate lobule
lóbulo frontal frontal lobe
lóbulo límbico limbic lobe
lóbulo occipital occipital lobe
lóbulo paracentral paracentral lobule
lóbulo parietal parietal lobe
lóbulo parietal posterior posterior parietal
    lobe
lóbulo piriforme pyriform lobe
lóbulo temporal temporal lobe
localización localization
localización auditiva auditory localization
localización binaural binaural localization
localización cerebral cerebral localization
localización de función localization of
    function
localización de función cortical cortical
    localization of function
localización de síntomas symptom
    localization
localización de sonido sound localization
localización estereotáctica stereotactic
    localization
localización estereotáxica stereotaxic
    localization
localización neumotáxica pneumotaxic
    localization
localización perceptiva perceptual localization
localizado localized

locomoción locomotion
locomoción bipedal bipedal locomotion
locomoción de grupo group locomotion
locomotor locomotor
loculación loculation
locura madness
locura de danza dancing madness
locus locus
locus coeruleus locus coeruleus
locus de control locus of control
locus de control interno internal locus of
    control
locus minoris resistentiae locus minoris
    resistentiae
logafasia logaphasia
logagnosia logagnosia
logagrafia logagraphia
logamnesia logamnesia
logarítmico logarithmic
logaritmo logarithm
logastenia logasthenia
lógica logic
lógica deductiva deductive logic
lógica indistinta fuzzy logic
lógica pervertida perverted logic
lógica transductiva transductive logic
lógico logical
logicogramatical logicogrammatical
logística logistics
logístico logistic
logoclonia logoclonia
logodiarrea logodiarrhea
logoespasmo logospasm
logofasia logophasia
logografía logography
logomanía logomania
logomonomanía logomonomania
logoneurosis logoneurosis
logopatía logopathy
logopedia logopedics
logoplejía logoplegia
logorrea logorrhea
logoterapia logotherapy
logro achievement
longevidad longevity
longilineal longilineal
longitípico longitypical
longitud de onda wavelength
longitud de onda dominante dominant
    wavelength
longitud focal focal length
longitud media de expresión mean length of
    utterance
longitudinal longitudinal
loprazolam loprazolam
lorazepam lorazepam
lordosis lordosis
loxapina loxapine
loxia loxia
lucidez lucidity
lucidificación lucidification
lúcido lucid
lúdico ludic
ludoterapia ludotherapy
lúes lues

lujuria lust
lumbago lumbago
lumbago isquémico ischemic lumbago
lumbar lumbar
lumbarización lumbarization
lumen lumen
luminancia luminance
luminosidad luminosity
luminosidad absoluta absolute luminosity
luminosidad fotópica photopic luminosity
luminosidad mesópica mesopic luminosity
luminoso luminous
lumpectomía lumpectomy
luna de miel honeymoon
lunático lunatic
lupinosis lupinosis
lupus lupus
lupus eritematoso lupus erythematosus
lupus eritematoso sistémico systemic lupus
     erythematosus
lúteo luteal
luto mourning
luto por niños mourning by children
lux lux
luz idiorretinal idioretinal light
luz lasérica laser light
luz obscura dark light
luz retinal retinal light

llaga por presión pressure sore
llanto crying
llanto inicial initial cry

macrencefalia macrencephaly
macroadenoma macroadenoma
macrobiótico macrobiotic
macrocefalia macrocephaly
macrocefálico macrocephalic
macrocéfalo macrocephalous
macrocosmo macrocosm
macrocráneo macrocranium
macroelectrodo macroelectrode
macroencéfalo macroencephalon
macroestereognosis macrostereognosis
macroestesia macroesthesia
macrófago macrophage
macrogenitosomía macrogenitosomia
macrogiria macrogyria
macroglobulinemia macroglobulinemia
macroglosia macroglossia
macrografía macrography
macrología macrology
macromanía macromania
macromastia macromastia
macropsia macropsia
macrosomatognosia macrosomatognosia
macrosquélico macroskelic
mácula acústica macula acusticae
mácula lútea macula lutea
mácula retinal retinal macula
maculocerebral maculocerebral
madre adicta a la heroína heroin-addicted
    mother
madre adicta al alcohol alcohol-addicted
    mother
madre adolescente adolescent mother
madre completa complete mother
**madre deprimida y el desarrollo afectivo de
    infante** depressed mother and infant's
    affective development
madre diabética diabetic mother
madre fálica phallic mother
madre hospedante host mother
madre sustituta surrogate mother
madre trabajadora working mother
maduración maturation
maduración anticipatoria anticipatory
    maturation
maduración cognitiva cognitive maturation
maduración desviada deviant maturation
maduración inhibitoria inhibitory maturation
maduración neurológica neurological
    maturation
maduración retardada retarded maturation
maduración sexual sexual maturation
maduración temprana contra tarde early
    versus late maturation

maduracional maturational
madurez maturity
madurez apropiada para la edad
    age-appropriate maturity
madurez biológica biological maturity
madurez emocional emotional maturity
madurez genital genital maturity
madurez intelectual intellectual maturity
madurez mental mental maturity
madurez sexual sexual maturity
madurez social social maturity
maduro mature
maestro de campo field teacher
maestro de recursos resource teacher
maestro itinerante itinerant teacher
magia magic
magia compulsiva compulsive magic
magia de comunicación communication
    magic
magia de imprecación cursing magic
mágico magical
Magna Mater Magna Mater
magnacidio magnacide
magnesio magnesium
magnesio sérico serum magnesium
magnetismo magnetism
magnetismo animal animal magnetism
magnetoencefalografía
    magnetoencephalography
magnetoencefalograma
    magnetoencephalogram
magnetómetro magnetometer
magnetotropismo magnetotropism
magnitud de respuesta magnitude of response
main d'accoucheur main d'accoucheur
main en crochet main en crochet
main en griffe main en griffe
mal de ojo evil eye
malapropismo malapropism
malaria malaria
malaria cerebral cerebral malaria
malaria terapéutica therapeutic malaria
maldición curse
maldición de Ondine Ondine's curse
maleación malleation
maleato maleate
malestar malaise
malévolo malevolent
malformación malformation
malformación congénita congenital
    malformation
malformación de Arnold-Chiari
    Arnold-Chiari malformation
malignidad malignancy
maligno malignant
maltrato de niños child maltreatment
maltrato psicológico psychological
    maltreatment
malum malum
malum minus malum minus
malum vertebrale suboccipitale malum
    vertebrale suboccipitale
mamalingus mammalingus
mamaria mammary
mancha tache

mancha cerebral tache cerebrale
mancha de café con leche cafe au lait spot
mancha de Graefe Graefe's spot
mancha de temperatura temperature spot
mancha espinal tache spinale
mancha hipnogénica hypnogenic spot
mancha meníngea tache meningeale
mandato paradójico paradoxical injunction
mandíbula jaw
mandíbula trabada lockjaw
mandibular mandibular
manía mania
manía absorta absorbed mania
manía adolescente adolescent mania
manía aguda acute mania
manía atípica atypical mania
manía constitucional constitutional mania
manía crónica chronic mania
manía de Bell Bell's mania
manía de comidas food faddism
manía de copiarse copying mania
manía de danza dancing mania
manía de morder biting mania
manía de razonamiento reasoning mania
manía de recomenzar recommencement
    mania
manía de refunfuñar grumbling mania
manía delirante delirious mania
manía delusoria delusional mania
manía depresiva depressive mania
manía efímera ephemeral mania
manía estuporosa stuporous mania
manía fantástica infantil mania phantastica
    infantilis
manía incrédula doubting mania
manía inhibida inhibited mania
manía posparto postpartum mania
manía reactiva reactive mania
manía religiosa religious mania
manía secundaria secondary mania
manía transitoria mania transitoria
manía unipolar unipolar mania
maníaco (adj) maniacal
maníaco (n) maniac
maniacodepresivo manic-depressive
maniafobia maniaphobia
manicia manicy
manicomio bedlam
manierismo mannerism
manierismo de ciego blindism
manifestación manifestation
manifestación conductual behavioral
    manifestation
manifestación neurótica neurotic
    manifestation
manifestación psicofisiológica
    psychophysiologic manifestation
manifestación psicótica psychotic
    manifestation
manifiesto manifest
maniobra maneuver
maniobra de Buzzard Buzzard's maneuver
maniobra de Jendrassik Jendrassik's
    maneuver
maniobra de Kohnstamm Kohnstamm

maneuver
manipulación manipulation
manipulación ambiental environmental
    manipulation
manipulativo manipulative
manitol mannitol
mano de escritor writing hand
mano de partero accoucheur's hand
mano en garra clawhand
mano obstétrica obstetrical hand
mano suculenta de Marinesco Marinesco's
    succulent hand
manoptoscopio manoptoscope
manosidosis mannosidosis
manta de seguridad security blanket
mantenimiento maintenance
mantenimiento corporal body maintenance
mantenimiento de metadona methadone
    maintenance
mantenimiento de salud health maintenance
mantenimiento fisiológico physiological
    maintenance
mantenimiento perceptivo perceptual
    maintenance
mantenimiento profiláctico prophylactic
    maintenance
mantra mantra
manual manual
manualismo manualism
mapa cognitivo cognitive map
mapa genético genetic map
maprotilina maprotiline
maquiavelismo Machiavellism
máquina de enseñanza teaching machine
máquina de escribir sonora talking
    typewriter
máquina de Turing Turing machine
máquina influyente influencing machine
marásmico marasmic
marasmo marasmus
maratón marathon
marcador marker
marcador de genes gene marker
marcador genético genetic marker
marcapasos pacemaker
marcapasos cardíaco cardiac pacemaker
marcapasos cerebral cerebral pacemaker
marcapasos talámico thalamic pacemaker
marco frame
marco de orientación frame of orientation
marco de referencia frame of reference
marcha gait
marcha atáxica ataxic gait
marcha cerebelosa cerebellar gait
marcha de Charcot Charcot's gait
marcha de estepaje steppage gait
marcha de estepaje alto high-steppage gait
marcha de propulsión propulsion gait
marcha en tijeras scissor gait
marcha equina equine gait
marcha espástica spastic gait
marcha festinante festinant gait
marcha helicópoda helicopod gait
marcha hemipléjica hemiplegic gait
marcha jacksoniana jacksonian march

mareamiento dizziness
mareo aéreo airsickness
margen margin
margen de atención margin of attention
margen de conciencia margin of
  consciousness
marginal marginal
marihuana marihuana
marijuana marijuana
mariposia mariposia
marital marital
masa mass
masa aperceptiva apperceptive mass
masa intermedia massa intermedia
masaje massage
masaje de puntas de nervios nerve-point
  massage
máscara mask
máscara de Hutchinson Hutchinson's mask
masculinidad masculinity
masculinizar masculinize
masculino masculine
masivo massive
masoquismo masochism
masoquismo en masa mass masochism
masoquismo erotogénico erotogenic
  masochism
masoquismo femenino feminine masochism
masoquismo ideal ideal masochism
masoquismo mental mental masochism
masoquismo moral moral masochism
masoquismo primario primary masochism
masoquismo sexual sexual masochism
masoquismo social social masochism
masoquismo verbal verbal masochism
masoquismo psíquico psychic masochism
masoquista (adj) masochistic
masoquista (n) masochist
masoterapia massotherapy
mastectomía mastectomy
mastectomía radical radical mastectomy
mastectomía simple simple mastectomy
mastectomía simple modificada modified
  simple mastectomy
masticatorio masticatory
mastigofobia mastigophobia
mastodinia mastodynia
masturbación masturbation
masturbación anal anal masturbation
masturbación compulsiva compulsive
  masturbation
masturbación de niñez childhood
  masturbation
masturbación doble dual masturbation
masturbación falsa false masturbation
masturbación infantil infantile masturbation
masturbación mutua mutual masturbation
masturbación psíquica psychic masturbation
masturbación simbólica symbolic
  masturbation
masturbación y culpabilidad masturbation
  and guilt
masturbar masturbate
matemagénico mathemagenic
matemático mathematical

materia blanca white matter
material corriente current material
material de práctica practice material
material de relleno filler material
material genético genetic material
materialismo materialism
materialización histérica hysterical
  materialization
maternal maternal
maternidad maternity
matices de colores color shades
matices invariables invariable hues
matiz hue
matiz espectral spectral hue
matiz extraespectral extraspectral hue
matiz primario primary hue
matiz puro pure hue
matiz único unique hue
matoide mattoid
matriarcado matriarchy
matriarcal matriarchal
matricidio matricide
matrilineal matrilineal
matrilocal matrilocal
matrimonio marriage
matrimonio abierto open marriage
matrimonio concertado arranged marriage
matrimonio de ensayo trial marriage
matrimonio de grupo group marriage
matrimonio de primos cousin marriage
matrimonio en grupo cluster marriage
matrimonio entre parientes intermarriage
matrimonio experimental experimental
  marriage
matrimonio homosexual homosexual
  marriage
matrimonio mixto intermarriage
matrimonio plural plural marriage
matrimonio simbiótico symbiotic marriage
matrimonio tradicional traditional marriage
matrimonios secuenciales sequential
  marriages
matriz matrix
matriz de correlación correlation matrix
matriz de creencias-valores belief-value
  matrix
matriz de decisiones decision matrix
matriz estructural structural matrix
matriz factorial factor matrix
matriz terapéutica therapeutic matrix
máximas conversacionales conversational
  maxims
maximización del ego ego maximization
máximo maximum
mayeusiofobia maieusiophobia
meato meatus
meato auditivo externo external auditory
  meatus
mecánico mechanical
mecanismo mechanism
mecanismo adaptivo adaptive mechanism
mecanismo compensatorio compensatory
  mechanism
mecanismo de ajuste adjustment mechanism
mecanismo de asociación association

mechanism
mecanismo de aumento de despertamiento
arousal boost mechanism
mecanismo de autoestimulación
self-stimulation mechanism
mecanismo de cancelación cancellation
mechanism
mecanismo de correlación cruzada
cross-correlation mechanism
mecanismo de chivo expiatorio scapegoat
mechanism
mecanismo de defensa defense mechanism
mecanismo de defensa del ego ego defense
mechanism
mecanismo de desconexión periódica gating
mechanism
mecanismo de dolor pain mechanism
mecanismo de enfoque focusing mechanism
mecanismo de entrada-salida input-output
mechanism
mecanismo de escape escape mechanism
mecanismo de inhibición inhibition
mechanism
mecanismo de Poliana Pollyanna mechanism
mecanismo de reducción de despertamiento
arousal reduction mechanism
mecanismo de reparación repair mechanism
mecanismo de retroalimentación feedback
mechanism
mecanismo de uvas verdes sour grapes
mechanism
mecanismo del ego ego mechanism
mecanismo inadaptivo maladaptive
mechanism
mecanismo liberador releasing mechanism
mecanismo liberador heredado inherited
releasing mechanism
mecanismo liberador innato innate releasing
mechanism
mecanismo mental mental mechanism
mecanismo neural neural mechanism
mecanismo olfativo smell mechanism
mecanismo para bregar coping mechanism
mecanismos de adaptación adaptation
mechanisms
mecanismos de alerta alerting mechanisms
mecanismos de mediación mediation
mechanisms
mecanismos de psicoterapia en grupo
mechanisms of group psychotherapy
mecanismos neurales de aprendizaje neural
mechanisms of learning
**mecanismos para bregar en trastorno de
personalidad fronterizo** coping
mechanisms in borderline personality
disorder
mecanístico mechanistic
mecanofobia mechanophobia
mecanorreceptor mechanoreceptor
mecanorreflejo mechanoreflex
meclofenoxato meclofenoxate
meclozina meclozine
meconismo meconism
medazepam medazepam
media mean

media aritmética arithmetic mean
media armónica harmonic mean
media asumida assumed mean
media cuadrática mean square
media dorada golden mean
media geométrica geometric mean
media logarítmica logarithmic mean
media obtenida obtained mean
media parental midparent
media vida half-life
mediación mediation
mediación cognitiva cognitive mediation
mediación de conflicto conflict mediation
mediación genética genetic mediation
mediador mediator
medial medial
mediana median
mediar mediate
mediato mediate
medicación medication
medicación antiansiedad antianxiety
medication
medicación broncodilatador bronchodilator
medication
medicación para dolor crónico medication
for chronic pain
medicina medicine
medicina conductual behavioral medicine
medicina constitucional constitutional
medicine
medicina de rehabilitación rehabilitation
medicine
medicina física physical medicine
medicina forense forensic medicine
medicina holísitica holistic medicine
medicina legal legal medicine
medicina preventiva preventive medicine
medicina psicosomática psychosomatic
medicine
medición measurement
medición absoluta absolute measurement
medición conjunta conjoint measurement
medición de actitudes attitude measurement
medición de trastornos afectivos
measurement of affective disorders
medición directa direct measurement
medición educacional educational
measurement
medición fotométrica photometric
measurement
medición indirecta indirect measurement
medición interactiva interactive measurement
medición mental mental measurement
médico de cuidado primario primary care
physician
médico primario primary physician
medicolegal medicolegal
medicopsicología medicopsychology
medida measure
medida de dispersión measure of dispersion
medida de partición partition measure
medida de tendencia central measure of
central tendency
medida de variación measure of variation
medida discreta discrete measure

medida estándar standard measure
medida psicológica psychological measure
medida reactiva reactive measure
medida representativa representative
    measure
medidas ambientales environmental measures
medidas biológicas biological measures
medidas de creatividad creativity measures
medidas de criterio criterion measures
medidas de inteligencia intelligence measures
medidas de precisión accuracy measures
medidas de tendencia central central
    tendency measures
medidas sociológicas sociological measures
medidor de intensidad de sonido sound-level
    meter
medio medium
medio espectáculo half-show
medios means
medios de comunicación mass media
meditación meditation
meditación ansiosa brooding
meditación ansiosa obsesiva obsessional
    brooding
meditación transcendental transcendental
    meditation
meditar ansiosamente brood
médula adrenal adrenal medulla
médula espinal spinal cord
médula oblonga medulla oblongata
médula ósea bone marrow
medular medullary
medulectomía medullectomy
meduloblastoma medulloblastoma
meduloepitelioma medulloepithelioma
medulomioblastoma medullomyoblastoma
mefenesina mephenesin
mefenitoína mephenytoin
mefexamida mefexamide
mefenoxalona mephenoxalone
mefobarbital mephobarbital
megacefalia megacephaly
megacefálico megacephalic
megacéfalo megacephalous
megacolon psicogénico psychogenic
    megacolon
megadosis megadose
megalgia megalgia
megalocefalia megalocephaly
megaloencefalia megaloencephaly
megaloencefálico megaloencephalic
megaloencéfalo megaloencephalon
megaloesplácnico megalosplanchnic
megalofobia megalophobia
megalografía megalographia
megalomanía megalomania
megalomaníaco megalomaniac
megalopia megalopia
megalopia histérica megalopia hysterica
megalopsia megalopsia
megavitamina megavitamin
meiosis meiosis
meiótico meiotic
mejor ajuste best fit
mejora improvement

mejora de transferencia transference
    improvement
mel mel
melancolía melancholia
melancolía abdominal abdominal melancholia
melancolía agitada melancholia agitata
melancolía climatérica climacteric
    melancholia
melancolía hipocondríaca hypochondriacal
    melancholia
melancolía involutiva involutional
    melancholia
melancolía paranoide paranoid melancholia
melancólico melancholic
melanocito melanocyte
melanoma melanoma
melanosis melanosis
melanosis neurocutánea neurocutaneous
    melanosis
melatonina melatonin
meliorístico melioristic
melisofobia melissophobia
melitracen melitracen
melomanía melomania
membrana membrane
membrana aracnoidea arachnoid membrane
membrana basilar basilar membrane
membrana de Corti Corti's membrane
membrana de Reissner Reissner's membrane
membrana hialina hyaline membrane
membrana mucosa mucous membrane
membrana neuronal neuronal membrane
membrana reticular reticular membrane
membrana tectorial tectorial membrane
membrana timpánica tympanic membrane
membrana vestibular vestibular membrane
membranectomía membranectomy
memoria memory
memoria a corto plazo short-term memory
memoria a corto plazo activo active
    short-term memory
memoria a largo plazo long-term memory
memoria afectiva affect memory
memoria anterógrada anterograde memory
memoria asociativa associative memory
memoria auditiva auditory memory
memoria autobiográfica autobiographical
    memory
memoria automática automatic memory
memoria biológica biological memory
memoria categórica categorical memory
memoria constructiva constructive memory
memoria cubriente cover memory
memoria de hábitos habit memory
memoria de lámpara de destello flashbulb
    memory
memoria de reconocimiento recognition
    memory
memoria de reemplazo replacement memory
memoria de referencia reference memory
memoria del pasado reciente recent past
    memory
memoria dependiente del estado
    state-dependent memory
memoria durante sueño memory during sleep

memoria e inteligencia artificial memory and artificial intelligence
memoria ecoica echoic memory
memoria episódica episodic memory
memoria episódica y enfermedad de Alzheimer episodic memory and Alzheimer's disease
memoria evocadora evocative memory
memoria excepcional exceptional memory
memoria filogenética phylogenetic memory
memoria fisiológica physiological memory
memoria fotográfica photographic memory
memoria genética genetic memory
memoria hiperestética hyperesthetic memory
memoria holográfica holographic memory
memoria icónica iconic memory
memoria implícita implicit memory
memoria inaccesible inaccessible memory
memoria incidental incidental memory
memoria inconsciente unconscious memory
memoria inmediata immediate memory
memoria intermedia buffer memory
memoria léxica lexical memory
memoria motora motor memory
memoria panorámica panoramic memory
memoria permanente permanent memory
memoria perturbadora disturbing memory
memoria primaria primary memory
memoria productiva productive memory
memoria reciente recent memory
memoria reconstructiva reconstructive memory
memoria redintegrativa redintegrative memory
memoria remota remote memory
memoria reproductiva reproductive memory
memoria retentiva retentive memory
memoria retrógrada retrograde memory
memoria secuencial sequential memory
memoria secundaria secondary memory
memoria selectiva selective memory
memoria semántica semantic memory
memoria senil senile memory
memoria sensorial sensory memory
memoria sensorial auditiva auditory sensory memory
memoria señalada cued memory
memoria serial serial memory
memoria significativa meaningful memory
memoria subconsciente subconscious memory
memoria temprana early recollection
memoria trabajadora working memory
memoria verbal verbal memory
memoria visual visual memory
memoria y amnesia memory and amnesia
memoria y atención memory and attention
memoria y daño cerebral memory and brain damage
memoria y enfermedad de Alzheimer memory and Alzheimer's disease
memorizar memorize
ménage à trois ménage à trois
menarca menarche
mendacidad mendacity

mendeliano mendelian
mendelismo mendelism
mendicidad patológica pathological mendicancy
mendigo emocional emotional beggar
meneo vertical bobbing
meneo vertical ocular ocular bobbing
meníngeo meningeal
meningeorrafia meningeorrhaphy
meninges meninges
meningioma meningioma
meningioma cutáneo cutaneous meningioma
meningioma psamomatoso psammomatous meningioma
meningiomatosis meningiomatosis
meningismo meningismus
meningítico meningitic
meningitis meningitis
meningitis bacterial bacterial meningitis
meningitis basilar basilar meningitis
meningitis cerebroespinal cerebrospinal meningitis
meningitis cerebroespinal epidémica epidemic cerebrospinal meningitis
meningitis epidural epidural meningitis
meningitis espinal spinal meningitis
meningitis externa external meningitis
meningitis interna internal meningitis
meningitis meningocócica meningococcal meningitis
meningitis neoplásica neoplastic meningitis
meningitis neumocócica pneumococcal meningitis
meningitis oclusiva occlusive meningitis
meningitis otítica otitic meningitis
meningitis serosa serous meningitis
meningitis tuberculosa tuberculous meningitis
meningitofobia meningitophobia
meningnoencefalitis biondulante biundulant meningoencephalitis
meningocele meningocele
meningocele espurio spurious meningocele
meningocele traumático traumatic meningocele
meningoencefalitis meningoencephalitis
meningoencefalitis amebiana primaria primary amebic meningoencephalitis
meningoencefalitis de paperas mumps meningoencephalitis
meningoencefalitis eosinófila eosinophilic meningoencephalitis
meningoencefalitis hemorrágica primaria aguda acute primary hemorrhagic meningoencephalitis
meningoencefalitis herpética herpetic meningoencephalitis
meningoencefalitis sifilítica syphilitic meningoencephalitis
meningoencefalocele meningoencephalocele
meningoencefalomielitis meningoencephalomyelitis
meningoencefalopatía meningoencephalopathy
meningomielitis meningomyelitis
meningomielocele meningomyelocele

meningorradiculitis meningoradiculitis
meningorragia meningorrhagia
menopausia menopause
menopausia masculina male menopause
menopáusico menopausal
menor emancipado emancipated minor
menorragia menorrhagia
menoscabo disparagement
mens rea mens rea
mensaje message
mensaje de dos lados two-sided message
mensajero messenger
mensajero químico externo external chemical
   messenger
mensajeros químicos chemical messengers
menstruación menstruation
menstrual menstrual
menstruo menses
mensuración mensuration
mentación mentation
mentación del sueño sleep mentation
mentación subjetiva subjective mentation
mental mental
mentalidad mentality
mentalidad dominante dominant mentality
mentalidad primitiva primitive mentality
mentalismo mentalism
mentalmente mentally
mentanfetamina methamphetamine
mente mind
mente de grupo group mind
mente miniatura miniature mind
mente popular folk mind
mente prelógica prelogical mind
mente social social mind
mente subconsciente subconscious mind
menticidio menticide
mentir lying
mentir no patológico nonpathological lying
mentir patológico pathological lying
mentira lie
mentira de vida life lie
mentiroso liar
mentismo mentism
meperidina meperidine
meprobamato meprobamate
meralgia meralgia
meralgia paraestésica meralgia paraesthetica
mercadeo marketing
mercado gris gray market
merergasia merergasia
mericismo merycism
merogonia merogony
merorraquisquisis merorrhachischisis
merosmia merosmia
mescalina mescaline
mesencefálico mesencephalic
mesencefalitis mesencephalitis
mesencéfalo mesencephalon
mesencefalotomía mesencephalotomy
meseta plateau
mesial mesial
mesilato mesylate
mesmerismo mesmerism
mesmerizar mesmerize

mesocefalia mesocephaly
mesocefálico mesocephalic
mesocúrtico mesokurtic
mesocurtosis mesokurtosis
mesodermo mesoderm
mesoesquélico mesoskelic
mesomorfia mesomorphy
mesomórfico mesomorphic
mesomorfo mesomorph
mesoneuritis mesoneuritis
mesoneuritis nodular nodular mesoneuritis
mesópico mesopic
mesoridazina mesoridazine
mesorraquisquisis mesorrhachischisis
mesosomático mesosomatic
metaanálisis meta-analysis
metabólico metabolic
metabolismo metabolism
metabolismo basal basal metabolism
metabolismo cerebral brain metabolism
metabolismo de aminoácidos amino acid
   metabolism
metabolismo de carbohidratos carbohydrate
   metabolism
metabolismo mental mental metabolism
metabolito neurotransmisor neurotransmitter
   metabolite
metacomunicación metacommunication
metacontraste metacontrast
metacualona methaqualone
metadona methadone
metaerotismo metaerotism
metaestético metaesthetic
metaevaluación metaevaluation
metafase metaphase
metafísica metaphysics
metafísico metaphysical
metáfora metaphor
metáfora computacional computational
   metaphor
metáfora de computadora computer
   metaphor
metafórico metaphoric
metafrenia metaphrenia
metagnosis metagnosis
metalenguaje metalanguage
metálico metallic
metalingüística metalinguistics
metalofobia metallophobia
metaloscopia metalloscopy
metamérico metameric
metámeros metamers
metamorfopsia metamorphopsia
metamorfosis metamorphosis
metamorfosis conductual behavioral
   metamorphosis
metamorfosis sexual paranoide
   metamorphosis sexualis paranoica
metamotivación metamotivation
metanecesidades metaneeds
metapatología metapathology
metapirileno methapyrilene
metapramina metapramine
metapsicoanálisis metapsychoanalysis
metapsicología metapsychology

metapsicológico metapsychological
metapsiquiatría metapsychiatry
metástasis metastasis
metatálamo metathalamus
metatarsalgia metatarsalgia
metateoría metatheory
metatético metathetic
metatropismo metatropism
metempírico metempirical
metempsicosis metempsychosis
metencefalina metenkephalin
metencéfalo metencephalon
meteorofobia meteorophobia
metildopa methyldopa
metilepsia methilepsia
metilfenidato methylphenidate
metilfenobarbital methylphenobarbital
metiprilona methyprylon
metisergida methysergide
metocarbamol methocarbamol
metoclopramida metoclopramide
método method
método anecdótico anecdotal method
método aristotélico Aristotelian method
método bifactorial bifactor method
método biográfico biographical method
método centroide centroid method
método científico scientific method
método cinestésico kinesthetic method
método clínico clinical method
método correlacional correlational method
método de ajuste adjustment method
método de alternación alternation method
método de Anel Anel's method
método de anticipación anticipation method
método de anticipación serial
    serial-anticipation method
método de Antyllus Antyllus' method
método de aprendizaje completo
    complete-learning method
método de aproximaciones method of
    approximations
método de aproximaciones sucesivas
    successive-approximations method
método de asociación association method
método de Barany Barany method
método de bisección halving method
método de Brasdor Brasdor's method
método de camada dividida split-litter
    method
método de cambio mínimo minimal-change
    method
método de casos case method
método de casos iguales y desiguales equal
    and unequal cases method
método de cifra cipher method
método de clasificación classification method
método de comparación factorial
    factor-comparison method
método de comparaciones emparejadas
    paired-comparisons method
método de componente principal
    principal-component method
método de componentes de trabajo
    job-component method

método de conducta behavior method
método de conferencia lecture method
método de conferencias conference method
método de contracepción de retirada
    withdrawal method of contraception
método de correlación correlation method
método de Delfos Delphi method
método de descubrimiento discovery method
método de destrucción destruction method
método de diario diary method
método de diferencias escasamente notables
    just noticeable differences method
método de discusión discussion method
método de documentos personales
    personal-document method
método de Donders Donders' method
método de enseñanza inductivo inductive
    teaching method
método de equivalentes equivalents method
método de escalera staircase method
método de estimulación stimulation method
método de estímulos constantes
    constant-stimuli method
método de exploración serial
    serial-exploration method
método de expresión expression method
método de Fere Fere method
método de Fernald Fernald method
método de frecuencias frequency method
método de graduación gradation method
método de Hilton Hilton's method
método de impedancia impedance method
método de impresión impression method
método de informe parcial partial-report
    method
método de interacción familiar family
    interaction method
método de intervalos aparentemente iguales
    equal-appearing-intervals method
método de intervalos sucesivos
    successive-intervals method
método de Lamaze Lamaze method
método de Leboyer Leboyer method
método de límites method of limits
método de masticación chewing method
método de Monte Carlo Monte Carlo method
método de Montessori Montessori method
método de Moore Moore's method
método de Muller-Urban Muller-Urban
    method
método de Nissl Nissl method
método de obstrucción obstruction method
método de palabra clave key-word method
método de palabra completa whole-word
    method
método de palabras word method
método de pares asociados paired-associates
    method
método de Pavlov Pavlov method
método de preferencias preference method
método de producción production method
método de proyecto project method
método de prueba-estudio-prueba
    test-study-test method
método de prueba-reprueba test-retest

method
método de Purmann Purmann's method
método de práctica sucesiva
    successive-practice method
método de reaprendizaje relearning method
método de recitación recitation method
método de reconocimiento recognition
    method
método de reconstrucción reconstruction
    method
método de recordación recall method
método de reproducción reproduction method
método de ritmo rhythm method
método de ritmo de contracepción rhythm
    method of contraception
método de Scarpa Scarpa's method
método de serie de sueños dream-series
    method
método de substracción subtraction method
método de Tadoma Tadoma method
método de terminación de oraciones
    sentence-completion method
método de videocinta videotape method
método de Vincent Vincent method
método de vista sight method
método de Wardrop Wardrop's method
método deductivo matemático
    mathematico-deductive method
método dialéctico dialectical method
método directo direct method
método en masa mass method
método exosomático exosomatic method
método experimental experimental method
método familiar family method
método fenomenológico phenomenological
    method
método fonético phonetic method
método fónico phonic method
método genético genetic method
método hipotético-deductivo
    hypothetical-deductive method
método histórico historical method
método indirecto de terapia indirect method
    of therapy
método introspectivo introspective method
método longitudinal longitudinal method
método manual manual method
método motocinestésico motokinesthetic
    method
método multisensorial multisensory method
método no experimental nonexperimental
    method
método observacional observational method
método oral oral method
método postulacional postulational method
método proyectivo projective method
método Q Q method
método transcultural cross-cultural method
método transversal cross-sectional method
metodología methodology
metodología Q Q methodology
métodos confrontantes confrontational
    methods
métodos criogénicos cryogenic methods
métodos de evaluación assessment methods

métodos de investigación empírica empirical
    research methods
métodos de investigación normativos
    normative research methods
métodos expresivos expressive methods
métodos métricos metric methods
métodos psicofísicos psychophysical methods
metonimia metonymy
metopón metopon
metopoplastia metopoplasty
metoprolol metoprolol
metotrimeprazina methotrimeprazine
metoxamina methoxamine
métrico metric
metromanía metromania
metronoscopio metronoscope
metsuximida methsuximide
mezcla mixture
mezcla aditiva additive mixture
mezcla auditiva auditory blending
mezcla de casos case mix
mezcla de colores color mixture
mezcla de colores aditiva additive color
    mixture
mezcla retinal retinal mixture
mialgia myalgia
mianserina mianserin
miastenia myasthenia
miastenia grave myasthenia gravis
miasténico myasthenic
miatonía myatonia
miatonía congénita myatonia congenita
micetismo mycetismus
micetismo cerebral mycetismus cerebralis
micoplasma mycoplasma
micosis micosis
micosis paralítica paralytic micosis
micrencefalia micrencephaly
micrencéfalo micrencephalous
microadenoma microadenoma
microangiopatía microangiopathy
microbiofobia microbiophobia
microcefalia microcephaly
microcefalia encefaloclástica encephaloclastic
    microcephaly
microcefalia esquizencefálica schizencephalic
    microcephaly
microcefalia familiar familial microcephaly
microcefalia primaria primary microcephaly
microcefalia pura pure microcephaly
microcefálico microcephalic
microcirugía microsurgery
microcosmo microcosm
microdisgenesia microdysgenesia
microelectrodo microelectrode
microencefalia microencephaly
microentrenamiento microtraining
microesplácnico microsplanchnic
microfobia microphobia
microfonía microphonia
microfónico microphonic
microfónicos cocleares cochlear microphonics
microgenia microgeny
microgiria microgyria
microglia microglia

microglioma microglioma
microgliomatosis microgliomatosis
microgliosis microgliosis
microglosia microglossia
micrognatia micrognathia
micrografía micrography
micromanía micromania
micromastia micromastia
micromelia micromelia
micromilímetro micromillimeter
micrón micron
microorganismo microorganism
microorquidismo microorchidism
microorquidismo primario primary microorchidism
micropsia micropsia
micropsicofisiología micropsychophysiology
micropsicosis micropsychosis
microscópico microscopic
microscopio microscope
microscopio operatorio operating microscope
microscopio quirúrgico surgical microscope
microsemo microseme
microsocial microsocial
microsoma microsome
microsomático microsomatic
microsomatognosia microsomatognosia
microsomía microsomia
microsueño microsleep
microsutura microsuture
micrótomo microtome
microvascular microvascular
micrúrgico micrurgical
micturición micturition
midazolam midazolam
midriasis mydriasis
midriasis alternante alternating mydriasis
midriasis espasmódica spasmodic mydriasis
midriasis espástica spastic mydriasis
midriasis paralítica paralytic mydriasis
midriático mydriatic
mielapoplejía myelapoplexy
mielatelia myelatelia
mielauxia myelauxe
mielencéfalo myelencephalon
mielina myelin
mielinación myelination
mielinización myelinization
mielinoclasis myelinoclasis
mielinólisis myelinolysis
mielinólisis pontina central central pontine myelinolysis
mielítico myelitic
mielitis myelitis
mielitis aguda acute myelitis
mielitis ascendente ascending myelitis
mielitis bulbar bulbar myelitis
mielitis de Foix-Alajouanine Foix-Alajouanine myelitis
mielitis funicular funicular myelitis
mielitis necrotizante subaguda subacute necrotizing myelitis
mielitis por concusión concussion myelitis
mielitis sistémica systemic myelitis
mielitis transversal transverse myelitis

mielitis transversal aguda acute transverse myelitis
mieloarquitectura myeloarchitecture
mielocele myelocele
mielocistocele myelocystocele
mielocistomeningocele myelocystomeningocele
mielodiastasia myelodiastasis
mielodisplasia myelodysplasia
mielodisplasia oculta occult myelodysplasia
mielografía myelography
mielograma myelogram
mieloide myeloid
mielólisis myelolysis
mieloma múltiple multiple myeloma
mielomalacia myelomalacia
mielomalacia angiodisgenética angiodysgenetic myelomalacia
mielomeningocele myelomeningocele
mielón myelon
mieloneuritis myeloneuritis
mieloparálisis myeloparalysis
mielopatía myelopathy
mielopatía carcinomatosa carcinomatous myelopathy
mielopatía compresiva compressive myelopathy
mielopatía diabética diabetic myelopathy
mielopatía paracarcinomatosa paracarcinomatous myelopathy
mielopatía por radiación radiation myelopathy
mielopático myelopathic
mielópeto myelopetal
mieloplejía myeloplegia
mieloquiste myelocyst
mieloquístico myelocystic
mielorradiculitis myeloradiculitis
mielorradiculodisplasia myeloradiculodysplasia
mielorradiculopatía myeloradiculopathy
mielorradiculopolineuronitis myeloradiculopolyneuronitis
mielorrafia myelorrhaphy
mielorragia myelorrhagia
mielosífilis myelosyphilis
mielosiringosis myelosyringosis
mielosis myelosis
mielosis funicular funicular myelosis
mielosquisis myeloschisis
mielotísico myelophthisic
mielotisis myelophthisis
mielotomía myelotomy
mielotomía comisural commissural myelotomy
mielotomía de Bischof Bischof's myelotomy
mielotomía en T T myelotomy
mielótomo myelotome
mielotomografía myelotomography
miembro member
miembro fantasma phantom limb
miembro masculino male member
miembro viril membrum virile
miestesia myesthesia
migración migration

migraña migraine
migraña abdominal abdominal migraine
migraña cervical cervical migraine
migraña clásica classic migraine
migraña común common migraine
migraña de Harris Harris' migraine
migraña fulgurante fulgurating migraine
migraña hemipléjica hemiplegic migraine
migraña oftálmica ophthalmic migraine
migraña oftalmopléjica ophthalmoplegic
  migraine
mililambert millilambert
milimicrón millimicron
mimesis mimesis
mimético mimetic
mímica mimicry
mímico mimic
mineralocorticoide mineralocorticoid
miniatura miniature
minimización minimization
mínimo minimum
mínimo de mantenimiento maintenance
  minimum
minusvalía handicap
minusvalía emocional emotional handicap
minusvalía física physical handicap
minusvalía mental mental handicap
minusválido emocionalmente emotionally
  handicapped
minusválido mentalmente mentally
  handicapped
minusválido perceptivamente perceptually
  handicapped
mioblastoma myoblastoma
mioblastoma de células granulares granular
  cell myoblastoma
miobradia myobradia
miocelialgia myocelialgia
mioclonía myoclonia
mioclonía fibrilar fibrillary myoclonia
mioclónico myoclonic
mioclono myoclonus
mioclono múltiple myoclonus multiplex
mioclono nocturno nocturnal myoclonus
mioclono palatal palatal myoclonus
mioclono sensitivo a estímulos stimulus
  sensitive myoclonus
miodinia myodynia
miodistonía myodystony
miodistrofia myodystrophy
mioedema myoedema
mioespasmo myospasm
mioespasmo cervical cervical myospasm
mioestesia myoesthesia
mioestesis myoesthesis
miofascia myofascia
miogénico myogenic
mioglobina myoglobin
mioglobinuria myoglobinuria
miografía myography
miógrafo myograph
miograma myogram
mioneuralgia myoneuralgia
mioneuralgia postural postural myoneuralgia
mioneurastenia myoneurasthenia

mioneuroma myoneuroma
miopalmo myopalmus
mioparálisis myoparalysis
mioparesia myoparesis
miopatía myopathy
miopatía alcohólica alcoholic myopathy
miopatía alcohólica aguda acute alcoholic
  myopathy
miopatía carcinomatosa carcinomatous
  myopathy
miopatía hereditaria hereditary myopathy
miopatía menopáusica menopausal myopathy
miopatía nemalínica nemaline myopathy
miopatía ocular ocular myopathy
miopatía tirotóxica thyrotoxic myopathy
miopático myopathic
miopía myopia
miopía crómica chromic myopia
miopía prodromal prodromal myopia
miopía progresiva progressive myopia
miopragia miopragia
mioquimia myokymia
mioquimia hereditaria hereditary myokymia
miorritmia myorhythmia
miosalgia myosalgia
mioseísmo myoseism
miosina myosin
miosis miosis
miosis espástica spastic miosis
miosis paralítica paralytic miosis
miositis myositis
miositis cervical cervical myositis
miositis múltiple multiple myositis
miotáctico myotactic
miotenotomía myotenotomy
miotonía myotonia
miotonía adquirida myotonia acquisita
miotonía atrófica myotonia atrophica
miotonía congénita myotonia congenita
miotonía distrófica myotonia dystrophica
miotonía neonatal myotonia neonatorum
miotónico myotonic
miotono myotonus
miotonoide myotonoid
mirada fija gaze, stare
mirada fija de ping-pong ping-pong gaze
mirada fija fascinante fascinating gaze
miriaquita myriachit
miringotomía myringotomy
misandria misandry
misantropía misanthropy
miserotia miserotia
misocainia misocainia
misofilia mysophilia
misofobia mysophobia
misogamia misogamy
misoginia misogyny
misología misology
misoneísmo misoneism
misopedia misopedy
misticismo mysticism
mito myth
mito personal personal myth
mitocondria mitochondria
mitofobia mythophobia

mitomanía mythomania
mitos sobre hipnotismo myths about hypnotism
mitosis mitosis
mitral mitral
mixedema myxedema
mixedema infantil infantile myxedema
mixoneuroma myxoneuroma
mixoneurosis myxoneurosis
mixoscopia mixoscopia
mixoscopia bestial mixoscopia bestialis
mixovariación mixovariation
mixto mixed
mnema mneme
mnemónico mnemenic
mnémico mnemic
mnemismo mnemism
mnemónica mnemonics
mnemónico mnemonic
mnemonista mnemonist
moción motion
moción absoluta absolute motion
moción alfa alpha motion
moción aparente apparent motion
moción beta beta motion
moción de fondo background motion
moción delta delta motion
moción en arco bow motion
moción épsilon epsilon motion
moción estroboscópica stroboscopic motion
moción fenomenal phenomenal motion
moción gama gamma motion
moción ilusoria illusory motion
moción inducida induced motion
moción phi phi motion
moción real real motion
moción relativa relative motion
moco mucus
moda fashion
modal modal
modalidad modality
modalidad sensorial sensory modality
modelado modeling
modelado abstracto abstract modeling
modelado conductual behavioral modeling
modelado de arcilla en hipnosis clay-modeling in hypnosis
modelado de conducta behavior modeling
modelado encubierto covert modeling
modelamiento shaping
modelo model
modelo activo-pasivo active-passive model
modelo adverso adversary model
modelo aleatorio random model
modelo atenuador attenuator model
modelo biológico biological model
modelo biomédico biomedical model
modelo biopsicosocial biopsychosocial model
modelo cerebral brain model
modelo cognitivo cognitive model
modelo conceptual conceptual model
modelo conductual behavioral model
modelo conductual del desarrollo behavioral model of development
modelo continuo continuous model

modelo de amistad friendship model
modelo de amplificación amplification model
modelo de análisis por síntesis analysis by synthesis model
modelo de aprendizaje learning model
modelo de asesoramiento-cooperación guidance-cooperation model
modelo de ayuda helping model
modelo de canal único single-channel model
modelo de características feature model
modelo de características de trabajo job-characteristics model
modelo de componentes de varianza components of variance model
modelo de computadora computer model
modelo de confluencia confluence model
modelo de conformidad a fricción friction-conformity model
modelo de contingencia contingency model
modelo de correlación correlation model
modelo de costo-recompensa cost-reward model
modelo de déficit deficit model
modelo de desconexión periódica gating model
modelo de discriminación discrimination model
modelo de educación-socialización education-socialization model
modelo de enfermedad disease model
modelo de enriquecimiento ambiental environmental enrichment model
modelo de enseñanza teaching model
modelo de enseñanza no directivo nondirective teaching model
modelo de enseñanza del desarrollo developmental teaching model
modelo de entrenamiento de conciencia awareness training model
modelo de entrenamiento de indagación inquiry training model
modelo de estrés-descompensación stress-decompensation model
modelo de estructura de intelecto structure-of-intellect model
modelo de fin de evaluación goal model of evaluation
modelo de historial de vida life history model
modelo de idiosincrasia-crédito idiosyncrasy-credit model
modelo de indagación social social-inquiry model
modelo de ingeniería engineering model
modelo de integración-desintegración social social integration-disintegration model
modelo de logro de fin goal-attainment model
modelo de método de laboratorio laboratory method model
modelo de necesidad-impulso-incentivo need-drive-incentive model
modelo de operador lineal linear-operator model
modelo de papel role model
modelo de participación mutua mutual participation model

modelo de potencial humano human-potential model
modelo de red network model
modelo de salud pública public health model
modelo de sistemas ecológicos ecological systems model
modelo de sobrecarga de estrés overload model of stress
modelo de todo o nada all-or-none model
modelo del desarrollo model of development
modelo del ego ego model
modelo del logro de conceptos concept-attainment model
modelo dependiente dependent model
modelo ecológico ecological model
modelo egoísta de altruísmo egoistic model of altruism
modelo estructural structural model
modelo etológico del espacio personal ethological model of personal space
modelo fijo fixed model
modelo hidraulico hydraulic model
modelo homeostático homeostatic model
modelo integrado integrated model
modelo maestro-estudiante teacher-student model
modelo matemático mathematical model
modelo médico medical model
modelo médico de enfermedad medical model of disease
modelo médico de psicoterapia medical model of psychotherapy
modelo metabólico-nutricional metabolic-nutritional model
modelo mixto mixed model
modelo multifactorial multifactorial model
modelo ontoanalítico ontoanalytic model
modelo psicoeducativo psychoeducational model
modelo psicosocial psychosocial model
modelo psicosocial del desarrollo psychosocial model of development
modelo socialmente íntimo socially intimate model
modelo sociotécnico sociotechnical model
modelo topográfico topographical model
modelos diacrónicos contra sincrónicos diachronic versus synchronic models
moderado moderate
moderador moderator
modificación modification
modificación ambiental environmental modification
modificación de agresión modification of aggression
modificación de ambiente environment modification
modificación de conducta behavior modification
modificación de conducta cognitiva cognitive behavior modification
modificación de conducta no aversiva nonaversive behavior modification
modificación intraocular intraocular modification

modificado modified
modificador modifier
modo mode
modo activo de conciencia active mode of consciousness
modo de cognición de campo field-cognition mode
modo de herencia mode of inheritance
modo icónico iconic mode
modo paratáxico parataxic mode
modo pasivo de conciencia passive mode of consciousness
modo prototáxico prototaxic mode
modo simbólico symbolic mode
modo sintáxico syntaxic mode
modorra drowsiness
modorra en infancia drowsiness in infancy
modorra patológica pathological drowsiness
modos de herencia mendelianos mendelian modes of inheritance
modismo idiom
modulador modulator
módulo module
modus operandi modus operandi
mogiartría mogiarthria
mogifonía mogiphonia
mogigrafía mogigraphia
mogilalia mogilalia
molar molar
molecular molecular
molecularismo molecularism
molestador annoyer
molilalia molilalia
molimen molimen
molimen menstrual menstrual molimen
molindona molindone
molismofobia molysmophobia
molisofobia molysophobia
molusco molluscum
molusco fibroso molluscum fibrosum
momento moment
momento psicológico psychological moment
mónada monad
monatetosis monathetosis
monaural monaural
monema funcional functional moneme
moniliasis moniliasis
monismo monism
monismo cultural cultural monism
monismo natural natural monism
monístico monistic
monitor monitor
monitorización monitoring
monitorización corporal body monitoring
monitorización electrónica electronic monitoring
monitorizar monitor
monoamina monoamine
monoamina oxidasa monoamine oxidase
monoblepsia monoblepsia
monocigosidad monozygosity
monocigótico monozygotic
monocigoto monozygote
monocorea monochorea
monocromacia monochromacy

monocromatismo monochromatism
monocromato monochromat
monocromia monochromia
monocular monocular
monoespasmo monospasm
monoestético monesthetic
monoetilamida de ácido lisérgico lysergic
    acid monoethylamide
monofagismo monophagism
monofasia monophasia
monofásico monophasic
monofobia monophobia
monogamia monogamy
monogamia serial serial monogamy
monogonia monogony
monohíbrido monohybrid
monoideísmo monoideism
monomanía monomania
monomanía afectiva affective monomania
monomanía homicida homicidal monomania
monomanía instintiva instinctive monomania
monomanía intelectual intellectual
    monomania
monomaníaco monomaniac
monomátrico monomatric
monomioplejía monomyoplegia
mononeuralgia mononeuralgia
mononeuritis mononeuritis
mononeuritis múltiple mononeuritis multiplex
mononeuropatía mononeuropathy
mononeuropatía múltiple mononeuropathy
    multiplex
mononoea mononoea
mononucleosis infecciosa infectious
    mononucleosis
monopagia monopagia
monoparesia monoparesis
monoparestesia monoparesthesia
monopatofobia monopathophobia
monoplejía monoplegia
monoplejía masticatoria monoplegia
    masticatoria
monóptico monoptic
monórquido monorchid
monorrínico monorhinic
monosináptico monosynaptic
monosintomático monosymptomatic
monosomía monosomy
monosomía de grupo G group G monosomy
monótico monotic
monotónico monotonic
monótono monotonous
monotrópico monotropic
monóxido de carbono carbon monoxide
montículo axónico axon hillock
moral (adj) moral
moral (n) morale
moral de grupo group morale
moralidad morality
moralidad autónoma autonomous morality
moralidad coordinada coordinate morality
moralidad de constreñimiento morality of
    constraint
moralidad de cooperación morality of
    cooperation

moralidad esfintérica sphincter morality
moralidad interpersonal interpersonal
    morality
moratoria moratorium
moratoria psicosexual psychosexual
    moratorium
moratoria psicosocial psychosocial
    moratorium
mórbido morbid
morbilidad morbidity
morbilidad perinatal perinatal morbidity
morder de dedos finger-biting
morder de labios lip-biting
mordisco bite
morfema morpheme
morfina morphine
morfinismo morphinism
morfinomanía morphinomania
morfofonémica morphophonemics
morfogénesis morphogenesis
morfología morphology
morfológico morphological
morfosíntesis morphosynthesis
moria moria
morsicatio buccarum morsicatio buccarum
morsicatio labiorum morsicatio labiorum
mortal deadly
mortalidad mortality
mortalidad de infantes infant mortality
mortalidad reproductiva reproductive
    mortality
mortido mortido
mórula morula
mosaico mosaic
mosaiquismo mosaicism
motilina motilin
motivación motivation
motivación adulta adult motivation
motivación aprendida learned motivation
motivación conjuntiva conjunctive motivation
motivación de competencia competence
    motivation
motivación de crecimiento growth motivation
motivación de logro achievement motivation
motivación de niñez childhood motivation
motivación de trabajo work motivation
motivación del ser being motivation
motivación disyuntiva disjunctive motivation
motivación extrínseca extrinsic motivation
motivación inconsciente unconscious
    motivation
motivación intrínseca intrinsic motivation
motivación personal personal motivation
motivación por deficiencia deficiency
    motivation
motivación positiva positive motivation
motivación primaria primary motivation
motivación secundaria secondary motivation
motivación sexual sexual motivation
motivacional motivational
motivado motivated
motivar motivate
motivo motive
motivo adquirido acquired motive
motivo competitivo competitive motive

motivo cooperativo cooperative motive
motivo de abundancia abundancy motive
motivo de dominio mastery motive
motivo de efectancia effectance motive
motivo de logro achievement motive
motivo de prestigio prestige motive
motivo de seguridad safety motive
motivo fisiológico physiological motive
motivo personal-social personal-social motive
motivo por deficiencia deficiency motive
motivo psicogénico psychogenic motive
motivo psicológico psychological motive
motivo psicológico específico de cultura
    culture-specific psychological motive
motivo social social motive
motivos psicológicos individuales individual
    psychological motives
motocinestésico motokinesthetic
motoneurona motoneuron
motoneuronas intrafusales intrafusal
    motoneurons
motor motor
motor fino fine motor
móvil mobile
movilidad mobility
movilidad de libido mobility of libido
movilidad gástrica gastric motility
movilidad gastrointestinal gastrointestinal
    motility
movilidad hacia abajo downward mobility
movilidad horizontal horizontal mobility
movilidad intergeneracional intergenerational
    mobility
movilidad psíquica psychic mobility
movilidad social social mobility
movilidad vertical vertical mobility
movilización mobilization
movimiento movement
movimiento aleatorio random movement
movimiento alfa alpha movement
movimiento aparente apparent movement
movimiento asociado associated movement
movimiento autocinético autokinetic
    movement
movimiento beta beta movement
movimiento centrífugo centrifugal swing
movimiento compensatorio compensatory
    movement
movimiento conjugado conjugate movement
movimiento coreico choreic movement
movimiento coreiforme choreiform
    movement
movimiento corporal body movement
movimiento de crecimiento humano
    human-growth movement
movimiento de encuentro encounter
    movement
movimiento de hospicios hospice movement
movimiento de motor fino fine motor
    movement
movimiento de motor grueso gross motor
    movement
movimiento de trombón de Magnan
    Magnan's trombone movement
movimiento delta delta movement

movimiento distónico dystonic movement
movimiento en arco bow movement
movimiento en masa mass movement
movimiento en sueño movement in sleep
movimiento épsilon epsilon movement
movimiento espontaneo spontaneous
    movement
movimiento estereotipado stereotyped
    movement
movimiento gama gamma movement
movimiento hacia el asesoramiento de niños
    child-guidance movement
movimiento humano human movement
movimiento ilusorio illusory movement
movimiento inducido induced movement
movimiento involuntario involuntary
    movement
movimiento mioclónico myoclonic movement
movimiento neurobiotáctico neurobiotactic
    movement
movimiento ocular sacádico saccadic eye
    movement
movimiento posterior aftermovement
movimiento reflejo reflex movement
movimiento sacádico saccadic movement
movimiento semiótico semiotic movement
movimiento social social movement
movimiento torsional ocular ocular torsional
    movement
movimiento voluntario voluntary movement
movimiento de potencial humano
    human-potential movement
movimiento pedestre pedestrian movement
movimientos de cabeza head movements
movimientos de ojo eye movements
movimientos de ojo involuntarios involuntary
    eye movements
movimientos de ojos de rastreo pursuit eye
    movements
movimientos expresivos expressive
    movements
movimientos oculares no rápidos non-rapid
    eye movement
movimientos oculares rápidos rapid eye
    movement
mucopolisacárido mucopolysaccharide
mucopolisacaridosis mucopolysaccharidosis
mucoso mucous
mucoviscidosis mucoviscidosis
muchedumbre mob
mudanza de familia household move
mudo mute
mueca grimace
muerte death
muerte cerebral cerebral death
muerte con autopsia negativa autopsy
    negative death
muerte de cónyuge death of spouse
muerte de ser querido death of loved one
muerte en cuna crib death
muerte fetal fetal death
muerte intencional intentional death
muerte neonatal neonatal death
muerte no intencionada unintentional death
muerte parental parental death

muerte por agotamiento exhaustion death
muerte por fenotiazina phenothiazine death
muerte resultante de abuso de niños death
    resulting from child abuse
muerte resultante de negligencia de niños
    death resulting from child neglect
muestra sample
muestra adecuada adequate sample
muestra aleatoria random sample
muestra apareada matched sample
muestra de estandarización standardization
    sample
muestra de trabajo work sample
muestra del tiempo time sample
muestra estratificada stratified sample
muestra representativa representative sample
muestra sesgada biased sample
muestreo sampling
muestreo con reemplazo replacement
    sampling
muestreo controlado controlled sampling
muestreo de conducta behavior sampling
muestreo de confiabilidad reliability
    sampling
muestreo de probabilidades probability
    sampling
muestreo de vellosidades coriónicas
    chorionic villus sampling
muestreo doble double sampling
muestreo doméstico domal sampling
muestreo en bloques block sampling
muestreo estratificado stratified sampling
muestreo fortuito haphazard sampling
muestreo horizontal horizontal sampling
muestreo mixto mixed sampling
muestreo por áreas area sampling
muestreo por cuotas quota sampling
muestreo representativo representative
    sampling
muestreo sesgado biased sampling
muestreo sin reemplazo sampling without
    replacement
muestreo sistemático systematic sampling
muestreo situacional situational sampling
muestreo vertical vertical sampling
mujer castrante castrating woman
mujer fálica phallic woman
mujer golpeada battered woman
muleta crutch
multiaxial multiaxial
multicultural multicultural
multideterminación multidetermination
multideterminado multidetermined
multidimensional multidimensional
multidisciplinario multidisciplinary
multifactorial multifactorial
multifásico multiphasic
multiminusválido multihandicapped
multimodal multimodal
multípara multiparous
múltiple multiple
multiplicación de personalidad multiplication
    of personality
multiplicidad multiplicity
multipolaridad multipolarity

multisensorial multisensory
multitud crowd
multivariado multivariate
muñeca de amputación amputation doll
muñeco de terapia therapy puppet
muñón stump
murmullo murmur
murmullo cerebral brain murmur
muscarina muscarine
muscular muscular
músculo muscle
músculo bulbocavernoso bulbocavernosus
    muscle
músculo bulboesponjoso bulbospongiosus
    muscle
músculo cardíaco cardiac muscle
músculo ciliar ciliary muscle
músculo esqueletal skeletal muscle
músculo estriado striate muscle
músculo flexor flexor muscle
músculo frontal frontalis muscle
músculo voluntario voluntary muscle
musculoespiral musculospiral
musculoesquelético musculoskeletal
músculos antagónicos antagonistic muscles
músculos de ojo eye muscles
músculos de ojo extrínsecos extrinsic eye
    muscles
músculos de ojo intrínsecos intrinsic eye
    muscles
músculos involuntarios involuntary muscles
músculos paréticos paretic muscles
musicoterapia musicotherapy
musitación mumbling
muslo de conductor driver's thigh
muslo de Heilbronner Heilbronner's thigh
musofobia musophobia
mutación mutation
mutación de gen gene mutation
mutación de punto point mutation
mutagénico mutagenic
mutágeno mutagen
mutante mutant
mutilación mutilation
mutilación genital genital mutilation
mutismo mutism
mutismo acinético akinetic mutism
mutismo electivo elective mutism
mutismo psicogénico psychogenic mutism
mutismo voluntario voluntary mutism
mutualidad mutuality
mutualismo mutualism
mutuamente mutually
mutuamente exclusivo mutually exclusive
mutuo mutual
Mycobacterium leprae Mycobacterium leprae

N

naciente nascent
nacimiento birth
nacimiento anal anal birth
nacimiento prematuro premature birth
nadolol nadolol
nafta naphtha
nalbufina nalbuphine
nalorfina nalorphine
naloxona naloxone
naltrexona naltrexone
nanismo nanism
nanómetro nanometer
nanosmia primordial primordial nanosmia
naproxeno naproxen
napsilato napsylate
narcisismo narcissism
narcisismo del ego ego narcissism
narcisismo por enfermedad disease
    narcissism
narcisismo corporal body narcissism
narcisismo primario primary narcissism
narcisismo primitivo primitive narcissism
narcisismo secundario secondary narcissism
narcisista narcissistic
narcoanálisis narcoanalysis
narcocatarsis narcocatharsis
narcohipnia narcohypnia
narcohipnosis narcohypnosis
narcolepsia narcolepsy
narcoléptico narcoleptic
narcomanía narcomania
narcosíntesis narcosynthesis
narcosis narcosis
narcosis continua continuous narcosis
narcosis por nitrógeno nitrogen narcosis
narcosugestión narcosuggestion
narcoterapia narcotherapy
narcótico narcotic
narcótico sintético synthetic narcotic
narcotismo narcotism
narcotización narcotization
nares nares
narratofilia narratophilia
nasal nasal
nasofaringe nasopharynx
nasomental nasomental
nativismo nativism
nativo native
natural natural
naturaleza nature
naturaleza contra crianza nature versus
    nurture
naturaleza de relaciones nature of
    relationships

naturaleza humana human nature
naturalista naturalistic
náusea nausea
náusea anticipatoria anticipatory nausea
náusea y vómitos anticipatorios anticipatory
    nausea and vomiting
nautomanía nautomania
navaja clasp-knife
navaja de Occam Occam's razor
nebulosidad cloudiness
necesidad need
necesidad afiliativa affiliative need
necesidad básica basic need
necesidad cognitiva cognitive need
necesidad convencional conventional need
necesidad de abatimiento abasement need
necesidad de afiliación affiliation need
necesidad de amor love need
necesidad de aprobación approval need
necesidad de castigo need for punishment
necesidad de conocimiento cognizance need
necesidad de construcción construction need
necesidad de contrarrestar counteraction
    need
necesidad de crianza nurturance need
necesidad de culpa blame need
necesidad de deferencia deference need
necesidad de determinante determinant need
necesidad de dominancia dominance need
necesidad de estado alto status need
necesidad de estima esteem need
necesidad de evitación de daño
    harm-avoidance need
necesidad de existencia existence need
necesidad de exposición exposition need
necesidad de identidad identity need
necesidad de instinto instinct need
necesidad de logro achievement need
necesidad de marco de orientación frame of
    orientation need
necesidad de reclusión seclusion need
necesidad de seguridad safety need
necesidad de socorro succorance need
necesidad de sueño need for sleep
necesidad de sueño de movimientos oculares
    no rápidos need for non-rapid eye
    movement sleep
necesidad de sueños need for dreams
necesidad derivada derived need
necesidad exhibicionista exhibitionistic need
necesidad fisiológica physiological need
necesidad primaria primary need
necesidad psicogénica psychogenic need
necesidad psicológica psychological need
necesidad psicológica para soñar
    psychological need for dreaming
necesidad social social need
necesidad somatogénica somatogenic need
necesidades biológicas biological needs
necesidades comunitarias community needs
necesidades de dependencia dependency
    needs
necesidades del crecimiento growth needs
necesidades del ego ego needs
necesidades fundamentales fundamental

needs
necesidades instintoides instinctoid needs
necesidades intermedias intermediate needs
necesidades neuróticas neurotic needs
necesidades por deficiencia deficiency needs
necrofilia necrophilia
necrofílico necrophilic
necrofilismo necrophilism
necrofobia necrophobia
necromanía necromania
necromimesis necromimesis
necropsia necropsy
necrosadismo necrosadism
necrosis necrosis
necrosis cortical laminar laminar cortical
    necrosis
necrotizante necrotizing
nefrectomía nephrectomy
nefrectomía abdominal abdominal
    nephrectomy
nefrectomía paraperitoneal paraperitoneal
    nephrectomy
nefrectomía posterior posterior nephrectomy
nefritis intersticial interstitial nephritis
nefrona nephron
negación denial
negación de hechos denial of facts
negación de implicaciones denial of
    implications
negación de realidad reality denial
negativamente negatively
negativamente batmotrópico negatively
    bathmotropic
negativismo negativism
negativismo activo active negativism
negativismo ante mandatos command
    negativism
negativismo catatónico catatonic negativism
negativismo sexual sexual negativism
negativo negative
negligencia neglect
negligencia de niño neglect of child
negligencia de niños child neglect
negligencia del deber neglect of duty
negligencia maternal maternal neglect
negligencia profesional malpractice
negligencia sensorial sensory neglect
negligencia unilateral unilateral neglect
negociación negotiation
neo-freudiano neo-freudian
neoanalista neoanalyst
neoasociacionismo neoassociationism
neoatavismo neoatavism
neocerebelo neocerebellum
neoconductismo neobehaviorism
neoconductual neobehavioral
neoconexionismo neoconnectionism
neocorteza neocortex
neoencéfalo neencephalon
neoestriado neostriatum
neofasia neophasia
neofasia políglota polyglot neophasia
neofilia neophilia
neofobia neophobia
neofobia dietética dietary neophobia

neofrenia neophrenia
neografía neography
neografismo neographism
neolalia neolalia
neolalismo neolallism
neolocal neolocal
neología neology
neologismo neologism
neomimismo neomimism
neomnesis neomnesis
neonatal neonatal
neonato neonate
neopalio neopallium
neoplásico neoplastic
neoplasma neoplasm
neoplasma benigno benign neoplasm
neoplasma maligno malignant neoplasm
neopsicoanálisis neopsychoanalysis
neopsicoanalítico neopsychoanalytical
neopsíquico neopsychic
neosueño neosleep
neotenia neoteny
nervimoción nervimotion
nervimotor nervimotor
nervimovilidad nervimotility
nervina nervine
nervio nerve
nervio abducente abducent nerve
nervio accesorio accessory nerve
nervio accesorio espinal spinal accessory
    nerve
nervio acústico acoustic nerve
nervio auditivo auditory nerve
nervio autónomo autonomic nerve
nervio centrífugo centrifugal nerve
nervio coclear cochlear nerve
nervio depresor depressor nerve
nervio estatoacústico statoacoustic nerve
nervio facial facial nerve
nervio frénico phrenic nerve
nervio genital-femoral genital-femoral nerve
nervio glosofaríngeo glossopharyngeal nerve
nervio gustatorio gustatory nerve
nervio hipogástrico hypogastric nerve
nervio hipogloso hypoglossal nerve
nervio iliohipogástrico iliohypogastric nerve
nervio ilioinguinal ilioinguinal nerve
nervio lingual lingual nerve
nervio lumbar lumbar nerve
nervio motor motor nerve
nervio neumogástrico pneumogastric nerve
nervio oculomotor oculomotor nerve
nervio olfatorio olfactory nerve
nervio óptico optic nerve
nervio patético pathetic nerve
nervio pudendo pudendal nerve
nervio sacral sacral nerve
nervio sensorial sensory nerve
nervio torácico thoracic nerve
nervio trigeminal trigeminal nerve
nervio troclear trochlear nerve
nervio trocular trocular nerve
nervio vago vagus nerve
nervio vestibular vestibular nerve
nervio vestibulococlear vestibulocochlear

nerve
nervios cervicales cervical nerves
nervios craneales cranial nerves
nervios espinales spinal nerves
nerviosidad nervousness
nervioso nervous
neumatocele pneumatocele
neumatocele extracraneal extracranial
pneumatocele
neumatocele intracraneal intracranial
pneumatocele
neumatorraquis pneumatorrhachis
neumocardiógrafo pneumocardiograph
neumocefalia pneumocephalus
neumocele pneumocele
neumocele extracraneal extracranial
pneumocele
neumocele intracraneal intracranial
pneumocele
neumocráneo pneumocranium
neumoencefalografía
pneumoencephalography
neumoencefalograma pneumoencephalogram
neumofonía pneumophonia
neumogástrico pneumogastric
neumógrafo pneumograph
neumonía pneumonia
neumoorbitografía pneumoorbitography
neumorraquis pneumorrhachis
neumotáxico pneumotaxic
neumoterapia pneumotherapy
neumotórax pneumothorax
neumoventrículo pneumoventricle
neuradinamia neuradynamia
neuragmia neuragmia
neural neural
neuralgia neuralgia
neuralgia alucinatoria hallucinatory neuralgia
neuralgia ciática sciatic neuralgia
neuralgia de Fothergill Fothergill's neuralgia
neuralgia de Hunt Hunt's neuralgia
neuralgia de Morton Morton's neuralgia
neuralgia de muñón stump neuralgia
neuralgia epileptiforme epileptiform
neuralgia
neuralgia facial facial neuralgia
neuralgia facial atípica atypical facial
neuralgia
neuralgia geniculada geniculate neuralgia
neuralgia glosofaríngea glossopharyngeal
neuralgia
neuralgia idiopática idiopathic neuralgia
neuralgia intercostal intercostal neuralgia
neuralgia mamaria mammary neuralgia
neuralgia migrañosa periódica periodic
migrainous neuralgia
neuralgia occipital occipital neuralgia
neuralgia reminiscente reminiscent neuralgia
neuralgia roja red neuralgia
neuralgia sintomática symptomatic neuralgia
neuralgia suboccipital suboccipital neuralgia
neuralgia supraorbitaria supraorbital
neuralgia
neuralgia trifacial trifacial neuralgia
neuralgia trigeminal trigeminal neuralgia

neuralgia trigeminal atípica atypical
trigeminal neuralgia
neurálgico neuralgic
neuralgiforme neuralgiform
neuranagénesis neuranagenesis
neurapraxia neurapraxia
neurastenia neurasthenia
neurastenia angioparalítica angioparalytic
neurasthenia
neurastenia angiopática angiopathic
neurasthenia
neurastenia experimental experimental
neurasthenia
neurastenia gástrica gastric neurasthenia
neurastenia grave neurasthenia gravis
neurastenia precoz neurasthenia precox
neurastenia primaria primary neurasthenia
neurastenia profesional professional
neurasthenia
neurastenia pulsátil pulsating neurasthenia
neurastenia sexual sexual neurasthenia
neurastenia traumática traumatic
neurasthenia
neurasténico neurasthenic
neurastenoide neurasthenoid
neuraxis neuraxis
neuraxón neuraxon
neurecotmía neurectomy
neurecotmía presacra presacral neurectomy
neurecotmía retrogasseriana retrogasserian
neurectomy
neurectasia neurectasy
neurectasis neurectasis
neurectopia neurectopy
neuremia neuremia
neurérgico neurergic
neurexéresis neurexeresis
neuriatría neuriatry
neurilema neurilemma
neurilemoma neurilemoma
neurilemoma acústico acoustic neurilemoma
neurilemoma tipo A de Antoni Antoni type A
neurilemoma
neurilemoma tipo B de Antoni Antoni type B
neurilemoma
neurilidad neurility
neurimotor neurimotor
neurimovilidad neurimotility
neurina neurin
neurinoma neurinoma
neurinoma acústico acoustic neurinoma
neurinomatosis neurinomatosis
neurítico neuritic
neuritis neuritis
neuritis adventicia adventitial neuritis
neuritis ascendente ascending neuritis
neuritis axial axial neuritis
neuritis braquial brachial neuritis
neuritis central central neuritis
neuritis ciática sciatic neuritis
neuritis de Eichhorst Eichhorst's neuritis
neuritis de Falopio Fallopian neuritis
neuritis de Leyden Leyden's neuritis
neuritis descendiente descending neuritis
neuritis endémica endemic neuritis

neuritis intersticial interstitial neuritis
neuritis intraocular intraocular neuritis
neuritis múltiple multiple neuritis
neuritis occipital occipital neuritis
neuritis óptica optic neuritis
neuritis parenquimatosa parenchymatous
   neuritis
neuritis retrobulbar retrobulbar neuritis
neuritis segmentaria segmental neuritis
neuritis suboccipital suboccipital neuritis
neuritis tóxica toxic neuritis
neuritis traumática traumatic neuritis
neuroadaptación neuroadaptation
neuroalergia neuroallergy
neuroanálisis neuroanalysis
neuroanastomosis neuroanastomosis
neuroanatomía neuroanatomy
neuroanatomía química chemical
   neuroanatomy
neuroartritismo neuroarthritism
neuroartropatía neuroarthropathy
neuroaumento neuroaugmentation
neuroaxonal neuroaxonal
neurobiotáctico neurobiotactic
neurobiotaxis neurobiotaxis
neuroblasto neuroblast
neuroblastoma neuroblastoma
neuroblastoma olfatorio olfactory
   neuroblastoma
neurocardíaco neurocardiac
neurocentral neurocentral
neurociencia neuroscience
neurocirculatorio neurocirculatory
neurocirugía neurosurgery
neurocirugía funcional functional
   neurosurgery
neurocirujano neurosurgeon
neurocito neurocyte
neurocitólisis neurocytolysis
neurocitoma neurocytoma
neurocladismo neurocladism
neuroconductual neurobehavioral
neurocoriorretinitis neurochorioretinitis
neurocoroiditis neurochoroiditis
neurocristopatía neurocristopathy
neurocutáneo neurocutaneous
neurodermatitis neurodermatitis
neurodinia neurodynia
neuroectomía neuroectomy
neuroefector neuroeffector
neuroencefalomielopatía
   neuroencephalomyelopathy
neuroendocrino neuroendocrine
neuroendocrinología neuroendocrinology
neuroespasmo neurospasm
neuroestimulador neurostimulator
neuroetología neuroethology
neurofarmacología neuropharmacology
neurofibrilar neurofibrillary
neurofibrilla neurofibril
neurofibroma neurofibroma
neurofibroma plexiforme plexiform
   neurofibroma
neurofibromatosis neurofibromatosis
neurofibromatosis abortivo abortive

neurofibromatosis
neurofibromatosis incompleta incomplete
   neurofibromatosis
neurofílico neurophillic
neurofisinas neurophysins
neurofisiología neurophysiology
neurofisiológico neurophysiological
neurofrenia neurophrenia
neuroftalmología neurophthalmology
neurogénesis neurogenesis
neurogenético neurogenetic
neurogénico neurogenic
neurógeno neurogenous
neuroglia neuroglia
neuroglial neuroglial
neurogliomatosis neurogliomatosis
neurografía neurography
neurograma neurogram
neurohipnosis neurohypnosis
neurohipófisis neurohypophysis
neurohormona neurohormone
neurohumor neurohumor
neurohumoral neurohumoral
neuroinducción neuroinduction
neurolema neurolemma
neuroléptico neuroleptic
neurolinfomatosis neurolymphomatosis
neurolingüística neurolinguistics
neurolingüítico neurolinguistic
neurólisis neurolysis
neurolítico neurolytic
neurología neurology
neurología conductual behavioral neurology
neurológico neurological
neurólogo neurologist
neuroma neuroma
neuroma acústico acoustic neuroma
neuroma cutáneo neuroma cutis
neuroma de amputación amputation neuroma
neuroma de Verneuil Verneuil's neuroma
neuroma falso false neuroma
neuroma fibrilar fibrillary neuroma
neuroma plexiforme plexiform neuroma
neuroma telangiectásico neuroma
   telangiectodes
neuroma traumático traumatic neuroma
neuromalacia neuromalacia
neuromatosis neuromatosis
neuromelanina neuromelanin
neuromensajero neuromessenger
neurométrica neurometrics
neuromiastenia neuromyasthenia
neuromiastenia epidémica epidemic
   neuromyasthenia
neuromielitis neuromyelitis
neuromielitis óptica neuromyelitis optica
neuromimesis neuromimesis
neuromiopatía neuromyopathy
neuromiopatía carcinomatosa carcinomatous
   neuromyopathy
neuromiositis neuromyositis
neuromodulador neuromodulator
neuromuscular neuromuscular
neurona neuron
neurona autonómica posganglionar

postganglionic autonomic neuron
neurona autonómica preganglionar
  preganglionic autonomic neuron
neurona bipolar bipolar neuron
neurona colinérgica cholinergic neuron
neurona de asociación association neuron
neurona de Golgi Golgi neuron
neurona dopaminérgica dopaminergic neuron
neurona internuncial internuncial neuron
neurona motora motor neuron
neurona motora gama gamma motor neuron
neurona motora inferior lower motor neuron
neurona motora superior upper motor
  neuron
neurona multipolar multipolar neuron
neurona noradrenérgica noradrenergic
  neuron
neurona sensorial sensory neuron
neurona serotonérgica serotonergic neuron
neurona tipo I de Golgi Golgi type I neuron
neurona tipo II de Golgi Golgi type II neuron
neurona unipolar unipolar neuron
neuronal neuronal
neuronas aferentes afferent neurons
neuronitis neuronitis
neuronixis neuronyxis
neuronofagia neuronophagy
neuronófago neuronophage
neuronopatía neuronopathy
neuronopatía sensorial sensory neuronopathy
neurooftalmología neuroopthalmalogy
neurooncología neurooncology
neurootología neurootology
neuropapilitis neuropapillitis
neuroparálisis neuroparalysis
neuroparalítico neuroparalytic
neurópata neuropath
neuropatía neuropathy
neuropatía alcohólica alcoholic neuropathy
neuropatía amiloide familiar familial
  amyloid neuropathy
neuropatía axonal gigante giant axonal
  neuropathy
neuropatía de entrampamiento entrapment
  neuropathy
neuropatía del plexo braquial brachial plexus
  neuropathy
neuropatía diabética diabetic neuropathy
neuropatía diftérica diphtheritic neuropathy
neuropatía distal simétrica symmetric distal
  neuropathy
neuropatía en bulbo de cebolla onion bulb
  neuropathy
neuropatía gástrica gastric neuropathy
neuropatía hipertrófica hereditaria
  hereditary hypertrophic neuropathy
neuropatía intersticial hipertrófica
  hypertrophic interstitial neuropathy
neuropatía leprosa leprous neuropathy
neuropatía motora asimétrica asymmetric
  motor neuropathy
neuropatía motora por dapsona motor
  dapsone neuropathy
neuropatía óptica isquémica ischemic optic
  neuropathy

neuropatía periférica peripheral neuropathy
neuropatía por isoniazida isoniazid
  neuropathy
neuropatía por plomo lead neuropathy
neuropatía por vitamina B-12 vitamin B-12
  neuropathy
neuropatía radicular sensorial hereditaria
  hereditary sensory radicular neuropathy
neuropatía segmentaria segmental
  neuropathy
**neuropatía sensorial congénita con
  anhidrosis** congenital sensory neuropathy
  with anhidrosis
neuropático neuropathic
neuropatogénesis neuropathogenesis
neuropatología neuropathology
neuropatológico neuropathological
neuropéptido neuropeptide
neurópilo neuropil
neuroplasma neuroplasm
neuroplastia neuroplasty
neuroplégico neuroplegic
neuroplexo neuroplexus
neuropsicodiagnóstico neuropsychodiagnosis
neuropsicofarmacología
  neuropsychopharmacology
neuropsicología neuropsychology
neuropsicológico neuropsychological
neuropsicopatía neuropsychopathy
neuropsicopático neuropsychopathic
neuropsicosis neuropsychosis
neuropsicosis de defensa defense
  neuropsychosis
neuropsicotrópico neuropsychotropic
neuropsiquiatría neuropsychiatry
neuroquímica neurochemistry
neuroquímica conductual behavioral
  neurochemistry
neuroquímica del sueño neurochemistry of
  sleep
neuroquímico neurochemical
neurorrafia neurorrhaphy
neurorreceptor neuroreceptor
neurorrecidiva neurorecidive
neurorrecurrencia neurorecurrence
neurorrelapso neurorelapse
neurorretinitis neuroretinitis
neurosarcocleisis neurosarcocleisis
neurosarcoidosis neurosarcoidosis
neuroschwannoma neuroschwannoma
neurosecretorio neurosecretory
neurosífilis neurosyphilis
neurosífilis asintomática asymptomatic
  neurosyphilis
neurosífilis intersticial interstitial
  neurosyphilis
neurosífilis parenquimatosa parenchymatous
  neurosyphilis
neurosis neurosis
neurosis analítica analytic neurosis
neurosis artificial artificial neurosis
neurosis cardíaca cardiac neurosis
neurosis compulsiva compulsive neurosis
neurosis de accidentes accident neurosis
neurosis de ama de casa housewife's neurosis

neurosis de ansiedad anxiety neurosis
neurosis de asociación association neurosis
neurosis de calambre cramp neurosis
neurosis de combate battle neurosis
neurosis de compensación compensation
    neurosis
neurosis de compulsión compulsion neurosis
neurosis de contratransferencia
    countertransference neurosis
neurosis de despersonalización
    depersonalization neurosis
neurosis de despersonalización ansiosa
    anxiety depersonalization neurosis
neurosis de destino fate neurosis
neurosis de domingo Sunday neurosis
neurosis de ejecución performance neurosis
neurosis de expectación expectation neurosis
neurosis de fin de semana weekend neurosis
neurosis de histeria de conversión
    conversion hysteria neurosis
neurosis de impulsos impulse neurosis
neurosis de indemnidad indemnity neurosis
neurosis de lo infinito infinity neurosis
neurosis de muerte death neurosis
neurosis de niñez childhood neurosis
neurosis de pensión pension neurosis
neurosis de prisión prison neurosis
neurosis de promoción promotion neurosis
neurosis de regresión regression neurosis
neurosis de retiro retirement neurosis
neurosis de síntomas symptom neurosis
neurosis de situación situation neurosis
neurosis de torsión torsion neurosis
neurosis de transferencia transference
    neurosis
neurosis de transferencia regresiva
    regressive transference neurosis
neurosis del carácter character neurosis
neurosis del ego ego neurosis
neurosis del éxito success neurosis
neurosis del quizás perhaps neurosis
neurosis depresiva depressive neurosis
neurosis descompensativa decompensative
    neurosis
neurosis edípica oedipal neurosis
neurosis esofagal esophageal neurosis
neurosis existencial existential neurosis
neurosis experimental experimental neurosis
neurosis familiar family neurosis
neurosis fóbica phobic neurosis
neurosis hipocondríaca hypochondriacal
    neurosis
neurosis histérica hysterical neurosis
neurosis institucional institutional neurosis
neurosis maligna malignant neurosis
neurosis mixta mixed neurosis
neurosis monosintomática monosymptomatic
    neurosis
neurosis motora motor neurosis
neurosis narcisista narcissistic neurosis
neurosis neurasténica neurasthenic neurosis
neurosis noogénica noogenic neurosis
neurosis nuclear nuclear neurosis
neurosis obsesiva obsessional neurosis
neurosis obsesiva-compulsiva

    obsessive-compulsive neurosis
neurosis oclusal occlusal neurosis
neurosis ocupacional occupational neurosis
neurosis oral oral neurosis
neurosis posconcusión postconcussion
    neurosis
neurosis postraumática posttraumatic
    neurosis
neurosis profesional professional neurosis
neurosis real actual neurosis
neurosis seudoesquizofrénica
    pseudoschizophrenic neurosis
neurosis situacional situational neurosis
neurosis tardía neurosis tarda
neurosis traumática traumatic neurosis
neurosis vegetativa vegetative neurosis
neurosis visceral visceral neurosis
neurosis orgánica organ neurosis
neurostenia neurosthenia
neurosutura neurosuture
neurotabes neurotabes
neurotabes periférico de Dejerine Dejerine's
    peripheral neurotabes
neurotensina neurotensin
neurotensión neurotension
neurotequeoma neurothekeoma
neuroterapéutica neurotherapeutics
neuroterapia neurotherapy
neuroticismo neuroticism
neurótico neurotic
neurotigénesis neurotigenesis
neurotigénico neurotigenic
neurotización neurotization
neurotizar neurotize
neurotlipsia neurothlipsia
neurotlipsis neurothlipsis
neurotmesis neurotmesis
neurotología neurotology
neurotomía neurotomy
neurotomía retrogasseriana retrogasserian
    neurotomy
neurótomo neurotome
neurotonía neurotony
neurotónico neurotonic
neurotoxicidad inducida por el plomo
    asintomática asymptomatic lead-induced
    neurotoxicity
neurotóxico neurotoxic
neurotoxina neurotoxin
neurotransmisión neurotransmission
neurotransmisor neurotransmitter
neurotrauma neurotrauma
neurotripsia neurotripsy
neurotrofia neurotrophy
neurotrófico neurotrophic
neurotropía neurotropy
neurotrópico neurotropic
neurotropismo neurotropism
neurotrosis neurotrosis
neurovaricosidad neurovaricosity
neurovaricosis neurovaricosis
neurovascular neurovascular
neurulación neurulation
neutral neutral
neutralidad neutrality

neutralización neutralization
neutralizador neutralizer
nevo nevus
nevoide nevoid
nexo nexus
niacina niacin
nialamida nialamide
nicotina nicotine
nicotínico nicotinic
nictación nictation
nictalgia nyctalgia
nictalopía nyctalopia
nictitación nictitation
nictitante nictitating
nictofilia nyctophilia
nictofobia nyctophobia
nictofonía nyctophonia
nicho ecológico ecological niche
nido vacío empty nest
niebla mental mental fog
nigroestriado nigrostriatal
nihilismo nihilism
nihilismo terapéutico therapeutic nihilism
nihilístico nihilistic
nimetazepam nimetazepam
ninfolepsia nympholepsy
ninfomanía nymphomania
ninfomaníaca nymphomaniac
ninfomaníaco nymphomaniacal
niñera nanny
niñez childhood
niñez temprana early childhood
niño child
niño abusable abusable child
niño abusado abused child
niño adaptado adapted child
niño adoptado adopted child
niño adoptivo adoptive child
niño ansioso-ambivalente anxious-ambivalent
  child
niño ansioso-evitante anxious-avoidant child
niño atípico atypical child
niño autista autistic child
niño consentido spoiled child
niño de ático attic child
niño difícil difficult child
niño dotado gifted child
niño especial special child
niño excepcional exceptional child
niño fácil easy child
niño feral feral child
niño golpeado battered child
niño inadaptado maladjusted child
niño lesionado cerebralmente brain-injured
  child
niño problema problem child
niño prodigio child prodigy
niño retardado del habla speech-retarded
  child
niño vulnerable vulnerable child
niños a riesgo children at risk
niños como testigos children as witnesses
niños preescolares preschool children
nirvana nirvana
nistagmo nystagmus

nistagmo calórico caloric nystagmus
nistagmo compensatorio compensatory
  nystagmus
nistagmo congénito congenital nystagmus
nistagmo de Bekhterev Bekhterev's
  nystagmus
nistagmo de retracción retraction nystagmus
nistagmo fisiológico physiological nystagmus
nistagmo hacia abajo down-beat nystagmus
nistagmo inverso inverse nystagmus
nistagmo optocinético optokinetic nystagmus
nistagmo palatal palatal nystagmus
nistagmo posrotacional postrotational
  nystagmus
nit nit
nitrato de potasio potassium nitrate
nitrazepam nitrazepam
nitrito de amilo amyl nitrite
nitrógeno ureico sanguíneo blood urea
  nitrogen
nivel level
nivel alfa alpha level
nivel beta beta level
nivel convencional conventional level
nivel convencional del desarrollo moral
  conventional level of moral development
nivel de actividad activity level
nivel de adaptación adaptation level
nivel de andrógeno androgen level
nivel de apego level of attachment
nivel de aptitud fitness level
nivel de aspiración aspiration level
nivel de atención attention level
nivel de cafeína sérico serum caffeine level
nivel de comparación comparison level
nivel de conciencia level of consciousness
nivel de conciencia cognitiva
  cognitive-awareness level
nivel de confianza level of confidence
nivel de cuidado level of care
nivel de descentración level of decentration
nivel de droga drug level
nivel de emoción conductual-expresiva
  behavioral-expressive level of emotion
nivel de incertidumbre uncertainty level
nivel de irrealidad irreality level
nivel de logro level of achievement
nivel de mantenimiento maintenance level
nivel de operaciones concretas concrete
  operations level
nivel de presión de sonido sound-pressure
  level
nivel de resistencia basal basal resistance
  level
nivel de riesgo risk level
nivel de sensación sensation level
nivel de significación significance level
nivel de tolerancia tolerance level
nivel del desarrollo level of development
nivel fálico phallic level
nivel genital genital level
nivel hedónico hedonic level
nivel mental mental level
nivel microscópico microscopic level
nivel ocupacional occupational level

nivel operante operant level
nivel operatorio formal formal operatory level
nivel plasmático plasma level
nivel posconvencional postconventional level
nivel posconvencional del desarrollo moral postconventional level of moral development
nivel preconvencional preconventional level
nivel preconvencional del desarrollo moral preconventional level of moral development
nivel preedípico preoedipal level
nivel pregenital pregenital level
nivel preoperatorio preoperatory level
nivel sanguíneo blood level
nivel sensorimotor sensory-motor level
nivel sérico serum level
nivel vegetativo vegetative level
nivelación leveling
nivelación-agudización leveling-sharpening
niveles de procesamiento levels of processing
niveles del desarrollo developmental levels
no aditivo nonadditive
no afectivo nonaffective
no agresivo nonaggressive
no aprendido unlearned
no aversivo nonaversive
no cetónico nonketonic
no clasificado en otra parte not elsewhere classified
no complementario noncomplementary
no comunicante noncommunicating
no contingente noncontingent
no directivo nondirective
no disyunción nondisjunction
no dominante nondominant
no especificado unspecified
no especificado de otra manera not otherwise specified
no específico nonspecific
no estructurado unstructured
no experimental nonexperimental
no fluente nonfluent
no fóbico nonphobic
no intermitente nonintermittent
no invasor noninvasive
no lineal nonlinear
no métrico nonmetric
no paramétrico nonparametric
no participante nonparticipant
no patológico nonpathological
no ponderado unweighted
no preferido nonpreferred
no psicótico nonpsychotic
no psicotrópic nonpsychotropic
no racional nonrational
no reactivo nonreactive
no recombinante nonrecombinant
no reconocimiento nonrecognition
no reproductivo nonreproductive
no resuelto unresolved
no sistemático nonsystematic
no social nonsocial
no tradicional nontraditional
no verbal nonverbal

no yo not me
nociceptivo nociceptive
nociceptor nociceptor
nocifensor nocifensor
nociinfluencia nociinfluence
nocipercepción nociperception
nocivo noxious
noctambulación noctambulation
noctifobia noctiphobia
nocturia nocturia
nocturno nocturnal
noche de boda wedding night
nodal nodal
nodular nodular
nódulo nodule
nódulo de Ranvier Ranvier's node
nódulo de Schmorl Schmorl's nodule
nódulos de Durck Durck's nodes
noemático noematic
noesis noesis
noético noetic
nomadismo nomadism
nomatofobia nomatophobia
nombramiento naming
nombre genérico generic name
nomenclatura nomenclature
nomifensina nomifensine
nominal nominal
nominalismo nominalism
nomógrafo nomograph
nomograma nomogram
nomograma de d'Ocagne d'Ocagne nomogram
nomológico nomological
nomotético nomothetic
non compos mentis non compos mentis
non sequitur non sequitur
noogénico noogenic
noología noology
nootrópico nootropic
noradrenalina noradrenaline
noradrenérgico noradrenergic
nordazepam nordazepam
norepinefrina norepinephrine
norma norm
norma de edad age norm
norma de grado grade norm
norma de grupo group norm
norma de reciprocidad reciprocity norm
norma de responsabilidad social social-responsibility norm
norma del desarrollo developmental norm
norma ocupacional occupational norm
norma percentil percentile norm
norma psíquica psychic norm
norma social social norm
normalidad normality
normalización normalization
normalizar normalize
normas culturales cultural norms
normas de competencia competence standards
normas de iluminación illumination standards
normativo normative
normotenso normotensive

normotimótico normothymotic
normotípico normotypical
normotipo normotype
normotónico normotonic
nortriptilina nortriptyline
nosocomial nosocomial
nosocomio nosocomium
nosofilia nosophilia
nosofobia nosophobia
nosogénesis nosogenesis
nosogenia nosogeny
nosografía nosography
nosología nosology
nosología psiquiátrica psychiatric nosology
nosológico nosological
nosomanía nosomania
nostalgia nostalgia
nostofobia nostophobia
nostomanía nostomania
notanencefalia notanencephalia
notocordio notochord
notogénesis notogenesis
noumenal noumenal
nous nous
novedad novelty
noveno nervio craneal ninth cranial nerve
noviciado apprenticeship
noxa noxa
nuclear nuclear
núcleo nucleus
núcleo abducente abducens nucleus
núcleo anterior anterior nucleus
núcleo anterior ventral ventral anterior
    nucleus
núcleo arqueado arcuate nucleus
núcleo caudado caudate nucleus
núcleo celular cell nucleus
núcleo cervical lateral lateral cervical nucleus
núcleo corticobulbar corticobulbar nucleus
núcleo corticopontino corticopontine nucleus
núcleo cuneiforme cuneate nucleus
núcleo de Edinger-Westphal
    Edinger-Westphal nucleus
núcleo del rafe nucleus of the raphe
núcleo dentado dentate nucleus
núcleo dorsal lateral lateral dorsal nucleus
núcleo dorsal medial medial dorsal nucleus
núcleo dorsolateral dorsolateral nucleus
núcleo dorsomedial dorsomedial nucleus
núcleo geniculado lateral lateral geniculate
    nucleus
núcleo geniculado medial medial geniculate
    nucleus
núcleo globoso nucleus globosus
núcleo grácil gracilis nucleus
núcleo lateral ventral ventral lateral nucleus
núcleo lenticular lenticular nucleus
núcleo mesencefálico mesencephalic nucleus
núcleo neurótico neurotic nucleus
núcleo oculomotor oculomotor nucleus
núcleo olivar olivary nucleus
núcleo olivar superior superior olivary
    nucleus
núcleo paraventricular paraventricular
    nucleus

núcleo pontino pontine nucleus
núcleo posterior posterior nucleus
núcleo posterior lateral lateral posterior
    nucleus
núcleo posterior ventral ventral posterior
    nucleus
núcleo posventral postventral nucleus
núcleo pulposo nucleus pulposus
núcleo reticular reticular nucleus
núcleo trigeminal trigeminal nucleus
núcleo trigeminal espinal spinal trigeminal
    nucleus
núcleo rojo red nucleus
núcleo subtalámico subthalamic nucleus
núcleo supraquiasmático suprachiasmatic
    nucleus
núcleo talámico thalamic nucleus
núcleo talámico lateral lateral thalamic
    nucleus
núcleo tectal tectal nucleus
núcleo tegmental central central tegmental
    nucleus
núcleo torácico nucleus thoracicus
núcleo ventromedial ventromedial nucleus
nucleófugo nucleofugal
nucléolo nucleolus
nucleópeto nucleopetal
núcleos anteriores del tálamo anterior nuclei
    of thalamus
núcleos cocleares cochlear nuclei
núcleos de asociación association nuclei
núcleos del ego ego nuclei
nucleótido nucleotide
nudismo nudism
nudo en la garganta lump in the throat
nulípara nulliparous
nulo null
numérico numerical
número aleatorio random number
número cromosómico chromosome number
número diploide diploid number
número haploide haploid number
número índice index number
nutación nutation
nutrición nutrition
nutricional nutritional
nutrimento emocional emotional nutriment

O

obdormición obdormition
obediencia obedience
obediencia a la autoridad obedience to authority
obediencia automática automatic obedience
obediencia destructiva destructive obedience
obediencia diferida deferred obedience
obesidad obesity
obesidad hipertrófica hypertrophic obesity
obesidad hipotalámica hypothalamic obesity
objetivación objectivation
objetividad objectivity
objetivismo objectivism
objetivo objective
objeto object
objeto bueno good object
objeto de amor love object
objeto de ansiedad anxiety object
objeto de estímulo stimulus object
objeto de instinto object of instinct
objeto de selección narcisista narcissistic object-choice
objeto fin goal object
objeto malo bad object
objeto percibido perceived object
objeto primario primary object
objeto sexual sexual object
objeto social social object
objeto transicional transitional object
objeto de medios means object
oblatividad oblativity
oblicuo oblique
oblicuo inferior inferior oblique
obligación moral moral obligation
obligaciones de pacientes patient obligations
obligaciones de terapeuta therapist obligations
obligatorio obligatory
oblongo oblongata
obnubilación obnubilation
obscenidad obscenity
obscurantismo obscurantism
observación observation
observación aleatoria random observation
observación conductual behavioral observation
observación de participante participant observation
observación directa direct observation
observación en masa mass observation
observación naturalista naturalistic observation
observacional observational
observaciones sistemáticas systematic observations

observador observer
observador de proceso process observer
observador escondido hidden observer
observador estándar standard observer
observador ideal ideal observer
observador ingenuo naive observer
observador participante participant observer
observador no participante nonparticipant observer
obsesión obsession
obsesión de contaminación contamination obsession
obsesión de contar counting obsession
obsesión de lavarse las manos hand-washing obsession
obsesión enmascarada masked obsession
obsesión impulsiva impulsive obsession
obsesión inhibitoria inhibitory obsession
obsesión pura pure obsession
obsesión somática somatic obsession
obsesiones y compulsiones obsessions and compulsions
obsesivo obsessive
obsesivo-compulsivo obsessive-compulsive
obsolescencia de papel role obsolescence
obstétrico obstetrical
obstinadamente obstinately
obstinado obstinate
obstipación obstipation
obstrucción obstruction
obstrucción de pensamientos thought obstruction
obstructivo obstructive
obtenido obtained
obturación obturation
obturador obturator
obtusión obtusion
obtuso obtuse
ocasional occasional
occipital occipital
ocio leisure
oclofobia ochlophobia
oclusión occlusion
oclusión glotal glottal stop
oclusivo occlusive
octava octave
ocular ocular
oculista oculist
oculocefálico oculocephalic
oculocefalógiro oculocephalogyric
oculocerebral oculocerebral
oculocerebrorrenal oculocerebrorenal
oculoencefálico oculoencephalic
oculógiro oculogyric
oculomotor oculomotor
ocultismo occultism
oculto occult
ocupación occupation
ocupación estimulante stimulating occupation
ocupación sedante sedative occupation
ocupacional occupational
odaxesmo odaxesmus
odaxético odaxetic
odinofobia odynophobia

odinómetro odynometer
odio hatred
odio propio self-hate
odogénesis odogenesis
odonterismo odonterism
odontofobia odontophobia
odontoneuralgia odontoneuralgia
odorífero odoriferous
odorimetría odorimetry
ofensa sexual sexual offense
ofensor sexual sex offender
ofensor sexual adolescente adolescent sex
 offender
ofidiofilia ophidiophilia
ofidiofobia ophidiophobia
ofriosis ophryosis
oftalmía ophthalmia
oftalmía eléctrica electric ophthalmia
oftalmía neonatal ophthalmia neonatorum
oftalmía neuroparalítica neuroparalytic
 ophthalmia
oftálmico ophthalmic
oftalmología ophthalmology
oftalmómetro ophthalmometer
oftalmoplejía ophthalmoplegia
oftalmoplejía de Parinaud Parinaud's
 ophthalmoplegia
oftalmoplejía externa ophthalmoplegia
 externa
oftalmoplejía fascicular fascicular
 ophthalmoplegia
oftalmoplejía infecciosa infectious
 ophthalmoplegia
oftalmoplejía interna ophthalmoplegia interna
oftalmoplejía internuclear ophthalmoplegia
 internuclearis
oftalmoplejía nuclear nuclear
 ophthalmoplegia
oftalmoplejía orbitaria ophthalmoplegia
 orbital
oftalmoplejía parcial ophthalmoplegia
 partialis
oftalmoplejía progresiva ophthalmoplegia
 progressiva
oftalmoplejía total ophthalmoplegia totalis
oftalmopléjico ophthalmoplegic
oftalmoscopia ophthalmoscopy
oftalmoscopia métrica metric
 ophthalmoscopy
oftalmoscopio ophthalmoscope
ofuscación obfuscation
oicofobia oikophobia
oicofugaz oikofugic
oicomanía oikomania
oicotrópico oikotropic
oído externo external ear
oído interno internal ear
oído medio middle ear
oinomanía oinomania
oiquiofobia oikiophobia
ojiva ogive
ojo compuesto compound eye
ojo de cíclope cyclopean eye
ojo de mapache raccoon eye
ojo de nautilo nautilus eye

ojo dominante leading eye
ojos contra cámaras eyes versus cameras
ojos danzantes dancing eyes
olfacción olfaction
olfato smell
olfatofobia olfactophobia
olfatometría olfactometry
olfatómetro olfactometer
olfatómetro de Zwaardemaker
 Zwaardemaker olfactometer
olfatorio olfactory
oligodactilia oligodactyly
oligodendroblastoma oligodendroblastoma
oligodendrocito oligodendrocyte
oligodendroglia oligodendroglia
oligodendroglioma oligodendroglioma
oligoencefalia oligoencephaly
oligofrenia oligophrenia
oligofrenia fenilpirúvica phenylpyruvic
 oligophrenia
oligofrenia polidistrófica polydystrophic
 oligophrenia
oligohidramnios oligohydramnios
oligologia oligologia
oligomenorrea oligomenorrhea
oligoria oligoria
oligospermia oligospermia
oligotimia oligothymia
olivar olivary
olivopontocerebeloso olivopontocerebellar
olofonía olophonia
olor odor
olor corporal body odor
olvidar forget
olvidar en la vida tardía late life forgetting
olvidar intencional intentional forgetting
olvidar motivado motivated forgetting
olvido forgetfulness
omatidio ommatidium
omatofobia ommatophobia
ombrofobia ombrophobia
ombudsman ombudsman
omega omega
ómicron omicron
omisión omission
omisión del deber omission of duty
omnipotencia omnipotence
omnipotencia de pensamiento omnipotence
 of thought
omnipotencia del id id omnipotence
omnipotencia mágica magic omnipotence
omofagia omophagia
onanismo onanism
oncocitoma oncocytoma
oncogen oncogene
oncología oncology
onda wave
onda alfa alpha wave
onda beta beta wave
onda de Berger Berger wave
onda de dientes de sierra sawtooth waves
onda de excitación wave of excitation
onda de sonido sound wave
onda delta delta wave
onda en huso spindle wave

onda senoidal sine wave
onda theta theta wave
ondas aleatorias random waves
ondas cerebrales brain waves
ondas de tope plano flat top waves
ondas gama gamma waves
ondas kappa kappa waves
ondas ultrasónicas ultrasonic waves
onicofagia onychophagy
oniomanía oniomania
onírico oneiric
onirismo oneirism
onirocrítico oneirocritical
onirodelirio oneirodelirium
onirodinia oneirodynia
onirodinia activa oneirodynia activa
onirodinia grave oneirodynia gravis
onirofrenia oneirophrenia
onirogma oneirogmus
onirogonorrea oneirogonorrhea
onirología oneirology
oniromancia oneiromancy
onironoso oneironosus
oniroscopia oneiroscopy
onología onology
onomatofobia onomatophobia
onomatomanía onomatomania
onomatopeya onomatopoeia
onomatopoyesis onomatopoesis
ontoanálisis ontoanalysis
ontoanalítico ontoanalytic
ontogénesis ontogenesis
ontogenético ontogenetic
ontogenia ontogeny
ontología ontology
oocito oocyte
oocito secundario secondary oocyte
ooforectomía oophorectomy
oogénesis oogenesis
oogonio oogonuim
opacidad opacity
opaco opaque
operación operation
operación de Ball Ball's operation
operación de Cotte Cotte's operation
operación de Dana Dana's operation
operación de Dandy Dandy operation
operación de descompresión decompression
    operation
operación de Frazier-Spiller Frazier-Spiller
    operation
operación de Hunter Hunter's operation
operación de Keen Keen's operation
operación de Koerte-Ballance
    Koerte-Ballance operation
operación de Leriche Leriche's operation
operación de Matas Matas' operation
operación de Mikulicz Mikulicz operation
operación de Ogura Ogura operation
operación de Smith-Robinson
    Smith-Robinson operation
operación de Stoffel Stoffel's operation
operación de Stookey-Scarff Stookey-Scarff
    operation
operación simulada sham operation

operacional operational
operacionalismo operationalism
operaciones cognitivas cognitive operations
operaciones concretas concrete operations
operaciones de seguridad security operations
operaciones formales formal operations
operaciones intelectuales intellectual
    operations
operacionismo operationism
operador operator
operante operant
operante discriminado discriminated operant
operante libre free operant
operativo operative
operatorio operatory
opiáceo opiate
opinión opinion
opinión privada private opinion
opinión pública public opinion
opio opium
opioide opioid
opioide endógeno endogenous opioid
opiomanía opiomania
opipramol opipramol
opistoporeia opisthoporeia
opistótónico opisthotonic
opistotonoide opisthotonoid
opistótonos opisthotonos
oportunidades educacionales educational
    opportunities
oposición de pulgar thumb opposition
oposicional oppositional
opoterapia opotherapy
opsina opsin
opsoclono opsoclonus
opsomanía opsomania
óptica optics
óptica ecológica ecological optics
óptico optical
opticofacial opticofacial
optimismo optimism
optimismo terapéutico therapeutic optimism
óptimo optimum
optocinético optokinetic
optograma optogram
optometría optometry
optometrista optometrist
opuestos polares polar opposites
oración anómala anomalous sentence
oración de Babcock Babcock sentence
oraciones incompletas incomplete sentences
oraciones internalizadas internalized
    sentences
oral-agresivo oral-aggressive
oral-incorporativo oral-incorporative
oral-pasivo oral-passive
oral-receptivo oral-receptive
oralidad orality
oralismo oralism
orbicular orbicularis
orbital orbital
orbitomedial orbitomedial
orden order
orden compulsivo compulsive orderliness
orden de magnitud order of magnitude

orden de mérito order of merit
orden de nacimiento birth order
orden de rango rank order
orden social social order
ordenación array
ordenada ordinate
ordinal ordinal
oréctico orectic
oreja artificial artificial ear
orexia orexia
orexis orexis
organelo organelle
organicidad organicity
organicismo organicism
organicista organicist
orgánico organic
organigrama flow chart
organísmico organismic
organismo organism
organismo social social organism
organismo vacío empty organism
organización organization
organización cerebral cerebral organization
organización columnar de la corteza
    columnar organization of cortex
organización comunitaria community
    organization
organización de libido libido organization
organización de mantenimiento de salud
    health maintenance organization
organización de pacientes mentales mental
    patient organization
organización de personalidad personality
    organization
organización de personalidad fronteriza
    borderline personality organization
organización de proveedores preferidos
    preferred provider organization
organización de rasgos trait organization
organización formal formal organization
organización informal informal organization
organización jerárquica hierarchical
    organization
organización perceptiva perceptual
    organization
organización pregenital pregenital
    organization
organización sensorial sensory organization
organización social social organization
organización somatotópica somatotopic
    organization
organización subjetiva subjective
    organization
organización tonotópica tonotopic
    organization
organización topográfica topographical
    organization
organización visual visual organization
organizativo organizational
órgano organ
órgano de Corti organ of Corti
órgano de Jacobson Jacobson's organ
órgano ejecutivo executive organ
órgano objetivo target organ
órgano sensorial sense organ

órgano tendinoso de Golgi Golgi tendon
    organ
órgano terminal end organ
órgano terminal de Ruffini Ruffini end organ
órgano terminal encapsulado encapsulated
    end organ
organogénesis organogenesis
organogenético organogenetic
organogénico organogenic
organoléptico organoleptic
órganos sexuales sex organs
organoterapia organotherapy
orgásmico orgasmic
orgasmo orgasm
orgasmo alimenticio alimentary orgasm
orgasmo aneyaculatorio anejaculatory
    orgasm
orgasmo clitoral clitoral orgasm
orgasmo farmacogénico pharmacogenic
    orgasm
orgasmo femenino inhibido inhibited female
    orgasm
orgasmo masculino inhibido inhibited male
    orgasm
orgasmo paradójico paradoxical orgasm
orgasmo seco dry orgasm
orgasmo sexual sexual orgasm
orgasmo vaginal vaginal orgasm
orgástico orgastic
orgía orgy
orgiástico orgiastic
orgón orgone
orgonomía orgonomy
orgullo pride
orgullo bruto brute pride
orgullo domesticado domesticated pride
orgullo fálico phallic pride
orgullo moral moral pride
orgullo neurótico neurotic pride
orgullo real real pride
orientación orientation
orientación autopsíquica autopsychic
    orientation
orientación de fin goal orientation
orientación de género gender orientation
orientación de ley y orden law-and-order
    orientation
orientación de mercadeo marketing
    orientation
orientación de realidad reality orientation
orientación derecha-izquierda right-left
    orientation
orientación doble double orientation
orientación espacial space orientation
orientación explotadora exploitative
    orientation
orientación hedonística hedonistic orientation
orientación instrumental-relativista
    instrumental-relativist orientation
orientación legalista legalistic orientation
orientación objetiva objective orientation
orientación oral oral orientation
orientación productiva productive orientation
orientación receptiva receptive orientation
orientación sexual sexual orientation

orientación subjetiva subjective orientation
orientación temporal temporal orientation
orientado a respuestas response oriented
orientado hacia tarea task-oriented
origen del habla speech origin
origen del lenguaje language origin
original original
originalidad originality
orina urine
orina sucia dirty urine
ornitinemia ornithinemia
ornitofobia ornithophobia
orofacial orofacial
orofaringe oropharynx
orogenital orogenital
orquiectomía orchiectomy
ortergasia orthergasia
ortobiosis orthobiosis
ortocorea orthochorea
ortofrenia orthophrenia
ortogénesis orthogenesis
ortogénica orthogenics
ortogenital orthogenital
ortognatia orthognathia
ortogonal orthogonal
ortógrado orthograde
ortografía orthography
ortomolecular orthomolecular
ortonasia orthonasia
ortopédico orthopedic
ortopnea orthopnea
ortopsiquiatría orthopsychiatry
ortóptica orthoptics
ortosimpático orthosympathetic
ortostático orthostatic
ortótica-prostética orthotics-prosthetics
ortótonos orthotonos
oscilación oscillation
oscilación conductual behavioral oscillation
oscilación retinal retinal oscillation
oscilógrafo oscillograph
oscilómetro oscillometer
osciloscopio oscilloscope
osfresia osphresia
osfresiofilia osphresiophilia
osfresiofobia osphresiophobia
osfresiolagnia osphresiolagnia
osfresis osphresis
osículo ossicle
osículos auditivos auditory ossicles
osificar ossify
osmoceptor osmoceptor
osmodisforia osmodysphoria
osmofobia osmophobia
osmorreceptor osmoreceptor
osmoterapia osmotherapy
osteítis osteitis
osteítis deformante osteitis deformans
osteítis fibrosa quística osteitis fibrosa cystica
ostensivo ostensive
osteoartritis osteoarthritis
osteodiastasis osteodiastasis
osteogénesis osteogenesis
osteogénesis imperfecta osteogenesis
   imperfecta

osteoma osteoma
osteomalacia osteomalacia
osteomalacia puerperal puerperal
   osteomalacia
osteomalacia senil senile osteomalacia
osteomielitis osteomyelitis
osteopático osteopathic
osteopetrosis osteopetrosis
osteopetrosis infantil infantile osteopetrosis
osteoplástico osteoplastic
osteoporosis osteoporosis
osteoporosis craneal circunscripta
   osteoporosis circumscripta cranii
osteoporosis postraumática posttraumatic
   osteoporosis
osteosarcoma osteosarcoma
osteotomía osteotomy
ostomía ostomy
otalgia otalgia
otalgia geniculada geniculate otalgia
ótico otic
otítico otitic
otitis otitis
otitis externa otitis externa
otitis interna otitis interna
otitis media otitis media
otitis media adhesiva adhesive otitis media
otitis media aguda acute otitis media
otitis media serosa serous otitis media
otocerebritis otocerebritis
otoencefalitis otoencephalitis
otoesclerosis otosclerosis
otogénico otogenic
otohemineurastenia otohemineurasthenia
otolaringología otolaryngology
otolito otolith
otología otology
otoneuralgia otoneuralgia
otopalatodigital otopalatodigital
otorrea otorrhea
otorrea del líquido cerebroespinal
   cerebrospinal fluid otorrhea
otra circunstancia familiar especificada
   other specified family circumstance
otra conducta other behavior
otra dependencia de sustancia especificada
   other specified substance dependence
otra disfunción sexual femenina other female
   sexual dysfunction
otra disfunción sexual masculina other male
   sexual dysfunction
otro generalizado generalized other
otro relevante relevant other
otro significante significant other
otro trastorno other disorder
otro trastorno afectivo especificado other
   specified affective disorder
otro trastorno psicosexual other psychosexual
   disorder
otro trastorno sexual other sexual disorder
otros problemas interpersonales other
   interpersonal problems
ovárico ovarian
ovariectomía ovariectomy
ovario ovary

ovariotomía ovariotomy
ovulación ovulation
ovulación paracíclica paracyclic ovulation
óvulo ovum
oxazepam oxazepam
oxazolam oxazolam
oxiacoia oxyacoia
oxiafia oxyaphia
oxicefalia oxycephaly
oxicefálico oxycephalic
oxicéfalo oxycephalous
oxicodona oxycodone
óxido nitroso nitrous oxide
oxiestesia oxyesthesia
oxigeusia oxygeusia
oxiosfresia oxyosphresia
oxiosmia oxyosmia
oxipertina oxypertine
oxitócico oxytocic
oxitocina oxytocin

P

pabellón ward
pabellón abierto open ward
pabellón cerrado con llave locked ward
paciente patient
paciente analítico analytic patient
paciente externo outpatient
paciente internado inpatient
paciente mental mental patient
paciente objetivo target patient
pacientes cardíacos cardiac patients
pacificación pacification
padre adolescente adolescent father
padre sustituto surrogate father
padres de fin de semana weekend parents
pagofagia pagophagia
paidología paidology
palabra completa full word
palabra de contenido content word
palabra de estímulo stimulus word
palabra de forma form word
palabra de función function word
palabra de vista sight word
palabra gramatical grammatical word
palabra híbrida portmanteau word
palabra relacional relational word
palabra vacía empty word
palabras abiertas open words
paladar palate
paladar blando soft palate
paladar duro hard palate
paladar hendido cleft palate
palanestesia pallanesthesia
palatal palatal
palatino palatine
palatoplejía palatoplegia
paleocerebelo paleocerebellum
paleocorteza paleocortex
paleoencéfalo paleencephalon
paleoespinotalámico paleospinothalamic
paleoestriado paleostriatum
paleoestriatal paleostriatal
paleofrenia paleophrenia
paleológico paleologic
paleomnesis paleomnesis
paleopsicología paleopsychology
paleopsíquico paleopsychic
paleosensación paleosensation
paleosímbolo paleosymbol
palestesia pallesthesia
palestético pallesthetic
paliativo palliative
palicinesia palikinesia
palidal pallidal
palidectomía pallidectomy

pálido pallidum
palidoamigdalotomía pallidoamygdalotomy
palidoansotomía pallidoansotomy
palidohipotalámico pallidohypothalamic
palidotomía pallidotomy
palifrasia paliphrasia
paligrafia paligraphia
palilalia palilalia
palilexia palilexia
palilogia palilogia
palindrómico palindromic
palíndromo palindrome
palinfrasia palinphrasia
palingrafia palingraphia
palinlexia palinlexia
palinopia palinopia
palinopsia palinopsia
palio pallium
paliopsia paliopsy
paliza battering
palmar palmar
palmestesia palmesthesia
palmestesis palmesthesis
pálmico palmic
palmo palmus
palmódico palmodic
palmomandibular palmomandibular
palmomentoniano palmomental
palpebral palpebral
palpitación palpitation
pamoato pamoate
panansiedad pananxiety
panarteritis panarteritis
pancreático pancreatic
pancreatitis pancreatitis
pancrestón panchreston
pandémico pandemic
pandiculación pandiculation
pandilla gang
pandilla escolar school gang
panel panel
panel continuo continuous panel
panencefalitis panencephalitis
panencefalitis esclerosante subaguda
subacute sclerosing panencephalitis
panencefalitis nodular nodular
panencephalitis
panestesia panesthesia
panfobia panphobia
panglosia panglossia
pánico panic
pánico de agresión aggression panic
pánico de insania insanity panic
pánico de insania neurótica neurotic insanity
panic
pánico en fuegos panic in fires
pánico homosexual homosexual panic
pánico prepsicótico prepsychotic panic
pánico primordial primordial panic
panmixia panmixia
panneuritis panneuritis
panneuritis endémica panneuritis endemica
panneurosis panneurosis
panódico panodic
panofobia panophobia

panplejía panplegia
panpsiquismo panpsychism
pansexualismo pansexualism
pantafobia pantaphobia
pantalgia pantalgia
pantalla screen
pantalla de reducción reduction screen
pantalla de sueños dream screen
pantalla en blanco blank screen
pantalla tangente tangent screen
pantanencefalia pantanencephaly
pantódico panthodic
pantofobia pantophobia
pantomima pantomime
papel role
papel administrativo managerial role
papel alcanzado achieved role
papel alternante alternating role
papel altruista altruistic role
papel atribuido ascribed role
papel complementario complementary role
papel comunitario community role
**papel de atractividad física en atracción
interpersonal** role of physical
attractiveness in interpersonal attraction
papel de enfermo sick role
papel de espectador spectator role
papel de estado status role
papel de género gender role
papel de grupo group role
papel de liderazgo leadership role
papel estereotípico stereotypical role
papel explícito explicit role
papel falso counterfeit role
papel fijo fixed role
papel implícito implicit role
papel maternal maternal role
papel no complementario noncomplementary
role
papel sexual sex role
papel sexual andrógeno androgynous sex role
papel social social role
papel terapéutico therapeutic role
papeles recíprocos reciprocal roles
papila papilla
papila acústica acoustic papilla
papila circunvalada circumvallate papilla
papila filiforme filiform papilla
papila lingual lingual papilla
papila óptica optic papilla
papilas del gusto taste buds
papilas fungiformes fungiform papillae
papiledema papilledema
papiloma papilloma
papiloma de células basales basal cell
papilloma
papiloma neuropático papilloma
neuropathicum
papiloma neurótico papilloma neuroticum
paquigiria pachygyria
paquileptomeningitis pachyleptomeningitis
paquimeninge pachymeninx
paquimeningitis pachymeningitis
paquimeningitis cervical hipertrófica
hypertrophic cervical pachymeningitis

paquimeningitis externa pachymeningitis
externa
paquimeningitis hemorrágica hemorrhagic
pachymeningitis
paquimeningitis interna pachymeningitis
interna
paquimeningitis piógena pyogenic
pachymeningitis
paquimeningopatía pachymeningopathy
par apareado matched pair
par de genes gene pair
par mínimo minimal pair
para parous
parabalismo paraballism
parabiosis parabiosis
parabiótico parabiotic
parablepsia parablepsia
parabulia parabulia
paracarcinomatoso paracarcinomatous
paracenestesia paracenesthesia
paracentral paracentral
paraciesis paracyesis
paracinesia parakinesia
paracinesis parakinesis
paracontraste paracontrast
paracromatopsia parachromatopsia
paracromopsia parachromopsia
paracusia paracusia
paracusis paracusis
paradigma paradigm
paradigma de aprendizaje learning paradigm
paradigma de inhibición asociativa paradigm
of associative inhibition
paradigma diátesis-estrés diathesis-stress
paradigm
paradigma estadística statistical paradigm
paradigma fisiológico physiological paradigm
paradigmático paradigmatic
paradipsia paradipsia
paradoja paradox
paradoja de Aubert-Fleischl Aubert-Fleischl
paradox
paradoja de Fechner Fechner's paradox
paradoja de similitud similarity paradox
paradoja neurótica neurotic paradox
paradójico paradoxical
paraequilibrio paraequilibrium
paraerotismo paraerotism
paraestesia paraesthesia
parafasia paraphasia
parafasia literal literal paraphasia
parafasia temática thematic paraphasia
parafasia verbal verbal paraphasia
parafásico paraphasic
parafemia paraphemia
parafia paraphia
parafilia paraphilia
parafilia atípica atypical paraphilia
parafílico paraphilic
parafisial paraphysial
parafobia paraphobia
parafonía paraphonia
paráfora paraphora
parafovea parafovea
parafrasia paraphrasia

parafrasia semántica semantic paraphrasia
paráfrasis paraphrase
parafrenia paraphrenia
parafrenia involutiva involutional
paraphrenia
parafrenia tardía late paraphrenia
paraganglioma paraganglioma
paraganglioma no cromafínico
nonchromaffin paraganglioma
paragenital paragenital
parageusia parageusia
paragéusico parageusic
paragnomen paragnomen
paragnosia paragnosia
paragrafía paragraphia
paragramatismo paragrammatism
parahipnosis parahypnosis
parahipófisis parahypophysis
paralaje parallax
paralaje binocular binocular parallax
paralaje de convergencia convergence
parallax
paralaje de moción motion parallax
paralalia paralalia
paralalia literal paralalia literalis
paraldehído paraldehyde
paralelismo parallelism
paralelismo cultural cultural parallelism
paralelismo formal formal parallelism
paralelismo psicofísico psychophysical
parallelism
paralelismo psiconeural psychoneural
parallelism
paralelo parallel
paralenguaje paralanguage
paraleprosis paraleprosis
paralepsia paralepsy
paralexia paralexia
paralgesia paralgesia
paralgia paralgia
paralingüística paralinguistics
paralingüístico paralinguistic
paralipofobia paralipophobia
parálisis paralysis, palsy
parálisis agitante paralysis agitans
parálisis ascendente ascending paralysis
parálisis ascendente aguda acute ascending
paralysis
parálisis atrófica aguda acute atrophic
paralysis
parálisis bulbar bulbar paralysis
parálisis bulbar progresiva progressive
bulbar palsy
parálisis central central paralysis
parálisis cerebral cerebral palsy
parálisis cerebral catatónica catatonic
cerebral paralysis
parálisis conjugada conjugate paralysis
parálisis cruzada crossed paralysis
parálisis de Bell Bell's palsy
parálisis de Brown-Sequard
Brown-Sequard's paralysis
parálisis de conversión conversion paralysis
parálisis de Duchenne Duchenne's paralysis
parálisis de Duchenne-Erb Duchenne-Erb

paralysis
parálisis de Erb Erb's paralysis
parálisis de escritor scrivener's palsy
parálisis de Fereol-Graux Fereol-Graux palsy
parálisis de Gubler Gubler's paralysis
parálisis de inmovilización immobilization
paralysis
parálisis de jengibre ginger paralysis
parálisis de Klumpke Klumpke's paralysis
parálisis de Kussmaul-Landry
Kussmaul-Landry paralysis
parálisis de Landry Landry's paralysis
parálisis de nacimiento birth palsy
parálisis de Pott Pott's paralysis
parálisis de Todd Todd's paralysis
parálisis de trabajo work paralysis
parálisis de Zenker Zenker's paralysis
parálisis degenerante wasting palsy
parálisis del sueño sleep paralysis
parálisis diftérica diphtheritic paralysis
parálisis espástica spastic paralysis
parálisis espinal spinal paralysis
parálisis espinal de Erb Erb's spinal paralysis
parálisis espinal espástica spastic spinal
paralysis
parálisis facial facial paralysis
parálisis faucial faucial paralysis
parálisis fláccida flaccid paralysis
parálisis general general paralysis
parálisis general juvenil juvenile general
paralysis
parálisis global global paralysis
parálisis glosolabiofaríngea
glossolabiopharyngeal paralysis
parálisis glosolabiolaríngeo
glossolabiolaryngeal paralysis
parálisis histérica hysterical paralysis
parálisis infantil infantile paralysis
parálisis inmunológica immunological
paralysis
parálisis labial labial paralysis
parálisis mimética mimetic paralysis
parálisis miogénica myogenic paralysis
parálisis mixta mixed paralysis
parálisis motora motor paralysis
parálisis muscular seudohipertrófica
pseudohypertrophic muscular paralysis
parálisis musculoespiral musculospiral
paralysis
parálisis natal braquial brachial birth palsy
parálisis nocturna nocturnal paralysis
parálisis obstétrica obstetrical paralysis
parálisis ocular ocular paralysis
parálisis ocupacional craft palsy
parálisis orgánica organic paralysis
parálisis periódica periodic paralysis
parálisis periódica familiar familial periodic
paralysis
parálisis periódica hiperpotasémica
hyperkalemic periodic paralysis
parálisis periódica hipopotasémica
hypokalemic periodic paralysis
parálisis periódica normopotasémica
normokalemic periodic paralysis
parálisis periódica responsiva al sodio

sodium-responsive periodic paralysis
parálisis por compresión compression
paralysis
parálisis por decúbito decubitus paralysis
parálisis por garrapata tick paralysis
parálisis por muletas crutch paralysis
parálisis por plomo lead palsy
parálisis por presión pressure paralysis
parálisis posdiftérica postdiphtheritic
paralysis
parálisis posepiléptica de Todd Todd's
postepileptic paralysis
parálisis póstica posticus paralysis
parálisis progresiva creeping palsy
parálisis psíquica psychic paralysis
parálisis sensorial sensory paralysis
parálisis seudobulbar pseudobulbar paralysis
parálisis seudogeneral saturnina saturnine
pseudogeneral paralysis
parálisis supranuclear supranuclear paralysis
parálisis supranuclear progresiva
progressive supranuclear palsy
parálisis tegmental medular medullary
tegmental paralysis
parálisis temblorosa trembling palsy
paralítico paralytic
paralizante paralyzing
paralizar paralyze
paralogía paralogia
paralogía metafórica metaphoric paralogia
paralogía temática thematic paralogia
paralogismo paralogism
parálogo paralog
parametadiona paramethadione
paramétrico parametric
parametrismo parametrismus
parámetro parameter
paramimia paramimia
paramimismo paramimism
paramioclono paramyoclonus
paramiotonía paramyotonia
paramiotonía atáxica ataxic paramyotonia
paramiotonía congénita congenital
paramyotonia
paramiotonía sintomática symptomatic
paramyotonia
paramiotono paramyotonus
paramnesia paramnesia
paramnesia reduplicativa reduplicative
paramnesia
paramusia paramusia
paranalgesia paranalgesia
paraneoplásico paraneoplastic
paraneural paraneural
paranoia paranoia
paranoia alcohólica alcoholic paranoia
paranoia alucinatoria aguda acute
hallucinatory paranoia
paranoia amorosa amorous paranoia
paranoia cargada de afecto affect-laden
paranoia
paranoia clásica classical paranoia
paranoia conyugal conjugal paranoia
paranoia erótica erotic paranoia
paranoia exaltada exalted paranoia

paranoia litigiosa litigious paranoia
paranoia originaria paranoia originaria
paranoia quejumbrosa paranoia querulans
paranoia senil paranoia senilis
paranoico paranoiac
paranoide paranoid
paranomasia paranomasia
paranomia paranomia
paranormal paranormal
paranósico paranosic
paranosis paranosis
paraparesia paraparesis
paraparético paraparetic
parapatía parapathy
paraperitoneal paraperitoneal
parapitimia parapithymia
parapléctico paraplectic
paraplejía paraplegia
paraplejía atáxica ataxic paraplegia
paraplejía de Pott Pott's paraplegia
paraplejía dolorosa painful paraplegia
paraplejía en extensión paraplegia in
   extension
paraplejía en flexión paraplegia in flexion
paraplejía espástica spastic paraplegia
paraplejía espástica congénita congenital
   spastic paraplegia
paraplejía espástica hereditaria hereditary
   spastic paraplegia
paraplejía espástica infantil infantile spastic
   paraplegia
paraplejía senil senile paraplegia
paraplejía superior superior paraplegia
paraplejía tetanoide tetanoid paraplegia
parapléjico paraplegic
parapoplejía parapoplexy
parapraxia parapraxia
parapraxis parapraxis
paraprofesional paraprofessional
parapsia parapsia
parapsicología parapsychology
parapsicosis parapsychosis
pararreacción parareaction
pararreflexia parareflexia
parasagital parasagittal
parasexualidad parasexuality
parasimpático parasympathetic
parasimpaticolítico parasympatholytic
parasimpaticomimético parasympathomimetic
parasimpaticotonía parasympathicotonia
parasítico parasitic
parasitismo parasitism
parásito parasite
parasitofobia parasitophobia
parasocial parasocial
parasomnia parasomnia
parasuicidio parasuicide
parataxia parataxia
paratáxico parataxic
parataxis parataxis
parateresiomanía parateresiomania
parathormona parathormone
paratimia parathymia
paratípico paratypic
paratipo paratype

paratiroideo parathyroid
paratiroidismo parathyroidism
paratiroprivo parathyroprival
paratonía paratonia
paravariación paravariation
paraverbal paraverbal
paraverterbral paravertebral
paraxial paraxial
parcial partial
parcialidad partiality
parcialismo partialism
parcialización partialization
parecido asumido assumed similarity
parectropia parectropia
paregórico paregoric
pareidolia pareidolia
pareja couple
pareja sexual sexual partner
pareja sexual sustituta surrogate sexual
   partner
pareja sustituta surrogate partner
parencefalia parencephalia
parencefalitis parencephalitis
parencefalocele parencephalocele
parencefaloso parencephalous
parénquima parenchyma
parénquima neural neural parenchyma
parenquimatoso parenchymatous
parens patriae parens patriae
parental parental
parentela kin
parenteral parenteral
parentesco kinship
pareo matching
pareo a muestra matching to sample
pareo de colores color matching
pareo de modalidades cruzadas
   cross-modality matching
pareo de probabilidades probability matching
pareo metafórico metaphoric matching
parepitimia parepithymia
pareretisis parerethisis
parergasia parergasia
parerosia parerosia
pares asociados paired associates
paresia paresis
paresia general general paresis
paresia histérica hysterical paresis
paresia infantil infantile paresis
paresia juvenil juvenile paresis
paresia tipo Lissauer Lissauer type paresis
parestesia paresthesia
parestesia de Berger Berger's paresthesia
parestésico paresthetic
parético paretic
pargilina pargyline
pariente relative
parietal parietal
parietooccipital parietooccipital
paritario peer
parkinsoniano parkinsonian
parkinsonismo parkinsonism
parkinsonismo inducido por drogas
   drug-induced parkinsonism
parkinsonismo inducido por neuroléptico

neuroleptic-induced parkinsonism
parkinsonismo primario primary
　parkinsonism
paro locomotor locomotor arrest
parofresia parophresia
paroniria paroniria
parorexia parorexia
parosfresia parosphresia
parosfresis parosphresis
parosmia parosmia
paroxismo paroxysm
paroxístico paroxysmal
parpadeo blinking
parricidio parricide
parricidio simbólico symbolic parricide
pars pro toto pars pro toto
parsimonia parsimony
parte del cuerpo artificial artificial body part
partenofobia parthenophobia
partenogénesis parthenogenesis
partición partition
participación participation
participante participant
particular particular
particularismo particularism
parto parturition
parto natural natural childbirth
parto normal normal delivery
parto preparado prepared childbirth
parturifobia parturiphobia
paruresis paruresis
pasión passion
pasional passional
pasividad passivity
pasivismo passivism
pasivo passive
pasivo-agresivo passive-aggressive
paso de Hoffding Hoffding step
pata de mono monkey-paw
patemático pathematic
patergasia pathergasia
paternal paternal
paternalismo paternalism
paternidad paternity
patético pathetic
patetismo pathetism
pático pathic
patobiografía pathobiography
patobiología pathobiology
patocinesis pathokinesis
patoclisis pathoclisis
patocura pathocure
patodixia pathodixia
patofisiología pathophysiology
patofisiológico pathophysiological
patofobia pathophobia
patofórmico pathoformic
patofrenesis pathophrenesis
patogénesis pathogenesis
patogenia pathogeny
patogénico pathogenic
patógeno pathogen
patógeno conductual behavioral pathogen
patognomía pathognomy
patognómico pathognomic

patognomónico pathognomonic
patognóstico pathognostic
patografía pathography
patohisteria pathohysteria
patolesia patholesia
patología pathology
patología auditiva auditory pathology
patología cerebral brain pathology
patología del habla speech pathology
patología del lenguaje language pathology
patología focal focal pathology
patología social social pathology
patológico pathological
patomimesis pathomimesis
patomímica pathomimicry
patomiosis pathomiosis
patomorfismo pathomorphism
patoneurosis pathoneurosis
patoplastia pathoplasty
patopsicología pathopsychology
patopsicosis pathopsychosis
patosis pathosis
patriarcal patriarchal
patricidio patricide
patrilineal patrilineal
patriofobia patriophobia
patroiofobia patroiophobia
patrón pattern
patrón afectomotor affectomotor pattern
patrón cultural culture pattern
patrón de acción fija fixed-action pattern
patrón de activación activation pattern
patrón de alimentación feeding pattern
patrón de comunicación communication
　pattern
patrón de conducta behavior pattern
patrón de despertamiento erótico
　erotic-arousal pattern
patrón de emociones pattern of emotions
patrón de estímulo stimulus pattern
**patrón de factores ambientales apremiantes
　y necesidades** press-need pattern
patrón de juego play pattern
**patrón de pensamiento desviado en
　delincuencia** deviant thinking pattern in
　delinquency
patrón de puntas positivas positive spike
　pattern
patrón de reacción reaction pattern
patrón del desarrollo developmental pattern
patrón demográfico demographic pattern
patrón dinámico específico specific dynamic
　pattern
patrón expresivo expressive pattern
patrón familiar family pattern
patrón familiar patogénico pathogenic family
　pattern
patrón fenomenal phenomenal pattern
patrón patofisiológico pathophysiological
　pattern
patrón repetitivo repetitive pattern
patrón respiratorio respiratory pattern
patrón temporal seasonal pattern
patrón tonal tonal pattern
patrones de cortejo humanos human

courtship patterns
patrones de empleo employment patterns
patrones del sueño sleep patterns
patrones del sueño en autismo sleep patterns
   in autism
patrones del sueño en depresión sleep
   patterns in depression
pausa pause
pausa apneica apneic pause
pausa de fijación fixation pause
pausa de hesitación hesitation pause
pausa rellenada filled pause
pausa respiratoria respiratory pause
pausa silenciosa silent pause
pauta guideline
pautas para el uso de hipnosis guidelines for
   use of hypnosis
pavlovianismo pavlovianism
pavloviano pavlovian
pavor diurno pavor diurnus
pavor nocturno pavor nocturnus
pecatifobia peccatiphobia
pectoral pectoral
pectoralgia pectoralgia
pecho breast
pecho bueno good breast
pecho carinado pectus carinatum
pecho fantasma phantom breast
pecho malo bad breast
pedagogía pedagogy
pederasta pederast
pederastia pederasty
pederosis pederosis
pediatría pediatrics
pediátrico pediatric
pedicación pedication
pediculofobia pediculophobia
pediofobia pediophobia
pedionalgia pedionalgia
pedioneuralgia pedioneuralgia
pedofilia pedophilia
pedofilia adolescente adolescent pedophilia
pedofilia bisexual bisexual pedophilia
pedofilia en edad madura middle age
   pedophilia
pedofilia heterosexual heterosexual
   pedophilia
pedofilia homosexual homosexual pedophilia
pedofilia senescente senescent pedophilia
pedofilia y padres incrédulos pedophilia and
   unbelieving parents
pedofílico pedophilic
pedofobia pedophobia
pedolalia pedolalia
pedología pedology
pedólogo pedologist
pedomorfismo pedomorphism
pedomorfosis pedomorphosis
pedotrofia pedotrophy
peduncular peduncular
pedúnculo peduncle
pedunculotomía pedunculotomy
pelagra pellagra
película film
peligro danger

peligros de hipnotismo dangers of hypnotism
peligrosidad dangerousness
pelos de irritación de Frey Frey's irritation
   hairs
pelvifemoral pelvifemoral
pemolina pemoline
penalidad penalty
pendiente slope
pene penis
pene artificial artificial penis
pene cautivo penis captivus
penetración penetration, insight
penetración analítica analytic insight
penetración derivada derivative insight
penetración deteriorada impaired insight
penetración emocional emotional insight
penetración intelectual intellectual insight
penetración súbita sudden insight
penetración verdadera true insight
penetrancia penetrance
penfluridol penfluridol
peniafobia peniaphobia
peniano penile
penilingus penilingus
penología penology
pensamiento thinking, thought
pensamiento abstracto abstract thinking
pensamiento alusivo allusive thinking
pensamiento animístico animistic thinking
pensamiento antropomórfico
   anthropomorphic thinking
pensamiento arcaico archaic thought
pensamiento arcaico-paralógico
   archaic-paralogical thinking
pensamiento asindético asyndetic thinking
pensamiento asociativo associative thinking
pensamiento audible audible thought
pensamiento autista autistic thinking
pensamiento automático automatic thought
pensamiento categórico categorical thought
pensamiento concreto concrete thinking
pensamiento convergente convergent thinking
pensamiento creativo creative thinking
pensamiento crítico critical thinking
pensamiento de computadora computer
   thought
pensamiento de todo o nada all-or-nothing
   thinking
pensamiento deductivo deductive thinking
pensamiento dereístico dereistic thinking
pensamiento deseoso wishful thinking
pensamiento dicotómico dichotomous
   thinking
pensamiento dirigido directed thinking
pensamiento divergente divergent thinking
pensamiento egocéntrico egocentric thinking
pensamiento espontaneo spontaneous thought
pensamiento fantásmico fantasmic thinking
pensamiento fenomenístico phenomenistic
   thought
pensamiento fisionómico physiognomic
   thinking
pensamiento formal formal thought
pensamiento janoniano Janusian thinking
pensamiento lateral lateral thinking

pensamiento lógico abstracto abstract logical thought
pensamiento mágico magical thinking
pensamiento medieval medieval thinking
pensamiento operacional operational thought
pensamiento operatorio operatory thought
pensamiento operatorio concreto concrete operatory thought
pensamiento operatorio formal formal operatory thought
pensamiento oposicional oppositional thinking
pensamiento paleológico paleologic thinking
pensamiento pervertido perverted thinking
pensamiento preconsciente preconscious thinking
pensamiento predicativo predicative thinking
pensamiento prelógico prelogical thinking
pensamiento preoperacional preoperational thinking
pensamiento preoperatorio preoperatory thought
pensamiento primario primary thinking
pensamiento primitivo primitive thinking
pensamiento productivo productive thinking
pensamiento psicótico psychotic thinking
pensamiento realista realistic thinking
pensamiento reproductivo reproductive thinking
pensamiento simbólico symbolic thinking
pensamiento sin imagen imageless thought
pensamiento sincrético syncretic thought
pensamiento sintáxico syntaxic thought
pensamiento tangencial tangential thinking
pensamiento verbal verbal thought
pensamientos obsesivos obsessional thoughts
pentatónico pentatonic
pentazocina pentazocine
pentetrazol pentetrazol
pentilenotetrazol pentylenetetrazol
pentobarbital pentobarbital
penuria económica economic hardship
peña clique
peña sociométrica sociometric clique
peonaje peonage
peonaje institucional institutional peonage
peotilomanía peotillomania
pepsina pepsin
pepsinógeno pepsinogen
péptico peptic
peptidérgico peptidergic
péptido peptide
péptido cardioexcitatorio cardioexcitatory peptide
péptido inducidor de sueño sleep-inducing peptide
péptido intestinal vasoactivo vasoactive intestinal peptide
pequeño mal petit mal
perazina perazine
percentila percentile
percepción perception
percepción-alucinación perception-hallucination
percepción auditiva auditory perception
percepción automórfica automorphic

perception
percepción básica sentience
percepción binocular binocular perception
percepción categórica categorical perception
percepción consciente conscious perception
percepción cruzada crossed perception
percepción cutánea cutaneous perception
percepción de borde edge perception
percepción de calor perception of heat
percepción de color color perception
percepción de color de infantes infant perception of color
percepción de distancia distance perception
percepción de enfermedad perception of illness
percepción de espacio auditivo auditory space perception
percepción de figura-fondo figure-ground perception
percepción de formas form perception
percepción de infantes infant perception
percepción de melodía melody perception
percepción de moción motion perception
percepción de patrón pattern perception
percepción de personas person perception
percepción de profundidad depth perception
percepción de relaciones espaciales perception of spatial relations
percepción de rotación rotation perception
percepción de tamaño size perception
percepción del albedo albedo perception
percepción del gusto taste perception
percepción del habla speech perception
percepción del tiempo time perception
percepción dermoóptica dermooptical perception
percepción directa direct perception
percepción ecológica ecological perception
percepción endopsíquica endopsychic perception
percepción espacial space perception
percepción extrasensorial extrasensory perception
percepción facial facial perception
percepción fisionómica physiognomic perception
percepción háptica haptic perception
percepción intermodal intermodal perception
percepción interpersonal interpersonal perception
percepción intersensorial intersensory perception
percepción mente-cuerpo mind-body perception
percepción multimodal multimodal perception
percepción obligatoria obligatory perception
percepción persistente afterperception
percepción preferencial preferential perception
percepción remota remote perception
percepción selectiva selective perception
percepción sensorial sense perception
percepción social social perception
percepción subliminal subliminal perception

percepción táctil tactile perception
percepción visual visual perception
percepciones abstractas abstract perceptions
perceptividad perceptivity
perceptivo perceptive
percepto percept
percepto corporal body percept
perceptor percipient
perceptualización perceptualization
percibido perceived
percibir perceive
percutáneo percutaneous
pérdida loss
pérdida de afecto loss of affect
pérdida de audición hearing loss
pérdida de audición no organica nonorganic
    hearing loss
pérdida de audición sensorineural
    sensorineural hearing loss
pérdida de control loss of control
pérdida de embarazo pregnancy loss
pérdida de identidad personal loss of
    personal identity
pérdida de objeto object loss
pérdida del límite del ego ego-boundary loss
pérdida hemisensorial hemisensory loss
pérdida múltiple multiple loss
pérdida real real loss
pérdida simbólica symbolic loss
pérdida y aflicción loss and grief
pérdida y conducta suicida loss and suicidal
    behavior
perdurable enduring
perencefalia perencephaly
perfeccionismo perfectionism
perfenazina perphenazine
perfil profile
perfil de modalidad modality profile
perfil de personalidad personality profile
perfil de prueba test profile
perfil de rasgos trait profile
perfil estructural structural profile
perfil metapsicológico metapsychological
    profile
perforador perforator
performativo performative
pergolida pergolide
periarterial periarterial
periblepsia periblepsis
pericárdico pericardial
pericareia perichareia
pericarion perikaryon
periciazina periciazine
pericranitis pericranitis
periencefalitis periencephalitis
periespondilitis perispondylitis
periferalismo peripheralism
periferia periphery
periferia de la rétina periphery of the retina
periférico peripheral
perilinfa perilymph
perimacular perimacular
perimeningitis perimeningitis
perimetría perimetry
perimetría de sonido sound perimetry

perímetro perimeter
perinatal perinatal
perineural perineural
perineuritis perineuritis
periodicidad periodicity
periódico periodic
periodo period
periodo adicional latente latent additional
    period
periodo crítico critical period .
periodo de adaptación adaptation period
periodo de calentamiento warm-up period
periodo de descanso rest period
periodo de fantasía fantasy period
periodo de gestación gestation period
periodo de latencia latency period
periodo de mamar oral oral sucking period
periodo de morder oral oral biting period
periodo de neurona subnormal subnormal
    period of neuron
periodo de operaciones concretas concrete
    operations period
periodo de práctica practice period
periodo del desarrollo developmental period
periodo edípico oedipal period
periodo embriónico embryonic period
periodo fetal fetal period
periodo germinativo germinal period
periodo homosexual natural natural
    homosexual period
periodo involutivo involutional period
periodo juvenil juvenile period
periodo latente latent period
periodo negativo negative period
periodo neonatal neonatal period
periodo operatorio formal formal operatory
    period
periodo perinatal perinatal period
periodo pospartal postpartal period
periodo prelingüístico prelinguistic period
periodo prenatal prenatal period
periodo preoperatorio preoperatory period
periodo refractario refractory period
periodo refractario absoluto absolute
    refractory period
periodo refractario psicológico psychological
    refractory period
periodo refractario relativo relative
    refractory period
periodo sensitivo sensitive period
periodo sensorimotor sensorimotor period
periodo silencioso silent period
periodo supernormal supernormal period
perióstico periosteal
peripaquimeningitis peripachymeningitis
peripatólogo peripathologist
perístasis peristasis
peritoneal peritoneal
peritonismo peritonism
peritonitis peritonitis
periventricular periventricular
permanencia permanence
permanencia de objeto object permanence
permanente permanent
permeabilidad permeability

permeable permeable
permisividad permissiveness
permisividad parental parental permissiveness
permisivo permissive
pernicioso pernicious
peroneo peroneal
perplejidad perplexity
perplejidad mórbida morbid perplexity
perplejidad parental parental perplexity
perplejo perplexed
perro guía guide dog
persecución persecution
persecución de ideas idea chase
persecutorio persecutory
perseveración perseveration
perseveración infantil infantile perseveration
perseveración motora motor perseveration
perseverancia perseverance
perseverante perseverative
persistencia persistence
persistencia de visión persistence of vision
persistencia motora motor persistence
persistente persistent
persona persona
persona compleja complex person
persona completamente en funcionamiento fully functioning person
persona compuesta composite person
persona de recursos resource person
persona dirigida hacia el exterior outer-directed person
persona dirigida hacia otros other-directed person
persona en el paciente person in the patient
persona golpeada battered person
personal (adj) personal
personal (n) personnel
personal apoyador supportive personnel
personal de cuidado diurno day care personnel
personalidad personality
personalidad acaparadora hoarding personality
personalidad acromegaloide acromegaloid personality
personalidad adictiva addictive personality
personalidad alotrópica allotropic personality
personalidad alternante alternating personality
personalidad anal anal personality
personalidad anal-expulsiva anal-expulsive personality
personalidad anal-retentiva anal-retentive personality
personalidad anancástica anancastic personality
personalidad antisocial antisocial personality
personalidad asténica asthenic personality
personalidad autoritaria authoritarian personality
personalidad básica basic personality
personalidad ciclotímica cyclothymic personality
personalidad como sí as if personality

personalidad compulsiva compulsive personality
personalidad de mercadeo marketing personality
personalidad de migraña migraine personality
personalidad de vida lifetime personality
personalidad dependiente dependent personality
personalidad depresiva depressive personality
personalidad disocial dyssocial personality
personalidad dividida split personality
personalidad doble double personality
personalidad dramática dramatic personality
personalidad encerrada shut-in personality
personalidad epiléptica epileptic personality
personalidad esquizofrénica schizophrenic personality
personalidad esquizoide schizoid personality
personalidad esquizotímica schizothymic personality
personalidad esquizotípica schizotypal personality
personalidad evitante avoidant personality
personalidad explosiva explosive personality
personalidad explotadora exploitative personality
personalidad fronteriza borderline personality
personalidad hiperestética hyperaesthetic personality
personalidad hipomaníaca hypomanic personality
personalidad histérica hysterical personality
personalidad histriónica histrionic personality
personalidad impulsiva impulsive personality
personalidad inadecuada inadequate personality
personalidad independiente independent personality
personalidad inestable emocionalmente emotionally unstable personality
personalidad infantil infantile personality
personalidad inmadura immature personality
personalidad intraconsciente intraconscious personality
personalidad introvertida introverted personality
personalidad maniacodepresiva manic-depressive personality
personalidad masoquista masochistic personality
personalidad melancólica melancholic personality
personalidad múltiple multiple personality
personalidad narcisista narcissistic personality
personalidad neurótica neurotic personality
personalidad obsesiva obsessive personality
personalidad obsesiva-compulsiva obsessive-compulsive personality
personalidad oral oral personality
personalidad paranoide paranoid personality
personalidad pasiva-agresiva

passive-aggressive personality
personalidad pasiva-dependiente
   passive-dependent personality
personalidad premórbida premorbid
   personality
personalidad prepsicótica prepsychotic
   personality
personalidad pretraumática pretraumatic
   personality
personalidad primaria primary personality
personalidad productiva productive
   personality
personalidad propensa a accidentes
   accident-prone personality
personalidad psicopática psychopathic
   personality
personalidad receptiva receptive personality
personalidad represiva repressive personality
personalidad sádica sadistic personality
personalidad saludable healthy personality
personalidad secundaria secondary
   personality
personalidad seudoindependiente
   pseudoindependent personality
personalidad sintónica syntonic personality
personalidad sociopática sociopathic
   personality
personalidad subconsciente subconscious
   personality
personalidad tipo A A-type personality
personalidad tipo B B-type personality
personalidad tormentosa stormy personality
personalidad ulcerosa ulcer personality
personalismo personalism
personalista personalistic
personalización personalization
personalizado personalized
personificación personification
personificación eidética eidetic
   personification
personificado personified
personología personology
perspectiva perspective
perspectiva aérea aerial perspective
perspectiva alternante alternating perspective
perspectiva atmosférica atmospheric
   perspective
perspectiva biológica biological view
perspectiva biológica de delincuencia
   biological view of delinquency
perspectiva de Laingian Laingian view
perspectiva de moción motion perspective
perspectiva de movimiento movement
   perspective
perspectiva del tiempo time perspective
perspectiva ecológica ecological perspective
perspectiva ecológica del desarrollo
   ecological perspective of development
perspectiva extraspectiva extraspective
   perspective
perspectiva humanística humanistic
   perspective
perspectiva lineal linear perspective
perspectiva reversible reversible perspective
perspectiva temporal temporal perspective

persuasión persuasion
persuasión coercitiva coercive persuasion
persuasivo persuasive
perturbación ácido-base acid-base
   disturbance
perturbador disturbing
perversión perversion
perversión polimorfa polymorphous
   perversion
perversión sexual sexual perversion
perverso perverse
pervertido (adj) perverted
pervertido (n) pervert
pervigilium pervigilium
pesadilla nightmare
pesadilla ansiosa anxiety nightmare
pesadilla despierta daymare
pesimismo pessimism
pesimismo oral oral pessimism
pesimismo terapéutico therapeutic pessimism
peso weight
peso beta beta weight
peso corporal body weight
peso de nacimiento birth weight
peso de regresión regression weight
peso efectivo effective weight
peso factorial factor weight
peso nominal nominal weight
petrifacción petrifaction
petrificación petrification
petrositis petrositis
peyote peyote
phi phi
piamadre pia mater
piamadre craneal cranial pia mater
piamadre espinal spinal pia mater
piaracnitis piaarachnitis
piblokto piblokto
pica pica
pica de papel paper pica
pícnico pyknic
picnodisostosis pyknodysostosis
picnoepilepsia pyknoepilepsy
picnofrasia pyknophrasia
picnolepsia pyknolepsy
picrotoxina picrotoxin
pictofilia pictophilia
pictograma pictogram
pie en garra clawfoot
pie plano flat foot
pie terminal end foot
pie zambo clubfoot
piel brillante glossy skin
pielonefritis pyelonephritis
piencéfalo pyencephalus
pierna inquieta restless leg
piesestesia piesesthesia
pigmalionismo pygmalionism
pigmento pigment
píldora contraceptiva contraceptive pill
píldora contraceptiva oral oral contraceptive
   pill
pilocarpina pilocarpine
piloerección piloerection
piloide piloid

pilomotor pilomotor
piloyección pilojection
piminodina piminodine
pimozida pimozide
pinazepam pinazepam
pineal pineal
pinealectomía pinealectomy
pinealoma pinealoma
pinealoma ectópico ectopic pinealoma
pinealoma extrapineal extrapineal pinealoma
pinealopatía pinealopathy
pineoblastoma pineoblastoma
pinna pinna
pinocitosis pinocytosis
pintura con dedos finger painting
piocefalia pyocephalus
piocefalia externa external pyocephalus
piocefalia interna internal pyocephalus
piocéfalo circunscrito circumscribed
     pyocephalus
piógeno pyogenic
piojo louse
piojos lice
pipamperona pipamperone
piperacetazina piperacetazine
piperazina piperazine
piperidina piperidine
pipotiazina pipotiazine
pipradrol pipradrol
piramidal pyramidal
pirámide pyramid
pirámide de color color pyramid
pirámide social social pyramid
piramidotomía pyramidotomy
piramidotomía espinal spinal pyramidotomy
piramidotomía medular medullary
     pyramidotomy
pirazolona pyrazolone
pirexeofobia pyrexeophobia
pirexiofobia pyrexiophobia
piridostigmina pyridostigmine
piridoxina pyridoxine
pirofobia pyrophobia
pirógeno pyrogen
pirolagnia pyrolagnia
piromanía pyromania
piromanía erótica erotic pyromania
piromaníaco pyromaniac
piroptotimia pyroptothymia
pirosis pyrosis
pitiatismo pithiatism
pitiátrico pithiatric
pito de Galton Galton whistle
pituicitoma pituicytoma
pituitaria pituitary
pituitaria anterior anterior pituitary
pituitarismo pituitarism
placa plaque
placa cribiforme cribiform plate
placa neural neural plate
placa neurítica neuritic plaque
placa senil senile plaque
placa terminal end plate
placa terminal motora motor end plate
placas argentófilas argentophilic plaques

placas argirófilas argyrophilic plaques
placebo placebo
placenta placenta
placenta previa placenta praevia
placentario placental
placentero pleasant
placentitis placentitis
placer pleasure
placer de actividad activity pleasure
placer de función function pleasure
placer estético esthetic pleasure
placer final end pleasure
placer orgánico organ pleasure
placer previo forepleasure
placer vicario vicarious pleasure
plan de educación individualizada
     individualized education plan
plan de Keller Keller plan
plan de precio por servicio fee-for-service
     plan
plan de Scanlon Scanlon plan
plan de tratamiento treatment plan
plan de vida life plan
plan instruccional instructional plan
planes de educación individualizada y
     traslación a la corriente principal
     individualized education plans and
     mainstreaming
planificación planning
planificación de carrera career planning
planificación de política social social policy
     planning
planificación estratégica strategic planning
planificación familiar family planning
planificación operacional operational
     planning
planificación permanente permanent planning
planificado planned
plano plane
plano ecuatorial equatorial plane
plano horizontal horizontal plane
plano medial medial plane
plano medio median plane
planofrasia planophrasia
planomanía planomania
planotopocinesia planotopokinesia
plantalgia plantalgia
plantar plantar
plantígrado plantigrade
plaqueta platelet
plasma plasma
plasma germinativo germ plasm
plasmaféresis plasmapheresis
plásmido plasmid
plasticidad plasticity
plasticidad cerebral brain plasticity
plasticidad conductual behavioral plasticity
plasticidad de descerebración decerebrate
     plasticity
plasticidad funcional functional plasticity
plasticidad neuronal neuronal plasticity
plataforma de saltos de Lashley Lashley
     jumping stand
plataforma orgásmica orgasmic platform
platibasia platybasia

platicefalia platycephaly
platicefálico platycephalic
platicúrtico platykurtic
platicurtosis platykurtosis
platillo volador flying saucer
platonización platonization
platonizar platonize
pleiotropía pleiotropy
pleiotrópico pleiotropic
plenilocuencia pleniloquence
pleocitosis pleocytosis
pleonasmo pleonasm
pleonexia pleonexia
pletismógrafo plethysmograph
pletismógrafo peniano penile plethysmograph
pleurotótonos pleurothotonos
plexectomía plexectomy
plexiforme plexiform
plexitis plexitis
plexo plexus
plexo coroideo choroid plexus
pliege neural neural fold
plomo lead
plumbismo plumbism
pluralismo pluralism
pluralismo cultural cultural pluralism
pluralista pluralistic
plutomanía plutomania
pnigofobia pnigophobia
población population
población de estímulo stimulus population
población de muestreo sampling population
pobreza poverty
pobreza de contenido del habla poverty of
    content of speech
pobreza de ideas poverty of ideas
pobreza del habla poverty of speech
poder power
poder de policía police power
poder de resolución resolving power
poder discriminante discriminating power
podismo podismus
podoespasmo podospasm
poiesis poiesis
poinefobia poinephobia
poiquilotimia poikilothymia
polaquiuria pollakiuria
polaridad polarity
polaridad ego-objeto ego-object polarity
polarización polarization
polarización en masa mass polarization
polarización sexual sexual polarization
poliandria polyandry
policiesis polycyesis
policinematosomnografía
    polycinematosomnography
policlonía polyclonia
policomental pollicomental
policratismo polycratism
policromático polychromatic
policromato polychromate
polidactilismo polydactylism
polidáctilo polydactyl
polidipsia polydipsia
polidipsia histérica hysterical polydipsia

polidipsia nocturna psicogénica psychogenic
    nocturnal polydipsia
polidipsia psicogénica psychogenic polydipsia
poliestesia polyesthesia
poliestro polyestrous
polifagia polyphagia
polifálico polyphallic
polifarmacia polypharmacy
polifásico polyphasic
polifobia polyphobia
polifonía polyphony
polifrasia polyphrasia
poligamia polygamy
poligamia serial serial polygamy
poligénico polygenic
poliginia polygyny
poligiria polygyria
polígloto polyglot
polígono polygon
polígono de frecuencias frequency polygon
polígrafo polygraph
polígrafo de Keeler Keeler polygraph
polihíbrido polyhybrid
poliléptico polyleptic
polilogia polylogia
polimátrico polymatric
polimialgia polymyalgia
polimialgia arterítica polymyalgia arteritica
polimialgia reumática polymyalgia
    rheumatica
polimioclono polymyoclonus
polimiositis polymyositis
polimorfismo polymorphism
polimorfo polymorphous
polineuralgia polyneuralgia
polineurítico polyneuritic
polineuritis polyneuritis
polineuritis aguda acute polyneuritis
polineuritis eritredema erythredema
    polyneuritis
polineuritis familiar crónica chronic familial
    polyneuritis
polineuritis idiopática aguda acute idiopathic
    polyneuritis
polineuritis infecciosa infectious polyneuritis
polineuronitis polyneuronitis
polineuropatía polyneuropathy
polineuropatía nutricional nutritional
    polyneuropathy
polineuropatía sensorial sensory
    polyneuropathy
polineuropatía urémica uremic
    polyneuropathy
polio polio
polioclástico polioclastic
poliodistrofia poliodystrophy
poliodistrofia cerebral infantil progresiva
    progressive infantile cerebral
    poliodystrophy
poliodistrofia cerebral progresiva
    progressive cerebral poliodystrophy
polioencefalitis polioencephalitis
polioencefalitis hemorrágica superior
    superior hemorrhagic polioencephalitis
polioencefalitis infecciosa polioencephalitis

infectiva
polioencefalitis inferior inferior
   polioencephalitis
polioencefalitis superior superior
   polioencephalitis
polioencefalomeningomielitis
   polioencephalomeningomyelitis
polioencefalomielitis polioencephalomyelitis
polioencefalopatía polioencephalopathy
poliomielencefalitis poliomyelencephalitis
poliomielitis poliomyelitis
poliomielitis anterior aguda acute anterior
   poliomyelitis
poliomielitis anterior crónica chronic anterior
   poliomyelitis
poliomielitis bulbar bulbar poliomyelitis
poliomielitis bulbar aguda acute bulbar
   poliomyelitis
poliomielitis bulboespinal bulbospinal
   poliomyelitis
poliomielitis espinal spinal poliomyelitis
poliomieloencefalitis poliomyeloencephalitis
poliomielopatía poliomyelopathy
polionomía polyonomy
poliopía polyopia
poliopsia polyopsia
poliórquido polyorchid
poliparesia polyparesis
polipéptido polypeptide
polipéptido neuronal neuronal polypeptide
poliplejía polyplegia
polipnea polypnea
pólipo polyp
poliposia polyposia
poliposis polyposis
polipsiquismo polypsychism
polirradiculitis polyradiculitis
polirradiculomiopatía polyradiculomyopathy
polirradiculoneuritis polyradiculoneuritis
polirradiculoneuropatía
   polyradiculoneuropathy
polirradiculopatía polyradiculopathy
polisemia polysemy
polisensorial polysensory
poliserositis polyserositis
polisináptico polysynaptic
polisomnografía polysomnography
polisomnograma polysomnogram
polisteráxico polysteraxic
política de puerta giratoria revolving-door
   policy
política de puertas abiertas open-door policy
política de salud health policy
politoxicomaníaco polytoxicomaniac
poliuria polyuria
polódico pollodic
polución del humo de cigarrillo
   cigarette-smoke pollution
ponderación weighting
ponderación de artículo item weighting
ponderado weighted
ponofobia ponophobia
ponopatía ponopathy
pons pons
pontino pontine

pontocerebeloso pontocerebellar
popularidad popularity
porencefalia porencephaly
porencefálico porencephalic
porencefalitis porencephalitis
porencéfalo porencephalous
porfiria porphyria
porfiria aguda acute porphyria
porfiria aguda intermitente intermittent acute
   porphyria
porfiria hepática hepatic porphyria
porfirinuria porphyrinuria
porfirismo porphyrismus
porfobilinógeno porphobilinogen
poriomanía poriomania
poriomaníaco poriomanic
pornerástico pornerastic
pornografía pornography
pornografía de niños child pornography
pornografomanía pornographomania
pornolagnia pornolagnia
porosis porosis
porosis cerebral cerebral porosis
porropsia porropsia
portador carrier
portador de rasgo trait carrier
portador de síntomas symptom bearer
posalucinógeno posthallucinogen
posambivalencia postambivalence
posapopléctico postapoplectic
poscentral postcentral
posconcusión postconcussion
poscontracción aftercontraction
poscorriente aftercurrent
posdesastre postdisaster
posdiftérico postdiphtheritic
posdivorcio postdivorce
posdormital postdormital
posdormitum postdormitum
posedípico postoedipal
posempleo postemployment
posencefalítico postencephalitic
posencefalitis postencephalitis
posepiléptico postepileptic
posesión possession
posesión demoníaca demonic possession
posesividad possessiveness
posesivo possessive
posesquizofrénico postschizophrenic
posexperimental postexperimental
posexpulsión afterexpulsion
posganglionar postganglionic
poshemipléjico posthemiplegic
poshipnótico posthypnotic
posición position
posición coital coital position
posición de ojo eye position
posición de optimización de información
   information-optimization position
posición depresiva depressive position
posición esquizoide schizoid position
posición ordinal ordinal position
posición paranoide-esquizoide
   paranoid-schizoid position
posición relativa relative position

posictal postictal
posiomanía posiomania
positivamente positively
positivamente batmotrópico positively
  bathmotropic
positivismo positivism
positivismo lógico logical positivism
positivo positive
positrón positron
posmadurez postmaturity
posmaduro postmature
posmeningítico postmeningitic
posmortem postmortem
posnatal postnatal
posneurítico postneuritic
posinfeccioso postinfectious
posoperatorio postoperative
posparalítico postparalytic
pospartal postpartal
posparto postpartum
pospotencial afterpotential
post hoc post hoc
posterior posterior
posterolateral posterolateral
póstico posticus
postión posthion
postración prostration
postraumático posttraumatic
postremidad postremity
postseparación postseparation
postsináptico postsynaptic
postulado postulate
postulados conversacionales conversational
  postulates
postura posture
posturación posturing
posturación catatónica catatonic posturing
postural postural
posturología posturology
posvacunal postvaccinal
potamofobia potamophobia
potasio potassium
potasio sérico serum potassium
potencia potency
potencia orgástica orgastic potency
potencia sexual sexual potency
potenciación a largo plazo long-term
  potentiation
potenciación postetánica posttetanic
  potentiation
potencial potential
potencial académico academic potential
potencial bioeléctrico bioelectric potential
potencial cerebral brain potential
potencial cerebral relacionado a evento
  event-related brain potential
potencial cutáneo skin potential
potencial de acción action potential
potencial de acción muscular muscle-action
  potential
potencial de aprendizaje learning potential
potencial de demarcación demarcation
  potential
potencial de generador generator potential
potencial de lesión injury potential

potencial de placa terminal end-plate
  potential
potencial de placa terminal miniatura
  miniature end-plate potential
potencial de punta spike potential
potencial de reacción reaction potential
potencial de reacción efectivo effective
  reaction potential
potencial de receptor receptor potential
potencial de reposo resting potential
potencial de vértice vertex potential
potencial endolinfático endolymphatic
  potential
potencial evocado evoked potential
potencial evocado auditivo auditory evoked
  potential
potencial evocado de campo lejano far-field
  evoked potential
potencial evocado sensorial sensory-evoked
  potential
potencial evocado somatosensorial
  somatosensory evoked potential
potencial evocado somatosensorial extremo
  extreme somatosensory evoked potential
potencial evocado visual visual evoked
  potential
potencial excitatorio excitatory potential
potencial graduado graded potential
potencial humano human potential
potencial inhibitorio inhibitory potential
potencial inhibitorio generalizado
  generalized inhibitory potential
potencial local local potential
potencial postsináptico postsynaptic potential
potencial postsináptico excitatorio
  excitatory-postsynaptic potential
potencial postsináptico inhibitorio inhibitory
  postsynaptic potential
potencial relacionado a evento event-related
  potential
potencial subumbral subthreshold potential
potenciales corticales cortical potentials
potencialidad potentiality
potente potent
práctica practice
práctica de grupo group practice
práctica distribuida distributed practice
práctica independiente independent practice
práctica negativa negative practice
práctica programada programmed practice
practicar repetidamente drill
prácticas de empleo employment practices
prácticas en la crianza de niños child-rearing
  practices
pragmatagnosia pragmatagnosia
pragmatamnesia pragmatamnesia
pragmática pragmatics
pragmático pragmatic
pragmatismo pragmatism
prandial prandial
praxiología praxiology
praxis praxis
praxis ideocinética ideokinetic praxis
praxiterapéutica praxitherapeutics
prazepam prazepam

preadaptivo preadaptive
preadolescencia preadolescence
preambivalencia preambivalence
preatáxico preataxic
precentro precenter
precipicio visual visual cliff
precipitante (adj) precipitating
precipitante (n) precipitant
precisión precision
precisión de estereotipo stereotype accuracy
precisión de proceso precision of process
precisión de prueba test accuracy
precisión del ajuste goodness of fit
precisión diferencial differential accuracy
preclínico preclinical
precocidad precocity
precodificación precoding
precognición precognition
preconcepción preconception
preconcepto preconcept
precondicionamiento preconditioning
precondicionamiento sensorial sensory
    preconditioning
preconsciente preconscious
preconvencional preconventional
preconvulsivo preconvulsive
precoz precocious
precúneo precuneus
precursor precursor
predatismo predation
predatorio predatory
predemencia predementia
predemencia precoz predementia praecox
predesastre predisaster
predestinación predestination
predeterminismo predeterminism
predicación predication
predicción prediction
predicción clínica clinical prediction
predicción de conducta prediction of
    behavior
predicción de mortalidad prediction of
    mortality
predicción de violencia violence prediction
predicción estadística contra clínica clinical
    versus statistical prediction
predictivo predictive
predictor predictor
predisposición predisposition
predisposición biológica biological
    predisposition
predisposición de estímulo stimulus set
predisposición de perseveración
    perseveration set
predisposición de respuesta response set
predisposición determinante determining set
predisposición genética genetic predisposition
predisposición hereditaria hereditary
    predisposition
predisposición mental mental set
predisposición motora motor set
predisposición objetiva objective set
predisposición para aprendizaje learning set
predisposición para una situación situation
    set

predisposición perceptiva perceptual set
predisposición postural postural set
predisposición preparatoria preparatory set
predivorcio predivorce
predormital predormital
predormitum predormitum
preeclampsia preeclampsia
preedípico preoedipal
preescolar preschool
preesquizofrénico preschizophrenic
prefálico prephallic
preferencia preference
preferencia de color color preference
preferencia de género gender preference
preferencia de marca brand preference
preferencia de ojo eye preference
preferencia de posición position preference
preferencia de secuencia sequence preference
preferencia global global preference
preferencia ojo-mano eye-hand preference
preferencia sexual sexual preference
preferencial preferential
preferencias auditivas auditory preferences
preferencias de comida food preferences
preformismo preformism
prefrontal prefrontal
preganglionar preganglionic
pregenital pregenital
pregunta question
pregunta clave key question
pregunta con alternativas fijas closed-ended
    question
pregunta con cola tag question
pregunta de Molyneux Molyneux's question
pregunta de Pigem Pigem's question
pregunta de sí-no yes-no question
pregunta posexperimental postexperimental
    inquiry
pregunta sin alternativas fijas open-ended
    question
prehabla prespeech
prehemipléjico prehemiplegic
preictal preictal
prejuicio prejudice
prejuicio racial race prejudice
prelingüístico prelinguistic
prelógico prelogical
premadurez prematurity
premaníaco premaniacal
premarital premarital
prematuro premature
premeditación premeditation
premenstrual premenstrual
premisa premise
premoralidad premorality
premórbido premorbid
premotor premotor
prenatal prenatal
prensil prehensile
prensión prehension
preocupación preoccupation
preocupación sexual sexual concern
preocupación somática somatic concern
preoperacional preoperational
preoperatorio preoperatory

preóptico preoptic
preorgásmico preorgasmic
preparación preparation
preparación aguda acute preparation
preparación biológica biological preparedness
preparación crónica chronic preparation
preparación nervio-músculo nerve-muscle preparation
preparación para hospitalización preparation for hospitalization
preparación parabiótica parabiotic preparation
preparado prepared
preparalítico preparalytic
preparatorio preparatory
prepartal prepartal
prepercepción preperception
preperiodo foreperiod
prepotente prepotent
preprogramación preprogramming
preprueba pretest
prepsicótico prepsychotic
prepuberal prepuberal
prepubertad prepuberty
prepubertal prepubertal
prepubescencia prepubescence
prepucio prepuce
prepucio del clítoris prepuce of clitoris
prepucio del pene prepuce of penis
presacro presacral
presbiacusis presbyacusis
presbicusis presbycusis
presbiofrenia presbyophrenia
presbiopía presbyopia
preselección de sexo sex preselection
presenil presenile
presenilidad presenility
presenium presenium
presentación presentation
presentación de caso case presentation
presentación de instinto instinct presentation
presente especioso specious present
presináptico presynaptic
presión pressure
presión acústica acoustic pressure
presión audible mínima minimum audible pressure
presión cerebroespinal cerebrospinal pressure
presión de actividad pressure of activity
presión de grupo group pressure
presión de grupo paritario peer-group pressure
presión de ideas pressure of ideas
presión de pensamientos thought pressure
presión del habla pressure of speech
presión intracraneal intracranial pressure
presión intraocular intraocular pressure
presión paritaria peer pressure
presión paritaria y beber peer pressure and drinking
presión paritaria y fumar peer pressure and smoking
presión paritaria y uso de drogas peer pressure and drug use
presión sanguínea blood pressure

presión sanguínea alta high blood pressure
presión sanguínea diastólica diastolic blood pressure
presión sanguínea e ira blood pressure and anger
presión sanguínea sistólica systolic blood pressure
presión social social pressure
presolución presolution
presorreceptor pressoreceptor
prestigio prestige
presuperego presuperego
presuposición presupposition
presupuestación funcional functional budgeting
pretraumático pretraumatic
prevalencia prevalence
prevalencia de depresión depression prevalence
prevalencia de periodo period prevalence
prevalencia de problemas de conducta prevalence of behavior problems
prevalencia de punto point prevalence
prevalencia de trastornos del comer prevalence of eating disorders
prevalencia de vida lifetime prevalence
prevalencia transversal cross-sectional prevalence
prevalencia tratada treated prevalence
prevención prevention
prevención de abuso de niños prevention of child abuse
prevención de abuso sexual de niños prevention of child sexual abuse
prevención de alcoholismo alcoholism prevention
prevención de ansiedad prevention of anxiety
prevención de crímenes crime prevention
prevención de crímenes mediante asesoramiento crime prevention by counseling
prevención de crímenes mediante castigo crime prevention by punishing
prevención de delincuencia delinquency prevention
prevención de recaída relapse prevention
prevención de respuestas response prevention
prevención de suicidios suicide prevention
prevención de trastornos del comer prevention of eating disorders
prevención primaria primary prevention
prevención primaria de psicopatología primary prevention of psychopathology
prevención secundaria secondary prevention
prevención terciaria tertiary prevention
prevención de accidentes accident prevention
preventivo preventive
preverbal preverbal
prevocacional prevocational
priapismo priapism
prima facie prima facie
primacía primacy
primacía fálica phallic primacy
primacía genital genital primacy
primacía oral oral primacy

primal primal
primario primary
primate primate
primer ataque first attack
primer momento first moment
primer plano foreground
primer sistema de señalamiento first
  signaling system
primera admisión first admission
primera causa first cause
primera fase de represión first phase of
  repression
primera fase negativa first negative phase
primera impresión first impression
primeras palabras first words
primeros auxilios first aid
primeros movimientos fetales percibidos
  quickening
primidona primidone
primípara primipara
primitivación primitivation
primitivización primitivization
primitivo primitive
primordial primordial
principal principal
principio principle
principio de autoridad authority principle
principio de cierre closure principle
principio de comunión communion principle
principio de congruencia congruence
  principle
principio de constancia principle of
  constancy
principio de contraste máximo principle of
  maximum contrast
principio de cuadrados mínimos
  least-squares principle
principio de distancia mínima minimum
  distance principle
principio de dolor pain principle
principio de dolor-placer pain-pleasure
  principle
principio de eco echo principle
principio de economía principle of economy
principio de equipotencialidad principle of
  equipotentiality
principio de estimulación óptima
  optimal-stimulation principle
principio de generalización de respuestas
  response-generalization principle
principio de inercia inertia principle
principio de intimidad intimacy principle
principio de Jackson Jackson's principle
principio de la consistencia consistency
  principle
principio de la contigüidad contiguity
  principle
principio de la explicación contemporánea
  contemporaneous explanation principle
principio de lo más reciente principle of
  recency
principio de maduración anticipatoria
  anticipatory-maturation principle
principio de Morgan Morgan's principle
principio de nirvana nirvana principle

principio de pertenencia principle of
  belongingness
principio de placer-dolor pleasure-pain
  principle
principio de postremidad postremity
  principle
principio de Pragnanz principle of Pragnanz
principio de Premack Premack's principle
principio de primacía principle of primacy
principio de proximidad proximity principle
principio de realidad reality principle
principio de relajación relaxation principle
principio de reorganización reorganization
  principle
principio de repetición-compulsión
  repetition-compulsion principle
principio de situaciones dinámicas
  dynamic-situations principle
principio de todo o nada all-or-nothing
  principle
principio de von Domarus von Domarus
  principle
principio del crecimiento growth principle
principio del desuso disuse principle
principio del esfuerzo mínimo least-effort
  principle
principio del impulso irresistible principle of
  the irresistible impulse
principio del placer pleasure principle
principio del talión talion principle
principio descriptivo descriptive principle
principio epigenético epigenetic principle
principio filogenético phylogenetic principle
principio homeopático homeopathic principle
principio homeostático homeostatic principle
principio isopático isopathic principle
principio moral moral principle
principio utilitario utilitarian principle
principios éticos ethical principles
prisión prison
prisma prism
prisma de Henning Henning's prism
prisma de olores odor prism
prisma olfativa smell prism
privacidad privacy
privación deprivation
privación ambiental environmental
  deprivation
privación cultural cultural deprivation
privación de actividad activity deprivation
privación de comidas food deprivation
privación de movimientos oculares rápidos
  rapid eye movement deprivation
privación de movimientos oculares rápidos y
  esquizofrenia rapid eye movement
  deprivation and schizophrenia
privación de papel role deprivation
privación de pensamientos thought
  deprivation
privación de potasio potassium deprivation
privación de privilegios deprivation of
  privileges
privación del sueño sleep deprivation
privación emocional emotional deprivation
privación-gratificación relativa relative

deprivation-gratification
privación maternal maternal deprivation
privación psicosocial psychosocial deprivation
privación sensorial sensory deprivation
privación social social deprivation
privado private
privilegio privilege
proactivo proactive
probabilidad probability
probabilidad condicional conditional
    probability
probabilidad conjunta joint probability
probabilidad de dos colas two-tailed
    probability
probabilidad de respuesta probability of
    response
probabilidad de una cola one-tailed
    probability
probabilidad máxima maximum likelihood
probabilidad subjetiva subjective probability
probabilidad transicional transitional
    probability
probabilismo probabilism
probabilístico probabilistic
probable probable
probando proband
probarbital probarbital
probenecid probenecid
problema problem
problema académico academic problem
problema conductual behavioral problem
problema cuerpo-mente body-mind problem
problema de aculturación acculturation
    problem
problema de alimentación feeding problem
problema de alternación doble
    double-alternation problem
problema de aprendizaje learning problem
problema de barrera barrier problem
problema de circunstancia de vida life
    circumstance problem
problema de conducta behavior problem
problema de desvíos detour problem
problema de direccionalidad directionality
    problem
problema de fase de vida phase of life
    problem
problema de identidad identity problem
problema de intensidad de afecto affect
    intensity problem
problema de personalidad personality
    problem
problema de rareza oddity problem
problema de tercera variable third-variable
    problem
problema del lenguaje language problem
problema escolar school problem
problema espiritual spiritual problem
problema gastrointestinal gastrointestinal
    problem
problema interpersonal interpersonal
    problem
problema nuclear nuclear problem
problema ocupacional occupational problem
problema psicoeducativo psychoeducational

problem
problema raíz root problem
problema relacionado con abuso problem
    related to abuse
problema relacionado con negligencia
    problem related to neglect
problema relacional relational problem
problema relacional de hermanos sibling
    relational problem
problema relacional de pareja partner
    relational problem
**problema relacional relacionado a condición
    médica general** relational problem related
    to general medical condition
**problema relacional relacionado a trastorno
    mental** relational problem related to
    mental disorder
problema religioso religious problem
problema sexual sexual problem
problema social social problem
problemas con la audición problems with
    hearing
problemas conductuales sexuales sexual
    behavioral problems
problemas de agregación aggregation
    problems
problemas de audición hearing problems
problemas de conducta y abuso de niños
    behavior problems and child abuse
problemas de escritura handwriting problems
problemas escolares y familia school
    problems and family
problemas éticos ethical problems
problemas maritales marital problems
problemático problematic
procaína procaine
procedimiento procedure
procedimiento clínico clinical procedure
procedimiento de alimentación simulada
    sham feeding procedure
procedimiento de comparación comparison
    procedure
procedimiento de conciencia sensorial
    sensory-awareness procedure
procedimiento de cuidado y protección care
    and protection proceedings
procedimiento de dar de alta discharge
    procedure
procedimiento de desensibilización
    desensitization procedure
procedimiento de enfoque de atención
    attention-focusing procedure
procedimiento de grupo apareado
    matched-group procedure
procedimiento de grupos equivalentes
    equivalent groups procedure
procedimiento de Monte Carlo Monte Carlo
    procedure
procedimiento de rastreo rotatorio
    rotary-pursuit procedure
procedimiento de reconocimiento recognition
    procedure
procedimiento de reproducción reproduction
    procedure
procedimiento de tiempo fuera time-out

procedure
procedimiento demorado delayed procedure
procedimiento diagnóstico diagnostic
  procedure
procedimiento para establecer competencia
  procedure for establishing competency
procedimientos antianalíticos antianalytic
  procedures
procedimientos cognitivos cognitive
  procedures
procedimientos de admisión admission
  procedures
procedimientos de evaluación conductual
  behavioral assessment procedures
procedimientos de mamar no nutritivos
  nonnutritive sucking procedures
procesador processor
procesamiento processing
procesamiento activo active processing
procesamiento acústico acoustic processing
procesamiento analítico analytic processing
procesamiento auditivo auditory processing
procesamiento automático automatic
  processing
procesamiento controlado controlled
  processing
procesamiento de información information
  processing
procesamiento de información humano
  human information processing
procesamiento de información y cognición
  information processing and cognition
procesamiento de información y percepción
  information processing and perception
procesamiento del fondo hacia arriba
  bottom-up processing
procesamiento del tope hacia abajo
  top-down processing
procesamiento distribuido distributed
  processing
procesamiento distribuido paralelo parallel
  distributed processing
procesamiento global global processing
procesamiento intermitente intermittent
  processing
procesamiento paralelo parallel processing
procesamiento perceptivo perceptual
  processing
procesamiento sensorial sensory processing
procesamiento serial serial processing
proceso process
proceso adictivo addictive process
proceso automático automatic process
proceso central central process
proceso cerebral brain process
proceso cerebral vicario vicarious brain
  process
proceso cognitivo inconsciente unconscious
  cognitive process
proceso cultural cultural process
proceso de asesoramiento counseling process
proceso de cambio switch process
proceso de dar y tomar give-and-take process
proceso de difusión diffusion process
proceso de entrada de información

information-input process
proceso de entrevista interview process
proceso de grupo group process
proceso de grupo de acción action group
  process
proceso de Markov Markov process
proceso de pensamiento thought process
proceso de reacción reaction process
proceso de reactivación reactivation process
proceso de socialización socialization process
proceso de vinculación bonding process
proceso elemental elementary process
proceso ergotrópico ergotropic process
proceso inconsciente unconscious process
proceso inhibitorio inhibitory process
proceso interpersonal interpersonal process
proceso latente latent process
proceso mental mental process
proceso nervioso nerve process
proceso neural neural process
proceso neurótico neurotic process
proceso predominante regnant process
proceso primario primary process
proceso psi psi process
proceso psíquico primario primary psychic
  process
proceso secundario secondary process
proceso sensorial sensory process
proceso sensorimotor sensorimotor process
proceso simbólico symbolic process
proceso social social process
proceso voluntario voluntary process
procesos adaptivos adaptive processes
procesos cognitivos cognitive processes
procesos conductuales behavioral processes
procesos conscientes conscious processes
procesos corticales cortical processes
procesos de ajuste adjustment processes
procesos de aprendizaje complejos complex
  learning processes
procesos de comunicación communication
  processes
procesos de innovación innovation processes
procesos de Lenhossek Lenhossek's
  processes
procesos de mediación mediation processes
procesos de oponentes opponent process
procesos de respuesta fundamentales
  fundamental response processes
procesos emotivos emotive processes
procesos episódicos episodic processes
procesos excitatorios-inhibitorios
  excitatory-inhibitory processes
procesos imitativos imitative processes
procesos mentales superiores higher mental
  processes
procesos perceptivos perceptual processes
prociclidina procyclidine
proclorperazina prochlorperazine
procrastinación procrastination
proctalgia proctalgia
proctalgia fugaz proctalgia fugax
proctoespasmo proctospasm
proctofobia proctophobia
proctoparálisis proctoparalysis

proctoplejía proctoplegia
procursivo procursive
prodigio prodigy
prodromal prodromal
prodrómico prodromic
pródromo prodrome
producción production
producción de imagen imaging
producción de imagen cerebral brain imaging
producción de imagen cerebral dinámica cerebral dynamic imaging
producción de imagen óptica optical imaging
producción de imagen por resonancia magnética magnetic resonance imaging
producción de imagen superficial surface imaging
producción de imágenes nuclear nuclear imaging
producción de magnitud magnitude production
producción de proporciones ratio production
producción del habla speech production
productividad productivity
productividad de empleado employee productivity
productividad en lenguaje productiveness in language
productivo productive
producto product
producto de reacción reaction product
proespermia prospermia
proestro proestrus
profase prophase
profecía autorrealizante self-fulfilling prophecy
profesión profession
profesión de ayuda helping profession
profesional professional
profesional aliado a la salud allied health professional
profesional de salud health professional
profético prophetic
profiláctico prophylactic
profilaxis prophylaxis
profundidad depth
profundidad de procesamiento depth of processing
profundidad del humor depth of mood
profundo deep
progeria progeria
progesterona progesterone
progestina progestin
progestógeno progestogen
prognosis prognosis
prognosis de daño cerebral brain damage prognosis
prognosis de dirección direction prognosis
programa program
programa bifurcado branching program
programa comunitario community program
programa conjuntivo conjunctive schedule
programa cribador screening program
programa de abuso de sustancias substance abuse program

programa de acción social social-action program
programa de alimentación por demanda propia self-demand schedule of feeding
programa de asesoramiento guidance program
programa de bienestar social social welfare program
programa de cuidado diurno day care program
programa de cuidado nocturno night-care program
programa de demanda propia self-demand schedule
programa de educación individualizada individualized education program
programa de enriquecimiento enrichment program
programa de entrenamiento transcultural cross-cultural training program
programa de entrevistas estandarizada standardized interview schedule
programa de estimulación de infantes infant-stimulation program
programa de evitación de Sidman Sidman avoidance schedule
programa de intervalo fijo fixed-interval schedule
programa de intervalo variable variable-interval schedule
programa de intervalos interval schedule
programa de mantenimiento maintenance schedule
programa de razón fija fixed-ratio schedule
programa de razón variable variable-ratio schedule
programa de reestructuración de actitudes sexuales sexual attitude restructuring program
programa de refuerzo reinforcement schedule
programa de refuerzo aperiódico aperiodic reinforcement schedule
programa de refuerzo continuo continuous reinforcement schedule
programa de refuerzo de intervalo fijo fixed-interval reinforcement schedule
programa de refuerzo de intervalo variable variable-interval reinforcement schedule
programa de refuerzo de razón fija fixed-ratio reinforcement schedule
programa de refuerzo de razón variable variable-ratio reinforcement schedule
programa de refuerzo múltiple multiple-reinforcement schedule
programa de refuerzo no intermitente nonintermittent reinforcement schedule
programa de rehabilitación rehabilitation program
programa de salud mental mental-health program
programa de salud mental comunitario community mental health program
programa de terapeutas padres parent therapist program

programa educacional educational program
programa encadenado chained schedule
programa entrelazado interlocking schedule
programa individual individual program
programa intermitente intermittent schedule
programa lineal linear program
programa mixto mixed schedule
programa preescolar preschool program
programa psicoeducativo psychoeducational
program
programa transicional transitional program
programación programming
programación genética genetic programming
programación genotípica genotypic
programming
programado programmed
programas concurrentes concurrent
schedules
programas de computadora computer
software
**programas de educación individualizada y
traslación a la corriente principal**
individualized education programs and
mainstreaming
progresión progression
progresión obstinada obstinate progression
progresivo progressive
prohibido prohibited
prohormona prohormone
prolactina prolactin
prolactina sérica serum prolactin
prolactinoma prolactinoma
prolapso prolapse
proliferación proliferation
proliferativo proliferative
promazina promazine
promedio average
promedio descriptivo descriptive average
prometazina promethazine
prominencia salience
promiscuidad promiscuity
promiscuo promiscuous
pronación pronation
prono prone
pronosticación forecasting
pronosticador prognostic
pronóstico prognosis
propagación propagation
propagación del efecto spread of effect
propaganda propaganda
propedéutico propaedeutic
propensión propensity
propensión a los accidentes accident
proneness
propensión al aburrimiento boredom
proneness
propenso a accidentes accident-prone
propenso a ansiedad anxiety-prone
propenso a coronaria coronary-prone
propiedad derivada derived property
propiedades de cables cable properties
propiedades de campo field properties
propiedades integrantes integrative
properties
propincuidad propinquity

propiocepción proprioception
propioceptivo proprioceptive
propioceptor proprioceptor
propiomazina propiomazine
proporción proportion
proporción de dadas de alta discharge rate
proposición proposition
propósito purpose
propositus propositus
propoxifeno propoxyphene
propranolol propranolol
propulsión propulsion
prosencéfalo prosencephalon
prosocial prosocial
prosodia prosody
prosódico prosodic
prosopagnosia prosopagnosia
prosopalgia prosopalgia
prosopálgico prosopalgic
prosoplejía prosoplegia
prosopodiplejía prosopodiplegia
prosopoespasmo prosopospasm
prosoponeuralgia prosoponeuralgia
prosopoplejía prosopoplegia
prosopopléjico prosopoplegic
prospectivo prospective
prostaglandina prostaglandin
prostatectomía prostatectomy
prosternación prosternation
prosteta prosthetist
prostitución prostitution
prostitución de homosexuales masculinos
male homosexual prostitution
prostitución de niños child prostitution
protanomalía protanomaly
protanopía protanopia
proteasa protease
protección protection
protección por remoción removal protection
proteína protein
proteína sérica serum protein
protensidad protensity
protensión protension
prótesis prosthesis
prótesis conductual behavioral prosthesis
protesta protest
protesta corporal body protest
protesta masculina masculine protest
protético prothetic
protimia prothymia
protipendilo prothipendyl
protocolo protocol
protoespasmo protospasm
protofálico protophallic
protomasoquismo protomasochism
protopático protopathic
protoplasma protoplasm
protoplásmico protoplasmic
prototáxico prototaxic
prototaxis prototaxis
prototeoría prototheory
prototipo prototype
protriptilina protriptyline
protrombina prothrombin
proveedor de cuidado de salud health care

provider
provisional provisional
provocación sexual sexual provocation
proxémica proxemics
proxibarbal proxibarbal
proximal proximal
proximidad proximity
proximidad madre-infante mother-infant
proximity
proximoataxia proximoataxia
proximodistal proximodistal
proyección projection
proyección excéntrica eccentric projection
proyección impersonal impersonal projection
proyección óptica optical projection
proyección visual visual projection
proyectivo projective
proyecto project
prueba test, proof
prueba a posteriori a posteriori test
prueba a priori a priori test
prueba adaptiva adaptive test
prueba administrada por computadora
computer-administered test
prueba anecdótica anecdotal evidence
prueba autoadministrada self-administered
test
prueba binomial binomial test
prueba cara-mano face-hand test
prueba ceruloplasmina ceruloplasmin test
prueba cíclica cycle test
prueba circunstancial circumstantial evidence
prueba colectiva omnibus test
prueba computerizada computerized test
prueba cribadora screening test
prueba de absurdidades absurdities test
**prueba de acceso por retiro de dióxido de
carbono** carbon dioxide withdrawal
seizure test
prueba de agudeza acuity test
prueba de Akerfeldt Akerfeldt test
prueba de aleatorización randomization test
prueba de alfabetismo literacy test
prueba de alternación demorada
delayed-alternation test
prueba de analogías analogies test
prueba de anclaje anchor test
prueba de anomalías de pinturas
picture-anomalies test
prueba de antónimos antonym test
prueba de aprovechamiento achievement test
prueba de aprovechamiento académico
academic achievement test
prueba de aprovechamiento escolástico
scholastic achievement test
prueba de aptitud aptitude test
prueba de aptitud académica academic
aptitude test
prueba de aptitud general general aptitude
test
prueba de aptitud mecánica
mechanical-aptitude test
prueba de aptitud profesional professional
aptitude test
prueba de aptitud vocacional

vocational-aptitude test
prueba de aptitudes especiales
special-aptitude test
prueba de aptitudes múltiples
multiple-aptitude test
prueba de articulación articulation test
prueba de asociación association test
prueba de asociación de palabras
word-association test
prueba de asociación remota
remote-association test
prueba de audición hearing test
prueba de aula classroom test
prueba de Aussage Aussage test
prueba de autoclasificación self-rating test
prueba de autoconcepto self-concept test
prueba de Barany Barany test
prueba de bien y mal good-and-evil test
prueba de bola y campo ball-and-field test
prueba de Broadbent Broadbent test
prueba de caída de cabeza head-dropping
test
prueba de cancelación cancellation test
prueba de características-perfil
feature-profile test
prueba de categorías category test
prueba de causa y efecto cause-and-effect
test
prueba de clasificación sorting test
prueba de clasificación de colores color
sorting test
prueba de clasificación de objetos object
sorting test
prueba de clasificar cartas card-sorting test
prueba de cloruro férrico ferric chloride test
prueba de cociente de inteligencia
intelligence quotient test
prueba de codificaciones coding test
prueba de códigos code test
prueba de colecistoquinina cholecystokinin
test
prueba de colocación placement test
prueba de comprensión comprehension test
prueba de cómputos calculation test
prueba de concentración concentration test
prueba de conducción de aire air conduction
test
prueba de conocimientos knowledge test
prueba de conteo de bloques block-counting
test
prueba de Coombs Coombs' test
prueba de creatividad creativity test
prueba de dedo-nariz finger-nose test
prueba de destreza dexterity test
prueba de destrezas de oficina
clerical-aptitude test
prueba de dibujo drawing test
prueba de dibujo con espejo mirror-drawing
test
prueba de dibujo de figuras figure-drawing
test
prueba de direcciones directions test
prueba de diseños con bloques block-design
test
prueba de distorsión visual visual-distortion

test
prueba de doblar papel paper-folding test
prueba de doblar papel mental mental paper-folding test
prueba de dominancia dominance test
prueba de dominancia de Wada Wada dominance test
prueba de dominio mastery test
prueba de dos colas two-tailed test
prueba de Duncan Duncan test
prueba de Durham Durham test
prueba de Ebbinghaus Ebbinghaus test
prueba de ejecución performance test
prueba de empleo employment test
prueba de encuesta survey test
prueba de ensamblaje de objetos object-assembly test
prueba de ensayo essay test
prueba de espontaneidad spontaneity test
prueba de estación station test
prueba de estrés stress test
prueba de estrés situacional situational-stress test
prueba de extensión del brazo arm extension test
prueba de fábulas fables test
prueba de factibilidad feasibility test
prueba de figuras encerradas embedded-figures test
prueba de figuras escondidas hidden-figure test
prueba de Finckh Finckh test
prueba de Fisher Fisher's test
prueba de Folling Folling's test
prueba de formación de conceptos concept-formation test
prueba de fotometrazol photometrazol test
prueba de funcionamiento tiroide thyroid function test
prueba de Funkenstein Funkenstein test
prueba de Goldscheider Goldscheider's test
prueba de golpecito de talón heel-tap test
prueba de grupo group test
prueba de Guthrie Guthrie test
prueba de habilidad ability test
prueba de Hejna Hejna test
prueba de hiperventilación hyperventilation test
prueba de hipoglucemia insulínica insulin hypoglycemia test
prueba de hipótesis test of hypothesis
prueba de hipótesis no direccional nondirectional test of hypothesis
prueba de Hollander Hollander test
prueba de Holmgren Holmgren test
prueba de honradez honesty test
prueba de identificación identification test
prueba de impulsos irresistibles irresistible impulse test
prueba de indicios escondidos hidden-clue test
prueba de inducción induction test
prueba de infante infant test
prueba de infusión de metacolina methacholine infusion test

prueba de inhalación de dióxido de carbono carbon dioxide inhalation test
prueba de integridad orgánica organic integrity test
prueba de inteligencia intelligence test
prueba de inteligencia de grupo group intelligence test
prueba de intereses interest test
prueba de interpretación de pinturas picture-interpretation test
prueba de inventario inventory test
prueba de inversión de objetos object reversal test
prueba de Ishihara Ishihara test
prueba de Janet Janet's test
prueba de ji cuadrada chi square test
prueba de Kahn Kahn test
prueba de Kohnstamm Kohnstamm test
prueba de Kolomogorov-Smirnov Kolomogorov-Smirnov test
prueba de Kruskal-Wallis Kruskal-Wallis test
prueba de la mejor razón best reason test
prueba de la mejor respuesta best answer test
prueba de laboratorio laboratory test
prueba de Lange Lange's test
prueba de lapso de dígitos digit-span test
prueba de lectura reading test
prueba de lectura de mapa map-reading test
prueba de Lichtheim Lichtheim's test
prueba de lo correcto e incorrecto right-and-wrong test
prueba de lo correcto o incorrecto right-or-wrong test
prueba de localización de punto point-localization test
prueba de manchas de tinta inkblot test
prueba de McNemar McNemar test
prueba de melatonina melatonin test
prueba de monedas coin test
prueba de monitor de Holter Holter monitor test
prueba de mosaico mosaic test
prueba de mundo en pintura picture world test
prueba de Nalline Nalline test
prueba de nicotina nicotine test
prueba de objetos object test
prueba de opuestos opposites test
prueba de oración desarreglada disarranged sentence test
prueba de oraciones incompletas incomplete sentences test
prueba de ordenación de pinturas picture-arrangement test
prueba de organicidad organicity test
prueba de Pachon Pachon's test
prueba de papel y lápiz paper and pencil test
prueba de pareo matching test
prueba de pareo demorado delayed-matching test
prueba de partes faltantes missing-parts test
prueba de Patrick Patrick's test
prueba de personalidad personality test

prueba de pinturas incompletas incomplete pictures test
prueba de poder power test
prueba de polígrafo polygraph test
prueba de precisión accuracy test
prueba de preferencia preference test
prueba de preparación readiness test
prueba de proverbios proverbs test
prueba de psicopenetración psychopenetration test
prueba de punteo dotting test
prueba de puntería aiming test
prueba de Queckensiedt-Stookey Queckenstedt-Stookey test
prueba de rastreo rotatorio rotary-pursuit test
prueba de realidad reality test
prueba de reconocimiento recognition test
prueba de recordación recall test
prueba de recordación de cuento story-recall test
prueba de relaciones sociales social relations test
prueba de reloj watch test
prueba de repetición de oraciones sentence-repetition test
prueba de responsabilidad criminal test of criminal responsibility
prueba de respuestas alternas alternate-response test
prueba de respuestas cortas short-answer test
prueba de respuestas forzadas forced-response test
prueba de respuestas libres free-response test
prueba de ritmo rhythm test
prueba de Romberg Romberg test
prueba de Rorschach Rorschach test
prueba de Rosanoff Rosanoff test
prueba de Rosenbach-Gmelin Rosenbach-Gmelin test
prueba de Scheffe Scheffe test
prueba de selección selection test
prueba de selecciones forzadas forced-choice test
prueba de significación test of significance
prueba de significado de párrafo paragraph-meaning test
prueba de signos sign test
prueba de símbolos-dígitos symbol-digit test
prueba de similitudes similarities test
prueba de sinónimos-antónimos synonym-antonym test
prueba de situación situation test
prueba de Snellen Snellen test
prueba de Stilling Stilling test
prueba de Stroop Stroop test
prueba de Student Student's test
prueba de sudación sweating test
prueba de supresión de dexametasona dexamethasone suppression test
prueba de supresión de dexametasona y diagnóstico de depresión dexamethasone suppression test and depression diagnosis

prueba de supresión de dexametasona y suicidio dexamethasone suppression test and suicide
prueba de sustitución substitution test
prueba de sustitución de símbolos symbol-substitution test
prueba de tabla de formas formboard test
prueba de tabla de multiplicación multiplication table test
prueba de talón a rodilla heel-to-knee test
prueba de tendencia trend test
prueba de terminación completion test
prueba de terminación de números number-completion test
prueba de terminación de oraciones sentence-completion test
prueba de terminación de pinturas picture-completion test
prueba de tolerancia tolerance test
prueba de tolerancia de glucosa glucose-tolerance test
prueba de tumescencia peniana nocturna nocturnal penile tumescence test
prueba de Turing Turing's test
prueba de umbral de presión pressure-threshold test
prueba de una cola one-tailed test
prueba de usos alternos alternate-uses test
prueba de varillas de Maddox Maddox rod test
prueba de velocidad speed test
prueba de vocabulario vocabulary test
prueba de Vygotsky Vygotsky test
prueba de Wada Wada test
prueba de Weber Weber test
prueba de Wilcoxon Wilcoxon test
prueba del laboratorio de investigación de enfermedades venéreas venereal disease research laboratory test
prueba del lenguaje language test
prueba del personal personnel test
prueba del reflejo cocleopalpebral cochleopalpebral reflex test
prueba del sentido del tiempo time sense test
prueba diagnóstica diagnostic test
prueba direccional de hipótesis directional test of hypothesis
prueba educacional educational test
prueba educativa diagnóstica diagnostic educational test
prueba empírica empirical test
prueba espectrográfica spectrographic evidence
prueba espiral spiral test
prueba estadística statistical test
prueba estandarizada standardized test
prueba exacta de Fisher Fisher exact test
prueba F F test
prueba final end test
prueba individual individual test
prueba informal informal test
prueba libre de clases class-free test
prueba mental mental test
prueba motora motor test
prueba no verbal nonverbal test

prueba objetiva objective test
prueba ocupacional occupational test
prueba oral oral test
prueba paramétrica de significación
   parametric test of significance
prueba planificada planned test
prueba posterior post-test
prueba pronosticadora prognostic test
prueba proyectiva projective test
prueba psicoacústica psychoacoustic test
prueba psicológica psychological test
prueba psicomotora psychomotor test
prueba Q Q test
prueba-reprueba test-retest
prueba saturada saturated test
prueba secuencial sequential test
prueba sensorial sensory test
prueba sensorial-perceptiva
   sensory-perceptual test
prueba sin sesgo cultural culture-free test
prueba situacional situational test
prueba sociométrica sociometric test
prueba subjetiva subjective test
prueba táctil dicotómica dichotomous tactile
   test
prueba transcultural cross-cultural test
prueba verbal verbal test
pruebas cumulativas cumulative tests
pruebas de arte art tests
pruebas de disfunción cerebral cerebral
   dysfunction tests
pruebas de Fournier Fournier tests
pruebas de infantes y preescolares infant and
   preschool tests
pruebas de inteligencia alternativas
   alternative intelligence tests
pruebas de ji cuadrada de Pearson Pearson
   chi square tests
pruebas de Kendall Kendall tests
pruebas de masculinidad-feminidad
   masculinity-femininity tests
pruebas de Seashore Seashore tests
prurito pruritus
prurito psicogénico psychogenic pruritus
psamocarcinoma psammocarcinoma
psamoma psammoma
psamoma de Virchow Virchow's psammoma
psamomatoso psammomatous
psamoso psammous
pselafesia pselaphesia
pselismo psellism
psi psi
psicagogía psychagogy
psicalgalia psychalgalia
psicalgia psychalgia
psicalia psychalia
psicanopsia psychanopsia
psicastenia psychasthenia
psicataxia psychataxia
psicauditivo psychauditory
psicoactivo psychoactive
psicoacústica psychoacoustics
psicoacústico psychoacoustic
psicoalergia psychoallergy
psicoanaléptica psychoanaleptica

psicoanaléptico psychoanaleptic
psicoanálisis psychoanalysis
psicoanálisis activo active psychoanalysis
psicoanálisis adleriano adlerian
   psychoanalysis
psicoanálisis aplicado applied psychoanalysis
psicoanálisis clásico classical psychoanalysis
psicoanálisis directo direct psychoanalysis
psicoanálisis existencial existential
   psychoanalysis
psicoanálisis freudiano freudian
   psychoanalysis
psicoanálisis histórico historical
   psychoanalysis
psicoanálisis jungiano jungian psychoanalysis
psicoanálisis no directivo nondirective
   psychoanalysis
psicoanálisis ortodoxo orthodox
   psychoanalysis
psicoanalista psychoanalyst
psicoanalítico psychoanalytic
psicoastenia psychoasthenia
psicoasténica psychoasthenics
psicoataxia psychoataxia
psicoauditivo psychoauditory
psicobioanálisis psychobioanalysis
psicobiograma psychobiogram
psicobiología psychobiology
psicobiología del desarrollo developmental
   psychobiology
psicobiológico psychobiological
psicocardíaco psychocardiac
psicocatarsis psychocatharsis
psicociencia psychoscience
psicocinesia psychokinesis
psicocirugía psychosurgery
psicocortical psychocortical
psicocromestesia psychochromesthesia
psicocromo psychochrome
psicocultural psychocultural
psicodélico psychedelic
psicodiagnóstica psychodiagnostics
psicodiagnóstico psychodiagnosis
psicodietética psychodietetics
psicodinámica psychodynamics
psicodinámico psychodynamic
psicodometría psychodometry
psicodómetro psychodometer
psicodrama psychodrama
psicoeducación psychoeducation
psicoeducativo psychoeducational
psicoendocrinología psychoendocrinology
psicoestimulante psychostimulant
psicoexploración psychoexploration
psicofarmacéutico psychopharmaceutical
psicofarmacología psychopharmacology
psicofarmacología clínica clinical
   psychopharmacology
psicofarmacología geriátrica geriatric
   psychopharmacology
psicofarmacología pediátrica pediatric
   psychopharmacology
psicofarmacología preclínica preclinical
   psychopharmacology
psicofarmacológico psychopharmacological

psicofarmacoterapia psychopharmacotherapy
psicofísica psychophysics
psicofísico psychophysical
psicofisiología psychophysiology
psicofisiología cognitiva cognitive psychophysiology
psicofisiología sensorial sensory psychophysiology
psicofisiología social social psychophysiology
psicofisiológico psychophysiological
psicofobia psychophobia
psicogalvánico psychogalvanic
psicogalvanómetro psychogalvanometer
psicogénero psychogender
psicogénesis psychogenesis
psicogenética psychogenetics
psicogenético psychogenetic
psicogenia psychogeny
psicogénico psychogenic
psicogeriatría psychogeriatrics
psicogerontología psychogerontology
psicogéusico psychogeusic
psicognosia psychognosia
psicogógico psychogogic
psicogonia psychogony
psicogónico psychogonical
psicografía psychography
psicográfica psychographics
psicográfico psychographic
psicógrafo psychograph
psicograma psychogram
psicohistoria psychohistory
psicoinfantilismo psychoinfantilism
psicoinmunología psychoimmunology
psicolagnia psycholagny
psicolegal psycholegal
psicolepsia psycholepsy
psicolepsis psycholepsis
psicoléptica psycholeptica
psicolingüística psycholinguistics
psicolingüística del desarrollo developmental psycholinguistics
psicolingüístico psycholinguistic
psicolítico psycholytic
psicología psychology
psicología adleriana adlerian psychology
psicología administrativa managerial psychology
psicología agrícola agricultural psychology
psicología ambiental environmental psychology
psicología analítica analytic psychology
psicología animal animal psychology
psicología anormal abnormal psychology
psicología aplicada applied psychology
psicología atomística atomistic psychology
psicología centralista centralist psychology
psicología científica scientific psychology
psicología clínica clinical psychology
psicología clínica ocupacional occupational clinical psychology
psicología cognitiva cognitive psychology
psicología comparativa comparative psychology
psicología comunitaria community

psychology
psicología comunitaria correccional correctional community psychology
psicología conductual behavioral psychology
psicología constitucional constitutional psychology
psicología consultora consulting psychology
psicología contractual contractual psychology
psicología correccional correctional psychology
psicología criminal criminal psychology
psicología de anuncios advertising psychology
psicología de asesoramiento counseling psychology
psicología de contenido content psychology
psicología de actos act psychology
psicología de deportes sports psychology
psicología de ejercicio exercise psychology
psicología de estímulo-respuesta stimulus-response psychology
psicología de factores humanos human-factors psychology
psicología de facultades faculty psychology
psicología de ingeniería engineering psychology
psicología de Janet Janet's psychology
psicología de jurado jury psychology
psicología de la sala del tribunal courtroom psychology
psicología de muchedumbre mob psychology
psicología de niños child psychology
psicología de personalidad personality psychology
psicología de salud health psychology
psicología de seguridad safety psychology
psicología de servicio público public-service psychology
psicología de ventas sales psychology
psicología de víctima victim psychology
psicología del consumidor consumer psychology
psicología del desarrollo developmental psychology
psicología del desarrollo psicoanalítico psychoanalytic development psychology
psicología del ego ego psychology
psicología del id id psychology
psicología del personal personnel psychology
psicología descriptiva descriptive psychology
psicología dialéctica dialectical psychology
psicología diferencial differential psychology
psicología dinámica dynamic psychology
psicología ecológica ecological psychology
psicología educacional educational psychology
psicología en masa mass psychology
psicología escolar school psychology
psicología espacial space psychology
psicología especulativa speculative psychology
psicología estadística statistical psychology
psicología estructural structural psychology
psicología existencial existential psychology
psicología experimental experimental psychology

psicología filosófica philosophical psychology
psicología fisiológica physiological psychology
psicología forense forensic psychology
psicología funcional functional psychology
psicología general general psychology
psicología genética genetic psychology
psicología geriátrica geriatric psychology
psicología gerontológica gerontological psychology
psicología gestalt gestalt psychology
psicología herbartiana Herbartian psychology
psicología holísitca holistic psychology
psicología hórmica hormic psychology
psicología humanística humanistic psychology
psicología ideográfica ideographic psychology
psicología individual individual psychology
psicología industrial industrial psychology
psicología industrial-organizacional industrial-organizational psychology
psicología intencionada purposive psychology
psicología interconductual interbehavioral psychology
psicología jungiana jungian psychology
psicología legal legal psychology
psicología matemática mathematical psychology
psicología médica medical psychology
psicología objetiva objective psychology
psicología organísmica organismic psychology
psicología organizativa organizational psychology
psicología pediátrica pediatric psychology
psicología perceptiva perceptual psychology
psicología personalista personalistic psychology
psicología popular folk psychology
psicología profunda depth psychology
psicología racional rational psychology
psicología refleja reflex psychology
psicología social social psychology
psicología subjetiva subjective psychology
psicología teorética theoretical psychology
psicología topográfica topographical psychology
psicología topológica topological psychology
psicología transaccional transactional psychology
psicología transcultural cross-cultural psychology
psicología transpersonal transpersonal psychology
psicologías alternativas alternative psychologies
psicológico psychological
psicologismo psychologism
psicólogo psychologist
psicólogo clínico clinical psychologist
psicólogo consultor consulting psychologist
psicólogo correccional correctional psychologist
psicólogo de asesoramiento counseling psychologist
psicólogo de prisión prison psychologist

psicólogo de rehabilitación rehabilitation psychologist
psicólogo de salud health psychologist
psicólogo del desarrollo developmental psychologist
psicólogo educacional educational psychologist
psicólogos correccionales como consultores correctional psychologists as consultants
psicometría psychometry
psicométrica psychometrics
psicométrico psychometric
psicometrista psychometrician
psicomimético psychomimetic
psicomímico psychomimic
psicomotor psychomotor
psicomovilidad psychomotility
psicomúsica psychomusic
psiconeumatología psychopneumatology
psiconeural psychoneural
psiconeuroide psychoneuroid
psiconeuroinmunología psychoneuroimmunology
psiconeurosis psychoneurosis
psiconeurosis compulsiva-obsesiva compulsive-obsessive psychoneurosis
psiconeurosis de defensa defense psychoneurosis
psiconeurosis maídica psychoneurosis maidica
psiconeurosis obsesiva-compulsiva obsessive-compulsive psychoneurosis
psiconeurótico psychoneurotic
psiconocivo psychonoxious
psiconomía psychonomy
psiconómica psychonomics
psiconómico psychonomic
psiconosología psychonosology
psicooncología psychooncology
psicoparesia psychoparesis
psicópata psychopath
psicópata constitucional constitutional psychopath
psicópata criminal criminal psychopath
psicopatía psychopathy
psicopatía autista autistic psychopathy
psicopático psychopathic
psicopatista psychopathist
psicopatología psychopathology
psicopatología del desarrollo developmental psychopathology
psicopatología en adolescencia psychopathology in adolescence
psicopatológico psychopathological
psicopatólogo psychopathologist
psicopedagogía psychopedagogy
psicopedia psychopedics
psicopenetración psychopenetration
psicoplejía psychoplegia
psicopolítica psychopolitics
psicoprofilaxis psychoprophylaxis
psicoquímica psychochemistry
psicoquimo psychokym
psicórmico psychormic
psicorrea psychorrhea

psicorreacción psychoreaction
psicorrelajación psychorelaxation
psicorritmia psychorhythmia
psicosensorial psychosensory
psicosexual psychosexual
psicosexualidad psychosexuality
psicosíntesis psychosynthesis
psicosis psychosis
psicosis acinética akinetic psychosis
psicosis afectiva affective psychosis
psicosis alcohólica alcoholic psychosis
psicosis alternante alternating psychosis
psicosis amnésica amnestic psychosis
psicosis anfetamina amphetamine psychosis
psicosis arterioesclerótica arteriosclerotic
   psychosis
psicosis artiopática senil senile artiopathic
   psychosis
psicosis atípica atypical psychosis
psicosis autista autistic psychosis
psicosis autoscópica autoscopic psychosis
psicosis biógena biogenic psychosis
psicosis cardíaca cardiac psychosis
psicosis Cheyne-Stokes Cheyne-Stokes
   psychosis
psicosis cicloide cycloid psychosis
psicosis circular circular psychosis
psicosis circulatoria circulatory psychosis
psicosis climatérica climacteric psychosis
psicosis colectiva collective psychosis
psicosis comunicada communicated psychosis
psicosis con arterioesclerosis cerebral
   psychosis with cerebral arteriosclerosis
psicosis con enfermedad cardiorrenal
   psychosis with cardiorenal disease
psicosis con retardo mental psychosis with
   mental retardation
psicosis constitucional constitutional
   psychosis
psicosis conyugal conjugal psychosis
psicosis crónica inducida por sustancia
   substance-induced chronic psychosis
psicosis de agotamiento exhaustion psychosis
psicosis de alcohol alcohol psychosis
psicosis de ambigüedad de género gender
   ambiguity psychosis
psicosis de ancianos elderly psychosis
psicosis de ansiedad-elación anxiety-elation
   psychosis
psicosis de asociación psychosis of association
psicosis de bufonería buffoonery psychosis
psicosis de cannabis cannabis psychosis
psicosis de confusión confusion psychosis
psicosis de choque agudo acute shock
   psychosis
psicosis de degeneración degeneration
   psychosis
psicosis de grupo group psychosis
psicosis de infección-agotamiento
   infection-exhaustion psychosis
psicosis de intervalo interval psychosis
psicosis de Korsakoff Korsakoff's psychosis
psicosis de Korsakoff no alcohólica
   nonalcoholic Korsakoff psychosis
psicosis de migración migration psychosis

psicosis de movilidad motility psychosis
psicosis de niñez childhood psychosis
psicosis de niñez atípica atypical childhood
   psychosis
psicosis de prisión prison psychosis
psicosis de proceso process psychosis
psicosis de protesta protest psychosis
psicosis de septicemia septicemia psychosis
psicosis de sífilis psychosis of syphilis
psicosis de vergüenza embarrassment
   psychosis
psicosis degenerativa degenerative psychosis
psicosis delusoria aguda acute delusional
   psychosis
psicosis depresiva depressive psychosis
psicosis desintegrante disintegrative psychosis
psicosis deteriorativa deteriorative psychosis
psicosis dismnésica dysmnesic psychosis
psicosis en privación de sueño psychosis in
   sleep deprivation
psicosis epiléptica epileptic psychosis
psicosis esquizoafectiva schizoaffective
   psychosis
psicosis esquizofrénica schizophrenic
   psychosis
psicosis esquizofreniforme schizophreniform
   psychosis
psicosis étnica ethnic psychosis
psicosis exótica exotic psychosis
psicosis familiar familial psychosis
psicosis febril febrile psychosis
psicosis fronteriza borderline psychosis
psicosis funcional functional psychosis
psicosis gestacional gestational psychosis
psicosis heredofamiliar heredofamilial
   psychosis
psicosis hipocondríaca hypochondriacal
   psychosis
psicosis hipocondríaca monosintomática
   monosymptomatic hypochondriacal
   psychosis
psicosis histérica hysterical psychosis
psicosis iatrogénica iatrogenic psychosis
psicosis incipiente incipient psychosis
psicosis inducida induced psychosis
psicosis inducida por drogas drug-induced
   psychosis
psicosis infantil simbiótica symbiotic infantile
   psychosis
psicosis intermitente intermittent psychosis
psicosis involutiva involutional psychosis
psicosis latente latent psychosis
psicosis maligna malignant psychosis
psicosis maniacodepresiva manic-depressive
   psychosis
psicosis maniacodepresiva unipolar unipolar
   manic-depressive psychosis
psicosis marginal marginal psychosis
psicosis modelo model psychosis
psicosis monosintomática monosymptomatic
   psychosis
psicosis orgánica organic psychosis
psicosis paranoide paranoid psychosis
psicosis paranoide reactiva reactive paranoid
   psychosis

psicosis parética paretic psychosis
psicosis periódica de pubertad periodic psychosis of puberty
psicosis polineurítica polyneuritic psychosis
psicosis por drogas drug psychosis
psicosis poshipnótica posthypnotic psychosis
psicosis posinfecciosa postinfectious psychosis
psicosis posparto postpartum psychosis
psicosis postraumática posttraumatic psychosis
psicosis prepsicótica prepsychotic psychosis
psicosis psicogénica psychogenic psychosis
psicosis puerperal puerperal psychosis
psicosis reactiva reactive psychosis
psicosis reactiva breve brief reactive psychosis
psicosis semántica semantic psychosis
psicosis senil senile psychosis
psicosis simbiótica symbiotic psychosis
psicosis sintomática symptomatic psychosis
psicosis situacional situational psychosis
psicosis tabética tabetic psychosis
psicosis tóxica toxic psychosis
psicosis traumática traumatic psychosis
psicosis unipolar unipolar psychosis
psicosocial psychosocial
psicosocialmente psychosocially
psicosoma psychosoma
psicosomático psychosomatic
psicosomimético psychosomimetic
psicotécnica psychotechnics
psicotécnico psychotechnician
psicotecnología psychotechnology
psicoterapeuta psychotherapist
psicoterapéutica psychotherapeutics
psicoterapéutico psychotherapeutic
psicoterapia psychotherapy
psicoterapia a corto plazo short-term psychotherapy
psicoterapia a largo plazo long-term psychotherapy
psicoterapia adolescente adolescent psychotherapy
psicoterapia ambulatoria ambulatory psychotherapy
psicoterapia anaclítica anaclitic psychotherapy
psicoterapia analítica analytic psychotherapy
psicoterapia analítica activa active analytic psychotherapy
psicoterapia analítica de grupo group analytic psychotherapy
psicoterapia apoyadora supportive psychotherapy
psicoterapia apoyadora-expresiva supportive-expressive psychotherapy
psicoterapia autónoma autonomous psychotherapy
psicoterapia biétnica biethnic psychotherapy
psicoterapia birracial biracial psychotherapy
psicoterapia breve brief psychotherapy
psicoterapia breve para niños brief psychotherapy for children
psicoterapia centrada en el cliente client-centered psychotherapy

psicoterapia cognitiva-conductual cognitive-behavioral psychotherapy
psicoterapia con carbamatos carbamate psychotherapy
psicoterapia conductual behavioral psychotherapy
psicoterapia contractual contractual psychotherapy
psicoterapia de apoyo adaptiva de realidad reality-adaptive supportive psychotherapy
psicoterapia de dietilamida de ácido lisérgico lysergic acid diethylamide psychotherapy
psicoterapia de emergencia emergency psychotherapy
psicoterapia de grupo group psychotherapy
psicoterapia de grupo analítica analytic group psychotherapy
psicoterapia de grupo de actividad activity group psychotherapy
psicoterapia de grupo de entrevista interview group psychotherapy
psicoterapia de grupo de entrevista de actividad activity-interview group psychotherapy
psicoterapia de grupo de intervención de crisis crisis-intervention group psychotherapy
psicoterapia de grupo de juego play-group psychotherapy
psicoterapia de grupo de maratón marathon group psychotherapy
psicoterapia de grupo directiva directive group psychotherapy
psicoterapia de grupo interaccional estructurada structured interactional group psychotherapy
psicoterapia de grupo psicoanalítica psychoanalytic group psychotherapy
psicoterapia de inhibición recíproca reciprocal-inhibition psychotherapy
psicoterapia de niños child psychotherapy
psicoterapia del ego ego psychotherapy
psicoterapia diádica dyadic psychotherapy
psicoterapia dinámica dynamic psychotherapy
psicoterapia dinámica breve brief dynamic psychotherapy
psicoterapia dinámica limitada por tiempo time-limited dynamic psychotherapy
psicoterapia directiva directive psychotherapy
psicoterapia ecléctica eclectic psychotherapy
psicoterapia eidética eidetic psychotherapy
psicoterapia existencial existential psychotherapy
psicoterapia experiencial experiential psychotherapy
psicoterapia experimental experimental psychotherapy
psicoterapia feminista feminist psychotherapy
psicoterapia filosófica philosophical psychotherapy
psicoterapia focal focal psychotherapy
psicoterapia heterónoma heteronomous psychotherapy

psicoterapia hipnótica hypnotic
  psychotherapy
psicoterapia individual individual
  psychotherapy
psicoterapia intensiva intensive
  psychotherapy
psicoterapia interactiva interactional
  psychotherapy
psicoterapia interpersonal interpersonal
  psychotherapy
psicoterapia limitada por tiempo
  time-limited psychotherapy
psicoterapia médica medical psychotherapy
psicoterapia no directiva nondirective
  psychotherapy
psicoterapia objetiva objective psychotherapy
psicoterapia orientada a la penetración
  insight-oriented psychotherapy
psicoterapia orientada a la penetración
  exploratoria exploratory insight-oriented
  psychotherapy
psicoterapia para niños psychotherapy for
  children
psicoterapia por inhibiciones recíprocas
  psychotherapy by reciprocal inhibitions
psicoterapia provocante de ansiedad a corto
  plazo short-term anxiety-provoking
  psychotherapy
psicoterapia proyectiva projective
  psychotherapy
psicoterapia psicoanalítica psychoanalytic
  psychotherapy
psicoterapia psicodinámica psychodynamic
  psychotherapy
psicoterapia racional rational psychotherapy
psicoterapia reconstructiva reconstructive
  psychotherapy
psicoterapia sugestiva suggestive
  psychotherapy
psicoterapia transaccional transactional
  psychotherapy
psicoterapia transcultural cross-cultural
  psychotherapy
psicoterapias innovadoras innovative
  psychotherapies
psicoterapias alternativas alternative
  psychotherapies
psicoticismo psychoticism
psicótico psychotic
psicotogénico psychotogenic
psicotógeno psychotogen
psicotomimético psychotomimetic
psicotoxicomanía psychotoxicomania
psicotrópico psychotropic
psicroalgia psychroalgia
psicroestesia psychroesthesia
psicrofobia psychrophobia
psilocibina psilocybin
psilocina psilocin
psiquefórico psychephoric
psiquehórmico psychehormic
psiqueismo psycheism
psiquelítico psychelytic
psiquentonía psychentonia
psiqueplástico psycheplastic

psiquiatra psychiatrist
psiquiatra certificado por junta board
  certified psychiatrist
psiquiatra correccional correctional
  psychiatrist
psiquiatra mono monkey psychiatrist
psiquiatría psychiatry
psiquiatría administrativa administrative
  psychiatry
psiquiatría adolescente adolescent psychiatry
psiquiatría analítica analytic psychiatry
psiquiatría biológica biological psychiatry
psiquiatría clínica clinical psychiatry
psiquiatría comparativa comparative
  psychiatry
psiquiatría comunitaria community
  psychiatry
psiquiatría conductual behavioral psychiatry
psiquiatría contractual contractual psychiatry
psiquiatría correccional correctional
  psychiatry
psiquiatría criminal criminal psychiatry
psiquiatría cultural cultural psychiatry
psiquiatría de consultación-coordinación
  consultation-liaison psychiatry
psiquiatría de coordinación liaison psychiatry
psiquiatría de grupo minoritario
  minority-group psychiatry
psiquiatría de infantes infant psychiatry
psiquiatría de niños child psychiatry
psiquiatría de sentido común common-sense
  psychiatry
psiquiatría descriptiva descriptive psychiatry
psiquiatría dinámica dynamic psychiatry
psiquiatría ecológica ecological psychiatry
psiquiatría existencial existential psychiatry
psiquiatría forense forensic psychiatry
psiquiatría geriátrica geriatric psychiatry
psiquiatría gerontológica gerontological
  psychiatry
psiquiatría industrial industrial psychiatry
psiquiatría interpersonal interpersonal
  psychiatry
psiquiatría legal legal psychiatry
psiquiatría molecular molecular psychiatry
psiquiatría ocupacional occupational
  psychiatry
psiquiatría ortomolecular orthomolecular
  psychiatry
psiquiatría política political psychiatry
psiquiatría popular folk psychiatry
psiquiatría preventiva preventive psychiatry
psiquiatría psicoanalítica psychoanalytic
  psychiatry
psiquiatría social social psychiatry
psiquiatría sociocultural sociocultural
  psychiatry
psiquiatría transcultural transcultural
  psychiatry
psiquiátrico psychiatric
psiquiatrismo psychiatrism
psiquicismo psychicism
psíquico psychic
psiquinosis psychinosis
psiquis psyche

psiquismo psychism
psitacismo psittacism
psofolalia psopholalia
psoriasis psoriasis
pteronofobia pteronophobia
ptialismo ptyalism
ptosis ptosis
ptosis simpática ptosis sympathetica
puberal puberal
puberismo puberism
puberismo persistente persistent puberism
pubertad puberty
pubertad precoz precocious puberty
pubertad seudoprecoz pseudoprecocious
 puberty
pubertal pubertal
pubes pubes
pubescencia pubescence
pubescente pubescent
púbico pubic
pubis pubis
publicidad advertising
público public
pudenda pudenda
pudendo pudendal
puente hacia la realidad bridge to reality
pueril puerile
puerilismo puerilism
puerperal puerperal
puerperio puerperium
puerta espinal spinal gate
pulmón lung
pulmón de hierro iron lung
pulmonar pulmonary
pulmónico pulmonic
pulmonocoronario pulmonocoronary
pulso pulse
pulvinar pulvinar
punción puncture
punción cisternal cisternal puncture
punción de Bernard Bernard's puncture
punción de Quincke Quincke's puncture
punción de ventrículo ventricle puncture
punción diabética diabetic puncture
punción espinal spinal tap
punción esternal sternal puncture
punción lumbar lumbar puncture
punción suboccipital suboccipital puncture
punitivo punitive
punta de la lengua tip-of-the-tongue
puntación reducida reduced score
punteado punctate
punto point
punto apofisario apophysary point
punto cercano near point
punto cercano de convergencia near-point of
 convergence
punto ciego blind spot
punto ciego mental mental blind spot
punto crítico critical point
punto de cambio change point
punto de dolor pain spot
punto de fijación fixation point
punto de fusión de centelleo flicker fusion
 point

punto de gatillo trigger point
punto de igualdad subjetiva point of
 subjective equality
punto de indiferencia indifference point
punto de inflexión inflection point
punto de mirada point of regard
punto de presión pressure point
punto de selección choice point
punto de Trousseau Trousseau's point
punto de Valleix Valleix's point
punto de vista biológico biological viewpoint
punto de vista neoconductual neobehavioral
 viewpoint
punto de vista orgánico organic viewpoint
punto doloroso painful point
punto fijo set point
punto frío cold spot
punto histerogénico hysterogenic spot
punto lejano far point
punto medio midpoint
punto motor motor point
punto nodal nodal point
punto sensible tender point
punto sensitivo a presión pressure-sensitive
 spot
punto vascular punctum vasculosum
puntos congruentes congruent points
puntos de anclaje anchor points
puntos idénticos identical points
puntos retinales congruentes congruent
 retinal points
puntos retinales correspondientes
 corresponding retinal points
puntos retinales dispares disparate retinal
 points
puntos retinales idénticos identical retinal
 points
puntuación score
puntuación bruta gross score
puntuación compuesta composite score
puntuación cortante cutting score
puntuación crítica critical score
puntuación cuantitativa quantitative score
puntuación cumulativa cumulative score
puntuación de Apgar Apgar score
puntuación de banda band score
puntuación de criterio criterion score
puntuación de desviación deviation score
puntuación de edad age score
puntuación de optimidad obstétrica
 obstetrical optimality score
puntuación de optimidad obstétrica y
 desarrollo cognitivo obstetrical optimality
 score and cognitive development
puntuación de prueba test score
puntuación del lenguaje language score
puntuación del tiempo time score
puntuación derivada derived score
puntuación en bruto raw score
puntuación estándar standard score
puntuación estandarizada standardized score
puntuación ipsativa ipsative score
puntuación media midscore
puntuación normativa normative score
puntuación obtenida obtained score

puntuación original original score
puntuación percentil percentile score
puntuación representativa representative
  score
puntuación sigma sigma score
puntuación transformada transformed score
puntuaciones igualadas equated scores
pupila pupil
pupila artificial artificial pupil
pupila de Adie Adie's pupil
pupila de Argyll Robertson Argyll Robertson
  pupil
pupila de Holmes-Adie Holmes-Adie pupil
pupila de Hutchinson Hutchinson's pupil
pupila de Robertson Robertson pupil
pupila fija fixed pupil
pupila paradójica paradoxical pupil
pupila rígida rigid pupil
pupila tónica tonic pupil
pupila tónica de Adie tonic pupil of Adie
pupilar pupillary
pupilomotor pupillomotor
pupiloplejía pupilloplegia
pupilotonía pupillotonia
pupilotónico pupillotonic
puritano puritan
puro pure
puromicina puromycin
púrpura purple
putamen putamen
pútrido putrid

Q

que forma hábito habit-forming
queilitis cheilitis
queilofagia cheilophagia
queimafobia cheimaphobia
queiroespasmo keirospasm
queja complaint
queja de hábito habit complaint
queja principal chief complaint
quejumbroso complaining
quelación chelation
quemado burned-out, burnt
quemadura de primer grado first-degree
  burn
quemaduras burns
quenofobia kenophobia
queratitis keratitis
queratitis neuroparalítica neuroparalytic
  keratitis
queratosis keratosis
queratosis actínica actinic keratosis
queratosis faríngea pharyngeal keratosis
queratosis senil senile keratosis
queraunofobia keraunophobia
queraunoneurosis keraunoneurosis
querofobia cherophobia
queromanía cheromania
quiasma chiasma
quiasma óptico optic chiasm
quilofagia chilophagia
quimera chimera
química mental mental chemistry
químico chemical
quimiodectoma chemodectoma
quimionucleólisis chemonucleolysis
quimiopalidectomía chemopallidectomy
quimiopalidotalamectomía
  chemopallidothalamectomy
quimiopalidotomía chemopallidotomy
quimiopsiquiatría chemopsychiatry
quimiorreceptor chemoreceptor
quimiorreflejo chemoreflex
quimiotáctico chemotactic
quimiotalamectomía chemothalamectomy
quimiotalamotomía chemothalamotomy
quimiotaxis chemotaxis
quimioterapia chemotherapy
quimiotropismo chemotropism
quionofobia chionophobia
quirobraquialgia cheirobrachialgia
quirocinestesia cheirokinesthesia
quirocinestésico cheirokinesthetic
quiroespasmo cheirospasm
quirognóstico cheirognostic
quiromancia palmistry

quiste cyst
quiste apopléctico apoplectic cyst
quiste aracnoideo arachnoid cyst
quiste cerebeloso cerebellar cyst
quiste de Rathke Rathke's cyst
quiste de Tarlov Tarlov's cyst
quiste ependimario ependymal cyst
quiste hendido de Rathke Rathke's cleft cyst
quiste leptomeníngeo postraumático
    posttraumatic leptomeningeal cyst
quiste neural neural cyst
quiste parafisial paraphysial cyst
quiste pineal pineal cyst
quiste suprasclar suprasellar cyst

R

rabdofobia rhabdophobia
rabdomancia dowsing
rabia rage, rabies
rabia simulada sham rage
rabieta tantrum
racional rational
racionalidad rationality
racionalidad limitada bounded rationality
racionalismo rationalism
racionalización rationalization
racionalizar rationalize
racismo racism
racismo aversivo aversive racism
racha incrédula doubting spell
rachas de meditación ansiosa brooding spells
radiación radiation
radiación acústica acoustic radiation
radiación electromagnética electromagnetic
    radiation
radiación ionizante ionizing radiation
radiación óptica optic radiation
radiactivo radioactive
radial radial
radiancia radiance
radical radical
radicalismo radicalism
radicotomía radicotomy
radiculalgia radiculalgia
radicular radicular
radiculectomía radiculectomy
radiculitis radiculitis
radiculitis braquial brachial radiculitis
radiculitis braquial aguda acute brachial
    radiculitis
radiculoganglionitis radiculoganglionitis
radiculomeningomielitis
    radiculomeningomyelitis
radiculomielopatía radiculomyelopathy
radiculoneuropatía radiculoneuropathy
radiculopatía radiculopathy
radioautografía radioautography
radiobicipital radiobicipital
radiofobia radiophobia
radiografía radiograph
radiograma radiogram
radioinmunoanálisis radioimmunoassay
radioisótopo radioisotope
radiológico radiologic
radiómetro radiometer
radiomimético radiomimetic
radioneuritis radioneuritis
radionúclido radionuclide
radioperióstico radioperiosteal
radiorreceptor radioreceptor

radioterapia radiotherapy
radix radix
rafe raphe
raíz root
raíz anterior anterior root
raíz del pene crus penis
raíz dorsal dorsal root
raíz espinal spinal root
raíz nerviosa nerve root
raíz posterior posterior root
raíz sensorial sensory root
raíz ventral ventral root
rami communicantes rami communicantes
ramicotomía ramicotomy
ramisección ramisection
ramitis ramitis
ramus ramus
rango rank
rango percentil percentile rank
rápido quick
rapport rapport
rapport psicológico psychological rapport
raptus raptus
raptus melancholicus raptus melancholicus
raquicentesis rachicentesis
raquígrafo rachigraph
raquílisis rachilysis
raquiocentesis rachiocentesis
raquioescoliosis rachioscoliosis
raquiómetro rachiometer
raquiopatía rachiopathy
raquioplejía rachioplegia
raquioquisis rachiochysis
raquiotomía rachiotomy
raquiótomo rachiotome
raquisquisis rachischisis
raquisquisis parcial rachischisis partialis
raquisquisis posterior rachischisis posterior
raquisquisis total rachischisis totalis
raquitismo rickets
raquitomía rachitomy
raquítomo rachitome
rareza oddity
rarezas de conducta oddities of behavior
rasero doble double standard
rasgo trait
rasgo adquirido acquired trait
rasgo anal-erótico anal-erotic trait
rasgo cardenal cardinal trait
rasgo compensatorio compensatory trait
rasgo compuesto composite trait
rasgo común common trait
rasgo cultural culture trait
rasgo de molde ambiental
　　environmental-mold trait
rasgo de personalidad personality trait
rasgo del carácter character trait
rasgo dominante dominant trait
rasgo érgico ergic trait
rasgo fuente source trait
rasgo heredado inherited trait
rasgo latente latent trait
rasgo neurótico neurotic trait
rasgo ortogonal orthogonal trait
rasgo patológico pathological trait

rasgo recesivo recessive trait
rasgo superficial surface trait
rasgo único unique trait
rasgos centrales central traits
rasgos de personalidad histriónica histrionic
　　personality traits
rasgos neuropáticos neuropathic traits
rasgos poligénicos polygenic traits
rastreo tracking
rastreo ocular ocular pursuit
rastreo visual visual tracking
rastro de estímulo stimulus trace
rastro de memoria memory trace
rastro mnemónico mnemonic trace
rastro perseverante perseverative trace
ratimia rhathymia
Rauwolfia Rauwolfia
raza race
razón reason, ratio
razón afectiva affective ratio
razón binuaral binaural ratio
razón crítica critical ratio
razón de asociación-sensación
　　association-sensation ratio
razón de Brunswik Brunswik ratio
razón de correlación correlation ratio
razón de edad age ratio
razón de extinción extinction ratio
razón de heredabilidad heritability ratio
razón de inspiración-expiración
　　inspiration-expiration ratio
razón de probabilidades probability ratio
razón de recuperación recovery ratio
razón de señal a ruido signal-to-noise ratio
razón de Thouless Thouless ratio
razón estándar standard ratio
razón F F ratio
razón fija fixed ratio
razón fundamental rationale
razón mendeliana mendelian ratio
razón sexual sex ratio
razonamiento reasoning
razonamiento analógico analogical reasoning
razonamiento causal causal reasoning
razonamiento circular circular reasoning
razonamiento deductivo deductive reasoning
razonamiento dialéctico dialectical reasoning
razonamiento dinámico dynamic reasoning
razonamiento evaluativo evaluative reasoning
razonamiento funcional functional reasoning
razonamiento general general reasoning
razonamiento hipotético-deductivo
　　hypothetical-deductive reasoning
razonamiento inductivo inductive reasoning
razonamiento lógico logical reasoning
razonamiento moral moral reasoning
razonamiento moral durante adolescencia
　　moral reasoning during adolescence
razonamiento moral exonerativo exonerative
　　moral reasoning
razonamiento silogístico syllogistic reasoning
razonamiento transductivo transductive
　　reasoning
reacción reaction
reacción a desastre reaction to disaster

reacción adrenérgica adrenergic reaction
reacción ansiosa anxiety reaction
reacción antisocial antisocial reaction
reacción cardiovascular psicofisiológica
  psychophysiologic cardiovascular reaction
reacción catastrófica catastrophic reaction
reacción circular circular reaction
reacción circular primaria primary circular
  reaction
reacción circular secundaria secondary
  circular reaction
reacción circular terciaria tertiary circular
  reaction
reacción compleja complex reaction
reacción compuesta compound reaction
reacción conductual behavioral reaction
reacción confirmante confirming reaction
reacción de abandono abandonment reaction
reacción de adaptación general general
  adaptation reaction
reacción de aflicción grief reaction
reacción de aflicción maníaca maniacal grief
  reaction
reacción de aflicción patológica pathological
  grief reaction
reacción de ajuste adjustment reaction
reacción de ajuste de adolescencia
  adjustment reaction of adolescence
reacción de ajuste de infancia adjustment
  reaction of infancy
reacción de ajuste de la postrimería
  adjustment reaction of later life
reacción de ajuste de niñez adjustment
  reaction of childhood
reacción de alargamiento lengthening
  reaction
reacción de alarma alarm reaction
reacción de aniversario anniversary reaction
reacción de arteriola arteriole reaction
reacción de aversión aversion reaction
reacción de catástrofe de civil civilian
  catastrophe reaction
reacción de conversión conversion reaction
reacción de defensa defense reaction
reacción de degeneración reaction of
  degeneration
reacción de despertamiento arousal reaction
reacción de detención arrest reaction
reacción de dolor pain reaction
reacción de eco echo reaction
reacción de enderezamiento righting reaction
reacción de estrés stress reaction
reacción de estrés aguda acute stress reaction
reacción de estrés enorme gross stress
  reaction
reacción de evitación defensiva defensive
  avoidance reaction
reacción de golpecito de talón heel-tap
  reaction
reacción de Herxheimer Herxheimer reaction
reacción de hipersensibilidad hypersensitivity
  reaction
reacción de imán magnet reaction
reacción de Jarisch-Herxheimer
  Jarisch-Herxheimer reaction

reacción de Jolly Jolly's reaction
reacción de mano a boca hand-to-mouth
  reaction
reacción de movilización mobilization
  reaction
reacción de niño consentido spoiled-child
  reaction
reacción de niños a amputación children's
  reaction to amputation
reacción de niños a desastres children's
  reaction to disasters
reacción de niños a divorcio children's
  reaction to divorce
reacción de niños a enfermedad children's
  reaction to illness
reacción de niños a hospitalización
  children's reaction to hospitalization
reacción de Pandy Pandy's reaction
reacción de pelea-fuga fight-flight reaction
reacción de piel galvánica galvanic skin
  reaction
reacción de piel psicofisiológica
  psychophysiologic skin reaction
reacción de piel psicogalvánica
  psychogalvanic skin reaction
reacción de rastreo pursuit reaction
reacción de repetición repetition reaction
reacción de retiro withdrawal reaction
reacción de seguir following reaction
reacción de selección choice reaction
reacción de sentido especial psicofisiológica
  psychophysiologic special sense reaction
reacción de síntoma especial
  special-symptom reaction
reacción de sobresalto startle reaction
reacción de somatización somatization
  reaction
reacción de transferencia transference
  reaction
reacción de Wernicke Wernicke's reaction
reacción defensiva defensive reaction
reacción del sistema nervioso psicofisiológica
  psychophysiologic nervous system reaction
reacción delirante delirious reaction
reacción demorada delayed reaction
reacción depresiva depressive reaction
reacción depresiva psiconeurótica
  psychoneurotic depressive reaction
reacción depresiva psicótica psychotic
  depressive reaction
reacción diabética diabetic reaction
reacción diferida deferred reaction
reacción disocial dyssocial reaction
reacción disociativa dissociative reaction
reacción distónica dystonic reaction
reacción disyuntiva disjunctive reaction
reacción duplicativa duplicative reaction
reacción emocional emotional reaction
reacción emocional de niños al divorcio
  emotional reaction of children to divorce
reacción endocrina psicofisiológica
  psychophysiologic endocrine reaction
reacción esquizofrénica schizophrenic
  reaction
reacción fantasma phantom reaction

reacción fóbica phobic reaction
reacción gastrointestinal psicofisiológica
psychophysiologic gastrointestinal reaction
reacción gemistocítica gemistocytic reaction
reacción genitourinaria psicofisiológica
psychophysiologic genitourinary reaction
reacción hémica y linfática psicofisiológica
psychophysiologic hemic and lymphatic
reaction
reacción hipercinética de niñez hyperkinetic
reaction of childhood
reacción histérica hysterical reaction
reacción idiosincrásica idiosyncratic reaction
reacción maniacodepresiva manic-depressive
reaction
reacción miasténica myasthenic reaction
reacción musculoesquelética psicofisiológica
psychophysiologic musculoskeletal reaction
reacción negativa negative reaction
reacción neurótica-depresiva
neurotic-depressive reaction
reacción orgánica organic reaction
reacción orientada hacia tarea task-oriented
reaction
reacción paradójica paradoxical reaction
reacción paranoide aguda acute paranoid
reaction
reacción políglota polyglot reaction
reacción primaria primary reaction
reacción psicogalvánica psychogalvanic
reaction
reacción psicótica involutiva involutional
psychotic reaction
reacción pupilar miotónica myotonic
pupillary reaction
reacción respiratoria psicofisiológica
psychophysiologic respiratory reaction
reacción Rh Rh reaction
reacción situacional situational reaction
reacción situacional adulta adult situational
reaction
reacción situacional aguda acute situational
reaction
reacción socializada agresiva aggressive
socialized reaction
reacción socializada no agresiva
nonaggressive socialized reaction
reacción subsocializada agresiva aggressive
undersocialized reaction
reacción subsocializada no agresiva
nonaggressive undersocialized reaction
reacción terapéutica therapeutic reaction
reacción terapéutica negativa negative
therapeutic reaction
reaccional reactional
reacciones al cáncer cancer reactions
reacciones antígeno-anticuerpo
antigen-antibody reactions
reacciones cardíacas cardiac reactions
reacciones de deshidratación dehydration
reactions
reacciones de droga adversas adverse drug
reactions
reacciones de hambre starvation reactions
reacciones de infantes a divorcio parental
infant reactions to parental divorce
reacciones de infantes a enfermedad infant
reactions to illness
reacciones de infantes a hospitalización
infant reactions to hospitalization
reacciones de pacientes dentales dental
patient reactions
reacciones individuales a desastres individual
reactions to disasters
reactancia reactance
reactancia psicológica psychological
reactance
reactivación reactivation
reactivación de memoria reactivation of
memory
reactividad reactivity
reactividad autónoma autonomic reactivity
reactivo reactive
readhesión reattachment
readmisión readmission
reaferencia reafference
real real
realidad reality
realidad compartida shared reality
realidad fenomenológica phenomenological
reality
realidad objetiva objective reality
realidad percibida perceived reality
realidad psíquica psychic reality
realidad social social reality
realineamiento circadiano circadian
realignment
realismo realism
realismo directo direct realism
realismo ecológico ecological realism
realismo experimental experimental realism
realismo ingenuo naive realism
realismo moral moral realism
realismo mundano mundane realism
realismo nominal nominal realism
realista realistic
realización fulfillment
realización de sueño wish fulfillment
realización simbólica symbolic realization
realzado ambiental environmental
enhancement
realzado de sueños dream enhancement
reaprendizaje relearning
reasignación de género gender reassignment
reasignación sexual sex reassignment
reasociación reassociation
rebelde rebellious
rebeldía rebelliousness
rebeldía neurótica neurotic rebelliousness
rebosamiento overflow
rebosamiento motor adventicio adventitious
motor overflow
recaída relapse
recapitulación recapitulation
recapitulación sexual pubertal pubertal
sexual recapitulation
recatexis recathexis
recelo suspiciousness
receptividad receptivity
receptivo receptive

receptoma receptoma
receptor receptor
receptor a distancia distance receptor
receptor alfa alpha receptor
receptor beta beta receptor
receptor colinérgico cholinergic receptor
receptor cutáneo skin receptor
receptor de dolor pain receptor
receptor de dopamina dopamine receptor
receptor de estiramiento stretch receptor
receptor de norepinefrina norepinephrine receptor
receptor de opiáceos opiate receptor
receptor de opioide opioid receptor
receptor de presión pressure receptor
receptor de serotonina serotonin receptor
receptor de vibraciones vibration receptor
receptor neurotransmisor neurotransmitter receptor
receptor proximal proximal receptor
receptor serotonérgico serotonergic receptor
receptor somático somatic receptor
receptor táctil tactile receptor
receptor vestibular vestibular receptor
receptores de acetilcolina acetylcholine receptors
receptores de color color receptors
recesividad genética genetic recessiveness
recesivo recessive
receso recess
recibidor receiver
recidiva recidivation
recidivismo recidivism
recidivismo de víctima victim recidivism
recidivista recidivist
recién nacido newborn
recipiomotor recipiomotor
reciprocidad reciprocity
recíproco reciprocal
recitación propia self-recitation
reclamación neurótica neurotic claim
reclusión seclusion
reclutamiento recruitment
reclutamiento coclear cochlear recruitment
reclutamiento por cultos recruitment by cults
recolección de datos data collection
recolección de información information gathering
recombinación recombination
recompensa reward
recompensa de fichas token reward
recompensa demorada delayed reward
recompensa extrínseca extrinsic reward
recompensa intrínseca intrinsic reward
recompensa negativa negative reward
recompensa por el superego reward by the superego
recompensa positiva positive reward
recompensa secundaria secondary reward
recompensación recompensation
reconciliación reconciliation
recondicionamiento reconditioning
recondicionamiento orgásmico orgasmic reconditioning
reconocimiento recognition

reconocimiento de caras face recognition
reconocimiento de monedas coin recognition
reconocimiento de palabras word recognition
reconocimiento de patrón pattern recognition
reconocimiento falso false recognition
reconocimiento social social recognition
reconstitución reconstitution
reconstrucción reconstruction
reconstructivo reconstructive
recordación recall
recordación de sueños dream recall
recordación de sueños y ansiedad dream recall and anxiety
recordación demorada delayed recall
recordación libre free recall
recordación mecánica rote recall
recordación serial serial recall
recorte clipping
recorte de picos peak-clipping
recorte del centro center-clipping
recorte delantero front-clipping
recorte trasero back-clipping
recreación recreation
recreación activa active recreation
recreación pasiva passive recreation
recreación terapéutica therapeutic recreation
recreativo recreational
rectal rectal
rectilíneo rectilinear
recto inferior inferior rectus
recto interno internal rectus
recto lateral lateral rectus
recto medial medial rectus
rectocardíaco rectocardiac
rectofobia rectophobia
rectolaríngeo rectolaryngeal
recumbente recumbent
recuperación recovery
recuperación de capacidad limitada limited-capacity retrieval
recuperación de función recovery of function
recuperación espontanea spontaneous recovery
recuperación social social recovery
recuperación y reorganización recovery and reorganization
recurrente recurrent
recurso resource
recurso mental mental resource
recursos comunitarios community resources
rechazo rejection
rechazo de injerto graft rejection
rechazo de tejido tissue rejection
rechazo maternal maternal rejection
rechazo parental parental rejection
rechazo social social rejection
rechinamiento gnashing
red network
red de Purkinje Purkinje network
red neural neural network
red psicológica psychological network
red semántica semantic network
red social social network
redes asociativas associative networks
redes de comunicación communication

network
redintegración redintegration
redintegrativo redintegrative
reducción cromática chromatic dimming
reducción de accidentes accident reduction
reducción de estrés stress reduction
reducción de impulso drive reduction
reducción de necesidad need reduction
reducción de señal cue reduction
reducción de tensión tension reduction
reducción del ego ego retrenchment
reduccionismo reductionism
reducido reduced
reductivo reductive
redundancia redundancy
redundancia correlacional correlational
    redundancy
redundancia distribucional distributional
    redundancy
redundancia genética genetic redundancy
reeducación reeducation
reeducación emocional emotional reeducation
reeducación hipnótica hypnotic reeducation
reeducativo reeducative
reemplazo replacement
reemplazo de cadera hip replacement
reentrada reentry
reestructuración cognitiva cognitive
    restructuring
reestructuración perceptiva perceptual
    restructuring
reestructuración racional sistemática
    systematic rational restructuring
reestructurar restructure
reevaluación reevaluation
referencia reference
referencia de memoria memory reference
referente referent
referido referred
reflectividad-impulsividad
    reflectivity-impulsivity
reflejado reflected
reflejar reflect
reflejo reflex
reflejo abdominal abdominal reflex
reflejo abdominal profundo deep abdominal
    reflex
reflejo acromial acromial reflex
reflejo acústico acoustic reflex
reflejo acusticopalpebral acousticopalpebral
    reflex
reflejo adquirido acquired reflex
reflejo aductor adductor reflex
reflejo afectivo agudo acute affective reflex
reflejo aliado allied reflex
reflejo anal anal reflex
reflejo aponeurótico aponeurotic reflex
reflejo articular basal basal joint reflex
reflejo auditivo auditory reflex
reflejo auriculopalpebral auriculopalpebral
    reflex
reflejo auropalpebral auropalpebral reflex
reflejo axónico axon reflex
reflejo Bezold-Jarisch Bezold-Jarisch reflex
reflejo braquiorradial brachioradial reflex

reflejo bregmocardíaco bregmocardiac reflex
reflejo bulbocavernoso bulbocavernosus
    reflex
reflejo bulbomímico bulbomimic reflex
reflejo cefálico cephalic reflex
reflejo cefalopalpebral cephalopalpebral
    reflex
reflejo cilioespinal ciliospinal reflex
reflejo cocleoestapedio cochleostapedial
    reflex
reflejo cocleoorbicular cochleoorbicular
    reflex
reflejo cocleopalpebral cochleopalpebral
    reflex
reflejo cocleopupilar cochleopupillary reflex
reflejo condicionado conditioned reflex
reflejo condicionado positivo positive
    conditioned reflex
reflejo condicional conditional reflex
reflejo conjuntival conjunctival reflex
reflejo consensual consensual reflex
reflejo contralateral contralateral reflex
reflejo convulsivo convulsive reflex
reflejo coordinado coordinated reflex
reflejo costopectoral costopectoral reflex
reflejo craneal cranial reflex
reflejo craneocardíaco craniocardiac reflex
reflejo cremastérico cremasteric reflex
reflejo cruzado crossed reflex
reflejo cruzado del pelvis crossed reflex of
    pelvis
reflejo cuboidodigital cuboidodigital reflex
reflejo cutáneo skin reflex
reflejo cutáneo-muscular skin-muscle reflex
reflejo cutáneo-pupilar skin-pupillary reflex
reflejo darwiniano darwinian reflex
reflejo de abrazo embrace reflex
reflejo de acomodación accommodation
    reflex
reflejo de actitud attitudinal reflex
reflejo de agarre grasp reflex
reflejo de agarre forzado forced grasping
    reflex
reflejo de agarre palmar palmar grasp reflex
reflejo de ahogamiento gag reflex
reflejo de Aquiles Achilles reflex
reflejo de atención attention reflex
reflejo de Babinski Babinski reflex
reflejo de Babkin Babkin reflex
reflejo de Barkman Barkman's reflex
reflejo de Bechterew-Mendel
    Bechterew-Mendel reflex
reflejo de Bekhterev-Mendel
    Bekhterev-Mendel reflex
reflejo de Benedek Benedek's reflex
reflejo de biceps femoral biceps femoris
    reflex
reflejo de Bing Bing's reflex
reflejo de Brain Brain's reflex
reflejo de Brissaud Brissaud's reflex
reflejo de castañeteo snapping reflex
reflejo de Chaddock Chaddock reflex
reflejo de Chodzko Chodzko's reflex
reflejo de conducta behavior reflex
reflejo de cuello neck reflex

reflejo de defecación defecation reflex
reflejo de defensa defense reflex
reflejo de deglución deglutition reflex
reflejo de Dejerine Dejerine's reflex
reflejo de enderezamiento righting reflex
reflejo de enderezamiento corporal body
  righting reflex
reflejo de enderezamiento laberíntico
  labyrinthine righting reflex
reflejo de enderezamiento óptico optical
  righting reflex
reflejo de enderezamiento visual visual
  righting reflex
reflejo de estiramiento stretch reflex
reflejo de extensión extension reflex
reflejo de extensión cruzada crossed
  extension reflex
reflejo de eyección de leche milk-ejection
  reflex
reflejo de flexión flexion reflex
reflejo de Galant Galant's reflex
reflejo de Geigel Geigel's reflex
reflejo de Gifford Gifford's reflex
reflejo de golpecito frontal front-tap reflex
reflejo de golpecito plantar sole tap reflex
reflejo de Gordon Gordon reflex
reflejo de Guillain-Barre Guillain-Barre
  reflex
reflejo de guiño wink reflex
reflejo de Hering-Breuer Hering-Breuer
  reflex
reflejo de hociquear rooting reflex
reflejo de Hoffmann Hoffmann's reflex
reflejo de imán magnet reflex
reflejo de Jacobson Jacobson's reflex
reflejo de Joffroy Joffroy's reflex
reflejo de Kisch Kisch's reflex
reflejo de la barbilla chin reflex
reflejo de la risa laughter reflex
reflejo de Landau Landau reflex
reflejo de Liddell-Sherrington
  Liddell-Sherrington reflex
reflejo de Loven Loven reflex
reflejo de luz light reflex
reflejo de luz consensual consensual light
  reflex
reflejo de llanto cry reflex
reflejo de mano a boca hand-to-mouth reflex
reflejo de Mayer Mayer's reflex
reflejo de McCarthy McCarthy's reflex
reflejo de Mendel Mendel's reflex
reflejo de Mendel-Bechterew
  Mendel-Bechterew reflex
reflejo de micturición micturition reflex
reflejo de Mondonesi Mondonesi's reflex
reflejo de Moro Moro reflex
reflejo de nariz-ojo nose-eye reflex
reflejo de nariz-puente-párpado
  nose-bridge-lid reflex
reflejo de natación swimming reflex
reflejo de navaja clasp-knife reflex
reflejo de ojos consensual consensual eye
  reflex
reflejo de Oppenheim Oppenheim's reflex
reflejo de orientación orienting reflex

reflejo de palanca bar reflex
reflejo de paracaidas parachute reflex
reflejo de parpadeo blink reflex
reflejo de Perez Perez reflex
reflejo de Phillipson Phillipson's reflex
reflejo de piel galvánico galvanic skin reflex
reflejo de piel psicogalvánico psychogalvanic
  skin reflex
reflejo de Piltz Piltz reflex
reflejo de pupila cutáneo cutaneous pupil
  reflex
reflejo de rabia rage reflex
reflejo de rascarse scratch reflex
reflejo de Remak Remak's reflex
reflejo de retiro withdrawal reflex
reflejo de rodilla knee reflex
reflejo de rodilla cruzado crossed knee reflex
reflejo de Roger Roger's reflex
reflejo de Rossolimo Rossolimo's reflex
reflejo de sacudida de rodilla knee-jerk
  reflex
reflejo de Schaffer Schaffer's reflex
reflejo de sobresalto startle reflex
reflejo de sobresalto acústico acoustic startle
  reflex
reflejo de Starling Starling's reflex
reflejo de Strumpell Strumpell's reflex
reflejo de succión sucking reflex
reflejo de supinación supination reflex
reflejo de tragar swallowing reflex
reflejo de Tromner Tromner's reflex
reflejo de vómito vomiting reflex
reflejo de Weingrow Weingrow's reflex
reflejo de zambullida diving reflex
reflejo dedo-pulgar finger-thumb reflex
reflejo del aductor cruzado crossed adductor
  reflex
reflejo del arco costal costal arch reflex
reflejo del biceps biceps reflex
reflejo del cierre de ojo eye-closure reflex
reflejo del clono de muñeca wrist clonus
  reflex
reflejo del codo elbow reflex
reflejo del corazón heart reflex
reflejo del cuadríceps quadriceps reflex
reflejo del cuello tónico tonic neck reflex
reflejo del dedo del pie toe reflex
reflejo del dedo gordo del pie great toe reflex
reflejo del dorso del pie back of foot reflex
reflejo del empeine de Mendel Mendel's
  instep reflex
reflejo del iris iris reflex
reflejo del olécranon olecranon reflex
reflejo del pulgar thumb reflex
reflejo del seno carotídeo carotid sinus reflex
reflejo del supinador supinator reflex
reflejo del supinador largo supinator longus
  reflex
reflejo del tendón de Aquiles Achilles tendon
  reflex
reflejo del tendón rotuliano patellar tendon
  reflex
reflejo del tobillo ankle reflex
reflejo del tríceps triceps reflex
reflejo del tríceps paradójico paradoxical

triceps reflex
reflejo del tríceps sural triceps surae reflex
reflejo del trocánter trochanter reflex
reflejo demorado delayed reflex
reflejo difuso diffused reflex
reflejo digital digital reflex
reflejo directo direct reflex
reflejo dorsal dorsal reflex
reflejo en cadena chain reflex
reflejo en masa mass reflex
reflejo enterogástrico enterogastric reflex
reflejo entrenado trained reflex
reflejo epigástrico epigastric reflex
reflejo erector-espinal erector-spinal reflex
reflejo escapular scapular reflex
reflejo escapulohumeral scapulohumeral
    reflex
reflejo escapuloperióstico scapuloperiosteal
    reflex
reflejo esofagosalival esophagosalivary reflex
reflejo espinal spinal reflex
reflejo espinoaductor spinoadductor reflex
reflejo espinoaductor cruzado crossed
    spino-adductor reflex
reflejo estático static reflex
reflejo estatocinético statokinetic reflex
reflejo estatotónico statotonic reflex
reflejo esternobraquial sternobrachial reflex
reflejo estilorradial styloradial reflex
reflejo extensor cuadripedal quadripedal
    extensor reflex
reflejo extensor paradójico paradoxical
    extensor reflex
reflejo facial facial reflex
reflejo faríngeo pharyngeal reflex
reflejo fásico phasic reflex
reflejo faucial faucial reflex
reflejo femoral femoral reflex
reflejo femoroabdominal femoroabdominal
    reflex
reflejo flexor flexor reflex
reflejo flexor paradójico paradoxical flexor
    reflex
reflejo gastrocólico gastrocolic reflex
reflejo gastroileal gastroileal reflex
reflejo glúteo gluteal reflex
reflejo gustatorio-sudorífico
    gustatory-sudorific reflex
reflejo H H reflex
reflejo heterónimo heteronymous reflex
reflejo hipocondrial hypochondrial reflex
reflejo hipogástrico hypogastric reflex
reflejo homónimo homonymous reflex
reflejo incondicionado unconditioned reflex
reflejo incondicional unconditional reflex
reflejo inhibitorio inhibitory reflex
reflejo innato innate reflex
reflejo interescapular interscapular reflex
reflejo intrínseco intrinsic reflex
reflejo invertido inverted reflex
reflejo investigador investigatory reflex
reflejo ipsilateral ipsilateral reflex
reflejo irítico iritic reflex
reflejo laberíntico labyrinthine reflex
reflejo labial lip reflex

reflejo lagrimal lacrimal reflex
reflejo lagrimo-gustatorio lacrimo-gustatory
    reflex
reflejo laríngeo laryngeal reflex
reflejo laríngeo protector protective
    laryngeal reflex
reflejo laringoespástico laryngospastic reflex
reflejo latente latent reflex
reflejo mandibular mandibular reflex
reflejo masetérico masseter reflex
reflejo mediopúbico mediopubic reflex
reflejo metacarpohipotenar
    metacarpohypothenar reflex
reflejo metacarpotenar metacarpothenar
    reflex
reflejo metatarsiano metatarsal reflex
reflejo miotático myotatic reflex
reflejo muscular muscular reflex
reflejo muscular plantar plantar muscle
    reflex
reflejo nasomental nasomental reflex
reflejo nociceptivo nociceptive reflex
reflejo nocifensor nocifensor reflex
reflejo oblicuo externo external oblique reflex
reflejo oculocardíaco oculocardiac reflex
reflejo oculocefálico oculocephalic reflex
reflejo oculocefalógiro oculocephalogyric
    reflex
reflejo oculógiro auditivo auditory oculogyric
    reflex
reflejo opticofacial opticofacial reflex
reflejo orbicular de los ojos orbicularis oculi
    reflex
reflejo orbicular visual visual orbicularis
    reflex
reflejo óseo bone reflex
reflejo palatal palatal reflex
reflejo palatino palatine reflex
reflejo palma-barbilla palm-chin reflex
reflejo palmar palmar reflex
reflejo palmomandibular palmomandibular
    reflex
reflejo palmomentoniano palmomental reflex
reflejo paradójico paradoxical reflex
reflejo pectoral pectoral reflex
reflejo pericárdico pericardial reflex
reflejo perióstico periosteal reflex
reflejo perióstico abdominal inferior lower
    abdominal periosteal reflex
reflejo perióstico abdominal superior upper
    abdominal periosteal reflex
reflejo pilomotor pilomotor reflex
reflejo plantar plantar reflex
reflejo policomental pollicomental reflex
reflejo postural postural reflex
reflejo prepotente prepotent reflex
reflejo presorreceptor pressoreceptor reflex
reflejo profundo deep reflex
reflejo pronador pronator reflex
reflejo propioceptivo proprioceptive reflex
reflejo psicocardíaco psychocardiac reflex
reflejo psicogalvánico psychogalvanic reflex
reflejo pulmonocoronario pulmonocoronary
    reflex
reflejo pupilar pupillary reflex

reflejo pupilar cutáneo cutaneous pupillary reflex
reflejo pupilar de Haab Haab's pupillary reflex
reflejo pupilar de Westphal Westphal's pupillary reflex
reflejo pupilar orbicular orbicularis pupillary reflex
reflejo pupilar paradójico paradoxical pupillary reflex
reflejo radial radial reflex
reflejo radial invertido inverted radial reflex
reflejo radiobicipital radiobicipital reflex
reflejo radioperióstico radioperiosteal reflex
reflejo rectoanal rectoanal reflex
reflejo rectocardíaco rectocardiac reflex
reflejo rectolaríngeo rectolaryngeal reflex
reflejo rotuliano patellar reflex
reflejo rotuliano paradójico paradoxical patellar reflex
reflejo rotuloaductor patelloadductor reflex
reflejo semimembranoso semimembranosus reflex
reflejo semitendinoso semitendinosus reflex
reflejo sexual sexual reflex
reflejo sincrónico synchronous reflex
reflejo sinusal sinus reflex
reflejo superficial superficial reflex
reflejo supraorbitario supraorbital reflex
reflejo suprarrotuliano suprapatellar reflex
reflejo suprasegmentario suprasegmental reflex
reflejo supraumbilical supraumbilical reflex
reflejo tarsofalángico tarsophalangeal reflex
reflejo tendinoso tendon reflex
reflejo timpánico tympanic reflex
reflejo tónico tonic reflex
reflejo trigeminofacial trigeminofacial reflex
reflejo ulnar ulnar reflex
reflejo urinario urinary reflex
reflejo utricular utricular reflex
reflejo vasopresor vasopressor reflex
reflejo venorrespiratorio venorespiratory reflex
reflejo vesical vesical reflex
reflejo vestibuloespinal vestibulospinal reflex
reflejo viscerogénico viscerogenic reflex
reflejo visceromotor visceromotor reflex
reflejo viscerosensorial viscerosensory reflex
reflejos antagónicos antagonistic reflexes
reflejos posturales de Magnus de Kleyn Magnus de Kleyn postural reflexes
reflexión reflection
reflexión de sensación reflection of feeling
reflexión difusa diffuse reflection
reflexión factorial factor reflection
reflexófilo reflexophile
reflexogénico reflexogenic
reflexógeno reflexogenous
reflexógrafo reflexograph
reflexología reflexology
reflexómetro reflexometer
reflexoterapia reflexotherapy
reflujo reflux
reflujo gastroesofágico gastroesophageal

reflux
reforma social social reform
reforzador reinforcer
reforzador condicionado conditioned reinforcer
reforzador generalizado generalized reinforcer
reforzador negativo negative reinforcer
reforzador positivo positive reinforcer
reforzador primario primary reinforcer
reforzador secundario secondary reinforcer
reforzante reinforcing
reforzar reinforce
refracción refraction
refractario refractory
refuerzo reinforcement
refuerzo accidental accidental reinforcement
refuerzo adventicio adventitious reinforcement
refuerzo alternativo alternative reinforcement
refuerzo aperiódico aperiodic reinforcement
refuerzo autoadministrado self-managed reinforcement
refuerzo autogénico autogenic reinforcement
refuerzo concurrente concurrent reinforcement
refuerzo conjugado conjugate reinforcement
refuerzo conjuntivo conjunctive reinforcement
refuerzo continuado continued reinforcement
refuerzo continuo continuous reinforcement
refuerzo de contingencia contingency reinforcement
refuerzo de intervalo interval reinforcement
refuerzo de intervalo variable variable-interval reinforcement
refuerzo de Jendrassik Jendrassik reinforcement
refuerzo de proporciones ratio reinforcement
refuerzo de razón variable variable-ratio reinforcement
refuerzo de ritmo diferencial differential rate reinforcement
refuerzo demorado delayed reinforcement
refuerzo diferencial differential reinforcement
refuerzo diferencial de otras conductas differential reinforcement of other behavior
refuerzo diferencial de respuestas en ritmo differential reinforcement of paced responses
refuerzo diferencial de ritmo alto differential reinforcement of high rate
refuerzo diferencial de ritmo bajo differential reinforcement of low rate
refuerzo en tándem tandem reinforcement
refuerzo encadenado chained reinforcement
refuerzo encubierto covert reinforcement
refuerzo entrelazado interlocking reinforcement
refuerzo fijo fixed reinforcement
refuerzo homogéneo homogeneous reinforcement
refuerzo intermitente intermittent reinforcement

refuerzo interpolado interpolated
  reinforcement
refuerzo mixto mixed reinforcement
refuerzo múltiple multiple reinforcement
refuerzo negativo negative reinforcement
refuerzo neural neural reinforcement
refuerzo no contingente noncontingent
  reinforcement
refuerzo parcial partial reinforcement
refuerzo periódico periodic reinforcement
refuerzo positivo positive reinforcement
refuerzo predemora predelay reinforcement
refuerzo primario primary reinforcement
refuerzo reactivo reactive reinforcement
refuerzo secundario secondary reinforcement
refuerzo sistemático systematic reinforcement
refuerzo social social reinforcement
refuerzo terminal terminal reinforcement
refuerzo variable variable reinforcement
refunfuñar grumble
refunfuñon grumbling
regateo bargaining
regeneración regeneration
regeneración aberrante aberrant regeneration
regeneración de fibras ópticas optic fiber
  regeneration
regeneración de nervios regeneration of
  nerves
régimen regimen
región region
región crítica critical region
región de rechazo region of rejection
región incidente incident region
región perceptiva-motora perceptual-motor
  region
región personal interna inner-personal region
región vecina neighboring region
regional regional
registrador cumulativo cumulative recorder
registro record, registration, recording
registro anecdótico anecdotal record
registro cumulativo cumulative record
registro de actividad activity record
registro de caso case register
registro de casos psiquiátricos psychiatric
  case register
registro de conducta behavior record
registro de conducta de espécimen
  behavior-specimen recording
registro de espécimen specimen record
registro de puntas múltiples multiple-spike
  recording
registro de unidad única single-unit
  recording
registro en profundidad depth recording
registro médico medical record
registro orientado a problemas
  problem-oriented record
registro sensorial sensory register
registros clínicos automatizados automated
  clinical records
regla básica basic rule
regla de abstinencia abstinence rule
regla de Durham Durham rule
regla de Jackson Jackson's rule

regla de M'Naghten M'Naghten rule
regla de Pitres Pitres' rule
regla de transformación transformation rule
regla disyuntiva disjunctive rule
regla fundamental fundamental rule
regla práctica rule of thumb
reglas analíticas analytic rules
reglas de decisiones decision rules
reglas de despliegue display rules
reglas de herencia mendelianas mendelian
  rules of inheritance
reglas de Kundt Kundt's rules
reglas del juego rules of the game
regresión regression
regresión curvilínea curvilinear regression
regresión de edad age regression
regresión espontanea spontaneous regression
regresión estadística statistical regression
regresión fenomenal phenomenal regression
regresión filial filial regression
regresión hacia la media regression toward
  the mean
regresión hipnótica hypnotic regression
regresión lineal linear regression
regresión múltiple multiple regression
regresión oral oral regression
regresión parcial partial regression
regresión teleológica teleological regression
regresión teleológica progresiva progressive
  teleological regression
regresivo regressive
regulación regulation
regulación de calcio calcium regulation
regulación de consumo de comida
  food-intake regulation
regulación de emoción regulation of emotion
regulación de hambre regulation of hunger
regulación de impulso drive regulation
regulación de límites interpersonales
  interpersonal boundary regulation
regulación de oxígeno oxygen regulation
regulación de peso weight regulation
regulación de respiración durante sueño
  regulation of breathing during sleep
regulación del sistema inmune immune
  system regulation
regulación recíproca reciprocal regulation
regulación sexual sexual regulation
regulador regulatory
regularidad regularity
regurgitación regurgitation
rehabilitación rehabilitation
rehabilitación de daño cerebral brain
  damage rehabilitation
rehabilitación del habla speech rehabilitation
rehabilitación geriátrica geriatric
  rehabilitation
rehabilitación ocupacional occupational
  rehabilitation
rehabilitación psicológica psychological
  rehabilitation
rehabilitación psiquiátrica psychiatric
  rehabilitation
rehabilitación sexual sex rehabilitation
rehabilitación social social rehabilitation

rehabilitación vocacional vocational rehabilitation
rehabilitar rehabilitate
rehospitalización rehospitalization
reinervación reinnervation
reintegración reintegration
rejilla de agudeza acuity grating
rejuvenecimiento rejuvenation
relación relation, intercourse
relación anal anal intercourse
relación binaria binary relation
relación bucal buccal intercourse
relación calamitosa calamitous relationship
relación causa-efecto cause-effect relationship
relación contingente contingent relationship
relación curvilínea curvilinear relationship
relación de asesoramiento counseling relationship
relación de ayuda helping relationship
relación de dosis-respuesta dose-response relationship
relación de forma-función form-function relation
relación de hermanos sibling relationship
relación de inversión inversion relationship
relación de objeto object relationship
relación de relajar joking relationship
relación de significación de signos sign-significance relation
relación diádica dyadic relationship
relación doctor-paciente doctor-patient relationship
relación dolorosa painful intercourse
relación evitada avoided relationship
relación extramarital extramarital intercourse
relación fiduciaria fiduciary relation
relación funcional functional relation
relación genital genital intercourse
relación hipnótica hypnotic relationship
relación impersonal impersonal relationship
relación interpersonal interpersonal relationship
relación íntima intimate relationship
relación inversa inverse relationship
relación logarítmica logarithmic relationship
relación maestro-estudiante teacher-student relationship
relación marital marital relationship
relación masticación-habla chewing-speech relationship
relación negativa perfecta perfect negative relationship
relación no lineal nonlinear relationship
relación parental parental intercourse
relación paritaria peer relationship
relación personal personal relationship
relación positiva perfecta perfect positive relationship
relación psicofísica psychophysical relationship
relación requerida required relationship
relación sadomasoquista sadomasochistic relationship
relación secundaria secondary relationship
relación sexual sexual intercourse

relación simbiótica symbiotic relationship
relación social-sexual social-sexual relationship
relación espacial spatial relationship
relación terapéutica therapeutic relationship
relacionado con la edad age-related
relacionado al alcohol alcohol-related
relacional relational
relaciones de amistad friendship relationships
relaciones de dominancia-subordinación dominance-subordination relationships
relaciones de grupo group relations
relaciones de objetos object relations
relaciones humanas human relations
relaciones interpersonales interpersonal relations
relaciones medios-fin means-end relations
relaciones paritarias peer relations
relaciones paritarias y ansiedad peer relations and anxiety
relajación relaxation
relajación diferencial differential relaxation
relajación progresiva progressive relaxation
relajamiento muscular muscle relaxation
relajamiento terapéutico therapeutic relaxation
relajante muscular muscle relaxant
relatividad relativity
relatividad de realidad relativity of reality
relatividad lingüística linguistic relativity
relativismo relativism
relativismo cultural cultural relativism
relativismo moral moral relativism
relativo relative
relevante relevant
reloj clock
reloj biológico biological clock
reloj endógeno endogenous clock
relleno filler
remediador remedial
remembranza remembrance
reminiscencia reminiscence
reminiscente reminiscent
remisión remission
remisión completa full remission
remisión de transferencia transference remission
remisión espontanea spontaneous remission
remisión parcial partial remission
remitente remitting
remordimiento remorse
remordimiento anticipatorio anticipatory regret
remotivación remotivation
remoto remote
renacimiento rebirth
renal renal
rendición surrender
rendición esquizofrénica schizophrenic surrender
rendición psicótica psychotic surrender
renunciación renunciation
renunciación instintiva instinctual renunciation
reobase rheobase

reoencefalografía rheoencephalography
reoencefalograma rheoencephalogram
reorganización reorganization
reorganización conductual behavioral reorganization
reorganización neural neural reorganization
reotaxis rheotaxis
reotropismo rheotropism
reparación reparation
repertorio repertoire
repertorio conductual behavioral repertoire
repetición repetition
repetición compulsiva compulsive repetition
repetición inmediata shadowing
repetidor de accidentes accident repeater
repetitivo repetitive
replicación replication
replicación conceptual conceptual replication
replicación exacta exact replication
replicación modificada modified replication
replicar replicate
reportaje de sueños dream reporting
reportando abuso de niños reporting child abuse
represado damned-up
represalia retaliation
represamiento damming-up
representación representation
representación cognitiva cognitive representation
representación como sí as if performance
representación de coito coitus representation
representación de concepto concept representation
representación de objeto object representation
representación doble double representation
representación icónica iconic representation
representación interna internal representation
representación mental mental representation
representación representativa enactive representation
representación simbólica symbolic representation
representación tonotópica tonotopic representation
representar represent
representativo representative
represión repression
represión orgánica organic repression
represión primal primal repression
represión primaria primary repression
represión-resistencia repression-resistance
represión secundaria secondary repression
represivo repressive
represor repressor
reprimido repressed
reprimir repress
reproducción reproduction
reproducción consanguínea inbreeding
reproducción en cadena chain reproduction
reproducción no consanguínea outbreeding
reproducción sexual sexual reproduction
reproducciones sucesivas successive reproductions

reproductivo reproductive
reprueba retest
repugnancia disgust
repulsión repulsion
requerido required
requisitos de ejecución performance requirements
requisitos de trabajo job requirements
resaca hangover
resbalamiento cognitivo cognitive slippage
reserpina reserpine
reserva reserve
reserva operante operant reserve
reserva refleja reflex reserve
reservorio reservoir
reservorio de Ommaya Ommaya reservoir
residencia de grupo group residence
residencial residential
residente resident
residual residual
residuo residue
residuo arcaico archaic residue
residuo cultural cultural residue
residuo nocturno night residue
residuos del día day residue
resignación resignation
resignación neurótica neurotic resignation
resimbolización resymbolization
resinoso resinous
resistencia resistance
resistencia a extinción resistance to extinction
resistencia a tentación resistance to temptation
resistencia al estrés resistance to stress
resistencia cardiorespiratoria cardiorespiratory endurance
resistencia consciente conscious resistance
resistencia de dolor pain endurance
resistencia de transferencia transference resistance
resistencia del ego ego resistance
resistencia del id id resistance
resistencia del superego superego resistance
resistencia inconsciente unconscious resistance
resistencia mínima least resistance
resistencia palmar palmar resistance
resistencia sináptica synaptic resistance
resistencia social social resistance
resistente resistant
resocialización resocialization
resolución resolution
resolución de ansiedad anxiety resolution
resolución de conflicto conflict resolution
resolución de crisis crisis resolution
resolución de problemas problem solving
resolución de problemas de grupo group problem-solving
resolución de problemas inductiva inductive problem solving
resolución de problemas racional rational problem-solving
resolución factorial factor resolution
resonador resonator
resonancia acústica acoustic resonance

resonancia magnética nuclear nuclear magnetic resonance
respeto propio self-respect
respiración respiration
respiración apnéustica apneustic breathing
respiración controlada controlled breathing
respiración de Biot Biot's respiration
respiración de Cheyne-Stokes Cheyne-Stokes respiration
respiración de tejidos tissue respiration
respiración electrofrénica electrophrenic respiration
respiración interna internal respiration
respiración por difusión diffusion respiration
respirador respirator
respiratorio respiratory
respirógrafo respirograph
respondiente respondent
responsabilidad responsibility, liability
responsabilidad criminal criminal responsibility
responsabilidad criminal y defensa de insania criminal responsibility and insanity defense
responsabilidad descriptiva descriptive responsibility
responsabilidad limitada limited responsibility
responsabilidad social social responsibility
responsabilidad del paciente patient responsibility
responsivo responsive
respuesta response
respuesta a color acromático achromatic color response
respuesta acromática achromatic response
respuesta adelantada antedating response
respuesta alfa alpha response
respuesta anticipatoria anticipatory response
respuesta apetitiva condicionada conditioned appetitive response
respuesta aprendida learned response
respuesta autofónica autophonic response
respuesta autónoma autonomic response
respuesta beta beta response
respuesta biopsicosocial a los accidentes biopsychosocial response to accidents
respuesta condicionada conditioned response
respuesta condicionada demorada delayed conditioned response
respuesta condicional conditional response
respuesta conductual behavioral response
respuesta consumatoria consummatory response
respuesta cromática chromatic response
respuesta de acercamiento approach response
respuesta de ansiedad-alivio anxiety-relief response
respuesta de artículo item response
respuesta de aversión aversion response
respuesta de barrera barrier response
respuesta de conductancia cutánea skin conductance response
respuesta de Cushing Cushing response
respuesta de escape condicionado

conditioned escape response
respuesta de evitación avoidance response
respuesta de evitación condicionada conditioned avoidance response
respuesta de fin goal response
respuesta de fin adelantado fraccional fractional antedating goal response
respuesta de frustración frustration response
respuesta de fuga o pelea flight or fight response
respuesta de intrusión intrusion response
respuesta de la comunidad a desastres community response to disasters
respuesta de la madre al llanto mother's response to crying
respuesta de Moro Moro response
respuesta de orientación orienting response
respuesta de parpadeo blink response
respuesta de penetración penetration response
respuesta de piel galvánica galvanic skin response
respuesta de piel psicogalvánica psychogalvanic skin response
respuesta de reclutamiento recruiting response
respuesta de relajación relaxation response
respuesta de sobresalto startle response
respuesta de temor fear response
respuesta demorada delayed response
respuesta diferencial differential response
respuesta distal distal response
respuesta electrodérmica electrodermal response
respuesta emocional emotional response
respuesta emocional condicionada conditioned emotional response
respuesta en el vacío vacuum response
respuesta encadenada chained response
respuesta encubierta covert response
respuesta estática static response
respuesta estatocinética statokinetic response
respuesta evocada evoked response
respuesta evocada auditiva auditory evoked response
respuesta evocada cortical cortical-evoked response
respuesta evocada del tallo cerebral brainstem evoked response
respuesta evocada somatosensorial somatosensory evoked response
respuesta evocada visual visual evoked response
respuesta fetal fetal response
respuesta fija fixated response
respuesta fisiológica physiological response
respuesta habituada habituated response
respuesta hemisférica hemispheric response
respuesta hostil-agresiva al estrés hostile-aggressive response to stress
respuesta implícita implicit response
respuesta impunitiva impunitive response
respuesta inadaptiva maladaptive response
respuesta incompatible incompatible response
respuesta incondicionada unconditioned

response
respuesta incondicional unconditional
   response
respuesta individual individual response
respuesta instrumental instrumental response
respuesta intropunitiva intropunitive
   response
respuesta involuntaria involuntary response
respuesta irrelevante irrelevant answer
respuesta libre free response
respuesta manifiesta overt response
respuesta miotípica myotypical response
respuesta motora motor response
respuesta negativa negative response
respuesta objetivo target response
respuesta oculomotora oculomotor response
respuesta operante operant response
respuesta original original response
respuesta palmar palmar response
respuesta paradójica paradoxical response
respuesta pilomotora pilomotor response
respuesta popular popular response
respuesta preparatoria preparatory response
respuesta prepotente prepotent response
respuesta proximal proximal response
respuesta psicogalvánica psychogalvanic
   response
respuesta rojo-verde red-green response
respuesta selectiva selective response
respuesta serial serial response
respuesta sexual sexual response
respuesta sonomotora sonomotor response
respuesta voluntaria voluntary response
respuestas a patrones en círculos
   circular-pattern responses
respuestas hostiles-agresivas en niños
   hostile-aggressive responses in children
restitución restitution
restitucional restitutional
restricción restriction
restricción de intervalo range restriction
restringido restricted
resultado nulo null result
resultados de tratamiento treatment outcome
resultantes creativos creative resultants
retardado mental educable educable mentally
   retarded
retardado mentalmente mentally retarded
retardo retardation
retardo de lectura reading retardation
retardo del desarrollo developmental
   retardation
retardo del lenguaje language retardation
retardo familiar familial retardation
retardo mental mental retardation
retardo mental contra autismo mental
   retardation versus autism
retardo mental cultural-familiar
   cultural-familial mental retardation
retardo mental familiar familial mental
   retardation
retardo mental fronterizo borderline mental
   retardation
retardo mental leve mild mental retardation
retardo mental moderado moderate mental

retardation
retardo mental no especificado unspecified
   mental retardation
retardo mental profundo profound mental
   retardation
retardo mental y aprendizaje mental
   retardation and learning
retardo mental y derechos legales mental
   retardation and legal rights
retardo mental y disfunción cerebral mental
   retardation and brain dysfunction
retardo mental y función cognitiva mental
   retardation and cognitive function
retardo mental y lenguaje mental retardation
   and language
retardo metal severo severe mental
   retardation
retardo moderado moderate retardation
retardo orgánico organic retardation
retardo psicomotor psychomotor retardation
retardo psicosocial psychosocial retardation
retención retention
retención anal anal retention
retención de afecto retention of affect
retención de memoria memory retention
retención de respiración breath-holding
retención selectiva selective retention
reticular reticular
retículo endoplásmico endoplasmic reticulum
reticulotomía reticulotomy
retifismo retifism
retina retina
retina desprendida detached retina
retina neural neural retina
retinal retinal
retineno retinene
retinitis retinitis
retinoblastoma retinoblastoma
retinocerebral retinocerebral
retinodiencefálico retinodiencephalic
retinopatía diabética diabetic retinopathy
retinoscopio retinoscope
retirada withdrawal
retirada apática apathetic withdrawal
retirada de pensamientos thought withdrawal
retirada social social withdrawal
retirada social y abuso de niños social
   withdrawal and child abuse
retiro withdrawal, retirement, retreat
retiro de alcohol alcohol withdrawal
retiro de alcohol no complicado
   uncomplicated alcohol withdrawal
retiro de anfetaminas amphetamine
   withdrawal
retiro de ansiolítico anxiolytic withdrawal
retiro de barbituratos barbiturate withdrawal
retiro de cocaína cocaine withdrawal
retiro de hipnótico hypnotic withdrawal
retiro de la realidad retreat from reality
retiro de morfina morphine withdrawal
retiro de nicotina nicotine withdrawal
retiro de opioide opioid withdrawal
retiro de otra sustancia other substance
   withdrawal
retiro de sedante sedative withdrawal

retiro de sustancia substance withdrawal
retiro de sustancia desconocida unknown substance withdrawal
retiro de sustancia psicoactiva psychoactive substance withdrawal
retiro de tabaco tobacco withdrawal
retiro narcótico de infante infant narcotic withdrawal
retiro simpatomimético sympathomimetic withdrawal
retiro vegetativo vegetative retreat
reto de lactato lactate challenge
retracción retraction
retroacción positiva positive retroaction
retroactivo retroactive
retroalimentación feedback
retroalimentación auditiva auditory feedback
retroalimentación auditiva demorada delayed auditory feedback
retroalimentación de ampliación de desviación deviation-amplification feedback
retroalimentación de información information feedback
retroalimentación fisiológica physiological feedback
retroalimentación interna internal feedback
retroalimentación negativa negative feedback
retroalimentación positiva positive feedback
retroalimentación sensorial sensory feedback
retroalimentación social social feedback
retrobulbar retrobulbar
retrococlear retrocochlear
retrocólico retrocollic
retrocolis retrocollis
retrocruzamiento backcross
retrocursivo retrocursive
retroflexión retroflexion
retrogasseriano retrogasserian
retrogénesis retrogenesis
retrógrado retrograde
retrografía retrography
retrogresión retrogression
retropulsión retropulsion
retropulsivo retropulsive
retrospección retrospection
retrospectivo retrospective
reubicación relocation
reubicación institucional institutional relocation
reumático rheumatic
reumatismo rheumatism
reumatismo lumbar lumbar rheumatism
reumatoide rheumatoid
reverberación neural neural reverberation
reversibilidad reversibility
reversible reversible
reversión reversion
revisión review
revisión concurrente concurrent review
revisión de estadía continuada continued stay review
revisión de estadía extendida extended-stay review
revisión de reclamaciones claims review

revisión de utilización utilization review
revisión médica medical review
revisión paritaria peer review
revisión secundaria secondary revision
revocación undoing
ribonucleasa ribonuclease
ribosoma ribosome
riesgo risk
riesgo atribuible attributable risk
riesgo biológico biohazard
riesgo coronario coronary risk
riesgo de abuso abuse liability
riesgo de administración management risk
riesgo de descubrimiento discovery risk
riesgo empírico empirical risk
riesgo mínimo minimal risk
riesgo moral moral hazard
riesgo relativo relative risk
riesgo relativo en epidemología relative risk in epidemology
riesgos ambientales environmental hazards
rigidez rigidity
rigidez afectiva affective rigidity
rigidez catatónica catatonic rigidity
rigidez cerebelosa cerebellar rigidity
rigidez de descerebración decerebrate rigidity
rigidez de grupo group rigidity
rigidez de navaja clasp-knife rigidity
rigidez de tubo de plomo lead-pipe rigidity
rigidez en rueda dentada cogwheel rigidity
rigidez hipnótica hypnotic rigidity
rigidez intelectual intellectual rigidity
rigidez midriática mydriatic rigidity
rígido rigid
rigosis rhigosis
rigótico rhigotic
rinencéfalo rhinencephalon
rinolalia rhinolalia
rinorrea rhinorrhea
rinorrea del líquido cerebroespinal cerebrospinal fluid rhinorrhea
ripofagia rhypophagy
ripofobia rhypophobia
risa laughter
risa compulsiva compulsive laughter
ritmicidad rhythmicity
rítmico rhythmic
ritmo rhythm
ritmo alfa alpha rhythm
ritmo beta beta rhythm
ritmo biológico biological rhythm
ritmo cardíaco heart rate
ritmo cardíaco en el sueño de infantes heart rate in infants sleep
ritmo circadiano circadian rhythm
ritmo circanual circannual rhythm
ritmo de Berger Berger rhythm
ritmo de respiración respiration rate
ritmo de sueño monofásico monophasic sleep rhythm
ritmo de sueño polifásico polyphasic sleep rhythm
ritmo de vida life rhythm
ritmo del sueño sleep rhythm

ritmo delta delta rhythm
ritmo diurno diurnal rhythm
ritmo endógeno endogenous rhythm
ritmo infradiano infradian rhythm
ritmo interno internal rhythm
ritmo rápido fast rhythm
ritmo sensorimotor sensorimotor rhythm
ritmo theta theta rhythm
ritmo ultradiano ultradian rhythm
ritmo y periodicidad rhythm and periodicity
ritmos conductuales humanos human
    behavioral rhythms
ritmos nocturnos nocturnal rhythms
rito rite
ritos coribantes corybantic rites
ritos de crisis crisis rites
ritos de pubertad puberty rites
ritos púbicos pubic rites
ritual ritual
ritual reproductivo reproductive ritual
rituales a la hora de acostarse bedtime
    rituals
rituales de evitación avoidance rituals
ritualista ritualistic
rivalidad rivalry
rivalidad binocular binocular rivalry
rivalidad de hermanos sibling rivalry
rivalidad interaural interaural rivalry
rivalidad perceptiva perceptual rivalry
rivalidad retinal retinal rivalry
rivalidad sexual sexual rivalry
rizomélico rhizomelic
rizomeningomielitis rhizomeningomyelitis
rizotomía rhizotomy
rizotomía anterior anterior rhizotomy
rizotomía posterior posterior rhizotomy
rizotomía trigeminal trigeminal rhizotomy
robo compulsivo compulsive stealing
robótica robotics
rodado de cabeza head-rolling
rodonalgia rodonalgia
rodopsina rhodopsin
romance de memoria memory romance
romance familiar family romance
rombencéfalo rhombencephalon
rombergismo rombergism
rombocele rhombocele
romboidal rhomboidal
rompimiento disengagement
rompimiento del ego ego splitting
rompimiento psicótico agudo acute psychotic
    break
roseta rosette
rostral rostral
rotación rotation
rotación de cabeza head rotation
rotación factorial factor rotation
rotación mental mental rotation
rotación oblicua oblique rotation
rotación ortogonal orthogonal rotation
rotatorio rotatory
rótula patella
rotuliano patellar
rotulómetro patellometer
rubéola rubella

rubor caliente hot flash
ruborizarse blush
ruborozo blushing
rudimento rudiment
rueda de actividad activity wheel
rueda de colores color wheel
rueda dentada cogwheel
ruido noise
ruido aleatorio random noise
ruido ambiental environmental noise
ruido blanco white noise
ruido coloreado colored noise
ruido congelado frozen noise
ruido de fondo background noise
ruido rosado pink noise
ruido visual visual noise
rumbo cultural cultural drift
rumbo genético genetic drift
rumiación rumination
ruminativo ruminative
rumor rumor
rupofobia rupophobia
rutina routine

S

sabiduría wisdom
sabor flavor
sabotaje masoquista masochistic sabotage
sabuloso sabulous
sacádico saccadic
saciedad satiation
saciedad semántica semantic satiation
sacral sacral
sacrificar sacrifice
sacrificio sacrifice
sacro sacrum
sacrolistesis sacrolisthesis
sacudida jerk
sacudida cruzada crossed jerk
sacudida de la barbilla chin jerk
sacudida de rodilla knee jerk
sacudida de rodilla cruzada crossed knee
  jerk
sacudida de rodilla pendular pendular knee
  jerk
sacudida del aductor cruzada crossed
  adductor jerk
sacudida del codo elbow jerk
sacudida del supinador supinator jerk
sacudida del talón heel jar
sacudida del tobillo ankle jerk
sacudida mandibular jaw jerk
sáculo saccule
sádico sadistic
sadismo sadism
sadismo anal anal sadism
sadismo del id id sadism
sadismo del superego superego sadism
sadismo fálico phallic sadism
sadismo infantil infantile sadism
sadismo invertido inverted sadism
sadismo larval larval sadism
sadismo oral oral sadism
sadismo sexual sexual sadism
sadista sadist
sadomasoquismo sadomasochism
sadomasoquismo sexual sexual
  sadomasochism
sadomasoquista sadomasochistic
safismo sapphism
sagital sagittal
sala de emergencia emergency room
salbutamol salbutamol
salicilato salicylate
salicilato sérico serum salicylate
salivación salivation
salpingectomía salpingectomy
saltación saltation
saltador jumper

saltatorio saltatory
salud health
salud mental mental health
salud mental comunitaria community mental
  health
salud mental de infantes infant mental health
salud psicológica psychological health
salud pública public health
salud sexual sexual health
saludable healthy
salvaje savage
salvamento de apariencias face saving
sanable sanable
sanatorio sanatorium
sanción sanction
sanción social social sanction
sangre blood
sanguíneo sanguineous
sarampión alemán German measles
sarcasmo sarcasm
sarcoma sarcoma
sarcoma angiolítico angiolithic sarcoma
sarcoma leucocítico leukocytic sarcoma
sarmasación sarmassation
satanofobia satanophobia
satélite satellite
satelitosis satellitosis
satiriasis satyriasis
satirismo satyrism
satisfacción satisfaction
satisfacción de instintos satisfaction of
  instincts
satisfacción de trabajo job satisfaction
satisfacción vicaria vicarious satisfaction
saturación saturation
saturnino saturnine
scala media scala media
scala tympani scala tympani
scala vestibuli scala vestibuli
schwannoma schwannoma
schwannoma acústico acoustic schwannoma
schwannosis schwannosis
sección section
sección cesárea cesarean section
sección coronal coronal section
sección craneal desprendida detached cranial
  section
sección craneal unida attached cranial section
sección del tallo pituitario pituitary stalk
  section
sección dorada golden section
sección horizontal horizontal section
sección lateral lateral section
sección sagital sagittal section
sección transversal cross-section
secobarbital secobarbital
secreción psíquica psychic secretion
secretina secretin
secta sect
secuela sequela
secuencia sequence
secuencia de embudo funnel sequence
secuencia de estados status sequence
secuencia de eventos event sequence
secuencia de fase phase sequence

secuencia del desarrollo developmental
  sequence
secuencia genética genetic sequence
secuencial sequential
secuestro kidnapping
secuestro subclavio subclavian steal
secular secular
secundario secondary
secundinas afterbirth
sed thirst
sed extracelular extracellular thirst
sed mórbida morbid thirst
sedación sedation
sedante sedative
sedante-hipnótico sedative-hypnotic
sedante no barbiturato nonbarbiturate
  sedative
sedativismo sedativism
sedimentación sedimentation
seducción seduction
seducción infantil infantile seduction
seductivo seductive
segmentación segmentation
segmentario segmental
segmento fonético phonetic segment
segregación segregation
segregación perceptiva perceptual segregation
seguimiento follow-up
seguimiento del desarrollo developmental
  follow-up
segunda fase negativa second negative phase
segundo nervio craneal second cranial nerve
seguridad security
seguridad de trabajo job security
seguridad emocional emotional security
seguro secure
seguro de responsabilidad civil liability
  insurance
seguro de salud health insurance
sejunción sejunction
selafobia selaphobia
selección selection
selección adversa adverse selection
selección anaclítica anaclitic choice
selección artificial artificial selection
selección binaria binary choice
selección de artículo item selection
selección de carrera career choice
selección de cónyuge spouse selection
selección de jurado jury selection
selección de neurosis choice of neurosis
selección de objeto object choice
selección de objeto anaclítico anaclitic object
  choice
selección de prueba test selection
selección de síntoma symptom choice
selección del personal personnel selection
selección ejecutiva executive selection
selección forzada forced choice
selección natural natural selection
selección ocupacional occupational choice
selección sexual sexual selection
selección social social selection
selección vocacional vocational selection
seleccionismo selectionism

selectividad motivacional motivational
  selectivity
selectivo selective
semana de trabajo de cuatro días four-day
  workweek
semantena semantene
semántica semantics
semántica cuantitativa quantitative semantics
semántica general general semantics
semántica generativa generative semantics
semanticidad semanticity
semántico semantic
semantogénico semantogenic
semasiografía semasiography
semejanza familiar family resemblance
semen semen
semenuria semenuria
semicoma semicoma
semicomatoso semicomatose
semiconsciente semiconscious
semiconsonante semiconsonant
semimembranoso semimembranosus
seminación semination
seminal seminal
semiología semiology
semiopático semiopathic
semiosis semiosis
semiótica semiotics
semiótico semiotic
semitendinoso semitendinous
semitono semitone
semivocal semivowel
senescencia senescence
senescente senescent
senil senile
senilidad senility
senilismo senilism
senium senium
senium praecox senium praecox
seno sinus
seno carotídeo carotid sinus
seno romboidal rhomboidal sinus
seno sagital superior superior sagittal sinus
sensación sensation
sensación afectiva affective sensation
sensación asténica asthenic feeling
sensación atáxica ataxic feeling
sensación comunal communal feeling
sensación comunitaria community feeling
sensación de cincho cincture sensation
sensación de miembro fantasma phantom
  limb sensation
sensación de presión pressure sensation
sensación del ego corporal bodily ego feeling
sensación demorada delayed sensation
sensación en cinturón girdle sensation
sensación epicrítica epicritic sensation
sensación especial special sensation
sensación general general sensation
sensación muscular muscle sensation
sensación negativa negative sensation
sensación objetiva objective sensation
sensación oceánica oceanic feeling
sensación orgánica organic sensation
sensación persistente aftersensation

sensación primaria primary sensation
sensación referida referred sensation
sensación refleja reflex sensation
sensación secundaria secondary sensation
sensación sensorial sense feeling
sensación sexual sexual sensation
sensación subjetiva subjective sensation
sensación táctil tactile sensation
sensación táctil simultánea simultaneous
  tactile sensation
sensación táctil simultánea doble double
  simultaneous tactile sensation
sensación transferida transferred sensation
sensación visceral visceral sensation
sensacionalismo sensationalism
sensaciones de superioridad superiority
  feelings
sensaciones sexuales sex sensations
sensibilidad sensitivity
sensibilidad absoluta absolute sensitivity
sensibilidad articular articular sensibility
sensibilidad auditiva auditory sensitivity
sensibilidad común common sensibility
sensibilidad cortical cortical sensibility
sensibilidad cósmica cosmic sensitivity
sensibilidad cutánea cutaneous sensitivity
sensibilidad de centelleo flicker sensitivity
sensibilidad de contraste contrast sensitivity
sensibilidad de disociación dissociation
  sensibility
sensibilidad de luz light sensitivity
sensibilidad de presión profunda
  deep-pressure sensitivity
sensibilidad de receptor de dopamina
  dopamine receptor sensitivity
sensibilidad dermal dermal sensitivity
sensibilidad diferencial differential sensitivity
sensibilidad direccional directional sensitivity
sensibilidad electromuscular electromuscular
  sensibility
sensibilidad epicrítica epicritic sensibility
sensibilidad espectral spectral sensitivity
sensibilidad esplacnestésica splanchnesthetic
  sensibility
sensibilidad fótica photic sensitivity
sensibilidad mesoblástica mesoblastic
  sensibility
sensibilidad olfatoria olfactory sensitivity
sensibilidad ósea bone sensibility
sensibilidad palestética pallesthetic sensibility
sensibilidad profunda deep sensitivity
sensibilidad propioceptiva proprioceptive
  sensibility
sensibilidad protopática protopathic
  sensibility
sensibilidad social social sensitivity
sensibilidad subcutánea subcutaneous
  sensibility
sensibilidad térmica thermal sensitivity
sensibilidad vibratoria vibratory sensibility
sensibilidad visual absoluta absolute visual
  sensitivity
sensibilización sensitization
sensibilización encubierta covert sensitization
sensibilización manifiesta overt sensitization

sensibilización perceptiva perceptual
  sensitization
sensibilización refleja reflex sensitization
sensibilizador sensitizer
sensible sensible
sensífero sensiferous
sensígeno sensigenous
sensímetro sensimeter
sensitivo sensitive
sensomóvil sensomobile
sensomovilidad sensomobility
sensor sensor
sensorial sensory
sensoriglandular sensoriglandular
sensorimotor sensorimotor
sensorimuscular sensorimuscular
sensorineural sensorineural
sensorio sensorium
sensorio claro clear sensorium
sensorio enturbado clouded sensorium
sensorivascular sensorivascular
sensorivasomotor sensorivasomotor
sensual sensual
sensualidad sensuality
sensualismo sensualism
sentido sense
sentido articular joint sense
sentido cinestésico kinesthetic sense
sentido común common sense
sentido cutáneo skin sense
sentido de culpabilidad sense of guilt
sentido de dolor pain sense
sentido de equilibrio sense of equilibrium
sentido de identidad sense of identity
sentido de identidad propia sense of self
sentido de movimiento movement sense
sentido de obstáculos obstacle sense
sentido de posición position sense
sentido de postura posture sense
sentido de presión pressure sense
sentido de temperatura temperature sense
sentido de vibraciones vibration sense
sentido del humor sense of humor
sentido del tacto touch sense
sentido del tiempo time sense
sentido dermal dermal sense
sentido espacial space sense
sentido especial special sense
sentido estático static sense
sentido externo external sense
sentido interoceptivo interoceptive sense
sentido laberíntico labyrinthine sense
sentido magnético magnetic sense
sentido motor motor sense
sentido muscular muscular sense
sentido químico común common chemical
  sense
sentido sistémico systemic sense
sentido somático somatic sense
sentido táctil tactile sense
sentido térmico thermal sense
sentido vestibular vestibular sense
sentido vibratorio vibratory sense
sentido visceral visceral sense
sentidos corporales body senses

sentidos eléctricos electric senses
sentidos internos internal senses
sentidos químicos chemical senses
sentimentalismo sentimentality
sentimiento sentiment
sentimiento de grupo group feeling
sentimiento propio self-sentiment
sentimientos de culpabilidad guilt feelings
sentimientos de inferioridad inferiority
 feelings
sentimientos de irrealidad feelings of
 unreality
señal signal, cue
señal acústica acoustic cue
señal binocular binocular cue
señal cognitiva cognitive marker
señal contextual contextual cue
señal de fase phase cue
señal de profundidad binocular binocular
 depth cue
señal de profundidad monocular monocular
 depth cue
señal mínima minimal cue
señal monocular monocular cue
señal reducida reduced cue
señal sensorial sensory cue
señal social social cue
señalado signaled
señalamiento signaling
señalamiento ideomotor ideomotor signaling
señalamiento ideosensorial ideosensory
 signaling
señalamiento intraceptivo intraceptive
 signaling
señales auditivas auditory signals
señales binaurales binaural cues
señales condicionadas conditioned cues
señales de categorías category cues
señales de distancia distance cues
señales de localización cues to localization
señales naturales natural cues
señales perceptivas perceptual cues
señales producidas por respuestas
 response-produced cues
separación separation
separación afectiva affective separation
separación breve brief separation
separación-individuación
 separation-individuation
separación neonatal neonatal separation
separación parental parental separation
separación paritaria peer separation
sepsis sepsis
sepsis intestinal intestinal sepsis
septal septal
septicemia septicemia
séptico septic
séptimo nervio craneal seventh cranial nerve
séptimo sentido seventh sense
septum septum
septum pellucidum septum pellucidum
ser social social being
serendipismo serendipity
seriación seriation
serial serial

serialización serialization
serie series
serie aritmética arithmetic series
serie ascendente-descendente
 ascending-descending series
serie del tiempo time series
serie experimental experimental series
serie geométrica geometric series
seroso serous
serotonérgico serotonergic
serotonina serotonin
servicio de apoyo telefónico telephone
 support service
servicio de línea de emergencia hot-line
 service
servicio sexual sex service
servicios ambulatorios ambulatory services
servicios centrados en pacientes
 patient-centered services
servicios comunitarios community services
servicios de asesoramiento counseling
 services
servicios de ayuda múltiple mutual-help
 services
servicios de extensión outreach services
servicios de pacientes externos outpatient
 services
servicios de pacientes internados inpatient
 services
servicios de salud mental correccionales
 correctional mental health services
servicios educacionales educational services
servicios humanos human services
servicios posempleo postemployment services
servicios psiquiátricos psychiatric services
servicios vocacionales vocational services
servicios centrados en el ambiente
 environment-centered services
servicios de emergencia emergency services
servicios sociales social services
servomecanismo servomechanism
sesgo bias
sesgo antitecnología antitechnology bias
sesgo cultural cultural bias
sesgo cultural en pruebas cultural bias in
 tests
sesgo de beneficio propio self-serving bias
sesgo de confirmación confirmation bias
sesgo de consenso falso false-consensus bias
sesgo de deseabilidad social
 social-desirability bias
sesgo de jurado juror bias
sesgo de muestra sample bias
sesgo de prueba test bias
sesgo de respuestas response bias
sesgo de selección selection bias
sesgo de ubicación location bias
sesgo de voluntarios volunteer bias
sesgo del contexto context bias
sesgo del entrevistador interviewer bias
sesgo del experimentador experimenter bias
sesgo emocional emotional bias
sesgo exótico exotic bias
sesgo experimental experimental bias
sesgo inferencial en memoria inferential bias

in memory
sesgo intersensorial intersensory bias
sesgo por barruntamiento guessing bias
sesión session
sesión de aprendizaje learning session
sesión de grupo alternativo alternative group
session
sesión de maratón marathon session
sesión diádica dyadic session
sesión espiritista seance
seudoacceso pseudoseizure
seudoafectivo pseudoaffective
seudoafia pseudaphia
seudoagrafia pseudoagraphia
seudoagramatismo pseudoagrammatism
seudoagresión pseudoaggression
seudoalucinación pseudohallucination
seudoalucinación percibida perceived
pseudohallucination
seudoamnesia pseudoamnesia
seudoangina pseudoangina
seudoanhedonia pseudoanhedonia
seudoapoplejía pseudoapoplexy
seudoapraxia pseudoapraxia
seudoataxia pseudoataxia
seudoatetosis pseudoathetosis
seudoautenticidad pseudoauthenticity
seudoblepsia pseudoblepsia
seudoblepsis pseudoblepsis
seudobulbar pseudobulbar
seudocatatonía pseudocatatonia
seudocatatonía traumática traumatic
pseudocatatonia
seudocefalocele pseudocephalocele
seudociencia pseudoscience
seudociesis pseudocyesis
seudoclono pseudoclonus
seudocolinesterasa pseudocholinesterase
seudocolusión pseudocollusion
seudocoma pseudocoma
seudocomunicación pseudocommunication
seudocomunidad pseudocommunity
seudocondicionamiento pseudoconditioning
seudocondroplasia pseudochondroplasia
seudoconversación pseudoconversation
seudoconvulsión pseudoconvulsion
seudocopulación pseudocopulation
seudocorea pseudochorea
seudocromestesia pseudochromesthesia
seudodemencia pseudodementia
seudodemencia histérica hysterical
pseudodementia
seudoepilepsia pseudoepilepsy
seudoesclerosis pseudosclerosis
seudoesclerosis de Westphal Westphal's
pseudosclerosis
seudoesclerosis de Westphal-Strumpell
Westphal-Strumpell pseudosclerosis
seudoesquizofrenia pseudoschizophrenia
seudoesquizofrénico pseudoschizophrenic
seudoestesia pseudoesthesia
seudofamilia pseudofamily
seudoflexibilitas pseudoflexibilitas
seudófono pseudophone
seudofotestesia pseudophotesthesia

seudoganglio pseudoganglion
seudogeusestesia pseudogeusesthesia
seudogeusia pseudogeusia
seudografia pseudographia
seudohermafrodismo pseudohermaphrodism
seudohermafrodita pseudohermaphrodite
seudohidrocefalia pseudohydrocephaly
seudohidrofobia pseudohydrophobia
seudohipersexualidad pseudohypersexuality
seudohipertrófico pseudohypertrophic
seudohipnosis pseudohypnosis
seudohipoparatiroidismo
pseudohypoparathyroidsm
seudohomosexual pseudohomosexual
seudohomosexualidad pseudohomosexuality
seudoidentificación pseudoidentification
seudoindependiente pseudoindependent
seudoinsomnio pseudoinsomnia
seudoisocromático pseudoisochromatic
seudolalia pseudolalia
seudología pseudologia
seudología fantástica pseudologia phantastica
seudomaduro pseudomature
seudomalignidad pseudomalignancy
seudomanía pseudomania
seudomasturbación pseudomasturbation
seudomemoria pseudomemory
seudomeningitis pseudomeningitis
seudomnesia pseudomnesia
seudomotivación pseudomotivation
seudomuscular pseudomuscular
seudomutualidad pseudomutuality
seudonarcotismo pseudonarcotism
seudonecrofilia pseudonecrophilia
seudoneoplasma pseudoneoplasm
seudoneurogénico pseudoneurogenic
seudoneuroma pseudoneuroma
seudoneurótico pseudoneurotic
seudonomanía pseudonomania
seudoparálisis pseudoparalysis
seudoparálisis atónica congénita congenital
atonic pseudoparalysis
seudoparálisis general artrítica arthritic
general pseudoparalysis
seudoparámetro pseudoparameter
seudoparanoia pseudoparanoia
seudoparaplejía pseudoparaplegia
seudoparaplejía de Basedow Basedow's
pseudoparaplegia
seudoparesia pseudoparesis
seudoparesia alcohólica alcoholic
pseudoparesis
seudoparkinsonismo pseudoparkinsonism
seudoperitonitis pseudoperitonitis
seudopersonalidad pseudopersonality
seudoplejía pseudoplegia
seudoprecoz pseudoprecocious
seudoprodigio pseudoprodigy
seudopsia pseudopsia
seudopsicología pseudopsychology
seudopsicopático pseudopsychopathic
seudopsicosis pseudopsychosis
seudorretardo pseudoretardation
seudorretroalimentación pseudofeedback
seudorroseta pseudorosette

seudoscopio pseudoscope
seudosenilidad pseudosenility
seudosexualidad pseudosexuality
seudosmia pseudosmia
seudotabes pseudotabes
seudotabes pupilotónica pupillotonic
    pseudotabes
seudotransferencia pseudotransference
seudotumor pseudotumor
seudotumor cerebral pseudotumor cerebri
seudoventrículo pseudoventricle
severidad severity
sexismo sexism
sexo biológico biological sex
sexo coercitivo coercive sex
sexo de grupo group sex
sexo extramarital extramarital sex
sexo forzado forced sex
sexo genital genital sex
sexo intermedio intermediate sex
sexología sexology
sexológico sexological
sexopatía sexopathy
sexto nervio craneal sixth cranial nerve
sexto sentido sixth sense
sexualidad sexuality
sexualidad del contenido de sueños sexuality
    of dream content
sexualidad en adolescencia sexuality in
    adolescence
sexualidad humana human sexuality
sexualidad infantil infantile sexuality
sexualidad perversa polimorfa polymorphous
    perverse sexuality
sexualismo sexualism
sexualización sexualization
sexualizar sexualize
sexualmente sexually
sialidosis sialidosis
sialoaerofagia sialoaerophagy
sialorrea sialorrhea
sibilante sibilant
sicasia sicchasia
SIDA AIDS
sideración sideration
siderodromofobia siderodromophobia
siderofobia siderophobia
sierra de Gigli Gigli's saw
sífilis syphilis
sífilis cerebral cerebral syphilis
sífilis congénita congenital syphilis
sífilis meníngea meningeal syphilis
sífilis meningovascular meningovascular
    syphilis
sifilítico syphilitic
sifilofobia syphilophobia
sifiloma syphiloma
sigma sigma
sigmación sigmation
sigmatismo sigmatism
sigmatismo interdental interdental sigmatism
significación significance
significación estadística statistical significance
significado meaning
significado connotativo connotative meaning

significado de palabras meaning of words
significado de sueños meaning of dreams
significado denotativo denotative meaning
significado en el lenguaje meaning in
    language
significado mnemónico de sueños mnemonic
    meaning of dreams
significado puro pure meaning
significado social social meaning
significante significant
significar signify
significativo meaningful
signo sign
signo contralateral contralateral sign
signo de Abadie Abadie's sign
signo de abanico fan sign
signo de Babinski Babinski's sign
signo de Bamberger Bamberger's sign
signo de Barre Barre's sign
signo de Battle Battle's sign
signo de Bechterew Bechterew's sign
signo de Beevor Beevor's sign
signo de Biernacki Biernacki's sign
signo de Bonhoeffer Bonhoeffer's sign
signo de Brudzinski Brudzinski's sign
signo de Bruns Bruns' sign
signo de Cantelli Cantelli's sign
signo de Castellani-Low Castellani-Low sign
signo de Chaddock Chaddock sign
signo de Chvostek Chvostek's sign
signo de Crichton-Browne
    Crichton-Browne's sign
signo de cuello neck sign
signo de Dejerine Dejerine's sign
signo de Duchenne Duchenne's sign
signo de eco echo sign
signo de Erb Erb's sign
signo de Erb-Westphal Erb-Westphal sign
signo de Escherich Escherich's sign
signo de espejo mirror sign
signo de Froment Froment's sign
signo de Gordon Gordon's sign
signo de Gorlin Gorlin's sign
signo de Graefe Graefe's sign
signo de Grasset Grasset's sign
signo de guiño mandibular jaw-winking sign
signo de Hoffmann Hoffmann's sign
signo de Jackson Jackson's sign
signo de Joffroy Joffroy's sign
signo de Kernig Kernig's sign
signo de Lasegue Lasegue's sign
signo de Legendre Legendre's sign
signo de Leichtenstern Leichtenstern's sign
signo de Leri Leri's sign
signo de Lhermitte Lhermitte's sign
signo de Lichtheim Lichtheim's sign
signo de Litten Litten's sign
signo de los dedos del pie de Goldstein
    Goldstein's toe sign
signo de Macewen Macewen's sign
signo de Magendie-Hertwig
    Magendie-Hertwig sign
signo de Magnan Magnan's sign
signo de Mannkopf Mannkopf's sign
signo de mano extraña strange-hand sign

signo de Marcus Gunn Marcus Gunn sign
signo de Masini Masini's sign
signo de Neri Neri's sign
signo de ojos de muñeca doll's eye sign
signo de pestañas eyelash sign
signo de Pfuhl Pfuhl's sign
signo de Piltz Piltz sign
signo de Pitres Pitres' sign
signo de Pool-Schlesinger Pool-Schlesinger
  sign
signo de Remak Remak's sign
signo de Revilliod Revilliod's sign
signo de Romberg Romberg's sign
signo de Rosenbach Rosenbach's sign
signo de Rossolimo Rossolimo's sign
signo de Rumpf Rumpf's sign
signo de Russell Russell's sign
signo de Saenger Saenger's sign
signo de Schlesinger Schlesinger's sign
signo de Schultze Schultze's sign
signo de Seeligmuller Seeligmuller's sign
signo de Siegert Siegert's sign
signo de Signorelli Signorelli's sign
signo de Simon Simon's sign
signo de Stewart-Holmes Stewart-Holmes
  sign
signo de Stiller Stiller's sign
signo de Straus Straus' sign
signo de Tinel Tinel's sign
signo de Trousseau Trousseau's sign
signo de Uhthoff Uhthoff sign
signo de von Graefe von Graefe's sign
signo de Weber Weber's sign
signo de Weiss Weiss' sign
signo de Wernicke Wernicke's sign
signo de Westphal Westphal's sign
signo de Westphal-Erb Westphal-Erb sign
signo del orbicular sign of the orbicularis
signo del rodado de ojo eye-roll sign
signo espinal spine sign
signo icónico iconic sign
signo indicativo indexical sign
signo local local sign
signo maleolar externo external malleolar
  sign
signo piramidal pyramid sign
signo seudo-Graefe pseudo-Graefe sign
signos convencionales conventional signs
signos de Hoover Hoover's signs
signos patognomónicos pathognomonic signs
signos vitales vital signs
sílaba syllable
sílaba disparatada nonsense syllable
sílaba medial medial syllable
silabario syllabary
silencio silence
silencio electrocerebral electrocerebral
  silence
silencioso silent
silogismo syllogism
silogismo categórico categorical syllogism
silogismo disyuntivo disjunctive syllogism
silogismo hipotético hypothetical syllogism
silla de ruedas wheelchair
simbionte symbiont

simbiosis symbiosis
simbiosis diádica dyadic symbiosis
simbiosis triádica triadic symbiosis
simbiótico symbiotic
simbolia symbolia
simbólico symbolic
simbolismo symbolism
simbolismo abstracto abstract symbolism
simbolismo anagógico anagogic symbolism
simbolismo criptofórico cryptophoric
  symbolism
simbolismo criptogénico cryptogenic
  symbolism
simbolismo de sueños dream symbolism
simbolismo metafórico metaphoric symbolism
simbolización symbolization
símbolo symbol
símbolo de estado status symbol
símbolo fálico phallic symbol
símbolo individual individual symbol
símbolo universal universal symbol
simbolofobia symbolophobia
símbolos arbitrarios arbitrary symbols
simetría symmetry
simétrico symmetrical
similitud similarity
simpatectomía sympathectomy
simpatectomía periarterial periarterial
  sympathectomy
simpatectomía presacra presacral
  sympathectomy
simpatectomía química chemical
  sympathectomy
simpatetectomía sympathetectomy
simpatetoblastoma sympathetoblastoma
simpatía sympathy
simpaticectomía sympathicectomy
simpaticoblastoma sympathicoblastoma
simpaticogonioma sympathicogonioma
simpaticoneuritis sympathiconeuritis
simpaticopatía sympathicopathy
simpaticotonía sympathicotonia
simpaticotónico sympathicotonic
simpaticotripsia sympathicotripsy
simpatina sympathin
simpatismo sympathism
simpatista sympathist
simpatizar sympathize
simpatizante sympathizer
simpatoblastoma sympathoblastoma
simpatogonioma sympathogonioma
simpatolítico sympatholytic
simpatomimético sympathomimetic
simulación simulation
simulación de enfermo malingering
simulación por computadora computer
  simulation
simulado simulated
simulador simulator
simular simulate
simularse enfermo malinger
simultagnosia simultagnosia
simultanagnosia simultanagnosia
simultaneidad simultaneity
simultáneo simultaneous

sin hogar homeless
sin imagen imageless
sin líder leaderless
sin propósito purposeless
sinafoceptores synaphoceptors
sinalgia synalgia
sinálgico synalgic
sinapsis synapse
sinapsis adrenérgica adrenergic synapse
sinapsis axoaxónica axoaxonic synapse
sinapsis axodendrítica axodendritic synapse
sinapsis axosomática axosomatic synapse
sinapsis colinérgica cholinergic synapse
sinapsis dopaminérgica dopaminergic
    synapse
sinapsis excitatoria excitatory synapse
sinapsis inhibitoria inhibitory synapse
sinapsis noradrenérgica noradrenergic
    synapse
sinapsis serotonérgica serotonergic synapse
sináptico synaptic
sincinesia synkinesia
sincinesis synkinesis
sinclónico synclonic
sinclono synclonus
sincopal syncopal
síncope syncope
síncope de micturición micturition syncope
síncope del seno carotídeo carotid sinus
    syncope
síncope histérico hysterical syncope
síncope laríngeo laryngeal syncope
síncope local local syncope
síncope postural postural syncope
síncope vasovagal vasovagal syncope
sincópico syncopic
sincrético syncretic
sincretismo syncretism
sincronía synchrony
sincronía bilateral bilateral synchrony
sincronía interactiva interactional synchrony
sincrónico synchronous
sincronismo synchronism
sincronización synchronization
sincronizado synchronized
síndrome syndrome
síndrome abúlico-acinético abulic-akinetic
    syndrome
síndrome adaptacional general general
    adaptational syndrome
síndrome adiposogenital adiposogenital
    syndrome
síndrome adrenogenital adrenogenital
    syndrome
síndrome afectivo orgánico organic affective
    syndrome
síndrome agresivo orgánico organic
    aggressive syndrome
síndrome amnésico amnesic syndrome
síndrome amnésico de alcohol alcohol
    amnesic syndrome
síndrome amotivacional amotivational
    syndrome
síndrome anticolinérgico anticholinergic
    syndrome

síndrome anticolinérgico central central
    anticholinergic syndrome
síndrome antimotivacional antimotivational
    syndrome
síndrome apálico apallic syndrome
síndrome arterial cerebeloso inferior
    posterior posterior inferior cerebellar
    artery syndrome
síndrome arterial cerebeloso superior
    superior cerebellar artery syndrome
síndrome autoscópico autoscopic syndrome
síndrome barbital fetal fetal barbital
    syndrome
síndrome cerebeloso cerebellar syndrome
síndrome cerebral brain syndrome
síndrome cerebral alcohólico alcoholic brain
    syndrome
síndrome cerebral crónico chronic brain
    syndrome
síndrome cerebral intermedio debido al
    alcohol intermediate brain syndrome due
    to alcohol
síndrome cerebral orgánico organic brain
    syndrome
síndrome cerebral orgánico atípico atypical
    organic brain syndrome
síndrome cerebrohepatorrenal
    cerebrohepatorenal syndrome
síndrome cianótico de Scheid cyanotic
    syndrome of Scheid
síndrome confabulatorio amnésico amnesic
    confabulatory syndrome
síndrome coreatiforme choreatiform
    syndrome
síndrome costoclavicular costoclavicular
    syndrome
síndrome criptoftálmico cryptophthalmos
    syndrome
síndrome de abstinencia abstinence syndrome
síndrome de abstinencia neonatal neonatal
    abstinence syndrome
síndrome de Acosta Acosta's syndrome
síndrome de acroparestesia acroparesthesia
    syndrome
síndrome de Adams-Stokes Adams-Stokes
    syndrome
síndrome de adaptación adaptation syndrome
síndrome de adaptación de Selye adaptation
    syndrome of Selye
síndrome de Adie Adie's syndrome
síndrome de agotamiento burnout syndrome
síndrome de Aicardi Aicardi's syndrome
síndrome de aislamiento social
    social-isolation syndrome
síndrome de Alajouanine Alajouanine's
    syndrome
síndrome de Almaric Almaric's syndrome
síndrome de Alport Alport's syndrome
síndrome de Alstrom Alstrom's syndrome
síndrome de Alstrom-Hallgren
    Alstrom-Hallgren syndrome
síndrome de alucinación visual de negación
    denial visual hallucination syndrome
síndrome de ama de casa housewife's
    syndrome

síndrome de amante fantasma　phantom-lover syndrome

síndrome de Angelucci　Angelucci's syndrome

síndrome de ansiedad　anxiety syndrome

síndrome de ansiedad orgánica　organic anxiety syndrome

síndrome de Anton　Anton's syndrome

síndrome de apatía　apathy syndrome

síndrome de Apert　Apert's syndrome

síndrome de aplastamiento　crush syndrome

síndrome de Arnold-Chiari　Arnold-Chiari syndrome

síndrome de atrofia-ataxia óptico　optic atrophy-ataxia syndrome

síndrome de atropina　atropine syndrome

síndrome de Avellis　Avellis' syndrome

síndrome de Babinski　Babinski's syndrome

síndrome de Babinski-Nageotte　Babinski-Nageotte syndrome

síndrome de Balint　Balint's syndrome

síndrome de Bamatter　Bamatter's syndrome

síndrome de Barany　Barany's syndrome

síndrome de Bardet-Biedl　Bardet-Biedl syndrome

síndrome de Barre-Lieou　Barre-Lieou syndrome

síndrome de Bartschi-Rochaix　Bartschi-Rochaix's syndrome

síndrome de Bassen-Kornzweig　Bassen-Kornzweig syndrome

síndrome de Batten-Steinert　Batten-Steinert syndrome

síndrome de Beck　Beck's syndrome

síndrome de Beckwith-Widemann　Beckwith-Widemann syndrome

síndrome de Behcet　Behcet's syndrome

síndrome de Behr　Behr's syndrome

síndrome de Benedikt　Benedikt's syndrome

síndrome de Bernard-Horner　Bernard-Horner syndrome

síndrome de Bernhardt-Roth　Bernhardt-Roth syndrome

síndrome de Beuren　Beuren syndrome

síndrome de Bianchi　Bianchi's syndrome

síndrome de Biemond　Biemond's syndrome

síndrome de Blocq　Blocq's syndrome

síndrome de Bogorad　Bogorad's syndrome

síndrome de Bonnier　Bonnier's syndrome

síndrome de Borjeson-Forssman-Lehmann　Borjeson-Forssman-Lehmann syndrome

síndrome de Briquet　Briquet's syndrome

síndrome de Brissaud-Marie　Brissaud-Marie syndrome

síndrome de Brissaud-Meige　Brissaud-Meige syndrome

síndrome de Brown-Sequard　Brown-Sequard's syndrome

síndrome de Bruns　Bruns' syndrome

síndrome de Brushfield-Wyatt　Brushfield-Wyatt syndrome

síndrome de cabello ensortijado　kinky-hair syndrome

síndrome de caos dietético　dietary chaos syndrome

síndrome de Capgras　Capgras' syndrome

síndrome de cápsula interna　internal capsule syndrome

síndrome de Carpenter　Carpenter's syndrome

síndrome de cauda equina　cauda equina syndrome

síndrome de Cestan-Chenais　Cestan-Chenais syndrome

síndrome de Charcot　Charcot's syndrome

síndrome de Charcot-Weiss-Baker　Charcot-Weiss-Baker syndrome

síndrome de Chavany-Brunhes　Chavany-Brunhes syndrome

síndrome de Chiari II　Chiari II syndrome

síndrome de Chotzen　Chotzen's syndrome

síndrome de Citelli　Citelli's syndrome

síndrome de Claude　Claude's syndrome

síndrome de Clerambault　Clerambault's syndrome

síndrome de Clerambault-Kandinski　Clerambault-Kandinski syndrome

síndrome de Cobb　Cobb syndrome

síndrome de Cockayne　Cockayne's syndrome

síndrome de Cogan　Cogan's syndrome

síndrome de colapso social　social breakdown syndrome

síndrome de Collet-Sicard　Collet-Sicard syndrome

síndrome de comer nocturno　night-eating syndrome

síndrome de compresión cervical　cervical compression syndrome

síndrome de conducta por daño cerebral　brain-damage behavior syndrome

síndrome de conejo　rabbit syndrome

síndrome de Conn　Conn's syndrome

síndrome de contaminación del aire　air pollution syndrome

síndrome de convexidad　convexity syndrome

síndrome de convexidad dorsolateral　dorsolateral convexity syndrome

síndrome de Cornelia de Lange　Cornelia de Lange syndrome

síndrome de costilla cervical　cervical rib syndrome

síndrome de Cotard　Cotard's syndrome

síndrome de covada　couvade syndrome

síndrome de cráneo en hoja de trébol　cloverleaf skull syndrome

síndrome de craneosinostosis　craniosynostosis syndrome

síndrome de cresta neural　neural crest syndrome

síndrome de Crigler-Najjar　Crigler-Najjar syndrome

síndrome de cuello torcido　wryneck syndrome

síndrome de cuidado intensivo　intensive-care syndrome

síndrome de Curschmann-Batten-Steinert　Curschmann-Batten-Steinert syndrome

síndrome de Cushing　Cushing's syndrome

síndrome de D'Acosta　D'Acosta's syndrome

síndrome de Da Costa　Da Costa's syndrome

síndrome de Dalila　Delilah syndrome

síndrome de Dana Dana's syndrome
síndrome de Dandy-Walker Dandy-Walker syndrome
síndrome de de Clerambault de Clerambault's syndrome
síndrome de de Lange de Lange syndrome
síndrome de de Morsier de Morsier's syndrome
síndrome de de Sanctis-Cacchione de Sanctis-Cacchione syndrome
síndrome de Debre-Semelaigne Debre-Semelaigne syndrome
síndrome de deficiencia inmune immune deficiency syndrome
síndrome de Dejerine-Klumpke Dejerine-Klumpke syndrome
síndrome de Dejerine-Roussy Dejerine-Roussy syndrome
síndrome de Dejerine-Thomas Dejerine-Thomas syndrome
síndrome de denegación escolar school refusal syndrome
síndrome de dependencia dependency syndrome
síndrome de dependencia de alcohol alcohol dependence syndrome
síndrome de Dercum Dercum's syndrome
síndrome de desastre disaster syndrome
síndrome de desconexión disconnection syndrome
síndrome de descontrol dyscontrol syndrome
síndrome de descontrol episódico episodic dyscontrol syndrome
síndrome de desinhibición disinhibition syndrome
síndrome de desmayo parcial gray-out syndrome
síndrome de despersonalización depersonalization syndrome
síndrome de dificultad respiratoria respiratory-distress syndrome
síndrome de Diógenes Diogenes syndrome
síndrome de discapacidad disability syndrome
síndrome de discapacidad social social disability syndrome
síndrome de disociación dissociation syndrome
síndrome de disparates nonsense syndrome
síndrome de Dollinger-Bielschowsky Dollinger-Bielschowsky syndrome
síndrome de dolor pain syndrome
síndrome de dolor relampagueante flashing pain syndrome
síndrome de Doose Doose syndrome
síndrome de Down Down's syndrome
síndrome de Down de translocación translocation Down's syndrome
síndrome de Down e interacciones madre-infante Down's syndrome and mother-infant interactions
síndrome de Duchenne Duchenne's syndrome
síndrome de Eagle Eagle syndrome
síndrome de Eaton-Lambert Eaton-Lambert

syndrome
síndrome de Edward Edward's syndrome
síndrome de Ehret Ehret's syndrome
síndrome de Eisenlohr Eisenlohr's syndrome
síndrome de Ekbom Ekbom syndrome
síndrome de Ellis-van Creveld Ellis-van Creveld syndrome
síndrome de encefalopatía por diálisis dialysis encephalopathy syndrome
síndrome de energía temporal seasonal energy syndrome
síndrome de Erb-Goldflam Erb-Goldflam syndrome
síndrome de esfuerzo effort syndrome
síndrome de esposa golpeada battered wife syndrome
síndrome de Estocolmo Stockholm syndrome
síndrome de estrés demorado delayed stress syndrome
síndrome de estrés postraumático posttraumatic stress syndrome
síndrome de estrés premenstrual premenstrual-stress syndrome
síndrome de Fahr Fahr's syndrome
síndrome de fase del sueño demorado delayed sleep phase syndrome
síndrome de feminización testicular testicular feminization syndrome
síndrome de feriado holiday syndrome
síndrome de Figueira Figueira's syndrome
síndrome de Fisch-Renwick Fisch-Renwick syndrome
síndrome de Fisher Fisher's syndrome
síndrome de Flynn-Aird Flynn-Aird syndrome
síndrome de Foster Kennedy Foster Kennedy's syndrome
síndrome de Foville Foville's syndrome
síndrome de fracaso en crecer failure to grow syndrome
síndrome de fracaso en medrar failure to thrive syndrome
síndrome de Frey Frey's syndrome
síndrome de Frohlich Frohlich's syndrome
síndrome de Froin Froin's syndrome
síndrome de fusión cervical cervical fusion syndrome
síndrome de Ganser Ganser's syndrome
síndrome de Gardner-Diamond Gardner-Diamond syndrome
síndrome de Gelineau Gelineau's syndrome
síndrome de Gerstmann Gerstmann's syndrome
síndrome de Gerstmann-Straussler Gerstmann-Straussler syndrome
síndrome de Gilles de la Tourette Gilles de la Tourette's syndrome
síndrome de Gjessing Gjessing's syndrome
síndrome de Goldenhar Goldenhar's syndrome
síndrome de Goltz Goltz syndrome
síndrome de Gowers Gowers syndrome
síndrome de Gradenigo Gradenigo's syndrome
síndrome de Gubler Gubler's syndrome

síndrome de Guillain-Barre Guillain-Barre
syndrome
síndrome de guiño mandibular jaw-winking
syndrome
síndrome de Gunn Gunn's syndrome
síndrome de Gunther-Waldenstrom
Gunther-Waldenstrom syndrome
síndrome de Hallermann-Streiff
Hallermann-Streiff syndrome
síndrome de Hallervorden Hallervorden
syndrome
síndrome de Hallervorden-Spatz
Hallervorden-Spatz syndrome
síndrome de Hand-Christian-Schuller
Hand-Christian-Schuller syndrome
síndrome de Harris Harris' syndrome
síndrome de Heller Heller's syndrome
síndrome de Herrmann Herrmann's
syndrome
síndrome de Hinman Hinman syndrome
síndrome de hiperabducción hyperabduction
syndrome
síndrome de hipercalcemia hypercalcemia
syndrome
síndrome de hiperventilación
hyperventilation syndrome
síndrome de hiperventilación crónica
chronic hyperventilation syndrome
síndrome de hipopigmentación oculocerebral
oculocerebral-hypopigmentation syndrome
síndrome de Holmes-Adie Holmes-Adie
syndrome
síndrome de Horner Horner's syndrome
síndrome de Hughlings Jackson Hughlings
Jackson's syndrome
síndrome de Hunt Hunt's syndrome
síndrome de Hunter Hunter's syndrome
síndrome de Hurler Hurler's syndrome
síndrome de ictiosis-hipogonadismo
ichthyosis-hypogonadism syndrome
síndrome de imidazol imidazole syndrome
síndrome de impostor impostor syndrome
síndrome de indiferencia al dolor
indifference to pain syndrome
síndrome de inmunodeficiencia adquirida
acquired immunodeficiency syndrome
síndrome de insensibilidad a andrógenos
androgen-insensitivity syndrome
síndrome de intestino irritable irritable
bowel syndrome
síndrome de Jackson Jackson's syndrome
síndrome de Jahnke Jahnke's syndrome
síndrome de Joubert Joubert's syndrome
síndrome de Kahlbaum-Wernicke
Kahlbaum-Wernicke syndrome
síndrome de Kallmann Kallmann's syndrome
síndrome de Kanner Kanner's syndrome
síndrome de Kearns-Sayre Kearns-Sayre
syndrome
síndrome de Kennedy Kennedy's syndrome
síndrome de Kleine-Levin Kleine-Levin
syndrome
síndrome de Klinefelter Klinefelter's
syndrome
síndrome de Klippel-Feil Klippel-Feil

syndrome
síndrome de Klumpke-Dejerine
Klumpke-Dejerine syndrome
síndrome de Kluver-Bucy Kluver-Bucy
syndrome
síndrome de Kocher-Debre-Semelaigne
Kocher-Debre-Semelaigne syndrome
síndrome de Koerber-Salus-Elschnig
Koerber-Salus-Elschnig syndrome
síndrome de Korsakoff Korsakoff's
syndrome
síndrome de Krabbe Krabbe's syndrome
**síndrome de la articulación
temporomandibular** temporomandibular
joint syndrome
síndrome de lágrimas de cocodrilo crocodile
tears syndrome
síndrome de Lambert-Eaton Lambert-Eaton
syndrome
síndrome de Landau-Kleffner
Landau-Kleffner syndrome
síndrome de Landry Landry's syndrome
síndrome de Landry-Guillain-Barre
Landry-Guillain-Barre syndrome
síndrome de Lasegue Lasegue's syndrome
síndrome de Laurence-Biedl Laurence-Biedl
syndrome
síndrome de Laurence-Moon
Laurence-Moon syndrome
síndrome de Laurence-Moon-Bardet-Biedl
Laurence-Moon-Bardet-Biedl syndrome
síndrome de Laurence-Moon-Biedl
Laurence-Moon-Biedl syndrome
síndrome de Lawford Lawford's syndrome
síndrome de Lennox Lennox syndrome
síndrome de Lennox-Gastaut
Lennox-Gastaut syndrome
síndrome de Lesch-Nyhan Lesch-Nyhan
syndrome
síndrome de lisencefalia lissencephaly
syndrome
síndrome de lóbulo frontal frontal lobe
syndrome
síndrome de lóbulo temporal temporal-lobe
syndrome
síndrome de loculación loculation syndrome
síndrome de Loeffler Loeffler's syndrome
síndrome de Louis-Bar Louis-Bar syndrome
síndrome de Magendie-Hertwig
Magendie-Hertwig syndrome
síndrome de Main Main's syndrome
síndrome de malformación cerebelomedular
cerebellomedullary malformation
syndrome
síndrome de Malin Malin syndrome
síndrome de Marcus Gunn Marcus Gunn
syndrome
síndrome de Marfan Marfan's syndrome
síndrome de Marie-Robinson
Marie-Robinson syndrome
síndrome de Marin Amat Marin Amat's
syndrome
síndrome de Marinesco-Garland
Marinesco-Garland syndrome
síndrome de Marinesco-Sjogren

Marinesco-Sjogren syndrome
síndrome de Maroteaux-Lamy
 Maroteaux-Lamy syndrome
síndrome de Mast Mast syndrome
síndrome de May-White May-White
 syndrome
síndrome de Meckel Meckel's syndrome
síndrome de Meige Meige syndrome
síndrome de Melkersson-Rosenthal
 Melkersson-Rosenthal syndrome
síndrome de Menkes Menkes' syndrome
síndrome de Midas Midas syndrome
síndrome de Millard-Gubler Millard-Gubler
 syndrome
síndrome de Milles Milles' syndrome
síndrome de Mobius Mobius' syndrome
síndrome de Monakow Monakow's syndrome
síndrome de Morel Morel's syndrome
síndrome de Morgagni Morgagni's syndrome
síndrome de Morgagni-Adams-Stokes
 Morgagni-Adams-Stokes syndrome
síndrome de motivación aberrante aberrant
 motivational syndrome
síndrome de muerte de infante súbita
 sudden infant death syndrome
síndrome de mujer airada angry woman
 syndrome
síndrome de Munchausen Munchausen
 syndrome
**síndrome de muñeca con meneo vertical de
 cabeza** head-bobbing doll syndrome
síndrome de muñeco feliz happy puppet
 syndrome
síndrome de Naffziger Naffziger syndrome
síndrome de narcolepsia-catalepsia
 narcolepsy-catalepsy syndrome
síndrome de necrosis pituitaria posparto
 postpartum pituitary necrosis syndrome
síndrome de Nelson Nelson syndrome
síndrome de neuroma mucoso múltiple
 multiple mucosal neuroma syndrome
síndrome de nido vacío empty-nest syndrome
síndrome de niño desplazado displaced child
 syndrome
síndrome de niño golpeado battered child
 syndrome
síndrome de niño hiperactivo hyperactive
 child syndrome
síndrome de niño torpe clumsy-child
 syndrome
síndrome de niño vulnerable vulnerable-child
 syndrome
síndrome de Noonan Noonan's syndrome
síndrome de Nothnagel Nothnagel's
 syndrome
síndrome de ojo de gato cat's eye syndrome
síndrome de Oppenheim Oppenheim's
 syndrome
síndrome de Otelo Othello syndrome
síndrome de Pancoast Pancoast syndrome
síndrome de Parinaud Parinaud's syndrome
síndrome de Parry-Romberg Parry-Romberg
 syndrome
síndrome de Pepper Pepper syndrome
síndrome de persecución persecution

syndrome
síndrome de persona muy importante very
 important person syndrome
síndrome de personalidad personality
 syndrome
síndrome de personalidad orgánico organic
 personality syndrome
síndrome de Pfaundler-Hurler
 Pfaundler-Hurler syndrome
síndrome de Pfeiffer Pfeiffer's syndrome
síndrome de Pick Pick's syndrome
síndrome de Pickwick pickwickian syndrome
síndrome de piernas inquietas restless leg
 syndrome
síndrome de Pierre Robin Pierre Robin's
 syndrome
síndrome de Pinel-Haslam Pinel-Haslam
 syndrome
síndrome de Pisa Pisa syndrome
síndrome de placa negra black-patch
 syndrome
síndrome de pobreza clínica clinical poverty
 syndrome
síndrome de polidipsia nocturna psicogénica
 psychogenic nocturnal polydipsia
 syndrome
síndrome de Potzl Potzl syndrome
síndrome de Prader-Labhart-Willi
 Prader-Labhart-Willi syndrome
síndrome de Prader-Willi Prader-Willi
 syndrome
síndrome de privación maternal maternal
 deprivation syndrome
síndrome de privación social social
 deprivation syndrome
síndrome de Putnam-Dana Putnam-Dana
 syndrome
síndrome de quiasma chiasma syndrome
síndrome de Ramsay Hunt Ramsay Hunt's
 syndrome
síndrome de rapto de la profundidad
 rapture-of-the-deep syndrome
síndrome de referencia olfatoria olfactory
 reference syndrome
síndrome de Refsum Refsum's syndrome
síndrome de Reiter Reiter's syndrome
síndrome de Renpenning Renpenning's
 syndrome
síndrome de respuesta al estrés stress
 response syndrome
síndrome de respuestas aproximadas
 syndrome of approximate answers
**síndrome de respuestas relevantes
 aproximadas** syndrome of approximate
 relevant answers
síndrome de respuestas relevantes tortuosas
 syndrome of deviously relevant answers
síndrome de retiro withdrawal syndrome
síndrome de retiro prolongado protracted
 withdrawal syndrome
síndrome de Rett Rett's syndrome
síndrome de Reye Reye's syndrome
síndrome de Richards-Rundel
 Richards-Rundel syndrome
síndrome de Rieger Rieger's syndrome

síndrome de Riley-Day Riley-Day syndrome
síndrome de Robert Robert's syndrome
síndrome de Romano-Ward Romano-Ward
  syndrome
síndrome de Romberg Romberg's syndrome
síndrome de Rothmund-Thomson
  Rothmund-Thomson syndrome
síndrome de Roussy-Levy Roussy-Levy
  syndrome
síndrome de rubéola congénita congenital
  rubella syndrome
síndrome de Rubinstein-Taybi
  Rubinstein-Taybi syndrome
síndrome de Russell Russell's syndrome
síndrome de Sandifer Sandifer's syndrome
síndrome de Sanfilippo Sanfilippo's
  syndrome
síndrome de Saunders-Sutton
  Saunders-Sutton syndrome
síndrome de Scheie Scheie's syndrome
síndrome de Schirmer Schirmer's syndrome
síndrome de Schmidt Schmidt's syndrome
**síndrome de secreción inapropiada de
  hormona antidiurética** syndrome of
  inappropriate secretion of antidiuretic
  hormone
síndrome de secuestro subclavio subclavian
  steal syndrome
síndrome de Sheehan Sheehan's syndrome
síndrome de Shy-Drager Shy-Drager
  syndrome
síndrome de Silver Silver's syndrome
síndrome de Silver-Russell Silver-Russell
  syndrome
síndrome de Sjogren-Larsson
  Sjogren-Larsson syndrome
síndrome de Sluder Sluder's syndrome
síndrome de Smith-Lemli-Opitz
  Smith-Lemli-Opitz syndrome
síndrome de Sneddon Sneddon's syndrome
síndrome de Sohval-Soffer Sohval-Soffer
  syndrome
síndrome de sombrerero loco Mad Hatter
  syndrome
síndrome de somnolencia por radiación
  radiation somnolence syndrome
síndrome de Sotos Sotos syndrome
síndrome de Spens Spens' syndrome
síndrome de Steele-Richardson-Olszewski
  Steele-Richardson-Olszewski syndrome
síndrome de Stevens-Johnson
  Stevens-Johnson syndrome
síndrome de Stewart-Morel Stewart-Morel
  syndrome
síndrome de Stokes-Adams Stokes-Adams
  syndrome
síndrome de Strauss Strauss' syndrome
síndrome de Sturge-Kalischer-Weber
  Sturge-Kalischer-Weber syndrome
síndrome de Sturge-Weber Sturge-Weber
  syndrome
síndrome de sudación gustatoria gustatory
  sweating syndrome
síndrome de Sudeck Sudeck's syndrome
síndrome de superviviente survivor

  syndrome
síndrome de Tapia Tapia's syndrome
síndrome de tensión cervical cervical tension
  syndrome
síndrome de tensión premenstrual
  premenstrual-tension syndrome
síndrome de Tolosa-Hunt Tolosa-Hunt
  syndrome
síndrome de Torsten Sjogren Torsten
  Sjogren's syndrome
síndrome de Tourette Tourette's syndrome
síndrome de trauma de violación rape
  trauma syndrome
síndrome de Treacher Collins Treacher
  Collins' syndrome
síndrome de triple X triple-X syndrome
síndrome de trisomia trisomy syndrome
síndrome de trisomia 21 trisomy 21
  syndrome
síndrome de Trousseau Trousseau's
  syndrome
síndrome de Turcot Turcot syndrome
síndrome de Turner Turner's syndrome
síndrome de van Buchem van Buchem's
  syndrome
síndrome de Vernet Vernet's syndrome
síndrome de Vogt Vogt syndrome
síndrome de von Gierke von Gierke's
  syndrome
síndrome de von Hippel-Lindau von
  Hippel-Lindau syndrome
síndrome de Waardenburg Waardenburg's
  syndrome
síndrome de Wallenberg Wallenberg's
  syndrome
síndrome de Weber Weber's syndrome
síndrome de Werner Werner's syndrome
síndrome de Wernicke Wernicke's syndrome
síndrome de Wernicke-Korsakoff
  Wernicke-Korsakoff syndrome
síndrome de West West's syndrome
síndrome de Westphal-Leyden
  Westphal-Leyden syndrome
síndrome de Wildervanck Wildervanck's
  syndrome
síndrome de Williams Williams syndrome
síndrome de Wilson Wilson's syndrome
síndrome de Wyburn-Mason Wyburn-Mason
  syndrome
síndrome de X frágil fragile X syndrome
síndrome de Zange-Kindler Zange-Kindler
  syndrome
síndrome de Zanoli-Vecchi Zanoli-Vecchi
  syndrome
síndrome de Zappert Zappert's syndrome
síndrome del alcohol fetal fetal alcohol
  syndrome
síndrome del ángulo cerebelopontino
  cerebellopontine angle syndrome
síndrome del ángulo pontocerebeloso
  pontocerebellar-angle syndrome
síndrome del cayado aórtico aortic arch
  syndrome
síndrome del cordón central central cord
  syndrome

síndrome del cuerpo calloso corpus callosum syndrome

síndrome del disco disk syndrome

síndrome del disco cervical cervical disc syndrome

síndrome del escaleno anterior scalenus anterior syndrome

síndrome del humor orgánico organic mood syndrome

síndrome del maullido de gato cat-cry syndrome

síndrome del nervio auriculotemporal auriculotemporal nerve syndrome

síndrome del retiro de alcohol alcohol withdrawal syndrome

síndrome del retiro de esteroides steroid withdrawal syndrome

síndrome del seno carotídeo carotid sinus syndrome

síndrome del seno cavernoso cavernous sinus syndrome

síndrome del síndrome de la China China Syndrome syndrome

síndrome del túnel carpiano carpal tunnel syndrome

síndrome del túnel tarsiano tarsal tunnel syndrome

síndrome delusorio delusional syndrome

síndrome delusorio orgánico organic delusional syndrome

síndrome depresivo orgánico organic depressive syndrome

síndrome diencefálico de infancia diencephalic syndrome of infancy

síndrome dismnésico dysmnesic syndrome

síndrome disociativo dissociative syndrome

síndrome endogenomórfico endogenomorphic syndrome

síndrome específico de cultura culture-specific syndrome

síndrome extrapiramidal extrapyramidal syndrome

síndrome fronterizo borderline syndrome

síndrome hemibulbar hemibulbar syndrome

síndrome hipercinético hyperkinetic syndrome

síndrome hipercinético infantil infantile hyperkinetic syndrome

síndrome hipertónico-discinético hypertonic-dyskinetic syndrome

síndrome hipocinético hypokinetic syndrome

síndrome hipofisario hypophysial syndrome

síndrome hipofisioesfenoidal hypophysio-sphenoidal syndrome

síndrome hipotalámico hypothalamic syndrome

síndrome hipotalámico lateral lateral hypothalamic syndrome

síndrome hipotalámico ventromedial ventromedial hypothalamic syndrome

síndrome hombro-cinturón shoulder-girdle syndrome

síndrome hombro-mano shoulder-hand syndrome

síndrome inducido por sustancia

substance-induced syndrome

síndrome infeccioso-exhaustivo infectious-exhaustive syndrome

síndrome limitado a una cultura culture-bound syndrome

síndrome maligno malignant syndrome

síndrome maligno neuroléptico neuroleptic malignant syndrome

síndrome maníaco manic syndrome

síndrome maníaco orgánico organic manic syndrome

síndrome masticatorio bucolingual buccolingual masticatory syndrome

síndrome médico medical syndrome

síndrome medular lateral lateral medullary syndrome

síndrome mental orgánico organic mental syndrome

síndrome neurocirculatorio de Labbe Labbe's neurocirculatory syndrome

síndrome neuroconductual neurobehavioral syndrome

síndrome neurocutáneo neurocutaneous syndrome

síndrome neuroléptico neuroleptic syndrome

síndrome neuroléptico maligno malignant neuroleptic syndrome

síndrome neurótico neurotic syndrome

síndrome oculocerebrorrenal oculocerebrorenal syndrome

síndrome oral-facial-digital oral-facial-digital syndrome

síndrome orbitomedial orbitomedial syndrome

síndrome orgánico organic syndrome

síndrome otopalatodigital otopalatodigital syndrome

síndrome paleoestriatal paleostriatal syndrome

síndrome palidal pallidal syndrome

síndrome paratrigeminal de Raeder Raeder's paratrigeminal syndrome

síndrome por vibraciones vibration syndrome

síndrome posadrenalectomía postadrenalectomy syndrome

síndrome posconcusión postconcussion syndrome

síndrome posencefalitis postencephalitis syndrome

síndrome postraumático posttraumatic syndrome

síndrome premenstrual premenstrual syndrome

síndrome premotor premotor syndrome

síndrome psicogénico psychogenic syndrome

síndrome psicomímico psychomimic syndrome

síndrome psicótico infantil simbiótico symbiotic infantile psychotic syndrome

síndrome radicular radicular syndrome

síndrome rígido-acinético rigid-akinetic syndrome

síndrome seudomaduro pseudomature syndrome

síndrome sincinético de Gunn Gunn's

synkinetic syndrome
síndrome talámico thalamic syndrome
síndrome tegmental tegmental syndrome
síndrome teratogénico teratogenic syndrome
síndrome tirohipofisario thyrohypophysial syndrome
síndrome vascular encefalotrigeminal encephalotrigeminal vascular syndrome
síndrome vasovagal vasovagal syndrome
sineidesis syneidesis
sinencefalocele synencephalocele
sinergía synergy
sinérgico synergistic
sinergismo synergism
sinergismo sexual sexual synergism
sinestesia synesthesia
sinestesia álgica synesthesia algica
sinestesia auditiva auditory synesthesia
sinestesialgia synesthesialgia
singamia syngamy
singulto singultus
sinistral sinistral
sinistralidad sinistrality
sinistropedal sinistropedal
sinografía sinography
sinónimo synonym
sinóptico synoptic
sinorquidismo synorchidism
sinorquismo synorchism
sinostosis synostosis
sinostosis tribasilar tribasilar synostosis
sinqueiria syncheiria
sinquiria synchiria
sintáctica syntactics
sintáctico syntactic
sintalidad syntality
sintaxis syntax
síntesis synthesis
síntesis creativa creative synthesis
síntesis de proteína protein synthesis
síntesis figural figural synthesis
síntesis mental mental synthesis
síntesis perceptiva perceptual synthesis
síntesis silábica syllabic synthesis
síntesis simbólica symbolic synthesis
sintético synthetic
sintetizador del habla speech synthesizer
síntoma symptom
síntoma bifásico biphasic symptom
síntoma de abstinencia abstinence symptom
síntoma de conversión conversion symptom
síntoma de conversión motor motor conversion symptom
síntoma de conversión sensorial sensory conversion symptom
síntoma de Epstein Epstein's symptom
síntoma de Frenkel Frenkel's symptom
síntoma de Gordon Gordon's symptom
síntoma de Haenel Haenel's symptom
síntoma de homónimo homonym symptom
síntoma de Kerandel Kerandel's symptom
síntoma de Macewen Macewen's symptom
síntoma de Romberg Romberg's symptom
síntoma de Romberg-Howship Romberg-Howship symptom

síntoma de Schneider schneiderian symptom
síntoma de Trendelenburg Trendelenburg's symptom
síntoma de Wartenberg Wartenberg's symptom
síntoma eclámptico pospartal postpartal eclamptic symptom
síntoma eclámptico prepartal prepartal eclamptic symptom
síntoma filogenético phylogenetic symptom
síntoma fundamental fundamental symptom
síntoma negativo negative symptom
síntoma prodromal prodromal symptom
síntoma productivo productive symptom
síntoma vegetativo vegetative symptom
síntomas accesorios accessory symptoms
síntomas cardíacos cardiac symptoms
síntomas de defensas secundarias secondary defense symptoms
síntomas de déficit deficit symptoms
síntomas de depresión symptoms of depression
síntomas de primer rango first-rank symptoms
síntomas de primer rango de Schneider Schneider's first-rank symptoms
síntomas de retiro withdrawal symptoms
síntomas eclámpticos eclamptic symptoms
síntomas primarios primary symptoms
síntomas secundarios secondary symptoms
sintomático symptomatic
sintonía syntonia
sintónico syntonic
síntono syntone
sintropía syntropy
sintrópico syntropic
sinusoidal sinusoidal
siringobulbia syringobulbia
siringocele syringocele
siringoencefalomielia syringoencephalomyelia
siringoide syringoid
siringomeningocele syringomeningocele
siringomielia syringomyelia
siringomiélico syringomyelic
siringomielo syringomyelus
siringomielocele syringomyelocele
siringopontia syringopontia
sistáltico systaltic
sistema system
sistema abierto open system
sistema activante reticular reticular activating system
sistema adrenérgico adrenergic system
sistema anabólico anabolic system
sistema anterolateral anterolateral system
sistema antirrecompensa antireward system
sistema auditivo auditory system
sistema biofísico biophysical system
sistema biopsicosocial biopsychosocial system
sistema cardiovascular cardiovascular system
sistema centrencefálico centrencephalic system
sistema cerebral psicodinámico psychodynamic cerebral system
sistema cerebroespinal cerebrospinal system

sistema cerrado closed system
sistema colinérgico cholinergic system
sistema conductual behavioral system
sistema craneosacro craniosacral system
sistema de acción action system
sistema de actividad activity system
sistema de adquisición del lenguaje language acquisition system
sistema de alerta alerting system
sistema de alimentación feeding system
sistema de apoyo de decisiones decision support system
sistema de apoyo informal informal support system
sistema de casitas de campo cottage plan
sistema de codificación conductual behavioral coding system
sistema de colores color system
sistema de colores de Munsell Munsell color system
sistema de colores de Ostwald Ostwald color system
sistema de colores de Ridgway Ridgway color system
sistema de condicionamiento sensorial sensory-conditioning system
sistema de conducta behavior system
sistema de control control system
sistema de coordenadas cartesianas Cartesian coordinate system
sistema de Crocker-Henderson Crocker-Henderson system
sistema de cuidado de salud health care system
sistema de defensa psicológico psychological defense system
sistema de defensas neurótico neurotic defense system
sistema de delusiones delusion system
sistema de despertamiento central central arousal system
sistema de Holt Holt system
sistema de incentivos incentive system
sistema de información information system
sistema de información ejecutiva executive information system
sistema de límites boundary system
sistema de memoria memory system
sistema de Muller Mullerian system
sistema de olfato de Zwaardemaker Zwaardemaker smell system
sistema de pareo de perfiles profile-matching system
sistema de Pinel Pinel's system
sistema de primera señal first signal system
sistema de proyección talámica difusa diffuse thalamic projection system
sistema de realidad reality system
sistema de reclutamiento recruiting system
sistema de recompensa reward system
sistema de respuesta innata innate response system
sistema de respuestas response system
sistema de retroalimentación feedback system

sistema de retroalimentación de ciclo cerrado closed-loop feedback system
sistema de rotación rotation system
sistema de segundas señales second signal system
sistema de señalamiento signaling system
sistema de señales secundario secondary signaling system
sistema de signos sign system
sistema de signos diacríticos diacritical marking system
sistema de valores value system
sistema de valores sexual sexual value system
sistema del yo self-system
sistema delusorio delusional system
sistema digestivo digestive system
sistema dinámico dynamic system
sistema epicrítico epicritic system
sistema ergotrópico ergotropic system
sistema estesiódico esthesiodic system
sistema extrapiramidal extrapyramidal system
sistema inmune immune system
sistema inmune y estrés immune system and stress
sistema intralaminar intralaminar system
sistema lemniscal lemniscal system
sistema límbico limbic system
sistema lineal linear system
sistema métrico metric system
sistema miniatura miniature system
sistema motor motor system
sistema motor extrapiramidal extrapyramidal motor system
sistema motor piramidal pyramidal motor system
sistema musculoesquelético musculoskeletal system
sistema nervioso nervous system
sistema nervioso autónomo autonomic nervous system
sistema nervioso central central nervous system
sistema nervioso conceptual conceptual nervous system
sistema nervioso parasimpático parasympathetic nervous system
sistema nervioso periférico peripheral nervous system
sistema nervioso simpático sympathetic nervous system
sistema nervioso somático somatic nervous system
sistema nervioso vegetativo vegetative nervous system
sistema nervioso voluntario voluntary nervous system
sistema neural neural system
sistema neuromuscular neuromuscular system
sistema neurovegetativo neurovegetative system
sistema no específico nonspecific system
sistema numérico binario binary number system

sistema olfatorio olfactory system
sistema piramidal pyramidal system
sistema portal hipotalámico-hipofisario
hypothalamic-hypophysial portal system
sistema protopático protopathic system
sistema psicofísico balanceado balanced
psychophysical system
sistema psicosocial psychosocial system
sistema regulador regulatory system
sistema reticular ascendente ascending
reticular system
sistema reticular descendente descending
reticular system
sistema sensorial sensory system
sistema somatosensorial somatosensory
system
sistema somestésico somesthetic system
sistema toracolumbar thoracolumbar system
sistema ventricular ventricular system
sistema vertebrobasilar vertebrobasilar
system
sistema vestibular vestibular system
sistema vestibuloespinal vestibulospinal
system
sistema visual visual system
sistema visual artificial artificial visual
system
sistemas conceptuales conceptual systems
sistemas de control conductual behavioral
control systems
sistemas de creencias belief systems
sistemas educativos alternativos alternative
education systems
sistemático systematic
sistematización systematization
sistémico systemic
sístole systole
sitio de receptor receptor site
sitio de reconocimiento recognition site
sitio de resistencia mínima least-resistance
site
sitofobia sitophobia
situación situation
situación Asch Asch situation
situación de estímulo stimulus situation
situación de estrés stress situation
situación de medios means situation
situación de peligro danger situation
situación de señales abiertas open-cue
situation
situación edípica oedipal situation
situación psicoanalítica psychoanalytic
situation
situación social social situation
situacional situational
situacionalismo situationalism
soborno bribe
sobreactividad overactivity
sobreansioso overanxious
sobreapiñamiento overcrowding
sobreaprendizaje overlearning
sobrecalentamiento overheating
sobrecarga overload
sobrecarga de atención attention overload
sobrecarga de estímulo stimulus overload

sobrecarga de hierro iron overloading
sobrecarga de información information
overload
sobrecompensación overcompensation
sobrecontrolado overcontrolled
sobrecorrección overcorrection
sobredependiente overdependent
sobredeterminación overdetermination
sobredosis overdose
sobredosis de heroína heroin overdose
sobreestimulación overstimulation
sobreexclusión overexclusion
sobreextensión overextension
sobregeneralización overgeneralization
sobreinclusión overinclusion
sobremovilización overmobilization
sobrenatural supernatural
sobrepeso overweight
sobreposición overlay
sobreposición emocional emotional overlay
sobreproducción overproduction
sobreprotección overprotection
sobrerreacción overreaction
sobrerrendimiento overachievement
sobrerrespuesta overresponse
sobresalto startle
sobreventilación overbreathing
sociabilidad sociability
sociable sociable
social social
socialización socialization
socialización de individuos socialization of
individuals
socialización de infantes infant socialization
socializado socialized
socializar socialize
socialmente socially
sociedad society
sociedad de insectos insect society
sociedad intrapsíquica intrapsychic society
sociedad no agresiva nonaggressive society
societal societal
sociobiología sociobiology
sociobiología animal animal sociobiology
sociocéntrico sociocentric
sociocentrismo sociocentrism
sociocentro sociocenter
sociocognitivo sociocognitive
sociocosmo sociocosm
sociocultural sociocultural
sociocusis sociocusis
sociodrama sociodrama
socioeconómico socioeconomic
socioempatía socioempathy
sociogénesis sociogenesis
sociogenética sociogenetics
sociogénico sociogenic
sociograma sociogram
sociograma de observador observer
sociogram
sociograma intuitivo intuitive sociogram
sociograma objetivo objective sociogram
sociograma perceptivo perceptual sociogram
sociolingüística sociolinguistics
sociología sociology

sociología clínica clinical sociology
sociológico sociological
sociomédico sociomedical
sociometría sociometry
sociométrica sociometrics
sociométrico sociometric
socionomía socionomics
sociópata sociopath
sociópata neurótico neurotic sociopath
sociópata primario primary sociopath
sociopatía sociopathy
sociopático sociopathic
sociopatología sociopathology
sociosexual sociosexual
sociotaxis sociotaxis
sociotécnico sociotechnical
socioterapia sociotherapy
sodio sérico serum sodium
sodomía sodomy
sodomista sodomist
sodomita sodomite
sofisma sophism
sofistería sophistry
sofisticación de prueba test sophistication
sofomanía sophomania
solapo recíproco reciprocal overlap
soledad solitude
solidaridad solidarity
solidaridad de grupo group solidarity
sólido de color color solid
solipsismo solipsism
solitario solitary
solución solution
solución auxiliar auxiliary solution
solución comprensiva comprehensive solution
solución mayor major solution
solución neurótica neurotic solution
solución oblicua oblique solution
solución ortogonal orthogonal solution
soluciones del fondo hacia arriba bottom-up
    solutions
soma soma
somatagnosia somatagnosia
somatalgia somatalgia
somatestesia somatesthesia
somatestético somatesthetic
somático somatic
somatista somatist
somatización somatization
somatobiología somatobiology
somatoforme somatoform
somatofrenia somatophrenia
somatogénesis somatogenesis
somatogénico somatogenic
somatognosia somatognosia
somatometría somatometry
somatopático somatopathic
somatoplasma somatoplasm
somatopsicología somatopsychology
somatopsicosis somatopsychosis
somatopsíquico somatopsychic
somatosensorial somatosensory
somatosentido somatosense
somatosexual somatosexual
somatosexualidad somatosexuality

somatostatina somatostatin
somatoterapia somatotherapy
somatotipo somatotype
somatotipología somatotypology
somatotonía somatotonia
somatotónico somatotonic
somatotopagnosia somatotopagnosia
somatotopagnosis somatotopagnosis
somatotopia somatotopy
somatotópico somatotopic
somatotrófico somatotrophic
somatotropina somatotropin
sombra de sonido sound shadow
somestesia somesthesia
somestésico somesthetic
somestesis somesthesis
somita somite
somnial somnial
somnifaciente somnifacient
somnífero somniferous
somnífico somnific
somnífugo somnifugous
somnilocuencia somniloquence
somniloquia somniloquy
somniloquismo somniloquism
somniloquista sleeptalker
somnípata somnipathist
somnipatía somnipathy
somniquista somniloquist
somnocinematografía somnocinematography
somnocinematógrafo somnocinematograph
somnolencia somnolence
somnolencia diurna excesiva excessive
    daytime sleepiness
somnolencia excesiva excessive somnolence
somnolencia patológica pathological
    sleepiness
somnolescente somnolescent
somnoliento somnolent
somnolismo somnolism
sonambulancia somnambulance
sonambulismo somnambulism
sonambulístico somnambulistic
sonámbulo somnambulist
sonante sonant
sonda probe
sonido sound
sonido de coco coconut sound
sonido de voz voice sound
sonido persistente aftersound
sonio sone
sonoencefalograma sonoencephalogram
sonografía sonography
sonograma sonogram
sonómetro sonometer
sonomotor sonomotor
sonoridad loudness
sonoridad más cómoda most comfortable
    loudness
sonrisa endógena endogenous smile
sonrisa exógena exogenous smile
soñar global global dreaming
sopor sopor
soporífero soporiferous
soporífico soporific

soporoso soporous
sordera deafness
sordera adventicia adventitious deafness
sordera central central deafness
sordera ceruminosa ceruminous deafness
sordera congénita congenital deafness
sordera cortical cortical deafness
sordera de conducción conduction deafness
sordera de frecuencias altas high-frequency deafness
sordera de palabras word deafness
sordera de percepción perception deafness
sordera de tono tone deafness
sordera funcional functional deafness
sordera histérica hysterical deafness
sordera mesencefálica midbrain deafness
sordera mixta mixed deafness
sordera nerviosa nerve deafness
sordera neural neural deafness
sordera por exposición exposure deafness
sordera psicogénica psychogenic deafness
sordera retrococlear retrocochlear deafness
sordera sensorineural sensorineural deafness
sordo deaf
sordo-ciego deaf-blind
sordo-mudo deaf-mute
sordomudez surdimutism
sororato sororate
sospecha suspicion
sospechoso suspicious
sotalol sotalol
spasmus spasmus
spasmus agitans spasmus agitans
spasmus caninus spasmus caninus
spasmus coordinatus spasmus coordinatus
spasmus nictitans spasmus nictitans
spasmus nutans spasmus nutans
stafiloplejía staphyloplegia
suavidad softness
subafectivo subaffective
subagudo subacute
subaracnoideo subarachnoid
subcalloso subcallosal
subcepción subception
subclavio subclavian
subclínico subclinical
subcoma subcoma
subsconsciencia subconsciousness
subconsciente subconscious
subcontrolado undercontrolled
subcortical subcortical
subcultura subculture
subcutáneo subcutaneous
subchoque subshock
subdelirante subdelirious
subdelirio subdelirium
subdespertamiento underarousal
subdeterminado underdetermined
subdural subdural
subependimoma subependymoma
subestimulación understimulation
subfalcial subfalcial
subfecundidad subfecundity
subfin subgoal
subgaleal subgaleal

subgeneralización undergeneralization
subgrundación subgrundation
súbito sudden
subjetividad subjectivity
subjetivismo subjectivism
subjetivo subjective
sublimación sublimation
sublimar sublimate
subliminal subliminal
subluxación de cadera congénita congenital hip subluxation
submanía submania
subnormal subnormal
subnormal educativamente educationally subnormal
suboccipital suboccipital
subordinación subordination
subprueba subtest
subpsiquis subpsyche
subrendimiento underachievement
subrendimiento académico academic underachievement
subsocializado undersocialized
subsultus subsultus
subsultus clonus subsultus clonus
subsultus tendinum subsultus tendinum
subtalámico subthalamic
subtálamo subthalamus
subtemporal subtemporal
subtetánico subtetanic
subtipo de alcoholismo masculino male alcoholism subtype
subumbral subthreshold
subvocal subvocal
subvocalización subvocalization
succinilcolina succinylcholine
sucesivo successive
súcubo succubus
sudorífero sudoriferous
sueño sleep, dream
sueño activado activated sleep
sueño activo active sleep
sueño alfa alpha sleep
sueño ansioso anxiety dream
sueño artificial artificial dream
sueño con emisión wet dream
sueño contra deseo counter-wish dream
sueño crepuscular twilight sleep
sueño D D sleep
sueño de castigo punishment dream
sueño de consolación consolation dream
sueño de examinación examination dream
sueño de movimientos oculares no rápidos non-rapid eye movement sleep
sueño de movimientos oculares rápidos rapid eye movement sleep
sueño de movimientos oculares rápidos en infantes rapid eye movement sleep in infants
sueño de movimientos oculares rápidos en recién nacidos rapid eye movement sleep in newborns
sueño de ondas delta delta-wave sleep
sueño de ondas lentas slow-wave sleep
sueño de terror terror dream

sueño de vergüenza embarrassment dream
sueño delta delta sleep
sueño dentro de un sueño dream within a
  dream
sueño desincronizado desynchronized sleep
sueño eléctrico electrical sleep
sueño electroterapéutico electrotherapeutic
  sleep
sueño en crescendo crescendo sleep
sueño hipnótico hypnotic sleep
sueño interrumpido interrupted dream
sueño liviano light sleep
sueño lúcido lucid dream
sueño ortodoxo orthodox sleep
sueño paradójico paradoxical sleep
sueño paralelo parallel dream
sueño paroxístico paroxysmal sleep
sueño perenne perennial dream
sueño pontino pontine sleep
sueño prodrómico prodromic dream
sueño profético prophetic dream
sueño profundo deep sleep
sueño recurrente recurrent dream
sueño rombencefálico rhombencephalic sleep
sueño sincronizado synchronized sleep
sueño telencefálico telencephalic sleep
sueño telepático telepathic dream
sueños a colores color dreams
sueños comparados con cuentos de hadas
  dreams compared to fairy tales
sueños de conveniencia convenience dreams
sueños de homosexualidad dreams of
  homosexuality
sueños de los ciegos dreams of the blind
sueños de los incapacitados físicamente
  dreams of the physically disabled
sueños de los sordos dreams of the deaf
sueños de muerte dreams of death
sueños de niños dreams of children
sueños y hora de la noche dreams and time
  of night
suero serum
suero de la verdad truth serum
sufrimiento suffering
sufrimiento del ego ego suffering
sufrir suffer
sugestibilidad suggestibility
sugestión suggestion
sugestión afectiva affective suggestion
sugestión contingente contingent suggestion
sugestión de prestigio prestige suggestion
sugestión de sueño dream suggestion
sugestión directa direct suggestion
sugestión negativa negative suggestion
sugestión poshipnótica posthypnotic
  suggestion
sugestionable suggestible
sugestivo suggestive
sui generis sui generis
suicida suicidal
suicidio suicide
suicidio adolescente adolescent suicide
suicidio altruista altruistic suicide
suicidio anómico anomic suicide
suicidio copión copycat suicide

suicidio egoísta egoistic suicide
suicidio egotista egotistic suicide
suicidio en adolescencia suicide in
  adolescence
suicidio focal focal suicide
suicidio psicosomático psychosomatic suicide
suicidio psíquico psychic suicide
suicidios en grupo cluster suicides
suicidogénico suicidogenic
suicidología suicidology
suigenerismo suigenderism
sujeción subjection
sujeto subject
sujeto del ego ego subject
sujetos ingenuos naive subjects
sulfatidosis sulfatidosis
sulfato sulfate
sulpirida sulpiride
suma de cuadrados sum of squares
sumación summation
sumación binocular binocular summation
sumación espacial spatial summation
sumación temporal temporal summation
sumidero conductual behavioral sink
suminstros emocionales emotional supplies
sumisión submission
sumisión autoritaria authoritarian submission
superación overcoming
superación del temor overcoming of fear
superar overcome
superego superego
superego de grupo group superego
superego doble double superego
superego heterónomo heteronomous superego
superego parasítico parasitic superego
superego primitivo primitive superego
superexcitación superexcitation
superfecundación superfecundation
superfetación superfetation
superficial superficial
superficialidad de afecto shallowness of
  affect
superficie de color color surface
superficie escondida hidden surface
supergen supergene
superior superior
supermovilidad supermotility
supernormal supernormal
superpoblación overpopulation
supersónico supersonic
superstición superstition
supersticioso superstitious
supervisión supervision
supervivencia del más apto survival of the
  fittest
supinación supination
suposición supposition
supraclinoideo supraclinoid
supraliminal supraliminal
supranuclear supranuclear
supraorbitario supraorbital
suprarrenal suprarenal
suprarrenalectomía suprarenalectomy
suprarrotuliano suprapatellar
suprasegmentario suprasegmental

supraselar suprasellar
supratentorial supratentorial
supraumbilical supraumbilical
supresión suppression
supresión binocular binocular suppression
supresión condicionada conditioned
　suppression
supresión monocular monocular suppression
supresor suppressor
supresor de apetito appetite suppressant
supurativo suppurative
surco sulcus
surco calloso callosal sulcus
surco central central sulcus
surco cingulado cingulate sulcus
surco hipotalámico hypothalamic sulcus
surco lateral lateral sulcus
surco longitudinal longitudinal sulcus
surco marginal marginal sulcus
surco neural neural groove
surco olfatorio olfactory sulcus
surco paracentral paracentral sulcus
surco parietooccipital parietooccipital sulcus
surgencia surgency
sursunversión sursumversion
susceptibilidad hipnótica hypnotic
　susceptibility
susceptibilidad teratogénica conductual
　behavioral teratogenic susceptibility
suspiro sigh
sustancia substance
sustancia controlada controlled substance
sustancia cromófila chromophil substance
sustancia gelatinosa substantia gelatinosa
sustancia gris gray matter
sustancia K substance K
sustancia negra substantia nigra
sustancia neurotóxica neurotoxic substance
sustancia P substance P
sustancia pineal pineal substance
sustancia psicoactiva psychoactive substance
sustancia transmisora transmitter substance
sustitución substitution
sustitución de estímulo stimulus substitution
sustitución de síntoma symptom substitution
sustituta de madre mother substitute
sustituto substitute, surrogate
sustituto de humano human surrogate
sustituto del padre father substitute
sustituto sexual sexual surrogate
sustrato substrate
sutura suture
sutura de nervio nerve suture
suturectomía suturectomy

T

tabaco tobacco
tabes tabes
tabes diabética tabes diabetica
tabes dorsal tabes dorsalis
tabes ergótica tabes ergotica
tabes espasmódica tabes spasmodica
tabes espinal tabes spinalis
tabes juvenil juvenile tabes
tabes periférica peripheral tabes
tabético tabetic
tabetiforme tabetiform
tábico tabic
tábido tabid
tabla de contingencias contingency table
tabla de correlación correlation table
tabla de doble entrada double-entry table
tabla de formas formboard
tabla de números aleatorios random-number
　table
tabla de probabilidades probability table
tabla de vida life table
tabla rasa tabula rasa
tablero de clavijas pegboard
taboparesia taboparesis
tabú taboo
tabú de incesto incest taboo
tabulaciones cruzadas cross-tabulations
tacañería stinginess
tacción taction
tácito tacit
táctico tactic
táctil tactile
tacto persistente aftertouch
tactoagnosia tactoagnosia
tactómetro tactometer
tafefobia taphephobia
tafofilia taphophilia
tafofobia taphophobia
talamectomía thalamectomy
talámico thalamic
tálamo thalamus
tálamo extrínseco extrinsic thalamus
tálamo posterior posterior thalamus
talamotomía thalamotomy
talasofobia thalassophobia
talbutal talbutal
talectomía thalectomy
talento talent
talidomida thalidomide
talión talion
talipes talipes
talipes espasmódico talipes spasmodicus
talón heel
taller de carrera career workshop

taller de empleo employment workshop
taller refugiado sheltered workshop
tallo cerebral brain stem
tamaño aparente apparent size
tamaño cerebral brain size
tamaño de clase class size
tamaño de grupo óptimo optimal group size
tamaño de objeto object size
tamaño relativo relative size
tamaño retinal retinal size
tambalear stagger
tambor tambour
tambor del oído ear drum
tanatofobia thanatophobia
tanatografía thanatography
tanatología thanatology
tanatomanía thanatomania
tanatopsia thanatopsy
tanatos thanatos
tanatótico thanatotic
tándem tandem
tangencial tangential
tangencialidad tangentiality
tanifonía tanyphonia
tanteo scoring
tanteo diferencial differential scoring
tanteo objetivo objective scoring
tanteo subjetivo subjective scoring
tanteo vicario vicarious trial and error
tapetum tapetum
taquiatetosis tachyathetosis
taquicardia tachycardia
taquifagia tachyphagia
taquifasia tachyphasia
taquifemia tachyphemia
taquifilaxis tachyphylaxis
taquifrasia tachyphrasia
taquifrenia tachyphrenia
taquilalia tachylalia
taquilogia tachylogia
taquipnea tachypnea
taquipragia tachypragia
taquistoscopio tachistoscope
taquitrofismo tachytrophism
tarantismo tarantism
taraxeína taraxein
tarea task
tarea adaptiva modal modal adaptive task
tarea cognitiva cognitive task
tarea compuesta compound task
tarea de clasificar cartas card-sorting task
tarea de decisión léxica lexical-decision task
tarea de detección detection task
tarea de detección de señales signal-detection task
tarea de discriminación discrimination task
tarea de motivos mixtos mixed-motive task
tarea de recordación libre free-recall task
tarea de Sternberg Sternberg task
tarea del desarrollo developmental task
tarea funcional functional task
tarea perceptiva perceptual task
tarea primaria primary task
tarea propedéutica propaedeutic task
tareas concurrentes concurrent tasks

tareas continuas continuous tasks
tarsofalángico tarsophalangeal
tartamudear stutter, stammer
tartamudeo stutter, stammer, stammering, stuttering
tartamudez stuttering, stammering
tartamudez primaria primary stuttering
tartamudez secundaria secondary stuttering
tartamudez urinaria urinary stuttering
tartrato tartrate
tasa rate
tasa base base rate
tasa de cambio rate of change
tasa de concordancia concordance rate
tasa de fertilidad fertility rate
tasa de incidencia incidence rate
tasa de mejora improvement rate
tasa de morbilidad morbidity rate
tasa de mortalidad mortality rate
tasa de mutación mutation rate
tasa de natalidad birth rate
tasa de ocurrencia rate of occurrence
tasa de primeras admisiones rate of first admission
tasa de recaídas relapse rate
tasa de recidivismo recidivism rate
tasa de residencia residence rate
tasa de respuestas response rate
tasa de sedimentación de eritrocitos erythrocyte sedimentation rate
tasa de vibraciones vibration rate
taurina taurine
tautófono tautophone
tautología tautology
taxis taxis
taxonomía taxonomy
taxonomía biológica biological taxonomy
taxonómico taxonomic
tebaína thebaine
técnica technique
técnica activa active technique
técnica adaptiva adaptive technique
técnica antiexpectación antiexpectation technique
técnica clásica classical technique
técnica conductual behavioral technique
técnica de adhesión bandwagon technique
técnica de alimentación feeding technique
técnica de asociación de palabras word-association technique
técnica de azotar al caballo muerto flogging the dead horse technique
técnica de ballet ballet technique
técnica de cartas perdidas lost-letter technique
técnica de cerebro dividido split-brain technique
técnica de Cornell Cornell technique
técnica de Delfos Delphi technique
técnica de distractor distractor technique
técnica de embudo funnel technique
técnica de encuesta de ventas sales-survey technique
técnica de enmascaramiento hacia atrás backward masking technique

técnica de ensueño activo active daydream technique
técnica de espejo mirror technique
técnica de estimación de parámetros parameter-estimation technique
técnica de estímulos breves brief-stimuli technique
técnica de exposición controlada controlled-exposure technique
técnica de Hartel Hartel technique
técnica de incidentes críticos critical incident technique
técnica de intervención intervention technique
técnica de la puerta en la cara door-in-the-face technique
técnica de Leboyer Leboyer technique
técnica de Luria Luria technique
técnica de microelectrodo microelectrode technique
técnica de nominación nominating technique
técnica de observación observation technique
técnica de pares-nones odd-even technique
técnica de presión squeeze technique
técnica de psicoterapia psychotherapy technique
técnica de reatribución reattribution technique
técnica de reconocimiento recognition technique
técnica de reflexión corneal corneal reflection technique
técnica de selecciones forzadas forced-choice technique
técnica de silla vacía empty-chair technique
técnica de tiempo fuera time-out technique
técnica de variable única single-variable technique
técnica de ventajas-desventajas assets-liabilities technique
técnica de visualización visualization technique
técnica del jurado de consumidores consumer-jury technique
técnica del pie en la puerta foot-in-the-door technique
técnica esfuerzo-forma effort-shape technique
técnica estereotáxica stereotaxic technique
técnica exosomática exosomatic technique
técnica grafomotora graphomotor technique
técnica O O technique
técnica P P technique
técnica paradójica paradoxical technique
técnica proyectiva projective technique
técnica Q Q technique
técnicas de amortiguamiento capping techniques
técnicas de autodominio self-control techniques
técnicas de deceleración deceleration techniques
técnicas de evaluación assessment techniques
técnicas de extinción extinction techniques
técnicas de individuación individuation techniques
técnicas de medición measurement techniques

técnicas de refuerzo diferencial differential reinforcement techniques
técnicas de video video techniques
técnicas manipulativas manipulative techniques
técnicas para fortalecimiento del ego ego strengthening techniques
técnico de laboratorio médico medical laboratory technician
técnico histológico histologic technician
tecnología genética genetic technology
tecnología social social technology
tecnólogo nuclear-médico nuclear-medical technologist
tecnólogo radiológico radiologic technologist
tecnonimia teknonymy
tecnopsicología technopsychology
tectal tectal
tectorial tectorial
tectum tectum
tefrilómetro tephrylometer
tefromalacia tephromalacia
tegmental tegmental
tegmento mesencefálico mesencephalic tegmentum
tegmentotomía tegmentotomy
tegmentum tegmentum
teicopsia teichopsia
tejido tissue
tejido nervioso nerve tissue
telalgia telalgia
telangiectasia telangiectasia
telangiectasia cefalooculocutánea cephalooculocutaneous telangiectasia
telangiectásico telangiectatic
telangiectasis telangiectasis
telarca thelarche
telebinocular telebinocular
teleceptor teleceptor
telecinesia telekinesis
telegnosis telegnosis
telencefálico telencephalic
telencefalización telencephalization
telencéfalo telencephalon
teleología teleology
teleológico teleologic
teleonomía teleonomy
teleonómico teleonomic
teleopsia teleopsia
teleorreceptor teleoreceptor
teleoterapéutica teleotherapeutics
telepatía telepathy
telepatía mental mental telepathy
telepático telepathic
telergía telergy
telerreceptor telereceptor
telesis telesis
telestereoscopio telestereoscope
telestesia telesthesia
teletactor teletactor
teletractor teletractor
televisión y agresión television and aggression
télico telic
telodendria telodendria
telodendrón telodendron

telofase telophase
temático thematic
temazepam temazepam
temblor tremor
temblor alternante alternating tremor
temblor arsenical arsenical tremor
temblor cerebeloso agudo acute cerebellar tremor
temblor cerebral progresivo progressive cerebral tremor
temblor cinético kinetic tremor
temblor continuo continuous tremor
temblor de acción action tremor
temblor de aleteo flapping tremor
temblor de Chvostek Chvostek's tremor
temblor de Hunt Hunt's tremor
temblor de intención intention tremor
temblor esencial essential tremor
temblor esencial benigno benign essential tremor
temblor estático static tremor
temblor fibrilar fibrillary tremor
temblor fino fine tremor
temblor grueso coarse tremor
temblor hereditario benigno benign hereditary tremor
temblor heredofamiliar heredofamilial tremor
temblor mercurial mercurial tremor
temblor metálico metallic tremor
temblor pasivo passive tremor
temblor persistente persistent tremor
temblor postural postural tremor
temblor postural inducido por medicación medication-induced postural tremor
temblor psicológico psychological tremor
temblor saturnino saturnine tremor
temblor senil senile tremor
temblor transitorio transient tremor
temblor volitivo volitional tremor
tembloroso trembling
temor fear
temor a alturas fear of heights
temor a animales fear of animals
temor a cadáveres fear of corpses
temor a comer fear of eating
temor a comida fear of food
temor a confinamiento fear of confinement
temor a contaminación fear of contamination
temor a cuerpos desnudos fear of naked bodies
temor a deformidad fear of deformity
temor a demonios fear of demons
temor a enfermedad fear of disease
temor a enfermedad mental fear of brain disease
temor a enfermedad venérea fear of venereal disease
temor a estar solo fear of being alone
temor a extraños fear of strangers
temor a fantasmas fear of ghosts
temor a gatos fear of cats
temor a genitales femeninos fear of female genitals
temor a genitales masculinos fear of male genitals
temor a gente fear of people
temor a hombres fear of men
temor a innovación fear of innovation
temor a insania fear of insanity
temor a insectos fear of insects
temor a justicia fear of justice
temor a la eternidad fear of eternity
temor a la medicina fear of medicine
temor a la muerte fear of death
temor a la noche fear of night
temor a la obscuridad fear of darkness
temor a la sangre fear of blood
temor a la soledad fear of loneliness
temor a ladrones fear of burglars
temor a lesión fear of injury
temor a los genitales femeninos female-genitals fear
temor a mujeres fear of women
temor a multitudes fear of crowds
temor a olores fear of odors
temor a penes penis fear
temor a perros fear of dogs
temor a ratones fear of mice
temor a relámpagos fear of lightning
temor a ser encerrado fear of being enclosed
temor a ser enterrado vivo fear of being buried alive
temor a ser tocado fear of being touched
temor a todo fear of everything
temor a volar fear of flying
temor adquirido acquired fear
temor al cambio fear of change
temor al castigo fear of punishment
temor al coito coitus fear
temor al confinamiento confinement fear
temor al dolor fear of pain
temor al éxito fear of success
temor al fracaso fear of failure
temor al fuego fear of fire
temor al matrimonio fear of marriage
temor al parto fear of childbirth
temor al placer fear of pleasure
temor al rechazo fear of rejection
temor al sexo fear of sex
temor al sueño fear of sleep
temor al veneno fear of poison
temor condicionado conditioned fear
temor contra ansiedad fear versus anxiety
temor de castración castration fear
temor de desmembración fear of dismemberment
temor de vida life fear
temor flotante free-floating fear
temor obsesivo obsessive fear
temores de niñez childhood fears
temores de niños children's fears
temores normales de infantes normal fears of infants
temperado temperate
temperamento temperament
temperamento flemático phlegmatic temperament
temperamento hipogenital hypogenital temperament

temperamento somatotónico somatotonic temperament

temperamento viscerotónico viscerotonic temperament

temperamento y conducta suicida temperament and suicidal behavior

temperancia temperance

temperatura temperature

temperatura corporal body temperature

temperatura corporal basal basal body temperature

temperatura efectiva effective temperature

tempo conceptual conceptual tempo

tempo impulsivo impulsive tempo

temporal temporal

temprano early

tendencia tendency

tendencia anagógica anagogic tendency

tendencia central central tendency

tendencia configuracional configurational tendency

tendencia de acción tendency of action

tendencia de observadores observer drift

tendencia del pensamiento trend of thought

tendencia determinante determining tendency

tendencia estadística statistical trend

tendencia final final tendency

tendencia neurótica neurotic trend

tendencia paranoide paranoid trend

tendencia parietal parietal drift

tendencia perniciosa pernicious trend

tendencia psiquiátrica psychiatric trend

tendencia suicida suicide tendency

tenesmo tenesmus

teniofobia taeniophobia

tenofobia taenophobia

tensión tension

tensión de estímulo stimulus tension

tensión de grupo group tension

tensión de necesidad need tension

tensión emocional emotional tension

tensión mental mental tension

tensión motora motor tension

tensión premenstrual premenstrual tension

tensión psíquica psychic tension

tensión sexual sexual tension

tensión social social tension

tenso tense

tensor timpánico tensor tympani

tentación temptation

tentaciones horrendas horrific temptations

tentorium tentorium

tentorium cerebelli tentorium cerebelli

teofobia theophobia

teomanía theomania

teorema theorem

teorema de Bayes Bayes' theorem

teorema del límite central central limit theorem

teorético theoretical

teoría theory

teoría algorítmica-heurística algorithmic-heuristic theory

teoría bifactorial de condicionamiento bifactorial theory of conditioning

teoría biológica biological theory

teoría biosocial biosocial theory

teoría cadena-asociativa associative-chain theory

teoría centrada en la persona person-centered theory

teoría cibernética del envejecimiento cybernetic theory of aging

teoría clásica classical theory

teoría cloacal cloacal theory

teoría cognitiva cognitive theory

teoría cognitiva-fisiológica cognitive-physiological theory

teoría conductual de depresión behavioral theory of depression

teoría conductual de rumiación behavioral theory of rumination

teoría constitucional constitutional theory

teoría constitucional de Sheldon Sheldon's constitutional theory

teoría constitucional de Sheldon de personalidad Sheldon's constitutional theory of personality

teoría control control theory

teoría cuántica quantum theory

teoría de accesibilidad accessibility theory

teoría de acción en masa mass action theory

teoría de actitud específica specific attitude theory

teoría de actitudes attitude theory

teoría de activación de emoción activation theory of emotion

teoría de agresión theory of aggression

teoría de ajuste social social-adjustment theory

teoría de alternación de respuesta alternation of response theory

teoría de ansiedad theory of anxiety

teoría de apego attachment theory

teoría de aprendizaje learning theory

teoría de aprendizaje ambiental environmental-learning theory

teoría de aprendizaje cognitiva cognitive theory of learning

teoría de aprendizaje de irradiación irradiation theory of learning

teoría de aprendizaje estadística statistical-learning theory

teoría de aprendizaje matemática mathematical learning theory

teoría de aprendizaje observacional observational learning theory

teoría de aprendizaje social social learning theory

teoría de apuro doble de esquizofrenia double bind theory of schizophrenia

teoría de arpa harp theory

teoría de asimilación-contraste assimilation-contrast theory

teoría de asociación association theory

teoría de atención attention theory

teoría de atracción de ganancia-pérdida gain-loss theory of attraction

teoría de atribución attribution theory

teoría de audición de patrón de sonido

    sound-pattern theory of hearing

teoría de audición de teléfono telephone
    theory of hearing

teoría de autismo theory of autism

teoría de autopercepción self-perception
    theory

teoría de balance balance theory

teoría de bloque de hielo iceblock theory

teoría de Burn y Rand Burn and Rand theory

teoría de cambios rápidos rapid-change
    theory

teoría de campo field theory

teoría de cancelación cancellation theory

teoría de Cannon Cannon's theory

teoría de Cannon-Bard Cannon-Bard theory

teoría de Cannon talámica thalamic theory of
    Cannon

teoría de carga ambiental environmental-load
    theory

teoría de catástrofe catastrophe theory

teoría de ciclos de vida life cycle theory

teoría de codificaciones coding theory

teoría de cognición theory of cognition

teoría de comparación social
    social-comparison theory

teoría de competencia conductual behavioral
    competition theory

teoría de conducta behavior theory

teoría de conflictos focales focal-conflict
    theory

teoría de congruencia congruity theory

teoría de constreñimiento de conducta
    behavior constraint theory

teoría de constructo personal personal
    construct theory

teoría de contingencias contingency theory

teoría de continuidad continuity theory

teoría de continuidad del aprendizaje
    continuity theory of learning

teoría de continuidad del envejecimiento
    continuity theory of aging

teoría de control de puerta gate-control
    theory

teoría de control de puerta del dolor
    gate-control theory of pain

teoría de crisis crisis theory

teoría de decisiones decision theory

teoría de delincuencia theory of delinquency

teoría de depresión cognitiva cognitive
    theory of depression

teoría de depresión de impotencia aprendida
    learned helplessness theory of depression

teoría de despertamiento arousal theory

teoría de despertamiento doble dual-arousal
    theory

teoría de detección detection theory

teoría de detección de señales
    signal-detection theory

teoría de diferenciación differentiation theory

teoría de diseño de dos factores two-factor
    design theory

teoría de doble aspecto double aspect theory

teoría de elementos idénticos identical
    elements theory

teoría de emergencia emergency theory

teoría de emergencia de emociones
    emergency theory of emotions

teoría de emoción cognitiva cognitive theory
    of emotion

teoría de emoción de Cannon-Bard
    Cannon-Bard theory of emotion

teoría de emoción de James-Lange
    James-Lange theory of emotion

teoría de emoción de MacLean MacLean's
    theory of emotion

teoría de emoción de Papez Papez theory of
    emotion

teoría de emoción talámica thalamic theory
    of emotion

teoría de emociones theory of emotion

teoría de emociones diferencial differential
    emotions theory

teoría de enlaces cruzados cross-linkage
    theory

teoría de envejecimiento aging theory

teoría de envejecimiento de actividad
    activity theory of aging

teoría de épocas culturales culture-epoch
    theory

teoría de equidad equity theory

teoría de equidad de atracción equity theory
    of attraction

teoría de estímulo-respuesta
    stimulus-response theory

teoría de estrés stress theory

teoría de estrés adaptada adapted stress
    theory

teoría de estrés ambiental
    environmental-stress theory

teoría de estrés de eventos de la vida
    life-event stress theory

teoría de etapas stage theory

teoría de etapas múltiples multistage theory

teoría de etiquetaje labeling theory

teoría de evaluación cognitiva
    cognitive-appraisal theory

teoría de eversión eversion theory

teoría de eversión de envejecimiento
    eversion theory of aging

teoría de evolución evolution theory

teoría de exclamación exclamation theory

teoría de expectación expectancy theory

teoría de expectaciones-valores
    expectancy-value theory

teoría de filtro filter theory

teoría de Flourens Flourens' theory

teoría de frecuencias frequency theory

teoría de frecuencias de audición frequency
    theory of hearing

teoría de Freud Freud's theory

teoría de Fromm Fromm's theory

teoría de género gender theory

teoría de grupo de referencia
    reference-group theory

teoría de guauguau bow-wow theory

teoría de Hebb Hebb's theory

teoría de Hebb de aprendizaje perceptivo
    Hebb's theory of perceptual learning

teoría de Hering Hering theory

teoría de Hering de visión de colores Hering

theory of color vision
teoría de hipersensibilidad hypersensitivity theory
teoría de identidad identity theory
teoría de identidad de tipo type-identity theory
teoría de impulso secundario secondary-drive theory
teoría de impulsos drive theory
teoría de incentivos incentive theory
teoría de individualidad individuality theory
teoría de infección infection theory
teoría de información information theory
teoría de instinto doble dual-instinct theory
teoría de intercambio exchange theory
teoría de intercambio social social exchange theory
teoría de interferencia interference theory
teoría de interferencia de olvidar interference theory of forgetting
teoría de interjección interjection theory
teoría de irradiación irradiation theory
teoría de James-Lange James-Lange theory
teoría de jerarquía de necesidades need-hierarchy theory
teoría de la cloaca cloaca theory
teoría de la comunicación communication theory
teoría de la consistencia consistency theory
teoría de la contigüidad contiguity theory
teoría de la degeneración degeneracy theory
teoría de la discontinuidad discontinuity theory
teoría de la discontinuidad de aprendizaje discontinuity theory of learning
teoría de la disonancia cognitiva cognitive dissonance theory
teoría de la duplicidad duplicity theory
teoría de la emoción hipotalámica de Cannon Cannon hypothalamic theory of emotion
teoría de Ladd-Franklin Ladd-Franklin theory
teoría de Land de visión de color Land theory of color vision
teoría de libido libido theory
teoría de liderazgo leadership theory
teoría de liderazgo de contingencias contingency theory of leadership
teoría de lugar place theory
teoría de lugar de audición place theory of hearing
teoría de Malthus Malthusian theory
teoría de mapa cognitivo cognitive map theory
teoría de Maslow de motivación humana Maslow's theory of human motivation
teoría de mediación mediation theory
teoría de memoria doble dual-memory theory
teoría de mosaico de percepción mosaic theory of perception
teoría de motivación humana human-motivation theory
teoría de muestras pequeñas small-sample theory
teoría de muestreo sampling theory

teoría de muestreo de estímulos stimulus-sampling theory
teoría de necesidades y factores ambientales apremiantes need-press theory
teoría de origen del lenguaje origin-of-language theory
teoría de papeles de personalidad role theory of personality
teoría de patrón de sonido sound-pattern theory
teoría de percepción clásica classical perception theory
teoría de percepción indirecta indirect theory of perception
teoría de percepción transaccional transactional theory of perception
teoría de periodicidad periodicity theory
teoría de personalidad personality theory
teoría de personalidad de interacción interaction theory of personality
teoría de personalidad implícita implicit personality theory
teoría de piano piano theory
teoría de piano de audición piano theory of hearing
teoría de práctica del juego practice theory of play
teoría de probabilidades probability theory
teoría de procesamiento de información information-processing theory
teoría de proceso doble dual-process theory
teoría de procesos de oponentes de motivación opponent-process theory of motivation
teoría de procesos de oponentes de motivación adquirida opponent-process theory of acquired motivation
teoría de procesos de oponentes de visión de color opponent-process theory of color vision
teoría de rasgo trait theory
teoría de rasgo de personalidad personality-trait theory
teoría de rasgo latente latent trait theory
teoría de ratificación ratification theory
teoría de reacción específica specific-reaction theory
teoría de reacción societal societal-reaction theory
teoría de reactancia reactance theory
teoría de recapitulación recapitulation theory
teoría de reducción de impulso drive-reduction theory
teoría de reducción de tensión tension-reduction theory
teoría de reflejos clásico classical reflex theory
teoría de refuerzo reinforcement theory
teoría de relaciones de grupo group-relations theory
teoría de relaciones de grupo de Allport Allport's group relations theory
teoría de relaciones de objetos object relations theory
teoría de reorganización reorganization

theory
teoría de reproducción reproduction theory
teoría de resonancia resonance theory
teoría de resonancia de audición resonance
   theory of hearing
teoría de saciedad de comida food-satiation
   theory
teoría de Semon-Hering Semon-Hering
   theory
teoría de sensibilización refleja reflex
   sensitization theory
teoría de sentimientos de tres dimensiones
   feeling theory of three dimensions
teoría de sistema dinámico dynamical system
   theory
teoría de sistemas systems theory
teoría de sistemas de familia family systems
   theory
teoría de sistemas generales general systems
   theory
teoría de sobrecarga overload theory
teoría de subestimulación understimulation
   theory
teoría de transformación de ansiedad
   transformation theory of anxiety
teoría de tres colores three-color theory
teoría de tres componentes three-component
   theory
teoría de visión de color de Granit Granit
   theory of color vision
teoría de visión de colores theory of color
   vision
teoría de vulnerabilidad vulnerability theory
teoría de Wollaston Wollaston's theory
teoría de Young-Helmholtz Young-Helmholtz
   theory
teoría de Young-Helmholtz de visión de color
   Young-Helmholtz theory of color vision
teoría del álter ego ego-alter theory
teoría del aprendizaje clásica classical
   learning theory
teoría del aprendizaje cognitivo cognitive
   learning theory
teoría del contexto context theory
teoría del contexto del significado context
   theory of meaning
teoría del desarrollo theory of development
teoría del desarrollo emocional cognitiva
   cognitive theory of emotional development
teoría del deterioro decay theory
teoría del deterioro de olvidar decay theory
   of forgetting
teoría del estrés prestado borrowed stress
   theory
teoría del estrés social social-stress theory
teoría del habla speech theory
teoría del juego game theory
teoría del medio instrumentality theory
teoría del nivel de adaptación adaptation
   level theory
teoría del rompimiento disengagement theory
teoría del rompimiento de envejecimiento
   disengagement theory of aging
teoría diátesis-estrés de la esquizofrenia
   diathesis-stress theory of schizophrenia

teoría dinámica dynamic theory
teoría ecológica ecological theory
teoría ecológica de percepción ecological
   theory of perception
teoría epigenética epigenetic theory
teoría estereoquímica stereochemical theory
teoría estereoquímica del olfato
   stereochemical theory of smell
teoría estérica de olores steric theory of odor
teoría evolutiva evolutionary theory
teoría factorial factor theory
teoría factorial de aprendizaje factor theory
   of learning
teoría factorial de personalidad factor theory
   of personality
teoría formativa formative theory
teoría formativa de personalidad formative
   theory of personality
teoría freudiana freudian theory
teoría freudiana de personalidad freudian
   theory of personality
teoría genética genetic theory
teoría germinativa germ theory
teoría gestalt gestalt theory
teoría glucoestática glucostatic theory
teoría hidraulica hydraulic theory
teoría hidraulica de audición hydraulic
   theory of hearing
teoría hipotalámica de Cannon hypothalamic
   theory of Cannon
teoría humanística humanistic theory
teoría humoral humoral theory
teoría infrarroja del olfato infrared theory of
   smell
teoría instruccional instructional theory
teoría interjeccional interjectional theory
teoría interpersonal interpersonal theory
teoría jerárquica hierarchical theory
teoría jerárquica del instinto hierarchical
   theory of instinct
teoría lamarckiana lamarckian theory
teoría local de sed local theory of thirst
teoría mecanística mechanistic theory
teoría mnémica mnemic theory
teoría motora motor theory
teoría motora de conciencia motor theory of
   consciousness
teoría motora de percepción del habla motor
   theory of speech perception
teoría motora del pensamiento motor theory
   of thought
teoría multimodal de inteligencia multimodal
   theory of intelligence
teoría nativista nativistic theory
teoría psicoanalítica psychoanalytic theory
teoría psicoanalítica del apego psychoanalytic
   theory of attachment
teoría psicodinámica psychodynamic theory
teoría psicosocial psychosocial theory
teoría sensorimotora sensorimotor theory
teoría tetracromática tetrachromatic theory
teoría topográfica topographical theory
teoría transaccional transactional theory
teoría tricromática trichromatic theory
teoría visuomotora visuomotor theory

teorías de audición hearing theories
teorías de color color theories
teorías del desarrollo developmental theories
teorías del lenguaje language theories
teorías éticas ethical theories
teorías infantiles de nacimiento
  infantile-birth theories
teorizante del desarrollo developmental
  theorist
teoterapia theotherapy
terapeusis therapeusis
terapeuta therapist
terapeuta activo active therapist
terapeuta adjunto adjunctive therapist
terapeuta auxiliar auxiliary therapist
terapeuta compañero companion-therapist
terapeuta correctivo corrective therapist
terapeuta de artes manuales manual arts
  therapist
terapeuta de voz voice therapist
terapeuta educacional educational therapist
terapeuta físico physical therapist
terapeuta mono monkey therapist
terapeuta ocupacional occupational therapist
terapeuta pasivo passive therapist
terapéutica therapeutics
terapéutica sugestiva suggestive therapeutics
terapéutico therapeutic
terapia therapy
terapia a corto plazo short-term therapy
terapia racional-emotiva rational-emotive
  therapy
terapia activa active therapy
terapia adyuvante adjuvant therapy
terapia ambiental environmental therapy
terapia anaclítica anaclitic therapy
terapia analítica analytic therapy
terapia antiandrógena antiandrogen therapy
terapia apoyadora supportive therapy
terapia artística art therapy
terapia aversiva aversive therapy
terapia biofuncional biofunctional therapy
terapia biológica biological therapy
terapia biomédica biomedical therapy
terapia centrada en el asesor
  counselor-centered therapy
terapia centrada en el cliente client-centered
  therapy
terapia centrada en el cuerpo body-centered
  therapy
terapia cognitiva cognitive therapy
terapia colaboradora collaborative therapy
terapia combinada combined therapy
terapia computerizada computerized therapy
terapia con dióxido de carbono carbon
  dioxide therapy
terapia con el modelado de arcilla
  clay-modeling therapy
terapia concurrente concurrent therapy
terapia conductual behavioral therapy
terapia conductual cognitiva cognitive
  behavioral therapy
terapia conductual cognitiva para abuso de
  niños cognitive behavioral therapy for
  child abuse

terapia conductual cognitiva para ansiedad
  cognitive behavioral therapy for anxiety
terapia conductual cognitiva para depresión
  cognitive behavioral therapy for depression
terapia conductual cognitiva para problemas
  psicosomáticos cognitive behavioral
  therapy for psychosomatic problems
terapia conductual cognitiva para trastornos
  del comer cognitive behavioral therapy for
  eating disorders
terapia conductual-directiva
  behavioral-directive therapy
terapia conductual para autismo behavioral
  therapy for autism
terapia conductual para retardo mental
  behavioral therapy for mental retardation
terapia conjunta conjoint therapy
terapia convulsiva convulsive therapy
terapia cooperativa cooperative therapy
terapia corporal body therapy
terapia corticosteroide corticosteroid therapy
terapia cuadrangular quadrangular therapy
terapia de actitudes attitude therapy
terapia de actividad activity therapy
terapia de actividad-juego activity-play
  therapy
terapia de actualización actualizing therapy
terapia de aflicción grief therapy
terapia de ajuste limitado a fin goal-limited
  adjustment therapy
terapia de artes gráficas graphic-arts therapy
terapia de artes plásticas plastic-arts therapy
terapia de autodominio self-control therapy
terapia de aversión aversion therapy
terapia de aversión eléctrica electric aversion
  therapy
terapia de aversión para abuso de alcohol
  aversion therapy for alcohol abuse
terapia de aversión química chemical
  aversion therapy
terapia de aversión verbal verbal aversion
  therapy
terapia de aversión y ansiedad aversion
  therapy and anxiety
terapia de ayudante helper therapy
terapia de beber controlado
  controlled-drinking therapy
terapia de bombardeo sensorial rítmica
  rhythmic sensory-bombardment therapy
terapia de cambio mínimo minimum-change
  therapy
terapia de coma insulínico insulin-coma
  therapy
terapia de comida food therapy
terapia de comunicación communication
  therapy
terapia de condicionamiento conditioning
  therapy
terapia de conducta behavior therapy
terapia de conducta cognitiva cognitive
  behavior therapy
terapia de conducta con personalidades tipo
  A behavior therapy with type A
  personalities
terapia de conducta de ansiedad no fóbica

nonphobic anxiety behavior therapy
terapia de conducta dialéctica dialectical behavior therapy
terapia de conducta multimodal multimodal behavior therapy
terapia de conducta para dejar de fumar behavior therapy for quitting smoking
terapia de conducta para problemas del comer behavior therapy for eating problems
terapia de convulsión eléctrica electric convulsion therapy
terapia de corticoides corticoid therapy
terapia de crisis crisis therapy
terapia de choque insulínico insulin-shock therapy
terapia de choques shock therapy
terapia de choques convulsivos convulsive shock therapy
terapia de choques eléctricos electric shock therapy
terapia de danza dance therapy
terapia de decisiones directas direct decision therapy
terapia de demora delay therapy
terapia de desensibilización desensitization therapy
terapia de drama drama therapy
terapia de droga de mantenimiento maintenance drug therapy
terapia de drogas drug therapy
terapia de electrochoques electroshock therapy
terapia de electrochoques regresiva regressive electroshock therapy
terapia de electrosueño electrosleep therapy
terapia de empuje total total push therapy
terapia de entrevista interview therapy
terapia de espectador spectator therapy
terapia de espontaneidad spontaneity therapy
terapia de estímulo breve brief-stimulus therapy
terapia de evitación avoidance therapy
terapia de familia extendida extended-family therapy
terapia de familia múltiple multiple family therapy
terapia de grupo group therapy
terapia de grupo apoyador supportive group therapy
terapia de grupo breve brief group therapy
terapia de grupo conductual behavioral group therapy
terapia de grupo de actividad activity group therapy
terapia de grupo de aprendizaje social social learning group therapy
terapia de grupo de inspiración inspiration group therapy
terapia de grupo de parejas couples group therapy
terapia de grupo de parejas conductual behavioral couples group therapy
terapia de grupo de parejas maritales marital couples group therapy

terapia de grupo de psicodrama psychodrama group therapy
terapia de grupo de realidad reality group therapy
terapia de grupo didáctica didactic group therapy
terapia de grupo familiar family group therapy
terapia de grupo para autismo group therapy for autism
terapia de grupo para niños group therapy for children
terapia de grupo para niños de padres divorciados group therapy for children of divorced parents
terapia de grupo para padres group therapy for parents
terapia de grupo para trastornos de aprendizaje group therapy for learning disorders
terapia de grupo paritario peer-group therapy
terapia de grupo racional rational group therapy
terapia de grupo sin líder leaderless-group therapy
terapia de imagen corporal body image therapy
terapia de imaginería imagery therapy
terapia de implosión implosion therapy
terapia de inhalación inhalation therapy
terapia de inhibición recíproca reciprocal-inhibition therapy
terapia de instigación instigation therapy
terapia de interacción social social interaction therapy
terapia de juego play therapy
terapia de juego directivo directive-play therapy
terapia de juego no directivo nondirective play therapy
terapia de liberación release therapy
terapia de liderazgo doble dual-leadership therapy
terapia de litio lithium therapy
terapia de mantenimiento maintenance therapy
terapia de mantenimiento de continuación continuation maintenance therapy
terapia de megavitamina megavitamin therapy
terapia de Morita Morita therapy
terapia de movimiento movement therapy
terapia de música music therapy
terapia de orgón orgone therapy
terapia de papel fijo fixed-role therapy
terapia de papel mayor major role therapy
terapia de parejas couples therapy
terapia de penetración insight therapy
terapia de pérdida de peso weight loss therapy
terapia de persuasión persuasion therapy
terapia de programación psicológica psychological programming therapy
terapia de proyección projection therapy

terapia de radiación radiation therapy
terapia de Rankian Rankian therapy
terapia de realidad reality therapy
terapia de recondicionamiento reconditioning therapy
terapia de red network therapy
terapia de red social social network therapy
terapia de reemplazo replacement therapy
terapia de reflejos condicionados conditioned-reflex therapy
terapia de relación relationship therapy
terapia de relajación relaxation therapy
terapia de relajación progresiva progressive-relaxation therapy
terapia de replicación replication therapy
terapia de resolución de conflicto conflict resolution therapy
terapia de restauración restoration therapy
terapia de restricción del sueño sleep restriction therapy
terapia de sexo doble dual-sex therapy
terapia de subchoques subshock therapy
terapia de sueño continuo continuous sleep therapy
terapia de sueño electroterapéutico electrotherapeutic sleep therapy
terapia de sueño prolongado prolonged-sleep therapy
terapia de sugestión suggestion therapy
terapia de tercera fuerza third-force therapy
terapia de tiempo extendido time-extended therapy
terapia de trabajador manual blue-collar therapy
terapia de trabajo work therapy
terapia de transferencia doble dual-transference therapy
terapia de tres esquinas three-cornered therapy
terapia de voluntad will therapy
terapia del habla speech therapy
terapia del lenguaje language therapy
terapia diádica dyadic therapy
terapia didáctica didactic therapy
terapia directiva directive therapy
terapia disuasiva deterrent therapy
terapia disyuntiva disjunctive therapy
terapia doble dual therapy
terapia electroconvulsiva electroconvulsive therapy
terapia emotiva emotive therapy
terapia en grupos therapy in groups
terapia estructural structural therapy
terapia estructural-estratégica structural-strategic therapy
terapia evocadora evocative therapy
terapia existencial existential therapy
terapia existencial-humanística existential-humanistic therapy
terapia expresiva expressive therapy
terapia familiar family therapy
terapia familiar estratégica strategic family therapy
terapia familiar estructurada structured family therapy

terapia familiar estructural structural family therapy
terapia familiar para abuso de hijos family therapy for child abuse
terapia familiar para delincuencia family therapy for delinquency
terapia familiar para problemas psicosomáticos family therapy for psychosomatic problems
terapia familiar para problemas sexuales family therapy for sexual problems
terapia familiar para trastornos del comer family therapy for eating disorders
terapia familiar sistemática systematic family therapy
terapia feminista feminist therapy
terapia física physical therapy
terapia fisiodinámica physiodynamic therapy
terapia focal focal therapy
terapia gestalt gestalt therapy
terapia hipnodélica hypnodelic therapy
terapia humanística humanistic therapy
terapia humanística-existencial humanistic-existential therapy
terapia implosiva implosive therapy
terapia individual individual therapy
terapia industrial industrial therapy
terapia interpersonal interpersonal therapy
terapia interpretativa interpretative therapy
terapia limitada a fin goal-limited therapy
terapia marital marital therapy
terapia marital conjunta conjoint marital therapy
terapia matrimonial marriage therapy
terapia multimodal multimodal therapy
terapia múltiple multiple therapy
terapia musical musical therapy
terapia no directiva nondirective therapy
terapia no verbal nonverbal therapy
terapia nutricional nutritional therapy
terapia ocupacional occupational therapy
terapia orgánica organic therapy
terapia ortomolecular orthomolecular therapy
terapia paradójica paradoxical therapy
terapia paraverbal paraverbal therapy
terapia pasiva passive therapy
terapia persuasiva persuasive therapy
terapia polivitamínica polyvitamin therapy
terapia preventiva preventive therapy
terapia primal primal therapy
terapia profunda depth therapy
terapia psicoanalítica psychoanalytic therapy
terapia psicodélica psychedelic therapy
terapia psicolítica psycholytic therapy
terapia psicosexual psychosexual therapy
terapia psicosocial psychosocial therapy
terapia racional rational therapy
terapia radical radical therapy
terapia recreativa recreational therapy
terapia reeducativa reeducative therapy
terapia refleja reflex therapy
terapia remediadora remedial therapy
terapia respiratoria respiratory therapy
terapia retroactiva retroactive therapy
terapia semántica semantic therapy

terapia sexual sex therapy
terapia sexual de parejas couples sex therapy
terapia situacional situational therapy
terapia social social therapy
terapia somática somatic therapy
terapia superficial surface therapy
terapia supresora suppressive therapy
terapia triádica triadic therapy
terapia triangular triangular therapy
terapia ultrasónica ultrasonic therapy
terapia vitamínica vitamin therapy
terapia de asignación assignment therapy
terapias aborígenes aboriginal therapies
terapias innovadoras innovative therapies
teratofobia teratophobia
teratogénesis teratogenesis
teratogénesis conductual behavioral
    teratogenesis
teratogénico teratogenic
teratógeno teratogen
teratógeno conductual behavioral teratogen
teratógeno físico physical teratogen
teratógeno psicológico psychological
    teratogen
teratología teratology
teratológico teratological
tercer nervio craneal third cranial nerve
tercer ventrículo third ventricle
tercera dimensión third dimension
tercera oreja third ear
tercero pagador third party payer
terciario tertiary
terebración terebration
terebrante terebrant
teriomorfismo theriomorphism
termalgesia thermalgesia
termalgia thermalgia
termanalgesia thermanalgesia
termanestesia thermanesthesia
termestesia thermesthesia
termestesiómetro thermesthesiometer
térmico thermal
terminación anuloespiral anulospiral ending
terminación de acto act ending
terminación de Ruffini Ruffini ending
terminación nerviosa nerve ending
terminación opcional optional stopping
terminación papilar de Ruffini Ruffini
    papillary ending
terminaciones en cesta basket endings
terminaciones nerviosas encapsuladas
    encapsulated nerve endings
terminaciones nerviosas libres free nerve
    endings
terminal terminal
terminal axónico axon terminal
termistor thermistor
termoalgesia thermoalgesia
termoanalgesia thermoanalgesia
termoanestesia thermoanesthesia
termocoagulación thermocoagulation
termoestesia thermoesthesia
termoestesiómetro thermoesthesiometer
termofobia thermophobia
termografía thermography

termohiperalgesia thermohyperalgesia
termohiperestesia thermohyperesthesia
termohipestesia thermohypesthesia
termohipoestesia thermohypoesthesia
termoneurosis thermoneurosis
termorreceptor thermoreceptor
termorregulación thermoregulation
termotaxis thermotaxis
termotropismo thermotropism
teroide theroid
territorialidad territoriality
territorio territory
territorio de interacción interaction territory
territorio primario primary territory
territorio público public territory
territorio secundario secondary territory
terror terror
tesis thesis
testes testes
testicular testicular
testículo testicle
testículo ectópico ectopic testis
testículo irritable irritable testis
testigo hipnotizado hypnotized witness
testigo ocular eyewitness
testigo perito expert witness
testimonio de testigo ocular eyewitness
    testimony
testis testis
testitis testitis
testosterona testosterone
testosterona sérica serum testosterone
tetania tetany
tetania duradera duration tetany
tetania epidémica epidemic tetany
tetania gástrica gastric tetany
tetania hipoparatiroidea hypoparathyroid
    tetany
tetania infantil infantile tetany
tetania latente latent tetany
tetania manifiesta manifest tetany
tetania neonatal neonatal tetany
tetania paratiroidea parathyroid tetany
tetania paratiropriva parathyroprival tetany
tetania por alcalosis tetany of alkalosis
tetania por hiperventilación hyperventilation
    tetany
tetania posoperatoria postoperative tetany
tetania reumática rheumatic tetany
tetánico tetanic
tetaniforme tetaniform
tetanígeno tetanigenous
tetanilla tetanilla
tetanismo tetanism
tetanización tetanization
tetanizante tetanizing
tetanizar tetanize
tetánodo tetanode
tetanoide tetanoid
tetanómetro tetanometer
tetanomotor tetanomotor
tétanos tetanus
tétanos anticus tetanus anticus
tétanos apirético apyretic tetanus
tétanos benigno benign tetanus

tétanos cefálico cephalic tetanus
tétanos cefálico de Rose Rose's cephalic
   tetanus
tétanos cerebral cerebral tetanus
tétanos completo tetanus completus
tétanos de cabeza head tetanus
tétanos de Ritter Ritter's tetanus
tétanos dorsal tetanus dorsalis
tétanos extensor extensor tetanus
tétanos flexor flexor tetanus
tétanos generalizado generalized tetanus
tétanos hidrofóbico hydrophobic tetanus
tétanos imitativo imitative tetanus
tétanos intermitente intermittent tetanus
tétanos local local tetanus
tétanos neonatal tetanus neonatorum
tétanos por drogas drug tetanus
tétanos posticus tetanus posticus
tétanos tóxico toxic tetanus
tétanos traumático traumatic tetanus
tetartanopía tetartanopia
tetrabenazina tetrabenazine
tetracloruro de carbono carbon tetrachloride
tetracromático tetrachromatic
tetracromatismo tetrachromatism
tétrada tetrad
tétrada narcoléptica narcoleptic tetrad
tetraedro de Henning Henning's tetrahedron
tetraedro del gusto taste tetrahedron
tetrahidrocannabinol tetrahydrocannabinol
tetraparesia tetraparesis
tetraplejía tetraplegia
tetrapléjico tetraplegic
tetrasomia tetrasomy
texto programado programmed text
textual textual
textura texture
textura causal causal texture
theta theta
tiamina thiamine
tiazida thiazide
tibamato tybamate
tic tic
tic convulsivo convulsive tic
tic de pensamiento tic de pensee
tic doloroso tic douloureux
tic espasmódico spasmodic tic
tic facial facial tic
tic glosofaríngeo glossopharyngeal tic
tic habitual habit tic
tic local local tic
tic mímico mimic tic
tic psíquico psychic tic
tic rotatorio rotatory tic
tics múltiples con coprolalia multiple tics
   with coprolalia
tiempo time
tiempo biológico biologic time
tiempo de acceso access time
tiempo de adaptación adaptation time
tiempo de articulación articulation time
tiempo de asociación association time
tiempo de asociación-reacción
   association-reaction time
tiempo de comienzo de voz voice onset time

tiempo de consolidación consolidation time
tiempo de discriminación-reacción
   discrimination-reaction time
tiempo de inercia inertia time
tiempo de percepción perception time
tiempo de protrombina prothrombin time
tiempo de reacción reaction time
tiempo de reacción compleja complex
   reaction time
tiempo de reacción compuesta compound
   reaction time
tiempo de reacción concurrente concurrent
   reaction time
tiempo de reacción de selección choice
   reaction time
tiempo de reconocimiento recognition time
tiempo de recuperación recovery time
tiempo de reflejo central central reflex time
tiempo de regresión regression time
tiempo de respuesta response time
tiempo de sueño sleep time
tiempo de verificación verification time
tiempo entre respuestas interresponse time
tiempo evaluado evaluated time
tiempo fuera time out
tiempo fuera de refuerzo time out from
   reinforcement
tiempo psicológico psychological time
tiempo real real time
tiempo reflejo reflex time
tiempo social social time
tierra de niñez land of childhood
tifomanía typhomania
tigmestesia thigmesthesia
tigretier tigretier
tigrólisis tigrolysis
tijeras de Smellie Smellie's scissors
timbre timbre
timectomía thymectomy
timidez shyness
timidez de carnada bait shyness
timina thymine
timiperona timiperone
timo thymus
timogénico thymogenic
timoléptico thymoleptic
timopatía thymopathy
timopático thymopathic
timopsiquis thymopsyche
timpánico tympanic
tímpano tympanum
timpanometría tympanometry
timpanoplastia tympanoplasty
tinnitus tinnitus
tintes de colores color tints
tiopental thiopental
tiopropazato thiopropazate
tioproperazina thioproperazine
tioridazina thioridazine
tiotixeno thiothixene
tiouracilo thiouracil
tioxanteno thioxanthene
tipicalidad typicality
típico typical
típico de especie species-typical

tipificación sexual sex-typing
tipo type
tipo A A-type
tipo acaparador hoarding type
tipo adenoide adenoid type
tipo agresivo aggressive type
tipo agresivo-predador aggressive-predator type
tipo agresivo solitario solitary aggressive type
tipo apopléctico apoplectic type
tipo asténico asthenic type
tipo atlético athletic type
tipo auditivo auditory type
tipo B B-type
tipo catatónico catatonic type
tipo celoso jealous type
tipo clínico clinical type
tipo colérico choleric type
tipo complejo complex type
tipo constitucional constitutional type
tipo corporal body type
tipo corporal mesomórfico mesomorphic body type
tipo criminal criminal type
tipo de carácter character type
tipo de conducta behavior type
tipo de depresión reclamante claiming type of depression
tipo de grupo group type
tipo de mercadeo marketing type
tipo de pensamiento thinking type
tipo de personalidad personality type
tipo de personalidad básica basic personality type
tipo de reacción reaction type
tipo de reacción activamente agresiva actively aggressive reaction type
tipo de reacción motora motor reaction type
tipo de reacción sensorial sensory-reaction type
tipo de sensación sensation type
tipo digestivo digestive type
tipo displástico dysplastic type
tipo eidético eidetic type
tipo erótico erotic type
tipo erotomaníaco erotomanic type
tipo esténico sthenic type
tipo explotador exploiting type
tipo extravertido extraverted type
tipo familiar family type
tipo físico physique type
tipo flemático phlegmatic type
tipo funcional functional type
tipo hipercompensatorio hypercompensatory type
tipo hipergenital hypergenital type
tipo hipertónico hypertonic type
tipo hipervegetativo hypervegetative type
tipo hipoafectivo hypoaffective type
tipo hipogenital hypogenital type
tipo introvertido introverted type
tipo intuitivo intuitive type
tipo irracional irrational type
tipo libidinal libidinal type
tipo lineal linear type

tipo macroesplácnico macrosplanchnic build
tipo melancólico melancholic type
tipo microesplácnico microsplanchnic type
tipo muscular muscular type
tipo narcisista narcissistic type
tipo normoesplácnico normosplanchnic type
tipo objetivo objective type
tipo obsesivo obsessional type
tipo oral-pasivo oral-passive type
tipo paranoide paranoid type
tipo pícnico pyknic type
tipo psicológico psychological type
tipo racional rational type
tipo reactivo reactive type
tipo reproductivo reproductive type
tipo sanguíneo blood type, sanguine type
tipo simple simple type
tipo sociable sociable type
tipo social social type
tipo visual visual type
tipografía typography
tipología typology
tipología de ansiedad anxiety typology
tipología de Carus Carus' typology
tipología de Kretschmer Kretschmer typology
tipos de funciones function types
tipos de Kretschmer Kretschmer types
tiramina tyramine
tiranismo tyrannism
tiritar shiver
tirohipofisario thyrohypophysial
tiroidectomía thyroidectomy
tiroides thyroid
tiroidismo thyroidism
tironeo de oreja ear pulling
tironeo de pelo hair pulling
tirosina tyrosine
tirotóxico thyrotoxic
tirotoxicosis thyrotoxicosis
tirotoxicosis endógena endogenous thyrotoxicosis
tirotrópico thyrotropic
tirotropina thyrotropin
tiroxina thyroxine
tisiofobia phthisiophobia
tisiomanía phthisiomania
titilación titillation
titubeo titubation
tobillo ankle
tocofobia tocophobia
tocomanía tocomania
todo o nada all-or-none
tolerancia tolerance
tolerancia a la competencia competition tolerance
tolerancia aguda acute tolerance
tolerancia aprendida learned tolerance
tolerancia crónica chronic tolerance
tolerancia cruzada cross-tolerance
tolerancia cruzada de drogas cross-tolerance of drugs
tolerancia de alcohol alcohol tolerance
tolerancia de ambigüedad tolerance of ambiguity

tolerancia de anfetaminas amphetamine tolerance
tolerancia de ansiedad anxiety tolerance
tolerancia de dolor pain tolerance
tolerancia de drogas drug tolerance
tolerancia de drogas condicionada conditioned drug tolerance
tolerancia de drogas crónica chronic drug tolerance
tolerancia de estrés stress tolerance
tolerancia de frustración frustration tolerance
tolerancia farmacodinámica pharmacodynamic tolerance
tolerancia inversa reverse tolerance
toma de decisiones decision making
toma de decisiones bajo estrés decision making under stress
toma de decisiones de administración management decision making
toma de decisiones de carrera career decision making
toma de decisiones por grupos decision making by groups
toma de historial history taking
toma de riesgos de grupo group risk-taking
tomografía tomography
tomografía axial computerizada computerized axial tomography
tomografía computerizada computerized tomography
tomografía de emisión de fotón único single photon emission tomography
tomografía de emisión de positrones positron-emission tomography
tomomanía tomomania
tonafasia tonaphasia
tonal tonal
tonalidad tonality
tonicidad tonicity
tónico tonic
tonicoclónico tonicoclonic
tonitofobia tonitophobia
tonitrofobia tonitrophobia
tono tone
tono absoluto absolute pitch
tono afectivo affective tone
tono complejo complex tone
tono compuesto compound tone
tono de combinación combination tone
tono de diferencia difference tone
tono de intermitencia intermittence tone
tono de interrupción interruption tone
tono de sentimientos feeling tone
tono de sumación summation tone
tono de Tartini Tartini's tone
tono emocional emotional tone
tono espinal spinal tonus
tono fundamental fundamental tone
tono hedónico hedonic tone
tono inducido induced tonus
tono muscular muscle tone
tono otogénico otogenic tone
tono parcial partial tone
tono perfecto perfect pitch
tono plástico plastic tonus

tono psíquico psychic tone
tono puro pure tone
tono relativo relative pitch
tono simple simple tone
tono subjetivo subjective tone
tonoclónico tonoclonic
tonogenia tonogeny
tonogénico tonogenic
tonometría tonometry
tonómetro tonometer
tonotopia tonotopy
tonotópico tonotopic
topagnosis topagnosis
topalgia topalgia
tope ceiling
topectomía topectomy
topestesia topesthesia
tópico topical
topoanestesia topoanesthesia
topofobia topophobia
topognosia topognosia
topognosis topognosis
topografagnosia topographagnosia
topografía topography
topografía mental mental topography
topográfico topographic
topología topology
topológico topological
toponarcosis toponarcosis
toponeurosis toponeurosis
toposcopio toposcope
topotermestesiómetro topothermesthesiometer
torácico thoracic
toracolumbar thoracolumbar
tórax thorax
tormenta de movimientos oculares rápidos rapid eye movement storm
tormenta emocional emotional storm
torneo staggers
torpe clumsy
torpeza clumsiness
torpor torpor
torsión torsion
torsionómetro torsionometer
torticolar torticollar
tortícolis torticollis
tortícolis dermatógeno dermatogenic torticollis
tortícolis distónico dystonic torticollis
tortícolis espasmódico spasmodic torticollis
tortícolis espástico torticollis spastica
tortícolis espurio spurious torticollis
tortícolis fijo fixed torticollis
tortícolis intermitente intermittent torticollis
tortícolis laberíntico labyrinthine torticollis
tortícolis ocular ocular torticollis
tortícolis psicogénico psychogenic torticollis
tortícolis reumático rheumatic torticollis
tortícolis sintomático symptomatic torticollis
toruloma toruloma
total marginal marginal total
total progresivo progressive total
tótem totem
totémico totemistic
totemismo totemism

toxemia toxemia
toxemia del embarazo toxemia of pregnancy
toxicidad toxicity
toxicidad conductual behavioral toxicity
toxicidad de cocaína cocaine toxicity
tóxico toxic
toxicofobia toxicophobia
toxicología de conducta behavior toxicology
toxicomanía toxicomania
toxicosis condicionada conditioned toxicosis
toxifobia toxiphobia
toxina toxin
toxinas ambientales environmental toxins
toxofobia toxophobia
toxoplasmosis toxoplasmosis
toxoplasmosis congénita congenital
    toxoplasmosis
trabajador de caso caseworker
trabajador de salud mental mental-health
    worker
trabajador en el cuidado de niños child-care
    worker
trabajador social social worker
trabajador social comunitario community
    social worker
trabajador social médico medical social
    worker
trabajador social psiquiátrico psychiatric
    social worker
trabajo clínico clinical work
trabajo de aflicción grief work
trabajo de campo field work
trabajo de casos sociales social case work
trabajo de grupo group work
trabajo del sueño dream-work
trabajo dental con hipnotismo dental work
    with hypnotism
trabajo en casos case work
trabajo en equipo teamwork
trabajo social social work
trabajo social familiar family social work
trabajo social psiquiátrico psychiatric social
    work
tracoma trachoma
tracto tract
tracto alimenticio alimentary tract
tracto colinérgico cholinergic tract
tracto corticoespinal corticospinal tract
tracto corticoespinal lateral lateral
    corticospinal tract
tracto de Lissauer Lissauer's tract
tracto del censo census tract
tracto dopaminérgico dopaminergic tract
tracto espinocerebeloso spinocerebellar tract
tracto espinotalámico spinothalamic tract
tracto espinotalámico lateral lateral
    spinothalamic tract
tracto extrapiramidal extrapyramidal tract
tracto intersegmentario intersegmental tract
tracto mesolímbico mesocortical
    mesolimbic-mesocortical tract
tracto olfatorio olfactory tract
tracto olfatorio lateral lateral olfactory tract
tracto óptico optic tract
tracto paleoespinotalámico

    paleospinothalamic tract
tracto palidohipotalámico
    pallidohypothalamic tract
tracto piramidal pyramidal tract
tracto rubroespinal rubrospinal tract
tracto serotonérgico serotonergic tract
tracto vocal vocal tract
tractotomía tractotomy
tractotomía anterolateral anterolateral
    tractotomy
tractotomía de Schwartz Schwartz
    tractotomy
tractotomía de Sjoqvist Sjoqvist tractotomy
tractotomía de Walker Walker tractotomy
tractotomía espinal spinal tractotomy
tractotomía espinotalámica spinothalamic
    tractotomy
tractotomía estereotáctica stereotactic
    tractotomy
tractotomía intramedular intramedullary
    tractotomy
tractotomía piramidal pyramidal tractotomy
tractotomía trigeminal trigeminal tractotomy
traducción translation
traducción por máquina machine translation
tragado de aire air swallowing
trampa social social trap
trancazo bends
trance trance
trance de muerte death trance
trance hipnótico hypnotic trance
trance inducido induced trance
trance liviano light trance
trance mediano medium trance
trance profundo deep trance
trance sonambulístico somnambulistic trance
tranilcipromina tranylcypromine
tranquilizante tranquilizer
tranquilizante mayor major tranquilizer
tranquilizante menor minor tranquilizer
transacción transaction
transaccional transactional
transaccionalismo perceptivo perceptual
    transactionalism
transaminasa glutámica-pirúvica sérica
    serum glutamic-pyruvic transaminase
transaminasa glutamil sérica serum glutamyl
    transaminase
transcendental transcendental
transcetolasa transketolase
transcortical transcortical
transcripción transcription
transcultural transcultural
transducción transduction
transducción sensorial sensory transduction
transductivo transductive
transductor transducer
transección transection
transección espinal spinal transection
transexual transsexual
transexual nuclear nuclear transsexual
transexualismo transsexualism
transferasa transferase
transferencia transfer, transference
transferencia afectuosa affectionate

transference
transferencia bilateral bilateral transfer
transferencia de aprendizaje transfer of learning
transferencia de entrenamiento transfer of training
transferencia de espejo mirror transference
transferencia de identificación identification transference
transferencia de información information transfer
transferencia de memoria memory transfer
transferencia de pensamientos thought transference
transferencia de pensamientos extrasensorial extrasensory thought transference
transferencia de principios transfer of principles
transferencia de principios generales general principles transfer
transferencia del fin aim transference
transferencia doble dual transference
transferencia erótica erotic transference
transferencia específica specific transfer
transferencia flotante floating transference
transferencia general general transfer
transferencia hostil hostile transference
transferencia institucional institutional transference
transferencia interhemisférica interhemispheric transfer
transferencia libidinal libidinal transference
transferencia negativa negative transference
transferencia por generalización transfer by generalization
transferencia positiva positive transference
transferencia transmodal cross-modal transfer
transformación transformation
transformación arco seno arc sine transformation
transformación de afecto transformation of affect
transformación malévola malevolent transformation
transformación perceptiva perceptual transformation
transformación Z de Fisher Fisher's Z-transformation
transformacional transformational
transformado transformed
transformismo transformism
transición transition
transición de intensidad alta high-intensity transition
transicional transitional
transináptico transsynaptic
transinstitucionalización transinstitutionalization
transitividad transitivity
transitivismo transitivism
transitorio transient
transituacional transsituational
translocación translocation
transmisible transmissible

transmisión transmission
transmisión cultural cultural transmission
transmisión de información information transmission
transmisión doble duplex transmission
transmisión genética genetic transmission
transmisión genética de depresión genetic transmission of depression
transmisión horizontal horizontal transmission
transmisión neural neural transmission
transmisión neuroefectora neuroeffector transmission
transmisión neurohumoral neurohumoral transmission
transmisión química chemical transmission
transmisión sináptica synaptic transmission
transmisión social social transmission
transmisión vertical vertical transmission
transmisor transmitter
transmisor falso false transmitter
transmisor químico chemical transmitter
transmodal cross-modal
transneuronal transneuronal
transorbitario transorbital
transparencia transparency
transpersonal transpersonal
transpersonalidad transpersonality
transplante cerebral brain transplant
transplante corneal corneal transplant
transporte activo active transport
transporte axonal axonal transport
transposición transposition
transposición de afecto transposition of affect
transposón transposon
transtentorial transtentorial
transversal transverse
transversectomía transversectomy
transvéstico transvestic
transvestismo transvestism
transvestismo fetichístico fetishistic cross-dressing
transvestista transvestite
transvestista marginal marginal transvestite
transvestista nuclear nuclear transvestite
traquelagra trachelagra
traquelismo trachelism
traquelocifosis trachelokyphosis
traquelocirtosis trachelocyrtosis
traquelodinia trachelodynia
traquelología trachelology
traquifonía trachyphonia
trascendencia del ego ego transcendence
traslación a la corriente principal mainstreaming
traslación a la corriente principal educacional educational mainstreaming
traslación a la corriente principal y currículo mainstreaming and curriculum
traslación a la corriente principal y destrezas sociales mainstreaming and social skills
traslación a la corriente principal y educación individualizada mainstreaming and individualized education
traslado de fase phase shift

traslocación recíproca reciprocal
  translocation
trasplante transplantation
trasplante de órgano organ transplant
trastornado disordered
trastorno disorder
trastorno afectivo affective disorder
trastorno afectivo adolescente adolescent
  affective disorder
trastorno afectivo atípico atypical affective
  disorder
trastorno afectivo bipolar bipolar affective
  disorder
trastorno afectivo crónico chronic affective
  disorder
trastorno afectivo mayor major affective
  disorder
trastorno afectivo temporal seasonal
  affective disorder
trastorno alucinógeno-afectivo
  hallucinogen-affective disorder
trastorno alucinógeno-delusorio
  hallucinogen-delusional disorder
trastorno amnésico amnesic disorder
trastorno amnésico de alcohol alcohol
  amnesic disorder
trastorno amnésico de barbituratos
  barbiturate amnesic disorder
trastorno amnésico de sustancia psicoactiva
  psychoactive substance amnestic disorder
trastorno amnésico orgánico organic
  amnestic disorder
trastorno amnésico persistente de alcohol
  alcohol persisting amnestic disorder
trastorno amnésico persistente de ansiolítico
  anxiolytic persisting amnestic disorder
trastorno amnésico persistente de hipnótico
  hypnotic persisting amnestic disorder
trastorno amnésico persistente de otra
  sustancia other substance persisting
  amnestic disorder
trastorno amnésico persistente de sedante
  sedative persisting amnestic disorder
trastorno amnésico persistente de sustancia
  desconocida unknown substance persisting
  amnestic disorder
trastorno anfetamina amphetamine disorder
trastorno aritmético arithmetic disorder
trastorno aritmético del desarrollo
  developmental arithmetic disorder
trastorno artificial artificial disorder
trastorno atípico atypical disorder
trastorno auditivo auditory disorder
trastorno autista autistic disorder
trastorno autónomo autonomic disorder
trastorno bipolar bipolar disorder
trastorno bipolar atípico atypical bipolar
  disorder
trastorno bipolar deprimido depressed
  bipolar disorder
trastorno bipolar familiar familial bipolar
  disorder
trastorno bipolar I bipolar I disorder
trastorno bipolar II bipolar II disorder
trastorno bipolar maníaco manic bipolar

  disorder
trastorno bipolar mixto mixed bipolar
  disorder
trastorno bipolar y depresión bipolar
  disorder and depression
trastorno cardíaco cardiac disorder
trastorno cardiovascular cardiovascular
  disorder
trastorno cerebral brain disorder
trastorno cerebral agudo acute brain disorder
trastorno cerebral arterioesclerótico
  arteriosclerotic brain disorder
trastorno cerebral crónico chronic brain
  disorder
trastorno cíclico cyclic disorder
trastorno ciclotímico cyclothymic disorder
trastorno coercitivo parafílico paraphilic
  coercive disorder
trastorno compulsivo compulsive disorder
trastorno conceptual conceptual disorder
trastorno conductual behavioral disorder
trastorno convulsivo convulsive disorder
trastorno cutáneo skin disorder
trastorno de abuso de sustancia substance
  abuse disorder
trastorno de afecto disorder of affect
trastorno de ajuste adjustment disorder
trastorno de ajuste con ansiedad adjustment
  disorder with anxiety
trastorno de ajuste con características
  atípicas adjustment disorder with atypical
  features
trastorno de ajuste con características
  emocionales mixtas adjustment disorder
  with mixed emotional features
trastorno de ajuste con disturbio de
  conducta adjustment disorder with
  disturbance of conduct
trastorno de ajuste con humor ansioso
  adjustment disorder with anxious mood
trastorno de ajuste con humor deprimido
  adjustment disorder with depressed mood
trastorno de ajuste con inhibición académica
  adjustment disorder with academic
  inhibition
trastorno de ajuste con inhibición de trabajo
  adjustment disorder with work inhibition
trastorno de ajuste con quejas físicas
  adjustment disorder with physical
  complaints
trastorno de ajuste con retirada adjustment
  disorder with withdrawal
trastorno de ajuste depresivo depressive
  adjustment disorder
trastorno de alimentación feeding disorder
trastorno de ansiedad anxiety disorder
trastorno de ansiedad anfetamina
  amphetamine anxiety disorder
trastorno de ansiedad atípico atypical anxiety
  disorder
trastorno de ansiedad de adolescencia
  anxiety disorder of adolescence
trastorno de ansiedad de alcohol alcohol
  anxiety disorder
trastorno de ansiedad de alucinógeno

hallucinogen anxiety disorder
trastorno de ansiedad de ansiolítico
anxiolytic anxiety disorder
trastorno de ansiedad de cannabis cannabis
anxiety disorder
trastorno de ansiedad de cocaína cocaine
anxiety disorder
trastorno de ansiedad de fenciclidina
phencyclidine anxiety disorder
trastorno de ansiedad de hipnótico hypnotic
anxiety disorder
trastorno de ansiedad de inhalante inhalant
anxiety disorder
trastorno de ansiedad de niñez childhood
anxiety disorder
trastorno de ansiedad de otra sustancia
other substance anxiety disorder
trastorno de ansiedad de sedante sedative
anxiety disorder
trastorno de ansiedad de separación
separation anxiety disorder
trastorno de ansiedad de separación de niñez
separation anxiety disorder of childhood
trastorno de ansiedad de sueños dream
anxiety disorder
**trastorno de ansiedad de sustancia
desconocida** unknown substance anxiety
disorder
**trastorno de ansiedad de sustancia
psicoactiva** psychoactive substance anxiety
disorder
**trastorno de ansiedad debido a condición
médica general** anxiety disorder due to
general medical condition
trastorno de ansiedad generalizada
generalized anxiety disorder
trastorno de ansiedad orgánica organic
anxiety disorder
trastorno de apego attachment disorder
trastorno de apego de infancia attachment
disorder of infancy
trastorno de apego reactivo reactive
attachment disorder
trastorno de apego reactivo de infancia
reactive attachment disorder of infancy
**trastorno de apego reactivo de niñez
temprana** reactive attachment disorder of
early childhood
trastorno de apetito appetite disorder
trastorno de articulación articulation disorder
trastorno de articulación del desarrollo
developmental articulation disorder
trastorno de Asperger Asperger's disorder
trastorno de atención attention disorder
trastorno de audición hearing disorder
trastorno de aversión sexual sexual aversion
disorder
trastorno de cognición cognition disorder
trastorno de comunicación communication
disorder
trastorno de conducta conduct disorder
trastorno de conducta agresiva aggressive
conduct disorder
trastorno de conducta agresiva socializada
socialized-aggressive conduct disorder

**trastorno de conducta agresiva
subsocializada**
undersocialized-aggressive-conduct
disorder
trastorno de conducta atípica atypical
conduct disorder
trastorno de conducta compulsiva
compulsive-conduct disorder
**trastorno de conducta contra trastorno
afectivo** conduct disorder versus affective
disorder
**trastorno de conducta de movimientos
oculares rápidos** rapid eye movement
behavior disorder
trastorno de conducta de tipo de grupo
group type conduct disorder
trastorno de conducta disruptiva disruptive
behavior disorder
trastorno de conducta e historial familiar
conduct disorder and family history
trastorno de conducta episódica
episodic-behavior disorder
**trastorno de conducta no agresiva
socializada** socialized-nonaggressive
conduct disorder
**trastorno de conducta no agresiva
subsocializada**
undersocialized-nonaggressive-conduct
disorder
trastorno de conducta primario primary
behavior disorder
trastorno de conducta subsocializada
undersocialized conduct disorder
trastorno de control de impulsos impulse
control disorder
trastorno de control de impulsos atípico
atypical impulse control disorder
**trastorno de control de impulsos no
clasificado en otra parte** disorder of
impulse control not elsewhere classified
trastorno de conversión conversion disorder
trastorno de coordinación coordination
disorder
trastorno de coordinación del desarrollo
developmental coordination disorder
trastorno de cromosoma sexual sex
chromosome disorder
trastorno de déficit de atención
attention-deficit disorder
**trastorno de déficit de atención con
hiperactividad** attention-deficit disorder
with hyperactivity
trastorno de déficit de atención de adultos
adult attention-deficit disorder
trastorno de déficit de atención hiperactiva
attention-deficit hyperactivity disorder
**trastorno de déficit de atención sin
hiperactividad** attention-deficit disorder
without hyperactivity
trastorno de dependencia dependence
disorder
trastorno de dependencia de sustancia
substance dependence disorder
trastorno de deseo sexual hipoactivo
hypoactive sexual desire disorder

trastorno de deseo sexual hipoactivo femenino female hypoactive sexual desire disorder

trastorno de deseo sexual hipoactivo femenino debido a condición médica general female hypoactive sexual desire disorder due to general medical condition

trastorno de deseo sexual hipoactivo masculino male hypoactive sexual desire disorder

trastorno de despersonalización depersonalization disorder

trastorno de despertamiento arousal disorder

trastorno de despertamiento sexual femenino female sexual arousal disorder

trastorno de destrezas académicas academic skills disorder

trastorno de destrezas motoras motor skills disorder

trastorno de dolor pain disorder

trastorno de dolor asociado con factores psicológicos pain disorder associated with psychological factors

trastorno de dolor psicogénico psychogenic pain disorder

trastorno de dolor psicosexual psychosexual pain disorder

trastorno de dolor sexual sexual pain disorder

trastorno de dolor somatoforme somatoform pain disorder

trastorno de eliminación elimination disorder

trastorno de emancipación emancipation disorder

trastorno de entrada input disorder

trastorno de escritura writing disorder

trastorno de espectro antisocial antisocial spectrum disorder

trastorno de espectro depresivo depressive spectrum disorder

trastorno de estereotipia stereotypy disorder

trastorno de estereotipia y hábito stereotypy and habit disorder

trastorno de estrés stress disorder

trastorno de estrés agudo acute stress disorder

trastorno de estrés postraumático posttraumatic stress disorder

trastorno de estrés postraumático agudo acute posttraumatic stress disorder

trastorno de expresión escrita disorder of written expression

trastorno de eyaculación ejaculation disorder

trastorno de fenilalanina phenylalanine disorder

trastorno de fluidez fluency disorder

trastorno de género cruzado cross-gender disorder

trastorno de género cruzado no transexual nontranssexual cross-gender disorder

trastorno de hábito habit disorder

trastorno de hipersomnia hypersomnia disorder

trastorno de hipersomnia primaria primary hypersomnia disorder

trastorno de hipersomnolencia hypersomnolence disorder

trastorno de identidad identity disorder

trastorno de identidad de género gender-identity disorder

trastorno de identidad de género atípico atypical gender identity disorder

trastorno de identidad de género de adolescencia gender-identity disorder of adolescence

trastorno de identidad de género de adultez gender-identity disorder of adulthood

trastorno de identidad de género de niñez childhood gender identity disorder

trastorno de identidad de niñez identity disorder of childhood

trastorno de identidad disociativa dissociative identity disorder

trastorno de impulsos impulse disorder

trastorno de impulsos hipercinéticos hyperkinetic impulse disorder

trastorno de iniciar y mantener el sueño disorder of initiating and maintaining sleep

trastorno de insomnio insomnia disorder

trastorno de intimidad intimacy disorder

trastorno de lectura reading disorder

trastorno de lectura del desarrollo developmental reading disorder

trastorno de marcha gait disorder

trastorno de memoria memory disorder

trastorno de movilidad motility disorder

trastorno de movimiento movement disorder

trastorno de movimiento estereotipado atípico atypical stereotyped movement disorder

trastorno de movimientos estereotipados stereotyped-movement disorder

trastorno de movimientos estereotípicos stereotypic-movement disorder

trastorno de movimientos inducido por medicación medication-induced movement disorder

trastorno de orgasmo orgasm disorder

trastorno de orientación orientation disorder

trastorno de pánico panic disorder

trastorno de pánico con agorafobia panic disorder with agoraphobia

trastorno de pánico sin agorafobia panic disorder without agoraphobia

trastorno de papel de género gender-role disorder

trastorno de papel de género de niñez gender-role disorder of childhood

trastorno de pensamiento esquizofrénico schizophrenic thought disorder

trastorno de pensamiento formal formal thought disorder

trastorno de pensamiento primario primary thought disorder

trastorno de pensamientos thought disorder

trastorno de percepción persistente de alucinógeno hallucinogen persisting perception disorder

trastorno de percepción posalucinógena posthallucinogen perception disorder

trastorno de personalidad personality
disorder
trastorno de personalidad antisocial
antisocial personality disorder
trastorno de personalidad atípica atypical
personality disorder
trastorno de personalidad autoderrotante
self-defeating personality disorder
trastorno de personalidad ciclotímica
cyclothymic personality disorder
trastorno de personalidad compulsiva
compulsive personality disorder
trastorno de personalidad dependiente
dependent personality disorder
trastorno de personalidad esquizoide
schizoid personality disorder
trastorno de personalidad esquizotípica
schizotypal personality disorder
trastorno de personalidad evitante avoidant
personality disorder
trastorno de personalidad explosiva
explosive personality disorder
trastorno de personalidad fronterizo
borderline personality disorder
**trastorno de personalidad fronterizo del
desarrollo** developmental borderline
personality disorder
**trastorno de personalidad fronterizo en
adolescencia** borderline personality
disorder in adolescence
**trastorno de personalidad fronterizo en
adultez** borderline personality disorder in
adulthood
**trastorno de personalidad fronterizo en
niños** borderline personality disorder in
children
**trastorno de personalidad fronterizo y
personalidad esquizoide** borderline
personality disorder and schizoid
personality
trastorno de personalidad histérica
hysterical personality disorder
trastorno de personalidad histriónica
histrionic personality disorder
trastorno de personalidad inmadura
immature personality disorder
trastorno de personalidad introvertida
introverted personality disorder
trastorno de personalidad lábil labile
personality disorder
trastorno de personalidad masoquista
masochistic personality disorder
trastorno de personalidad múltiple multiple
personality disorder
trastorno de personalidad narcisista
narcissistic personality disorder
**trastorno de personalidad
obsesivo-compulsivo**
obsessive-compulsive personality disorder
trastorno de personalidad oposicional
oppositional personality disorder
trastorno de personalidad orgánico organic
personality disorder
trastorno de personalidad paranoide
paranoid personality disorder

**trastorno de personalidad
paranoide-esquizotípico**
paranoid-schizotypal personality disorder
trastorno de personalidad pasiva-agresiva
passive-aggressive personality disorder
**trastorno de personalidad por sustancia
psicoactiva** psychoactive substance
personality disorder
trastorno de personalidad postraumática
posttraumatic personality disorder
trastorno de personalidad sádica sadistic
personality disorder
**trastorno de personalidad situacional
transitoria** transient situational personality
disorder
trastorno de personalidad sociopática
sociopathic personality disorder
trastorno de pesadillas nightmare disorder
trastorno de Rett Rett's disorder
trastorno de ritmo rhythm disorder
trastorno de rumiación de infancia
rumination disorder of infancy
trastorno de Schmidt Schmidt's disorder
trastorno de somatización somatization
disorder
trastorno de somnolencia excesiva disorder
of excessive somnolence
trastorno de sonambulismo sleepwalking
disorder
trastorno de subrendimiento académico
academic underachievement disorder
trastorno de terror del sueño sleep terror
disorder
trastorno de tic tic disorder
trastorno de tic atípico atypical tic disorder
trastorno de tic motor crónico chronic motor
tic disorder
trastorno de tic transitorio transient tic
disorder
trastorno de tic vocal crónico chronic vocal
tic disorder
trastorno de timidez shyness disorder
trastorno de Tourette Tourette's disorder
trastorno de uso de alcohol alcohol use
disorder
trastorno de uso de alucinógenos
hallucinogen use disorder
trastorno de uso de anfetaminas
amphetamine use disorder
trastorno de uso de ansiolítico anxiolytic use
disorder
trastorno de uso de cafeína caffeine use
disorder
trastorno de uso de cannabis cannabis use
disorder
trastorno de uso de cocaína cocaine use
disorder
trastorno de uso de fenciclidina
phencyclidine use disorder
trastorno de uso de hipnótico hypnotic use
disorder
trastorno de uso de inhalante inhalant use
disorder
trastorno de uso de nicotina nicotine use
disorder

trastorno de uso de opioide opioid use disorder

trastorno de uso de otra sustancia other substance use disorder

trastorno de uso de sedante sedative use disorder

trastorno de uso de sustancia substance use disorder

trastorno de uso de sustancia desconocida unknown substance use disorder

trastorno de uso de sustancia psicoactiva psychoactive substance use disorder

trastorno de voz voice disorder

trastorno de voz funcional functional voice disorder

trastorno del carácter character disorder

trastorno del comer eating disorder

trastorno del comer atípico atypical eating disorder

trastorno del comer en adolescencia eating disorder in adolescence

trastorno del comer en infancia eating disorder in infancy

trastorno del contenido de pensamientos content-thought disorder

trastorno del desarrollo developmental disorder

trastorno del desarrollo específico specific developmental disorder

trastorno del desarrollo específico mixto mixed specific developmental disorder

trastorno del deseo sexual sexual desire disorder

trastorno del despertamiento sexual sexual arousal disorder

trastorno del escribir expresivo del desarrollo developmental expressive writing disorder

trastorno del habla speech disorder

trastorno del habla funcional functional speech disorder

trastorno del horario de dormir-despertar sleep-wake schedule disorder

trastorno del humor mood disorder

trastorno del humor crónico chronic mood disorder

trastorno del humor de alucinógeno hallucinogen mood disorder

trastorno del humor de anfetaminas amphetamine mood disorder

trastorno del humor de ansiolítico anxiolytic mood disorder

trastorno del humor de cocaína cocaine mood disorder

trastorno del humor de fenciclidina phencyclidine mood disorder

trastorno del humor de hipnótico hypnotic mood disorder

trastorno del humor de inhalante inhalant mood disorder

trastorno del humor de opioide opioid mood disorder

trastorno del humor de otra sustancia other substance mood disorder

trastorno del humor de sedante sedative mood disorder

trastorno del humor de sustancia desconocida unknown substance mood disorder

trastorno del humor debido a condición médica general mood disorder due to general medical condition

trastorno del humor inducido por sustancia substance-induced mood disorder

trastorno del humor orgánico organic mood disorder

trastorno del humor por sustancia psicoactiva psychoactive substance mood disorder

trastorno del humor temporal seasonal mood disorder

trastorno del lenguaje language disorder

trastorno del lenguaje del desarrollo developmental language disorder

trastorno del lenguaje expresivo expressive language disorder

trastorno del lenguaje expresivo del desarrollo developmental expressive language disorder

trastorno del lenguaje por daño cerebral brain-damage language disorder

trastorno del lenguaje receptivo receptive language disorder

trastorno del lenguaje receptivo del desarrollo developmental receptive language disorder

trastorno del lenguaje receptivo-expresivo mixto mixed receptive-expressive language disorder

trastorno del lenguaje y habla language and speech disorder

trastorno del lenguaje y habla del desarrollo developmental language and speech disorder

trastorno del proceso de pensamientos thought-process disorder

trastorno del sistema nervioso central central nervous system disorder

trastorno del sueño sleep disorder

trastorno del sueño de alcohol alcohol sleep disorder

trastorno del sueño de anfetaminas amphetamine sleep disorder

trastorno del sueño de ansiolítico anxiolytic sleep disorder

trastorno del sueño de cafeína caffeine sleep disorder

trastorno del sueño de cocaína cocaine sleep disorder

trastorno del sueño de deterioro respiratorio respiratory impairment sleep disorder

trastorno del sueño de hipnótico hypnotic sleep disorder

trastorno del sueño de niñez childhood sleep disorder

trastorno del sueño de opioide opioid sleep disorder

trastorno del sueño de otra sustancia other substance sleep disorder

trastorno del sueño de ritmo circadiano

circadian rhythm sleep disorder

trastorno del sueño de sedante sedative sleep disorder

trastorno del sueño de sustancia desconocida unknown substance sleep disorder

trastorno del sueño debido a condición médica general sleep disorder due to general medical condition

trastorno del sueño inducido por sustancia substance-induced sleep disorder

trastorno del sueño mioclónico myoclonic sleep disorder

trastorno del sueño relacionado con la respiración breathing-related sleep disorder

trastorno del sueño secundario secondary sleep disorder

trastorno del tiempo y ritmo time and rhythm disorder

trastorno delusorio delusional disorder

trastorno delusorio anfetamina amphetamine delusional disorder

trastorno delusorio de alucinógeno hallucinogen delusional disorder

trastorno delusorio de cannabis cannabis delusional disorder

trastorno delusorio de cocaína cocaine delusional disorder

trastorno delusorio de fenciclidina phencyclidine delusional disorder

trastorno delusorio orgánico organic delusional disorder

trastorno delusorio persecutorio persecutory delusional disorder

trastorno delusorio por sustancia psicoactiva psychoactive substance delusional disorder

trastorno delusorio simpatomimético sympathomimetic delusional disorder

trastorno depresivo depressive disorder

trastorno depresivo mayor major depressive disorder

trastorno desafiante oposicional oppositional defiant disorder

trastorno desintegrante disintegrative disorder

trastorno desintegrante de niñez childhood disintegrative disorder

trastorno disfórico de fase lútea tardía late luteal phase dysphoric disorder

trastorno disfórico de fase perilútea periluteal phase dysphoric disorder

trastorno disfórico premenstrual premenstrual dysphoric disorder

trastorno dismórfico corporal body dysmorphic disorder

trastorno disociativo dissociative disorder

trastorno disociativo atípico atypical dissociative disorder

trastorno distímico dysthymic disorder

trastorno emocional emotional disorder

trastorno endocrino endocrine disorder

trastorno endocrinológico endocrinological disorder

trastorno enmascarado masked disorder

trastorno epiléptico epileptic disorder

trastorno episódico episodic disorder

trastorno eréctil masculino male erectile disorder

trastorno eréctil masculino debido a condición médica general male erectile disorder due to general medical condition

trastorno espacial spatial disorder

trastorno esquizoafectivo schizoaffective disorder

trastorno esquizofrénico schizophrenic disorder

trastorno esquizofreniforme schizophreniform disorder

trastorno esquizoide schizoid disorder

trastorno esquizoide de adolescencia schizoid disorder of adolescence

trastorno esquizoide de niñez schizoid disorder of childhood

trastorno esquizotípico schizotypal disorder

trastorno evitante avoidant disorder

trastorno evitante de adolescencia avoidant disorder of adolescence

trastorno evitante de niñez avoidant disorder of childhood

trastorno experimental experimental disorder

trastorno explosivo explosive disorder

trastorno explosivo aislado isolated explosive disorder

trastorno explosivo intermitente intermittent explosive disorder

trastorno extractivo extractive disorder

trastorno facticio factitious disorder

trastorno facticio atípico atypical factitious disorder

trastorno facticio con síntomas físicos factitious disorder with physical symptoms

trastorno facticio con síntomas psicológicos factitious disorder with psychological symptoms

trastorno físico physical disorder

trastorno fóbico phobic disorder

trastorno fonémico phonemic disorder

trastorno fonológico phonological disorder

trastorno fonológico del desarrollo developmental phonologic disorder

trastorno fronterizo borderline disorder

trastorno funcional functional disorder

trastorno gastrointestinal gastrointestinal disorder

trastorno genético genetic disorder

trastorno geriátrico geriatric disorder

trastorno heredado inherited disorder

trastorno hereditario hereditary disorder

trastorno hipomaníaco hypomanic disorder

trastorno hipotémico hypothemic disorder

trastorno histérico hysterical disorder

trastorno hormonal familiar familial hormonal disorder

trastorno iatrogénico iatrogenic disorder

trastorno inducido por sustancia substance-induced disorder

trastorno intersensorial intersensory disorder

trastorno intestinal bowel disorder

trastorno limitado a una cultura culture-bound disorder

trastorno logicogramatical logicogrammatical
disorder
trastorno maníaco manic disorder
trastorno maniacodepresivo
manic-depressive disorder
trastorno matemático mathematics disorder
trastorno menstrual menstrual disorder
trastorno mental mental disorder
trastorno mental debido a condición médica
general mental disorder due to general
medical condition
trastorno mental inducido por alcohol
alcohol-induced mental disorder
trastorno mental inducido por anfetaminas
amphetamine-induced mental disorder
trastorno mental no especificado unspecified
mental disorder
trastorno mental no psicótico nonpsychotic
mental disorder
trastorno mental orgánico organic mental
disorder
trastorno mental orgánico inducido por
alucinógenos hallucinogen-induced
organic mental disorder
trastorno mental orgánico inducido por
cafeína caffeine-induced organic mental
disorder
trastorno mental orgánico inducido por
cocaína cocaine-induced organic mental
disorder
trastorno mental orgánico inducido por
inhalante inhalant-induced organic mental
disorder
trastorno mental orgánico inducido por
nicotina nicotine-induced organic mental
disorder
trastorno mental orgánico inducido por
opioide opioid-induced organic mental
disorder
trastorno mental orgánico inducido por
sustancia substance-induced organic
mental disorder
trastorno mental orgánico inducido por
sustancia psicoactiva psychoactive
substance-induced organic mental disorder
trastorno mental orgánico por sustancia
psicoactiva psychoactive substance
organic mental disorder
trastorno miotónico myotonic disorder
trastorno motor motor disorder
trastorno neurológico neurological disorder
trastorno neuromuscular neuromuscular
disorder
trastorno neuropsicológico neuropsychologic
disorder
trastorno neurótico neurotic disorder
trastorno nutricional nutritional disorder
trastorno obsesivo obsessional disorder
trastorno obsesivo-compulsivo
obsessive-compulsive disorder
trastorno obsesivo-compulsivo contra
esquizofrenia obsessive-compulsive
disorder versus schizophrenia
trastorno oposicional oppositional disorder
trastorno orgánico organic disorder

trastorno orgásmico femenino female
orgasmic disorder
trastorno orgásmico masculino male
orgasmic disorder
trastorno ortopédico orthopedic disorder
trastorno paranoide paranoid disorder
trastorno paranoide agudo acute paranoid
disorder
trastorno paranoide atípico atypical paranoid
disorder
trastorno paranoide compartido shared
paranoid disorder
trastorno paranoide delusorio delusional
paranoid disorder
trastorno paranoide somático somatic
paranoid disorder
trastorno penetrante del desarrollo
pervasive developmental disorder
trastorno penetrante del desarrollo de
comienzo en niñez childhood-onset
pervasive developmental disorder
trastorno perceptivo perceptual disorder
trastorno perceptivo auditivo auditory
perceptual disorder
trastorno perceptivo de búsqueda visual
visual-search perceptual disorder
trastorno perceptivo frontal frontal
perceptual disorder
trastorno pituitario pituitary disorder
trastorno posoperatorio postoperative
disorder
trastorno postraumático posttraumatic
disorder
trastorno premenstrual premenstrual
disorder
trastorno propenso al dolor pain-prone
disorder
trastorno psicofisiológico psychophysiologic
disorder
trastorno psicogénico psychogenic disorder
trastorno psicomotor psychomotor disorder
trastorno psicosexual psychosexual disorder
trastorno psicosexual atípico atypical
psychosexual disorder
trastorno psicosomático psychosomatic
disorder
trastorno psicosomático y enfermedad
crónica psychosomatic disorder and
chronic illness
trastorno psicótico psychotic disorder
trastorno psicótico anfetamina amphetamine
psychotic disorder
trastorno psicótico anfetamina con
alucinaciones amphetamine psychotic
disorder with hallucinations
trastorno psicótico anfetamina con
delusiones amphetamine psychotic
disorder with delusions
trastorno psicótico breve brief psychotic
disorder
trastorno psicótico compartido shared
psychotic disorder
trastorno psicótico de alcohol alcohol
psychotic disorder
trastorno psicótico de alcohol con

alucinaciones alcohol psychotic disorder with hallucinations

trastorno psicótico de alcohol con delusiones alcohol psychotic disorder with delusions

trastorno psicótico de alucinógeno hallucinogen psychotic disorder

trastorno psicótico de alucinógeno con alucinaciones hallucinogen psychotic disorder with hallucinations

trastorno psicótico de alucinógeno con delusiones hallucinogen psychotic disorder with delusions

trastorno psicótico de ansiolítico anxiolytic psychotic disorder

trastorno psicótico de ansiolítico con alucinaciones anxiolytic psychotic disorder with hallucinations

trastorno psicótico de ansiolítico con delusiones anxiolytic psychotic disorder with delusions

trastorno psicótico de cannabis cannabis psychotic disorder

trastorno psicótico de cannabis con alucinaciones cannabis psychotic disorder with hallucinations

trastorno psicótico de cannabis con delusiones cannabis psychotic disorder with delusions

trastorno psicótico de cocaína cocaine psychotic disorder

trastorno psicótico de cocaína con alucinaciones cocaine psychotic disorder with hallucinations

trastorno psicótico de cocaína con delusiones cocaine psychotic disorder with delusions

trastorno psicótico de fenciclidina phencyclidine psychotic disorder

trastorno psicótico de fenciclidina con alucinaciones phencyclidine psychotic disorder with hallucinations

trastorno psicótico de fenciclidina con delusiones phencyclidine psychotic disorder with delusions

trastorno psicótico de hipnótico hypnotic psychotic disorder

trastorno psicótico de hipnótico con alucinaciones hypnotic psychotic disorder with hallucinations

trastorno psicótico de hipnótico con delusiones hypnotic psychotic disorder with delusions

trastorno psicótico de inhalante inhalant psychotic disorder

trastorno psicótico de inhalante con alucinaciones inhalant psychotic disorder with hallucinations

trastorno psicótico de inhalante con delusiones inhalant psychotic disorder with delusions

trastorno psicótico de opioide opioid psychotic disorder

trastorno psicótico de opioide con alucinaciones opioid psychotic disorder with hallucinations

trastorno psicótico de opioide con delusiones opioid psychotic disorder with delusions

trastorno psicótico de otra sustancia other substance psychotic disorder

trastorno psicótico de otra sustancia con alucinaciones other substance psychotic disorder with hallucinations

trastorno psicótico de otra sustancia con delusiones other substance psychotic disorder with delusions

trastorno psicótico de sedante sedative psychotic disorder

trastorno psicótico de sedante con alucinaciones sedative psychotic disorder with hallucinations

trastorno psicótico de sedante con delusiones sedative psychotic disorder with delusions

trastorno psicótico de sustancia desconocida unknown substance psychotic disorder

trastorno psicótico de sustancia desconocida con alucinaciones unknown substance psychotic disorder with hallucinations

trastorno psicótico de sustancia desconocida con delusiones unknown substance psychotic disorder with delusions

trastorno psicótico debido a condición médica general psychotic disorder due to general medical condition

trastorno psicótico inducido induced psychotic disorder

trastorno psiquiátrico psychiatric disorder

trastorno puerperal puerperal disorder

trastorno pulmonar pulmonary disorder

trastorno reactivo reactive disorder

trastorno relacionado al estrés stress related disorder

trastorno relacionado con sustancia substance-related disorder

trastorno respiratorio respiratory disorder

trastorno sanguíneo blood disorder

trastorno semantogénico semantogenic disorder

trastorno sensorial sensory disorder

trastorno sexual sexual disorder

trastorno simulado sham disorder

trastorno sobreansioso overanxious disorder

trastorno sobreansioso de niñez overanxious disorder of childhood

trastorno somático somatic disorder

trastorno somatoforme somatoform disorder

trastorno somatoforme atípico atypical somatoform disorder

trastorno somatoforme dismórfico dysmorphic somatoform disorder

trastorno somatoforme indiferenciado undifferentiated somatoform disorder

trastorno somatopsíquico somatopsychic disorder

trastorno somestésico somesthetic disorder

trastorno táctil-perceptivo tactile-perceptual disorder

trastorno temporal-perceptivo temporal-perceptual disorder

trastorno tóxico toxic disorder

trastorno traumático agudo acute traumatic disorder

trastorno traumático crónico chronic traumatic disorder
trastorno visceral visceral disorder
trastornos de conducta de niñez behavior disorders of childhood
trastornos del desarrollo de aquellos con lesiones cerebrales developmental disorders of the brain injured
trastornos del desarrollo y abuso de niños developmental disorders and child abuse
trastornos del yo disorders of the self
trastornos disociativos y reacción de conversión dissociative disorders and conversion reaction
trastornos mentales orgánicos alcohólicos alcoholic organic mental disorders
trastornos mentales orgánicos de cannabis cannabis organic mental disorders
trastornos mentales orgánicos inducidos por cannabis cannabis-induced organic mental disorders
trastornos por deficiencia de calcio calcium-deficiency disorders
tratamiento treatment
tratamiento ambulatorio ambulatory treatment
tratamiento arriesgado hazardous treatment
tratamiento biomédico biomedical treatment
tratamiento coercitivo coercive treatment
tratamiento cognitivo-lingüístico cognitive-linguistic treatment
tratamiento con envolturas calientes hot-pack treatment
tratamiento con envolturas frías cold-pack treatment
tratamiento conductual behavioral treatment
tratamiento convulsivo de inhalación inhalation convulsive treatment
tratamiento de acidificación acidification treatment
tratamiento de alcoholismo treatment of alcoholism
tratamiento de ansiedad treatment of anxiety
tratamiento de autismo treatment of autism
tratamiento de baño continuo continuous-bath treatment
tratamiento de coma insulínico insulin-coma treatment
tratamiento de choques shock treatment
tratamiento de delincuencia treatment of delinquency
tratamiento de depresión treatment of depression
tratamiento de discapacidades del aprendizaje treatment of learning disabilities
tratamiento de dolor de biorretroalimentación biofeedback treatment of pain
tratamiento de hipertransfusión hypertransfusion treatment
tratamiento de insulina insulin treatment
tratamiento de insulina ambulatoria ambulatory insulin treatment
tratamiento de insulina subcoma subcoma

insulin treatment
tratamiento de insulina subchoque subshock insulin treatment
tratamiento de maltrato psicológico treatment of psychological maltreatment
tratamiento de mantenimiento de metadona methadone maintenance treatment
tratamiento de Mitchell Mitchell's treatment
tratamiento de obesidad obesity treatment
tratamiento de Oppenheimer Oppenheimer treatment
tratamiento de pacientes externos outpatient treatment
tratamiento de pacientes internados inpatient treatment
tratamiento de sueño sleep treatment
tratamiento de sueño prolongado prolonged-sleep treatment
tratamiento de trastornos de conducta treatment of behavior disorders
tratamiento de trastornos del comer treatment of eating disorders
tratamiento de violencia doméstica treatment of domestic violence
tratamiento de Weir Mitchell Weir Mitchell treatment
tratamiento depletivo depletive treatment
tratamiento diurno day treatment
tratamiento electroconvulsivo electroconvulsive treatment
tratamiento ético ethical treatment
tratamiento ético de animales ethical treatment of animals
tratamiento forzado forced treatment
tratamiento holísitco holistic treatment
tratamiento institucional institutional treatment
tratamiento interdisciplinario interdisciplinary treatment
tratamiento intrusivo intrusive treatment
tratamiento invasor invasive treatment
tratamiento involuntario involuntary treatment
tratamiento moral moral treatment
tratamiento ordenado por tribunal court-ordered treatment
tratamiento ortomolecular orthomolecular treatment
tratamiento psicoanalítico psychoanalytic treatment
tratamiento residencial residential treatment
tratamiento residencial de cuidado diurno day care residential treatment
tratamiento sintomático symptomatic treatment
tratamiento social psiquiátrico psychiatric social treatment
traumatofilia traumatophilia
trauma trauma
trauma acústico acoustic trauma
trauma cerebral cerebral trauma
trauma de cabeza head trauma
trauma de cabeza agudo acute head trauma
trauma de nacimiento birth trauma
trauma de niñez childhood trauma

trauma externo external trauma
trauma neural neural trauma
trauma primal primal trauma
trauma psicosexual psychosexual trauma
trauma psíquico psychic trauma
trauma sexual sexual trauma
traumastenia traumasthenia
traumático traumatic
traumatismo traumatism
traumatización traumatization
traumatizar traumatize
traumatofílico traumatophilic
traumatofobia traumatophobia
traza trace
trazador radiactivo radioactive tracer
trazodona trazodone
trefina trephine
trefinación trephination
tremofobia tremophobia
tremógrafo tremograph
tremograma tremogram
tremor artuum tremor artuum
tremor opiophagorum tremor opiophagorum
tremor potatorum tremor potatorum
tremor tendinum tremor tendinum
trémulo tremulous
trepanación trepanation
trépano trepan
trepidación trepidation
trepidante trepidant
tríada triad
tríada anal anal triad
tríada cognitiva cognitive triad
triada de Charcot Charcot's triad
tríada de Sandler Sandler's triad
tríada oral oral triad
triádico triadic
triage triage
triangulación triangulation
triángulo de color color triangle
triazolam triazolam
tríbada tribade
tribadismo tribadism
tricalgia trichalgia
Trichomonas vaginalis Trichomonas vaginalis
tricíclico tricyclic
tricodinia trichodynia
tricoestesia trichoesthesia
tricofagia trichophagy
tricofobia trichophobia
tricología trichology
tricopatofobia trichopathophobia
tricosis trichosis
tricosis sensitiva trichosis sensitiva
tricotilomanía trichotillomania
tricotomía trichotomy
tricromacia trichromacy
tricrómata trichromat
tricromático trichromatic
tricromatismo trichromatism
tricromatismo anómalo anomalous trichromatism
tricromatopsia trichromatopsia
tricromia trichromia
trifacial trifacial

trifosfato de adenosina adenosine triphosphate
trigeminal trigeminal
trigeminofacial trigeminofacial
trígrafo trigraph
trigrama trigram
trigrama consonante consonant trigram
trihíbrido trihybrid
trilogía trilogy
trimetadiona trimethadione
trimipramina trimipramine
triolista triolist
triórquido triorchid
tripanosoma trypanosome
tripanosomiasis trypanosomiasis
tripanosomiasis aguda acute trypanosomiasis
tripanosomiasis crónica chronic trypanosomiasis
triplejía triplegia
triploide triploid
triptamina tryptamine
triptófano tryptophan
triscaidecafobia triskaidekaphobia
trisexualidad trisexuality
trísmico trismic
trismo trismus
trismo doloroso trismus dolorificus
trismo neonatal trismus neonatorum
trismo sardónico trismus sardonicus
trismoide trismoid
trisomia trisomy
trisomia 21 trisomy 21
trisomia del cromosoma 13 chromosome 13 trisomy
trisomia del cromosoma 18 chromosome 18 trisomy
trisomia del cromosoma 21 chromosome 21 trisomy
trisomia E E trisomy
tristeza sadness
tritanopía tritanopia
trocánter trochanter
troclear trochlear
trofesía trophesy
trofésico trophesic
troficidad trophicity
trófico trophic
trofismo trophism
trofodermatoneurosis trophodermatoneurosis
trofoneurosis trophoneurosis
trofoneurosis de Romberg Romberg's trophoneurosis
trofoneurosis facial facial trophoneurosis
trofoneurosis lingual lingual trophoneurosis
trofoneurosis muscular muscular trophoneurosis
trofoneurótico trophoneurotic
trofotrópico trophotropic
troilismo troilism
trombo thrombus
trombosis thrombosis
trombosis cerebral cerebral thrombosis
trombótico thrombotic
trompas de Falopio Fallopian tubes
trompo de Benham Benham's top

tronco nervioso nerve trunk
tropismo tropism
tropismo negativo negative tropism
tropismo positivo positive tropism
tropotaxis tropotaxis
tubectomía tubectomy
tubérculo grácil gracile tubercule
tuberculofobia tuberculophobia
tuberculoma tuberculoma
tuberculomanía tuberculomania
tuberculosis tuberculosis
tuberculosis cerebral cerebral tuberculosis
tuberculoso tuberculous
tuberoso tuberous
tubo neural neural tube
tubos de Quincke Quincke tubes
tubulización tubulization
túbulos seminíferos seminiferous tubules
tumefacción tumefaction
tumefacción aguda de Spielmeyer
    Spielmeyer's acute swelling
tumefacción cerebral brain swelling
tumefaciente tumefacient
tumescencia tumescence
tumescencia peniana penile tumescence
tumescencia peniana nocturna nocturnal
    penile tumescence
tumor tumor
tumor cerebral brain tumor
tumor cromafín chromaffin tumor
tumor de arena sand tumor
tumor de bolsa de Rathke Rathke's pouch
    tumor
tumor de células granulares granular cell
    tumor
tumor de Erdheim Erdheim tumor
tumor de Lindau Lindau's tumor
tumor de Nelson Nelson tumor
tumor de Pancoast Pancoast tumor
tumor de quimiorreceptor chemoreceptor
    tumor
tumor de surco pulmonar superior superior
    pulmonary sulcus tumor
tumor del ángulo cerebelopontino
    cerebellopontine angle tumor
tumor del ángulo pontino pontine angle
    tumor
tumor del ángulo pontocerebeloso
    pontocerebellar-angle tumor
tumor del cuerpo aórtico aortic body tumor
tumor del cuerpo carotídeo carotid body
    tumor
tumor del octavo nervio eighth nerve tumor
tumor edematoso de Pott Pott's puffy tumor
tumor en turbante turban tumor
tumor espinal spinal tumor
tumor intracraneal intracranial tumor
tumor perlado pearl tumor
tumor primario primary tumor
tumor secundario secondary tumor
tumulto turmoil
tunica dartos tunica dartos
túrbido turbid
turricefalia turricephaly
tusivo tussive

tutela guardianship

U

ubicación location
ubicación del lenguaje language localization
ubicación egocéntrica egocentric localization
úlcera ulcer
úlcera de decúbito aguda acute decubitus
  ulcer
úlcera péptica peptic ulcer
ulceración gastroduodenal gastroduodenal
  ulceration
ulegiria ulegyria
ulnar ulnar
ultradiano ultradian
ultrasónico ultrasonic
ultrasonocirugía ultrasonosurgery
ultravioleta ultraviolet
ultromotividad ultromotivity
ululación ululation
umbral threshold
umbral absoluto absolute threshold
umbral absoluto mínimo minimum absolute
  threshold
umbral auditivo auditory threshold
umbral de brillantez brightness threshold
umbral de conciencia threshold of
  consciousness
umbral de contraste contrast threshold
umbral de convulsivante convulsant threshold
umbral de desmayo blackout threshold
umbral de despertamiento arousal threshold
umbral de despertamiento auditivo auditory
  arousal threshold
umbral de detección detection threshold
umbral de diferencia difference threshold
umbral de dolor pain threshold
umbral de dos puntos two-point threshold
umbral de estímulo stimulus threshold
umbral de incremento increment threshold
umbral de lactato lactate threshold
umbral de punto doble double-point
  threshold
umbral de recepción del habla
  speech-reception threshold
umbral de respuesta response threshold
umbral de sedación sedation threshold
umbral de sensación sensation threshold
umbral diferencial differential threshold
umbral doble dual threshold
umbral emocional emotional threshold
umbral espacial spatial threshold
umbral excitatorio excitatory threshold
umbral relacional relational threshold
umbral superior upper threshold
umbral terminal terminal threshold
uncal uncal

uncinado uncinate
uncovertebral uncovertebral
uniaural uniaural
único unique
unidad unit
unidad básica basic unit
unidad conyugal conjugal unit
unidad cultural culturgen
unidad de análisis analysis unit
unidad de comunicación communication unit
unidad de crisis de vida life-crisis unit
unidad de cuidado continuado
  continuing-care unit
unidad de cuidado intensivo intensive-care
  unit
unidad de cuidado intensivo neonatal
  neonatal intensive care unit
unidad de iluminación illumination unit
unidad de quemaduras burn unit
unidad de respuesta superior higher
  response unit
unidad de seguridad máxima
  maximum-security unit
unidad de sensación sensation unit
unidad funcional functional unity
unidad motora motor unit
unidad polisensorial polysensory unit
unidad psiquiátrica psychiatric unit
unidad social primaria primary social unit
unidades de cambio de vida life-change units
unidextro unidextrous
unidimensional unidimensional
uniformidad uniformity
uniformidad racional rational uniformity
uniformismo uniformism
unilateral unilateral
unimodal unimodal
uniocular uniocular
unión de brecha gap junction
unión de neuroefector neuroeffector junction
unión mioneural myoneural junction
unión neuromuscular neuromuscular junction
uniovular uniovular
unipolar unipolar
unisex unisex
unisexual unisexual
universales lingüísticos linguistic universals
universalidad universality
universalismo universalism
upsilón upsilon
uracilo uracil
uraniscolalia uraniscolalia
uranismo uranism
uranofobia uranophobia
urémico uremic
uresis uresis
ureterólisis ureterolysis
uretra urethra
uretral urethral
uretrismo urethrism
uretritis urethritis
uretritis no específica nonspecific urethritis
uretroespasmo urethrospasm
urgencia urgency
urinálisis urinalysis

urinario urinary
uriposia uriposia
urocrisia urocrisia
urocrisis urocrisis
urofilia urophilia
urolagnia urolagnia
urorrea urorrhea
urticación urtication
urticado urticate
urticaria urticaria
urticaria gigante urticaria gigantea
urticaria tuberosa urticaria tuberosa
uso de alcohol y abuso de niños alcohol use and child abuse
uso de concepto concept use
uso de drogas drug use
uso de drogas recreativo recreational use of drugs
uso de tabaco tobacco use
uso selectivo de hipnosis selective use of hypnosis
uso terapéutico therapeutic use
usos forenses del hipnotismo forensic uses of hypnotism
uterino uterine
útero uterus
útero errante wandering uterus
uteroplacentario uteroplacental
utilidad utility
utilidad decreciente diminishing returns
utilidad esperada subjetiva subjective expected utility
utilitario utilitarian
utilitarismo hedonístico hedonistic utilitarianism
utilitarismo negativo negative utilitarianism
utilitarismo pluralista pluralistic utilitarianism
utilización utilization
utilización de evaluación evaluation utilization
utopía utopia
utricular utricular
utrículo utricle
uvas verdes sour grapes
uxoricidio uxoricide

vacío existencial existential vacuum
vacuna vaccine
vacunación vaccination
vacunofobia vaccinophobia
vagal vagal
vagina vagina
vagina dentada vagina dentata
vaginal vaginal
vaginalplastía vaginalplasty
vaginar vaginate
vaginismo vaginismus
vaginismo funcional functional vaginismus
vaginismo psíquico psychic vaginismus
vaginitis vaginitis
vagólisis vagolysis
vagolítico vagolytic
vagomimético vagomimetic
vagotomía vagotomy
vagotonía vagotonia
vagotónico vagotonic
vagotrópico vagotropic
vagovagal vagovagal
vaina de mielina myelin sheath
vaina de Schwann Schwann sheath
valencia valence
valencia cromática chromatic valence
valencia negativa negative valence
valencia positiva positive valence
valencia sustituta substitute valence
valeriana valerian
valgus valgus
validación validation
validación consensual consensual validation
validación cruzada cross-validation
validación discriminante discriminant validation
validez validity
validez a priori a priori validity
validez aparente face validity
validez concurrente concurrent validity
validez consensual consensual validity
validez convergente convergent validity
validez de artículo item validity
validez de contenido content validity
validez de criterio criterion validity
validez de detección de mentiras validity of lie detection
validez de discriminante discriminant validity
validez de estado status validity
validez de muestreo sampling validity
validez de prueba validity of test
validez de rasgo trait validity
validez de sentido común common-sense validity

validez del constructo construct validity
validez diferencial differential validity
validez ecológica ecological validity
validez empírica empirical validity
validez etiológica etiological validity
validez externa external validity
validez incremental incremental validity
validez interna internal validity
validez intrínseca intrinsic validity
validez predictiva predictive validity
validez sintética synthetic validity
validez y método experimental validity and
    experimental method
válido valid
valnoctamida valnoctamide
valor value
valor absoluto absolute value
valor crítico critical value
valor D D value
valor de color color value
valor de dificultad difficulty value
valor de discriminación discrimination value
valor de estímulo stimulus value
valor de resultados subjetivos
    subjective-outcome value
valor de supervivencia survival value
valor diagnóstico diagnostic value
valor escalar scale value
valor esperado expected value
valor estético esthetic value
valor numérico numerical value
valor predictivo predictive value
valor propio self-worth
valor representativo representative value
valor social social value
valor verdadero true value
valores concebidos conceived values
valores culturales cultural values
valores del ser being values
valproato valproate
válvula valve
válvula de Heyer-Pudenz Heyer-Pudenz
    valve
vandalismo vandalism
vandalismo sexual sexual vandalism
variabilidad variability
variabilidad conductual behavioral variability
variabilidad cotidiana quotidian variability
variabilidad de muestreo sampling variability
variabilidad de rasgo trait variability
variabilidad presolución presolution
    variability
variable variable
variable aleatoria random variable
variable aleatoria continua continuous
    random variable
variable autóctona autochthonous variable
variable continua continuous variable
variable control control variable
variable controlada controlled variable
variable cuantitativa quantitative variable
variable de criterio criterion variable
variable de estímulo stimulus variable
variable de respuesta response variable
variable de resultados outcome variable

variable de sujeto subject variable
variable de tratamiento treatment variable
variable dependiente dependent variable
variable discreta discrete variable
variable distal distal variable
variable experimental experimental variable
variable independiente independent variable
variable índice index variable
variable interviniente intervening variable
variable limitada a una cultura
    culture-bound variable
variable moderadora moderator variable
variable multidimensional multidimensional
    variable
variable orgánica organic variable
variable organísmica organismic variable
variable predictora predictor variable
variable supresora suppressor variable
variables experimentales en estudios de
    sueño experimental variables in sleep
    studies
variación variation
variación casual chance variation
variación concomitante concomitant variation
variación doble double variation
variación negativa contingente contingent
    negative variation
variación diurna diurnal variation
variador tonal tonal variator
variante variant
varianza variance
varianza de interacción interaction variance
varianza del desarrollo developmental
    variance
varianza entre grupos between-group
    variance
varianza entre sujetos between-subject
    variance
varicela varicella
varus varus
vas deferens vas deferens
vascular vascular
vasculomielinopatía vasculomyelinopathy
vasectomía vasectomy
vasoactivo vasoactive
vasoconstricción vasoconstriction
vasoconstrictor vasoconstrictor
vasodepresión vasodepression
vasodilatación vasodilatation
vasoespasmo vasospasm
vasoestimulante vasostimulant
vasogénico vasogenic
vasomotor vasomotor
vasoneuropatía vasoneuropathy
vasoneurosis vasoneurosis
vasopresina vasopressin
vasopresor vasopressor
vasorreflejo vasoreflex
vasovagal vasovagal
vector vector
vector de referencia reference vector
vegetativo vegetative
vejez old age
vejiga bladder
vejiga atónica atonic bladder

vejiga en cuerda cord bladder
vejiga irritable irritable bladder
vejiga nerviosa nervous bladder
vejiga neurogénica neurogenic bladder
vejiga neurogénica autónoma autonomic
  neurogenic bladder
vejiga neurogénica desinhibida uninhibited
  neurogenic bladder
vejiga neurogénica refleja reflex neurogenic
  bladder
vejiga seudoneurogénica pseudoneurogenic
  bladder
velar velar
velicación vellication
velicar vellicate
velocidad speed
velocidad de articulación articulation speed
velocidad de conducción de nervio nerve
  conduction velocity
velocidad de producción del habla rate of
  production of speech
velocidad perceptiva perceptual speed
vendaje bandage
vendaje en hamaca hammock bandage
venéreo venereal
venereofobia venereophobia
venganza revenge
venografía venography
venografía transósea transosseous
  venography
venografía vertebral vertebral venography
venorrespiratorio venorespiratory
ventaja inicial head start
ventaja por enfermedad advantage by illness
ventaja secundaria secondary advantage
ventana de Ames Ames window
ventana oval oval window
ventana redonda round window
ventana terapéutica therapeutic window
ventilación ventilation
ventral ventral
ventricular ventricular
ventriculitis ventriculitis
ventrículo ventricle
ventrículo lateral lateral ventricle
ventriculocisternostomía
  ventriculocisternostomy
ventriculografía ventriculography
ventriculograma ventriculogram
ventriculomastoidostomía
  ventriculomastoidostomy
ventriculopunción ventriculopuncture
ventriculoscopia ventriculoscopy
ventriculostomía ventriculostomy
ventriculotomía ventriculotomy
ventromedial ventromedial
verapamil verapamil
verbal verbal
verbalismo verbalism
verbalización verbalization
verbigeración verbigeration
verbigeración alucinatoria hallucinatory
  verbigeration
verbigerar verbigerate
verbocromia verbochromia

verbomanía verbomania
verboso verbose
vergencia vergence
verídico veridical
verificación verification
vermis vermis
vernáculo vernacular
vernier vernier
vertebral vertebral
vertebrectomía vertebrectomy
vertebrobasilar vertebrobasilar
vértice vertex
vertiginoso vertiginous
vértigo vertigo
vértigo crónico chronic vertigo
vértigo de alturas height vertigo
vértigo de Charcot Charcot's vertigo
vértigo de movimientos falsos
  sham-movement vertigo
vértigo epidémico epidemic vertigo
vértigo galvánico galvanic vertigo
vértigo gástrico gastric vertigo
vértigo horizontal horizontal vertigo
vértigo laríngeo laryngeal vertigo
vértigo lateral lateral vertigo
vértigo mecánico mechanical vertigo
vértigo nocturno nocturnal vertigo
vértigo objetivo objective vertigo
vértigo orgánico organic vertigo
vértigo paralítico endémico endemic paralytic
  vertigo
vértigo paralizante paralyzing vertigo
vértigo postural postural vertigo
vértigo rotatorio rotatory vertigo
vértigo sistemático systematic vertigo
vértigo subjetivo subjective vertigo
vértigo vertical vertical vertigo
vértigo voltaico voltaic vertigo
vesical vesical
vesículas seminales seminal vesicles
vestibular vestibular
vestíbulo vestibule
vestibulocerebeloso vestibulocerebellar
vestibulococlear vestibulocochlear
vestibuloequilibratorio vestibuloequilibratory
vestibuloespinal vestibulospinal
vestigio vestige
vestimenta dress
vestir dressing
vía pathway
vía auditiva auditory pathway
vía bioquímica biochemical pathway
vía común final final common path
vía de respuesta alfa alpha response pathway
vía dopaminérgica dopaminergic pathway
vía nerviosa nerve pathway
vía neural neural pathway
vía sensorial sensory pathway
viable viable
viaje malo bad trip
vías auditivas centrales central auditory
  pathways
vías de dolor pain pathways
vías del gusto centrales central taste pathways
vías descendientes descending pathways

vías olfatorias centrales central olfactory
    pathways
vías periféricas centrífugas centrifugal
    peripheral pathways
vibración simpática sympathetic vibration
vibrador vibrator
vicario vicarious
víctima victim
victimización victimization
victimología victimology
vida lifetime
vida de fantasía fantasy life
vida del ego de realidad reality life of ego
vida sexual sexual life
vigilambulismo vigilambulism
vigilancia vigilance
vigilancia congelada frozen watchfulness
vigilancia perceptiva perceptual vigilance
vigilia vigil
vigilia de coma coma vigil
vigilia fatigante fatiguing vigil
vigor de híbridos hybrid vigor
vileza moral moral turpitude
viloxazina viloxazine
vinbarbital vinbarbital
vinculación bonding
vinculación afiliativa affiliative bonding
vinculación en familias mezcladas bonding in
    blended families
vinculación y apego bonding and attachment
vínculo bond
vínculo afectivo affectional bond
vínculo asociativo associative bond
vínculo de apego attachment bond
vínculo de apego y ansiedad de separación
    attachment bond and separation anxiety
vínculo social social bond
vínculos incestuosos incestuous ties
violación rape
violación estatutaria statutory rape
violación homosexual homosexual rape
violación por acompañante date rape
violación por conocido acquaintance rape
violación por ira anger rape
violación por venganza revenge rape
violación sádica sadistic rape
violación y pornografía violenta rape and
    violent pornography
violencia violence
violencia catatímica catathymic violence
violencia doméstica domestic violence
violencia doméstica e incesto domestic
    violence and incest
violencia doméstica y abuso de niños
    domestic violence and child abuse
violencia doméstica y abuso del cónyuge
    domestic violence and spouse abuse
violencia doméstica y abuso sexual domestic
    violence and sexual abuse
violencia en televisión violence on television
violencia familiar family violence
violento violent
viraginidad viraginity
viraje del humor mood swing
viral viral

virgofrenia virgophrenia
virilescencia virilescence
virilismo virilism
virulento virulent
virus virus
virus convencional conventional virus
virus de Epstein-Barr Epstein-Barr virus
virus de inmunodeficiencia humana human
    immunodeficiency virus
virus del herpes simple herpes simplex virus
virus entérico enteric virus
virus huérfano orphan virus
virus lento slow virus
víscera viscus
visceral visceral
vísceras viscera
visceroceptor visceroceptor
viscerogénico viscerogenic
visceromotor visceromotor
viscerorreceptor visceroreceptor
viscerosensorial viscerosensory
viscerotonía viscerotonia
viscerotónico viscerotonic
viscosidad de libido viscosity of libido
visibilidad visibility
visión vision
visión alternante alternating vision
visión binocular binocular vision
visión central central vision
visión cercana near vision
visión crepuscular twilight vision
visión de bastoncillos rod vision
visión de color color vision
visión de distancia distance vision
visión de luz del día daylight vision
visión de túnel tunnel vision
visión desplazada displaced vision
visión doble double vision
visión escotópica scotopic vision
visión espacial spatial vision
visión estereoscópica stereoscopic vision
visión estereoscópica binocular binocular
    stereoscopic vision
visión facial facial vision
visión fotópica photopic vision
visión foveal foveal vision
visión hiperópica hyperopic vision
visión indirecta indirect vision
visión mesópica mesopic vision
visión monocular monocular vision
visión nocturna night vision
visión paracentral paracentral vision
visión periférica peripheral vision
visión perimacular perimacular vision
visión subjetiva subjective vision
visión temporal temporal vision
visita al hogar home visit
visitante de salud health visitor
vista sight
vista cercana nearsightedness
vista ciega blind sight
vista lejana farsightedness
vista parcial partial sight
visual visual
visual-motor visual-motor

visualización visualization
visualizar visualize
visuoauditivo visuoauditory
visuoespacial visuospatial
visuognosis visuognosis
visuomotor visuomotor
visuopsíquico visuopsychic
visuosensorial visuosensory
vital vital
vitalidad vitality
vitalismo vitalism
vitamina vitamin
vitamina A sérica serum vitamin A
vitamina B-12 sérica serum vitamin B-12
vitrectomía vitrectomy
vítreo vitreous
vivienda satélite satellite housing
vivir existencial existential living
vivir independiente independent living
vivir vicario vicarious living
vivisección vivisection
vocabulario vocabulary
vocabulario activo active vocabulary
vocabulario de reconocimiento recognition
    vocabulary
vocabulario de vista sight vocabulary
vocabulario pasivo passive vocabulary
vocación vocation
vocacional vocational
vocal vocal
vocalidad vocality
vocalización vocalization
volar volar
volátil volatile
volición volition
volitivo volitional
volubilidad volubility
volumen volume
volumen tonal tonal volume
voluntad will
voluntad de sobrevivir will to survive
voluntad de vivir will to live
voluntario voluntary
voluntarismo voluntarism
vómito vomiting
vómitos histéricos hysterical vomiting
vómitos nerviosos nervous vomiting
vómitos psicogénicos psychogenic vomiting
voyeur voyeur
voyeurismo voyeurism
voz voice
voz esofagal esophageal voice
vudú voodoo
vulnerabilidad vulnerability
**vulnerabilidad biológica a problemas de
    conducta** biological vulnerability to
    behavior problems
vulnerabilidad especial special vulnerability
vulnerabilidad genética genetic vulnerability
vulnerable vulnerable
vulva vulva
vulvectomía vulvectomy
vulvismo vulvismus

warfarina warfarin

xantina xanthine
xantocianopsia xanthocyanopsia
xantomatosis xanthomatosis
xantomatosis cerebrotendinosa
  cerebrotendinous xanthomatosis
xantomatosis familiar primario primary
  familial xanthomatosis
xantopsia xanthopsia
xenofobia xenophobia
xenógeno xenogenous
xenoglosia xenoglossia
xenoglosofilia xenoglossophilia
xenoglosofobia xenoglossophobia
xenorexia xenorexia
xerostomía xerostomia
xifodinia xiphodynia
xifoidalgia xiphoidalgia
xiroespasmo xyrospasm

yo self
yo bueno good me
yo cohesivo cohesive self
yo creativo creative self
yo de espejo looking-glass self
yo empírico empirical self
yo escondido hidden self
yo falso false self
yo fenomenal phenomenal self
yo glorificado glorified self
yo ideal self ideal
yo idealizado idealized self
yo malo bad me
yo percibido perceived self
yo personificado personified self
yo psicológico psychological me
yo real real self
yo social social self
yo subliminal subliminal self
yoga yoga
yohimbina yohimbine
yunque anvil
yuxtaposición juxtaposition

Z

zeitgeist zeitgeist
zeta zeta
zoantropía zoanthropy
zoantrópico zoanthropic
zona arqueada del cerebro arcuate zone of
    the brain
zona cortical primaria primary cortical zone
zona cortical secundaria secondary cortical
    zone
zona cortical terciaria tertiary cortical zone
zona de alcance catchment area
zona de amortiguamiento corporal body
    buffer zone
zona de disparo quimiorreceptor
    chemoreceptor trigger zone
zona de distancia personal personal-distance
    zone
zona de distancia pública public-distance
    zone
zona de gatillo trigger zone
zona de Marchant Marchant's zone
zona del lenguaje language zone
zona dendrítica dendritic zone
zona dermática zona dermatica
zona dolorogénica dolorogenic zone
zona epileptogénica epileptogenic zone
zona epitelioserosa zona epithelioserosa
zona erógena erogenous zone
zona erotogénica erotogenic zone
zona genital genital zone
zona íntima intimate zone
zona latente latent zone
zona motora motor zone
zona primaria primary zone
zona reflexogénica reflexogenic zone
zona retinal retinal zone
zona sensible tender zone
zona sensitiva sensitive zone
zona social social zone
zona trofotrópica de Hess trophotropic zone
    of Hess
zonas corticales cortical zones
zonas de color color zones
zonas de distancia distance zones
zonas de Head Head's zones
zonas histerogénicas hysterogenic zones
zonestesia zonesthesia
zonífugo zonifugal
zonípeto zonipetal
zooerastia zooerasty
zoofilia zoophilia
zoofílico zoophilic
zoofilismo zoophilism
zoofilismo erótico erotic zoophilism

zoófilo zoophile
zoofobia zoophobia
zoolagnia zoolagnia
zoomanía zoomania
zoomorfismo zoomorphism
zoopsia zoopsia
zoosadismo zoosadism
zurdo left-handed